Abbreviation	Derivation	Meaning
o.h.	omni hora	every hour
o.m.	omni mane	every morning
o.n.	omni nocte	every night
o.s.	oculus sinister	left eye
os	os	mouth
o.u.	oculus uterque	each eye
oz	uncia	ounce
p.c.	post cibum	after meals
per	per	through or by
pil.	pilula	pill
p.o.	per os	orally
p.r.		by rectum
p.r.n.	pro re nata	when required or as needed
q	quaque hora	every hour
q. 2 h.		every two hours
q. 3 h.		every three hours
q. 4 h.		every four hours
q. 5 h.		every five hours
q. 6 h.		every six hours
q.i.d.	quarter in die	four times a day
q.o.d		every other day
q.l.	quantum libet	as much as desired
q.n.	quaque nocte	every night
q.p.	quantum placeat	as much as desired
q.v.	quantum vis	as much as you please
q.s.	quantum sufficit	as much as is required
Rx	recipe	take
Rep.	repetatur	let it be repeated
s	sine	without
seq. luce.	sequenti luce	the following day
Sig. or S.	signa	write on lable
sl.		sublingual
s.o.s.	so opus sit	if necessary
sp.	spiritus	spirits
supp.		suppository
ss	semis	a half
stat.	statim	immediately
syr.	syrupus	syrup
t.d.s.	ter die sumendum	to be taken three times daily
t.i.d.	ter in die	three times a day
t.i.n.	ter in nocte	three times a night
tr. or tinct.	tincture	tincture
ung.	unguetum	ointment
ut. dict. or u.d.	ut dictum	as directed
vin.	vini	of wine

Adapted from Mosby's Medical, Nursing, & Allied Health Dictionary, ed 6, Revised Reprint, St. Louis, 2005, Mosby; Daniel SJ, Harfst SA: Mosby's Dental Hygiene 2004 Update, St. Louis, 2004, Mosby.

Mosby's 2007

DENTAL DRUG CONSULT

MOSBY
ELSEVIER

MOSBY
ELSEVIER

11830 Westline Industrial Drive
St. Louis, Missouri 63146

MOSBY'S 2007 DENTAL DRUG CONSULT ISBN-10: 0-323-03959-6
ISBN-13: 978-0-323-03959-8

Notice

Knowledge and best practice in this field are constantly changing. As new research and experience broaden our knowledge, changes in practice, treatment and drug therapy may become necessary or appropriate. Readers are advised to check the most current information provided (i) on procedures featured or (ii) by the manufacturer of each product to be administered, to verify the recommended dose or formula, the method and duration of administration, and contraindications. It is the responsibility of the practitioner, relying on their own experience and knowledge of the patient, to make diagnoses, to determine dosages and the best treatment for each individual patient, and to take all appropriate safety precautions. To the fullest extent of the law, neither the Publisher nor the Editors assume any liability for any injury and/or damage to persons or property arising out of or related to any use of the material contained in this book.

The Publisher

ISBN-10: 0-323-03959-6
ISBN-13: 978-0-323-03959-8

Publishing Director: Linda Duncan
Acquisitions Editor: John Dolan
Developmental Editor: John Dedeke
Drug Consult Editorial Director: A.M. Maheswaran
Drug Consult Associate Database Editor: Laura Kudowitz
Drug Consult Associate Database Editor: Robert D. Todd
Drug Consult Associate Database Editor: Gina Hopf
Publishing Services Manager: Melissa Lastarria
Project Manager: Kelly E.M. Steinmann
Designer: Paula Ruckenbrod

Printed in the United States of America

Last digit is the print number: 9 8 7 6 5 4 3 2 1

Special Content Experts

Tommy W. Gage, RPh, DDS, PhD
Professor Emeritus
Department of Oral and Maxillofacial Surgery and Pharmacology
Formerly Director of Curriculum
Academic Services
Baylor College of Dentistry
The Texas A&M University System Health Science Center
Dallas, Texas

James W. Little, DMD, MS
Professor Emeritus
University of Minnesota
School of Dentistry
Minneapolis, Minnesota; Naples, Florida

Drug Monograph Content Contributors*

Barbara B. Hodgson, RN, OCN
Cancer Institute
St. Joseph's Hospital
Tampa, Florida

Robert J. Kizior, BS, RPh
Education Coordinator
Department of Pharmacy
Alexian Brothers Medical Center
Elk Grove Village, Illinois

*Drug monograph content culled from the *Mosby's Drug Consult*™ database.

Preface

Dental care professionals face many challenges in today's environment, not the least of which is familiarity with the large number of medications available. New medications are being introduced, and new applications, dosage forms, and different routes of administration for existing medications are increasing at a rapid rate. This voluminous amount of drug information must be quickly integrated into the patient care environment.

This guide contains:

1. *Practice-oriented precautions and considerations.* Every drug entry provides extensive, practice-oriented precautions and considerations, putting essential drug facts directly into the context of your care.
2. *Prioritized side effects.* Each drug entry ranks side effects by frequency of occurrence, from most common to least common. Entries also include the percentage of frequency, when known. This information helps you focus your care by knowing which effects to monitor more closely.
3. *Highlights on serious adverse reactions.* In each drug entry, the book calls attention to dangerous or life-threatening reactions so that you can identify them easily and act on them promptly.
4. *Specialized dental care guidelines.* Suggested protocols for the treatment of medically compromised patients and the therapeutic management of common oral lesions.
5. *Combination drug guide.* Detailed index of combination drugs arranged by trade name.
6. *Herbal and nonherbal remedies.* Extensive clinical data and dental considerations for commonly used alternative remedies.
7. *Comprehensive appendices.* Ten ready-reference appendices give you easy access to additional vital drug-related information, such as the English-Spanish Drug Phrase Translator, and detailed sections concerning anesthetics, controlled substances, disorders and conditions, pregnancy and pediatrics, and example prescriptions.

A detailed guide to *Mosby's 2007 Dental Drug Consult:*

Mosby's 2007 Dental Drug Consult provides essential drug information in a user-friendly format. The bulk of this handbook contains an alphabetical listing of drug entries by generic name. Drug entries include the following:

Generic and Brand Names. Drug entries begin with the generic drug name, followed by its pronunciation and U.S., Canadian, and Australian brand names.

Category and Schedule. This section lists the drug's pregnancy risk category and, when appropriate, its controlled substance schedule or over-the-counter (OTC) status.

Mechanism of Action. This section clearly and concisely details the drug's mechanism of action and therapeutic effects.

Pharmacokinetics. Under this heading, a quick-reference chart outlines the drug's route, onset, peak, and duration, when known. This information is followed by a discussion of the drug's absorption, distribution, metabolism, excretion, and half-life.

Availability. This section identifies the forms that the drug comes in, such as tablets, sustained-release capsules, or an injectable solution. Available doses and concentrations are also listed.

Indications and Dosages. Here, you'll find the approved indications and routes, along with the dosage information for all age groups and populations, including adults, elderly patients, children, neonates, and those with preexisting conditions such as liver or kidney disease.

Contraindications. Each entry lists conditions in which use of the generic drug is contraindicated and should not be used.

Interactions. For drugs, herbal supplements, and food, this section supplies vital information about interactions with the topic drug.

Diagnostic Test Effects. Under the heading, you'll see a brief description of the drug's effects on laboratory and diagnostic test results, such as liver enzyme levels and electrocardiogram tracings.

Side Effects. Unlike other handbooks that mix common, deadly effects with rare, minor ones in a long, undifferentiated list, this book ranks side effects by frequency of occurrence by indicating expected, frequent, occasional, and rare. Within each frequency, effects are listed by highest to lowest percentage of occurrence, when known.

Serious Adverse Reactions. Because serious adverse reactions are life-threatening responses that require prompt intervention, this section highlights them, apart from other side effects, for easy identification.

Precautions and Considerations. Using a practice-oriented format and written specifically for dentistry, this section presents precautions and considerations for each drug entry.

Mosby's 2007 Dental Drug Consult is an easy-to-use source of the current drug information for a wide spectrum of dental care providers. When it comes to providing quality patient care, you'll need no other drug reference.

Contents

Contents

abacavir

ah-bah′-cah-veer
(Ziagen)

CATEGORY AND SCHEDULE

Pregnancy Risk Category: C

MECHANISM OF ACTION

An antiretroviral that inhibits the activity of HIV-1 reverse transcriptase by competing with the natural substrate deoxyguanosine-5′-triphosphate (dGTP) and by its incorporation into viral DNA. ***Therapeutic Effect:*** Inhibits viral DNA growth.

PHARMACOKINETICS

Rapidly and extensively absorbed after PO administration. Protein binding: 50%. Widely distributed, including to CSF and erythrocytes. Metabolized in the liver to inactive metabolites. Primarily excreted in urine. Unknown if removed by hemodialysis. ***Half-life:*** 1.5 hr.

AVAILABILITY

Tablets: 300 mg.
Oral Solution: 20 mg/ml.

INDICATIONS AND DOSAGES

▸ **HIV Infection (in combination with other antiretrovirals)**

PO

Adults. 300 mg twice a day.
Children (3 mo–16 yr). 8 mg/kg twice a day. Maximum: 300 mg twice a day.

▸ **Dosage in Hepatic Impairment**

Mild impairment: 200 mg 2 times/day.
Moderate to severe impairment: Not recommended.

CONTRAINDICATIONS

Hypersensitivity to abacavir or its components

INTERACTIONS

Drug

Alcohol: May increase abacavir blood concentration and half-life.

Herbal

St. John's wort: May decrease abacavir blood concentration and effect.

Food

None known.

Drug interactions of concern to dentistry

- None reported

DIAGNOSTIC TEST EFFECTS

May increase blood glucose and serum GGT, AST(SGOT), ALT(SGPT), and triglyceride levels.

SIDE EFFECTS

Adult

Frequent

Nausea (47%), nausea with vomiting (16%), diarrhea (12%), decreased appetite (11%)

Occasional

Insomnia (7%)

Children

Frequent

Nausea with vomiting (39%), fever (19%), headache, diarrhea (16%), rash (11%)

Occasional

Decreased appetite (9%)

SERIOUS REACTIONS

! A hypersensitivity reaction may be life threatening. Signs and symptoms include fever, rash, fatigue, intractable nausea and vomiting, severe diarrhea, abdominal pain, cough, pharyngitis, and dyspnea.

! Life-threatening hypotension may occur.

! Lactic acidosis and severe hepatomegaly may occur.

DENTAL CONSIDERATIONS

General:

• Examine for oral manifestation of opportunistic infection.
• Patient on chronic drug therapy may rarely have symptoms of blood dyscrasias, which include infection, bleeding, and poor healing.
• Avoid dental light in patient's eyes; offer dark glasses for patient comfort.
• Place on frequent recall because of oral side effects.
• Consider semisupine chair position for patient comfort if gastrointestinal (GI) side effects occur.

Consultations:

• In a patient with symptoms of blood dyscrasias, request a medical consultation for blood studies and postpone treatment until normal values are reestablished.
• Medical consultation may be required to assess disease control.

Teach Patient/Family:

• Importance of good oral hygiene to prevent soft tissue inflammation
• To prevent trauma when using oral hygiene aids
• To be alert for the possibility of secondary oral infection and the need to see dentist immediately if signs of infection occur

abarelix

ah-bar′-eh-lex
(Plenaxis)

CATEGORY AND SCHEDULE

Pregnancy Risk Category: X

MECHANISM OF ACTION

A luteinizing hormone-releasing hormone (LHRH) antagonist that inhibits gonadotropin and androgen production by blocking gonadotrop in releasing-hormone receptors in the pituitary. ***Therapeutic Effect:*** Suppresses luteinizing hormone, follicle stimulating hormone secretion, reducing the secretion of testosterone by the testes.

PHARMACOKINETICS

Slowly absorbed following intramuscular administration. Distributed extensively. Protein binding: 96%–99%. ***Half-life:*** 13.2 days.

AVAILABILITY

Powder for Injection: 113 mg kit containing 10 ml 0.9% NaCl, 18-gauge needle, 22-gauge needle.

INDICATIONS AND DOSAGES

▸ Prostate Cancer

IM

Adults, Elderly. 100 mg on days 1, 15, 29 and every 4 weeks thereafter. Treatment failure can be detected by obtaining serum testosterone concentration prior to abarelix administration, day 19 and every 8 weeks thereafter.

CONTRAINDICATIONS

This drug should not be used in women and children.

INTERACTIONS

Drug

None known.

Herbal

None known.

Food

None known.

Drug interactions of concern to dentistry

• Dental drug interactions have not been studied.

DIAGNOSTIC TEST EFFECTS

May increase serum transaminase, serum AST (SGOT), ALT (SGPT), and serum triglyceride levels. May slightly decrease blood hemoglobin concentrations. May decrease bone mineral density.

SIDE EFFECTS

Frequent (79%–30%)
Hot flashes, sleep disturbances, breast enlargement
Occasional (20%–11%)
Breast pain, nipple tenderness, back pain, constipation, peripheral edema, dizziness, upper respiratory tract infection, diarrhea
Rare (10%)
Fatigue, nausea, dysuria, micturition frequency, urinary retention, urinary tract infection

SERIOUS REACTIONS

! Immediate-onset systemic allergic reaction characterized by hypotension, urticaria, pruritus, periorbital and/or circumoral edema, shortness of breath, wheezing, and syncope may occur.
! Prolongation of the QT interval may occur. Tightening of throat, tongue swelling, wheezing, shortness of breath, and low blood pressure occur rarely.

DENTAL CONSIDERATIONS

General:
- If additional analgesia is required for dental pain, consider alternative analgesics (NSAIDs) in patients taking narcotics for acute or chronic pain.
- This drug may be used in the hospital or on an outpatient basis. Confirm the patient's disease and treatment status.

Consultations:
- Medical consultation may be required to assess disease control and patient's ability to tolerate stress.

Teach Patient/Family:
- Importance of good oral hygiene to prevent soft tissue inflammation
- To prevent trauma when using oral hygiene aids
- Importance of updating health and medication history if physician makes any changes in evaluation or drug regimens; include OTC, herbal, and nonherbal remedies in the update

abciximab

ab-six′-ih-mab
(c7E3 Fab, ReoPro)

CATEGORY AND SCHEDULE

Pregnancy Risk Category: C

MECHANISM OF ACTION

A glycoprotein IIb/IIIa receptor inhibitor that rapidly inhibits platelet aggregation by preventing the binding of fibrinogen to GP IIb/IIIa receptor sites on platelets.
Therapeutic Effect: Prevents closure of treated coronary arteries. Prevents acute cardiac ischemic complications.

PHARMACOKINETICS

Rapidly cleared from plasma. Initial-phase half-life is less than 10 min; second-phase half-life is 30 min. Platelet function generally returns within 48 hr.

AVAILABILITY

Injection: 2 mg/ml (5-ml vial).

INDICATIONS AND DOSAGES

▸ Percutaneous Coronary Intervention (PCI)
IV Bolus
Adults. 0.25 mg/kg 10–60 min before angioplasty or atherectomy, then 12-hr IV infusion of 0.125 mcg/kg/min. Maximum: 10 mcg/min.

▸ **PCI (unstable angina)**
IV Bolus
Adults. 0.25 mg/kg, followed by 18- to 24-hr infusion of 10 mcg/min, ending 1 hr after procedure.

CONTRAINDICATIONS

Active internal bleeding, arteriovenous malformation or aneurysm, cerebrovascular accident (CVA) with residual neurologic defect, history of CVA (within the past 2 years) or oral anticoagulant use within the past 7 days unless PT is less than 1.2 × control, history of vasculitis, intracranial neoplasm, prior IV dextran use before or during PTCA, recent surgery or trauma (within the past 6 weeks), recent (within the past 6 weeks or less) GI or GU bleeding, thrombocytopenia (< 100,000 cells/mcl), and severe uncontrolled hypertension

INTERACTIONS

Drug

Anticoagulants, including heparin: May increase risk of hemorrhage.
Platelet aggregation inhibitors (such as aspirin, dextran, thrombolytic agents): May increase risk of bleeding.

Herbal

None known.

Food

None known.

Drug interactions of concern to dentistry

- Increased risk of bleeding: drugs that interfere with coagulation or platelet function, such as NSAIDs and aspirin

DIAGNOSTIC TEST EFFECTS

Increases activated clotting time (ACT), aPTT, and PT. Decreases platelet count.

IV INCOMPATIBILITIES

Administer in separate line; no other medication should be added to infusion solution.

SIDE EFFECTS

Frequent

Nausea (16%), hypotension (12%)

Occasional (9%)

Vomiting

Rare (3%)

Bradycardia, confusion, dizziness, pain, peripheral edema, urinary tract infection

SERIOUS REACTIONS

! Major bleeding complications may occur. If complications occur, stop the infusion immediately.
! Hypersensitivity reaction may occur.
! Atrial fibrillation or flutter, pulmonary edema, and complete atrioventricular block occur occasionally.

DENTAL CONSIDERATIONS

General:

- Monitor vital signs at every appointment due to cardiovascular side effects.
- For use in hospitals or emergency rooms.
- Review patient's medical and drug history.
- Provide palliative emergency dental care only during drug use.
- Patients may be at risk of bleeding, check for oral signs.

Consultations:

- Medical consultation may be required to assess disease control and patient's ability to tolerate stress.
- Medical consultation should include routine blood counts including platelet counts and bleeding time.
- Avoid products that affect platelet function, such as aspirin and NSAIDs.

Teach Patient/Family:
- Importance of good oral hygiene to prevent soft tissue inflammation
- To prevent trauma when using oral hygiene aids
- To report oral lesions, soreness, or bleeding to dentist
- Importance of updating health and medication history if physician makes any changes in evaluation or drug regimens; include OTC, herbal, and nonherbal remedies in the update
- To use soft tooth brush to reduce risk of bleeding

acarbose

a-car′-bose
(Glucobay[AUS], Prandase[CAN], Precose)
Do not confuse Precose with PreCare.

CATEGORY AND SCHEDULE
Pregnancy Risk Category: B

MECHANISM OF ACTION
An alpha glucosidase inhibitor that delays glucose absorption and digestion of carbohydrates, resulting in a smaller rise in blood glucose concentration after meals.
Therapeutic Effect: Lowers postprandial hyperglycemia.

AVAILABILITY
Tablets: 25 mg, 50 mg, 100 mg.

INDICATIONS AND DOSAGES
▸ **Diabetes Mellitus**
PO
Adults, Elderly. Initially, 25 mg 3 times a day with first bite of each main meal. Increase at 4- to 8-wk intervals. Maximum: For patients weighing more than 60 kg, 100 mg 3 times a day; for patients weighing 60 kg or less, 50 mg 3 times a day.

CONTRAINDICATIONS
Chronic intestinal diseases associated with marked disorders of digestion or absorption, cirrhosis, colonic ulceration, conditions that may deteriorate as a result of increased gas formation in the intestine, diabetic ketoacidosis, hypersensitivity to acarbose, inflammatory bowel disease, partial intestinal obstruction or predisposition to intestinal obstruction, significant renal dysfunction (serum creatinine level greater than 2 mg/dl)

INTERACTIONS
Drug
Digestive enzymes, intestinal absorbents (such as charcoal): Reduces effects of acarbose.
Herbal
None known.
Food
None known.
Drug interactions of concern to dentistry
- None reported

DIAGNOSTIC TEST EFFECTS
May increase AST(SGOT) levels.

SIDE EFFECTS
Side effects diminish in frequency and intensity over time.
Frequent
Transient GI disturbances: flatulence (77%), diarrhea (33%), abdominal pain (21%)

SERIOUS REACTIONS
! None known.

DENTAL CONSIDERATIONS
General:
- Ensure that patient is following prescribed diet and takes medication regularly.

• Type 2 patients may also be using insulin. If symptomatic hypoglycemia occurs while taking this drug, use dextrose rather than sucrose because of interference with sucrose metabolism.
• Place on frequent recall to evaluate healing response.
• Patients with diabetes may be more susceptible to infection and have delayed wound healing.
• Question the patient about self-monitoring the drug's antidiabetic effect.
• Consider semisupine chair position for patient comfort if GI side effects occur.

Consultations:

• Medical consultation may be required to assess disease control and patient's ability to tolerate stress.

Teach Patient/Family:

• Importance of good oral hygiene to prevent soft tissue inflammation

acetaminophen

ah-seet′-ah-min-oh-fen
(Abenol[CAN], Apo-Acetaminophen[CAN], Atasol[CAN], Dymadon[AUS], Feverall, Panadol[AUS], Panamax[AUS], Paralgin[AUS], Setamol[AUS], Tempra, Tylenol)
Do not confuse with Fiorinal, Hycodan, Indocin, Percodan, or Tuinal.

CATEGORY AND SCHEDULE

Pregnancy Risk Category: B
OTC

MECHANISM OF ACTION

A central analgesic whose exact mechanism is unknown, but appears to inhibit prostaglandin synthesis in the central nervous system (CNS) and, to a lesser extent, block pain impulses through peripheral action. Acetaminophen acts centrally on hypothalamic heat-regulating center, producing peripheral vasodilation (heat loss, skin erythema, sweating).
Therapeutic Effect: Results in antipyresis. Produces analgesic effect. Results in antipyresis.

PHARMACOKINETICS

Route	Onset	Peak	Duration
PO	15–30 mins	1–1.5 hrs	4–6 hrs

Rapidly, completely absorbed from gastrointestinal (GI) tract; rectal absorption variable. Protein binding: 20%–50%. Widely distributed to most body tissues. Metabolized in liver; excreted in urine. Removed by hemodialysis. ***Half-life:*** 1–4 hrs (half-life is increased in those with liver disease, elderly, neonates; decreased in children).

AVAILABILITY

Caplet (Genapap, Tylenol): 500 mg.
Caplet, extended release (Mapap, Tylenol Arthritis Pain): 650 mg.
Capsule (Mapap): 500 mg.
Elixir: 160 mg/5 ml.
Liquid, oral (Tylenol Extra Strength): 500 mg/15 ml.
Solution, oral drops (Genapap Infant): 80 mg/0.8 ml.
Suppository, rectal (Feverall): 80 mg, *(Acephen, Feverall):* 120 mg, 325 mg, 650 mg.
Tablet (Genapap, Mapap, Tylenol): 325 mg, 500 mg.
Tablet, chewable (Genapap, Mapap, Tylenol): 80 mg.

INDICATIONS AND DOSAGES

▸ **Analgesia and Antipyresis**

PO

Adults, Elderly. 325–650 mg q4–6h or 1 g 3–4 times/day. Maximum: 4 g/day.

Children. 10–15 mg/kg/dose q4–6h as needed. Maximum: 5 doses/24 hrs.
Neonates. 10–15 mg/kg/dose q6–8h as needed.
RECTAL
Adults. 650 mg q4–6h. Maximum: 6 doses/24 hrs.
Children. 10–20 mg/kg/dose q4–6h as needed.
Neonates. 10–15 mg/kg/dose q6–8h as needed.

▸ **Dosage in Renal Impairment**

Creatinine Clearance	Frequency
10–50 ml/min	q6h
less than 10 ml/min	q8h

CONTRAINDICATIONS

Active alcoholism, liver disease, or viral hepatitis, all of which increase the risk of hepatotoxicity

INTERACTIONS

Drug

Alcohol (chronic use), hepatotoxic medications (e.g., phenytoin), liver enzyme inducers (e.g., cimetidine): May increase risk of hepatotoxicity with prolonged high dose or single toxic dose.
Warfarin: May increase the risk of bleeding with regular use.

Herbal

None known.

Food

None known.

Drug interactions of concern to dentistry

- Decreased effects: barbiturates, oral contraceptives, loop diuretics
- Nephrotoxicity: nonsteroidal antiinflammatory drugs (NSAIDs), salicylates (chronic, high-dose concurrent use)
- Liver toxicity: chronic use of hydantoins, chronic alcohol use, high-dose carbamazepine
- Possible increased effects of zidovudine
- Possible increased effects of acetaminophen: β-blockers, probenecid
- Increased bleeding: warfarin

DIAGNOSTIC TEST EFFECTS

May increase serum bilirubin, prothrombin time (may indicate hepatotoxicity), SGOT (AST), and SGPT (ALT). Therapeutic serum level: 10–30 mcg/ml; toxic serum level: greater than 200 mcg/ml.

SIDE EFFECTS

Rare

Hypersensitivity reaction

SERIOUS REACTIONS

! Acetaminophen toxicity is the primary serious reaction.
! Early signs and symptoms of acetaminophen toxicity include anorexia, nausea, diaphoresis, and generalized weakness within the first 12 to 24 hrs.
! Later signs of acetaminophen toxicity include vomiting, right upper quadrant tenderness, and elevated liver function tests within 48 to 72 hrs after ingestion.
! The antidote to acetaminophen toxicity is acetylcysteine.

DENTAL CONSIDERATIONS

General:

- Reports regarding the concomitant use of acetaminophen and warfarin seem to suggest a possible increase in anticoagulant effects, especially in patients with other diseases or contributing factors, diarrhea, age, debilitation, etc. Patients taking warfarin should be questioned about recent use of acetaminophen and current international normalized ratio (INR) values. Acetaminophen has been shown to increase the INR depending on the amount and duration of acetaminophen use. A new prothrombin time (PT) or INR value

may be required if surgical procedures are planned. Data from one study (*JAMA* 279:657–662, 1998) indicated that use of four regular-strength acetaminophen tablets (325 mg) qd for 1 wk can increase the INR values. It is important to closely monitor INR values with use of acetaminophen over a long duration and in higher doses.
• Avoid prolonged use with aspirin-containing products or NSAIDs.
• Determine why the patient is taking the drug.
• Patients on chronic drug therapy may rarely have symptoms of blood dyscrasias, which can include infection, bleeding, and poor healing.
• Question patient about the use of other drug products, including over-the-counter (OTC) products, that also contain acetaminophen because of risk of acetaminophen overdose

Consultations:
• In a patient with symptoms of blood dyscrasias, request a medical consult for blood studies and postpone dental treatment until normal values are reestablished.

acetazolamide

a-seat-a-zole′-a-mide
(Apo-Acetazolamide[CAN], Dazamide, Diamox, Diamox Sequels)
Do not confuse with acetohexamide.

CATEGORY AND SCHEDULE

Pregnancy Risk Category: C

MECHANISM OF ACTION

A carbonic anhydrase inhibitor that reduces formation of hydrogen and bicarbonate ions from carbon dioxide and water by inhibiting, in proximal renal tubule, the enzyme carbonic anhydrase, thereby promoting renal excretion of sodium, potassium, bicarbonate, water. Ocular: Reduces rate of aqueous humor formation, lowers intraocular pressure. ***Therapeutic Effect:*** Produces anticonvulsant activity.

PHARMACOKINETICS

Rapidly absorbed. Protein binding: 95%. Widely distributed throughout body tissues including erythrocytes, kidneys, and blood brain barrier. Not metabolized. Excreted unchanged in urine. Removed by hemodialysis. ***Half-life:*** 2.4–5.8 hrs.

AVAILABILITY

Capsules, sustained release: 500 mg (Diamox Sequels).
Powder for reconstitution: 500 mg.
Tablets: 125 mg, 250 mg (Diamox).

INDICATIONS AND DOSAGES

▸ **Glaucoma**

PO

Adults. 250 mg 1–4 times/day. Extended-Release: 500 mg 1–2 times/day usually given in morning and evening.

▸ **Secondary Glaucoma, Preop Treatment of Acute Congestive Glaucoma**

PO/IV

Adults. 250 mg q4h, 250 mg q12h; or 500 mg, then 125–250 mg q4h.

PO

Children. 10–15 mg/kg/day in divided doses.

IV

Children. 5–10 mg/kg q6h.

▸ **Edema**

IV

Adults. 25–375 mg once daily.
Children. 5 mg/kg or 150 mg/m^2 once daily.

Epilepsy

ORAL

Adults, Children. 375–1,000 mg/day in 1–4 divided doses.

Acute Mountain Sickness

PO

Adults. 500–1,000 mg/day in divided doses. If possible, begin 24–48 hrs before ascent; continue at least 48 hrs at high altitude.

Usual elderly dosage

PO

Initially, 250 mg 2 times/day; use lowest effective dose.

Dosage in Renal Impairment

Creatinine Clearance	Dosage Interval
10–50 ml/min	q12h
less than 10 ml/min	avoid use

OFF-LABEL USES

Urine alkalinization, respiratory stimulant in COPD

CONTRAINDICATIONS

Severe renal disease, adrenal insufficiency, hypochloremic acidosis, hypersensitivity to acetazolamide, to any component of the formulation, or to sulfonamides.

INTERACTIONS

Drug

Amphetamines: May increase effects and toxicity of amphetamines

Cyclosporine: May increase cyclosporine through concentrations and possible neprotoxicity and neurotoxicity.

Digoxin: May increase the risk of digoxin toxicity caused by hypokalemia.

Lithium: May increase lithium excretion and decrease serum levels.

Methenamine: May decrease effects of methenamine.

Phenytoin: May increase serum concentrations of phenytoin.

Primidone: May decrease serum concentrations of primidone.

Quinidine: May decrease urinary excretion of quinidine and increase effects.

Salicylates: May increase risk of acetazolamide accumulation and toxicity including CNS depression and metabolic acidosis.

Herbal

None known.

Food

None known.

Drug interactions of concern to dentistry

- Toxicity: salicylates (large doses)
- Hypokalemia: corticosteroids (systemic use)
- Crystalluria: ciprofloxacin

DIAGNOSTIC TEST EFFECTS

May increase ammonia, bilirubin, glucose, chloride, uric acid, calcium. May decrease bicarbonate, potassium.

IV INCOMPATIBILITIES

No drug incompatibilities reported.

IV COMPATIBILITIES

Cimetidine (Tagament), procaine, ranitidine (Zantac)

SIDE EFFECTS

Frequent

Unusually tired/weak, diarrhea, increased urination/frequency, decreased appetite/weight, altered taste (metallic), nausea, vomiting, numbness in extremities, lips, mouth

Occasional

Depression, drowsiness

Rare

Headache, photosensitivity, confusion, tinnitus, severe muscle weakness, loss of taste

SERIOUS REACTIONS

! Long-term therapy may result in acidotic state.

! Nephrotoxicity/hepatotoxicity occurs occasionally, manifested as dark urine/stools, pain in lower back, jaundice, dysuria, crystalluria, renal colic/calculi.
! Bone marrow depression may be manifested as aplastic anemia, thrombocytopenia, thrombocytopenic purpura, leukopenia, agranulocytosis, hemolytic anemia.

DENTAL CONSIDERATIONS

General:

- Patients on chronic drug therapy may rarely have symptoms of blood dyscrasias, which can include infection, bleeding, and poor healing.
- Assess salivary flow as a factor in caries, periodontal disease, and candidiasis.
- Avoid drugs that may exacerbate glaucoma (e.g., anticholinergics).

Consultations:

- In a patient with symptoms of blood dyscrasias, request a medical consultation for blood studies and postpone dental treatment until normal values are reestablished.
- Consultation may be required to assess disease control.

Teach Patient/Family:

- Importance of good oral hygiene to prevent soft tissue inflammation
- Caution to prevent injury when using oral hygiene aids
- *When chronic dry mouth occurs, advise patient:*
  - To avoid mouth rinses with high alcohol content because of drying effects
  - To use daily home fluoride products for anticaries effect
  - To use sugarless gum, frequent sips of water, or saliva substitutes

acetohexamide

a-seat-oh-hex′-a-mide
(Dymelor)
Do not confuse with acetazolamide.

CATEGORY AND SCHEDULE

Pregnancy Risk Category: D

MECHANISM OF ACTION

An intermediate acting sulfonylurea that promotes the release of insulin from beta cells of pancreas, increases insulin sensitivity at peripheral sites. ***Therapeutic Effect:*** Lowers blood glucose concentration.

PHARMACOKINETICS

Well absorbed from the gastrointestinal (GI) tract. Protein binding: 65–90%. Metabolized in liver. Excreted in urine.
Not removed by hemodialysis. ***Half-life:*** 1.3 hrs.

AVAILABILITY

Tablets: 250 mg, 500 mg (Dymelor).

INDICATIONS AND DOSAGES

▸ Diabetes Mellitus

PO

Adults, Elderly. Initially, 250 mg/day. Adjust dosage in 250- to 500-mg increments at intervals of 5–7 days. Maximum daily dose: 1.5 g. Elderly patients may be more sensitive and should be started at a lower dosage initially.

CONTRAINDICATIONS

Diabetic ketoacidosis with or without coma, Type 1 diabetes mellitus, hypersensitivity to acetohexamide or any component of the formulation

INTERACTIONS

Drug

Acarbose, clofibrate, fluoroquinolones, NSAIDs, thioctic acid: May increase risk of hypoglycemia.
Beta-blockers: May increase the hypoglycemic effect and mask signs of hypoglycemia.
Cotrimoxazole, MAOIs, sulfadiazine, sulfamethoxazole, sulfisoxazole: May increase the effects of acetohexamide.

Herbal

Bitter melon, eucalyptus, fenugreek, ginseng, guar gum, gymnema extracts, psyllium, St. John's wort: May increase risk of hypoglycemia.
Glucosamine, licorice: May decrease acetohexamide effectiveness.

Food

None known.

Drug interactions of concern to dentistry

- Increased hypoglycemic effects: salicylates (large doses)
- Decreased action: corticosteroids
- Disulfiram-like reaction: alcohol

DIAGNOSTIC TEST EFFECTS

None known.

SIDE EFFECTS

Frequent

Altered taste sensation, dizziness, drowsiness, weight gain, constipation, diarrhea, heartburn, nausea, vomiting, stomach fullness, headache.

Occasional

Increased sensitivity of skin to sunlight, peeling of skin, itching, rash.

SERIOUS REACTIONS

! Hypoglycemia may occur because of overdosage or insufficient food intake, especially with increased glucose demands.

! GI hemorrhage, cholestatic hepatic jaundice, leukopenia, thrombocytopenia, pancytopenia, agranulocytosis, aplastic or hemolytic anemia occurs rarely.

DENTAL CONSIDERATIONS

General:

- Monitor vital signs at every appointment because of cardiovascular effects of diabetes.
- Patients on chronic drug therapy may rarely have symptoms of blood dyscrasias, which can include infection, bleeding, and poor healing.
- Place on frequent recall to evaluate healing response.
- Ensure that patient is following prescribed diet and takes medication regularly.
- Question patient about self-monitoring of drug's antidiabetic effect, including self-monitored blood glucose (SMBG) values or finger-stick records.
- Avoid prescribing aspirin-containing products.
- Early-morning appointments and a stress reduction protocol may be required for anxious patients.
- Patients with diabetes may be more susceptible to infection and have delayed wound healing.

Consultations:

- In a patient with symptoms of blood dyscrasias, request a medical consultation for blood studies and postpone dental treatment until normal values are reestablished.
- Medical consultation may include data from patient's blood glucose monitoring, including glycosylated hemoglobin or hemoglobin A_{1c} (HbA_{1c}) testing.

Teach Patient/Family:

- Importance of good oral hygiene to prevent soft tissue inflammation

- Caution to prevent injury when using oral hygiene aids
- To avoid mouth rinses with high alcohol content

acetylcholine chloride

a-se-teel-koe′-leen
(Miochol-E, Miochol-E/Steri-Tags, Miochol-E System Pak)

CATEGORY AND SCHEDULE

Pregnancy Risk Category: C

MECHANISM OF ACTION

A cholinergic agonist that causes contraction of the sphincter muscles of the iris. ***Therapeutic Effect:*** Results in miosis and contraction of ciliary muscle, leading to accommodation spasm.

PHARMACOKINETICS

Rapid miosis of short duration.

AVAILABILITY

Powder for reconstitution (intraocular): 1% (Miochol-E, Miochol-E/Steri-Tags, Miochol-E System Pak).

INDICATIONS AND DOSAGES

▶ Production of Miosis

INTRAOCULAR

Adults, Elderly. 0.5–2 ml instilled into anterior chamber before or after securing one or more sutures.

CONTRAINDICATIONS

Acute iritis and acute inflammatory disease of the anterior chamber, hypersensitivity to acetylcholine chloride or any component of the formulation

INTERACTIONS

Drug

Flurbiprofen, suprofen (ophthalmic): May decrease the effects of acetylcholine.

Tacrine: May increase or prolong the effects of acetylcholine.

Thioridazine: May increase risk of cardiotoxicity.

Herbal

None known.

Food

None known.

Drug interactions of concern to dentistry

- None reported

DIAGNOSTIC TEST EFFECTS

None known.

SIDE EFFECTS

Rare

Corneal clouding, corneal decompensation

SERIOUS REACTIONS

! Systemic effects rarely occur. These effects include bradycardia, hypotension, flushing, breathing difficulties, and sweating.

DENTAL CONSIDERATIONS

General:

- Acute-use drug in selected types of eye surgery.
- Protect patient's eyes from accidental spatter during dental treatment.
- Avoid dental light in patient's eyes; offer dark glasses for patient comfort.

acetylcysteine

a-see-til-sis′-tay-een
(Acetadote, Mucomyst, Parvolex[CAN])
Do not confuse acetylcysteine with acetylcholine.

CATEGORY AND SCHEDULE

Pregnancy Risk Category: B

MECHANISM OF ACTION

An intratracheal respiratory inhalant that splits the linkage of mucoproteins, reducing the viscosity of pulmonary secretions. ***Therapeutic Effect:*** Facilitates the removal of pulmonary secretions by coughing, postural drainage, mechanical means. Protects against acetaminophen overdose-induced hepatotoxicity.

AVAILABILITY

Injection (Acedote): 20% (200 mg/ml).
Inhalation Solution (Mucomyst): 10% (100 mg/ml), 20% (200 mg/ml).

INDICATIONS AND DOSAGES

▸ Adjunctive Treatment of Viscid Mucus Secretions from Chronic Bronchopulmonary Disease and for Pulmonary Complications of Cystic Fibrosis

NEBULIZATION

Adults, Elderly, Children. 3–5 ml (20% solution) 3–4 times a day or 6–10 ml (10% solution) 3–4 times a day. Range: 1–10 ml (20% solution) q2–6h or 2–20 ml (10% solution) q2–6h.

Infants. 1–2 ml (20%) or 2–4 ml (10%) 3–4 times a day.

▸ Treatment of Viscid Mucus Secretions in Patients with a Tracheostomy

INTRATRACHEAL

Adults, Children. 1–2 ml of 10% or 20% solution instilled into tracheostomy q1–4h.

▸ Acetaminophen Overdose

PO (Oral solution 5%)

Adults, Elderly, Children. Loading dose of 140 mg/kg, followed in 4 hr by maintenance dose of 70 mg/kg q4h for 17 additional doses (unless acetaminophen assay reveals nontoxic level).

IV

Adults, Elderly, Children. 150 mg/kg infused over 15 minutes, then 50 mg/kg infused over 4 hr, then 100 mg/kg infused over 16 hr. See administration and handling. Repeat dose if emesis occurs within 1 hr of administration. Continue until all doses are given, even if acetaminophen plasma level drops below toxic range.

▸ Prevention of Renal Damage from Dyes Used During Certain Diagnostic Tests

PO (Oral solution 5%)

Adults, Elderly. 600 mg twice a day for 4 doses starting the day before the procedure.

OFF-LABEL USES

Prevention of renal damage from dyes given during certain diagnostic tests (such as CT scans)

CONTRAINDICATIONS

None known.

INTERACTIONS

Drug

None known.

Herbal

None known.

Food

None known.

Drug interactions of concern to dentistry

- None reported

DIAGNOSTIC TEST EFFECTS

None known.

SIDE EFFECTS

Frequent

Inhalation: Stickiness on face, transient unpleasant odor

Occasional

Inhalation: Increased bronchial secretions, throat irritation, nausea, vomiting, rhinorrhea

Rare

Inhalation: Rash

Oral: Facial edema, bronchospasm, wheezing

SERIOUS REACTIONS

! Large doses may produce severe nausea and vomiting.

DENTAL CONSIDERATIONS

General:

- Be aware that aspirin and/or sulfite preservatives in vasoconstrictor-containing products may exacerbate asthma.
- Acute asthmatic episodes may be precipitated in the dental office. A rapid-acting sympathomimetic inhalant (rescue inhaler) should be available for emergency use. Many patients may already have a prescribed rescue inhaler they normally use for acute asthmatic events.
- Consider semisupine chair position for patients with respiratory disease.
- Determine dose and duration of glucocorticoid therapy to assess for risk of stress tolerance and immunosuppression. Patients on chronic glucocorticoid therapy may require supplemental doses for dental treatment.
- Examine for oral manifestation of opportunistic infection.
- Evaluate respiration characteristics and rate.
- Short appointments and a stress reduction protocol may be required for anxious patients.
- Inquire about other drugs patients are using for respiratory disease.

Consultations:

- Consultation with physician may be necessary if sedation or general anesthesia is required.
- Consultation may be required to confirm glucocorticoid dose and duration of use.
- Medical consultation may be required to assess disease control and patient's ability to tolerate stress

Teach Patient/Family:

- Importance of good oral hygiene to prevent soft tissue inflammation
- Importance of updating health and medication history if physician makes any changes in evaluation or drug regimens; include OTC, herbal, and nonherbal remedies in the update
- Importance of gargling, rinsing mouth with water, and expectorating after each aerosol dose

acitretin

a-si-tre′-tin

(Soriatane)

CATEGORY AND SCHEDULE

Pregnancy Risk Category: X

MECHANISM OF ACTION

A second-generation retinoid that adjusts factors influencing epidermal proliferation, RNA/DNA synthesis, controls glycoprotein, and governs immune response. ***Therapeutic Effect:*** Regulates keratinocyte growth and differentiation.

PHARMACOKINETICS

Well absorbed from the gastrointestinal (GI) tract. Food increases rate of absorption. Protein binding: greater than 99%. Metabolized in liver. Excreted in bile and urine. Not removed by hemodialysis. ***Half-life:*** 49 hrs.

AVAILABILITY

Capsules: 10 mg, 25 mg (Soriatane).

INDICATIONS AND DOSAGES

▸ **Psoriasis**

PO

Adults, Elderly. 25–50 mg/day as a single dose with main meal. May increase to 75 mg/day if necessary and dose tolerated. Maintenance: 25–50 mg/day after the initial response is noted. Continue until lesions have resolved.

OFF-LABEL USES

Treatment of Darier's disease, palmoplantar pustulosis, lichen planus; children with lameliar ichthyosis, nonbullous and bullous ichthyosiform erythroderma, Sjogren-Larsson syndrome

CONTRAINDICATIONS

Pregnancy or those who intend to become pregnant within 3 years following discontinuation of therapy, severely impaired liver or kidney function, chronic abnormal elevated lipid levels, concomitant use of methotrexate or tetracyclines, ingestion of alcohol (in females of reproductive potential), hypersensitivity to acitretin, etretinate or other retinoids, sensitivity to parabenz (used as preservative in gelatin capsule)

INTERACTIONS

Drug

Alcohol: May prevent elimination of acitretin.

"Minipill" oral contraceptive: May interfere with contraceptive effect.

Methotrexate: May increase risk of hepatotoxicity.

Tetracyclines: May increase risk of increased intracranial pressure.

Herbal

St. John's Wort: May increase risk of unplanned pregnancy and birth defects.

Vitamin A: May increase risk of vitamin A toxicity.

Food

None known.

Drug interactions of concern to dentistry

- Avoid vitamin preparations containing vitamin A
- Avoid tetracyclines and other drugs that cause photosensitivity

DIAGNOSTIC TEST EFFECTS

May increase triglucerides, SGOT (AST), SGPT (ALT). May decrease LDH (high-density lipoprotein).

SIDE EFFECTS

Frequent

Lip inflammation, alopecia, skin peeling, shakiness, dry eyes, rash, hyperesthesia, paresthesia, sticky skin, dry mouth, epistaxis, dryness/thickening of conjunctiva

Occasional

Eye irritation, brow and lash loss, sweating, chills, sensation of cold, flushing, edema, blurred vision, diarrhea, nausea, thirst

SERIOUS REACTIONS

! Benign intracranial hypertension (pseudotumor cerebri) occurs rarely.

DENTAL CONSIDERATIONS

General:

- Determine why patient is taking the drug.
- Apply lubricant to dry lips for patient comfort before dental procedures.

- Assess salivary flow as factor in caries, periodontal disease, and candidiasis.
- Palliative medication may be required for management of oral side effects.
- Place on frequent recall because of oral side effects.
- Consider semisupine chair position for patient comfort if GI side effects occur.
- Avoid dental light in patient's eyes; offer dark glasses for patient comfort.

Consultations:

- Medical consultation may be required to assess disease control.

Teach Patient/Family:

- Importance of good oral hygiene to prevent soft tissue inflammation
- Caution patient to prevent trauma when using oral hygiene aids
- To report oral lesions, soreness, or bleeding to dentist
- *When chronic dry mouth occurs, advise patient:*
- To avoid mouth rinses with high alcohol content because of drying effects
- To use daily home fluoride products for anticaries effect
- To use sugarless gum, frequent sips of water, or saliva substitutes

acyclovir

ay-sye′-kloe-ver
(Aciclovir-BC IV[AUS], Acihexal[AUS], Acyclo-V[AUS], Avirax[CAN], Lovir[AUS], Zovirax, Zyclir[AUS])
Do not confuse with Zostrix, Zyvox.

CATEGORY AND SCHEDULE

Pregnancy Risk Category: B

MECHANISM OF ACTION

A synthetic nucleoside that converts to acyclovir triphosphate, becoming part of the DNA chain. ***Therapeutic Effect:*** Interferes with DNA synthesis and viral replication. Virustatic.

PHARMACOKINETICS

Poorly absorbed from the GI tract; minimal absorption following topical application. Protein binding: 9%–36%. Widely distributed. Partially metabolized in liver. Excreted primarily in urine. Removed by hemodialysis. ***Half-life:*** 2.5 hr (increased in impaired renal function).

AVAILABILITY

Capsules: 200 mg.
Tablets: 400 mg, 800 mg.
Injection, solution: 50 mg/ml.
Oral Suspension: 200 mg/5 ml.
Powder for Injection: 500 mg, 1,000 mg.
Ointment: 5%/50 mg.

INDICATIONS AND DOSAGES

▸ Genital Herpes (initial episode)

IV
Adults, Elderly, Children 12 yr and older. 5 mg/kg q8h for 5 days.
PO
Adults, Elderly, Children 12 yr and older. 200 mg q4h 5 times a day.

▸ Genital Herpes (recurrent)

Fewer than 6 episodes per year:
PO
Adults, Elderly, Children 12 yr and older. 200 mg q4h 5 times a day for 5 days.
6 episodes or more per year:
PO
Adults, Elderly, Children 12 yr and older. 400 mg 2 times a day or 200 mg 3–5 times a day for up to 12 months.

Herpes Simplex Mucocutaneous

IV

Adults, Elderly, Children 12 yr and older. 5 mg/kg/dose q8h for 7 days.
Children younger than 12 yr.
10 mg/kg q8h for 7 days.

Herpes Simplex Neonatal

IV

Children younger than 4 mo.
10 mg/kg q8h for 10 days.

Herpes Simplex Encephalitis

IV

Adults, Elderly, Children 12 yr and older. 10 mg/kg q8h for 10 days.
Children 3 mos - younger than 12 yr.
20 mg/kg q8h for 10 days.

Herpes Zoster (caused by varicella)

IV

Adults, Elderly, Children 12 yr and older. 10 mg/kg q8h for 7 days.
Children younger than 12 yr.
20 mg/kg q8h for 7 days.

Herpes Zoster (shingles)

PO

Adults, Elderly, Children 12 yr and older. 800 mg q4h 5 times a day for 7–10 days.

Topical

Adults, Elderly. Apply to affected area 3–6 times a day for 7 days.

Varicella (chickenpox)

PO

Adults, Elderly, Children older than 12 yr or children 2–12 yr, weighing 40 kg or more. 800 mg 4 times a day for 5 days.
Children 2–12 yr, weighing less than 40 kg. 20 mg/kg 4 times a day for 5 days. Maximum: 800 mg/dose.
Children younger than 2 yr.
80 mg/kg/day.

Dosage in Renal Impairment

Dosage and frequency are modified on the basis of severity of infection and degree of renal impairment.

PO

For creatinine clearance of 10 ml/min or less, dosage is 200 mg q12h.

IV

Creatinine Clearance	Dosage Percent	Dosage Interval
greater than 50 ml/min	100	8 hr
25–50 ml/min	100	12 hr
10–25 ml/min	100	24 hr
less than 10 ml/min	50	24 hr

OFF-LABEL USES

Treatment of herpes simplex ocular infections, infectious mononucleosis

CONTRAINDICATIONS

Use in neonates when acyclovir is reconstituted with bacteriostatic water containing benzyl alcohol.

INTERACTIONS

Drug

Nephrotoxic medications (such as aminoglycosides): May increase the nephrotoxicity of acyclovir.
Probenecid: May increase acyclovir half-life.

Herbal

None known.

Food

None known.

DIAGNOSTIC TEST EFFECTS

May increase BUN and serum creatinine concentrations.

IV INCOMPATIBILITIES

Aztreonam (Azactam), cefepime (Maxipime), diltiazem (Cardizem), dobutamine (Dobutrex), dopamine (Intropin), levofloxacin (Levaquin), meropenem (Merrem IV), ondansetron (Zofran), piperacillin and tazobactam (Zosyn)

IV COMPATIBILITIES

Allopurinol (Alloprim), amikacin (Amikin), ampicillin, cefazolin (Ancef), cefotaxime (Claforan), ceftazidime (Fortaz), ceftriaxone

(Rocephin), cimetidine (Tagamet), clindamycin (Cleocin), famotidine (Pepcid), fluconazole (Diflucan), gentamicin, heparin, hydromorphone (Dilaudid), imipenem (Primaxin), lorazepam (Ativan), magnesium sulfate, methylprednisolone (SoluMedrol), metoclopramide (Reglan), metronidazole (Flagyl), morphine, multivitamins, potassium chloride, propofol (Diprivan), ranitidine (Zantac), vancomycin

SIDE EFFECTS

Frequent
Parenteral (9%–7%): Phlebitis or inflammation at IV site, nausea, vomiting
Topical (28%): Burning, stinging

Occasional
Parenteral (3%): Pruritus, rash, urticaria
Oral (12%–6%): Malaise, nausea
Topical (4%): Pruritus

Rare
Oral (3%–1%): Vomiting, rash, diarrhea, headache
Parenteral (2%–1%): Confusion, hallucinations, seizures, tremors
Topical (less than 1%): Rash

SERIOUS REACTIONS

! Rapid parenteral administration, excessively high doses, or fluid and electrolyte imbalance may produce renal failure exhibited by such signs and symptoms as abdominal pain, decreased urination, decreased appetite, increased thirst, nausea, and vomiting.

! Toxicity has not been reported with oral or topical use.

DENTAL CONSIDERATIONS

General:
- Postpone dental treatment when oral herpetic lesions are present.

Teach Patient/Family:
- To dispose of toothbrush or other contaminated oral hygiene devices used during period of infection to prevent reinoculation of herpetic infection
- To apply with a finger cot or latex glove to prevent herpes infection on fingers
- To avoid mouth rinses with high alcohol content because of irritating effects

adalimumab

ah-dah-lim′-you-mab
(Humira)

CATEGORY AND SCHEDULE

Pregnancy Risk Category: B

MECHANISM OF ACTION

A monoclonal antibody that binds specifically to tumor necrosis factor (TNF) alpha, blocking its interaction with cell surface TNF receptors.
Therapeutic Effect: Reduces inflammation, tenderness, and swelling of joints; slows or prevents progressive destruction of joints in rheumatoid arthritis.

PHARMACOKINETICS

Half-life: 10–20 days.

AVAILABILITY

Injection: 40 mg/0.8 ml in prefilled syringes.

INDICATIONS AND DOSAGES

▸ Rheumatoid Arthritis
SUBCUTANEOUS
Adults, Elderly. 40 mg every other week. Dose may be increased to 40 mg/wk in those not taking methotrexate.

CONTRAINDICATIONS
Active infections

INTERACTIONS
Drug
Methotrexate: Reduces the absorption of adalimumab by 29%–40%, but dosage adjustment is unnecessary if given concurrently.
Herbal
None known.
Food
None known.
Drug interactions of concern to dentistry
- None reported

DIAGNOSTIC TEST EFFECTS
May increase levels of blood cholesterol, other lipids, and serum alkaline phosphatase

SIDE EFFECTS
Frequent (20%)
Injection site, erythema, pruritus, pain, and swelling
Occasional (12%–9%)
Headache, rash, sinusitis, nausea
Rare (7%–5%)
Abdominal or back pain, hypertension

SERIOUS REACTIONS
! Rare reactions include hypersensitivity reactions, malignancies, respiratory tract infections, bronchitis, UTIs, and more serious infections (such as pneumonia, tuberculosis, cellulitus, pyelonephritis, and septic arthritis).

DENTAL CONSIDERATIONS
General:
- Patient may need assistance in getting into and out of dental chair.
- Adjust chair position for patient comfort.
- Determine why patient is taking the drug.
- Question patient about other drugs being taken.
- Examine for oral manifestation of opportunistic infection.
- Report oral infections to patient's physician; treat infections aggressively.
- Consider semisupine chair position for patient comfort if GI side effects occur.

Consultations:
- Medical consultation may be required to assess disease control and patient's ability to tolerate stress.

Teach Patient/Family:
- Importance of good oral hygiene to prevent soft tissue inflammation
- To immediately report any signs or symptoms of oral infection

adapalene
a-dap′-pa-leen
(Differin)

CATEGORY AND SCHEDULE
Pregnancy Risk category: C

MECHANISM OF ACTION
Binds to retinoic acid receptors in cell nuclei modulating cell differentiation, keratinization. Possesses anti-inflammatory properties. ***Therapeutic effect:*** Normalizes differentiation of follicular epithelial cells.

PHARMACOKINETICS
Absorption through the skin is low. Trace amount found in plasma following topical application. Excreted primarily by biliary route.

AVAILABILITY
Gel: 0.1%
Cream: 0.1%
Pledget (solution): 0.1%

A

INDICATIONS AND DOSAGES

▸ **Acne Vulgaris**

TOPICAL

Adults, elderly, children > 12 years. Apply to affected area once daily at bedtime after washing.

CONTRAINDICATIONS

Hypersensitivity to adapalene, vitamin A or any one of its components.

INTERACTIONS

Drug

Quinolones (particularly sparfloxacin), phenothiazines, sulfonamides, sulfonylureas, tetracyclines, thiazide diuretics: Adapalene may increase the effects of these photosensitizing agents.

Benzoyl peroxide, salicylic acid, sulfur, resorcinol, alcohol: Additive local irritation when used with adapalene.

Herbal

None known.

Food

None known.

Drug interactions of concern to dentistry

- Avoid use of topical antiinfectives on same skin application site

DIAGNOSTIC TEST EFFECTS

None known.

SIDE EFFECTS

Frequent

Erythema, scaling, dryness, pruritis, burning (likely to occur first 2–4 weeks, lessens with continued use)

Occasional

Skin irritation, stinging, sunburn, acne flares, erythema, photosensitivity, pruritis, xerosis

SERIOUS REACTIONS

! Concurrent use of other potentially irritating topical products (soaps, cleansers, aftershave, cosmetics may produce severe topical irritation).

DENTAL CONSIDERATIONS

General:

- Advise patient if dental drugs prescribed have a potential for photosensitivity.
- Apply lubricant to dry lips for patient comfort prior to dental procedures
- Limit systemic vitamin A doses to no more than the RDA

Teach Patient/Family:

- To avoid getting in eyes or mouth, or on other mucous membranes.

adefovir

ah-deh′-foh-veer

(Hepsera)

CATEGORY AND SCHEDULE

Pregnancy Risk Category: C

MECHANISM OF ACTION

An antiviral that inhibits the enzyme DNA polymerase, causing DNA chain termination after its incorporation into viral DNA. ***Therapeutic Effect:*** Prevents cell replication of viral DNA.

PHARMACOKINETICS

Binds to proteins after PO administration. Excreted in urine. ***Half-life:*** 7 hr (increased in impaired renal function).

AVAILABILITY

Tablets: 10 mg.

INDICATIONS AND DOSAGES

▸ Chronic Hepatitis B in Patients with Normal Renal Function

PO

Adults, Elderly. 10 mg once a day.

▸ Chronic Hepatitis B in Patients with Impaired Renal Function

Adults, Elderly with creatinine clearance 20–49 ml/min. 10 mg q48h.
Adults, Elderly with creatinine clearance 10–19 ml/min. 10 mg q72h.
Adults, Elderly on hemodialysis. 10 mg every 7 days following dialysis.

CONTRAINDICATIONS

None known.

INTERACTIONS

Drug

Ibuprofen: Increases adefovir plasma concentration.

Herbal

None known.

Food

None known.

Drug interactions of concern to dentistry

- None reported

DIAGNOSTIC TEST EFFECTS

May increase serum amylase, creatinine, AST (SGOT) and ALT (SGPT) levels.

SIDE EFFECTS

Frequent (13%)

Asthenia

Occasional (9%–4%)

Headache, abdominal pain, nausea, flatulence

Rare (3%)

Diarrhea, dyspepsia

SERIOUS REACTIONS

! Nephrotoxicity (characterized by increased serum creatinine and decreased serum phosphorus levels) is a treatment-limiting toxicity of adefovir therapy.

! Lactic acidosis and severe hepatomegaly occur rarely, particularly in female patients.

DENTAL CONSIDERATIONS

General:

- Examine for oral manifestation of opportunistic infection.
- Determine why patient is taking the drug.
- Consider semisupine chair position for patient comfort if GI side effects occur.
- Do not provide treatment if clinician does not have seroconversion to protective antibodies to hepatitis B.

Consultations:

- Medical consultation may be required to assess disease control and patient's ability to tolerate stress.
- Patients who report feeling symptoms of lactic acidosis, such as weakness, malaise, with unusual muscle pain, difficulty breathing, stomach pain with nausea, cold feeling in arms or legs, dizziness or light-headedness, and irregular heartbeat, should be immediately referred to their physician.

Teach Patient/Family:

- Importance of good oral hygiene to prevent soft tissue inflammation
- To prevent trauma when using oral hygiene aids
- Importance of updating health and drug history if physician makes any changes in evaluation or drug regimens

adenosine

ah-den′-oh-seen
(Adenocard, Adenocor[AUS], Adenoscan)

CATEGORY AND SCHEDULE

Pregnancy Risk Category: C

MECHANISM OF ACTION

A cardiac agent that slows impulse formation in the SA node and conduction time through the AV node. Adenosine also acts as a diagnostic aid in myocardial perfusion imaging or stress echocardiography.

Therapeutic Effect: Depresses left ventricular function and restores normal sinus rhythm.

AVAILABILITY

Injection (Adenocard): 3 mg/ml in 2 ml, 4 ml syringes.
Injection (Adenoscan): 3 mg/ml in 20 ml, 30 ml vials.

INDICATIONS AND DOSAGES

▸ Paroxysmal Supraventricular Tachycardia (PSVT)

RAPID IV BOLUS

Adults, Elderly. Initially, 6 mg given over 1–2 sec. If first dose does not convert within 1–2 min, give 12 mg; may repeat 12-mg dose in 1–2 min if no response has occurred.
Children. Initially 0.1 mg/kg (maximum: 6 mg). If ineffective, may give 0.2 mg/kg (maximum: 12 mg).

▸ Diagnostic Testing

IV INFUSION

Adults. 140 mcg/kg/min for 6 min.

CONTRAINDICATIONS

Atrial fibrillation or flutter, second- or third-degree AV block or sick sinus syndrome (with functioning pacemaker), ventricular tachycardia

INTERACTIONS

Drug

Carbamazepine: May increase degree of heart block caused by adenosine.
Dipyridamole: May increase effect of adenosine.
Methylxanthines (e.g., caffeine, theophylline): May decrease effect of adenosine.

Herbal

None known.

Food

None known.

Drug interactions of concern to dentistry

- Increased risk of heart block: carbamazepine

DIAGNOSTIC TEST EFFECTS

None known.

IV INCOMPATIBILITIES

Any drug or solution other than 0.9% NaCl or D_5W.

SIDE EFFECTS

Frequent (18%–12%)

Facial flushing, dyspnea

Occasional (7%–2%)

Headache, nausea, light-headedness, chest pressure

Rare (less than or equal to 1%)

Numbness or tingling in arms; dizziness; diaphoresis; hypotension; palpitations; chest, jaw, or neck pain

SERIOUS REACTIONS

! May produce short-lasting heart block.

DENTAL CONSIDERATIONS

General:

- Acute-use drug for use in emergency rooms, hospitals, or cardiac testing labs. If a patient reports use of this drug in his/her medical history, question about cardiovascular disease and drugs he/she may be taking.
- Provide palliative emergency dental care only during drug use.

Consultations:

- Medical consultation may be required to assess disease control and patient's ability to tolerate stress.

albendazole

all-ben′-dah-zole
(Albenza)

CATEGORY AND SCHEDULE

Pregnancy Risk Category: C

MECHANISM OF ACTION

A benzimidazole carbamate anthelmintic that degrades parasite cytoplasmic microtubules, irreversibly blocks cholinesterase secretion, glucose uptake in helminth and larvae (depletes glycogen, decreases ATP production, depletes energy). Vermicidal. ***Therapeutic Effect:*** Immobilizes and kills worms.

PHARMACOKINETICS

Poorly and variable absorbed gastrointestinal (GI) tract. Widely distributed, cyst fluid and including cerebrospinal fluid (CSF). Protein binding: 70%. Extensively metabolized in liver. Primarily excreted in urine and bile. Not removed by hemodialysis. ***Half-life:*** 8–12 hrs.

AVAILABILITY

Tablets: 200 mg (Albenza).

INDICATIONS AND DOSAGES

▸ Neurocysticercosis

PO

Adults, Elderly more than 60 kg. 400 mg 2 times/day. Continue for 28 days, rest 14 days, repeat cycle 3 times.

Adults, Elderly less than 60 kg. 15 mg/kg/day. Continue for 28 days, rest 14 days, repeat cycle 3 times.

▸ Cystic Hydatid

PO

Adults, Elderly more than 60 kg. 400 mg 2 times/day. Continue for 8–30 days.

Adults, Elderly less than 60 kg. 15 mg/kg/day. Continue for 8–30 days.

OFF-LABEL USES

Angiostrongyliasis, cysticercosis, gnathostomiasis, liver flukes, trichuriasis

CONTRAINDICATIONS

Hypersensitivity to albendazole or any component of the formulation, pregnancy

INTERACTIONS

Drug

Dexamethasone, praziquantel: May increase albendazole concentration.

Theophylline: May increase risk of theophylline toxicity.

Herbal

Ginseng: May decrease intestinal concentration of active drug.

Food

Grapefruit juice: May increase risk of albendazole adverse effects.

Drug interactions of concern to dentistry

- Possible increase in blood levels: glucocorticoids, cimetidine

DIAGNOSTIC TEST EFFECTS

May decrease total white blood cell (WBC) count.

SIDE EFFECTS

Frequent

Neurocysticerosis: Nausea, vomiting, headache

Hydatid: Abnormal liver function tests, abdominal pain, nausea, vomiting

Occasional

Neurocysticerosis: Increased intracranial pressure, meningeal signs

Hydatid: Headache, dizziness, alopecia, fever

SERIOUS REACTIONS

! Pancytopenia occurs rarely.
! In presence of cysticercosis, drug may produce retinal damage in presence of retinal lesions.

DENTAL CONSIDERATIONS

General:

- Determine why patient is taking the drug.
- Patient on chronic drug therapy may rarely present with symptoms of blood dyscrasias, which can include infection, bleeding, and poor healing. If dyscrasia is present, caution patient to prevent oral tissue trauma when using oral hygiene aids.
- Question patients about other drugs they may be taking

Consultations:

- In a patient with symptoms of blood dyscrasias, request a medical consultation for blood studies and postpone treatment until normal values are reestablished

albuterol

al-byoo′-ter-ole
(AccuNeb, Airomir[AUS], Asmol CFC-Free[AUS], Epaq Inhaler[AUS], Novosalmol[CAN], Proventil, Proventil Repetabs, Respax[AUS], Ventolin, Ventolin CFC-Free[AUS], Volmax, Vospire ER)
Do not confuse albuterol with Albutein or atenolol, or Proventil with Prinivil.

CATEGORY AND SCHEDULE

Pregnancy Risk Category: C

MECHANISM OF ACTION

A sympathomimetic that stimulates beta_2-adrenergic receptors in the lungs, resulting in relaxation of bronchial smooth muscle.

Therapeutic Effect: Relieves bronchospasm and reduces airway resistance.

PHARMACOKINETICS

Route	Onset	Peak	Duration
PO	15–30 min	2–3 hr	4–6 hr
PO (extended-release)	30 min	2–4 hr	12 hr
Inhalation	5–15 min	0.5–2 hr	2–5 hr

Rapidly, well absorbed from the GI tract; gradually absorbed from the bronchi after inhalation. Metabolized in the liver. Primarily excreted in urine. ***Half-life:*** 2.7–5 hr (PO); 3.8 hr (inhalation).

AVAILABILITY

Syrup: 2 mg/5ml.
Tablet: 2 mg, 4 mg.
Tablet (Extended-Release [Proventil Repetabs]): 4 mg.
Tablets (Extended-Release [Volmax, VoSpire ER]): 4 mg, 8 mg.
Inhalation (Aerosol [Proventil, Ventolin]): 90 mcg/spray.
Inhalation (Solution [AccuNeb]): 0.75 mg/3 ml, 1.5 mg/3 ml.
Inhalation (Solution [Proventil]): 0.083%, 0.5%.

INDICATIONS AND DOSAGES

▸ Bronchospasm

PO
Adults, Children older than 12 yr. 2–4 mg 3–4 times a day. Maximum: 8 mg 4 times/day.
Elderly. 2 mg 3–4 times a day. Maximum: 8 mg 4 times a day.
Children 6–12 yr. 2 mg 3–4 times a day. Maximum: 24 mg/day.
PO (Extended-Release)
Adults, Children older than 12 yr. 4–8 mg q12h.

INHALATION
Adults, Elderly, Children older than 12 yr: 1–2 puffs by metered dose inhaler q4–6h as needed.
Children 4–12 yr: 1–2 puffs 4 times a day.
NEBULIZATION
Adults, Elderly, Children older than 12 yr: 2.5 mg 3–4 times a day.
Children 2–12 yr: 0.63–1.25 mg 3–4 times a day.

▸ **Exercise-Induced Bronchospasm**
INHALATION
Adults, Elderly, Children 4 yr and older: 2 puffs 15–30 min before exercise.

CONTRAINDICATIONS

History of hypersensitivity to sympathomimetics

INTERACTIONS

Drug

Beta blockers: Antagonize effects of albuterol.
Digoxin: May increase the risk of arrhythmias.
MAOIs, tricyclic antidepressants: May potentiate cardiovascular effects.

Herbal

None known.

Food

None known.

Drug interactions of concern to dentistry

- None reported

DIAGNOSTIC TEST EFFECTS

May increase blood glucose level. May decrease serum potassium level.

SIDE EFFECTS

Frequent

Headache (27%); nausea (15%); restlessness, nervousness, tremors (20%); dizziness (< 7%); throat dryness and irritation, pharyngitis (< 6%); BP changes, including hypertension (5%–3%); heartburn, transient wheezing (less than 5%)

Occasional (3%–2%)

Insomnia, asthenia, altered taste
Inhalation: Dry, irritated mouth or throat; cough; bronchial irritation

Rare

Somnolence, diarrhea, dry mouth, flushing, diaphoresis, anorexia

SERIOUS REACTIONS

! Excessive sympathomimetic stimulation may produce palpitations, extrasystole, tachycardia, chest pain, a slight increase in BP followed by a substantial decrease, chills, diaphoresis, and blanching of skin.
! Too-frequent or excessive use may lead to decreased bronchodilating effectiveness and severe, paradoxical bronchoconstriction.

DENTAL CONSIDERATIONS

General:

- Monitor vital signs at every appointment because of cardiovascular and respiratory side effects.
- Assess salivary flow as a factor in caries, periodontal disease, and candidiasis.
- Consider semisupine chair position for patients with respiratory disease.
- Midday appointments and a stress reduction protocol may be required for anxious patients.
- Be aware that aspirin or sulfite preservatives in vasoconstrictor-containing products can exacerbate asthma.
- Acute asthmatic episodes may be precipitated in the dental office. Sympathomimetic inhalants should be available for emergency use.

Consultations:

- Medical consultation may be required to assess disease control and patient's ability to tolerate stress.

Teach Patient/Family:

- For inhalation dosage forms, rinse mouth with water after each dose to prevent dryness
- *When chronic dry mouth occurs, advise patient:*
  - To avoid mouth rinses with high alcohol content because of drying effects
  - To use daily home fluoride products for anticaries effect
  - To use sugarless gum, frequent sips of water, or saliva substitutes

alclometasone

al-kloe-met′-a-sone
(Aclovate)

CATEGORY AND SCHEDULE

Pregnancy Risk Category: C

MECHANISM OF ACTION

Topical corticosteroids exhibit anti-inflammatory, antipruritic, and vasoconstrictive properties. Clinically, these actions correspond to decreased edema, erythema, pruritus, plaque formation, and scaling of the affected skin.

PHARMACOKINETICS

Approximately 3% is absorbed during an 8-hour period. Metabolized in the liver. Excreted in the urine.

AVAILABILITY

Cream: (Aclovate)
Ointment: (Aclovate)

INDICATIONS AND DOSAGES

▸ **Atopic Dermatitis, Contact Dermatitis, Dermatitis, Discoid Lupus Erythematosus, Eczema, Exfoliative Dermatitis, Granuloma Annulare, Lichen Planus, Lichen Simplex, Polymorphous Light Eruption, Pruritis, Psoriasis, Rhus Dermatitis, Seborrheic Dermatitis, Xerosis**

TOPICAL

Adults, adolescents, children 1 year and older. Apply a thin film to the affected area 2–3 times a day.

CONTRAINDICATIONS

Hypersensitivity to alclometasone, other corticosteroids, or any of its components.

INTERACTIONS

Drug

None known.

Herbal

None known.

Food

None known.

Drug interactions of concern to dentistry

- None reported

DIAGNOSTIC TEST EFFECTS

None known.

SIDE EFFECTS

Frequent

Burning, erythema, maculopapular rash, pruritis, skin irritation, xerosis

Occasional

Acneiform rash, contact dermatitis, folliculitis, glycosuria, growth inhibition, headache, hyperglycemia, infection, miliaria, papilledema, skin atrophy, skin hypopigmentation, skin ulcer, striae, telangiectasia

Rare

Adrenalcortical insufficiency, increased intracranial pressure, pseudotumor cerebri, impaired wound healing, Cushing's syndrome, HPA suppression, skin ulcers, tolerance, withdrawal, visual impairment, ocular hypertension, cataracts

DENTAL CONSIDERATIONS

General:

- Determine why patient is taking the drug.

Teach Patient/Family:

- Use on oral herpetic ulcerations is contraindicated

Interleukin-2 (aldesleukin)

in-tur-lew′-kin

(IL-2, Proleukin)

Do not confuse interleukin-2 with interferon 2.

CATEGORY AND SCHEDULE

Pregnancy Risk Category: C

MECHANISM OF ACTION

A biological response modifier that acts like human recombinant interleukin-2, promoting proliferation, differentiation, and recruitment of T and B cells, lymphokine-activated and natural cells, and thymocytes. ***Therapeutic Effect:*** Enhances cytolytic activity in lymphocytes.

PHARMACOKINETICS

Primarily distributed into plasma, lymphocytes, lungs, liver, kidney, and spleen. Metabolized to amino acids in the cells lining the kidneys. ***Half-life:*** 85 min.

AVAILABILITY

Powder for Injection: 22 million units (1.3 mg).

INDICATIONS AND DOSAGES

▸ **Metastatic Melanoma, Metastatic Renal Cell Carcinoma**

IV

Adults 18 yr and older.

600,000 units/kg q8h for 14 doses; followed by 9 days of rest, then another 14 doses for a total of 28 doses per course. Course may be repeated after rest period of at least 7 wk from date of hospital discharge.

OFF-LABEL USES

Treatment of colorectal cancer, Kaposi's sarcoma, non-Hodgkin's lymphoma.

CONTRAINDICATIONS

Abnormal pulmonary function or thallium stress test results, bowel ischemia or perforation, coma or toxic psychosis lasting longer than 48 hr, GI bleeding requiring surgery, intubation lasting more than 72 hr, organ allografts, pericardial tamponade, renal dysfunction requiring dialysis for longer than 72 hr, repetitive or difficult-to-control seizures; retreatment in those who experience any of the following toxicities: angina, MI, recurrent chest pain with EKG changes, sustained ventricular tachycardia, uncontrolled or unresponsive cardiac rhythm disturbances

INTERACTIONS

Drug

Antihypertensives: May increase hypotensive effect.

Cardiotoxic, hepatotoxic, myelotoxic, or nephrotoxic medications: May increase the risk of toxicity.

Glucocorticoids: May decrease the effects of interleukin-2.

Herbal

None known.

Food

None known.

Drug interactions of concern to dentistry

Possible reduction in antitumor efficacy: glucocorticoids

DIAGNOSTIC TEST EFFECTS
May increase BUN and serum alkaline phosphatase, bilirubin, creatinine, AST (SGOT), and ALT (SGPT) levels. May decrease serum calcium, magnesium, phosphorus, potassium, and sodium levels.

IV INCOMPATIBILITIES
Ganciclovir (Cytovene), pentamidine (Pentam), prochlorperazine (Compazine), promethazine (Phenergan)

IV COMPATIBILITIES
Calcium gluconate, dopamine (Intropin), heparin, lorazepam (Ativan), magnesium, potassium

SIDE EFFECTS
Side effects are generally self-limiting and reversible within 2–3 days after discontinuing therapy.

Frequent (89%–48%)
Fever, chills, nausea, vomiting, hypotension, diarrhea, oliguria or anuria, mental status changes, irritability, confusion, depression, sinus tachycardia, pain (abdominal, chest, back), fatigue, dyspnea, pruritus

Occasional (47%–17%)
Edema, erythema, rash, stomatitis, anorexia, weight gain, infection (UTI, injection site, catheter tip), dizziness

Rare (15%–4%)
Dry skin, sensory disorders (vision, speech, taste), dermatitis, headache, arthralgia, myalgia, weight loss, hematuria, conjunctivitis, proteinuria

SERIOUS REACTIONS
! Anemia, thrombocytopenia, and leukopenia occur commonly.
! GI bleeding and pulmonary edema occur occasionally.
! Capillary leak syndrome results in hypotension (systolic pressure less than 90 mm Hg or a 20-mm Hg drop from baseline systolic pressure), extravasation of plasma proteins and fluid into extravascular space, and loss of vascular tone. It may result in cardiac arrhythmias, angina, MI, and respiratory insufficiency.
! Other rare reactions include fatal malignant hyperthermia, cardiac arrest, CVA, pulmonary emboli, bowel perforation, gangrene, and severe depression leading to suicide.

DENTAL CONSIDERATIONS

General:
- Monitor vital signs at every appointment due to cardiovascular side effects.
- If additional analgesia is required for dental pain, consider alternative analgesics (NSAIDs) in patients taking narcotics for acute or chronic pain.
- Examine for oral manifestation of opportunistic infection.
- Avoid products that affect platelet function, such as aspirin and NSAIDs.
- Chlorhexidine mouth rinse prior to and during chemotherapy may reduce severity of mucositis.
- Patient on chronic drug therapy may rarely present with symptoms of blood dyscrasias, which can include infection, bleeding, and poor healing. If dyscrasia is present, caution patient to prevent oral tissue trauma when using oral hygiene aids.
- Palliative medication may be required for management of oral side effects.
- Short appointments and a stress reduction protocol may be required for anxious patients.
- Provide emergency dental care only during drug use.
- Patients may be at risk of bleeding, check for oral signs.
- Oral infections should be eliminated and/or treated aggressively.

Consultations:

- Medical consultation should include routine blood counts including platelet counts and bleeding time.
- Consult physician; prophylactic or therapeutic antiinfectives may be indicated if surgery or periodontal treatment is required.
- Medical consultation may be required to assess immunologic status during cancer chemotherapy and determine safety risk, if any, posed by the required dental treatment.
- Medical consultation may be required to assess disease control and patient's ability to tolerate stress.

Teach Patient/Family:

- Secondary oral infection may occur; need to see dentist immediately if infection occurs
- To be aware of oral side effects
- Importance of good oral hygiene to prevent soft tissue inflammation
- To report oral lesions, soreness, or bleeding to dentist
- To prevent trauma when using oral hygiene aids
- Importance of updating health and medication history if physician makes any changes in evaluation or drug regimens; include OTC, herbal, and nonherbal remedies in the update

alefacept

ale′-fah-cept
(Amevive)

CATEGORY AND SCHEDULE

Pregnancy Risk Category: B

MECHANISM OF ACTION

An immunologic agent that interferes with the activation of T lymphocytes by binding to the lymphocyte antigen, thus reducing the number of circulating T lymphocytes. ***Therapeutic Effect:*** Prevents T cells from becoming overactive, which may help reduce symptoms of chronic plaque psoriasis.

PHARMACOKINETICS

Half-life: 270 hr.

AVAILABILITY

Powder for Injection: 7.5 mg, 15 mg.

INDICATIONS AND DOSAGES

▸ **Plaque Psoriasis**

IV

Adults, Elderly. 7.5 mg once weekly for 12 wk.

IM

Adults, Elderly. 15 mg once weekly for 12 wk.

CONTRAINDICATIONS

History of systemic malignancy, concurrent use of immunosuppressive agents or phototherapy

INTERACTIONS

Drug

None known.

Herbal

None known.

Food

None known.

Drug interactions of concern to dentistry

- None reported

DIAGNOSTIC TEST EFFECTS

Decreases serum T-lymphocyte levels. May increase serum AST(SGOT) and ALT(SGPT) levels.

IV INCOMPATIBILITIES

Don't mix alefacept with any other medications. Don't reconstitute it with any diluent other than that supplied by the manufacturer.

SIDE EFFECTS

Frequent (16%)

Injection site pain and inflammation (with IM administration)

Occasional (5%)

Chills

Rare (2% or less)

Pharyngitis, dizziness, cough, nausea, myalgia

SERIOUS REACTIONS

! Rare reactions include hypersensitivity reactions, lymphopenia, malignancies, and serious infections requiring hospitalization (such as abscess, pneumonia, and postoperative wound infection).

! Coronary artery disease and MI occur in less than 1% of patients.

alemtuzumab

al-lem-two′-zoo-mab

(Campath)

CATEGORY AND SCHEDULE

Pregnancy Risk Category: C

MECHANISM OF ACTION

Binds to CD52, a cell surface glycoprotein, found on the surface of all B and T lymphocytes, most monocytes, macrophages, natural killer cells, and granulocytes. ***Therapeutic Effect:*** Produces cytotoxicity reducing tumor size.

PHARMACOKINETICS

Half-life: About 12 days. Peak and trough levels rise during first few weeks of therapy and approach steady state by about week 6.

AVAILABILITY

Solution for Injection: 30 mg/3 ml.

INDICATIONS AND DOSAGES

▸ Chronic Lymphocytic Leukemia

IV

Adults, Elderly. Initially, 3 mg/day as a 2-hr infusion. When the 3-mg daily dose is tolerated (with only low-grade or no infusion-related toxicities), increase daily dose to 10 mg. When the 10 mg/day dose is tolerated, maintenance dose may be initiated. Maintenance: 30 mg/day 3 times a week on alternate days (such as Monday, Wednesday, and Friday or Tuesday, Thursday, and Saturday) for up to 12 wk.

The increase to 30 mg/day is usually achieved in 3–7 days.

CONTRAINDICATIONS

Active systemic infections, history of hypersensitivity or anaphylactic reaction to the drug, immunosuppression

INTERACTIONS

Drug

Live-virus vaccines: May potentiate viral replication, increase side effects, and decrease the patient's antibody response to the vaccine.

Herbal

None known.

Food

None known.

Drug interactions of concern to dentistry

- None reported

DIAGNOSTIC TEST EFFECTS

May decrease Hgb level, platelet count, and WBC count.

IV INCOMPATIBILITIES

Don't mix alemtuzumab with any other medications.

SIDE EFFECTS

Frequent

Rigors, tremors (86%), fever (85%), nausea (54%), vomiting (41%), rash (40%), fatigue (34%), hypotension (32%), urticaria (30%), pruritus, skeletal pain, headache (24%), diarrhea (22%), anorexia (20%)

Occasional (less than 10%)
Myalgia, dizziness, abdominal pain, throat irritation, vomiting, neutropenia, rhinitis, bronchospasm, urticaria

SERIOUS REACTIONS

! Neutropenia occurs in 85% of patients, anemia occurs in 80% of patients, and thrombocytopenia occurs in 72% of patients.
! A rash occurs in 40% of patients.
! Respiratory toxicity, manifested as dyspnea, cough, bronchitis, pneumonitis, and pneumonia, occurs in 26%–16% of patients.

DENTAL CONSIDERATIONS

General:

• Monitor vital signs at every appointment due to cardiovascular side effects.
• Examine for oral manifestation of opportunistic infection.
• Avoid products that affect platelet function, such as aspirin and NSAIDs.
• This drug may be used in the hospital or on an outpatient basis. Confirm the patient's disease and treatment status.
• Chlorhexidine mouth rinse prior to and during chemotherapy may reduce severity of mucositis.
• Patient on chronic drug therapy may rarely present with symptoms of blood dyscrasias, which can include infection, bleeding, and poor healing. If dyscrasia is present, caution patient to prevent oral tissue trauma when using oral hygiene aids.
• Palliative medication may be required for management of oral side effects.
• Short appointments and a stress reduction protocol may be required for anxious patients.
• Patients may be taking a prophylactic antiinfective.
• Patients are at risk of bleeding, check for oral signs.
• Place on frequent recall due to oral side effects.

Consultations:

• Medical consultation should include routine blood counts including platelet counts and bleeding time.
• Consult physician; prophylactic or therapeutic antiinfectives may be indicated if surgery or periodontal treatment is required.
• Medical consultation may be required to assess immunologic status during cancer chemotherapy and determine safety risk, if any, posed by the required dental treatment.
• Medical consultation may be required to assess disease control and patient's ability to tolerate stress.

Teach Patient/Family:

• To inform dentist of unusual bleeding episodes following dental treatment
• Secondary oral infection may occur; need to see dentist immediately if infection occurs
• To be aware of oral side effects
• Importance of good oral hygiene to prevent soft tissue inflammation
• To report oral lesions, soreness, or bleeding to dentist
• To prevent trauma when using oral hygiene aids
• Importance of updating health and medication history if physician makes any changes in evaluation or drug regimens; include OTC, herbal, and nonherbal remedies in the update

alendronate sodium

a-len′-dro-nate
(Fosamax)
Do not confuse Fosamax with Flomax.

CATEGORY AND SCHEDULE

Pregnancy Risk Category: C

MECHANISM OF ACTION

A bisphosphonate that inhibits normal and abnormal bone resorption, without retarding mineralization. ***Therapeutic Effect:*** Leads to significantly increased bone mineral density; reverses the progression of osteoporosis.

PHARMACOKINETICS

Poorly absorbed after oral administration. Protein binding: 78%. After oral administration, rapidly taken into bone, with uptake greatest at sites of active bone turnover. Excreted in urine. ***Terminal Half-life:*** Greater than 10 yr (reflects release from skeleton as bone is resorbed).

AVAILABILITY

Tablets: 5 mg, 10 mg, 35 mg, 40 mg, 70 mg.
Oral Solution: 70 mg/75 ml.

INDICATIONS AND DOSAGES

▸ **Osteoporosis (in men)**

PO
Adults, Elderly. 10 mg once a day in the morning.

▸ **Glucocorticoid-Induced Osteoporosis**

PO
Adults, Elderly. 5 mg once a day in the morning.
Postmenopausal women not receiving estrogen. 10 mg once a day in the morning.

▸ **Postmenopausal Osteoporosis**

PO (treatment)
Adults, Elderly. 10 mg once a day in the morning or 70 mg weekly.
PO (prevention)
Adults, Elderly. 5 mg once a day in the morning or 35 mg weekly.

▸ **Paget's Disease**

PO
Adults, Elderly. 40 mg once a day in the morning.

OFF-LABEL USES

Treatment of breast cancer

CONTRAINDICATIONS

GI disease, including dysphagia, frequent heartburn, gastrointestinal reflux disease, hiatal hernia, and ulcers, inability to stand or sit upright for at least 30 minutes; renal impairment; sensitivity to alendronate
Carefully evaluate patients when considering the use of dental implants. Osteonecrosis of the jaw has been reported in patients following oral surgical procedures and who are also taking bisphosphonates.

INTERACTIONS

Drug

Aspirin: May increase GI disturbances.
IV ranitidine: May double the bioavailability of alendronate.

Herbal

None known.

Food

Beverages other than plain water, dietary supplements, food: May interfere with absorption of alendronate.

Drug interactions of concern to dentistry

- Increased risk of GI side effects in doses greater than 10 mg/day: Use NSAIDs, acetylsalicylic acid (ASA) with caution
- After administration, must wait at least 30 min before taking any other drug

DIAGNOSTIC TEST EFFECTS

Reduces serum calcium and serum phosphate concentrations. Significantly decreases serum alkaline phosphatase level in patients with Paget's disease.

SIDE EFFECTS

Frequent (8%–7%)
Back pain, abdominal pain
Occasional (3%–2%)
Nausea, abdominal distention, constipation, diarrhea, flatulence
Rare (< 2%)
Rash

SERIOUS REACTIONS

! Overdose causes hypocalcemia, hypophosphatemia, and significant GI disturbances.
! Esophageal irritation occurs if alendronate is not given with 6–8 ounces of plain water or if the patient lies down within 30 minutes of drug administration.

DENTAL CONSIDERATIONS

General:

- Be aware of oral manifestations of Paget's disease (macrognathia, alveolar pain).
- Consider semisupine chair position for patient comfort because of pain experienced in osteoporosis and GI side effects of drug.
- Consider short appointments for patient comfort.

Consultations:

- Medical consultation may be required to assess disease control and patient's ability to tolerate stress.

alfuzosin hydrochloride

ale-few-zoe′-sin
(Uroxatral)

CATEGORY AND SCHEDULE

Pregnancy Risk Category: B

MECHANISM OF ACTION

An $alpha_1$ antagonist that targets receptors around bladder neck and prostate capsule. ***Therapeutic Effect:*** Relaxes smooth muscle and improves urinary flow and symptoms of prostatic hyperplasia.

PHARMACOKINETICS

Rapidly absorbed and widely distributed. Protein binding: 90%. Extensively metabolized in the liver. Primarily excreted in urine. ***Half-life:*** 3–9 hr.

AVAILABILITY

Tablets (Extended-Release): 10 mg.

INDICATIONS AND DOSAGES

▸ Benign Prostatic Hyperplasia

PO
Adults. 10 mg once a day, approximately 30 min after same meal each day.

CONTRAINDICATIONS

History of hypersensitivity to alfuzosin

INTERACTIONS

Drug
Cimetidine: May increase alfuzosin blood concentration.
Other alpha blockers, such as doxazosin, prazosin, tamsulosin, and terazosin: May increase the alpha-blockade effects of both drugs.
Herbal
None known.
Food
None known.
Drug interactions of concern to dentistry

- Potential for hypotension: antihypertensives drugs, other adrenergic antagonists
- Contraindicated with ketoconazole, itraconazole

- Possible risk of orthostatic hypotension may be increased with conscious sedation techniques
- Opioids and anticholinergic drugs may enhance urinary retention in benign prostatic hypertrophy (BPH); use alternative analgesics (NSAIDs)
- Erythromycin is an inhibitor of CYP3A4, but no data reported for possible interaction: use with caution

DIAGNOSTIC TEST EFFECTS
None known.

SIDE EFFECTS
Frequent (7%–6%)
Dizziness, headache, malaise
Occasional (4%)
Dry mouth
Rare (3%–2%)
Nausea, dyspepsia (such as heartburn, and epigastric discomfort), diarrhea, orthostatic hypotension, tachycardia, drowsiness

SERIOUS REACTIONS
! Ischemia-related chest pain may occur rarely.

DENTAL CONSIDERATIONS
General:
- Monitor vital signs at every appointment because of cardiovascular side effects.
- Consider semisupine chair position for patient comfort if GI side effects occur.
- After supine positioning, have patient sit upright for at least 2 min before standing to avoid orthostatic hypotension.

alitretinoin
ah-lee-tret′-i-noyn
(Panretin)

CATEGORY AND SCHEDULE
Pregnancy Risk Category: D

MECHANISM OF ACTION
Binds to and activates all known retinoid receptors. Once activated, receptors act as transcription factors, regulating genes that control cellular differentiation and proliferation.
Therapeutic Effect: Inhibits growth of Kaposi's sarcoma cells.

PHARMACOKINETICS
Minimally absorbed following topical administration.

AVAILABILITY
Gel: 0.1% (Panretin).

INDICATIONS AND DOSAGES
▸ **Kaposi's Sarcoma (KS) Skin Lesions**
TOPICAL
Adults. Initially, apply 2 times per day to lesions. May increase to 3 to 4 times per day.

OFF-LABEL USES
Breast, cervical, ovarian, prostatic carcinomas; myelodysplastic syndrome; psoriasis

CONTRAINDICATIONS
When systemic therapy is required (>10 new KS lesions in previous month, symptomatic pulmonary KS, symptomatic visceral involvement, symptomatic lymphedema, hypersensitivity to retinoids or alitretinoin ingredients)

INTERACTIONS
Drug
DEET (component of insect repellent): May increase risk of toxicity to products containing DEET.
Herbal
None known.
Food
None known.

Drug interactions of concern to dentistry

- Risk of photosensitivity reaction: tetracyclines, fluoroquinolones, other photosensitizing drugs

DIAGNOSTIC TEST EFFECTS

None known.

SIDE EFFECTS

Frequent

Rash (erythema, scaling, irritation, redness, dermatitis), itching, exfoliative dermatitis (flaking, peeling, desquamation, exfolliation), stinging, tingling, edema skin disorders (scabbing, crusting, drainage)

SERIOUS REACTIONS

! Severe local skin reaction (intense erythema, edema, vesiculation) may limit treatment.

DENTAL CONSIDERATIONS

General:

- Patients will be taking antiviral drugs; note which drugs are being used because some have potential for significant drug interactions.
- Take a complete medical history, including a current drug history with doses and duration of therapy.

allopurinol

al-oh-pure′-i-nole
(Aloprim, Allohexal[AUS], Allosig[AUS], Apo-Allopurinol[CAN], Capurate[AUS], Progout[AUS] Purinol[CAN], Zyloprim)
Do not confuse with ZORprin.

CATEGORY AND SCHEDULE

Pregnancy Risk Category: C

MECHANISM OF ACTION

A xanthine oxidase inhibitor that decreases uric acid production by inhibiting xanthine oxidase, an enzyme. ***Therapeutic Effect:*** Reduces uric acid concentrations in both serum and urine.

PHARMACOKINETICS

Route	Onset	Peak	Duration
PO/IV	2–3 days	1–3 wk	1–2 wk

Well absorbed from the GI tract. Widely distributed. Metabolized in the liver to active metabolite. Excreted primarily in urine. Removed by hemodialysis. ***Half-life:*** 1–3 hr; metabolite, 12–30 hr.

AVAILABILITY

Tablets (Zyloprim): 100 mg, 300 mg.
Powder for Injection (Aloprim): 500 mg.

INDICATIONS AND DOSAGES

▸ **Chronic Gouty Arthritis**

PO

Adults, Children older than 10 yr. Initially, 100 mg/day; may increase by 100 mg/day at weekly intervals. Maximum: 800 mg/day. Maintenance: 100–200 mg 2–3 times a day or 300 mg/day.

▸ **To Prevent Uric Acid Nephropathy During Chemotherapy**

PO

Adults. Initially, 600–800 mg/day starting 2–3 days before initiation of chemotherapy or radiation therapy.
Children 6–10 yr. 100 mg 3 times a day or 300 mg once a day.
Children younger than 6 yr. 50 mg 3 times a day.

IV

Adults. 200–400 mg/m^2/day beginning 24–48 hr before initiation of chemotherapy.
Children. 200 mg/m^2/day. Maximum: 600 mg/day.

▸ **Prevention of Uric Acid Calculi**

PO

Adults. 100–200 mg 1–4 times a day or 300 mg once a day.

▸ **Recurrent Calcium Oxalate Calculi**

PO

Adults. 200–300 mg/day.

Elderly. Initially, 100 mg/day, gradually increased until optimal uric acid level is reached.

▸ **Dosage in Renal Impairment**

Dosage is modified on the basis of creatinine clearance.

Creatinine Clearance	Dosage Adjustment
10–20 ml/min	200 mg/day
3–9 ml/min	100 mg/day
Less than 3 ml/min	100 mg at extended intervals

OFF-LABEL USES

In mouthwash following fluorouracil therapy to prevent stomatitis

CONTRAINDICATIONS

Asymptomatic hyperuricemia

INTERACTIONS

Drug

Amoxicillin, ampicillin: May increase incidence of rash.

Azathioprine, mercaptopurine: May increase therapeutic effect and toxicity of azathioprine and mercaptopurine.

Oral anticoagulants: May increase anticoagulant effect.

Thiazide diuretics: May decrease the effect of allopurinol.

Herbal

None known.

Food

None known.

Drug interactions of concern to dentistry

- Increased risk of rash: ampicillin, amoxicillin, bacampicillin, hetacillin

DIAGNOSTIC TEST EFFECTS

May increase BUN, serum creatinine, serum alkaline phosphatase, AST(SGOT), and ALT(SGPT) levels.

IV INCOMPATIBILITIES

Amikacin (Amikin), carmustine (BiCNU), cefotaxime (Claforan), chlorpromazine (Thorazine), cimetidine (Tagamet), clindamycin (Cleocin), cytarabine (Ara-C), dacarbazine (DTIC), diphenhydramine (Benadryl), doxorubicin (Adriamycin), doxycycline (Vibramycin), droperidol (Inapsine), fludarabine (Fludara), gentamicin (Garamycin), haloperidol (Haldol), hydroxyzine (Vistaril), idarubicin (Idamycin), imipenem-cilastatin (Primaxin), meperidine (Demerol), methylprednisolone (Solu-Medrol), metoclopramide (Reglan), ondansetron (Zofran), prochlorperazine (Compazine), promethazine (Phenergan), streptozocin (Zanosar), tobramycin (Nebcin), vinorelbine (Navelbine)

IV COMPATIBILITIES

Bumetanide (Bumex), calcium gluconate, furosemide (Lasix), heparin, hydromorphone (Dilaudid), lorazepam (Ativan), morphine, potassium chloride

SIDE EFFECTS

Occasional

Oral: Somnolence, unusual hair loss
IV: Rash, nausea, vomiting

Rare

Diarrhea, headache

SERIOUS REACTIONS

! Pruritic maculopapular rash possibly accompanied by malaise, fever, chills, joint pain, nausea, and vomiting should be considered a toxic reaction.

! Severe hypersensitivity may follow appearance of rash.

! Bone marrow depression, hepatic toxicity, peripheral neuritis, and acute renal failure occur rarely.

DENTAL CONSIDERATIONS

General:

• Patients on chronic drug therapy may rarely have symptoms of blood dyscrasias, which can include infection, bleeding, and poor healing.

Consultations:

• In a patient with symptoms of blood dyscrasias, request a medical consult for blood studies and postpone dental treatment until normal values are reestablished.

• Medical consult may be required to assess disease control.

Teach Patient/Family:

• Importance of good oral hygiene to prevent soft tissue inflammation

• To avoid mouth rinses with high alcohol content because of drying effects

almotriptan malate

al-moe-trip′-tan
(Axert)

Do not confuse Axert with Antivert.

CATEGORY AND SCHEDULE

Pregnancy Risk Category: C

MECHANISM OF ACTION

A serotonin receptor agonist that binds selectively to vascular receptors, producing a vasoconstrictive effect on cranial blood vessels. ***Therapeutic Effect:*** Produces relief of migraine headache.

PHARMACOKINETICS

Well absorbed after PO administration. Metabolized by the liver, excreted in urine.
Half-life: 3–4 hr.

AVAILABILITY

Tablets: 6.5 mg, 12.5 mg.

INDICATIONS AND DOSAGES

▸ Migraine Headache

PO

Adults, Elderly. 6.25–12.5 mg. If headache improves but then returns, dose may be repeated after 2 hr. Maximum: 2 doses/24 hr.

▸ Dosage in Renal Impairment

For adult and elderly patients, recommended initial dose is 6.25 mg and maximum daily dose is 12.5 mg.

CONTRAINDICATIONS

Arrhythmias associated with conduction disorders, hemiplegic or basilar migraine, ischemic heart disease (including angina pectoris, history of MI, silent ischemia, and Prinzmetal's angina), uncontrolled hypertension, use within 24 hours of ergotamine-containing preparation or another serotonin receptor antagonist, use within 14 days of MAOIs, Wolff-Parkinson-White syndrome

INTERACTIONS

Drug

Ergotamine-containing medications: May produce a vasospastic reaction.

Erythromycin, itraconazole, ketoconazole, MAOIs, ritonavir: May increase the almotriptan plasma level.

Fluoxetine, fluvoxamine, paroxetine, sertraline: May produce weakness, hyperreflexia, and incoordination.

Herbal

None known.

Food

None known.

Drug interactions of concern to dentistry

• Avoid concurrent use of ketoconazole, itraconazole, erythromycin

DIAGNOSTIC TEST EFFECTS
None known.

SIDE EFFECTS
Frequent
Nausea, dry mouth, paresthesia, flushing
Occasional
Changes in temperature sensation, asthenia, dizziness

SERIOUS REACTIONS
! Excessive dosage may produce tremor, red extremities, reduced respirations, cyanosis, seizures, and chest pain.
! Serious arrhythmias occur rarely, particularly in patients with hypertension or diabetes, obese patients, smokers, and those with a strong family history of coronary artery disease.

DENTAL CONSIDERATIONS
General:
- This is an acute-use drug; it is doubtful that patients will undergo dental treatment during acute migraine attacks.
- Be aware of patient's disease, its severity, frequency when known.

Consultations:
- If treating chronic orofacial pain, consult with physician of record.
- Medical consultation may be required to assess disease control and patient's ability to tolerate stress.

Teach Patient/Family:
- That dryness of the mouth may occur when taking this drug; avoid mouth rinses with high alcohol content because of additional drying effects
- Importance of updating health and drug history if physician makes any changes in evaluation or drug regimens

alosetron
al-ohs′-eh-tron
(Lotronex)
Do not confuse Lotronex with Lovenox.

CATEGORY AND SCHEDULE
Pregnancy Risk Category: B

MECHANISM OF ACTION
A serotonin (5-HT_3) receptor antagonist that mediates abdominal pain, bloating, nausea, vomiting, peristalsis, and secretory reflexes. ***Therapeutic Effect:*** Alleviates diarrhea, reduces gastric pain.

PHARMACOKINETICS
Rapidly absorbed after PO administration. Extensively metabolized in liver. Excreted primarily in urine and, to a lesser extent, in feces. ***Half-life:*** 1.5 hr.

AVAILABILITY
Tablets: 1 mg.

INDICATIONS AND DOSAGES
▸ **Irritable Bowel Syndrome**
PO
Adults (Women older than 18 yr). 1 mg twice a day. Maximum: 2 mg/day.

OFF-LABEL USES
Treatment of carcinoid diarrhea, irritable bowel syndrome in men

CONTRAINDICATIONS
Breast-feeding; constipation; diverticulitis (active or history of); GI bleeding, obstruction, or perforation; history ischemic colitis, ulcerative colitis, or Crohn's disease; thrombophlebitis

INTERACTIONS

Drug

Hydralazine, isoniazid, procainamide: May alter the effects of these drugs.

Herbal

St. John's wort: May increase alosetron blood concentration.

Food

All foods: May decrease the absorption or delay the peak blood concentration of alosetron.

Drug interactions of concern to dentistry

- Does not appear to induce CYP450 isoenzymes; no interactions are documented
- Avoid use of drugs (opioids) that could lead to increased risk of constipation
- Use NSAIDs or acetaminophen for mild to moderate dental pain

DIAGNOSTIC TEST EFFECTS

May increase serum alkaline phosphatase, bilirubin, ALT (SGPT) and AST (SGOT) levels.

SIDE EFFECTS

Frequent (28%)
Constipation
Occasional (10%–2%)
Nausea, GI or abdominal discomfort or pain, dyspepsia, flatulence, hypertension, clinical depression
Rare
Sedation, abnormal dreams, anxiety

SERIOUS REACTIONS

! Acute ischemic colitis and serious complications of constipation have resulted in the need for blood transfusions and surgery.

DENTAL CONSIDERATIONS

General:

- Short appointments and a stress reduction protocol may be required for anxious patients.
- Consider semisupine chair position for patient comfort because of GI side effects of disease.
- Avoid drugs with anticholinergic activity, such as antihistamines, opioids, benzodiazepines, propantheline, atropine, and scopolamine.
- Question patient about tolerance of NSAIDs or aspirin related to GI disease.

Consultations:

- Consider consulting with physician before prescribing drugs that can cause constipation (opioids).
- Consultation with physician may be necessary if sedation or general anesthesia is required.
- Medical consultation may be required to assess disease control and patient's ability to tolerate stress.

Teach Patient/Family:

- Importance of updating health and drug history if physician makes any changes in evaluation or drug regimens

alprazolam

al-pray′-zoe-lam

SCHEDULE IV

(Apo-Alpraz[CAN], Kalma[AUS], Niravam, Novo-Alprazol[CAN], Xanax, Xanax XR)
Do not confuse alprazolam with lorazepam, or Xanax with Tenex or Zantac.

CATEGORY AND SCHEDULE

Pregnancy Risk Category: D
Controlled Substance: Schedule IV

MECHANISM OF ACTION

A benzodiazepine that enhances the action of the inhibitory neurotransmitter gamma-aminobutyric acid in the brain.

Therapeutic Effect: Produces anxiolytic effect from its CNS depressant action.

PHARMACOKINETICS

Well absorbed from GI tract. Protein binding: 80%. Metabolized in the liver. Primarily excreted in urine. Minimal removal by hemodialysis. ***Half-life:*** 11–16 hr.

AVAILABILITY

Oral Solution (Alprazolam Intensol): 1 mg/ml.
Tablets (Xanax): 0.25 mg, 0.5 mg, 1 mg, 2 mg.
Tablets (Extended-Release [Xanax XR]): 0.5 mg, 1 mg, 2 mg, 3 mg.
Tablets (Orally-Disintegrating [Niravam]): 0.25 mg, 0.5 mg, 1 mg, 2 mg.

INDICATIONS AND DOSAGES

▸ Anxiety Disorders

PO (Immediate-Release)
Adults. Initially, 0.25–0.5 mg 3 times a day. May titrate q3–4 days. Maximum: 4 mg/day in divided doses.
Elderly, Debilitated patients, Patients with hepatic disease or low serum albumin. Initially, 0.25 mg 2–3 times a day. Gradually increase to optimum therapeutic response.
PO (Orally-Disintegrating)
Adults. 0.25–0.5 mg 3 times a day. Maximum: 4 mg/day in divided doses.

▸ Anxiety with Depression

PO
Adults. 2.5–3 mg/day in divided doses.

▸ Panic Disorder

PO (Immediate-Release)
Adults. Initially, 0.5 mg 3 times a day. May increase at 3- to 4-day intervals. Range: 5–6 mg/day. Maximum: 10 mg/day.
Elderly. Initially, 0.125–0.25 mg twice a day. May increase in 0.125-mg increments until desired effect attained.
PO (Extended-Release)

▸ Alert
To switch from immediate-release to extended "release form, give total daily dose (immediate release) as a single daily dose of extended release form.
Adults. Initially, 0.5–1 mg once a day. May titrate at 3- to 4-day intervals. Range: 3–6 mg/day. Maximum: 10 mg/day.
Elderly. Initially, 0.5 mg once daily.
PO (Orally-Disintegrating)
Adults. Initially, 0.5 mg 3 times a day. May increase at 3- to 4-day intervals. Range: 5–6 mg/day. Maximum: 10 mg/day.

▸ Premenstrual Syndrome

PO
Adults. 0.25 mg 3 times a day.

OFF-LABEL USES

Management of premenstrual syndrome symptoms (mood disturbances, insomnia, and cramps), irritable bowel syndrome, treatment of agoraphobia, post-traumatic stress disorder, tremors, ethanol withdrawal, anxiety in children.

CONTRAINDICATIONS

Acute alcohol intoxication with depressed vital signs, acute angle-closure glaucoma, concurrent use of itraconazole or ketoconazole, myasthenia gravis, severe COPD

INTERACTIONS

Drug

Alcohol, other CNS depressants: Potentiate effects of alprazolam and may increase sedation.
Fluvoxamine, itraconazole, ketoconazole, nefazodone: May inhibit metabolism and increase serum concentrations of alprazolam.

Herbal

Kava kava, valerian: May increase CNS depressant effect of alprazolam.
St. John's wort: May reduce effectiveness of alprazolam.

Food

Grapefruit, grapefruit juice: May inhibit alprazolam's metabolism.

Drug interactions of concern to dentistry

- Increased central nervous system (CNS) depression: alcohol, other CNS depressants, clarithromycin, erythromycin, fluconazole, miconazole, fluoxetine, isoniazid, fluvoxamine, nefazodone, rifamycin; St. John's wort (herb), kava (herb)
- Contraindicated with ketoconazole, itraconazole, ritonavir, indinavir, saquinavir

DIAGNOSTIC TEST EFFECTS

None known.

SIDE EFFECTS

Frequent

Ataxia; lightheadedness; transient, mild somnolence; slurred speech (particularly in elderly or debilitated patients)

Occasional

Confusion, depression, blurred vision, constipation, diarrhea, dry mouth, headache, nausea

Rare

Behavioral problems such as anger, impaired memory, paradoxical reactions such as insomnia, nervousness, or irritability

SERIOUS REACTIONS

! Abrupt or too rapid withdrawal may result in pronounced restlessness, irritability, insomnia, hand tremors, abdominal and muscle cramps, diaphoresis, vomiting, and seizures.

! Overdose results in somnolence, confusion, diminished reflexes, and coma.

! Blood dyscrasias have been reported rarely.

DENTAL CONSIDERATIONS

General:

- Monitor vital signs at every appointment because of cardiovascular side effects.
- After supine positioning, have patient sit upright for at least 2 min to avoid orthostatic hypotension.
- Assess salivary flow as a factor in caries, periodontal disease, and candidiasis.
- Psychologic and physical dependence may occur with chronic administration.

Consultations:

- Medical consultation may be required to assess disease control.

Teach Patient/Family:

- *When chronic dry mouth occurs, advise patient:*
  - To avoid mouth rinses with high alcohol content because of drying effects
  - To use daily home fluoride products for anticaries effect
  - To use sugarless gum, frequent sips of water, or saliva substitutes

alprostadil (prostaglandin E_1, PGE_1)

al-pros′-ta-dil

(Caverject, Edex, Muse, Prostin VR Pediatric)

CATEGORY AND SCHEDULE

Pregnancy Risk Category: C

MECHANISM OF ACTION

A prostaglandin that directly affects vascular and ductus arteriosus smooth muscle and relaxes trabecular smooth muscle.

Therapeutic Effect: Causes vasodilation; dilates cavernosal arteries, allowing blood flow to and entrapment in the lacunar spaces of the penis.

AVAILABILITY

Injection (Prostin VR Pediatric): 500 mcg/ml.
Powder for Injection (Caverject, Edex): 10 mcg, 20 mcg, 40 mcg.
Urethral Pellet (Muse): 125 mcg, 250 mcg, 500 mcg, 1000 mcg.

INDICATIONS AND DOSAGES

▸ Maintain Patency of Ductus Arteriosus

IV INFUSION
Neonates. Initially, 0.05–0.1 mcg/kg/min. Maintenance: 0.01–0.4 mcg/kg/min. Maximum: 0.4 mcg/kg/min.

▸ Impotence

Pellet, Intracavernosal
Adults. Dosage is individualized.

OFF-LABEL USES

Treatment of atherosclerosis, gangrene, pain due to severe peripheral arterial occlusive disease

CONTRAINDICATIONS

Conditions predisposing to anatomic deformation of penis, hyaline membrane disease, penile implants, priapism, respiratory distress syndrome

INTERACTIONS

Drug

Anticoagulants, including heparin, thrombolytics: May increase risk of bleeding.
Sympathomimetics: May decrease effect of alprostadil.
Vasodilators: May increase risk of hypotension.

Herbal

None known.

Food

None known.

Drug interactions of concern to dentistry

- None reported

DIAGNOSTIC TEST EFFECTS

May increase blood bilirubin levels. May decrease glucose, serum calcium, and serum potassium levels.

IV INCOMPATIBILITIES

No information available.

SIDE EFFECTS

Frequent

Intracavernosal (4%–1%): Penile pain (37%), prolonged erection, hypertension, localized pain, penile fibrosis, injection site hematoma or ecchymosis, headache, respiratory infection, flu-like symptoms
Intraurethral (3%): Penile pain (36%), urethral pain or burning, testicular pain, urethral bleeding, headache, dizziness, respiratory infection, flu-like symptoms
Systemic (> 1%): Fever, seizures, flushing, bradycardia, hypotension, tachycardia, apnea, diarrhea, sepsis

Occasional

Intracavernosal (< 1%): Hypotension, pelvic pain, back pain, dizziness, cough, nasal congestion
Intraurethral (< 3%): Fainting, sinusitis, back and pelvic pain
Systemic (< 1%): Anxiety, lethargy, myalgia, arrhythmias, respiratory depression, anemia, bleeding, thrombocytopenia, hematuria

SERIOUS REACTIONS

! Overdose is manifested as apnea, flushing of the face and arms, and bradycardia.
! Cardiac arrest and sepsis occur rarely.

alteplase, recombinant

al-teep′-lase

(Activase, Actilyse[AUS], Cathflo Activase)

Do not confuse alteplase or Activase with Altace.

CATEGORY AND SCHEDULE

Pregnancy Risk Category: C

MECHANISM OF ACTION

A tissue plasminogen activator that acts as a thrombolytic by binding to the fibrin in a thrombus and converting entrapped plasminogen to plasmin. This process initiates fibrinolysis. ***Therapeutic Effect:*** Degrades fibrin clots, fibrinogen, and other plasma proteins.

PHARMACOKINETICS

Rapidly metabolized in the liver. Primarily excreted in urine. ***Half-life:*** 35 min.

AVAILABILITY

Powder for Injection (Cathflo Activase): 2 mg.
Powder for Injection(Activase): 50 mg, 100 mg.

INDICATIONS AND DOSAGES

▸ Acute MI

IV INFUSION

Adults weighing greater than 67 kg. 100 mg over 90 min, starting with 15-mg bolus over 1–2 min, then 50 mg over 30 min, then 35 mg over 60 min. Or a 3-hour infusion, giving 60 mg over first hr (6–10 mg as bolus over 1–2 min), 20 mg over second hr, and 20 mg over third hr.
Adults weighing 67 kg or less: 100 mg over 90 min, starting with 15-mg bolus, then 0.75 mg/kg over 30 min (maximum: 50 mg), then 0.5 mg/kg over 60 min (maximum: 35 mg). Or 3-hour infusion of 1.25 mg/kg giving 60% of dose over first hr (6%–10% as 1- to 2-min bolus), 20% over second hr, and 20% over third hr.

▸ Acute Pulmonary Emboli

IV INFUSION

Adults. 100 mg over 2 hr. Institute or reinstitute heparin near end or immediately after infusion when aPTT or thrombin time (TT) returns to twice normal or less.

▸ Acute Ischemic Stroke

IV INFUSION

Adults. 0.9 mg/kg over 60 min (10% total dose as initial IV bolus over 1 min).

▸ Central Venous Catheter Clearance

IV

Adults, Elderly. 2 mg; may repeat after 2 hr.

OFF-LABEL USES

Coronary thrombolysis, to decrease ischemic events in unstable angina

CONTRAINDICATIONS

Active internal bleeding, AV malformation or aneurysm, bleeding diathesis, intracranial neoplasm, intracranial or intraspinal surgery or trauma, recent (within past 2 months) cerebrovascular accident, severe uncontrolled hypertension

INTERACTIONS

Drug

Anticoagulants, including cefotetan, heparin, plicamycin, valproic acid: May increase risk of hemorrhage.
Platelet aggregation inhibitors, including aspirin, NSAIDs, ticlopidine: May increase risk of bleeding.

Herbal

None known.

Food
None known.
Drug interactions of concern to dentistry
• Increased risk of bleeding: drugs that interfere with coagulation or platelet function, such as NSAIDs and aspirin

DIAGNOSTIC TEST EFFECTS

Decreases plasminogen and fibrinogen levels during infusion, which decreases clotting time (and confirms the presence of lysis). Decreases Hgb and Hct.

IV INCOMPATIBILITIES

Dobutamine (Dobutrex), dopamine (Intropin), heparin, nitroglycerin

IV COMPATIBILITIES

Lidocaine, metoprolol (Lopressor), morphine, nitroglycerin, propranolol (Inderal)

SIDE EFFECTS

Frequent
Superficial bleeding at puncture sites, decreased BP
Occasional
Allergic reaction, such as rash or wheezing; bruising

SERIOUS REACTIONS

! Severe internal hemorrhage may occur.
! Lysis of coronary thrombi may produce atrial or ventricular arrhythmias or stroke.

DENTAL CONSIDERATIONS

General:
• An acute use drug for use in hospitals or emergency rooms.
• Patients are at risk of bleeding; check for oral signs.
• Avoid products that affect platelet function, such as aspirin and NSAIDs.
• Monitor vital signs every appointment due to cardiovascular side effects.
• Patients who have been treated with drug may present with cardiovascular disease or stroke; review medical and drug history.
Consultations:
• Consult should include data on bleeding time.
• Medical consult should include routine blood counts including platelet counts and bleeding time.
• In a patient with symptoms of blood dyscrasias, request a medical consult for blood studies and postpone treatment until normal values are reestablished.
• Medical consult may be required to assess disease control and patient's ability to tolerate stress.
Teach patient/family:
• Use soft tooth brush to reduce risk of bleeding
• Importance of good oral hygiene to prevent soft tissue inflammation
• To report oral lesions, soreness, or bleeding to dentist
• To prevent trauma when using oral hygiene aids
• Importance of updating health and medication history if physician makes any changes in evaluation/drug regimens; include OTC, herbal, and nonherbal remedies in the update

amantadine hydrochloride

a-man′-ta-deen
(Endantadine[CAN], PMS-Amantadine[CAN], Symmetrel)

CATEGORY AND SCHEDULE

Pregnancy Risk Category: C

MECHANISM OF ACTION

A dopaminergic agonist that blocks the uncoating of influenza A virus, preventing penetration into the host and inhibiting M2 protein in the assembly of progeny virions.

Amantadine also blocks the reuptake of dopamine into presynaptic neurons and causes direct stimulation of postsynaptic receptors. ***Therapeutic Effect:*** Antiviral and antiparkinsonian activity.

PHARMACOKINETICS

Rapidly and completely absorbed from the GI tract. Protein binding: 67%. Widely distributed. Primarily excreted in urine. Minimally removed by hemodialysis. ***Half-life:*** 11–15 hr (increased in the elderly, decreased in impaired renal function).

AVAILABILITY

Capsule: 100 mg.
Syrup: 50 mg/5 ml.
Tablets: 100 mg.

INDICATIONS AND DOSAGES

▸ Prevention and Symptomatic Treatment of Respiratory Illness due to Influenza A Virus

PO

Adults older than 64 yr. 100 mg/day.
Adults 13–64 yr. 200 mg/day.
Children 10–12 yr. 5 mg/kg/day up to 200 mg/day.
Children 1–9 yr. 5 mg/kg/day (up to 150 mg/day).

▸ Parkinson's Disease, Extrapyramidal Symptoms

PO

Adults, Elderly. 100 mg twice a day. May increase up to 300 mg/day in divided doses.

▸ Dosage in Renal Impairment

Dose and frequency are modified on the basis of creatinine clearance.

Creatinine Clearance	Dosage
30–50 ml/min	200 mg first day; 100 mg/day thereafter
15–29 ml/min	200 mg first day; 100 mg on alternate days
less than 15 ml/min	200 mg every 7 days

OFF-LABEL USES

Treatment of ADHD. Fatigue associated with multiple sclerosis

CONTRAINDICATIONS

None known.

INTERACTIONS

Drug

Alcohol: May increase CNS effects, including dizziness, confusion, lightheadedness, and orthostatic hypotension.
Anticholinergics, antihistamines, phenothiazine, tricyclic antidepressants: May increase anticholinergic effects of amantadine.
Hydrochlorothiazide, triamterene: May increase amantadine blood concentration and risk for toxicity.

Herbal

None known.

Food

None known.

Drug interactions of concern to dentistry

- Increased anticholinergic response: anticholinergic drugs
- Increased CNS depression: alcohol, other CNS depressants

DIAGNOSTIC TEST EFFECTS

None known.

SIDE EFFECTS

Frequent (10%–5%)

Nausea, dizziness, poor concentration, insomnia, nervousness

Occasional (5%–1%)

Orthostatic hypotension, anorexia, headache, livedo reticularis (reddish blue, netlike blotching of skin), blurred vision, urine retention, dry mouth or nose

Rare

Vomiting, depression, irritation or swelling of eyes, rash

SERIOUS REACTIONS

! CHF, leukopenia, and neutropenia occur rarely.

! Hyperexcitability, seizures, and ventricular arrhythmias may occur.

DENTAL CONSIDERATIONS

General:

• Monitor vital signs at every appointment because of cardiovascular side effects.
• Assess salivary flow as a factor in caries, periodontal disease, and candidiasis.
• After supine positioning, have patient sit upright for at least 2 min to avoid orthostatic hypotension.
• Avoid dental light in patient's eyes; offer dark glasses for patient comfort.
• Short appointments and stress reduction protocol may be required for anxious patients.
• Consider semisupine chair position for patients with respiratory distress.

Teach Patient/Family:

• To avoid mouth rinses with high alcohol content because of drying effects
• To use electric toothbrush if patient has difficulty holding conventional devices

ambenonium

am-be-noe′-nee-um
(Mytelase)

CATEGORY AND SCHEDULE

Pregnancy Risk Category: C

MECHANISM OF ACTION

A cholinesterase inhibitor that enhances and prolongs cholinergic function by increasing the concentration of acetylcholine through inhibition of the hydrolysis of acetylcholine. ***Therapeutic Effect:*** Increases muscle strength in myasthenia gravis.

PHARMACOKINETICS

Poorly absorbed after PO administration.

AVAILABILITY

Tablets: 10 mg (Mytelase).

INDICATIONS AND DOSAGES

▸ Myasthenia Gravis

PO

Adults. 5–25 mg 3 or 4 times a day. If well tolerated, after 1 or 2 days, may increase to 50–75 mg 3 times a day. Range: 5–200 mg/day in divided doses.

CONTRAINDICATIONS

Not recommended in patients receiving routine administration of atropine or other belladonna derivatives. Not recommended in patients receiving mecamylamine.

INTERACTIONS

Drug

Atropine: Suppresses the symptoms of ambenonium overdose.

Herbal

None known.

Food

None known.

Drug interactions of concern to dentistry

• Avoid drugs with anticholinergic activity and neuromuscular blocking agents
• Avoid systemic use of ester-type local anesthetics because of reduced plasma cholinesterase activity
• Use glucocorticoids with caution

DIAGNOSTIC TEST EFFECTS

None known.

SIDE EFFECTS

Frequent

Abdominal pain, diarrhea, increased salivation, miosis, sweating, and vomiting

Occasional

Anxiety, blurred vision, and urinary urgency

Rare
Trembling, difficulty moving or controlling movement of the tongue, neck, or arms

SERIOUS REACTIONS

! Overdosage may result in cholinergic crisis, characterized by severe nausea, vomiting, diarrhea, increased salivation, diaphoresis, bradycardia, hypotension, flushed skin, stomach pain, respiratory depression, seizures, and paralysis of muscles.
! Increasing muscle weakness of myasthenia gravis may occur. Antidote: 0.5-1mg IV atropine sulfate with other supportive treatment.

DENTAL CONSIDERATIONS

General:
• Control excessive salivary flow with rubber dam and suction.
• Avoid drugs that reduce salivary flow because they will antagonize this drug.
• Patient may be unable to keep mouth open for long periods because of disease; short appointments may be necessary.
• Monitor vital signs at every appointment because of cardiovascular side effects. Evaluate respiration characteristics and rate.
• Consider semisupine chair position for patient comfort if GI side effects occur.
• After supine positioning, have patient sit upright for at least 2 min to avoid orthostatic hypotension.

Consultations:
• Consultation with physician may be necessary if sedation or general anesthesia is required.
• Medical consultation may be required to assess disease control and patient's ability to tolerate stress.

Teach Patient/Family:
• Use of electric toothbrush if patient has difficulty holding conventional devices
• Importance of updating health and drug history, reporting changes in health status, drug regimen changes, or disease/treatment status

amcinonide

am-sin′-oh-nide
(Cylocort)

CATEGORY AND SCHEDULE

Pregnancy Risk Category: C

MECHANISM OF ACTION

Topical corticosteroids have anti-inflammatory, antipruritic, and vasoconstrictive properties. The exact mechanism of the anti-inflammatory process is unclear. ***Therapeutic Effect:*** Reduces or prevents tissue response to inflammatory process.

PHARMACOKINETICS

Well absorbed systemically. Large variation in absorption among sites: forearm 1%; scalp 4%, forehead 7%, scrotum 36%. Greatest penetration occurs at groin, axillae, and face. Protein binding in varying degrees. Metabolized in liver. Primarily excreted in urine.

AVAILABILITY

Lotion: 0.1% (Cylocort).
Cream: 0.1% (Cylocort).
Ointment: 0.1% (Cylocort).

INDICATIONS AND DOSAGES

▸ **Dermatoses**
TOPICAL
Adults, Elderly. Apply sparingly 2–3 times/day.

CONTRAINDICATIONS

History of hypersensitivity to amcinonide or other corticosteroids.

INTERACTIONS

Drug
None known.

Herbal
None known.
Food
None known.
Drug interactions of concern to dentistry
- None reported

DIAGNOSTIC TEST EFFECTS
None known.

SIDE EFFECTS
Frequent
Itching, redness, irritation, burning
Occasional
Dryness, folliculitis, hypertrichosis, acneiform eruptions, hypopigmentation, perioral dermatitis
Rare
Allergic contact dermatitis, maceration of the skin, secondary infection, skin atrophy.
Systemic: Absorption more likely with occlusive dressings or extensive application in young children.

SERIOUS REACTIONS
! The serious reactions of long-term therapy and the addition of occlusive dressings are reversible hypothalamic-pituitary-adrenal (HPA) axis suppression, manifestations of Cushing's syndrome, hyperglycemia and glucosuria.
! Abruptly withdrawing the drug after long-term therapy may require supplemental systemic corticosteroids.

DENTAL CONSIDERATIONS
General:
- Determine why patient is taking the drug.
- Side effects include a variety of skin lesions.

Teach Patient/Family:
- Use on oral herpetic ulcerations is contraindicated

amifostine
am-ih-fos′-teen
(Ethyol)
Do not confuse Ethyol with ethanol.

CATEGORY AND SCHEDULE
Pregnancy Risk Category: C

MECHANISM OF ACTION
An antineoplastic adjunct and cytoprotective agent that is converted to an active metabolite by alkaline phosphatase in tissues. The active metabolite binds to and detoxifies metabolites of cisplatin. These actions occur more readily in normal tissues than in tumor tissue. ***Therapeutic Effect:*** Reduces the toxic effect of the chemotherapeutic agent cisplatin.

PHARMACOKINETICS
Rapidly cleared from plasma. Converted in tissue to active free thiol metabolite. Tissue uptake highest in bone marrow, skin, GI mucosa, salivary glands. ***Half-life:*** less than 1 minute. Less than 10% remains in plasma 6 min after drug administration.

AVAILABILITY
Powder for Injection: 500 mg in a 10-ml single-use vial.

INDICATIONS AND DOSAGES
▸ **To Reduce Cumulative Renal Toxicity from Repeated Administration of Cisplatin in Patients with Advanced Ovarian Cancer**
IV
Adults. 910 mg/m^2 once a day as 15-min infusion, beginning 30 min before chemotherapy. A 15-min infusion is better tolerated than extended infusions. If the full dose can't be administered, dose for subsequent cycles should be 740 mg/m^2.

▸ **Treatment of Postoperative Radiation-Induced Xerostomia in Patients with Head and Neck Cancer**
IV
Adults. 200 mg/m² once a day as 3-min infusion, starting 15–30 min before radiation therapy.
SUBCUTANEOUS
Adults. 500 mg/day during radiation therapy.

OFF-LABEL USES

To protect lung fibroblasts from damaging effects of chemotherapeutic agent paclitaxel

CONTRAINDICATIONS

Sensitivity to aminothiol compounds or mannitol

INTERACTIONS

Drug

Antihypertensive medications or drugs that may potentiate hypotension: May increase the risk of hypotension.

Herbal

None known.

Food

None known.

Drug interactions of concern to dentistry

- None reported

DIAGNOSTIC TEST EFFECTS

May reduce serum calcium levels, especially in patients with nephrotic syndrome.

IV INCOMPATIBILITIES

Don't mix amifostine in any solution other than 0.9% NaCl.

IV COMPATIBILITIES

Mannitol, potassium chloride

SIDE EFFECTS

Frequent (62%)

Transient reduction in BP (usually starts 14 min into infusion, lasts about 6 min and returns to normal in 5–15 min); severe nausea, vomiting

Occasional (20%–10%)

Flushing or feeling of warmth or chills or feeling of coldness; dizziness, hiccups, sneezing, somnolence

Rare (<1%)

Clinically relevant hypocalcemia, mild rash

SERIOUS REACTIONS

! A pronounced drop in BP may require temporary cessation of amifostine and fluid resuscitation.

DENTAL CONSIDERATIONS

General:

- This is an in-hospital or outpatient chemotherapy-administered drug. Confirm the patient's disease and treatment status.
- Dental treatment may be provided if necessary during treatment.
- Monitor vital signs at every appointment because of cardiovascular side effects.
- Consider semisupine chair position for patient comfort if GI side effects occur.
- Patients taking opioids for acute or chronic pain should be given alternative analgesics for dental pain.
- Short appointments and a stress reduction protocol may be required for anxious patients.
- Palliative medication may be required for management of oral side effects caused by chemotherapeutic drugs.
- Assess salivary flow as a factor in caries, periodontal disease, and candidiasis.
- Chlorhexidine mouth rinse before and during chemotherapy may reduce severity of mucositis.
- Apply lubricant to dry lips for patient comfort before dental procedures.
- Examine for oral manifestation of opportunistic infection.

Consultations:
- Medical consultation may be required to assess immunologic status during cancer therapy and determine safety risks posed by dental treatment.
- Consultation with physician may be necessary if sedation or general anesthesia is required.

Teach Patient/Family:
- To prevent trauma when using oral hygiene aids
- Importance of good oral hygiene to prevent soft tissue inflammation, infection
- To report oral lesions, soreness, or bleeding to dentist
- *When chronic dry mouth occurs, advise patient:*
  - To avoid mouth rinses with high alcohol content because of drying effects
  - To use daily home fluoride products for anticaries effect
  - To use sugarless gum, frequent sips of water, or saliva substitutes
  - Importance of updating health and drug history, reporting changes in health status, drug regimen changes, or disease/treatment status

amiloride hydrochloride

a-mill′-oh-ride
(Kaluril[AUS], Midamor)
Do not confuse amiloride with amiodarone or amlodipine.

CATEGORY AND SCHEDULE
Pregnancy Risk Category: B
(D if used in pregnancy-induced hypertension)

MECHANISM OF ACTION
A guanidine derivative that acts as a potassium-sparing diuretic, antihypertensive, and antihypokalemic by directly interfering with sodium reabsorption in the distal tubule.
Therapeutic Effect: Increases sodium and water excretion and decreases potassium excretion.

PHARMACOKINETICS

Route	Onset	Peak	Duration
PO	2 hrs	6–10 hrs	24 hrs

Incompletely absorbed from the GI tract. Protein binding: Minimal. Primarily excreted in urine; partially eliminated in feces. ***Half-life:*** 6–9 hr.

AVAILABILITY
Tablets: 5 mg.

INDICATIONS AND DOSAGES
▸ **To Counteract Potassium Loss Induced by Other Diuretics**
PO
Adults, Children weighing more than 20 kg. 5–10 mg/day up to 20 mg.
Elderly. Initially, 5 mg/day or every other day.
Children weighing 6–20 kg. 0.625 mg/kg/day. Maximum: 10 mg/day.

▸ **Dosage in Renal Impairment**

Creatinine Clearance	Dosage
10–50 ml/min	50% of normal
less than 10 ml/min	avoid use

OFF-LABEL USES
Treatment of edema associated with CHF, liver cirrhosis, and nephrotic syndrome; treatment of hypertension, reduces lithium-induced polyuria, slows pulmonary function reduction in cystic fibrosis

CONTRAINDICATIONS
Acute or chronic renal insufficiency, anuria, diabetic nephropathy, patients on other potassium-sparing diuretics, serum potassium greater than 5.5 mEq/L

INTERACTIONS

Drug

ACE inhibitors, including captopril, and potassium-containing diuretics: May increase potassium levels.
Anticoagulants, including heparin: May decrease effect of anticoagulants, including heparin.
Lithium: May decrease lithium clearance and increase risk of amiloride toxicity.
NSAIDs: May decrease antihypertensive effect.

Herbal

None known.

Food

None known.

Drug interactions of concern to dentistry

- Decreased effects: corticosteroids, NSAIDs, indomethacin

DIAGNOSTIC TEST EFFECTS

May increase BUN, calcium excretion, and glucose, serum creatinine, serum magnesium, serum potassium, and uric acid levels. May decrease serum sodium levels.

SIDE EFFECTS

Frequent (8%–3%)
Headache, nausea, diarrhea, vomiting, decreased appetite
Occasional (3%–1%)
Dizziness, constipation, abdominal pain, weakness, fatigue, cough, impotence
Rare (< 1%)
Tremors, vertigo, confusion, nervousness, insomnia, thirst, dry mouth, heartburn, shortness of breath, increased urination, hypotension, rash

SERIOUS REACTIONS

! Severe hyperkalemia may produce irritability; anxiety; a feeling of heaviness in the legs; paresthesia of hands, face, and lips; hypotension; bradycardia; tented T waves; widening of QRS, and ST depression.

DENTAL CONSIDERATIONS

General:

- Monitor vital signs at every appointment because of cardiovascular side effects.
- Assess salivary flow as a factor in caries, periodontal disease, and candidiasis.
- After supine positioning, have patient sit upright for at least 2 min to avoid orthostatic hypotension.
- Patients on chronic drug therapy may rarely have symptoms of blood dyscrasias, which can include infection, bleeding, and poor healing.
- Limit use of sodium-containing products, such as saline IV fluids, for those patients with a dietary salt restriction.

Consultations:

- Medical consultation may be required to assess patient's ability to tolerate stress.
- Medical consultation may be required to assess disease control.
- In a patient with symptoms of blood dyscrasias, request a medical consultation for blood studies and postpone dental treatment until normal values are reestablished.

Teach Patient/Family:

- Importance of good oral hygiene to prevent soft tissue inflammation
- Caution to prevent injury when using oral hygiene aids
- *When chronic dry mouth occurs, advise patient:*
  - To avoid mouth rinses with high alcohol content because of drying effects
  - To use daily home fluoride products for anticaries effect
  - To use sugarless gum, frequent sips of water, or saliva substitutes

aminocaproic acid

a-mee-noe-ka-proe′-ik

(Amicar)

Do not confuse Amicar with amikacin or Amikin.

CATEGORY AND SCHEDULE

Pregnancy Risk Category: C

MECHANISM OF ACTION

A systemic hemostatic that acts as an antifibrinolytic and antihemorrhagic by inhibiting the activation of plasminogen activator substances. ***Therapeutic Effect:*** Prevents formation of fibrin clots.

AVAILABILITY

Syrup: 250 mg/ml.
Tablets: 500 mg.
Injection: 250 mg/ml.

INDICATIONS AND DOSAGES

▸ **Acute Bleeding**

PO, IV INFUSION

Adults, Elderly. 4–5 g over first hr; then 1–1.25 g/hr. Continue for 8 hr or until bleeding is controlled. Maximum: 30 g/24 hr.

Children. 3 g/m^2 over first hr; then 1 $g/m^2/hr$. Maximum: 18 $g/m^2/24$ hr.

▸ **Dosage in Renal Impairment**

Decrease dose to 25% of normal.

OFF-LABEL USES

Prevention of recurrence of subarachnoid hemorrhage, prevention of hemorrhage in hemophiliacs following dental surgery

CONTRAINDICATIONS

Evidence of active intravascular clotting process, disseminated intravascular coagulation without concurrent heparin therapy, hematuria of upper urinary tract origin (unless benefit outweighs risk); newborns (parenteral form).

INTERACTIONS

Drug

None known.

Herbal

None known.

Food

None known.

DIAGNOSTIC TEST EFFECTS

May elevate serum potassium level.

IV INCOMPATIBILITIES

Sodium lactate

SIDE EFFECTS

Occasional

Nausea, diarrhea, cramps, decreased urination, decreased BP, dizziness, headache, muscle fatigue and weakness, myopathy, bloodshot eyes

SERIOUS REACTIONS

! Too rapid IV administration produces tinnitus, rash, arrhythmias, unusual fatigue, and weakness.

! Rarely, a grand mal seizure occurs, generally preceded by weakness, dizziness, and headache.

DENTAL CONSIDERATIONS

General:

- Monitor vital signs at every appointment because of cardiovascular side effects.
- After supine positioning, have patient sit upright for at least 2 min to avoid orthostatic hypotension.
- Consider additional local hemostasis measures to prevent excessive bleeding in patients with hemophilia.
- Determine why the patient is taking the drug.
- Avoid drugs such as aspirin; NSAIDs may have the potential to prolong bleeding.

Consultations:

- Medical consultation may be required to assess disease control.

• Medical consultation may be required to assess patient's ability to tolerate stress.

Teach Patient/Family:

• Importance of good oral hygiene to prevent soft tissue inflammation

• Caution to prevent injury when using oral hygiene aids

aminoglutethimide

a-meen-noe-gloo-teth′-i-mide
(Cytadren)

CATEGORY AND SCHEDULE

Pregnancy Risk Category: D

MECHANISM OF ACTION

An antiadrenal agent that partially inhibits the conversion of cholesterol to pregnenolone in the adrenal glands and blocks the conversion of androstenedione to estrone and estradiol in peripheral tissues.
Therapeutic Effect: Suppresses adrenal function.

PHARMACOKINETICS

Rapidly and completely absorbed from the gastrointestinal (GI) tract. Protein binding: Low (20%–25%). Metabolized in the liver by acetylation. Primarily excreted in urine. ***Half-life:*** 12.5 hours.

AVAILABILITY

Tablets: 250 mg (Cytadren).

INDICATIONS AND DOSAGES

▸ **Cushing's Syndrome**

PO

Adults. Initially, 250 mg q6h. May increase by 250 mg daily every 1 to 2 weeks. Maximum: 2 g/day.

CONTRAINDICATIONS

Hypersensitivity to glutethimide or aminoglutethimide

INTERACTIONS

Drug

Dexamethasone, digitoxin, theophylline, warfarin: May decrease effectiveness of these drugs.
Medroxyprogesterone: May decrease medroxyprogesterone efficacy.
Tamoxifen: May decrease tamoxifen efficacy.

Herbal

None known.

Food

None known.

Drug interactions of concern to dentistry

• None reported

DIAGNOSTIC TEST EFFECTS

None known.

SIDE EFFECTS

Frequent

Drowsiness, rash, loss of appetite, nausea

Occasional

Dizziness, headache, fever, myalgia, hypotension, tachycardia, pruritus, depression

Rare

Neck tenderness, swelling, increased hair growth in females

SERIOUS REACTIONS

! Adrenal insufficiency, agranulocytosis, leucopenia, neutropenia, and pancytopenia may occur.

DENTAL CONSIDERATIONS

General:

• Determine why patient is taking the drug.

• Monitor vital signs at every appointment due to cardiovascular side effects.

• Determine dose and duration of glucocorticoid therapy to assess for risk of stress tolerance and immunosuppression. Patients on chronic glucocorticoid therapy may require

supplemental doses for dental treatment.
- Precaution if dental surgery is anticipated or general anesthesia is required.
- Patient on chronic drug therapy may rarely present with symptoms of blood dyscrasias, which can include infection, bleeding and poor healing. If dyscrasia is present, caution patient to prevent oral tissue trauma when using oral hygiene aids.
- After supine positioning, have patient sit upright for at least 2 min before standing to avoid orthostatic hypotension.
- Patient may need assistance in getting into and out of dental chair. Adjust chair position for patient comfort.
- Examine for oral manifestation of opportunistic infection.
- Caution: use of additional CNS depressants.
- If cancer is present, evaluate surgical, radiation, and chemotherapy history.

Consultations:
- Consultation may be required to confirm glucocorticoid dose and duration of use.
- Medical consultation may be required to assess disease control and patient's ability to tolerate stress.
- In a patient with symptoms of blood dyscrasias, request a medical consultation for blood studies and postpone treatment until normal values are reestablished.

Teach Patient/Family:
- Importance of updating health and medication history if physician makes any changes in evaluation or drug regimens; include OTC, herbal, and nonherbal remedies in the update
- To report oral lesions, soreness, or bleeding to dentist
- Caution patients about driving or performing other tasks requiring mental alertness
- Importance of good oral hygiene to prevent soft tissue inflammation
- To prevent trauma when using oral hygiene aids

aminophylline/ theophylline

am-in-off′-i-lin (aminophylline)
Phyllocontin(theophylline)
Elixophyllin, Quibron-T, Quibron-T/SR, Nuelin[AUS], Nuelin SR[AUS], Slo-Bid Gyrocaps, Theo-24, Thoechron, Theodur, Theolair, T-Phyl, Uniphyl
Do not confuse aminophylline with amitriptyline or ampicillin, or Slo-Bid with Dolobid.

CATEGORY AND SCHEDULE

Pregnancy Risk Category: C

MECHANISM OF ACTION

A xanthine derivative that acts as a bronchodilator by directly relaxing smooth muscle of the bronchial airways and pulmonary blood vessels. ***Therapeutic Effect:*** Relieves bronchospasm and increases vital capacity.

AVAILABILITY

Capsules (Extended-Release [Theo-24]): 100 mg, 200 mg, 300 mg, 400 mg.
Elixir (Elixophyllin): 80 mg/15 ml.
Oral Solution: 80 mg/15 ml.
Tablets (Controlled-Release [Quibron-T/SR]): 300 mg.
Tablets (Controlled-Release [Theochron]): 100 mg, 200 mg, 300 mg.
Tablets (Controlled-Release [Theolair-SR]): 300 mg, 500 mg.
Tablets (Controlled-Release [T-Phyl]): 200 mg.
Tablets (Controlled-Release [Uniphyl]): 400 mg, 600 mg.

Infusion (theophylline): 0.8 mg/ml, 1.6 mg/ml, 2 mg/ml, 3.2 mg/ml, 4 mg/ml.
Injection (aminophylline): 25 mg/ml.

INDICATIONS AND DOSAGES

▸ Chronic Bronchospasm

PO

Adults, Elderly, Children. 16 mg/kg or 400 mg/day (whichever is less) in 3–4 divided doses (8-hr intervals); may increase by 25% every 2–3 days. Maximum: 13 mg/kg/day (children 13–16 yr); 18 mg/kg/day (children 9–12 yr); 20 mg/kg/day (children 1–8 yr). Maximum dosages are based on serum theophylline concentrations, clinical condition, and presence of toxicity.

▸ Acute Bronchospasm in Patients not Currently Taking Theophylline

PO

Adults, Children older than 1 yr. Initially, loading dose of 5 mg/kg (theophylline); then maintenance dosage of theophylline based on patient group (shown below).

Patient Group	Maintenance Theophylline Dosage
Healthy, nonsmoking adults	3 mg/kg q8h
Elderly patients, patients with cor pulmonale	2 mg/kg q8h
Patients with CHF or hepatic disease	1–2 mg/kg q12h
Children 9–16 yr, young adult smokers	3 mg/kg q6h
Children 1–8 yr	4 mg/kg q6h

IV

Adults, Children older than 1 yr. Initially, loading dose of 6 mg/kg (aminophylline); maintenance dosage of aminophylline based on patient group (shown below).

Patient Group	Maintenance Aminophylline Dosage
Healthy, nonsmoking adults	0.7 mg/kg/hr
Elderly patients, patients with cor pulmonale, CHF, or hepatic impairment	0.25 mg/kg/hr
Children 13–16 yr	0.7 mg/kg/hr
Children 9–12 yr, young adult smokers	0.9 mg/kg/hr
Children 1–8 yr	1–1.2 mg/kg/hr
Children 6 mo–1 yr	0.6–0.7 mg/kg/hr
Children 6 wk–6 mo	0.5 mg/kg/hr
Neonates	5 mg/kg q12h

▸ Acute Bronchospasm in Patients Currently Taking Theophylline

PO, IV

Adults, children older than 1 yr. Obtain serum theophylline level. If not possible and patient is in respiratory distress and not experiencing toxic effects, may give 2.5 mg/kg dose. Maintenance: Dosage based on peak serum theophylline concentration, clinical condition, and presence of toxicity.

OFF-LABEL USES

Treatment of apnea in neonates

CONTRAINDICATIONS

History of hypersensitivity to caffeine or xanthine

INTERACTIONS

Drug

Beta blockers: May decrease the effects of aminophylline.
Cimetidine, ciprofloxacin, erythromycin, norfloxacin: May increase aminophylline blood concentration and risk of aminophylline toxicity.
Glucocorticoids: May produce hypernatremia.

Phenytoin, primidone, rifampin: May increase aminophylline metabolism.
Smoking: May decrease aminophylline blood concentration.

Herbal

None known.

Food

Charcoal-broiled foods; high-protein, low-carbohydrate diet: May decrease the theophylline blood level.

Drug interactions of concern to dentistry

- Increased action: erythromycin (macrolides), ciprofloxacin
- Cardiac dysrhythmia: CNS stimulants, hydrocarbon inhalation anesthetics
- Decreased effects: barbiturates, carbamazepine
- Decreased effects of benzodiazepines

DIAGNOSTIC TEST EFFECTS

None known.

IV INCOMPATIBILITIES

Amiodarone (Cordarone), ciprofloxacin (Cipro), dobutamine (Dobutrex), ondansetron (Zofran)

IV COMPATIBILITIES

Aztreonam (Azactam), ceftazidime (Fortaz), fluconazole (Diflucan), heparin, morphine, potassium chloride

SIDE EFFECTS

Frequent

Altered smell (during IV administration), restlessness, tachycardia, tremor

Occasional

Heartburn, vomiting, headache, mild diuresis, insomnia, nausea

SERIOUS REACTIONS

! Too-rapid IV administration may produce marked hypotension with accompanying faintness, lightheadedness, palpitations, tachycardia, hyperventilation, nausea, vomiting, angina-like pain, seizures, ventricular fibrillation, and cardiac standstill.

DENTAL CONSIDERATIONS

General:

- Monitor vital signs at every appointment because of cardiovascular and respiratory side effects.
- Consider semisupine chair position for patient comfort because of respiratory disease and GI side effects of drug.
- Midday appointments and a stress reduction protocol may be required for anxious patients.
- Be aware that aspirin or sulfite preservatives in vasoconstrictor-containing products can exacerbate asthma.
- Acute asthmatic episodes may be precipitated in the dental office. Sympathomimetic inhalants should be available for emergency use.

Consultations:

- Medical consultation may be required to assess disease control.

aminosalicylic acid

a-mee-noe-sal-i-sil-ik as-id
(Nemasol[CAN], Paser)

CATEGORY AND SCHEDULE

Pregnancy Risk Category: C

MECHANISM OF ACTION

An antitubercular agent active against M. tuberculosis. Thought to exhibit competitive antagonism of folic acid synthesis. ***Therapeutic Effect:*** Bacteriostatic activity in susceptible microorganisms.

PHARMACOKINETICS

Readily absorbed from the gastrointestinal (GI) tract. Protein binding: 50–60%. Widely distributed (including cerebrospinal fluid [CSF]). Metabolized in liver. Primarily excreted in urine. Removed by hemodialysis. ***Half-life:*** 1.1–1.62 hrs.

AVAILABILITY

Packet granules: 4 g/packet granules (Paser).
Tablets, enteric-coated: 7.7 grains (Paser).
Tablets, sustained-release: 500 mg (Paser).

INDICATIONS AND DOSAGES

▸ Tuberculosis

PO
Adults, Elderly. 4 g in divided doses 3 times/day.
Children. 150 mg/kg/day in divided doses 3 times/day. Maximum: 12 g/day.

OFF-LABEL USES

Crohn's disease, hyperlipidemia, ulcerative colitis

CONTRAINDICATIONS

End-stage renal disease, hypersensitivity to aminosalicylic acid products

INTERACTIONS

Drug

Cyanocobalamin: May decrease cyanocobalamin absorption.
Isoniazid: May increase isoniazid serum levels.

Herbal

None known.

Food

None known.

Drug interactions of concern to dentistry

- None reported

DIAGNOSTIC TEST EFFECTS

May alter bilirubin levels in urinalysis.

SIDE EFFECTS

Occasional

Abdominal pain, diarrhea, nausea, vomiting

Rare

Hypersensitivity reactions, hepatotoxicity, thrombocytopenia

SERIOUS REACTIONS

! Liver toxicity and hepatitis, blood dyscrasias occur rarely.
! Agranulocytosis, methemoglobinemia, thrombocytopenia have been reported.

DENTAL CONSIDERATIONS

General:

- Determine that noninfectious status exists by ensuring that (1) anti-tuberculosis (TB) drugs have been taken for more than 3 wk, (2) culture confirmed TB susceptibility to antiinfectives, (3) patient has had three consecutive negative sputum smears, and (4) patient is not in the coughing stage.
- Determine why patient is taking drug (i.e., for prophylaxis or active therapy).
- Explain importance of taking medication for full length of regimen to ensure effectiveness of treatment and to prevent the emergence of resistant strains.
- Patients on chronic drug therapy may rarely have symptoms of blood dyscrasias, which can include infection, bleeding, and poor healing.
- Consider semisupine chair position for patient comfort if GI side effects occur.

Consultations:

- Medical consultation may be required to assess disease control and patient's ability to tolerate stress.
- In a patient with symptoms of blood dyscrasias, request a medical consultation for blood studies and postpone treatment until normal values are reestablished.

Teach Patient/Family:
• Importance of updating health and drug history if physician makes any changes in evaluation or drug regimens
• To prevent trauma when using oral hygiene aids

amiodarone hydrochloride

a-mee′-oh-da-rone
(Aratac[AUS], Cordarone, Cordarone X[AUS], Pacerone)
Do not confuse amiodarone with amiloride or Cordarone with Cardura.

CATEGORY AND SCHEDULE

Pregnancy Risk Category: D

MECHANISM OF ACTION

A cardiac agent that prolongs duration of myocardial cell action potential and refractory period by acting directly on all cardiac tissue. Decreases AV and sinus node function. ***Therapeutic Effect:*** Suppresses arrhythmias.

PHARMACOKINETICS

Route	Onset	Peak	Duration
PO	3 days–3 wk	1 wk–5 mo	7–50 days after discontinuation

Slowly, variably absorbed from GI tract. Protein binding: 96%. Extensively metabolized in the liver to active metabolite. Excreted via bile; not removed by hemodialysis. ***Half-life:*** 26–107 days; metabolite, 61 days.

AVAILABILITY

Tablets (Cordarone): 200 mg.
Tablets (Pacerone): 100 mg, 200 mg, 400 mg.
Injection (Cordarone): 50 mg/ml.

INDICATIONS AND DOSAGES

▸ Life-Threatening Recurrent Ventricular Fibrillation or Hemodynamically Unstable Ventricular Tachycardia

PO

Adults, Elderly. Initially, 800–1,600 mg/day in 2–4 divided doses for 1–3 wk. After arrhythmia is controlled or side effects occur, reduce to 600–800 mg/day for about 4 wk. Maintenance: 200–600 mg/day.
Children. Initially, 10–15 mg/kg/day for 4–14 days, then 5 mg/kg/day for several wk. Maintenance: 2.5 mg/kg or lowest effective maintenance dose for 5 of 7 days/wk.

IV INFUSION

Adults. Initially, 1050 mg over 24 hr; 150 mg over 10 min, then 360 mg over 6 hr; then 540 mg over 18 hr. May continue at 0.5 mg/min for up to 2–3 wk regardless of age or renal or left ventricular function.

OFF-LABEL USES

Treatment and prevention of supraventricular arrhythmias and symptomatic atrial flutter refractory to conventional treatment

CONTRAINDICATIONS

Bradycardia-induced syncope (except in the presence of a pacemaker), second- and third-degree AV block, severe hepatic disease, severe sinus-node dysfunction

INTERACTIONS

Drug

Antiarrhythmics: May increase cardiac effects.
Beta blockers, oral anticoagulants: May increase effect of beta blockers and oral anticoagulants.

Digoxin, phenytoin: May increase drug concentration and risk of toxicity of digoxin and phenytoin.

Herbal

None known.

Food

None known.

Drug interactions of concern to dentistry

- Bradycardia, hypotension: inhalation anesthetics, lidocaine, anticholinergics, vasoconstrictors
- Increased photosensitization: tetracyclines
- Do not use with grapefruit juice, gatifloxacin, moxifloxacin, or sparfloxacin
- Amiodarone is both a substrate and an inhibitor of CYP3A4; potential interactions with strong inhibitors of CYP3A4 isoenzymes

DIAGNOSTIC TEST EFFECTS

May increase antinuclear antibody titers and AST (SGOT), ALT (SGPT), and serum alkaline phosphatase levels. May cause changes in ECG and thyroid function test results. Therapeutic serum level is 0.5–2.5 mcg/ml; toxic serum level has not been established.

IV INCOMPATIBILITIES

Aminophylline (theophylline), cefazolin (Ancef), heparin, sodium bicarbonate

IV COMPATIBILITIES

Dobutamine (Dobutrex), dopamine (Intropin), furosemide (Lasix), insulin (regular), labetalol (Normodyne), lidocaine, midazolam (Versed), morphine, nitroglycerin, norepinephrine (Levophed), phenylephrine (Neo-Synephrine), potassium chloride, vancomycin

SIDE EFFECTS

Expected

Corneal microdeposits are noted in almost all patients treated for more than 6 months (can lead to blurry vision).

Frequent (> 3%)

Parenteral: Hypotension, nausea, fever, bradycardia.

Oral: Constipation, headache, decreased appetite, nausea, vomiting, paresthesias, photosensitivity, muscular incoordination.

Occasional (< 3%)

Oral: Bitter or metallic taste; decreased libido; dizziness; facial flushing; blue-gray coloring of skin (face, arms, and neck); blurred vision; bradycardia; asymptomatic corneal deposits.

Rare (< 1%)

Oral: Rash, vision loss, blindness.

SERIOUS REACTIONS

! Serious, potentially fatal pulmonary toxicity (alveolitis, pulmonary fibrosis, pneumonitis, acute respiratory distress syndrome) may begin with progressive dyspnea and cough with crackles, decreased breath sounds, pleurisy, CHF, or hepatotoxicity.

! Amiodarone may worsen existing arrhythmias or produce new arrhythmias (called proarrhythmias).

DENTAL CONSIDERATIONS

General:

- Monitor vital signs at every appointment because of cardiovascular and respiratory side effects.
- Assess salivary flow as a factor in caries, periodontal disease, and candidiasis.
- Avoid dental light in patient's eyes; offer dark glasses for patient comfort.
- After supine positioning, have patient sit upright for at least 2 min before standing to avoid orthostatic hypotension.

A

- Use vasoconstrictors with caution, in low doses, and with careful aspiration. Avoid gingival retraction cord with epinephrine.
- Stress from dental procedures may compromise cardiovascular function; determine patient risk.
- Delay or avoid dental treatment if patient shows signs of cardiac symptoms or respiratory distress.

Consultations:

- Medical consultation may be required to assess patient's ability to tolerate stress.
- Medical consultation may be required to assess disease control.

Teach Patient/Family:

- Importance of updating health and drug history, reporting changes in health status, drug regimen changes, or disease/treatment status
- *When chronic dry mouth occurs, advise patient:*
  - To avoid mouth rinses with high alcohol content because of drying effects
  - To use daily home fluoride products for anticaries effect
  - To use sugarless gum, frequent sips of water, or saliva substitutes

amitriptyline hydrochloride

a-mee-trip′-ti-leen
(Apo-Amitriptyline[CAN], Elavil, Endep[AUS], Levate[CAN], Novo-Triptyn[CAN], Tryptanol[AUS])

Do not confuse amitriptyline with aminophylline or nortriptyline, or Elavil with Equanil or Mellaril.

CATEGORY AND SCHEDULE

Pregnancy Risk Category: C

MECHANISM OF ACTION

A tricyclic antidepressant that blocks the reuptake of neurotransmitters, including norepinephrine and serotonin, at presynaptic membranes, thus increasing their availability at postsynaptic receptor sites. Also has strong anticholinergic activity.
Therapeutic Effect: Relieves depression.

PHARMACOKINETICS

Rapidly and well absorbed from the GI tract. Protein binding: 90%. Undergoes first-pass metabolism in the liver. Primarily excreted in urine. Minimal removal by hemodialysis.
Half-life: 10–26 hr.

AVAILABILITY

Tablets: 10 mg, 25 mg, 50 mg, 75 mg, 100 mg, 150 mg.
Injection: 10 mg/ml.

INDICATIONS AND DOSAGES

▸ **Depression**

PO

Adults. 30–100 mg/day as a single dose at bedtime or in divided doses. May gradually increase up to 300 mg/day. Titrate to lowest effective dosage.
Elderly. Initially, 10–25 mg at bedtime. May increase by 10–25 mg at weekly intervals. Range: 25–150 mg/day.
Children 6–12 yr. 1–5 mg/kg/day in 2 divided doses.

IM

Adults. 20–30 mg 4 times a day.

▸ **Pain Management**

PO

Adults, Elderly. 25–100 mg at bedtime.

OFF-LABEL USES

Relief of neuropathic pain, such as that experienced by patients with diabetic neuropathy or postherpetic neuralgia; treatment of bulimia nervosa

CONTRAINDICATIONS

Acute recovery period after MI, use within 14 days of MAOIs

INTERACTIONS

Drug

Antithyroid agents: May increase the risk of agranulocytosis.
Cimetidine, valproic acid: May increase amitriptyline blood concentration and risk of toxicity.
Clonidine, guanadrel: May decrease the effects of these drugs.
CNS depressants (including alcohol, anticonvulsants, barbiturates, phenothiazines, and sedative-hypnotics): May increase CNS and respiratory depression and the hypotensive effects of amitriptyline.
MAOIs: May increase the risk of neuroleptic malignant syndrome, seizures, hypertensive crisis, and hyperpyresis.
Phenothiazines: May increase the sedative and anticholinergic effects of amitriptyline.
Sympathomimetics: May increase the risk of cardiac effects.

Herbal

None known.

Food

None known.

Drug interactions of concern to dentistry

- Increased anticholinergic effects: muscarinic blockers, antihistamines, phenothiazines
- Increased effects of direct-acting sympathomimetics (epinephrine, levonordefrin)
- Possible risk of increased CNS depression: alcohol, barbiturates, benzodiazepines, CNS depressants, antidepressants
- Possible increase in serum levels: fluconazole, ketoconazole, bupropion, fluvoxamine, paroxetine, sertraline
- Decreased antihypertensive effect: clonidine, guanadrel, guanethidine
- Possible decrease in serum levels: barbiturates, St. John's wort (herb)

DIAGNOSTIC TEST EFFECTS

May alter blood glucose levels and ECG readings. Therapeutic serum drug level is 120–250 ng/ml; toxic serum drug level is greater than 500 ng/ml.

SIDE EFFECTS

Frequent

Dizziness, somnolence, dry mouth, orthostatic hypotension, headache, increased appetite, weight gain, nausea, unusual fatigue, unpleasant taste

Occasional

Blurred vision, confusion, constipation, hallucinations, delayed micturition, eye pain, arrhythmias, fine muscle tremors, parkinsonian syndrome, anxiety, diarrhea, diaphoresis, heartburn, insomnia

Rare

Hypersensitivity, alopecia, tinnitus, breast enlargement, photosensitivity

SERIOUS REACTIONS

! Overdose may produce confusion, seizures, severe somnolence, arrhythmias, fever, hallucinations, agitation, dyspnea, vomiting, and unusual fatigue or weakness.

! Abrupt discontinuation after prolonged therapy may produce headache, malaise, nausea, vomiting, and vivid dreams.

! Blood dyscrasias and cholestatic jaundice occur rarely.

DENTAL CONSIDERATIONS

General:

- Take vital signs every appointment because of cardiovascular side effects.

- Assess salivary flow as a factor in caries, periodontal disease, and candidiasis.
- Patients on chronic drug therapy may rarely have symptoms of blood dyscrasias, which can include infection, bleeding, and poor healing.
- After supine positioning, have patient sit upright for at least 2 min to avoid orthostatic hypotension.
- Use vasoconstrictors with caution, in low doses, and with careful aspiration. Avoid use of gingival retraction cord with epinephrine.
- Place on frequent recall because of oral side effects.

Consultations:

- In a patient with symptoms of blood dyscrasias, request a medical consultation for blood studies and postpone dental treatment until normal values are reestablished.
- Medical consultation may be required to assess disease control.
- Physician should be informed if significant xerostomic side effects occur (e.g., increased caries, sore tongue, problems eating or swallowing, difficulty wearing prosthesis) so that a medication change can be considered.

Teach Patient/Family:

- Importance of good oral hygiene to prevent soft tissue inflammation
- Caution to prevent injury when using oral hygiene aids
- *When chronic dry mouth occurs, advise patient:*
  - To avoid mouth rinses with high alcohol content because of drying effects
  - To use daily home fluoride products for anticaries effect
  - To use sugarless gum, frequent sips of water, or saliva substitutes

amlexanox

am-lecks-ah-knocks
(Apthasol)
Do not confuse with Ambesol.

CATEGORY AND SCHEDULE

Pregnancy Risk Category: B

MECHANISM OF ACTION

A mouth agent that has anti-allergic and anti-inflammatory properties. Appears to inhibit formation and/or release of inflammatory mediators (e.g., histamine) from mast cells, neutrophils, mononuclear cells.
Therapeutic Effect: Alleviates signs and symptoms of aphthous ulcers.

PHARMACOKINETICS

After topical application, most systemic absorption occurs from the gastrointestinal (GI) tract. Metabolized to inactive metabolite. Excreted in urine. ***Half-life:*** 3.5 hrs.

AVAILABILITY

Paste: 5% (Apthasol).

INDICATIONS AND DOSAGES

▸ Aphthous Ulcers

TOPICAL

Adults, Elderly. Administer ¼ inch directly to ulcers 4 times/day (after meals and at bedtime) following oral hygiene.

CONTRAINDICATIONS

Hypersensitivity to amlexanox or any component of the formulation

INTERACTIONS

Drug
None known.
Herbal
None known.
Food
None known.

Drug interactions of concern to dentistry

- None reported

DIAGNOSTIC TEST EFFECTS

None known.

SIDE EFFECTS

Rare

Stinging, burning at administration site, transient pain, rash

SERIOUS REACTIONS

! Ingestion of a full tube would result in nausea, vomiting, and diarrhea.

DENTAL CONSIDERATIONS

General:

- Recurrent aphthous ulcers may be associated with systemic conditions; evaluate as needed if healing has not occurred after 10 days.

Teach Patient/Family:

- To apply paste as directed and wash hands immediately before and after each use
- To report oral lesions or soreness to dentist

amoxapine

a-moks-a-peen

(Ascendin)

Do not confuse with atomoxetine or atropine.

CATEGORY AND SCHEDULE

Pregnancy Risk Category: C

MECHANISM OF ACTION

A tricyclic antidepressant that blocks the reuptake of neurotransmitters, such as norepinephrine and serotonin, at central nervous system (CNS) presynaptic membranes, increasing their availability at postsynaptic receptor sites. The metabolite 7-OH-amoxapine has significant dopamine receptor blocking activity similar to haloperidol. ***Therapeutic Effect:*** Produces antidepressant effects.

PHARMACOKINETICS

Rapidly, well absorbed from the gastrointestinal (GI) tract. Protein binding: 90%. Metabolized in liver. Excreted in urine and feces. ***Half-life:*** 8 hrs.

AVAILABILITY

Tablets: 25 mg, 50 mg, 100 mg, 150 mg (Ascendin).

INDICATIONS AND DOSAGES

▸ Depression

PO

Adults. 25 mg 2–3 times/day. May increase to 100 mg 2–3 times/day.

Adolescents. Initially, 25–50 mg/day as single or divided doses. May increase to 100 mg/day.

Elderly. Initially, 25 mg at bedtime. May increase by 25 mg/day q3–7 days. Maximum: 400 mg/day (outpatient), 600 mg/day (inpatient).

OFF-LABEL USES

Panic disorder

CONTRAINDICATIONS

Acute recovery period following myocardial infarction (MI), within 14 days of MAOI ingestion, hypersensitivity to dibenzoxazepine compounds

INTERACTIONS

Drug

Alcohol, CNS depressants: May increase CNS and respiratory depression and amoxapine's hypotensive effects.

Antithyroid agents: May increase risk of agranulocytosis.

Cimetidine: May increase amoxapine blood concentration and risk of toxicity.

Clonidine, guanadrel: May decrease the effects of clonidine and guanadrel
Estrogens, SSRIs: May increase risk of amoxapine toxicity.
Fluoroquinolones, sympathomimetics: May increase cardiac effects.
MAOIs: May increase the risk of convulsions, hyperpyresis, and hypertensive crisis.
Nefopam: May increase risk of seizures.
Phenothiazines: May increase the anticholinergic and sedative effects of clomipramine.

Herbal

St. John's Wort: May increase risk of serotonin syndrome.

Food

None known.

Drug interactions of concern to dentistry

- Increased anticholinergic effects: muscarinic blockers, antihistamines, phenothiazines
- Increased effects of direct-acting sympathomimetics (epinephrine, levonordefrin)
- Potential risk of increased CNS depression: alcohol, barbiturates, benzodiazepines, CNS depressants
- Decreased antihypertensive effect: clonidine, guanadrel, guanethidine
- Avoid concurrent use with St. John's wort (herb)

DIAGNOSTIC TEST EFFECTS

None known.

SIDE EFFECTS

Frequent

Drowsiness, fatigue, xerostomia, constipation, weight gain

Occasional

Nausea, dizziness, headache, confusion, nervousness, restlessness, insomnia, edema, tremor, blurred vision, aggressiveness, muscle weakness

Rare

Paradoxical reactions (agitation, restlessness, nightmares, insomnia, extrapyramidal symptoms, particularly fine hand tremor), laryngitis, seizures

SERIOUS REACTIONS

! High dosage may produce cardiovascular effects, including severe postural hypotension, dizziness, tachycardia, palpitations, and arrhythmias, and seizures. High dosage may also result in altered temperature regulation, such as hyperpyrexia or hypothermia.
! Abrupt withdrawal from prolonged therapy may produce headache, malaise, nausea, vomiting, and vivid dreams.

DENTAL CONSIDERATIONS

General:

- Take vital signs every appointment because of cardiovascular side effects.
- Assess salivary flow as a factor in caries, periodontal disease, and candidiasis.
- Patients on chronic drug therapy may rarely have symptoms of blood dyscrasias, which can include infection, bleeding, and poor healing.
- After supine positioning, have patient sit upright for at least 2 min to avoid orthostatic hypotension.
- Use vasoconstrictors with caution, in low doses, and with careful aspiration. Avoid use of gingival retraction cord with epinephrine.
- Place on frequent recall because of oral side effects.

Consultations:

- In a patient with symptoms of blood dyscrasias, request a medical consultation for blood studies and postpone dental treatment until normal values are reestablished.

• Medical consultation may be required to assess disease control.
• Physician should be informed if significant xerostomic side effects occur (e.g., increased caries, sore tongue, problems eating or swallowing, difficulty wearing prosthesis) so that a medication change can be considered.

Teach Patient/Family:

• Importance of good oral hygiene to prevent soft tissue inflammation
• Caution to prevent injury when using oral hygiene aids
• *When chronic dry mouth occurs, advise patient:*
  • To avoid mouth rinses with high alcohol content because of drying effects
  • To use daily home fluoride products for anticaries effect
  • To use sugarless gum, frequent sips of water, or saliva substitutes

amoxicillin/ clavulanate potassium

a-mox′-i-sill-in clav-u-lan′-ate (Augmentin, Augmentin ES 600, Augmentin XR, Ausclay[AUS], Ausclay Duo Forte[AUS], Ausclay Duo 400[AUS], Clamoxyl[AUS], Clamoxyl Duo 400[AUS], Clamoxyl Duo Forte[AUS], Clavulin[CAN], Clavulin Duo Forte[AUS])

Do not confuse amoxicillin with amoxapine.

CATEGORY AND SCHEDULE

Pregnancy Risk Category: B

MECHANISM OF ACTION

Amoxicillin inhibits bacterial cell wall synthesis, while clavulanate inhibits bacterial beta-lactamase. ***Therapeutic Effect:*** Amoxicillin is bactericidal in susceptible microorganisms. Clavulanate protects amoxicillin from enzymatic degradation.

PHARMACOKINETICS

Well absorbed from the GI tract. Protein binding: 20%. Partially metabolized in the liver. Primarily excreted in urine. Removed by hemodialysis. ***Half-life:*** 1–1.3 hr (increased in impaired renal function).

AVAILABILITY

Powder for Oral Suspension (Augmentin): 125 mg-31.25 mg/5 ml, 200 mg-28.5 mg/5 ml, 250 mg-62.5 mg/5 ml, 400 mg-57 mg/5 ml, 600 mg-42.9 mg/5 ml.
Tablets (Augmentin): 250 mg-125 mg, 500 mg-125 mg, 875 mg-125 mg.
Tablets (Extended-Release [Augmentin XR]): 1,000 mg-62.5 mg.
Tablets (Chewable [Augmentin]): 125 mg-31.25 mg, 200 mg-28.5 mg, 250 mg-62.5 mg, 400 mg-57 mg.

INDICATIONS AND DOSAGES

▸ **Mild to Moderate Infections**

PO

Adults, Elderly. 500 mg q12h or 250 mg q8h.

▸ **Severe Infections, Respiratory Tract Infections**

PO

Adults, Elderly. 875 mg q12h or 500 mg q8h.

▸ **Community-Acquired Pneumonia, Sinusitis**

PO

Adults, Elderly. 2 g (extended-release tablets) q12h for 7–10 days.

▸ **Usual Pediatric Dosage**

PO

Children weighing 40 kg and less. 25–45 mg/kg/day (200 or 400 mg/5 ml powder or 200 or

400 chewable tablets) in 2 divided doses or 20–40 mg/kg/day (125 or 250 mg/5 ml powder or 125 or 250 mg chewable tablets) in 3 divided doses.

Otitis Media

PO

Children. 90 mg/kg/day (600 mg/5 ml suspension) in divided doses q12h for 10 days.

Usual Neonate Dosage

PO

Neonates, Children younger than 3 mos. 30 mg/kg/day (125 mg/5 ml suspension) in divided doses q12h.

Dosage in Renal Impairment

Dosage and frequency are modified on the basis of creatinine clearance.

Creatinine clearance 10–30 ml/min. 250–500 mg q12h.

Creatinine clearance less than 10 ml/min. 250–500 mg q24h.

OFF-LABEL USES

Treatment of bronchitis and chancroid

CONTRAINDICATIONS

Hypersensitivity to any penicillins, infectious mononucleosis

INTERACTIONS

Drug

Allopurinol: May increase incidence of rash.

Oral contraceptives: May decrease effects of oral contraceptives.

Probenecid: May increase amoxicillin and clavulanate blood concentration and risk of toxicity.

Herbal

None known.

Food

None known.

Drug interactions of concern to dentistry

- Decreased antimicrobial effectiveness: tetracyclines, erythromycins, lincomycins
- Increased amoxicillin concentrations: probenecid
- Increased risk of skin rashes: allopurinol
- *When used for dental infection:*
  - Oral contraceptives: advise patient of a potential risk for decreased contraceptive action, to maintain compliance with oral contraceptive use while using antibiotics, and to consider the use of additional nonhormonal contraception

DIAGNOSTIC TEST EFFECTS

May increase serum AST and ALT levels. May cause a positive Coombs' test.

SIDE EFFECTS

Frequent

GI disturbances (mild diarrhea, nausea, vomiting), headache, oral or vaginal candidiasis

Occasional

Generalized rash, urticaria

SERIOUS REACTIONS

! Antibiotic-associated colitis and other superinfections may result from altered bacterial balance.

! Severe hypersensitivity reactions including anaphylaxis and acute interstitial nephritis occur rarely.

DENTAL CONSIDERATIONS

General:

- Take precautions regarding allergy to medication.
- Determine why the patient is taking the drug.

Consultations:

- Medical consultation may be required to assess disease control.

Teach Patient/Family:

- Importance of good oral hygiene to prevent soft tissue inflammation
- Caution to prevent injury when using oral hygiene aids

- *When used for dental infection, advise patient:*
  - To report sore throat, oral burning sensation, fever, and fatigue, any of which could indicate superinfection
  - To take at prescribed intervals and complete dosage regimen
  - To immediately notify the dentist if signs or symptoms of infection increase

amphetamine

am-fet′-ah-meen

SCHEDULE II

CATEGORY AND SCHEDULE

Pregnancy Risk Category: C
Controlled substance: Schedule II

MECHANISM OF ACTION

A sympathomimetic amine that produces central nervous system (CNS) and respiratory stimulation, mydriasis, bronchodilation, a pressor response, and contraction of the urinary sphincter. Directly affects alpha and beta receptor sites in peripheral system. Enhances release of norepinephrine by blocking reuptake, inhibiting monoamine oxidase. ***Therapeutic Effect:*** Increases motor activity, mental alertness; decreases drowsiness, fatigue.

PHARMACOKINETICS

Well absorbed from the gastrointestinal (GI) tract. Protein binding: 20%. Widely distributed (including CSF). Metabolized in liver. Excreted in urine. Unknown if removed by hemodialysis. ***Half-life:*** 7–31 hrs.

AVAILABILITY

Tablets: 5 mg, 10 mg.

INDICATIONS AND DOSAGES

▸ Attention-Deficit Hyperactivity Disorder (ADHD)

PO

Adults. 5–20 mg 1–3 times/day.
Adults, Children older than 12 yrs. Initially, 5 mg twice a day. Increase by 10 mg at weekly intervals until therapeutic response achieved.
Children 6–12 yrs. Initially, 2.5 mg twice a day. Increase by 5 mg/day at weekly intervals until therapeutic response achieved.
Children 3–6 yrs. Initially, 2.5 mg twice a day. Increase by 2.5 mg/day at weekly intervals until therapeutic response achieved.

▸ Narcolepsy

PO

Adults. 5–20 mg 1–3 times/day.
Adults, Children older than 12 yrs. Initially, 5 mg twice a day. Increase by 10 mg at weekly intervals until therapeutic response achieved.
Children 6–12 yrs. Initially, 2.5 mg twice a day. Increase by 5 mg/day at weekly intervals until therapeutic response achieved.

OFF-LABEL USES

Depression, obsessive-compulsive disorder

CONTRAINDICATIONS

Advanced arteriosclerosis, agitated states, glaucoma, history of drug abuse, history of hypersensitivity to sympathomimetic amines, hyperthyroidism, moderate to severe hypertension, symptomatic cardiovascular disease, within 14 days following discontinuation of an MAOI

INTERACTIONS

Drug

Beta-blockers: May increase risk of bradycardia, heart block, and hypertension.

Central nervous system (CNS) stimulants: May increase the effects of amphetamine.
Digoxin: May increase the risk of arrhythmias with this drug.
MAOIs: May prolong and intensify the effects of amphetamine.
Meperidine: May increase the risk of hypotension, respiratory depression, seizures, and vascular collapse.
Thyroid hormones: May increase the effects of this drug and of amphetamine.
Tricyclic antidepressants: May increase cardiovascular effects.

Herbal

None known.

Food

None known.

Drug interactions of concern to dentistry

- Increased sensitivity to effects of sympathomimetics; increased risk of serotonin syndrome with selective serotonin reuptake inhibitors (SSRIs)
- Increased pressor response: tricyclic antidepressants

DIAGNOSTIC TEST EFFECTS

May increase plasma corticosteroid concentrations.

SIDE EFFECTS

Frequent

Irregular pulse, increased motor activity, talkativeness, nervousness, mild euphoria, insomnia

Occasional

Headache, chills, dry mouth, gastrointestinal (GI) distress, worsening depression in patients who are clinically depressed, tachycardia, palpitations, chest pain

SERIOUS REACTIONS

! Overdose may produce skin pallor or flushing, arrhythmias, and psychosis.

! Abrupt withdrawal following prolonged administration of high dosage may produce lethargy (may last for weeks).

! Prolonged administration to children with ADHD may produce a temporary suppression of normal weight and height patterns.

DENTAL CONSIDERATIONS

General:

- Monitor vital signs at every appointment because of cardiovascular side effects.
- Assess salivary flow as a factor in caries, periodontal disease, and candidiasis.
- Psychologic and physical dependence may occur with chronic use.
- Consider short appointments, frequent recall if patient becomes restless during a dental appointment.

Consultations:

- Medical consultation may be required to assess disease control and patient's ability to tolerate stress.

Teach Patient/Family:

- Importance of updating health and drug history, reporting changes in health status, drug regimen changes, or disease/treatment status
- Importance of good oral hygiene to prevent soft tissue inflammation, infection
- To prevent trauma when using oral hygiene aids
- *When chronic dry mouth occurs, advise patient:*
  - To avoid mouth rinses with high alcohol content because of drying effects
  - To use daily home fluoride products for anticaries effect
  - To use sugarless gum, frequent sips of water, or saliva substitutes

amphotericin B

am-foe-ter′-i-sin bee
(Abelcet, AmBisome, Amphocin, Amphotec, Fungizone)

CATEGORY AND SCHEDULE

Pregnancy Risk Category: B

MECHANISM OF ACTION

An antifungal and antiprotozoal that is generally fungistatic but may become fungicidal with high dosages or very susceptible microorganisms. This drug binds to sterols in the fungal cell membrane. ***Therapeutic Effect:*** Increases fungal cell-membrane permeability, allowing loss of potassium and other cellular components.

PHARMACOKINETICS

Protein binding: 90%. Widely distributed. Metabolic fate unknown. Cleared by nonrenal pathways. Minimal removal by hemodialysis. Amphotec and Abelcet are not dialyzable. ***Half-life:*** Fungizone, 24 hr (increased in neonates and children); Amphotec, 26–28 hr; Abelcet, 7.2 days; AmBisome, 100–153 hr.

AVAILABILITY

Cream (Fungizone): 3%.
Injection, Powder for Reconstitution: (Amphotec): 50 mg, 100 mg.
Injection, Powder for Reconstitution (AmBisome, Amphocin, Fungizone): 50 mg.
Injection, Suspension (Abelcet): 5 mg/ml.

INDICATIONS AND DOSAGES

▸ Cryptococcosis; Blastomycosis; Systemic Candidiasis; Disseminated Forms of Moniliasis, Coccidioidomycosis, and Histoplasmosis; Zygomycosis; Sporotrichosis; Aspergillosis

IV INFUSION (Fungizone)
Adults, Elderly. Dosage based on patient tolerance and severity of infection. Initially, 1-mg test dose is given over 20–30 min. If test dose is tolerated, 5-mg dose may be given the same day. Subsequently, dosage is increased by 5 mg q12–24h until desired daily dose is reached. Alternatively, if test dose is tolerated, 0.25 mg/kg is given on same day and 0.5 mg/kg on second day; then dosage is increased until desired daily dose reached. Total daily dose: 1 mg/kg/day up to 1.5 mg/kg every other day. Maximum: 1.5 mg/kg/day.
Children. Test dose of 0.1 mg/kg/dose (maximum 1 mg) is infused over 20–60 min. If test dose is tolerated, initial dose of 0.4 mg/kg may be given on same day; dosage is then increased in 0.25-mg/kg increments as needed. Maintenance dose: 0.25–1 mg/kg/day.

▸ Invasive Fungal Infections Unresponsive to or Intolerant of Fungizone

IV INFUSION (Abelcet)
Adults, Children. 5 mg/kg at rate of 2.5 mg/kg/hr.

▸ Empiric Treatment of Fungal Infections in Patients with Febrile Neutropenia; Aspergillosis, Candidiasis, or Cryptococcosis in Patients with Renal Impairment and Those Who Have Experienced Toxicity or Treatment Failure with Fungizone

IV INFUSION (AmBisome)
Adults, Children. 3–5 mg/kg over 1 hr.

▸ Invasive Aspergillosis in Patients with Renal Impairment and Those Who have Experienced Toxicity or Treatment Failure with Fungizone

IV INFUSION (Amphotec)
Adults, Children. 3–4 mg/kg over 2–4 hr.

▸ Cutaneous and Mucocutaneous Infections Caused by Candida Albicans, such as Paronychia, Oral Thrush, Perléche, Diaper Rash, and Intertriginous Candidiasis
TOPICAL
Adults, Elderly, Children. Apply liberally to affected area and rub in 2–4 times a day.

CONTRAINDICATIONS

Hypersensitivity to amphotericin B or sulfites

INTERACTIONS

Drug

Bone marrow depressants: May increase the risk of anemia.
Digoxin: May increase the risk of digoxin toxicity from hypokalemia.
Nephrotoxic medications: May increase the risk of nephrotoxicity.
Steroids: May cause severe hypokalemia.

Herbal

None known.

Food

None known.

Drug interactions of concern to dentistry

- None reported

DIAGNOSTIC TEST EFFECTS

May increase BUN, serum alkaline phosphatase, serum creatinine, serum AST(SGOT), and ALT(SGPT) levels. May decrease serum calcium, magnesium, and potassium levels.

IV INCOMPATIBILITIES

Abelcet, AmBisome, Amphotec: Don't mix with any other drug, diluent, or solution. Fungizone: Allopurinol (Aloprim), amifostine (Ethyol), aztreonam (Azactam), calcium gluconate, cefepime (Maxipime), cimetidine (Tagamet), ciprofloxacin (Cipro), docetaxel (Taxotere), dopamine (Intropin), doxorubicin (Adriamycin), enalapril (Vasotec), etoposide (VP-16), filgrastim (Neupogen), fluconazole (Diflucan), fludarabine (Fludara), foscarnet (Foscavir), gemcitabine (Gemzar), magnesium sulfate, meropenem (Merrem IV), ondansetron (Zofran), paclitaxel (Taxol), piperacillin and tazobactam (Zosyn), potassium chloride, propofol (Diprivan), vinorelbine (Navelbine)

IV COMPATIBILITIES

None known; don't mix with other medications or electrolytes.

SIDE EFFECTS

Frequent (> 10%)

Abelcet: Chills, fever, increased serum creatinine level, multiple organ failure
AmBisome: Hypokalemia, hypomagnesemia, hyperglycemia, hypocalcemia, edema, abdominal pain, back pain, chills, chest pain, hypotension, diarrhea, nausea, vomiting, headache, fever, rigors, insomnia, dyspnea, epistaxis, increased hepatic or renal function test results
Amphotec: Chills, fever, hypotension, tachycardia, increased serum creatinine level, hypokalemia, bilirubinemia
Fungizone: Fever, chills, headache, anemia, hypokalemia, hypomagnesemia, anorexia, malaise, generalized pain, nephrotoxicity
Topical: Local irritation, dry skin

Rare

Topical: Rash

SERIOUS REACTIONS

! Cardiovascular toxicity (as evidenced by hypotension, ventricular fibrillation, and anaphylaxis) occurs rarely.
! Altered vision and hearing, seizures, hepatic failure, coagulation defects, multiple organ failure, and sepsis may be noted.

DENTAL CONSIDERATIONS

General:

• Determine why the patient is taking the drug.
• Broad-spectrum antibiotics may contribute to oral *Candida* infections.

Teach Patient/Family:

• That long-term therapy may be necessary to clear infection; complete entire course of medication
• Not to use commercial mouthwashes for mouth infection unless prescribed by dentist
• That patient with removable dental appliance should soak appliance in antifungal agent overnight
• To prevent reinoculation of *Candida* infection by disposing of toothbrush or other contaminated oral hygiene devices used during period of infection

amphotericin B, lipid-based

am-foe-**ter**-i-sin bee
(Abelcet, Amphotec, AmBisome)

CATEGORY AND SCHEDULE

Pregnancy Risk Category: B

MECHANISM OF ACTION

An antifungal and antiprotozoal that is generally fungistatic but may become fungicidal with high dosages or very susceptible micro-organisms. This drug binds to sterols in the fungal cell membrane. ***Therapeutic Effect:*** Increases fungal cell-membrane permeability, allowing loss of potassium and loss of other cellular components.

PHARMACOKINETICS

Protein binding: 90%. Widely distributed. Metabolic fate unknown. Cleared by nonrenal pathways. Minimal removal by hemodialysis. Not dialyzable. ***Half-life:*** 7.2 days.

AVAILABILITY

Injection, Suspension: 5 mg/ml (Abelcet).

INDICATIONS AND DOSAGES

Invasive fungal infections unresponsive to, or intolerant of, Fungizone.
IV INFUSION
Adults, Children. 5 mg/kg at rate of 2.5 mg/kg/hr.

CONTRAINDICATIONS

Hypersensitivity to amphotericin B or sulfites

INTERACTIONS

Drug

Bone marrow depressants: May increase risk for anemia.
Digoxin: May increase risk of digoxin toxicity from hypokalemia.
Nephrotoxic medications: May increase risk of nephrotoxicity.
Steroids: May cause severe hypokalemia.

Herbal

None known.

Food

None known.

Drug interactions of concern to dentistry

• Risk of hypokalemia: glucocorticoids and mineralocorticoids

DIAGNOSTIC TEST EFFECTS

May increase BUN, serum alkaline phosphatase, serum creatinine, AST, and ALT levels. May decrease serum calcium, magnesium, and potassium levels.

IV INCOMPATIBILITIES

Do not mix with any other drug, diluent, or solution.

IV COMPATIBILITIES
None known; do not mix with other medications or electrolytes.

SIDE EFFECTS
Frequent (> 10%)
Chills, fever, increased serum creatinine, multiple organ failure
Occasional (10%–1%)
Nausea, hypotension, vomiting, dyspnea, diarrhea, headache, hypokalemia, abdominal pain, rash

SERIOUS REACTIONS
! Cardiovascular toxicity (as evidenced by hypotension, ventricular fibrillation, and anaphylaxis) occurs rarely.
! Altered vision and hearing, seizures, hepatic failure, coagulation defects, multiple organ failure, and sepsis may be noted.

DENTAL CONSIDERATIONS
General:
- Intended for serious systemic fungal infections; palliative emergency dental care only.
- Determine why patient is taking the drug.
- Patient on chronic drug therapy may rarely present with symptoms of blood dyscrasias, which can include infection, bleeding and poor healing. If dyscrasia is present, caution patient to prevent oral tissue trauma when using oral hygiene aids.
- Monitor vital signs at every appointment due to cardiovascular side effects.
- Avoid prescribing aspirin-containing products.

Consultations:
- In a patient with symptoms of blood dyscrasias, request a medical consultation for blood studies and postpone treatment until normal values are reestablished.
- Medical consultation may be required to assess disease control and patient's ability to tolerate stress.

Teach Patient/Family:
- Importance of good oral hygiene to prevent soft tissue inflammation
- To report oral lesions, soreness, or bleeding to dentist
- To prevent trauma when using oral hygiene aids

ampicillin
am′-pi-sill-in
(Alpovex[AUS], Amficot, Apo-Ampi[CAN], Novo-Ampicillin[CAN], Nu-Ampi[CAN], Omnipen, Omnipen-N, Polycillin, Polycillin-N, Principen, Totacillin, Totacillin-N)
Do not confuse with aminophylline, Imipenem, or Unipen.

CATEGORY AND SCHEDULE
Pregnancy Risk Category: B

MECHANISM OF ACTION
A penicillin that inhibits cell wall synthesis in susceptible microorganisms. ***Therapeutic Effect:*** Produces bactericidal effect.

PHARMACOKINETICS
Moderately absorbed from the gastrointestinal (GI) tract. Protein binding: 28%. Widely distributed. Partially metabolized in liver. Primarily excreted in urine. Removed by hemodialysis. ***Half-life:*** 1–1.9 hrs (half-life increased in impaired renal function).

AVAILABILITY
Capsules: 250 mg (Amficot), 500 mg (Omnipen, Principen, Totacillin).
Powder for PO Suspension: 100/ml (Polycillin), 125 mg/5 ml (Omnipen, Polycillin, Principen, Totacillin), 250 mg/5 ml (Omnipen, Polycillin, Principen, Totacillin), 500 mg/5 ml (Polycillin).

Powder for Injection: 125 mg (Omnipen-N, Polycillin-N), 250 mg (Omnipen-N, Polycillin-N, Totacillin-N), 500 mg (Omnipen-N, Polycillin-N, Totacillin-N), 1 g (Omnipen-N, Polycillin-N, Totacillin-N), 2 g (Omnipen-N, Polycillin-N, Totacillin-N), 10 g (Omnipen-N, Polycillin-N).

INDICATIONS AND DOSAGES

▸ Respiratory Tract, Skin/Skin-Structure Infections

PO

Adults, Elderly, Children weighing more than 20 kg. 250–500 mg q6h.
Children weighing less than 20 kg. 50 mg/kg/day in divided doses q6h.

IM/IV

Adults, Elderly, Children weighing more than 40 kg. 250–500 mg q6h.
Children weighing less than 40 kg. 25–50 mg/kg/day in divided doses q6–8h. Bacterial meningitis, septicemia

IM/IV

Adults, Elderly. 2 g q4h or 3 g q6h. Children. 100–200 mg/kg/day in divided doses q4h. Gonococcal infections

PO

Adults. 3.5 g one time with 1 g probenecid. Perioperative prophylaxis

IM/IV

Adults, Elderly. 2 g 30 min before procedure. May repeat in 8 hrs.
Children. 50 mg/kg using same dosage regimen. Usual neonate dosage

IM/IV

Neonates 7–28 days old.
75 mg/kg/day in divided doses q8h up to 200 mg/kg/day in divided doses q6h.
Neonates 0–7 days old.
50 mg/kg/day in divided doses q12h up to 150 mg/kg/day in divided doses q8h.

CONTRAINDICATIONS

Hypersensitivity to any penicillin, infectious mononucleosis

INTERACTIONS

Drug

Allopurinol: May increase incidence of rash.
Oral contraceptives: May decrease effectiveness of oral contraceptives.
Probenecid: May increase ampicillin blood concentration and risk of ampicillin toxicity.

Herbal

None known.

Food

None known.

Drug interactions of concern to dentistry

- Decreased antimicrobial effectiveness: tetracyclines, erythromycins, lincomycins
- Increased ampicillin concentrations: probenecid
- Increased skin rash: allopurinol
- Decreased effects of atenolol
- Suspected increased risk of methotrexate toxicity
- *When used for dental infection:*
  - Oral contraceptives: advise patient of a potential risk for decreased contraceptive action, to maintain compliance with oral contraceptive use while using antibiotics, and to consider the use of additional nonhormonal contraception

DIAGNOSTIC TEST EFFECTS

May increase SGOT (AST) and SGPT (ALT) levels. May cause positive Coombs' test.

IV INCOMPATIBILITIES

Amikacin (Amikin), gentamicin, diltiazem (Cardizem), midazolam (Versed)

IV COMPATIBILITIES
Calcium gluconate, cefepime (Maxipime), dopamine (Inotropin), famotidine (Pepcid), furosemide (Lasix), heparin, hydromorphone (Dilaudid), insulin (regular), levofloxacin (Levaquin), magnesium sulfate, morphine, multivitamins, potassium chloride, propofol (Diprivan)

SIDE EFFECTS
Frequent
Pain at IM injection site, GI disturbances, including mild diarrhea, nausea, or vomiting, oral or vaginal candidiasis
Occasional
Generalized rash, urticaria, phlebitis, thrombophlebitis with IV administration, headache
Rare
Dizziness, seizures, especially with IV therapy

SERIOUS REACTIONS
! Altered bacterial balance may result in potentially fatal superinfections and antibiotic-associated colitis as evidenced by abdominal cramps, watery or severe diarrhea, and fever.
! Severe hypersensitivity reactions including anaphylaxis and acute interstitial nephritis occur rarely.

DENTAL CONSIDERATIONS
General:
- Take precautions regarding allergy to medication.
- Determine why the patient is taking the drug.

Consultations:
- Medical consultation may be required to assess disease control.

Teach Patient/Family:
- Importance of good oral hygiene to prevent soft tissue inflammation
- Caution to prevent injury when using oral hygiene aids
- *When used for dental infection, advise patient:*
  - To report sore throat, oral burning sensation, fever, and fatigue, any of which could indicate superinfection
  - To take at prescribed intervals and complete dosage regimen
  - To immediately notify the dentist if signs or symptoms of infection increase

ampicillin sodium
am-pi-sill′-in soe′-dee-um
(Alphacin[AUS], Apo-Ampi[CAN], Novo-Ampicillin[CAN], Nu-Ampi[CAN], Polycillin, Principen)
Do not confuse ampicillin with aminophylline, Imipenem, or Unipen.

CATEGORY AND SCHEDULE
Pregnancy Risk Category: B

MECHANISM OF ACTION
A penicillin that inhibits cell wall synthesis in susceptible microorganisms. ***Therapeutic Effect:*** Bactericidal.

PHARMACOKINETICS
Moderately absorbed from the GI tract. Protein binding: 28%. Widely distributed. Partially metabolized in the liver. Primarily excreted in urine. Removed by hemodialysis. ***Half-life:*** 1–1.5 hr (increased in impaired renal function).

AVAILABILITY
Capsules: 250 mg, 500 mg.
Powder for Oral Suspension: 125 mg/5 ml, 250 mg/5 ml, 500 mg/5 ml.

Powder for Injection: 125 mg, 250 mg, 500 mg, 1 g, 2 g.

INDICATIONS AND DOSAGES

▸ Respiratory Tract, Skin and Skin-Structure Infections

PO

Adults, Elderly. 250–500 mg q6h.
Children. 50–100 mg/kg/day in divided doses q6h. Maximum: 3 g/day.

IV, IM

Adults, Elderly. 500 mg to 3 g q6h. Maximum: 14 g/day.
Children. 100–200 mg/kg/day in divided doses q6h
Neonates. 50–100 mg/kg/day in divided doses q6–12h.

▸ Meningitis

IV

Children. 200–400 mg/kg/day in divided doses q6h. Maximum: 12 g/day
Neonates. 100–200 mg/kg/day in divided doses q6–12h.

▸ Gonococcal Infections

PO

Adults. 3.5 g one time with 1 g probenecid.

▸ Perioperative Prophylaxis

IV, IM

Adults, Elderly. 2 g 30 min before procedure. May repeat in 8 hr.
Children. 50 mg/kg 30 min before procedure. May repeat in 8 hr.

▸ Dosage in Renal Impairment

Creatinine Clearance	% of Normal Dosage
10–30 ml/min	give q6–12h
less than 10 ml/min	give q12h

CONTRAINDICATIONS

Hypersensitivity to any penicillin, infectious mononucleosis

INTERACTIONS

Drug

Allopurinol: May increase incidence of rash.
Oral contraceptives: May decrease effectiveness of oral contraceptives.
Probenecid: May increase ampicillin blood concentration and risk of ampicillin toxicity.

Herbal

None known.

Food

None known.

Drug interactions of concern to dentistry

- Decreased antimicrobial effectiveness: tetracyclines, erythromycins, lincomycins
- Increased ampicillin concentrations: probenecid
- Increased skin rash: allopurinol
- Decreased effects of atenolol
- Suspected increased risk of methotrexate toxicity
- *When used for dental infection:*
  - Oral contraceptives: advise patient of a potential risk for decreased contraceptive action, to maintain compliance with oral contraceptive use while using antibiotics, and to consider the use of additional nonhormonal contraception

DIAGNOSTIC TEST EFFECTS

May increase AST (SGOT) and ALT (SGPT) levels. May cause a positive Coombs' test.

IV INCOMPATIBILITIES

Amikacin (Amikin), diltiazem (Cardizem), gentamicin, midazolam (Versed)

IV COMPATIBILITIES

Calcium gluconate, cefepime (Maxipime), dopamine (Intropin), famotidine (Pepcid), furosemide (Lasix), heparin, hydromorphone (Dilaudid), insulin (regular), levofloxacin (Levaquin), magnesium sulfate, morphine, multivitamins, potassium chloride, propofol (Diprivan)

SIDE EFFECTS

Frequent

Pain at IM injection site, GI disturbances (mild diarrhea, nausea, vomiting), oral or vaginal candidiasis

Occasional

Generalized rash, urticaria, phlebitis or thrombophlebitis (with IV administration), headache

Rare

Dizziness, seizures (especially with IV therapy)

SERIOUS REACTIONS

! Antibiotic-associated colitis and other superinfections may result from altered bacterial balance.

! Severe hypersensitivity reactions, including anaphylaxis and acute interstitial nephritis, occur rarely.

DENTAL CONSIDERATIONS

General:

- Take precautions regarding allergy to medication.
- Determine why the patient is taking the drug.

Consultations:

- Medical consultation may be required to assess disease control.

Teach Patient/Family:

- Importance of good oral hygiene to prevent soft tissue inflammation
- Caution to prevent injury when using oral hygiene aids
- *When used for dental infection, advise patient:*
  - To report sore throat, oral burning sensation, fever, and fatigue, any of which could indicate superinfection
  - To take at prescribed intervals and complete dosage regimen
  - To immediately notify the dentist if signs or symptoms of infection increase

ampicillin/sulbactam sodium

am′-pi-sill-in/sul-bac′-tam

(Unasyn)

CATEGORY AND SCHEDULE

Pregnancy Risk Category: B

MECHANISM OF ACTION

Ampicillin inhibits bacterial cell wall synthesis, while sulbactam inhibits bacterial beta-lactamase. ***Therapeutic Effect:*** Ampicillin is bactericidal in susceptible microorganisms. Sulbactam protects ampicillin from enzymatic degradation

PHARMACOKINETICS

Protein binding: 28%–38%. Widely distributed. Partially metabolized in the liver. Primarily excreted in urine. Removed by hemodialysis. ***Half-life:*** 1 hr (increased in impaired renal function).

AVAILABILITY

Powder for Injection: 1.5 g (ampicillin 1 g/sulbactam 500 g), 3 g (ampicillin 2 g/sulbactam 1 g).

INDICATIONS AND DOSAGES

▸ Skin and Skin-Structure, Intra-Abdominal, and Gynecologic Infections

IV, IM

Adults, Elderly. 1.5 g (1 g ampicillin/500 mg sulbactam) to 3 g (2 g ampicillin/1 g sulbactam) q6h.

▸ Skin and Skin-Structure Infections

IV

Children 1–12 yr. 150–300 mg/kg/day in divided doses q6h.

▸ Dosage in Renal Impairment

Dosage and frequency are modified based on creatinine clearance and the severity of the infection.

Creatinine Clearance	Dosage
greater than 30 ml/min	0.5–3 g q6–8h
15–29 ml/min	1.5–3 g q12h
5–14 ml/min	1.5–3 g q24h
less than 5 ml/min	Not recommended

CONTRAINDICATIONS
Hypersensitivity to any penicillin, infectious mononucleosis

INTERACTIONS
Drug
Allopurinol: May increase incidence of rash.
Oral contraceptives: May decrease effectiveness of oral contraceptives.
Probenecid: May increase ampicillin blood concentration and risk of ampicillin toxicity.
Herbal
None known.
Food
None known.
Drug interactions of concern to dentistry
- Decreased antimicrobial effectiveness: tetracyclines, erythromycins, lincomycins
- Increased ampicillin concentration: probenecid
- Increased skin rash: allpurinol
- Decreased effects of atenolol
- Suspected increased risk of methotrexate toxicity
- Increased risk of bleeding with anticoagulants: large IV doses of penicillins
- *When used for dental infection:*
  - Oral contraceptives: advise patient of a potential risk for decreased contraceptive action, to maintain compliance with oral contraceptive use while using antibiotics, and to consider the use of additional nonhormonal contraception

DIAGNOSTIC TEST EFFECTS
May increase serum LDH, alkaline phosphatase, creatinine, AST (SGOT), and ALT (SGPT) levels. May cause a positive Coombs' test.

IV INCOMPATIBILITIES
Diltiazem (Cardizem), idarubicin (Idamycin), ondansetron (Zofran), sargramostim (Leukine)

IV COMPATIBILITIES
Famotidine (Pepcid), heparin, insulin (regular), morphine

SIDE EFFECTS
Frequent
Diarrhea and rash (most common), urticaria, pain at IM injection site, thrombophlebitis with IV administration, oral or vaginal candidiasis
Occasional
Nausea, vomiting, headache, malaise, urine retention

SERIOUS REACTIONS
! Severe hypersensitivity reactions including anaphylaxis, acute interstitial nephritis, and blood dyscrasias may occur.
! Antibiotic-associated colitis and other superinfections may result from altered bacterial balance.
! Overdose may produce seizures.

DENTAL CONSIDERATIONS
General:
- For selected infections in the hospital setting; provide emergency dental treatment only.
- Caution regarding allergy to medication.
- Examine for oral manifestation of opportunistic infection.
- Determine why patient is taking the drug.
Consultations:
- Medical consultation may be required to assess disease control.
- Consult patient's physician if an acute dental infection occurs and another antiinfective is required.

Teach Patient/Family:

- Importance of good oral hygiene to prevent soft tissue inflammation
- To report oral lesions, soreness, or bleeding to dentist
- To prevent trauma when using oral hygiene aids
- Secondary oral infection may occur; need to see dentist immediately if infection occurs
- *When antibiotics are used for dental infection:*
  - Oral contraceptives: advise patient of a potential risk for decreased contraceptive action, to maintain compliance with oral contraceptive use while using antibiotics, and to consider the use of additional nonhormonal contraception
- *When used for dental infection, advise patient:*
  - To report sore throat, oral burning sensation, fever, or fatigue, any of which could indicate superinfection
  - To take at prescribed intervals and complete dosage regimen
  - To immediately notify the dentist if signs or symptoms of infection increase

amprenavir

am-prehn′-eh-veer

(Agenerase)

Do not confuse Agenerase with asparaginase.

CATEGORY AND SCHEDULE

Pregnancy Risk Category: C

MECHANISM OF ACTION

An antiretroviral that inhibits HIV-1 protease by binding to the enzyme's active site, thus preventing processing of viral precursors and resulting in the formation of immature, noninfectious viral particles. ***Therapeutic Effect:*** Impairs HIV replication and proliferation.

PHARMACOKINETICS

Rapidly absorbed after PO administration. Protein binding: 90%. Metabolized in the liver. Primarily excreted in feces. ***Half-life:*** 7.1–10.6 hr.

AVAILABILITY

Capsules: 50 mg.
Oral Solution: 15 mg/ml.

INDICATIONS AND DOSAGES

▸ HIV-1 Infection (in combination with other antiretrovirals)

PO

Adults, Children 13–16 yr. 1200 mg capsules twice a day.

Children 4–12 yr, and children 13–16 yr weighing less than 50 kg. 20 mg/kg twice a day or 15 mg/kg 3 times a day. Maximum: 2400 mg/day.

Oral solution

Adults. 1400 mg 2 times/day.

Children 4–12 yr, and children 13–16 yr weighing less than 50 kg. 22.5 mg/kg/day (1.5 ml/kg) oral solution twice a day or 17 mg/kg/day (1.1 ml/kg) 3 times a day. Maximum: 2800 mg/day.

▸ Dosage in Hepatic Impairment

Dosage and frequency are modified on the basis of the Child-Pugh score.

Child-Pugh Score	Capsules	Oral Solution
5–8	450 mg bid	513 mg bid
9–12	300 mg bid	342 mg bid

CONTRAINDICATIONS

None known.

INTERACTIONS

Drug

Amiodarone, bepridil, ergotamine, lidocaine, midazolam, oral

contraceptives, quinidine, triazolam, tricyclic antidepressants: May interfere with the metabolism of these drugs.
Antacids, didanosine: May decrease amprenavir absorption.
Carbamazepine, phenobarbital, phenytoin, rifampin: May decrease amprenavir blood concentration.
Clozapine, HMG-CoA reductase inhibitors (including statins), warfarin: May increase the blood concentration of these drugs.

Herbal

St. John's wort: May decrease amprenavir blood concentration.

Food

High-fat meals: May decrease amprenavir absorption.

Drug interactions of concern to dentistry

- Contraindicated with midazolam, triazolam, tricyclic antidepressants
- Increased plasma levels of erythromycin, clarithromycin, itraconazole, alprazolam, clorazepate, diazepam, carbamazepine, loratadine, flurazepam, ketoconazole, itraconazole; lidocaine (systemic use for cardiac arrhythmias)
- Decreased effectiveness: dexamethasone, St. John's wort (herb)
- Use with caution: sildenafil

DIAGNOSTIC TEST EFFECTS

May increase blood cholesterol, serum glucose, and triglyceride levels.

SIDE EFFECTS

Frequent

Diarrhea or loose stools (56%), nausea (38%), oral paresthesia (30%), rash (25%), vomiting (20%)

Occasional

Peripheral paresthesia (12%), depression (4%)

SERIOUS REACTIONS

! Severe hypersensitivity reactions or Stevens-Johnson syndrome as evidenced by blisters, peeling of the skin, loosening of skin and mucous membranes, and fever may occur.

DENTAL CONSIDERATIONS

General:

- Palliative medication may be required for management of oral side effects.
- Examine for oral manifestation of opportunistic infection.
- Patients on chronic drug therapy may rarely have symptoms of blood dyscrasias, which can include infection, bleeding, and poor healing.
- Consider semisupine chair position for patient comfort if GI side effects occur.

Consultations:

- In a patient with symptoms of blood dyscrasias, request a medical consultation for blood studies and postpone treatment until normal values are reestablished.
- Medical consultation may be required to assess disease control and patient's ability to tolerate stress.

Teach Patient/Family:

- Importance of good oral hygiene to prevent soft tissue inflammation
- To prevent trauma when using oral hygiene aids
- Importance of updating health and drug history if physician makes any changes in evaluation or drug regimens
- That secondary oral infection may occur; must see dentist immediately if infection occurs

amyl nitrite

am′-il nye′-trate
(Amyl Nitrite)
Do not confuse with Nicobid, Nicoderm, Nilstat, nitroprusside, Nizoral, or Nystatin.

CATEGORY AND SCHEDULE
Pregnancy Risk Category: C

MECHANISM OF ACTION
A nitrite vasodilator that relaxes smooth muscles. Reduces afterload and improves vascular supply to the myocardium. ***Therapeutic Effect:*** Dilates coronary arteries, improves blood flow to ischemic areas within myocardium. Following inhalation, systemic vasodilation occurs.

PHARMACOKINETICS
The vapors are absorbed rapidly through the pulmonary alveoli and metabolized rapidly. Partially excreted in the urine.

AVAILABILITY
Solution: 0.3 ml (Amyl Nitrite).

INDICATIONS AND DOSAGES
▸ Acute Relief of Angina Pectoris
Nasal inhalation
Adults, Elderly. Place crushed capsule to nostrils for 0.18–0.3 ml inhalation of vapors. Repeat at 5–10 min intervals. No more than 3 doses in 15–30 min period.

OFF-LABEL USES
Cyanide toxicity

CONTRAINDICATIONS
Closed-angle glaucoma, severe anemia, head injury, postural hypotension, pregnancy, hypersensitivity to nitrates

INTERACTIONS
Drug
Sildenafil: May increase hypotensive effects.
Herbal
None known.
Food
Ethanol: May increase hypotensive effects.
Drug interactions of concern to dentistry
• None reported

DIAGNOSTIC TEST EFFECTS
None known.

SIDE EFFECTS
Frequent
Headache (may be severe) occurs mostly in early therapy, diminishes rapidly in intensity, usually disappears during continued treatment; transient flushing of face and neck; dizziness (especially if patient is standing immobile or is in a warm environment); weakness; postural hypotension
Occasional
Nausea, rash vomiting
Rare
Involuntary passage of urine and feces, restlessness, weakness

SERIOUS REACTIONS
! Large doses may produce hemolytic anemia or methemoglobinemia.
! Severe postural hypotension manifested by fainting, pulselessness, cold or clammy skin, and profuse sweating may occur.
! Tolerance may occur with repeated, prolonged therapy.
! High dose tends to produce severe headache.

DENTAL CONSIDERATIONS
General:
• For emergency relief of acute angina; if angina is not relieved

call 911 for transfer of patient to a medical emergency facility.
- Prior to treatment, inquire about disease control and frequency of angina episodes.
- Ensure that patient's rescue antianginal drug is available for use.
- Monitor vital signs at every appointment due to cardiovascular side effects.
- Postpone elective dental treatment if patient shows signs of cardiac symptoms or respiratory distress.
- After supine positioning, have patient sit upright for at least 2 min before standing to avoid orthostatic hypotension.

Consultations:
- Medical consultation may be required to assess disease control and patient's ability to tolerate stress.

Teach Patient/Family:
- To report angina symptoms to physician
- Importance of updating health and medication history if physician makes any changes in evaluation or drug regimens; include OTC, herbal, and nonherbal remedies in the update
- Importance of good oral hygiene to prevent soft tissue inflammation

anagrelide

ah-na′- greh-lide
(Agrylin)

CATEGORY AND SCHEDULE

Pregnancy Risk Category: C

MECHANISM OF ACTION

A hematologic agent that reduces platelet production and prevents platelet shape changes caused by platelet aggregating agents.
Therapeutic Effect: Inhibits platelet aggregation.

PHARMACOKINETICS

After oral administration, plasma concentration peak within 1 hr. Extensively metabolized. Primarily excreted in urine. ***Half-life:*** About 3 days.

AVAILABILITY

Capsules: 0.5 mg, 1 mg.

INDICATIONS AND DOSAGES

▸ **Thrombocythemia**

PO

Adults, Elderly. Initially, 0.5 mg 4 times a day or 1 mg twice a day. Adjust to lowest effective dosage, increasing by up to 0.5 mg/day or less in any 1 wk. Maximum: 10 mg/day or 2.5 mg/dose.

CONTRAINDICATIONS

None known.

INTERACTIONS

Drug

None known.

Herbal

None known.

Food

None known.

Drug interactions of concern to dentistry
- Possible risk of hemorrhage: NSAIDs, aspirin

DIAGNOSTIC TEST EFFECTS

May increase hepatic enzymes levels (rare).

SIDE EFFECTS

Frequent (5% or more)

Headache, palpitations, diarrhea, abdominal pain, nausea, flatulence, bloating, asthenia, pain, dizziness

Occasional (< 5%)

Tachycardia, chest pain, vomiting, paresthesia, peripheral edema, anorexia, dyspepsia, rash

Rare

Confusion, insomnia

SERIOUS REACTIONS

! Angina, heart failure, and arrhythmias occur rarely.

DENTAL CONSIDERATIONS

General:

- Laboratory studies should include routine complete blood counts (CBCs).
- Patients have risk of thrombohemorrhagic complications; prolonged bleeding time, anemia, or splenomegaly may occur in some patients with this disease. However, thrombosis may also occur in some patients.
- Mucosal bleeding can be a symptom of disease.
- Patients with severe symptoms may be taking chemotherapy.
- Monitor vital signs at every appointment because of cardiovascular side effects.
- Consider semisupine chair position for patient comfort if GI side effects occur.

Consultations:

- Medical consultation with hematologist or physician directing therapy is essential before dental treatment.

Teach Patient/Family:

- To inform dentist of unusual bleeding episodes following dental treatment
- Importance of updating health and drug history if physician makes any changes in evaluation or drug regimens

anakinra

an-a-kin′-ra
(Kineret)

CATEGORY AND SCHEDULE

Pregnancy Risk Category: B

MECHANISM OF ACTION

An interleukin-1 (IL-1) receptor antagonist that blocks the binding of IL-1, a protein that is a major mediator of joint disease and is present in excess amounts in patients with rheumatoid arthritis.
Therapeutic Effect: Inhibits the inflammatory response.

PHARMACOKINETICS

No accumulation of anakinra in tissues or organs was observed after daily subcutaneous doses. Excreted in urine. ***Half-life:*** 4–6 hr.

AVAILABILITY

Solution: 100-mg syringe.

INDICATIONS AND DOSAGES

▸ Rheumatoid Arthritis

SUBCUTANEOUS
Adults, Children older than 18 yr, Elderly. 100 mg/day, given at same time each day.

CONTRAINDICATIONS

Known hypersensitivity to *Escherichia coli*-derived proteins, serious infection

INTERACTIONS

Drug

Live-virus vaccines: May cause the vaccines to be ineffective.

Herbal

None known.

Food

None known.

Drug interactions of concern to dentistry

- None reported

DIAGNOSTIC TEST EFFECTS

May increase the eosinophil count. May decrease WBC, platelet, and absolute neutrophil counts.

SIDE EFFECTS

Occasional

Injection site ecchymosis, erythema, and inflammation

Rare

Headache, nausea, diarrhea, abdominal pain

SERIOUS REACTIONS

! Infections, including upper respiratory tract infection, sinusitis, flu-like symptoms, and cellulitis, have been noted.

! Neutropenia may occur, particularly when anakinra is used in combination with tumor necrosis factor-blocking agents.

DENTAL CONSIDERATIONS

General:

- Question patient about other drugs or products he/she may be taking for arthritis.
- Patient may be at risk for infection.
- Oral infections should be eliminated and/or treated aggressively.
- Evaluate efficacy of oral hygiene home care; preventive instruction appointment may be necessary.
- Patient on chronic drug therapy may rarely present with symptoms of blood dyscrasias, which can include infection, bleeding and poor healing. If dyscrasia is present, caution patient to prevent oral tissue trauma when using oral hygiene aids.
- Patient may need assistance in getting into and out of dental chair. Adjust chair position for patient comfort.

Consultations:

- Medical consultation may be required to assess disease control.
- In a patient with symptoms of blood dyscrasias, request a medical consultation for blood studies and postpone treatment until normal values are reestablished.

Teach Patient/Family:

- Use of electric toothbrush if patient has difficulty holding conventional devices
- To prevent trauma when using oral hygiene aids
- Importance of good oral hygiene to prevent soft tissue inflammation
- Importance of updating health and medication history if physician makes any changes in evaluation or drug regimens; include OTC, herbal, and nonherbal remedies in the update

anastrozole

ah-nas′-trow-zole

(Arimidex)

Do not confuse Arimidex with Imitrex.

CATEGORY AND SCHEDULE

Pregnancy Risk Category: D

MECHANISM OF ACTION

Decreases the circulating estrogen level by inhibiting aromatase, the enzyme that catalyzes the final step in estrogen production. ***Therapeutic Effect:*** Inhibits the growth of breast cancers that are stimulated by estrogens.

PHARMACOKINETICS

Well absorbed into systemic circulation (absorption not affected by food). Protein binding: 40%. Extensively metabolized in the liver. Eliminated by biliary system and, to a lesser extent, kidneys. ***Mean Half-life:*** 50 hr in postmenopausal women. Steady-state plasma levels reached in about 7 days.

AVAILABILITY

Tablets: 1 mg.

INDICATIONS AND DOSAGES

▸ **Breast Cancer**

PO

Adults, Elderly. 1 mg once a day.

CONTRAINDICATIONS

None known.

INTERACTIONS

Drug

None known.

Herbal

None known.

Food

None known.

Drug interactions of concern to dentistry

- None reported

DIAGNOSTIC TEST EFFECTS

May elevate serum GGT level in patients with liver metastasis. May increase serum LDL, serum alkaline phosphate, AST (SGOT), ALT (SGPT), and total cholesterol levels.

SIDE EFFECTS

Frequent (16%–8%)

Asthenia, nausea, headache, hot flashes, back pain, vomiting, cough, diarrhea

Occasional (6%–4%)

Constipation, abdominal pain, anorexia, bone pain, pharyngitis, dizziness, rash, dry mouth, peripheral edema, pelvic pain, depression, chest pain, paresthesia

Rare (2%–1%)

Weight gain, diaphoresis

SERIOUS REACTIONS

! Thrombophlebitis, anemia, leukopenia, and vaginal hemorrhage occur rarely.

! Vaginal hemorrhage occurs rarely (2%).

DENTAL CONSIDERATIONS

General:

- Monitor vital signs at every appointment due to cardiovascular side effects.
- If additional analgesia is required for dental pain, consider alternative analgesics (NSAIDs) in patients taking narcotics for acute or chronic pain.
- Avoid products that affect platelet function, such as aspirin and NSAIDs.
- Consider semisupine chair position for patient comfort if GI side effects occur.
- Examine for oral manifestation of opportunistic infection.
- Patient on chronic drug therapy may rarely present with symptoms of blood dyscrasias, which can include infection, bleeding and poor healing. If dyscrasia is present, caution patient to prevent oral tissue trauma when using oral hygiene aids.
- Assess salivary flow as a factor in caries, periodontal disease, and candidiasis

Consultations:

- Consider consulting with physician before prescribing drugs that may cause constipation (narcotics).
- Consultation with physician may be necessary if sedation or general anesthesia is required.
- In a patient with symptoms of blood dyscrasias, request a medical consultation for blood studies and postpone treatment until normal values are reestablished.
- Medical consultation may be required to assess disease control and patient's ability to tolerate stress.

Teach Patient/Family:

- Importance of good oral hygiene to prevent soft tissue inflammation
- To prevent trauma when using oral hygiene aids

- *When chronic dry mouth occurs advise patient:*
  - To avoid mouth rinses with high alcohol content due to drying effects
  - To use daily home fluoride products for anticaries effect
  - To use sugarless gum, frequent sips of water, or saliva substitutes
  - Importance of updating health and medication history if physician makes any changes in evaluation or drug regimens; include OTC, herbal, and nonherbal remedies in the update

anthralin

anth-rah′-lin
(A-Fil, Anthra-Derm, Anthraforte[CAN], Anthranol[CAN], Anthrascalp[CAN], Dithrocream[AUS], Drithocreme, Dritho-Scalp, Micanol, Psoriatec)
(capsules, tablets, chewable tablets, syrup, elixir, cream, spray)
Do not confuse with Antagon, Antabuse, or Andriol.

CATEGORY AND SCHEDULE

Pregnancy Risk Category: C

MECHANISM OF ACTION

A topical agent that binds DNA, inhibiting synthesis of nucleic protein, and reduces mitotic activity.
Therapeutic Effect: Results in damage to DNA sugar and enhances membrane lipid peroxidation, which may play a critical role in the antipsoriatic action.

PHARMACOKINETICS

Poorly absorbed systemically, but excellent epidermal absorption. Auto-oxidized to inactive metabolites - danthrone and dianthrone. Rapid urinary excretion, so significant levels do not accumulate in the blood or other tissues. ***Half-life:*** 6 hrs.

AVAILABILITY

Cream: 0.1% (Drithocreme), 0.25% (Drithocreme, Dritho-Scalp), 0.5% (Drithocreme, Dritho-Scalp), 1% (Anthra-Derm).
Ointment: 0.1% (Anthra-Derm), 0.25% (Anthra-Derm), 0.5% (Anthra-Derm), 1% (Micanol, Psoriatec).

INDICATIONS AND DOSAGES

▸ Psoriasis
TOPICAL
Adults, Elderly. Apply in a thin layer to affected areas q12h or q24h.

OFF-LABEL USES

Inflammatory linear verrucous epidermal nevus

CONTRAINDICATIONS

Acute psoriasis where inflammation is present, erythroderma, hypersensitivity to anthralin

INTERACTIONS

Drug
None known.
Herbal
None known.
Food
None known.
Drug interactions of concern to dentistry
- None reported

SIDE EFFECTS

Frequent
Irritation
Rare
Neutrophilia, proteinuria, staining of the skin

SERIOUS REACTIONS

! Patients with renal disease should have routine urine tests for albuminuria.
! Hypersensitivity reaction, such as burning, erythema, and dermatitis, may occur.

DENTAL CONSIDERATIONS

General:

- Determine why patient is taking the drug.
- Arthritic symptoms may occur in some patients; inquire about use of other medications.

apraclonidine hydrochloride

ap-raa-kloe′-ni-deen

(Iodipine)

Do not confuse with Cetapred, clomiphene, Klonopin, or quinidine.

CATEGORY AND SCHEDULE

Pregnancy Risk Category: C

MECHANISM OF ACTION

An ocular alpha-adrenergic agent that is relatively selective for alpha$_2$ receptor agonist. ***Therapeutic Effect:*** Reduces intraocular pressure.

PHARMACOKINETICS

Onset of action occurs within 1 hour. The duration of a single dose is about 12 hours. ***Half-life:*** 8 hrs.

AVAILABILITY

Ophthalmic solution: 0.5%, 1% (Iodipine).

INDICATIONS AND DOSAGES

▸ **Glaucoma**

OPHTHALMIC

Adults, Elderly. Instill 1 drop of 0.5% solution to affected eye(s) 3 times daily.

▸ **Intraocular Hypertension, Post Laser Surgery**

OPHTHALMIC

Adults, Elderly. Instill 1 drop of 1% solution in operative eye(s) 1 hour before surgery and 1 drop postoperatively.

OFF-LABEL USES

Postcycloplegic intraocular pressure spikes, intraocular pressure from post-cataract surgery.

CONTRAINDICATIONS

Hypersensitivity to apraclonidine or clonidine or any component of the formulation.

INTERACTIONS

Drug

MAOIs: May potentiate effects of MAOIs.

Herbal

None known.

Food

None known.

Drug interactions of concern to dentistry

- No drug interactions have been reported; this is a new drug and data are lacking
- Avoid using drugs that can exacerbate glaucoma: anticholinergic drugs

DIAGNOSTIC TEST EFFECTS

None known.

SIDE EFFECTS

Frequent

Eye discomfort, dry mouth.

Occasional

Headache, constipation, redness around eye, conjunctivitis, changes in visual acuity, mydriasis, ocular inflammation.

Rare

Nasal decongestion.

SERIOUS REACTIONS

! Allergic reaction occurs rarely.

! Peripheral edema and arrhythmias have been reported

DENTAL CONSIDERATIONS

General:

- Protect patient's eyes from accidental spatter during dental treatment.

• Avoid dental light in patient's eyes; offer dark glasses for patient comfort.
• Determine why the patient is taking the drug.
• Assess salivary flow as a factor in caries, periodontal disease, and candidiasis.

Consultations:

• Medical consultation may be required to assess disease control.

Teach Patient/Family:

• *When chronic dry mouth occurs, advise patient:*
  • To avoid mouth rinses with high alcohol content because of drying effects
  • Of need for daily home fluoride to prevent caries
  • To use sugarless gum, frequent sips of water, or saliva substitutes

aprepitant

ah-prep′-ih-tant
(Emend)

CATEGORY AND SCHEDULE

Pregnancy Risk Category: B

MECHANISM OF ACTION

A selective human substance P and neurokinin-1 (NK_1) receptor antagonist that inhibits chemotherapy-induced nausea and vomiting centrally in the chemoreceptor trigger zone.
Therapeutic Effect: Prevents the acute and delayed phases of chemotherapy-induced emesis, including vomiting caused by high-dose cisplatin.

PHARMACOKINETICS

Crosses the blood-brain barrier. Extensively metabolized in the liver. Eliminated primarily by liver metabolism (not excreted renally).
Half-life: 9–13 hr.

AVAILABILITY

Capsules: 80 mg, 125 mg.

INDICATIONS AND DOSAGES

▸ Prevention of Chemotherapy-Induced Nausea and Vomiting

PO

Adults, Elderly. 125 mg 1 hr before chemotherapy on day 1 and 80 mg once a day in the morning on days 2 and 3.

CONTRAINDICATIONS

Breast-feeding, concurrent use of pimozide (Orap)

INTERACTIONS

Drug

Alprazolam, docetaxel, etoposide, ifosfamide, imatinib, irinotecan, midazolam, paclitaxel, triazolam, vinblastine, vincristine, vinorelbine: May increase the plasma concentrations of these drugs.
Antifungals, clarithromycin, diltiazem, nefazodone, nelfinavir, ritonavir: Increase aprepitant plasma concentration.
Carbamazepine, phenytoin, rifampin: Decrease aprepitant plasma concentration.
Contraceptives: May decrease the effectiveness of contraceptives.
Paroxetine: May decrease the effectiveness of either drug.
Steroids: Increases the blood levels and effects of steroids.
Warfarin: May decrease the effectiveness of warfarin.

Herbal

None known.

Food

None known.

Drug interactions of concern to dentistry

• Increased plasma concentrations of midazolam and other benzodiazepines metabolized by CYP3A4

- Increased plasma levels: concurrent use of drugs that inhibit CYP3A4 enzymes (fluconazole, itraconazole, ketoconazole, erythromycin, and clarithromycin)
- Decreased plasma levels: concurrent use of drugs that induce CYP3A4 enzymes (carbamazepine)

DIAGNOSTIC TEST EFFECTS

May increase BUN level and serum creatinine, AST (SGOT), and ALT (SGPT) levels. May produce proteinuria.

SIDE EFFECTS

Frequent (17%–10%)
Fatigue, nausea, hiccups, diarrhea, constipation, anorexia
Occasional (8%–4%)
Headache, vomiting, dizziness, dehydration, heartburn
Rare (3% or less)
Abdominal pain, epigastric discomfort, gastritis, tinnitus, insomnia

SERIOUS REACTIONS

! Neutropenia and mucous membrane disorders occur rarely.

DENTAL CONSIDERATIONS

General:

- Patients using this drug are also undergoing or have recently undergone cancer chemotherapy; take a complete health history.
- Chemotherapy patients may show stomatitis and ulceration; palliative therapy may be required.
- Consider semisupine chair position for patient comfort if GI side effects occur.
- Examine for oral manifestation of opportunistic infection.
- Short appointments and a stress reduction protocol may be required for anxious patients.
- Patients taking opioids for acute or chronic pain should be given alternative analgesics for dental pain.
- Patients on chronic drug therapy may rarely have symptoms of blood dyscrasias, which can include infection, bleeding, and poor healing.
- Consult physician; prophylactic or therapeutic antibiotics may be indicated to prevent or treat infection if surgery or periodontal debridement is required for patients undergoing chemotherapy.

Consultations:

- Medical consultation may be required to assess immunologic status during cancer therapy and determine safety risks posed by dental treatment.
- Consultation with physician may be necessary if sedation or general anesthesia is required.
- Medical consultation may be required to assess disease control and patient's ability to tolerate stress.

Teach Patient/Family:

- Importance of good oral hygiene to prevent soft tissue inflammation
- To prevent trauma when using oral hygiene aids
- Importance of updating health and drug history if physician makes any changes in evaluation or drug regimens

argatroban

ar-gat′-tro-ban
(Acova)
Do not confuse argatroban with Aggrestat or Orgaran.

CATEGORY AND SCHEDULE

Pregnancy Risk Category: B

MECHANISM OF ACTION

A direct thrombin inhibitor that reversibly binds to thrombin-active sites.

Inhibits thrombin-catalyzed or thrombin-induced reactions, including fibrin formation, activation of coagulant factors V, VIII, and XIII; also inhibits protein C formation; and platelet aggregation. ***Therapeutic Effect:*** Produces anticoagulation.

PHARMACOKINETICS

Following IV administration, distributed primarily in extracellular fluid. Protein binding: 54%. Metabolized in the liver. Primarily excreted in the feces, presumably through biliary secretion. ***Half-life:*** 39–51 min.

AVAILABILITY

Injection: 100 mg/ml.

INDICATIONS AND DOSAGES

▸ To Prevent and Treat Heparin-Induced Thrombocytopenia

IV INFUSION

Adults, Elderly. Initially, 2 mcg/kg/min administered as a continuous infusion. After initial infusion, dose may be adjusted until steady state aPTT is 1.5–3 times initial baseline value, not to exceed 100 sec.

▸ Percutaneous Coronary Intervention

IV INFUSION

Adults, Elderly. Initially, 25 mcg/kg/min and administer bolus of 350 mcg/kg over 3–5 min. ACT (activated clotting time) checked in 5–10 min following bolus. If ACT is less than 300 sec, give additional bolus 150 mcg/kg, increase infusion to 30 mcg/kg/min. If ACT is greater than 450 sec, decrease infusion to 15 mcg/kg/min. Once ACT of 300–450 sec achieved, proceed with procedure.

▸ Dosage in Hepatic Impairment

Adults, Elderly. Initially, 0.5 mcg/kg/min.

OFF-LABEL USES

Cerebral thrombosis, MI

CONTRAINDICATIONS

Overt major bleeding

INTERACTIONS

Drug

Antiplatelet agents, thrombolytics, other anticoagulants: May increase the risk of bleeding.

Herbal

Arnica, astragalus, bilberry, black currant, cat's claw, chaparral, dandelion, evening primrose, feverfew, garlic, ginger, ginkgo biloba, hawthorn, kava, licorice, tan-shen, vitamin A: May increase the risk of bleeding.

Food

None known.

Drug interactions of concern to dentistry

- Increased risk of bleeding: drugs that interfere with coagulation or platelet function, such as NSAIDs and aspirin

DIAGNOSTIC TEST EFFECTS

Increases aPTT, International Normalized Ratio, and PT

IV INCOMPATIBILITIES

Do not mix with other medications or solutions.

SIDE EFFECTS

Frequent (8%–3%)

Dyspnea, hypotension, fever, diarrhea, nausea, pain, vomiting, infection, cough

SERIOUS REACTIONS

! Ventricular tachycardia and atrial fibrillation occur occasionally.

! Major bleeding and sepsis occur rarely.

DENTAL CONSIDERATIONS

General:

- Patients are at risk of bleeding, check for oral signs.
- Delay elective dental treatment until patient completes parenteral anticoagulant therapy.
- Determine why patient is taking the drug.
- Avoid products that affect platelet function, such as aspirin and NSAIDs.
- Consider local hemostasis measures to prevent excessive bleeding.

Consultations:

- Medical consultation should include partial prothrombin time, prothrombin time, or INR
- Medical consultation should include routine blood counts including platelet counts and bleeding time.

Teach Patient/Family:

- Use soft tooth brush to reduce risk of bleeding
- Importance of good oral hygiene to prevent soft tissue inflammation
- To report oral lesions, soreness, or bleeding to dentist
- To prevent trauma when using oral hygiene aids
- Importance of updating health and medication history if physician makes any changes in evaluation or drug regimens; include OTC, herbal, and nonherbal remedies in the update
- To inform dentist of unusual bleeding episodes following dental treatment

aripiprazole

ara-pip′-rah-zole
(Abilify)

CATEGORY AND SCHEDULE

Pregnancy Risk Category: C

MECHANISM OF ACTION

An antipsychotic agent that provides partial agonist activity at dopamine and serotonin (5-HT_{1A}) receptors and antagonist activity at serotonin (5-HT_{2A}) receptors. ***Therapeutic Effect:*** Diminishes schizophrenic behavior.

PHARMACOKINETICS

Well absorbed through the GI tract. Protein binding: 99% (primarily albumin). Reaches steady levels in 2 wks. Metabolized in the liver. Eliminated primarily in feces and, to a lesser extent, in urine. Not removed by hemodialysis. ***Half-life:*** 75 hr.

AVAILABILITY

Tablets: 5 mg, 10 mg, 15 mg, 20 mg, 30 mg.

INDICATIONS AND DOSAGES

▸ **Schizophrenia, Bipolar Disorder**

PO

Adults, Elderly. Initially, 10–15 mg once a day. May increase up to 30 mg/day.

OFF-LABEL USES

Schizoaffective disorder

CONTRAINDICATIONS

None known.

INTERACTIONS

Drug

Carbamazepine: May decrease the aripiprazole blood concentration.
Fluoxetine, ketoconazole, quinidine, paroxetine: May increase the aripiprazole blood concentration.

Herbal

None known.

Food

None known.

Drug interactions of concern to dentistry

- Possible lowering of blood levels: carbamazepine and other inducers of CYP3A4 isoenzymes

• Increased blood levels: ketoconazole and other inhibitors of CYP3A4 or CYP2D6 isoenzymes
• Caution with CNS depressants and alcohol

DIAGNOSTIC TEST EFFECTS
None known.

SIDE EFFECTS
Frequent (11%–5%)
Weight gain, headache, insomnia, vomiting
Occasional (4%–3%)
Light-headedness, nausea, akathisia, somnolence
Rare (2% or less)
Blurred vision, constipation, asthenia or loss of energy and strength, anxiety, fever, rash, cough, rhinitis, orthostatic hypotension

SERIOUS REACTIONS
! Extrapyramidal symptoms and neuroleptic malignant syndrome occur rarely.

DENTAL CONSIDERATIONS
General:
• Assess for presence of extrapyramidal motor symptoms, such as tardive dyskinesia and akathisia. Extrapyramidal motor activity may complicate dental treatment.
• Consider semisupine chair position for patient comfort if GI side effects occur.
Consultations:
• Consultation with physician may be necessary if sedation or general anesthesia is required.
• Medical consultation may be required to assess disease control and patient's ability to tolerate stress.
Teach Patient/Family:
• To consult physician if signs of tardive dyskinesia or akathisia are present
• Importance of good oral hygiene to prevent soft tissue inflammation
• Use of electric toothbrush if patient has difficulty holding conventional devices
• Importance of updating health and drug history if physician makes any changes in evaluation or drug regimens

articaine hydrochloride
ar-ti-kane
(Astracaine[CAN], Astracaine Forte[CAN], Septocaine)

CATEGORY AND SCHEDULE
Pregnancy Risk Category: C

MECHANISM OF ACTION
An amide anesthetic that inhibits conduction of nerve impulses.
Therapeutic Effect: Causes temporary loss of feeling and sensation.

PHARMACOKINETICS
Onset of action occurs within 1–6 min depending on route of administration. Complete anesthesia lasts approximately 1 hr. Well absorbed. Protein binding: 60%–80%. Rapidly metabolized by plasma carboxyesterase to its primary metabolite, articainic acid, which is inactive. Excreted in urine. ***Half-life:*** 20–120 min.

AVAILABILITY
Injection (Septocaine): 4% articaine hydrochloride 1:10,0000 epinephrine.

INDICATIONS AND DOSAGES
These recommended doses serve only as a guide to the amount of anesthetic required for most routine procedures. The actual volumes to be used depend on a number of factors, such as type and extent of surgical

procedure, depth of anesthesia, degree of muscular relaxation, and condition of the patient.
Local, infiltrative, or conductive anesthesia in both simple and complex dental or periodontal procedures

INFILTRATION

Adults, Elderly, Children Older than 4 yr. 0.5–2.5 ml of a 4% solution, which corresponds to 20–100 mg. Maximum dose administered should not exceed 7 mg/kg (0.175 ml/kg) or 3.2 mg/lb (0.0795 ml/lb) of body weight.

CONTRAINDICATIONS

History of hypersensitivity to local anesthetics of the amide type or sodium metabisulfite

INTERACTIONS

Drug

MAOIs, tricyclic antidepressants: May produce severe, prolonged hypertension.

Herbal

None known.

Food

None known.

Drug interactions of concern to dentistry

- CNS depressants: increased risk of CNS depression with all CNS depressants, especially in children and when larger doses are used
- Avoid placing dental cartridges in disinfectant solutions with heavy metals or surface-active agents; may see release of metal ions into local anesthetic solutions with tissue irritation following injection
- Risk of cardiovascular side effects; rapid intravascular administration of local anesthetic containing vasoconstrictor, either alone or in patients taking tricyclic antidepressants, monoamine oxidase inhibitors (MAOIs), digitalis drugs, cocaine, phenothiazines, β-blockers, and in presence of halogenated hydrocarbon general anesthetics; use smallest effective vasoconstrictor dose and careful aspiration technique
- Avoid use of vasoconstrictors in patients with uncontrolled hyperthyroidism, diabetes, angina, or hypertension; refer these patients for medical treatment before elective dental procedures

DIAGNOSTIC TEST EFFECTS

None known.

IV INCOMPATIBILITIES

None known.

SIDE EFFECTS

Rare

Drowsiness, dizziness, disorientation, light-headedness, tremors, blurred or double vision, nausea, sensation of heat, cold, numbness

SERIOUS REACTIONS

Tachycardia or bradycardia, BP changes, syncope, cardiac arrest, and seizures have been observed in some patients during dental procedures.

DENTAL CONSIDERATIONS

General:

- Monitor vital signs at every appointment because of cardiovascular side effects.
- Apply lubricant to dry lips for patient comfort before dental procedures.
- Use vasoconstrictor with caution, in low doses, and with careful aspiration.

Teach Patient/Family:

- To use care to prevent injury while numbness exists and to not chew gum or eat following dental anesthesia
- To report any signs of infection, muscle pain, or fever to dentist when feeling returns

• To report any unusual soft tissue reactions

ascorbic acid (vitamin C)

a-skor′-bic
(Apo-C[CAN], Cecon, Cenolate, Pro-C[AUS], Redoxon[CAN])

CATEGORY AND SCHEDULE

Pregnancy Risk Category: A (C if used in doses above recommended daily allowance)
OTC

MECHANISM OF ACTION

Assists in collagen formation and tissue repair and is involved in oxidation reduction reactions and other metabolic reactions. ***Therapeutic Effect:*** Involved in carbohydrate use and metabolism, as well as synthesis of carnitine, lipids, and proteins. Preserves blood vessel integrity.

PHARMACOKINETICS

Readily absorbed from the GI tract. Protein binding: 25%. Metabolized in the liver. Excreted in urine. Removed by hemodialysis.

AVAILABILITY

Capsules (Controlled-Release): 500 mg.
Liquid: 500 mg/5 ml.
Oral Solution: 500 mg/5 ml.
Tablets: 100 mg, 250 mg, 500 mg, 1 g.
Tablets (Chewable): 100 mg, 250 mg, 500 mg.
Tablets (Controlled-Release): 500 mg, 1 g, 1,500 mg.
Injection: 250 mg/ml, 500 mg/ml.

INDICATIONS AND DOSAGES

▸ Dietary Supplement
PO
Adults, Elderly. 50–200 mg/day.
Children. 35–100 mg/day.

▸ Acidification of Urine
PO
Adults, Elderly. 4–12 g/day in 3–4 divided doses.
Children. 500 mg q6–8h.

▸ Scurvy
PO
Adults, Elderly. 100–250 mg 1–2 times a day.
Children. 100–300 mg/day in divided doses.

▸ Prevention and Reduction of Severity of Colds
PO
Adults, Elderly. 1–3 g/day in divided doses.

OFF-LABEL USES

Prevention of common cold, control of idiopathic methemoglobinemia, urine acidifier

CONTRAINDICATIONS

None known.

INTERACTIONS

Drug
Deferoxamine: May increase iron toxicity.
Herbal
None known.
Food
None known.
Drug interactions of concern to dentistry
• Increased urinary excretion: salicylates, barbiturates

DIAGNOSTIC TEST EFFECTS

May decrease serum bilirubin level and urinary pH. May increase urine uric acid and urine oxalate levels.

IV INCOMPATIBILITIES

No information available for Y-site administration.

IV COMPATIBILITIES

Calcium gluconate, heparin

SIDE EFFECTS

Rare

Abdominal cramps, nausea, vomiting, diarrhea, increased urination with doses exceeding 1 g
Parenteral: Flushing, headache, dizziness, sleepiness or insomnia, soreness at injection site.

SERIOUS REACTIONS

! Ascorbic acid may acidify urine, leading to crystalluria.
! Large doses of IV ascorbic acid may lead to deep vein thrombosis.
! Abrupt discontinuation after prolonged use of large doses may produce rebound ascorbic acid deficiency.

DENTAL CONSIDERATIONS

General:

• An increased incidence of caries and soft tissue injury has been reported with excessive use of chewable ascorbic acid tablets.

aspirin/acetylsalicylic acid/ASA

as′-pir-in

(Ascriptin, Aspro[AUS], Bayer, Bex[AUS], Bufferin, Disprin[AUS], Ecotrin, Entrophen[CAN], Halfprin, Novasen[CAN], Solprin[AUS], Spren[AUS])

Do not confuse aspirin or Ascriptin with Aricept, Afrin, or Asendin, or Ecotrin with Edecrin.

CATEGORY AND SCHEDULE

Pregnancy Risk Category: C (D if full dose used in third trimester of pregnancy)
OTC

MECHANISM OF ACTION

A nonsteroidal salicylate that inhibits prostaglandin synthesis, acts on the hypothalamus heat-regulating center, and interferes with the production of thromboxane A, a substance that stimulates platelet aggregation. ***Therapeutic Effect:*** Reduces inflammatory response and intensity of pain; decreases fever; inhibits platelet aggregation.

PHARMACOKINETICS

Route	Onset	Peak	Duration
PO	1 hr	2–4 hr	24 hr

Rapidly and completely absorbed from GI tract; enteric-coated absorption delayed; rectal absorption delayed and incomplete. Protein binding: High. Widely distributed. Rapidly hydrolyzed to salicylate. ***Half-life:*** 15–20 min (aspirin); 2–3 hr (salicylate at low dose); more than 20 hr (salicylate at high dose).

AVAILABILITY

Tablets (Bayer): 325 mg, 500 mg.
Tablets (Chewable [Bayer and St. Joseph]): 81 mg.
Tablets (Enteric-Coated [Bayer, Ecotrin, St. Joseph]): 81 mg, 325 mg, 500 mg, 650 mg.
Tablets (Halfprin): 162 mg.
Caplets (Bayer): 81 mg, 325 mg, 500 mg.
Gelcaps (Bayer): 325 mg, 500 mg.
Suppositories: 60 mg, 120 mg, 125 mg, 200 mg, 325 mg, 600 mg, 650 mg.

INDICATIONS AND DOSAGES

▸ **Analgesia, Fever**

PO, Rectal

Adults, Elderly. 325–1,000 mg q4–6h
Children. 10–15 mg/kg/dose q4–6h. Maximum: 4 g/day.

▸ **Anti-Inflammatory**
PO
Adults, Elderly. Initially, 2.4–3.6 g/day in divided doses; then 3.6–5.4 g/day.
Children. Initially, 60–90 mg/kg/day in divided doses; then 80–100 mg/kg/day.
▸ **Suspected MI**
PO
Adults, Elderly. 162 mg as soon as the MI is suspected, then daily for 30 days after the MI.
▸ **Prevention of MI**
PO
Adults, Elderly. 75–325 mg/day.
▸ **Prevention of Stroke after Transient Ischemic Attack**
PO
Adults, Elderly. 50–325 mg/day.
▸ **Kawasaki Disease**
PO
Children. 80–100 mg/kg/day in divided doses.

OFF-LABEL USES
Prevention of thromboembolism, treatment of Kawasaki disease

CONTRAINDICATIONS
Allergy to tartrazine dye, bleeding disorders, chickenpox or flu in children and teenagers, GI bleeding or ulceration, hepatic impairment, history of hypersensitivity to aspirin or NSAIDs

INTERACTIONS
Drug
Alcohol, NSAIDs: May increase the risk of adverse GI effects, including ulceration.
Antacids, urinary alkalinizers: Increase the excretion of aspirin.
Anticoagulants, heparin, thrombolytics: Increase the risk of bleeding.
Insulin, oral antidiabetics: May increase the effects of these drugs (with large doses of aspirin).
Methotrexate, zidovudine: May increase the risk of toxicity of these drugs.
Ototoxic medications, vancomycin: May increase the risk of ototoxicity.
Platelet aggregation inhibitors, valproic acid: May increase the risk of bleeding.
Probenecid, sulfinpyrazone: May decrease the effects of these drugs.
Herbal
None known.
Food
None known.
Drug interactions of concern to dentistry
- Increased risk of GI complaints and occult blood loss: alcohol, NSAIDs, corticosteroids
- *Buffered aspirin:* Decreased absorption of tetracycline
- Recent report indicated ibuprofen may block clot-preventing effects of aspirin
- *Interactions when used as a dental drug:*
  - Increased risk of bleeding: oral anticoagulants, valproic acid, dipyridamole
  - Increased risk of hypoglycemia: sulfonylureas
  - Increased risk of toxicity: methotrexate, lithium, zidovudine
  - Decreased effects of probenecid, sulfinpyrazone
  - Avoid prolonged or concurrent use with NSAIDs, corticosteroids, acetaminophen
  - Suspected reduction in antihypertensives and vasodilator effects of angiotensin-converting enzyme (ACE) inhibitors; monitor blood pressure if used concurrently

DIAGNOSTIC TEST EFFECTS
May alter serum alkaline phosphatase, uric acid, AST (SGOT), and ALT (SGPT) levels. May prolong PT and bleeding time.

May decrease serum cholesterol, serum potassium, and T_3 and T_4 levels.

SIDE EFFECTS

Occasional

GI distress (including abdominal distention, cramping, heartburn, and mild nausea); allergic reaction (including bronchospasm, pruritus, and urticaria)

SERIOUS REACTIONS

! High doses of aspirin may produce GI bleeding and gastric mucosal lesions.
! Dehydrated, febrile children may experience aspirin toxicity quickly. Reye's syndrome may occur in children with the chickenpox or the flu.
! Low-grade toxicity is characterized by tinnitus, generalized pruritus (possibly severe), headache, dizziness, flushing, tachycardia, hyperventilation, diaphoresis, and thirst.
! Market toxicity is characterized by hyperthermia, restlessness, seizures, abnormal breathing patterns, respiratory failure, and coma.

DENTAL CONSIDERATIONS

General:

- Patients on chronic drug therapy may rarely have symptoms of blood dyscrasias, which can include infection, bleeding, and poor healing.
- Avoid prescribing buffered aspirin-containing products if patient is on a sodium-restricted diet.
- Chewable forms of aspirin should not be used for 7 days following oral surgery because of possible soft tissue injury.
- Evaluate allergic reactions: rash, urticaria; patients with allergy to salicylates may not be able to take NSAIDs; drug may need to be discontinued.

Consultations:

- In a patient with symptoms of blood dyscrasias, request a medical consultation for blood studies and postpone dental treatment until normal values are reestablished.
- Take precautions if dental surgery is anticipated because of risk of increased bleeding; avoid prescribing aspirin before dental surgery.
- Tinnitus, ringing, roaring in ears after high-dose and long-term therapy necessitates referral for salicylism.

Teach Patient/Family:

- That aspirin or buffered aspirin tablets should not be placed directly on a tooth or mucosal surface because of the risk of chemical burn
- To read label on other OTC drugs; may contain aspirin
- To avoid alcohol ingestion; GI bleeding may occur

atazanavir sulfate

ah-tah-zan′-ah-veer
(Reyataz)
Do not confuse Reyataz with Retavase.

CATEGORY AND SCHEDULE

Pregnancy Risk Category: B

MECHANISM OF ACTION

An antiviral that acts as an HIV-1 protease inhibitor, selectively preventing the processing of viral precursors found in cells infected with HIV-1. ***Therapeutic Effect:*** Prevents the formation of mature HIV cells.

PHARMACOKINETICS

Rapidly absorbed after PO administration. Protein binding: 86%. Extensively metabolized in the liver.

Excreted primarily in urine and, to a lesser extent, in feces. ***Half-life:*** 5–8 hr.

AVAILABILITY

Capsules: 100 mg, 150 mg, 200 mg.

INDICATIONS AND DOSAGES

▸ HIV-1 Infection

PO

Adults, Elderly (antiretroviral-naive). 400 mg (2 capsules) once a day with food.

Adults, Elderly (antiretroviral-experienced). 300 mg and ritonavir (Norvir) 100 mg once a day.

▸ HIV-1 Infection (concurrent therapy with efavirenz)

PO

Adults, Elderly. 300 mg atazanavir, 100 mg ritonavir, and 600 mg efavirenz as a single daily dose with food.

▸ HIV-1 Infection (concurrent therapy with didanosine)

PO

Adults, Elderly. Give atazanavir with food 2 hours before or 1 hour after didanosine.

▸ HIV-1 Infection (concurrent therapy with tenofovir)

PO

Adults, Elderly. 300 mg atazanavir and 100 mg ritonavir and 300 mg tenofovir given as a single daily dose with food.

▸ HIV-1 Infection in Patients with Mild to Moderate Hepatic Impairment

PO

Adults, Elderly. 300 mg once a day with food.

CONTRAINDICATIONS

Concurrent use with ergot derivatives, midazolam, pimozide, or triazolam; severe hepatic insufficiency

INTERACTIONS

Drug

Antacids, H2 receptor antagonists, proton pump inhibitors, rifampin: May decrease atazanavir plasma concentrations.

Atorvastatin, calcium channel blockers, immunosuppressants, irinotecan, lovastatin, sildenafil, simvastatin, tricyclic antidepressants: May increase atazanavir plasma concentrations.

Herbal

St. John's wort: May decrease atazanavir plasma concentration.

Food

High-fat meals: May decrease atazanavir absorption.

Drug interactions of concern to dentistry

- Avoid drugs metabolized by CYP3A4 isoenzymes; however, the package insert notes that significant drug interactions are not expected with azithromycin, erythromycin, itraconazole, or ketoconazole; use with caution and monitor

DIAGNOSTIC TEST EFFECTS

May increase serum amylase, bilirubin, lipase, AST (SGOT), and ALT (SGPT) levels. May decrease blood Hgb level and neutrophil and platelet counts. May alter LDL and serum triglyceride levels.

SIDE EFFECTS

Frequent (16%–14%)

Nausea, headache

Occasional (9%–4%)

Rash, vomiting, depression, diarrhea, abdominal pain, fever

Rare (3% or less)

Dizziness, insomnia, cough, fatigue, back pain

SERIOUS REACTIONS

! A severe hypersensitivity reaction (marked by angioedema and chest pain) and jaundice may occur.

DENTAL CONSIDERATIONS

General:

- Short appointments and a stress reduction protocol may be required for anxious patients.
- Use precaution if sedation or general anesthesia is required; risk of hypotensive episode.
- Consider semisupine chair position for patient comfort if GI side effects occur.
- Patient history should include all medications and herbal or nonherbal remedies taken by the patient.
- Assess salivary flow as a factor in caries, periodontal disease, and candidiasis.
- Examine for oral manifestation of opportunistic infection.
- Palliative medication may be required for management of oral side effects.
- Advise patient if dental drugs prescribed have a potential for photosensitivity.
- Precaution if dental surgery is anticipated and general anesthesia required.
- Patients on chronic drug therapy may rarely have symptoms of blood dyscrasias, which can include infection, bleeding, and poor healing.

Consultations:

- Consultation with physician may be necessary if sedation or general anesthesia is required.
- Medical consultation may be required to assess disease control and patient's ability to tolerate stress.

Teach Patient/Family:

- To be aware of oral side effects and potential sequelae
- Importance of updating health and drug history, reporting changes in health status, drug regimen changes, or disease/treatment status
- Importance of good oral hygiene to prevent soft tissue inflammation, infection
- To prevent trauma when using oral hygiene aids

atenolol

a-ten′-oh-lol
(Apo-Atenol[CAN], AteHexal[AUS], Noten[AUS], Tenolin[CAN], Tenormin, Tensig[AUS])

Do not confuse atenolol with albuterol or timolol.

CATEGORY AND SCHEDULE

Pregnancy Risk Category: D

MECHANISM OF ACTION

A $beta_1$-adrenergic blocker that acts as an antianginal, antiarrhythmic, and antihypertensive agent by blocking $beta_1$-adrenergic receptors in cardiac tissue. ***Therapeutic Effect:*** Slows sinus node heart rate, decreasing cardiac output and BP. Decreases myocardial oxygen demand.

PHARMACOKINETICS

Route	Onset	Peak	Duration
PO	1 hr	2–4 hr	24 hr

Incompletely absorbed from the GI tract. Protein binding: 6%–16%. Minimal liver metabolism. Primarily excreted unchanged in urine. Removed by hemodialysis. ***Half-life:*** 6–7 hr (increased in impaired renal function).

AVAILABILITY

Tablets: 25 mg, 50 mg, 100 mg.
Injection: 5 mg/10 ml.

INDICATIONS AND DOSAGES

▸ Hypertension

PO

Adults. Initially, 25–50 mg once a day. May increase dose up to 100 mg once a day.
Elderly. Usual initial dose, 25 mg a day.
Children. Initially, 0.8–1 mg/kg/dose given once a day. Range: 0.8–1.5 mg/kg/day. **Maxiumum:** 2 mg/kg/day or 100 mg/day.

▸ Angina Pectoris

PO

Adults. Initially, 50 mg once a day. May increase dose up to 200 mg once a day.
Elderly. Usual initial dose, 25 mg a day.

▸ Acute MI

IV

Adults. Give 5 mg over 5 min; may repeat in 10 min. In those who tolerate full 10-mg IV dose, begin 50-mg tablets 10 min after last IV dose followed by another 50-mg oral dose 12 hr later. Thereafter, give 100 mg once a day or 50 mg twice a day for 6–9 days. Or, for those who do not tolerate full IV dose, give 50 mg orally twice a day or 100 mg once a day for at least 7 days.

▸ Dosage in Renal Impairment

Dosage interval is modified on the basis of creatinine clearance.

Creatinine Clearance	Dosage interval
15–35 ml/min	50 mg a day
less than 15 ml/min	50 mg every other day

OFF-LABEL USES

Improved survival in diabetics with heart disease; treatment of hypertrophic cardiomyopathy, pheochromocytoma, and syndrome of mitral valve prolapse; prevention of migraine, thyrotoxicosis, tremors

CONTRAINDICATIONS

Cardiogenic shock, overt heart failure, second- or third-degree heart block, severe bradycardia

INTERACTIONS

Drug

Cimetidine: May increase atenolol blood concentration.
Diuretics, other antihypertensives: May increase hypotensive effect of atenolol.
Insulin, oral hypoglycemics: May mask symptoms of hypoglycemia and prolong hypoglycemic effect of insulin and oral hypoglycemics.
NSAIDs: May decrease antihypertensive effect of atenolol.
Sympathomimetics, xanthines: May mutually inhibit effects.

Herbal

None known.

Food

None known.

Drug interactions of concern to dentistry

- Decreased antihypertensive effects: NSAIDs, indomethacin, salicylates
- May slow metabolism of lidocaine
- Decreased β-blocking effects (or decreased β-adrenergic effects) of epinephrine, levonordefrin, isoproterenol, and other sympathomimetics
- Reduced bioavailability suspected with ampicillin

DIAGNOSTIC TEST EFFECTS

May increase serum antinuclear antibody titer and BUN, serum creatinine, potassium, lipoprotein, triglyceride, and uric acid levels.

IV INCOMPATIBILITIES

Amphotericin complex (Abelcet, AmBisome, Amphotec)

SIDE EFFECTS

Atenolol is generally well tolerated, with mild and transient side effects.

Frequent

Hypotension manifested as cold extremities, constipation or diarrhea, diaphoresis, dizziness, fatigue, headache, and nausea

Occasional

Insomnia, flatulence, urinary frequency, impotence or decreased libido, depression

Rare

Rash, arthralgia, myalgia, confusion (especially in the elderly), altered taste

SERIOUS REACTIONS

! Overdose may produce profound bradycardia and hypotension.

! Abrupt atenolol withdrawal may result in diaphoresis, palpitations, headache, and tremors.

! Atenolol administration may precipitate CHF or MI in patients with cardiac disease; thyroid storm in those with thyrotoxicosis; and peripheral ischemia in those with existing peripheral vascular disease.

! Hypoglycemia may occur in patients with previously controlled diabetes.

! Thrombocytopenia, manifested as unusual bruising or bleeding, occurs rarely.

DENTAL CONSIDERATIONS

General:

- Monitor vital signs at every appointment because of cardiovascular and respiratory side effects.
- After supine positioning, have patient sit upright for at least 2 min before standing to avoid orthostatic hypotension.
- Patients on chronic drug therapy may rarely have symptoms of blood dyscrasias, which can include infection, bleeding, and poor healing.
- Assess salivary flow as a factor in caries, periodontal disease, and candidiasis.
- Stress from dental procedures may compromise cardiovascular function; determine patient risk.
- Short appointments and a stress reduction protocol may be required for anxious patients.
- Use vasoconstrictors with caution, in low doses, and with careful aspiration. Avoid use of gingival retraction cord with epinephrine.

Consultations:

- In a patient with symptoms of blood dyscrasias, request a medical consultation for blood studies and postpone dental treatment until normal values are reestablished.
- Medical consultation may be required to assess disease control and stress tolerance of patient.
- Use precautions if general anesthesia is required for dental surgery.

Teach Patient/Family:

- Importance of good oral hygiene to prevent soft tissue inflammation
- Caution to prevent injury when using oral hygiene aids
- *When chronic dry mouth occurs, advise patient:*
  - To avoid mouth rinses with high alcohol content because of drying effects
  - To use daily home fluoride products for anticaries effect
  - To use sugarless gum, frequent sips of water, or saliva substitutes

atomoxetine

auto-mox′-eh-teen

(Strattera)

CATEGORY AND SCHEDULE

Pregnancy Risk Category: C

MECHANISM OF ACTION

A norepinephrine reuptake inhibitor that enhances noradrenergic function by selective inhibition of the presynaptic norepinephrine transporter. ***Therapeutic Effect:*** Improves symptoms of attention-deficit hyperactivity disorder (ADHD).

PHARMACOKINETICS

Rapidly absorbed after PO administration. Protein binding: 98% (primarily to albumin). Eliminated primarily in urine and, to a lesser extent, in feces. Not removed by hemodialysis. ***Half-life:*** 4–5 hr in general population, 22 hr in 7% of Caucasians and 2% of African-Americans; (increased in moderate to severe hepatic insufficiency).

AVAILABILITY

Capsules: 10 mg, 18 mg, 25 mg, 40 mg, 60 mg.

INDICATIONS AND DOSAGES

▸ ADHD

PO

Adults, Children weighing 70 kg and more. 40 mg once a day. May increase after at least 3 days to 80 mg as a single daily dose or in divided doses. Maximum: 100 mg.

Children weighing less than 70 kg. Initially, 0.5 mg/kg/day. May increase after at least 3 days to 1.2 mg/kg/day. Maximum: 1.4 mg/kg/day or 100 mg.

▸ Dosage in Hepatic Impairment

Expect to administer 50% of normal atomoxetine dosage to patients with moderate hepatic impairment and 25% of normal dosage to those with severe hepatic impairment.

OFF-LABEL USES

Treatment of depression.

CONTRAINDICATIONS

Angle-closure glaucoma, use within 14 days of MAOIs

INTERACTIONS

Drug

Fluoxetine, paroxetine, quinidine: May increase atomoxetine blood concentration.

MAOIs: May increase the risk of toxic effects.

Herbal

None known.

Food

None known.

Drug interactions of concern to dentistry

- No dental drug interactions reported; however, drugs that inhibit CYP2D6 enzymes (paroxetine, fluoxetine) can increase plasma levels
- Albuterol and other β_2-agonists should be used with caution because of potential effects on the cardiovascular system

DIAGNOSTIC TEST EFFECTS

None known.

SIDE EFFECTS

Frequent

Headache, dyspepsia, nausea, vomiting, fatigue, decreased appetite, dizziness, altered mood

Occasional

Tachycardia, hypertension, weight loss, delayed growth in children, irritability

Rare

Insomnia, sexual dysfunction in adults, fever

SERIOUS REACTIONS

! Urine retention or urinary hesitance may occur.

! In overdose, gastric emptying and repeated use of activated charcoal may prevent systemic absorption.

DENTAL CONSIDERATIONS

General:

- Assess salivary flow as a factor in caries, periodontal disease, and candidiasis.
- Monitor vital signs at every appointment because of cardiovascular side effects.
- Consider semisupine chair position for patient comfort if GI side effects occur.
- Use vasoconstrictor with caution, in low doses, and with careful aspiration.

Consultations:

- Medical consultation may be required to assess disease control and patient's ability to tolerate stress.

Teach Patient/Family:

- Importance of good oral hygiene to prevent soft tissue inflammation, infection
- *When chronic dry mouth occurs, advise patient:*
  - To avoid mouth rinses with high alcohol content because of drying effects
  - To use daily home fluoride products for anticaries effect
  - To use sugarless gum, frequent sips of water, or saliva substitutes

atorvastatin

ah-tore-vah′-stah-tin
(Lipitor)
Do not confuse Lipitor with Levatol.

CATEGORY AND SCHEDULE

Pregnancy Risk Category: X

MECHANISM OF ACTION

An antihyperlipidemic that inhibits HMG-CoA reductase, the enzyme that catalyzes the early step in cholesterol synthesis. ***Therapeutic Effect:*** Decreases LDL and VLDL cholesterol, and plasma triglyceride levels; increases HDL cholesterol concentration.

PHARMACOKINETICS

Poorly absorbed from the GI tract. Protein binding: greater than 98%. Metabolized in the liver. Minimally eliminated in urine. Plasma levels are markedly increased in chronic alcoholic hepatic disease but are unaffected by renal disease.
Half-life: 14 hr.

AVAILABILITY

Tablets: 10 mg, 20 mg, 40 mg, 80 mg.

INDICATIONS AND DOSAGES

▸ Hyperlipidemia, Reduction of Risk of MI, Angina Revascularization Procedures

PO

Adults, Elderly. Initially, 10–40 mg a day given as a single dose. Dose range: Increase at 2- to 4-wk intervals to maximum of 80 mg/day.
Children 10–17 yr. Initially, 10 mg/day, may increase to 20 mg/day.

▸ Familial Hypercholesterolemia

PO

Children 10–17 yr. Initially, 10 mg/day. May increase to 20 mg/day.

CONTRAINDICATIONS

Active hepatic disease, lactation, pregnancy, unexplained elevated hepatic function test results

INTERACTIONS

Drug

Antacids, colestipol, propranolol: Decreases atorvastatin activity.
Cyclosporine, erythromycin, gemfibrozil, nicotinic acid: Increases the risk of acute renal failure and rhabdomyolysis with these drugs.

Digoxin, itraconazole, oral contraceptives, warfarin: May increase atorvastatin blood concentration, producing severe muscle inflammation, pain, and weakness.

Herbal

None known.

Food

None known.

Drug interactions of concern to dentistry

- Severe myopathy or rhabdomyolysis: erythromycin, niacin, itraconazole, ketoconazole
- Increase in plasma levels: erythromycin, itraconazole, alcohol, ketoconazole
- Suspected increase in midazolam effects when used in general anesthesia (*Anesthesia* 58:899–904, 2003)

DIAGNOSTIC TEST EFFECTS

May increase serum CK and transaminase concentrations.

SIDE EFFECTS

Atorvastatin is generally well tolerated. Side effects are usually mild and transient.

Frequent (16%)

Headache

Occasional (5%–2%)

Myalgia, rash or pruritus, allergy

Rare (2%–1%)

Flatulence, dyspepsia

SERIOUS REACTIONS

! Cataracts may develop, and photosensitivity may occur.

DENTAL CONSIDERATIONS

General:

- Consider semisupine chair position for patient comfort if GI side effects occur.

atropine sulfate

a′-troe-peen

(Atropine Sulfate, Atropt[AUS])

Do not confuse atropine sulfate with Akarpine or Aplisol.

CATEGORY AND SCHEDULE

Pregnancy Risk Category: C

MECHANISM OF ACTION

An acetylcholine antagonist that inhibits the action of acetylcholine by competing with acetylcholine for common binding sites on muscarinic receptors, which are located on exocrine glands, cardiac and smooth-muscle ganglia, and intramural neurons. This action blocks all muscarinic effects. ***Therapeutic Effect:*** Decreases GI motility and secretory activity, and GU muscle tone (ureter, bladder); produces ophthalmic cycloplegia, and mydriasis.

AVAILABILITY

Injection: 0.05 mg/ml, 0.1 mg/ml, 0.4 mg/0.5 ml, 0.4 mg/ml, 0.5 mg/ml, 1 mg/ml.

INDICATIONS AND DOSAGES

▸ **Asystole, Slow, Pulseless Electrical Activity**

IV

Adults, Elderly. 1 mg; may repeat q3–5min up to total dose of 0.04 mg/kg.

▸ **Pre-Anesthetic**

IV/IM/SUBCUTANEOUS

Adults, Elderly. 0.4–0.6 mg 30–60 min pre-op.

Children weighing 5 kg and more. 0.01–0.02 mg/kg/dose to maximum of 0.4 mg/dose.

Children weighing less than 5 kg. 0.02 mg/kg/dose 30–60 min pre-op.

A

▸ **Bradycardia**

IV

Adults, Elderly. 0.5–1 mg q5min not to exceed 2 mg or 0.04 mg/kg.
Children. 0.02 mg/kg with a minimum of 0.1 mg to a maximum of 0.5 mg in children and 1 mg in adolescents. May repeat in 5 min. Maximum total dose: 1 mg in children, 2 mg in adolescents.

CONTRAINDICATIONS

Bladder neck obstruction due to prostatic hypertrophy, cardiospasm, intestinal atony, myasthenia gravis in those not treated with neostigmine, narrow-angle glaucoma, obstructive disease of the GI tract, paralytic ileus, severe ulcerative colitis, tachycardia secondary to cardiac insufficiency or thyrotoxicosis, toxic megacolon, unstable cardiovascular status in acute hemorrhage

INTERACTIONS

Drug

Antacids, antidiarrheals: May decrease absorption of atropine.
Anticholinergics: May increase effects of atropine.
Ketoconazole: May decrease absorption of ketoconazole.
Potassium chloride: May increase severity of GI lesions (wax matrix).

Herbal

None known.

Food

None known.

Drug interactions of concern to dentistry

- Increased anticholinergic effects: tricyclic antidepressants, antihistamines, opioid analgesics, antipsychotic medications, or other drugs with anticholinergic activity
- Decreased absorption of ketoconazole

DIAGNOSTIC TEST EFFECTS

None known.

IV INCOMPATIBILITIES

Pentothal (Thiopental)

IV COMPATIBILITIES

Diphenhydramine (Benadryl), droperidol (Inapsine), fentanyl (Sublimaze), glycopyrrolate (Robinul), heparin, hydromorphone (Dilaudid), midazolam (Versed), morphine, potassium chloride, propofol (Diprivan)

SIDE EFFECTS

Frequent

Dry mouth, nose, and throat that may be severe; decreased sweating, constipation, irritation at subcutaneous or IM injection site

Occasional

Swallowing difficulty, blurred vision, bloated feeling, impotence, urinary hesitancy

Rare

Allergic reaction, including rash and urticaria; mental confusion or excitement, particularly in children, fatigue

SERIOUS REACTIONS

! Overdosage may produce tachycardia, palpitations, hot, dry or flushed skin, absence of bowel sounds, increased respiratory rate, nausea, vomiting, confusion, somnolence, slurred speech, dizziness, and CNS stimulation.

! Overdosage may also produce psychosis as evidenced by agitation, restlessness, rambling speech, visual hallucinations, paranoid behavior, and delusions, followed by depression.

DENTAL CONSIDERATIONS

General:

- Give PO dose 30–60 min before drying effects are required for dental procedures.

• Request that patient remove contact lenses before using drug because of possible drying effects in the eyes.
• Caution patients that they may feel a dry, burning sensation in the throat and experience blurred vision.
• This drug is intended for acute use, usually in single doses only; therefore chronic dry mouth should not be a concern.
• Avoid dental light in patient's eyes; offer dark glasses for patient comfort.

Consultations:

• Medical consultation is advisable before using this drug in patients with a history of GI disease, cardiac disease, or glaucoma.

ATROPIN SULFATE (OPTIC)

DENTAL CONSIDERATIONS

General:

• Avoid dental light in patient's eyes; offer dark glasses for patient comfort.

aurothioglucose/gold sodium thiomalate

(Gold-50[AUS], Solganal); (Myochrysine, Myocrisin[AUS])

CATEGORY AND SCHEDULE

Pregnancy Risk Category: C

MECHANISM OF ACTION

Aurothioglucose: A gold compound that alters cellular mechanisms, collagen biosynthesis, enzyme systems, and immune responses. ***Therapeutic Effect:*** Suppresses synovitis of the active stage of rheumatoid arthritis.
Gold sodium thiomalate: A gold compound whose mechanism of action is unknown. May decrease prostaglandin synthesis or alter cellular mechanisms by inhibiting sulfhydryl systems. ***Therapeutic Effect:*** Decreases synovial inflammation, retards cartilage and bone destruction, suppresses or prevents but does not cure, arthritis, synovitis.

PHARMACOKINETICS

Aurothioglucose (50% gold): Slow, erratic absorption after IM administration. Protein binding: 95%–99%. Primarily excreted in urine. ***Half-life:*** 3–27 days (half-life increased with increased number of doses).
Gold sodium thiomalate: Well absorbed. Protein binding: 95%. Widely distributed. Metabolized in liver. Excreted in urine and feces. Not removed by hemodialysis. ***Half-life:*** 5 days.

AVAILABILITY

Aurothioglucose
Injection: 50 mg/ml suspension (Solganal).
Gold sodium thiomalate
Injection: 50 mg/ml (Myochrysine)

INDICATIONS AND DOSAGES

▸ Rheumatoid Arthritis (Aurothioglucose)

IM
Adults, Elderly. Initially, 10 mg, then 25 mg for 2 doses, then 50 mg weekly thereafter until total dose of 0.8–1 g given. If patient is improved and there are no signs of toxicity, may give 50 mg at 3- to 4-wk intervals for many months.
Children. 0.25 mg/kg, may increase by 0.25 mg/kg each week. Maintenance: 0.75–1 mg/kg/dose. Maximum: 25-mg dose for total of 20 doses, then q2–4wks.

▸ Rheumatoid Arthritis (Gold sodium thiomalate)

IM
Adults, Elderly. Initially, 10 mg, then 25 mg for second dose.

Follow with 25–50 mg/wk until improvement noted or total of 1 g administered. Maintenance: 25–50 mg q2wks for 2–20 wks; if stable, may increase to q3–4wk intervals.
Children. Initially, 10 mg, then 1 mg/kg/wk. Maximum single dose: 50 mg. Maintenance: 1 mg/kg/dose at 2- to 4-wk intervals.

▸ Dosage in Renal Impairment

Creatinine Clearance	Dosage
50–80 ml/min	50% of usual dosage
less than 50 ml/min	not recommended

OFF-LABEL USES

Treatment of pemphigus, psoriatic arthritis

CONTRAINDICATIONS

Aurothioglucose
Bone marrow aplasia, history of gold-induced pathologies, including blood dyscrasias, exfoliative dermatitis, necrotizing enterocolitis, and pulmonary fibrosis, serious adverse effects with previous gold therapy, severe blood dyscrasias
Gold sodium thiomalate
Colitis, concurrent use of antimalarials, immunosuppressive agents, penicillamine, or phenylbutazone, congestive heart failure (CHF), exfoliative dermatitis, history of blood dyscrasias, severe liver or renal impairment, systemic lupus erythematosus

INTERACTIONS

Drug

Bone marrow depressants; hepatotoxic, nephrotoxic medications: May increase risk of aurothioglucose toxicity.
Penicillamine: May increase risk of hematologic or renal adverse effects of aurothioglucose.

Herbal

None known.

Food

None known.

Drug interactions of concern to dentistry

- None reported

DIAGNOSTIC TEST EFFECTS

May decrease Hgb, Hct, platelets, white blood cell (WBC) count. May alter liver function tests. May increase urine protein.

SIDE EFFECTS

Frequent

Aurothioglucose: Rash, stomatitis, diarrhea
Gold sodium thiomalate: Pruritic dermatitis, stomatitis, marked by erythema, redness, shallow ulcers of oral mucous membranes, sore throat, and difficulty swallowing, diarrhea or loose stools, abdominal pain, nausea

Occasional

Aurothioglucose: Nausea, vomiting, anorexia, abdominal cramps
Gold sodium thiomalate: Vomiting, anorexia, flatulence, dyspepsia, conjunctivitis, photosensitivity

Rare

Gold sodium thiomalate: Constipation, urticaria, rash

SERIOUS REACTIONS

! Gold toxicity is the primary serious reaction. Signs and symptoms of gold toxicity include decreased hemoglobin, leukopenia (WBC count less than 4,000/mm^3), reduced granulocyte counts ($< 150{,}000/mm^3$), proteinuria, hematuria, stomatitis (sores, ulcers and white spots in the mouth and throat), blood dyscrasias (anemia, leukopenia, thrombocytopenia and eosinophilia), glomerulonephritis, nephritic syndrome, and cholestatic jaundice.

DENTAL CONSIDERATIONS

General:

- Patients on chronic drug therapy may rarely have symptoms of blood dyscrasias, which can include infection, bleeding, and poor healing.
- Palliative medication may be required for management of oral side effects.
- Consider semisupine chair position for patient comfort because of arthritic disease.

Consultations:

- Medical consultation may be required to assess disease control and patient's ability to tolerate stress.
- In a patient with symptoms of blood dyscrasias, request a medical consultation for blood studies and postpone dental treatment until normal values are reestablished.

Teach Patient/Family:

- Importance of good oral hygiene to prevent soft tissue inflammation
- To be aware of the possibility of secondary oral infection and the need to see dentist immediately if infection occurs
- To report oral lesions, soreness, or bleeding to dentist
- To avoid mouth rinses with high alcohol content because of drying effects

azatadine maleate

a-za′-ta-deen mal′-ee-ate
(Optimine)

Do not confuse with azelastine or azacitidine.

CATEGORY AND SCHEDULE

Pregnancy Risk Category: B

MECHANISM OF ACTION

A piperazine-derivative antihistamine that has both anticholinergic and antiserotonin activity. Inhibits mediator release from mast cells and prevents calcium entry into mast cells through voltage-dependent calcium channels.
Therapeutic Effect: Relieves allergic conditions, including urticaria and pruritus. Anticholinergic effects cause drying of nasal mucosa.

PHARMACOKINETICS

Rapidly and extensively absorbed from the gastrointestinal (GI) tract. Protein binding: minimal. Metabolized in liver. Excreted in urine. ***Half-life:*** 8.7 hrs

AVAILABILITY

Tablets: 1 mg (Optimine).

INDICATIONS AND DOSAGES

▸ Allergic Rhinitis

PO

Adults, Elderly, Children 12 yrs or older. 1–2 mg 2 times a day.

CONTRAINDICATIONS

History of hypersensitivity to azatadine, antihistamines, or any other component of the formulation or to other related antihistamines including cyproheptadine, concomitant use of MAO inhibitors

INTERACTIONS

Drug

Alcohol, central nervous system (CNS) depressants, tricylic antidepressants, procarbazine: May increase CNS depression.

Herbal

None known.

Food

None known.

Drug interactions of concern to dentistry

- Increased CNS depression: all CNS depressants, alcohol
- Increased anticholinergic effect: anticholinergics

DIAGNOSTIC TEST EFFECTS
None known.

SIDE EFFECTS
Frequent
Slight to moderate drowsiness, thickening of bronchial secretions.
Rare
Headache, fatigue, nervousness, dizziness, appetite increase, weight gain, nausea, diarrhea, abdominal pain, dry mouth, arthralgia, pharyngitis.

SERIOUS REACTIONS
! Hepatitis, bronchospasm, and epistaxis have been reported.

DENTAL CONSIDERATIONS
General:
- Assess salivary flow as a factor in caries, periodontal disease, and candidiasis.
- Patients on chronic drug therapy may rarely have symptoms of blood dyscrasias, which can include infection, bleeding, and poor healing.
- Consider semisupine chair position for patient comfort because of respiratory disease.
- Monitor vital signs at every appointment because of cardiovascular side effects.

Consultations:
- In a patient with symptoms of blood dyscrasia, request a medical consultation for blood studies and postpone dental treatment until normal values are reestablished.

Teach Patient/Family:
- Importance of good oral hygiene to prevent soft tissue inflammation
- Caution to prevent injury when using oral hygiene aids
- *When chronic dry mouth occurs, advise patient:*
- To avoid mouth rinses with high alcohol content because of drying effects
- To use daily home fluoride products for anticaries effect
- To use sugarless gum, frequent sips of water, or saliva substitutes

azathioprine
ay-za-thye′-oh-preen
(Alti-Azathioprine[CAN], Azasan, Imuran, Thioprine[AUS])
Do not confuse azathioprine with Azulfidine or azatadine, or Imuran with Elmiron or Imferon.

CATEGORY AND SCHEDULE
Pregnancy Risk Category: D

MECHANISM OF ACTION
An immunologic agent that antagonizes purine metabolism and inhibits DNA, protein, and RNA synthesis. ***Therapeutic Effect:*** Suppresses cell-mediated hypersensitivities; alters antibody production and immune response in transplant recipients; reduces the severity of arthritis symptoms.

AVAILABILITY
Tablets (Azasan): 25 mg, 50 mg, 75 mg, 100 mg.
Tablets (Imuran): 50 mg.
Injection: 100-mg vial.

INDICATIONS AND DOSAGES
▸ Adjunct in Prevention of Renal Allograft Rejection
PO, IV
Adults, Elderly, Children.
2–5 mg/kg/day on day of transplant, then 1–3 mg/kg/day as maintenance dose.

▸ **Rheumatoid Arthritis**

PO

Adults. Initially, 1 mg/kg/day as a single dose or in 2 divided doses. May increase by 0.5 mg/kg/day after 6–8 wk at 4-wk intervals up to maximum of 2.5 mg/kg/day. Maintenance: Lowest effective dosage. May decrease dose by 0.5 mg/kg or 25 mg/day q4wk (while other therapies, such as rest, physiotherapy, and salicylates, are maintained).

Elderly. Initially, 1 mg/kg/day (50–100 mg); may increase by 25 mg/day until response or toxicity.

▸ **Dosage in Renal Impairment**

Dosage is modified on the basis of creatinine clearance.

Creatinine Clearance	Dose
10–50 ml/min	75% of usual dose
less than 10 ml/min	50% of usual dose

OFF-LABEL USES

Treatment of biliary cirrhosis, chronic active hepatitis, glomerulonephritis, inflammatory bowel disease, inflammatory myopathy, multiple sclerosis, myasthenia gravis, nephrotic syndrome, pemphigoid, pemphigus, polymyositis, systemic lupus erythematosus

CONTRAINDICATIONS

Pregnant patients with rheumatoid arthritis

INTERACTIONS

Drug

Allopurinol: May increase activity and risk of toxicity of azathioprine.

Bone marrow depressants: May increase myelosuppression.

Live-virus vaccines: May potentiate virus replication, increase the vaccine's side effects, and decrease the patient's antibody response to the vaccine.

Other immunosuppressants: May increase the risk of infection or neoplasms.

Herbal

None known.

Food

None known.

Drug interactions of concern to dentistry

• Increased blood dyscrasias: NSAIDs, especially phenylbutazone, dapsone, phenothiazines

• Increased immunosuppression, risk of infection: corticosteroids

DIAGNOSTIC TEST EFFECTS

May decrease serum albumin, Hgb, and serum uric acid levels. May increase serum alkaline phosphatase, amylase, bilirubin, AST(SGOT), and ALT(SGPT) levels.

IV INCOMPATIBILITIES

Methyl and propyl parabens, phenol

SIDE EFFECTS

Frequent

Nausea, vomiting, anorexia (particularly during early treatment and with large doses)

Occasional

Rash

Rare

Severe nausea and vomiting with diarrhea, abdominal pain, hypersensitivity reaction

SERIOUS REACTIONS

! Azathioprine use increases the risk of developing neoplasia (new abnormal-growth tumors).

! Significant leukopenia and thrombocytopenia may occur, particularly in those undergoing kidney transplant rejection.

! Hepatotoxicity occurs rarely.

DENTAL CONSIDERATIONS

General:

• Patients on chronic drug therapy may rarely have symptoms of blood dyscrasias, which can include infection, bleeding, and poor healing.
• To prevent infection if surgery or deep scaling is planned, prophylactic antibiotics may be indicated in patients who develop neutropenia.
• Determine why the patient is taking the drug.
• Alert the patient to the possibility of secondary oral infection; must see dentist immediately if infection occurs.

Consultations:

• In a patient with symptoms of blood dyscrasias, request a medical consultation for blood studies and postpone dental treatment until normal values are reestablished.
• Medical consultation may be required to assess disease control and patient's ability to tolerate stress.

Teach Patient/Family:

• Importance of good oral hygiene to prevent soft tissue inflammation
• Caution to prevent injury when using oral hygiene aids
• To avoid mouth rinses with high alcohol content because of drying effects and irritation of mucous membranes

azelaic acid

aye-zeh-**lay**-ick
(Azelex, Finacea, Finevin)

CATEGORY AND SCHEDULE

Pregnancy Risk Category: B

MECHANISM OF ACTION

The exact mechanism of action of azelaic acid is not known. Possesses antimicrobial activity against *Propionibacterium acnes* and *Staphylococcus epidermidis*.
Therapeutic Effect: Inhibits microbial cellular protein synthesis.

PHARMACOKINETICS

Minimal absorption after topical administration. Metabolized in liver. Excreted in urine as unchanged drug. ***Half-life:*** 12 hr.

AVAILABILITY

Cream (Azelex, Finevin): 20%.
Gel (Finacea): 15%.

INDICATIONS AND DOSAGES

▸ Mild to Moderate Acne

TOPICAL

Adults, Adolescents. Apply cream or gel to affected area twice daily (morning and evening).

UNLABELED USES

Melasma

CONTRAINDICATIONS

Hypersensitivity to azelaic acid or any component of the formulation

INTERACTIONS

Drug

None known.

Herbal

None known.

Food

None known.

Drug interactions of concern to dentistry

• None reported

DIAGNOSTIC TEST EFFECTS

None known.

SIDE EFFECTS

Occasional

Pruritus, stinging, burning, tingling, erythema, dryness, rash, peeling, irritation, contact dermatitis

Rare
Worsening of asthma, vitiligo depigmentation, small depigmented spots, hypertrichosis, reddening (signs of keratosis pilaris), exacerbation of recurrent cold sore, fever blister, or oral herpes simplex

SERIOUS EFFECTS
None reported.

DENTAL CONSIDERATIONS
General:
• Topical use rarely causes exacerbation of recurrent herpes labialis.
• Keep away from mouth and other mucous membranes; wash eyes if cream comes in contact; irritation can occur.

azelastine
a′-zel-ah-steen
(Astelin, Optivar)
Do not confuse Optivar with Optiray.

CATEGORY AND SCHEDULE
Pregnancy Risk Category: C

MECHANISM OF ACTION
An antihistamine that competes with histamine for histamine receptor sites on cells in the blood vessels, GI tract, and respiratory tract.
Therapeutic Effect: Relieves symptoms associated with seasonal allergic rhinitis such as increased mucus production and sneezing and symptoms associated with allergic conjunctivitis, such as redness, itching, and excessive tearing.

PHARMACOKINETICS
Route	Onset	Peak	Duration
Nasal spray	0.5–1 hr	2–3 hr	12 hr
Ophthalmic	N/A	3 min	8 hr

Well absorbed through nasal mucosa. Primarily excreted in feces. ***Half-life:*** 22 hr.

AVAILABILITY
Nasal Spray (Astelin): 137 mcg.
Ophthalmic Solution (Optivar): 0.05%.

INDICATIONS AND DOSAGES
▸ **Allergic Rhinitis**
NASAL
Adults, Elderly, Children 12 yr and older. 2 sprays in each nostril twice a day.
Children 5–11 yr. 1 spray in each nostril twice a day.
▸ **Allergic Conjunctivitis**
OPHTHALMIC
Adults, Elderly, Children 3 yr or older. 1 drop into affected eye twice a day.

CONTRAINDICATIONS
Breast-feeding women, history of hypersensitivity to antihistamines, neonates or premature infants, third trimester of pregnancy

INTERACTIONS
Drug
Alcohol, other CNS depressants: May increase CNS depression.
Cimetidine: May increase azelastine blood concentration.
Herbal
None known.
Food
None known.
Drug interactions of concern to dentistry
• None reported

DIAGNOSTIC TEST EFFECTS
May increase ALT(SGPT) levels.
May suppress flare and wheal reactions to antigen skin testing unless drug is discontinued 4 days before testing.

SIDE EFFECTS
Frequent (20%–15%)
Headache, bitter taste
Rare
Nasal burning, paroxysmal sneezing
Ophthalmic: Transient eye burning or stinging, bitter taste, headache

SERIOUS REACTIONS
! Epistaxis occurs rarely.

DENTAL CONSIDERATIONS
General:
• Protect patient's eyes from accidental spatter during dental treatment.

INTERACTIONS
Drug interactions of concern to dentistry
• Increased risk of anticholinergic effects: anticholinergics
• Possible additive sedation: alcohol, anxiolytics, opioid analgesics

DENTAL CONSIDERATIONS
General:
• Assess salivary flow as factor in caries, periodontal disease, and candidiasis.

Teach Patient/Family:
• *When chronic dry mouth occurs, advise patient:*
  • To avoid mouth rinses with high alcohol content because of drying effects
  • To use daily home fluoride products for anticaries effect
  • To use sugarless gum, frequent sips of water, or saliva substitutes

azithromycin
ay-zi-thro-mye′-sin
(Zithromax, Zithromax TRI-PAK, Zithromax Z-PAK)
Do not confuse azithromycin with erythromycin.

CATEGORY AND SCHEDULE
Pregnancy Risk Category: B

MECHANISM OF ACTION
A macrolide antibiotic that binds to ribosomal receptor sites of susceptible organisms, inhibiting RNA-dependent protein synthesis. ***Therapeutic Effect:*** Bacteriostatic or bactericidal, depending on the drug dosage.

PHARMACOKINETICS
Rapidly absorbed from the GI tract. Protein binding: 7%–50%. Widely distributed. Eliminated primarily unchanged by biliary excretion. ***Half-life:*** 68 hr.

AVAILABILITY
Oral Suspension: 100 mg/5 ml, 200 mg/5 ml.
Tablets: 250 mg, 500 mg, 600 mg.
Tri-Pak: 3×500 mg. Z-Pak: 6×250 mg.
Injection: 500 mg.

INDICATIONS AND DOSAGES
▸ Respiratory Tract, Skin, and Skin-Structure Infections
PO
Adults, Elderly. 500 mg once, then 250 mg/day for 4 days.
Children 6 mo and older. 10 mg/kg once (maximum 500 mg) then 5 mg/kg/day for 4 days (maximum 250 mg).

▸ Acute Bacterial Exacerbations of COPD
PO
Adults. 500 mg/day for 3 days.

▸ Otitis Media
PO
Children 6 mo and older. 10 mg/kg once (maximum 500 mg) then 5 mg/kg/day for 4 days (maximum 250 mg). Single dose: 30 mg/kg. Maximum: 1500 mg. Three day regimen: 10 mg/kg/day as single daily dose. Maximum: 500 mg/day.

▸ Pharyngitis, Tonsillitis
PO
Children older than 2 yr.
12 mg/kg/day (maximum 500 mg) for 5 days.

▸ **Chancroid**
PO
Adults, Elderly: 1 g as single dose.
Children: 20 mg/kg as single dose. Maximum: 1 g.

▸ **Treatment of *Mycobacterium avium* Complex (MAC)**
PO
Adults, Elderly. 500 mg/day in combination.
Children. 5 mg/kg/day (maximum 250 mg) in combination.

▸ **Prevention of MAC**
PO
Adults, Elderly. 1,200 mg/wk alone or with rifabutin.
Children. 5 mg/kg/day (maximum 250 mg) or 20 mg/kg/wk (maximum 1,200 mg) alone or with rifabutin.

▸ **Nongonococcal Urethritis and Cervicitis due to *Chlamydia trachomatis***
PO
Adults. 1 g as a single dose.

▸ **Usual Pediatric Dosage**
PO
Children older than 6 mo. 10 mg/kg once (maximum: 500 mg) then 5 mg/kg/day for 4 days (maximum 250 mg).

▸ **Usual Parenteral Dosage (Community-Acquired Pneumonia, PID)**
IV
Adults. 500 mg/day, followed by oral therapy.

OFF-LABEL USES

Chlamydial infections, gonococcal pharyngitis, uncomplicated gonococcal infections of the cervix, urethra, and rectum

CONTRAINDICATIONS

Hypersensitivity to azithromycin or other macrolide antibiotics

INTERACTIONS

Drug

Aluminum- or magnesium-containing antacids: May decrease azithromycin blood concentration.
Carbamazepine, cyclosporine, theophylline, warfarin: May increase the serum concentrations of these drugs.

Herbal

None known.

Food

None known.

Drug interactions of concern to dentistry

- Increased serum levels: carbamazepine, cyclosporine, pimozide
- Risk of severe myopathy, rhabdomyolysis: hydroxymethylglutaryl coenzyme A (HMG-CoA) reductase inhibitors (statins)
- Decreased action of clindamycin, penicillin, lincomycin
- Oral contraceptives: advise patient of a potential risk for decreased contraceptive action, to maintain compliance with oral contraceptive use while using antibiotics, and to consider the use of additional nonhormonal contraception
- Possible increase in anticoagulant effect: warfarin
- Increased serum levels of theophylline

DIAGNOSTIC TEST EFFECTS

May increase serum CK, AST (SGOT), and ALT (SGPT) levels.

IV INCOMPATIBILITIES

Information is not available.

IV COMPATIBILITIES

None known; don't mix with other medications.

SIDE EFFECTS

Occasional

Nausea, vomiting, diarrhea, abdominal pain

A

Rare
Headache, dizziness, allergic reaction

SERIOUS REACTIONS

! Antibiotic-associated colitis and other superinfections may result from altered bacterial balance.
! Acute interstitial nephritis and hepatotoxicity occur rarely.

DENTAL CONSIDERATIONS

General:
- An alternative drug of choice for mild infection caused by susceptible organisms in patients allergic to penicillin.
- Determine why the patient is taking the drug.
- Consider semisupine chair position for patient comfort if GI side effects occur.

Teach Patient/Family:
- *When used for dental infection, advise patient:*
  - To report sore throat, oral burning sensation, fever, and fatigue, any of which could indicate superinfection
  - To take at prescribed intervals and complete dosage regimen
  - To immediately notify the dentist if signs or symptoms of infection increase

aztreonam

az-tree′-oo-nam
(Azactam)

CATEGORY AND SCHEDULE

Pregnancy Risk Category: B

MECHANISM OF ACTION

A monobactam antibiotic that inhibits bacterial cell wall synthesis. ***Therapeutic Effect:*** Bactericidal.

PHARMACOKINETICS

Completely absorbed after IM administration. Protein binding: 56%–60%. Partially metabolized by hydrolysis. Primarily excreted unchanged in urine. Removed by hemodialysis. ***Half-life:*** 1.4–2.2 hr (increased in impaired renal or hepatic function).

AVAILABILITY

Injection Powder for Reconstitution: 500 mg, 1 g, 2 g.

INDICATIONS AND DOSAGES

▸ **UTIs**
IV, IM
Adults, Elderly. 500 mg-1 g q8–12h.

▸ **Moderate to Severe Systemic Infections**
IV, IM
Adults, Elderly. 1–2 g q8–12h.

▸ **Severe or Life-Threatening Infections**
IV
Adults, Elderly. 2 g q6–8h.

▸ **Cystic Fibrosis**
IV
Children. 50 mg/kg/dose q6–8h up to 200 mg/kg/day. Maximum: 8g/d.

▸ **Mild to Severe Infections in Children**
IV
Children. 30 mg/kg q6–8h. Maximum: 120 mg/kg/day.
Neonates. 60–120 mg/kg/day q6–12h.

▸ **Dosage in Renal Impairment**
Dosage and frequency are modified on the basis of creatinine clearance and the severity of the infection:

Creatinine Clearance	Dosage
10–30 ml/min	1–2 g initially, then usual dose at usual intervals
less than 10 ml/min	1–2 g initially; then usual dose at usual intervals

OFF-LABEL USES
Treatment of bone and joint infections

CONTRAINDICATIONS
None known.

INTERACTIONS
Drug
None known.
Herbal
None known.
Food
None known.
Drug interactions of concern to dentistry
- None reported

DIAGNOSTIC TEST EFFECTS
May increase serum alkaline phosphatase, creatinine, LDH, AST (SGOT), and ALT (SGPT) levels. Produces a positive Coombs' test.

IV INCOMPATIBILITIES
Acyclovir (Zovirax), amphotericin (Fungizone), daunorubicin (Cerubidine), ganciclovir (Cytovene), lorazepam (Ativan), metronidazole (Flagyl), vancomycin (Vancocin)

IV COMPATIBILITIES
Aminophylline, bumetanide (Bumex), calcium gluconate, cimetidine (Tagamet), diltiazem (Cardizem), dobutamine (Dobutrex), dopamine (Intropin), famotidine (Pepcid), furosemide (Lasix), heparin, hydromorphone (Dilaudid), insulin (regular), magnesium sulfate, morphine, potassium chloride, propofol (Diprivan)

SIDE EFFECTS
Occasional (< 3%)
Discomfort and swelling at IM injection site, nausea, vomiting, diarrhea, rash

Rare (< 1%)
Phlebitis or thrombophlebitis at IV injection site, abdominal cramps, headache, hypotension

SERIOUS REACTIONS
! Antibiotic-associated colitis and other superinfections may result from altered bacterial balance.
! Severe hypersensitivity reactions, including anaphylaxis, occur rarely.

DENTAL CONSIDERATIONS
General:
- For selected infections in the hospital setting.
- Provide palliative dental care for dental emergencies only.
- Caution regarding allergy to medication.
- Examine for oral manifestation of opportunistic infection.
- Determine why patient is taking the drug.

Consultations:
- Medical consultation may be required to assess disease control.
- Consult patient's physician if an acute dental infection occurs and another antiinfective is required.

Teach Patient/Family:
- Importance of good oral hygiene to prevent soft tissue inflammation
- To report oral lesions, soreness, or bleeding to dentist
- To prevent trauma when using oral hygiene aids

bacitracin

bass-i-tray′-sin
(Baciguent, Baci-IM, Bacitracin)
Do not confuse bacitracin with Bactrim or Bactroban.

CATEGORY AND SCHEDULE

Pregnancy Risk Category: C
OTC

MECHANISM OF ACTION

An antibiotic that interferes with plasma membrane permeability and inhibits bacterial cell wall synthesis in susceptible bacteria. ***Therapeutic Effect:*** Bacteriostatic.

AVAILABILITY

Powder for Irrigation: 50,000 units.
Ophthalmic Ointment. 500 units/g.
Topical Ointment. 500 units/g.

INDICATIONS AND DOSAGES

▸ **Superficial Ocular Infections**
OPHTHALMIC
Adults. ½-inch ribbon in conjunctival sac q3–4h.
▸ **Skin Abrasions, Superficial Skin Infections**
TOPICAL
Adults, Children. Apply to affected area 1–5 times a day.
▸ **Surgical Treatment and Prophylaxis**
IRRIGATION
Adults, Elderly. 50,000–150,000 units, as needed.

CONTRAINDICATIONS

None known.

INTERACTIONS

Drug
None known.
Herbal
None known.
Food
None known.
Drug interactions of concern to dentistry
• None reported

DIAGNOSTIC TEST EFFECTS

None known.

SIDE EFFECTS

Rare
Ophthalmic: Burning, itching, redness, swelling, pain
Topical: Hypersensitivity reaction (allergic contact dermatitis, burning, inflammation, pruritus)

SERIOUS REACTIONS

! Severe hypersensitivity reactions, including apnea and hypotension, occur rarely.

DENTAL CONSIDERATIONS

General:
• Use protective glove or finger cot to apply.
• Determine why patient is taking the drug.
Teach Patient/Family:
• To report burning, itching, or rash

baclofen

bak′-loe-fen
(Apo-Baclofen[CAN], Baclo[AUS], Clofen[AUS], Lioresal, Liotec[CAN], Novo-Baclofen[CAN], Nu-Baclofen[CAN], Stelax[AUS])
Do not confuse baclofen with Bactroban or Beclovent.

CATEGORY AND SCHEDULE

Pregnancy Risk Category: C

MECHANISM OF ACTION

A direct-acting skeletal muscle relaxant that inhibits transmission of reflexes at the spinal cord level. ***Therapeutic Effect:*** Relieves muscle spasticity.

PHARMACOKINETICS

Well absorbed from the GI tract. Protein binding: 30%. Partially metabolized in the liver. Primarily excreted in urine. ***Half-life:*** 2.5–4 hr; intrathecal: 1.5 hr.

AVAILABILITY

Tablets: 10 mg, 20 mg.
Intrathecal Injection: 50 mcg/ml, 500 mcg/ml, 2000 mcg/ml.

INDICATIONS AND DOSAGES

▸ Spasticity

PO

Adults. Initially, 5 mg 3 times a day. May increase by 15 mg/day at 3-day intervals. Range: 40–80 mg/day. Maximum: 80 mg/day.
Elderly. Initially, 5 mg 2–3 times a day. May gradually increase dosage.
Children. Initially, 10–15 mg/day in divided doses q8h. May increase by 5–15 mg/day at 3-day intervals. Maximum: 40 mg/day (children 2–7 yr); 60 mg/day (children 8 yr and older).

▸ Usual Intrathecal Dosage

Adults, Elderly, Children older than 12 yr. 300–800 mcg/day.
Children 12 yr and younger. 100–300 mcg/day.

OFF-LABEL USES

Treatment of bladder spasms, cerebral palsy, intractable hiccups or pain, Huntington's chorea, trigeminal neuralgia

CONTRAINDICATIONS

Skeletal muscle spasm due to cerebral palsy, Parkinson's disease, rheumatic disorders, CVA, cough, intractable hiccups, neuropathic pain

INTERACTIONS

Drug

Alcohol, other CNS depressants: May increase CNS depression.

Herbal

None known.

Food

None known.

Drug interactions of concern to dentistry

- Increased CNS depression: alcohol, all CNS depressants
- Muscle hypertonia: tricyclic antidepressants
- *When used in dentistry:*
  - Warn patient of sedative effects while taking medication

DIAGNOSTIC TEST EFFECTS

May increase blood glucose level and serum alkaline phosphatase, AST (SGOT), and ALT (SGPT) levels.

SIDE EFFECTS

Frequent (> 10%)

Transient somnolence, asthenia, dizziness, light-headedness, nausea, vomiting

Occasional (10%–2%)

Headache, paresthesia, constipation, anorexia, hypotension, confusion, nasal congestion

Rare (< 1%)

Paradoxical CNS excitement or restlessness, slurred speech, tremor, dry mouth, diarrhea, nocturia, impotence

SERIOUS REACTIONS

! Abrupt discontinuation of baclofen may produce hallucinations and seizures.

! Overdose results in blurred vision, seizures, myosis, mydriasis, severe

B

muscle weakness, strabismus, respiratory depression, and vomiting.

DENTAL CONSIDERATIONS

General:

- Monitor vital signs at every appointment because of cardiovascular side effects.
- Assess salivary flow as a factor in caries, periodontal disease, and candidiasis.
- After supine positioning, have patient sit upright for at least 2 min to avoid orthostatic hypotension.

Teach Patient/Family:

- *When chronic dry mouth occurs, advise patient:*
  - To avoid mouth rinses with high alcohol content because of drying effects
  - To use daily home fluoride products for anticaries effect
  - To use sugarless gum, frequent sips of water, or saliva substitutes

balsalazide

ball-sal′-a-zide

(Colazal)

CATEGORY AND SCHEDULE

Pregnancy Risk Category: B

MECHANISM OF ACTION

A 5–aminosalicylic acid derivative that changes intestinal microflora, altering prostaglandin production and inhibiting function of natural killer cells, mast cells, neutrophils, and macrophages. ***Therapeutic Effect:*** Diminishes inflammatory effect in colon.

AVAILABILITY

Capsules: 750 mg.

INDICATIONS AND DOSAGES

▸ Ulcerative Colitis

PO

Adults, Elderly. Three 750-mg capsules 3 times a day for 8 wk.

CONTRAINDICATIONS

Hypersensitivity to salicylates

INTERACTIONS

Drug interactions of concern to dentistry

- None reported

SIDE EFFECTS

Frequent (8%–6%)

Headache, abdominal pain, nausea, diarrhea

Occasional (4%–2%)

Vomiting, arthralgia, rhinitis, insomnia, fatigue, flatulence, coughing, dyspepsia

SERIOUS REACTIONS

! Liver toxicity occurs rarely.

DENTAL CONSIDERATIONS

General:

- Consider semisupine chair position for patient comfort because of GI side effects of disease.

Consultations:

- To reduce any potential risk of antibiotic-associated pseudomembranous colitis, a consultation is recommended before selecting an antibiotic for a dental infection.

becaplermin

beh-cap-lear-min

(Regranex)

CATEGORY AND SCHEDULE

Pregnancy Risk Category: C

MECHANISM OF ACTION

A platelet-derived growth factor that heals open wounds.

Therapeutic Effect: Stimulates body to grow new tissue.

PHARMACOKINETICS
None reported.

AVAILABILITY
Gel: 0.01% (Regranex).

INDICATIONS AND DOSAGES
▸ Ulcers

TOPICAL

Adults, Elderly. Apply once daily (spread evenly; cover with saline-moistened gauze dressing). After 12 hrs, rinse ulcer, re-cover with saline gauze.

CONTRAINDICATIONS
Neoplasms at site of application, hypersensitivity to becaplermin or any component of the formulation

INTERACTIONS
Drug

None known.

Herbal

None known.

Food

None known.

Drug interactions of concern to dentistry

- Unknown

DIAGNOSTIC TEST EFFECTS
None known.

SIDE EFFECTS
Occasional

Local rash near ulcer

SERIOUS REACTIONS
! None reported.

DENTAL CONSIDERATIONS
General:

- Patients requiring use of this medication probably will be limited in activities or bedridden.
- Determine why patient is taking the drug.
- Diabetes: question patient about self-monitoring of blood glucose values or finger-stick records.
- Diabetics may be more susceptible to infection and have delayed wound healing.
- Examine for oral manifestation of opportunistic infection.
- Patients with advanced diabetes should be questioned about any limitations in activities or stress tolerance. Some will also be receiving dialysis treatment if renal function is compromised. Dental treatment usually can be performed the day after dialysis.

Consultations:

- Medical consultation may be required to assess disease control and patient's ability to tolerate stress.
- Medical consultation may include data from patient's blood glucose monitoring, including glycosylated hemoglobin or HbA_{1c} testing
- Patients in dialysis may require antibiotic prophylaxis; determine need.

Teach Patient/Family:

- Importance of good oral hygiene to prevent soft tissue inflammation
- To prevent trauma when using oral hygiene aids
- Importance of updating health and drug history if physician makes any changes in evaluation or drug regimens

benazepril
be-naze′-a-pril

(Lotensin)

Do not confuse benazepril with Benadryl, or Lotensin with Loniten or lovastatin.

CATEGORY AND SCHEDULE
Pregnancy Risk Category: C (D if used in second or third trimester)

B

MECHANISM OF ACTION

An ACE inhibitor that decreases the rate of conversion of angiotensin I to angiotensin II, a potent vasoconstrictor. Reduces peripheral arterial resistance. ***Therapeutic Effect:*** Lowers BP.

PHARMACOKINETICS

Route	Onset	Peak	Duration
PO	1 hr	2–4 hr	24 hr

Partially absorbed from the GI tract. Protein binding: 97%. Metabolized in the liver to active metabolite. Primarily excreted in urine. Minimal removal by hemodialysis. ***Half-life:*** 35 min; metabolite 10–11 hr.

AVAILABILITY

Tablets: 5 mg, 10 mg, 20 mg, 40 mg.

INDICATIONS AND DOSAGES

▸ Hypertension (monotherapy)

PO

Adults. Initially, 10 mg/day. Maintenance: 20–40 mg/day as single or in 2 divided doses. Maximum: 80 mg/day.

Elderly. Initially, 5–10 mg/day. Range: 20–40 mg/day.

▸ Hypertension (combination therapy)

PO

Adults. Discontinue diuretic 2–3 days prior to initiating benazepril, then dose as noted above. If unable to discontinue diuretic, begin benazepril at 5 mg/day.

▸ Dosage in Renal Impairment

For adult patients with creatinine clearance less than 30 ml/min, initially, 5 mg/day titrated up to maximum of 40 mg/day.

OFF-LABEL USES

Treatment of CHF

CONTRAINDICATIONS

History of angioedema from previous treatment with ACE inhibitors

INTERACTIONS

Drug

Alcohol, antihypertensives, diuretics: May increase the effects of benazepril.

Lithium: May increase the lithium blood concentration and risk of lithium toxicity.

NSAIDs: May decrease the effects of benazepril.

Potassium-sparing diuretics, potassium supplements: May cause hyperkalemia.

Herbal

None known.

Food

None known.

Drug interactions of concern to dentistry

- Increased hypotension: alcohol, phenothiazines
- Decreased hypotensive effects: indomethacin and possibly other NSAIDs, sympathomimetics
- Suspected reduction in the antihypertensive and vasodilator effects by salicylates; monitor blood pressure if used concurrently

DIAGNOSTIC TEST EFFECTS

May increase BUN, serum alkaline phosphatase, serum bilirubin, serum potassium, AST(SGOT), and ALT (SGPT) levels. May decrease serum sodium levels. May cause positive antinuclear antibody titer.

SIDE EFFECTS

Frequent (6%–3%)

Cough, headache, dizziness

Occasional (2%)

Fatigue, somnolence or drowsiness, nausea

Rare (< 1%)
Rash, fever, myalgia, diarrhea, loss of taste

SERIOUS REACTIONS

! Excessive hypotension ("first-dose syncope") may occur in patients with CHF and in those who are severely salt or volume depleted.
! Angioedema (swelling of the face and lips) and hyperkalemia occur rarely.
! Agranulocytosis and neutropenia may be noted in those with collagen vascular disease, including scleroderma and systemic lupus erythematosus, and impaired renal function.
! Nephrotic syndrome may be noted in patients with history of renal disease.

DENTAL CONSIDERATIONS

General:

- Monitor vital signs at every appointment because of cardiovascular and respiratory side effects.
- After supine positioning, have patient sit upright for at least 2 min to avoid orthostatic hypotension.
- Patients on chronic drug therapy may rarely have symptoms of blood dyscrasias, which can include infection, bleeding, and poor healing.
- Assess salivary flow as a factor in caries, periodontal disease, and candidiasis.
- Limit use of sodium-containing products, such as saline IV fluids, for those patients with a dietary salt restriction.
- Use vasoconstrictors with caution, in low doses, and with careful aspiration.
- Stress from dental procedures may compromise cardiovascular function; determine patient risk.
- Short appointments and a stress reduction protocol may be required for anxious patients.

Consultations:

- Medical consultation may be required to assess disease control and patient's ability to tolerate stress.
- In a patient with symptoms of blood dyscrasias, request a medical consultation for blood studies and postpone dental treatment until normal values are reestablished.
- Take precautions if dental surgery is anticipated and sedation or general anesthesia is required; risk of hypotensive episode.

Teach Patient/Family:

- Importance of good oral hygiene to prevent soft tissue inflammation
- Caution to prevent injury when using oral hygiene aids
- *When chronic dry mouth occurs, advise patient:*
  - To avoid mouth rinses with high alcohol content because of drying effects
  - To use daily home fluoride products for anticaries effect
  - To use sugarless gum, frequent sips of water, or saliva substitutes

bendroflumethiazide

ben-droe-floo-meth-**igh**-ah-zide
(Naturetin-5)

CATEGORY AND SCHEDULE

Pregnancy Risk Category: C

MECHANISM OF ACTION

A benzothiadiazine derivative that acts as a thiazide diuretic and antihypertensive. As a diuretic blocks reabsorption of water, sodium, and potassium at cortical diluting segment of distal tubule. As an antihypertensive reduces plasma, extracellular fluid volume, peripheral vascular resistance by direct effect on blood vessels. ***Therapeutic Effect:*** Promotes diuresis, reduces BP.

B

PHARMACOKINETICS

Route	Onset	Peak	Duration
PO	2 hr	4 hr	6–12 hr

Variably absorbed from the GI tract. Primarily excreted unchanged in urine. Not removed by hemodialysis. ***Half-life:*** 5.6–14.8 hr.

AVAILABILITY

Tablets: 5 mg (Naturetin-5).

INDICATIONS AND DOSAGES

▸ **Edema**

PO

Adults. 5 mg/day, preferably given in the morning. To initiate therapy, doses up to 20 mg may be given once a day or divided into 2 doses.

▸ **Hypertension**

PO

Adults. 5–20 mg/day, preferably given the morning.
Maintenance: 2.5–15 mg/day.

UNLABELED USES

Treatment of diabetes insipidus, prevention of calcium-containing renal calculi

CONTRAINDICATIONS

Anuria, history of hypersensitivity to sulfonamides or thiazide diuretics

INTERACTIONS

Drug

Alcohol, barbiturates, narcotics: May increase the risk of orthostatic hypotension.
Amphotericin B, corticosteroids: May increase the risk of electrolyte imbalance, particularly hypokalemia.
Antidiabetic agents, insulin: May elevate blood glucose levels.
Antihypertensive agents: May potentiate the effects of these agents.
Calcium salts: May increase serum calcium levels.
Cholestyramine, colestipol: May decrease the absorption and effects of bendroflumethiazide.
Digoxin: May increase the risk of digoxin toxicity associated with bendroflumethiazide-induced hyperkalemia.
Lithium: May increase the risk of lithium toxicity.
MAOIs: May increase the hypotensive effects of MAOIs and bendroflumethiazide.
NSAIDs: May decrease the diuretic and antihypertensive effect of bendroflumethiazide.
Oral anticoagulants: May decrease the effects of these agents.

Herbal

None known.

Food

None known.

Drug interactions of concern to dentistry

- Decreased hypotensive response: NSAIDs, especially indomethacin

DIAGNOSTIC TEST EFFECTS

May increase blood glucose levels, serum cholesterol, low-density lipoprotein (LDL), bilirubin, calcium, creatinine, uric acid, and triglyceride levels. May decrease urinary calcium, and serum magnesium, potassium, and sodium levels.

SIDE EFFECTS

Expected

Increase in urine frequency and volume

Frequent

Potassium depletion

Occasional

Postural hypotension, headache, GI disturbances, photosensitivity reaction

SERIOUS REACTIONS

! Vigorous diuresis may lead to profound water and electrolyte depletion, resulting in hypokalemia, hyponatremia, and dehydration.
! Acute hypotensive episodes may occur.
! Hyperglycemia may be noted during prolonged therapy.
! Pancreatitis, blood dyscrasias, pulmonary edema, allergic pneumonitis, and dermatologic reactions occur rarely.
! Overdose can lead to lethargy and coma without changes in electrolytes or hydration.

DENTAL CONSIDERATIONS

- Monitor vital signs at every appointment due to cardiovascular side effects.
- Patient on chronic drug therapy may rarely present with symptoms of blood dyscrasias, which can include infection, bleeding, and poor healing. If dyscrasia is present, caution patient to prevent oral tissue trauma when using oral hygiene aids.
- After supine positioning, have patient sit upright for at least 2 min before standing to avoid orthostatic hypotension.
- Limit use of sodium-containing products, such as saline IV fluids, for patients with a dietary salt restriction.
- Stress from dental procedures may compromise cardiovascular function, determine patient risk.
- Short appointments and a stress reduction protocol may be required for anxious patients.
- Advise patient if dental drugs prescribed have a potential for photosensitivity.
- Patients taking diuretics should be monitored for serum K^+ levels.

Consultations:

- In a patient with symptoms of blood dyscrasias, request a medical consultation for blood studies and postpone treatment until normal values are reestablished.
- Medical consultation may be required to assess disease control and patient's ability to tolerate stress.

Teach Patient/Family:

- Importance of good oral hygiene to prevent soft tissue inflammation
- To prevent trauma when using oral hygiene aids
- Importance of updating health and medication history if physician makes any changes in evaluation or drug regimens; include OTC, herbal, and nonherbal remedies in the update

benzocaine

ben′-zoe-kane

(Americaine Anesthetic Lubricant, Americaine Otic, Anbesol, Anbesol Baby Gel, Anbesol Maximum Strength, Babee Teething, Benzodent, Cepacol, Cetacaine, Chiggerex, Chiggertox, Cylex, Dermoplast, Detaine, Foille, Foille Medicated First Aid, Foille Plus, HDA Toothache, Hurricane, Lanacane, Mycinettes, Omedia, Orabase-B, Orajel, Orajel Baby, Orajel Baby Nighttime, Orajel Maximum Strength, Orasol, Otricaine, Otocain, Retre-Gel, Solarcaine, Topicaine[AUS], Trocaine, Zilactin, Zilactin Baby)

CATEGORY AND SCHEDULE

Pregnancy Risk Category: C

MECHANISM OF ACTION

A local anesthetic that blocks nerve conduction in the autonomic, sensory, and motor nerve fibers. Competes with calcium ions for membrane binding. Reduces permeability of resting nerves to potassium and sodium ions.

B

Therapeutic Effect: Produces local analgesic effect.

PHARMACOKINETICS

Poorly absorbed by topical administration. Well absorbed from mucous membranes and traumatized skin. Metabolized in liver and by hydrolysis with cholinesterase. Minimal excretion in urine.

AVAILABILITY

Cream: 5%, 20% (Lanacane).
Lozenge: 10 mg (Cepacol, Trocaine), 15 mg (Cyclex, Mycinettes).
Oral Aerosol: 14% (Cetacaine), 20% (Hurricane).
Oral Gel: 6.3% (Anbesol), 6.5% (HDA Toothache), 7.5% (Anbesol Baby, Detaine, Orajel Baby), 10% (Orajel, Orajel Baby Nighttime, Zilactin-B, Zilactin Baby), 20% (Anbesol Maximum Strength, Hurricane).
Oral Liquid: 6.3% (Anbesol), 7.5% (Orajel Baby), 10% (Orajel), 20% (Anbesol Maximum Strength, Hurricane).
Oral Lotion: 2.5% (Babee Teething).
Oral Ointment: 20% (Benzadent).
Otic Solution: 20% (Americane Otic, Omedia, Oticaine, Otocain).
Paste: 20% (Orabase-B).
Topical Aerosol: 5%, (Foille, Foille Plus), 20% (Dermoplast), Solarcaine).
Topical Gel: 5% (Retre-Gel), 20% (Americaine Anesthetic Lubricant).
Topical Liquid: 2% (Chiggertox).
Topical Ointment: 2% (Chiggerex), 5% (Foille Medicated First Aid).

INDICATIONS AND DOSAGES

▸ **Canker Sores**
TOPICAL
Adults, Elderly, Children older than 2 yrs. Apply gel, liquid, or ointment to affected area. Maximum: 4 times/day.

▸ **Denture Irritation**
TOPICAL
Adults, Elderly. Apply thin layer of gel to affected area up to 4 times/day or until pain is relieved.

▸ **General Lubrication**
TOPICAL
Adults, Elderly, Children older than 2 yrs. Apply gel to exterior of tube or instrument prior to use.

▸ **Otitis Externa, Otitis Media**
OTIC
Adults, Elderly, Children older than 1 yr. Instill 4–5 drops into external ear canal of affected ears. Repeat q1–2h as needed.

▸ **Pain and Itching Associated with Sunburn, Insect Bites, Minor Cuts, Scrapes, Minor Burns, Minor Skin Irritations**
TOPICAL
Adults, Elderly, Children older than 2 yrs. Apply to affected area 3–4 times/day.

▸ **Pharyngitis**
PO
Adults, Elderly. 1 lozenge q2h. Maximum 8 lozenges/day.

▸ **Toothache/Teething Pain**
TOPICAL
Adults, Elderly, Children older than 2 yrs. Apply gel, liquid, or ointment to affected areas. Maximum: 4 times/day.

▸ **Anesthesia**
TOPICAL
Adults, Elderly. Apply aerosol, gel, ointment, liquid q4–12h as needed.

OFF-LABEL USES

Obesity, spasticity

CONTRAINDICATIONS

Hypersensitivity to benzocaine or ester-type local anesthetics, perforated tympanic membrane or ear discharge (otic preparations)

INTERACTIONS

Drug

Hyaluronidase: May increase incidence of systemic reaction to benzocaine.

Sulfonamides: May decrease the antibacterial effect of sulfonamides.

Herbal

St. John's Wort: May increase risk of cardiovascular collapse and delay effects of benzocaine.

Food

None known.

DIAGNOSTIC TEST EFFECTS

None known.

SIDE EFFECTS

Occasional

Burning, stinging, angioedema, contact dermatitis, taste disorders

SERIOUS REACTIONS

! Methemoglobinermia occurs rarely in infants and young children.

DENTAL CONSIDERATIONS

General:

- Do not use for topical anesthesia if medical history reveals allergy to procaine, PABA, parabens, or other ester-type local anesthetics.
- Use smallest effective amount in infants and children.
- Avoid applying to large denuded areas of mucosa to prevent excessive systemic absorption and potential toxicity.

benzonatate

ben-zoe′-na-tate

(Tessalon Perles)

CATEGORY AND SCHEDULE

Pregnancy Risk Category: C

MECHANISM OF ACTION

A non-narcotic antitussive that anesthetizes stretch receptors in respiratory passages, lungs, and pleura. ***Therapeutic Effect:*** Reduces cough production.

AVAILABILITY

Capsules: 100 mg, 200 mg.

INDICATIONS AND DOSAGES

▸ **Antitussive**

PO

Adults, Elderly, Children older than 10 yr. 100 mg 3 times a day or every 4 hours up to 600 mg/day.

CONTRAINDICATIONS

None known.

INTERACTIONS

Drug

CNS depressants: May increase the effects of benzonatate.

Herbal

None known.

Food

None known.

Drug interactions of concern to dentistry

- Increased CNS depression: slight risk of increased sedation with other CNS depressants

DIAGNOSTIC TEST EFFECTS

None known.

SIDE EFFECTS

Occasional

Mild somnolence, mild dizziness, constipation, GI upset, skin eruptions, nasal congestion

SERIOUS REACTIONS

! A paradoxical reaction, including restlessness, insomnia, euphoria, nervousness, and tremor, has been noted.

3

DENTAL CONSIDERATIONS

General:

- Elective dental treatment may not be possible with significant coughing episodes.

benzoyl peroxide

ben′-zoe-ill per-ox′-ide
(Acetoxyl[CAN], Benoxyl[CAN], Benzac, Benzac AC, Benzac AC Wash, Benzac W, Benzac W Wash, Benzagel, Benzagel Wash, Benzashave, Brevoxyl, Brevoxyl Cleansing, Brevoxyl Wash, Clearplex, Clinac BPO, Del Aqua, Desquam-E, Desquam-X, Exact Acne Medication, Fostex 10% BPO, Loroxide, Neutrogena Acne Mask, Neutrogena On The Spot Acne Treatment, Oxy[AUS], Oxy 10 Balanced Medicated Face Wash, Oxy 10 Balance Spot Treatment, Palmer's Skin Success Acne, Oxyderm[CAN], PanOxyl, PanOxyl-AQ, PanOxyl Aqua Gel, PanOxylBar, Seba-Gel, Solugel[CAN], Triaz, Triaz Cleanser, Zapzyt)

CATEGORY AND SCHEDULE

Pregnancy Risk Category: C
OTC

MECHANISM OF ACTION

A keratolytic agent that releases free-radical oxygen, which oxidizes bacterial proteins in the sebaceous follicles, decreasing the number of anaerobic bacteria and decreasing irritating-type free fatty acids.
Therapeutic Effect: Bactericidal action against Propionbacterium acnes and Staphlococcus epidermidis.

PHARMACOKINETICS

Minimal absorption through skin. Gel is more penetrating than cream. Metabolized to benzoic acid in skin. Excreted in urine as benzoate.

AVAILABILITY

Cream, topical: 2.5% (Neutrogena On The Spot Acne Treatment), 5% (Benzashave, Exact Acne Medication, Neutrogena Acne Mask), 10% (Benzashave).
Gel, topical: 2.5% (Benzac, Benzac AC, Benzac W, Desquam-E), 4% (Brevoxyl), 5% (Benzac, Benzac AC, Benzac W, Benzagel, Clearplex, Desquam-E, Desquam-X, Oxy 10 Balance Spot Treatment, PanOxyl, PanOxyl AQ, Seba-Gel), 6% (Triaz, Triaz Cleanser), 7% (Clinac BPO), 8% (Brevoxyl), 10% (Benzac, Benzac AC, Benzac W, Benzagel, Benzagel Wash, Clearplex, Desquam-E, Desquam-X, Fostex, Oxy 10 Balance Spot Treatment, PanOxyl, PanOxyl AQ, PanOxyl Aqua Gel, Seba-Gel, Triaz, Triaz Cleanser, Zapzyt).
Liquid, topical: 2.5% (Benzac AC Wash), 5% (Benzac AC Wash, Benzac W Wash, Del-Aqua, Desquam-X), 10% Benzac AC Wash, Benzac W Wash, Del-Aqua, Oxy-10 Balance Medicated Face Wash).
Lotion, topical: 4% (Brevoxyl Cleansing, Brevoxyl Wash), 5.5% (Loroxide), 8% (Brevoxyl Cleansing, Brevoxyl Wash), 10% (Fostex, Palmer's Skin Success Acne).
Soap bar, topical: 5% (PanOxyl Bar), 10% (Desquam-X, Fostex, PanOxyl Bar).

INDICATIONS AND DOSAGES

▸ **Acne**

TOPICAL

Adults. Apply 2.5%–10% concentration 1–2 times/day.

OFF-LABEL USES

Dermal ulcers, seborrheic dermatitis, surgical wounds, tinea pedis, tinea versicolor

CONTRAINDICATIONS
Hypersensitivity to benzoyl peroxide or any component of the formulation

INTERACTIONS
Drug
Sunscreens containing PABA: May cause skin to change color when both agents are used concomitantly.
Herbal
None known.
Food
None known.
Drug interactions of concern to dentistry
- None reported

DIAGNOSTIC TEST EFFECTS
None known.

SIDE EFFECTS
Occasional
Irritation, dryness, burning, peeling, stinging, contact dermatitis, bleaching of hair

SERIOUS REACTIONS
! Hypersensitivity reactions have been reported with benzoyl peroxide use.

DENTAL CONSIDERATIONS
General:
- Determine why patient is taking the drug.
- Advise patient if dental drugs prescribed have a potential for photosensitivity.
- Inquire about other drugs the patient may be using for acne.

Teach Patient/Family:
- To avoid application to eyes, nose, mouth and mucous membranes.
- Importance of updating health and medication history if physician makes any changes in evaluation or drug regimens; include OTC, herbal, and nonherbal remedies in the update

benzthiazide
benz-**thigh**-ah-zide
(Exna)

CATEGORY AND SCHEDULE
Pregnancy Risk Category: C

MECHANISM OF ACTION
Thiazide diuretic and antihypertensive. As a diuretic blocks reabsorption of water, sodium, and potassium at cortical diluting segment of distal tubule. As an antihypertensive reduces plasma, extracellular fluid volume, peripheral vascular resistance by direct effect on blood vessels.
Therapeutic Effect: Promotes diuresis, reduces BP.

PHARMACOKINETICS
Route	Onset	Peak	Duration
PO	2 hr	4 hr	6–12 hr

Variably absorbed from the GI tract. Primarily excreted unchanged in urine. Not removed by hemodialysis. ***Half-life:*** Unknown.

AVAILABILITY
Tablets: 50 mg (Exna).

INDICATIONS AND DOSAGES
▸ Edema
PO
Adults. Initially, 50–200 mg/day.
Maintenance: 50–150 mg/day.
▸ Hypertension
PO
Adults. Initially, 50–100 mg/day. Dosage should be adjusted according to the patient response, either upward to as much as 50 mg 4 times/day or downward to the minimal effective dosage level.

CONTRAINDICATIONS

Anuria, history of hypersensitivity to sulfonamide-derived drugs or thiazide diuretics

INTERACTIONS

Drug

Alcohol, barbiturates, narcotics: May increase the risk of orthostatic hypotension.
Amphotericin B, corticosteroids: May increase the risk of electrolyte imbalance, particularly hypokalemia.
Antidiabetic agents, insulin: May elevate blood glucose levels.
Antihypertensive agents: May potentiate the effects of these agents.
Calcium salts: May increase serum calcium levels.
Cholestyramine, colestipol: May decrease the absorption and effects of benzthiazide.
Digoxin: May increase the risk of digoxin toxicity associated with benzthiazide-induced hyperkalemia.
Lithium: May increase the risk of lithium toxicity.
MAOIs: May increase the hypotensive effects of MAOIs and benzthiazide.
NSAIDs: May decrease the diuretic and antihypertensive effect of benzthiazide.
Oral anticoagulants: May decrease the effects of these agents.

Herbal

None known.

Food

None known.

Drug interactions of concern to dentistry

- Decreased hypotensive response: NSAIDs, especially indomethacin

DIAGNOSTIC TEST EFFECTS

May increase blood glucose levels, serum cholesterol, LDL, bilirubin, calcium, creatinine, uric acid, and serum triglyceride levels. May decrease urinary calcium, and serum magnesium, potassium, and sodium levels.

SIDE EFFECTS

Expected

Increase in urine frequency and volume

Frequent

Potassium depletion

Occasional

Postural hypotension, headache, GI disturbances, photosensitivity reaction

SERIOUS REACTIONS

! Vigorous diuresis may lead to profound water and electrolyte depletion, resulting in hypokalemia, hyponatremia, and dehydration.
! Acute hypotensive episodes may occur.
! Hyperglycemia may be noted during prolonged therapy.
! Pancreatitis, blood dyscrasias, pulmonary edema, allergic pneumonitis, and dermatologic reactions occur rarely.
! Overdose can lead to lethargy and coma without changes in electrolytes or hydration.

DENTAL CONSIDERATIONS

- Monitor vital signs at every appointment due to cardiovascular side effects.
- Patient on chronic drug therapy may rarely present with symptoms of blood dyscrasias, which can include infection, bleeding and poor healing. If dyscrasia is present, caution patient to prevent oral tissue trauma when using oral hygiene aids.
- After supine positioning, have patient sit upright for at least 2 min before standing to avoid orthostatic hypotension.
- Limit use of sodium-containing products, such as saline IV fluids, for patients with a dietary salt restriction.

- Stress from dental procedures may compromise cardiovascular function, determine patient risk.
- Short appointments and a stress reduction protocol may be required for anxious patients.
- Advise patient if dental drugs prescribed have a potential for photosensitivity.
- Patients taking diuretics should be monitored for serum K^+ levels.

Consultations:

- In a patient with symptoms of blood dyscrasias, request a medical consultation for blood studies and postpone treatment until normal values are reestablished.
- Medical consultation may be required to assess disease control and patient's ability to tolerate stress.

Teach Patient/Family:

- Importance of good oral hygiene to prevent soft tissue inflammation
- To prevent trauma when using oral hygiene aids
- Importance of updating health and medication history if physician makes any changes in evaluation or drug regimens; include OTC, herbal, and nonherbal remedies in the update

benztropine mesylate

benz′-troe-peen
(Apo-Benztropine[CAN], Bentrop[AUS], Cogentin)
Do not confuse benztropine with bromocriptine.

CATEGORY AND SCHEDULE

Pregnancy Risk Category: C

MECHANISM OF ACTION

An antiparkinson agent that selectively blocks central cholinergic receptors, helping to balance cholinergic and dopaminergic activity. ***Therapeutic Effect:*** Reduces the incidence and severity of akinesia, rigidity, and tremor.

AVAILABILITY

Tablets: 0.5 mg, 1 mg, 2 mg.
Injection: 1 mg/ml.

INDICATIONS AND DOSAGES

▸ **Parkinsonism**

PO

Adults. 0.5–6 mg/day as a single dose or in 2 divided doses. Titrate by 0.5 mg at 5–6 day intervals.
Elderly. Initially, 0.5 mg once or twice a day. Titrate by 0.5 mg at 5–6 day intervals.
Maximum: 4 mg/day.

▸ **Drug-Induced Extrapyramidal Symptoms**

PO, IM

Adults. 1–4 mg once or twice a day.
Children older than 3 yr. 0.02–0.05 mg/kg/dose once or twice a day.

▸ **Acute Dystonic Reactions**

IV, IM

Adults. Initially, 1–2 mg; then 1–2 mg PO twice a day to prevent recurrence.

CONTRAINDICATIONS

Angle-closure glaucoma, benign prostatic hyperplasia, children younger than 3 years, GI obstruction, intestinal atony, megacolon, myasthenia gravis, paralytic ileus, severe ulcerative colitis

INTERACTIONS

Drug

Alcohol, other CNS depressants: May increase sedation.
Amantadine, anticholinergics, MAOIs: May increase the effects of benztropine.

Antacids, antidiarrheals: May decrease the absorption and effects of benztropine.

Herbal

None known.

Food

None known.

Drug interactions of concern to dentistry

- Increased anticholinergic effect: antihistamines, anticholinergics, and meperidine
- Decreased effects of phenothiazines

DIAGNOSTIC TEST EFFECTS

None known.

SIDE EFFECTS

Frequent

Somnolence, dry mouth, blurred vision, constipation, decreased sweating or urination, GI upset, photosensitivity

Occasional

Headache, memory loss, muscle cramps, anxiety, peripheral paresthesia, orthostatic hypotension, abdominal cramps

Rare

Rash, confusion, eye pain

SERIOUS REACTIONS

! Overdose may produce severe anticholinergic effects, such as unsteadiness, somnolence, tachycardia, dyspnea, skin flushing, and severe dryness of the mouth, nose, or throat.

! Severe paradoxical reactions, marked by hallucinations, tremor, seizures, and toxic psychosis, may occur.

DENTAL CONSIDERATIONS

General:

- Monitor vital signs at every appointment because of cardiovascular side effects.
- Assess salivary flow as a factor in caries, periodontal disease, and candidiasis.
- After supine positioning, have patient sit upright for at least 2 min to avoid orthostatic hypotension.
- Avoid dental light in patient's eyes; offer dark glasses for patient comfort.
- Do not use ingestible sodium bicarbonate products, such as the Prophy-Jet air polishing system, within 1 hr of taking benztropine.
- Place on frequent recall because of oral side effects.

Consultations:

- Medical consultation may be required to assess disease control and patient's ability to tolerate stress.

Teach Patient/Family:

- Importance of good oral hygiene to prevent soft tissue inflammation
- Use of electric toothbrush if patient has difficulty holding conventional devices
- *When chronic dry mouth occurs, advise patient:*
  - To avoid mouth rinses with high alcohol content because of drying effects
  - To use daily home fluoride products for anticaries effect
  - To use sugarless gum, frequent sips of water, or saliva substitutes

bepridil

beh′-prih-dill

(Bepadin, Vascor)

CATEGORY AND SCHEDULE

Pregnancy Risk Category: C

MECHANISM OF ACTION

A calcium channel blocker that inhibits calcium ion entry across cell membranes of cardiac and vascular smooth muscle; decreases heart rate, myocardial contractility, slows SA and AV conduction. ***Therapeutic Effect:*** Dilates coronary arteries, peripheral arteries/arterioles.

PHARMACOKINETICS

Rapidly, completely absorbed from GI tract. Undergoes first-pass metabolism in liver to active metabolite. Primarily excreted in urine. Not removed by hemodialysis. ***Half-life:*** less than 24 hrs.

AVAILABILITY

Tablets: 200 mg, 300 mg (Vascor).

INDICATIONS AND DOSAGES

▸ Chronic Stable Angina

PO

Adults, Elderly: Initially, 200 mg/day; after 10 days, dosage may be adjusted. Maintenance: 200–400 mg/day.

CONTRAINDICATIONS

Sick sinus syndrome/second- or third-degree AV block (except in presence of pacemaker), severe hypotension (90 mm Hg, systolic), history of serious ventricular arrhythmias, uncompensated cardiac insufficiency, congenital QT interval prolongation, use with other drugs prolonging QT interval

INTERACTIONS

Drug

Beta blockers: May have additive effect.

Digoxin: May increase digoxin concentration.

Procainamide, quinidine: May increase risk of QT interval prolongation.

Hypokalemia-producing agents: May increase risk of arrhythmias.

Herbal

None known.

Food

None known.

Drug interactions of concern to dentistry

- Decreased effect: indomethacin, possibly other NSAIDs, phenobarbital
- Increased effect: parenteral and inhalational general anesthetics or other drugs with hypotensive actions
- Increased effects of carbamazepine

DIAGNOSTIC TEST EFFECTS

QT interval may be increased.

SIDE EFFECTS

Frequent

Dizziness, lightheadedness, nervousness, headache, asthenia (loss of strength), hand tremor, nausea, diarrhea

Occasional

Drowsiness, insomnia, tinnitus, abdominal discomfort, palpitations, dry mouth, shortness of breath, wheezing, anorexia, constipation

Rare

Peripheral edema, anxiety, flatulence, nasal congestion, paresthesia.

SERIOUS REACTIONS

! CHF, second- and third-degree AV block occur rarely.

! Serious arrhythmias can be induced.

! Overdosage produces nausea, drowsiness, confusion, slurred speech, profound bradycardia.

DENTAL CONSIDERATIONS

General:

- Monitor cardiac status; take vital signs at every appointment because of cardiovascular side effects. Consider a stress reduction protocol to prevent stress-induced angina during the dental appointment.
- After supine positioning, have patient sit upright for at least 2 min to avoid orthostatic hypotension.

• Limit use of sodium-containing products, such as saline IV fluids, for those patients with a dietary salt restriction.
• Assess salivary flow as a factor in caries, periodontal disease, and candidiasis.

Consultations:
• Medical consultation may be required to assess disease control and stress tolerance of patient.

Teach Patient/Family:
• Need for frequent oral prophylaxis if gingival overgrowth occurs
• *When chronic dry mouth occurs, advise patient:*
  • To avoid mouth rinses with high alcohol content because of drying effects
  • To use daily home fluoride products for anticaries effect
  • To use sugarless gum, frequent sips of water, or saliva substitutes

betamethasone

bay-ta-meth′-a-sone
(Alphatrex, Betaderm[CAN], Betatrex, Beta-Val, Betnesol[CAN], Celestone, Diprolene, Luxiq, Maxivate)

CATEGORY AND SCHEDULE

Pregnancy Risk Category: C (D if used in first trimester)

MECHANISM OF ACTION

An adrenocortical steroid that controls the rate of protein synthesis, depresses the migration of polymorphonuclear leukocytes and fibroblasts, reduces capillary permeability and prevents or controls inflammation. ***Therapeutic Effect:*** Decreases tissue response to inflammatory process.

AVAILABILITY

Tablet (Celestone): 0.6 mg.
Cream (Alphatrex, Diprolene, Maxivate): 0.05%.
Cream (Betatrex, Beta-Val): 0.1%.
Foam (Luxiq): 0.12%.
Gel (Diprolene): 0.05%.
Lotion: (Alphatrex, Diprolene, Maxivate): 0.05%.
Lotion (Betatrex, Beta-Val): 0.1%.
Ointment (Alphatrex, Diprolene, Maxivate): 0.05%.
Ointment (Betatrex): 0.1%.
Syrup (Celestone): 0.6 mg/5 ml.
Injection (Celestone, Soluspan): 6 mg/ml.

INDICATIONS AND DOSAGES

▸ Anti-Inflammation, Immunosuppression, Corticosteroid Replacement Therapy
PO
Adults, Elderly. 0.6–7.2 mg/day.
Children. 0.063–0.25 mg/kg/day in 3–4 divided doses.

▸ Relief of Inflamed and Pruritic Dermatoses
TOPICAL
Adults, Elderly. 1–3 times a day.
Foam: Apply twice a day.

CONTRAINDICATIONS

Hypersensitivity to betamethasone, systemic fungal infections

INTERACTIONS

Drug

Amphotericin: May increase hypokalemia.
Digoxin: May increase digoxin toxicity secondary to hypokalemia.
Diuretics, insulin, oral hypoglycemics, potassium supplements: May decrease the effects of these drugs.
Hepatic enzyme inducers: May decrease the effect of betamethasone.
Live-virus vaccines: May decrease the patient's antibody response to

vaccine, increase vaccine side effects, and potentiate virus replication.

Herbal

None known.

Food

None known.

Drug interactions of concern to dentistry

- Decreased action: barbiturates
- Increased GI side effects: alcohol, salicylates, and other NSAIDs
- Increased action: ketoconazole, macrolide antibiotics

DIAGNOSTIC TEST EFFECTS

May increase blood glucose levels and serum lipids, amylase, and sodium levels. May decrease serum calcium, potassium, and thyroxine levels.

SIDE EFFECTS

Frequent

Systemic: Increased appetite, abdominal distention, nervousness, insomnia, false sense of well-being
Topical: Burning, stinging, pruritus

Occasional

Systemic: Dizziness, facial flushing, diaphoresis, decreased or blurred vision, mood swings
Topical: Allergic contact dermatitis, purpura or blood-containing blisters, thinning of skin with easy bruising, telangiectases or raised dark red spots on skin

SERIOUS REACTIONS

! Overdose may cause systemic hypercorticism and adrenal suppression.

DENTAL CONSIDERATIONS

General:

- Monitor vital signs at every appointment because of cardiovascular side effects.
- Patients on chronic drug therapy may rarely have symptoms of blood dyscrasias, which can include infection, bleeding, and poor healing.
- Symptoms of oral infections may be masked.
- Determine dose and duration of steroid therapy for each patient to assess risk for stress tolerance and immunosuppression.
- Avoid prescribing aspirin-containing products.
- Place on frequent recall to evaluate healing response.
- Prophylactic antibiotics may be indicated to prevent infection if surgery or deep scaling is planned.
- Patients who have been or are currently on chronic steroid therapy (>2 wk) may require supplemental steroids for dental treatment.

Consultations:

- In a patient with symptoms of blood dyscrasias, request a medical consultation for blood studies and postpone dental treatment until normal values are reestablished.
- Medical consultation may be required to assess disease control.
- Consultation may be required to confirm steroid dose and duration of use.

Teach Patient/Family:

- Importance of good oral hygiene to prevent soft tissue inflammation
- Caution to prevent injury when using oral hygiene aids

betaxolol

bay-tax′-oh-lol
(Betoptic[AUS], Betoptic-S, Betoquin[AUS], Kerlone)
Do not confuse betaxolol with bethanechol.

CATEGORY AND SCHEDULE

Pregnancy Risk Category: C (D if used in second or third trimester)

B

MECHANISM OF ACTION
An antihypertensive and antiglaucoma agent that blocks $beta_1$-adrenergic receptors in cardiac tissue. Reduces aqueous humor production. ***Therapeutic Effect:*** Slows sinus heart rate, decreases BP, and reduces intraocular pressure (IOP).

AVAILABILITY
Tablets (Kerlone): 10 mg, 20 mg.
Ophthalmic Solution (Betoptic-S): 0.5%.
Ophthalmic Suspension (Betoptic-S): 0.25%.

INDICATIONS AND DOSAGES
▸ Hypertension
PO
Adults. Initially, 5–10 mg/day. May increase to 20 mg/day after 7–14 days.
Elderly. Initially, 5 mg/day.
▸ Chronic Open-Angle Glaucoma and Ocular Hypertension
Ophthalmic (Eye Drops)
Adults, Elderly. 1 drop twice a day.
▸ Dosage in Renal Impairment
For adult and elderly patients who are on dialysis, initially give 5 mg/day; increase by 5 mg/day q2wk. Maximum: 20 mg/day.

OFF-LABEL USES
Treatment of angle-closure glaucoma during or after iridectomy, malignant glaucoma, secondary glaucoma; with miotics, to decrease IOP in acute and chronic angle-closure glaucoma

CONTRAINDICATIONS
Cardiogenic shock, overt cardiac failure, second- or third-degree heart block, sinus bradycardia

INTERACTIONS
Drug
Cimetidine: May increase betaxolol blood concentration.
Diuretics, other antihypertensives: May increase hypotensive effect of betaxolol.
Insulin, oral hypoglycemics: May prolong hypoglycemic effect of these drugs.
NSAIDs: May decrease antihypertensive effect.
Sympathomimetics, xanthines: May mutually inhibit hypotensive effects and may mask symptoms of hypoglycemia.
Herbal
None known.
Food
None known.
Drug interactions of concern to dentistry
- Decreased antihypertensive effects: NSAIDs, indomethacin
- May slow metabolism of lidocaine
- Decreased β-blocking effects (or decreased β-adrenergic effects) of epinephrine, levonordefrin, isoproterenol, and other sympathomimetics

DIAGNOSTIC TEST EFFECTS
May increase serum antinuclear antibody titer and BUN, serum lipoprotein, creatinine, potassium, uric acid, and triglyceride levels.

SIDE EFFECTS
Betaxolol is generally well tolerated, with mild and transient side effects.
Frequent
Systemic: Hypotension manifested as dizziness, nausea, diaphoresis, headache, fatigue, constipation or diarrhea, dyspnea
Ophthalmic: Eye irritation, visual disturbances
Occasional
Systemic: Insomnia, flatulence, urinary frequency, impotence or decreased libido
Ophthalmic: Increased light sensitivity, watering of eye

B

Rare
Systemic: Rash, arrhythmias, arthralgia, myalgia, confusion, altered taste, increased urination
Ophthalmic: Dry eye, conjunctivitis, eye pain

SERIOUS REACTIONS

! Overdose may produce profound bradycardia, hypotension, and bronchospasm.
! Abrupt withdrawal may result in diaphoresis, palpitations, headache, and tremors.
! Betaxolol administration may precipitate CHF or MI in patients with cardiac disease; thyroid storm in those with thyrotoxicosis; and peripheral ischemia in those with existing peripheral vascular disease.
! Hypoglycemia may occur in patients with previously controlled diabetes.
! Ophthalmic overdose may produce bradycardia, hypotension, bronchospasm, and acute cardiac failure.

DENTAL CONSIDERATIONS

General:
- Monitor vital signs at every appointment because of cardiovascular and respiratory side effects.
- After supine positioning, have patient sit upright for at least 2 min to avoid orthostatic hypotension.
- Assess salivary flow as a factor in caries, periodontal disease, and candidiasis.
- Stress from dental procedures may compromise cardiovascular function; determine patient risk.
- Short appointments and a stress reduction protocol may be required for anxious patients.
- Use vasoconstrictors with caution, in low doses, and with careful aspiration. Avoid use of gingival retraction cord with epinephrine.

Consultations:
- Medical consultation may be required to assess disease control and stress tolerance of patient.
- Use precautions if general anesthesia is required for dental surgery.

Teach Patient/Family:
- Importance of good oral hygiene to prevent soft tissue inflammation
- Caution to prevent injury when using oral hygiene aids
- *When chronic dry mouth occurs, advise patient:*
  - To avoid mouth rinses with high alcohol content because of drying effects
  - To use daily home fluoride products for anticaries effect
  - To use sugarless gum, frequent sips of water, or saliva substitutes

bethanechol chloride

be-than′-e-kole
(Duvoid[CAN], Myotonachol[CAN], Urecholine, Urocarb[AUS])
Do not confuse bethanechol with betaxolol.

CATEGORY AND SCHEDULE

Pregnancy Risk Category: C

MECHANISM OF ACTION

A cholinergic that acts directly at cholinergic receptors in the smooth muscle of the urinary bladder and GI tract. Increases detrusor muscle tone. ***Therapeutic Effect:*** May initiate micturition and bladder emptying. Improves gastric and intestinal motility.

AVAILABILITY

Tablets (Duvoid): 10 mg, 25 mg, 50 mg.

B

INDICATIONS AND DOSAGES

▶ **Postoperative and Postpartum Urine Retention, Atony of Bladder**

PO

Adults, Elderly. 10–50 mg 3–4 times a day. Minimum effective dose determined by giving 5–10 mg initially, then repeating same amount at 1-hr intervals until desired response is achieved, or maximum of 50 mg is reached.
Children. 0.6 mg/kg/day in 3–4 divided doses.

OFF-LABEL USES

Treatment of congenital megacolon, gastroesophageal reflux, postoperative gastric atony

CONTRAINDICATIONS

Active or latent bronchial asthma, acute inflammatory GI tract conditions, anastomosis, bladder wall instability, cardiac or coronary artery disease, epilepsy, hypertension, hyperthyroidism, hypotension, GI or urinary tract obstruction, parkinsonism, peptic ulcer, pronounced bradycardia, recent GI resection, vasomotor instability

INTERACTIONS

Drug

Cholinesterase inhibitors: May increase the effects and risk of toxicity of bethanechol.
Procainamide, quinidine: May decrease the effects of bethanechol.

Herbal

None known.

Food

None known.

Drug interactions of concern to dentistry

- Decreased effects: anticholinergics

DIAGNOSTIC TEST EFFECTS

May increase serum amylase, lipase, and AST(SGOT) levels.

SIDE EFFECTS

Occasional

Belching, blurred or changed vision, diarrhea, urinary urgency

SERIOUS REACTIONS

! Overdosage produces CNS stimulation (including insomnia, anxiety, and orthostatic hypotension), and cholinergic stimulation (such as headache, increased salivation diaphoresis, nausea, vomiting, flushed skin, abdominal pain, and seizures).

DENTAL CONSIDERATIONS

General:

- Monitor vital signs at every appointment because of cardiovascular and respiratory side effects.
- After supine positioning, have patient sit upright for at least 2 min to avoid orthostatic hypotension.

Consultations:

- For excessive, troublesome salivation, reassure patient that treatment duration usually is limited to a few days; otherwise consult to lower bethanechol dose.

bevacizumab

be-vah-ciz′-you-mab
(Avastin)

CATEGORY AND SCHEDULE

Pregnancy Risk Category: C

MECHANISM OF ACTION

An antineoplastic that binds to and inhibits vascular endothelial growth factor, a protein that plays a major role in the formation of new blood vessels to tumors. ***Therapeutic Effect:*** Inhibits metastatic disease progression.

PHARMACOKINETICS

Clearance varies by body weight, gender, and tumor burden. ***Half-life:*** 20 days (range, 11–50 days).

AVAILABILITY

Injection: 25-mg/ml vial.

INDICATIONS AND DOSAGES

▶ First-Line Treatment of Metastatic Carcinoma of the Colon or Rectum in Combination with 5-Fluorouracil (5-FU)

IV

Adults, Elderly. 5 mg/kg once every 14 days.

OFF-LABEL USES

Adjunctive therapy in breast cancer, renal cell carcinoma

CONTRAINDICATIONS

GI perforation, hypertensive crisis, nephrotic syndrome, recent hemoptysis, serious bleeding, wound dehiscence requiring medical intervention

INTERACTIONS

Drug

None known.

Herbal

None known.

Food

None known.

Drug interactions of concern to dentistry

- None reported

DIAGNOSTIC TEST EFFECTS

May decrease serum potassium, sodium, and hemoglobin levels; hematocrit; and WBC and platelet counts.

IV INCOMPATIBILITIES

Don't mix bevacizumab with dextrose solutions.

SIDE EFFECTS

Frequent (73%–25%)

Asthenia, vomiting, anorexia, hypertension, epistaxis, stomatitis, constipation, headache, dyspnea

Occasional (21%–15%)

Altered taste, dry skin, exfoliative dermatitis, dizziness, flatulence, excessive lacrimation, skin discoloration, weight loss, myalgia

Rare (8%–6%)

Nail disorder, skin ulcer, alopecia, confusion, abnormal gait, dry mouth

SERIOUS REACTIONS

! UTIs, manifested as urinary frequency or urgency and proteinuria, occur frequently.

! CHF, deep vein thrombosis, GI perforation, hypertensive crisis, nephrotic syndrome, and severe hemorrhage are the most serious reactions that occur.

! Anemia, neutropenia, and thrombocytopenia occur occasionally.

! Hypersensitivity reactions occur rarely.

DENTAL CONSIDERATIONS

General:

- Assess salivary flow as a factor in caries, periodontal disease, and candidiasis.
- If additional analgesia is required for dental pain, consider alternative analgesics (NSAIDs) in patients taking narcotics for acute or chronic pain.
- Avoid products that affect platelet function, such as aspirin and NSAIDs.
- This drug may be used in the hospital or on an outpatient basis. Confirm the patient's disease and treatment status.
- Consider semisupine chair position for patient comfort if GI side effects occur.
- Chlorhexidine mouth rinse prior to and during chemotherapy may reduce severity of mucositis.

• Patient on chronic drug therapy may rarely present with symptoms of blood dyscrasias, which can include infection, bleeding, and poor healing. If dyscrasia is present, caution patient to prevent oral tissue trauma when using oral hygiene aids.
• Palliative medication may be required for management of oral side effects.
• Short appointments and a stress reduction protocol may be required for anxious patients.
• Monitor vital signs at every appointment due to cardiovascular side effects.
• Patients may have received other chemotherapy or radiation; confirm medical and drug history.
• Patients may be taking a prophylactic antiinfective.
• Patients may be at risk of bleeding, check for oral signs.
• Oral infections should be eliminated and/or treated aggressively.
• Place on frequent recall due to oral side effects.

Consultations:
• Medical consultation should include routine blood counts including platelet counts and bleeding time.
• Consult physician; prophylactic or therapeutic antiinfectives may be indicated if surgery or periodontal treatment is required.
• Medical consultation may be required to assess immunologic status during cancer chemotherapy and determine safety risk, if any, posed by the required dental treatment.
• Medical consultation may be required to assess disease control and patient's ability to tolerate stress.

Teach Patient/Family:
• *When chronic dry mouth occurs advise patient:*
  • To avoid mouth rinses with high alcohol content due to drying effects
  • To use daily home fluoride products for anticaries effect
  • To use sugarless gum, frequent sips of water or saliva substitutes
• To inform dentist of unusual bleeding episodes following dental treatment
• To be aware of oral side effects
• Importance of good oral hygiene to prevent soft tissue inflammation
• To report oral lesions, soreness, or bleeding to dentist
• To prevent trauma when using oral hygiene aids
• Importance of updating health and medication history if physician makes any changes in evaluation or drug regimens; include OTC, herbal, and nonherbal remedies in the update
• If abdominal pain associated with constipation and/or vomiting occur, advise patient to consultation physician immediately

bexarotene

becks-**aye**-row-teen
(Targretin)

CATEGORY AND SCHEDULE

Pregnancy Risk Category: X

MECHANISM OF ACTION

Retinoid antineoplastic agent that binds to and activates retinoid X receptor subtypes, which regulate the genes that control cellular differentiation and proliferation. ***Therapeutic Effect:*** Inhibits growth of tumor cell lines of hematopoietic and squamous cell origin and induces tumor regression.

PHARMACOKINETICS

Moderately absorbed from the GI tract. Protein binding: greater than 99%. Metabolized in the liver. Primarily eliminated through the hepatobiliary system. ***Half-life:*** 7 hr.

AVAILABILITY

Capsules (Soft Gelatin): 75 mg (Targretin).

INDICATIONS AND DOSAGES

▸ Cutaneous T-cell Lymphoma Refractory to at Least One Prior Systemic Therapy

PO

Adults 300 mg/m2/day. If no response and initial dose is well tolerated, may be increased to 400 mg/m²/day. If not tolerated, may decrease to 200 mg/m²/day, then to 100 mg/m²/day.

TOPICAL

Adults. Initially, apply once every other day. May increase at weekly intervals up to 4 times/day.

UNLABELED USES

Treatment of diabetes mellitus; head, neck, lung, and renal cell carcinomas; Kaposi's sarcoma

CONTRAINDICATIONS

Hypersensitivity to bexarotene or any component of the formulation

INTERACTIONS

Drug

Antidiabetics: May enhance the effects of these drugs.

Erythromycin, itraconazole, ketoconazole: May increase bexarotene blood concentrations.

Phenytoin, rifampin: May decrease bexarotene blood concentrations.

Herbal

None known.

Food

Grapefruit, grapefruit juice: May increase bexarotene blood concentration and risk of toxicity.

DIAGNOSTIC TEST EFFECTS

May increase serum cholesterol, serum triglyceride, and total and LDL cholesterol levels. May increase CA-125 assay value in patients with ovarian cancer. May decrease serum HDL cholesterol levels. May produce abnormal liver function test results.

SIDE EFFECTS

Frequent

Hyperlipidemia (79%), headache (30%), hypothyroidism (29%), asthenia (20%)

Occasional

Rash (17%), nausea (15%), peripheral edema (13%), dry skin, abdominal pain (11%), chills, exfoliative dermatitis (10%), diarrhea (7%)

SERIOUS REACTIONS

! Pancreatitis, hepatic failure, and pneumonia occur rarely.

bicalutamide

by-kale-yew′-tah-myd

(Casodex, Cosudex[AUS])

CATEGORY AND SCHEDULE

Pregnancy Risk Category: X

MECHANISM OF ACTION

An antiandrogen antineoplastic agent that competitively inhibits androgen action by binding to androgen receptors in target tissue.

Therapeutic Effect: Decreases growth of prostatic carcinoma.

PHARMACOKINETICS

Well absorbed from the GI tract. Protein binding: 96%. Metabolized in the liver to inactive metabolite. Excreted in urine and feces. Not removed by hemodialysis. ***Half-life:*** 5.8 days.

AVAILABILITY

Tablets: 50 mg.

INDICATIONS AND DOSAGES

▸ **Prostatic Carcinoma**

PO

Adults, Elderly. 50–100 mg once a day in morning or evening, given concurrently with a luteinizing hormone-releasing hormone (LHRH) analogue or after surgical castration.

CONTRAINDICATIONS

None known.

INTERACTIONS

Drug

Warfarin: May increase warfarin's effects.

Herbal

None known.

Food

None known.

Drug interactions of concern to dentistry

- Avoid drugs that could exacerbate urinary retention, such as anticholinergics

DIAGNOSTIC TEST EFFECTS

May increase BUN level and serum alkaline phosphatase, bilirubin, AST (SGOT), and ALT (SGPT) levels. May decrease blood Hgb level and WBC count.

SIDE EFFECTS

Frequent

Hot flashes (49%), breast pain (38%), muscle pain (27%), constipation (17%), diarrhea (10%), asthenia (15%), nausea (11%)

Occasional (9%–8%)

Nocturia, abdominal pain, peripheral edema

Rare (7%–3%)

Vomiting, weight loss, dizziness, insomnia, rash, impotence, gynecomastia

SERIOUS REACTIONS

! Sepsis, CHF, hypertension, and iron deficiency anemia may occur.

DENTAL CONSIDERATIONS

General:

- Patients taking opioids for acute or chronic pain should be given alternative analgesics for dental pain.
- Palliative medication may be required for management of oral side effects.
- Assess salivary flow as a factor in caries, periodontal disease, and candidiasis.
- Monitor vital signs at every appointment because of cardiovascular and respiratory side effects.
- Short appointments may be required for patient comfort.
- Consider semisupine chair position for patient comfort because of disease and drug side effects.
- Place on frequent recall because of oral side effects.

Consultations:

- Medical consultation may be required to assess disease control and patient's ability to tolerate stress.

Teach Patient/Family:

- Importance of updating medical/drug record if physician makes any changes in evaluation or drug regimens
- *When chronic dry mouth occurs, advise patient:*
  - To avoid mouth rinses with high alcohol content because of drying effects
  - Of need for daily home fluoride to prevent caries
  - To use sugarless gum, frequent sips of water, or saliva substitutes

bimatoprost

bi-mat′-oh-prost

(Lumigan)

CATEGORY AND SCHEDULE

Category and Schedule

MECHANISM OF ACTION
A synthetic analog of prostaglandin with ocular hypotensive activity. ***Therapeutic Effect:*** Reduces intraocular pressure (IOP) by increasing the outflow of aqueous humor.

PHARMACOKINETICS
Absorbed through the cornea and hydrolyzed to the active free acid form. Protein binding: 88%. Moderately distributed into body tissues. Metabolized in liver. Primarily excreted in urine; some elimination in feces. ***Half-life:*** 45 min.

AVAILABILITY
Ophthalmic Solution: 0.03% (Lumigan).

INDICATIONS AND DOSAGES
▸ Glaucoma, Ocular Hypertension
OPHTHALMIC
Adults, Elderly. 1 drop in affected eye(s) once daily, in the evening.

CONTRAINDICATIONS
Hypersensitivity to bimatoprost or any other component of the formulation

INTERACTIONS
Drug
None known.
Herbal
None known.
Food
None known.
Drug interactions of concern to dentistry
- None reported

DIAGNOSTIC TEST EFFECTS
None known.

SIDE EFFECTS
Frequent
Conjunctival hyperemia, growth of eyelashes, and ocular pruritus
Occasional
Ocular dryness, visual disturbance, ocular burning, foreign body sensation, eye pain, pigmentation of the periocular skin, blepharitis, cataract, superficial punctate keratitis, eyelid erythema, ocular irritation, and eyelash darkening
Rare
Intraocular inflammation (iritis)

SERIOUS REACTIONS
! Systemic adverse events, including infections (colds and upper respiratory tract infections), headaches, asthenia, and hirsutism, have been reported

DENTAL CONSIDERATIONS
General:
- Avoid drugs with anticholinergic activity, such as antihistamines, opioids, benzodiazepines, propantheline, atropine, and scopolamine.
- Protect patient's eyes from accidental spatter during dental treatment.
- Avoid dental light in patient's eyes; offer dark glasses for patient comfort.

Consultations:
- Medical consultation may be required to assess disease control.

Teach Patient/Family:
- Importance of updating health and drug history if physician makes any changes in evaluation or drug regimens

biperiden
bye-per′-i-den
(Akineton HCl)

CATEGORY AND SCHEDULE
Pregnancy Risk Category: C

MECHANISM OF ACTION
A weak anticholinergic that exhibits competitive antagonism of

acetylcholine at cholinergic receptors in the corpus striatum, which restores balance. ***Therapeutic Effect:*** Antiparkinson activity.

PHARMACOKINETICS

Well absorbed from gastrointestinal (GI) tract. Protein binding: 23%–33%. Widely distributed.
Half-life: 18–24 hrs.

AVAILABILITY

Tablets: 2 mg (Akineton HCl).

INDICATIONS AND DOSAGES

▸ Extrapyramidal Symptoms

PO
Adults, Elderly. 2 mg 3–4 times/day. Dosage in renal impairment.

▸ Parkinsonism

PO
Adults, Elderly. 2 mg 1–3 times/day.

OFF-LABEL USES

Adjunct to methadone maintenance

CONTRAINDICATIONS

None known.

INTERACTIONS

Drug

Anticholinergics, antihistamines, phenothiazine, tricyclic antidepressants: May increase anticholinergic effects of biperiden.
Atenolol: May increase the bioavailability of atenolol.
Cholinergic agents: May decrease the effects of cholinergic agents.
Digoxin: May increase the amount of digoxin by delaying gastric emptying.
Levodopa: May increase the amount of levodopa by delaying gastric emptying.

Herbal

Betel nut: May decrease the anticholinergic effects of biperiden.

Food

None known.

Drug interactions of concern to dentistry

- Increased anticholinergic effect: antihistamines, anticholinergic-acting drugs, meperidine
- Increased CNS depression: alcohol, CNS depressants
- Decreased effects of phenothiazines

DIAGNOSTIC TEST EFFECTS

None known.

SIDE EFFECTS

Frequent

Orthostatic hypotension, anorexia, headache, blurred vision, urinary retention, dry mouth or nose

Occasional

Insomnia, agitation, euphoria

Rare

Vomiting, depression, irritation or swelling of eyes, rash

SERIOUS REACTIONS

! Overdosage may vary from severe anticholinergic effects, such as unsteadiness, severe drowsiness, dryness of mouth, nose, or throat, tachycardia, shortness of breath, and skin flushing.
! Also produces severe paradoxical reaction, marked by hallucinations, tremor, seizures, and toxic psychosis.

DENTAL CONSIDERATIONS

General:

- Monitor vital signs at every appointment because of cardiovascular side effects.
- After supine positioning, have patient sit upright for at least 2 min to avoid orthostatic hypotension.
- Assess salivary flow as a factor in caries, periodontal disease, and candidiasis.

• Avoid dental light in patient's eyes; offer dark glasses for patient comfort.

Consultations:

• Medical consultation may be required to assess disease control and patient's ability to tolerate stress.

Teach Patient/Family:

• To use electric toothbrush if patient has difficulty holding conventional devices
• Importance of good oral hygiene to prevent soft tissue inflammation
• *When chronic dry mouth occurs, advise patient:*
  • To avoid mouth rinses with high alcohol content because of drying effects
  • To use daily home fluoride products for anticaries effect
  • To use sugarless gum, frequent sips of water, or saliva substitutes

bisacodyl

bis-a-koe′-dill
(Alophen, Apo-Bisacodyl[CAN], Bisalax[AUS], Dulcolax, Femilax, Gentlax, Modane, Veracolate)
Do not confuse Veracolate with Accolate or Modane with Mudrane.

CATEGORY AND SCHEDULE

Pregnancy Risk Category: C
OTC

MECHANISM OF ACTION

A GI stimulant that has a direct effect on colonic smooth musculature by stimulating the intramural nerve plexi. ***Therapeutic Effect:*** Promotes fluid and ion accumulation in the colon increasing peristalsis and producing a laxative effect.

PHARMACOKINETICS

Route	Onset	Peak	Duration
PO	6–12 hr	N/A	N/A
Rectal	15–60 min	N/A	N/A

Minimal absorption following oral and rectal administration. Absorbed drug is excreted in urine; remainder is eliminated in feces.

AVAILABILITY

Tablets (Enteric-Coated): 5 mg.
Suppositories: 10 mg.

INDICATIONS AND DOSAGES

▸ **Treatment of Constipation**

PO

Adults, Children older than 12 yr. 5–15 mg as needed. Maximum: 30 mg.
Children 3–12 yr. 5–10 mg or 0.3 mg/kg at bedtime or after breakfast.
Elderly. Initially, 5 mg/day.

RECTAL

Adults, Children 12 yr and older. 10 mg to induce bowel movement.
Children 2–11 yr. 5–10 mg as a single dose.
Children younger than 2 yr. 5 mg.
Elderly. 5–10 mg/day.

CONTRAINDICATIONS

Abdominal pain, appendicitis, intestinal obstruction, nausea, undiagnosed rectal bleeding, vomiting

INTERACTIONS

Drug

Antacids, cimetidine, famotidine, ranitidine: May cause rapid dissolution of bisacodyl, producing abdominal cramping, and vomiting.
Oral medications: May decrease transit time of concurrently administered oral medications, decreasing absorption of bisacodyl.

B

Herbal
None known.
Food
Milk: May cause rapid dissolution of bisacodyl.
Drug interactions of concern to dentistry
- None reported; however, a decreased transit time may be expected for orally administered drugs

DIAGNOSTIC TEST EFFECTS
None known.

SIDE EFFECTS
Frequent
Some degree of abdominal discomfort, nausea, mild cramps, faintness
Occasional
Rectal administration: burning of rectal mucosa, mild proctitis

SERIOUS REACTIONS
! Long-term use may result in laxative dependence, chronic constipation, and loss of normal bowel function.
! Prolonged use or overdose may result in electrolyte or metabolic disturbances (such as hypokalemia, hypocalcemia, and metabolic acidosis or alkalosis), as well as persistent diarrhea, vomiting, muscle weakness, malabsorption, and weight loss.

DENTAL CONSIDERATIONS
General:
- Determine why patient is taking the drug.
- Consider semisupine chair position for patient comfort if GI side effects occur.
- Avoid the use of drugs that may exacerbate constipation.

bismuth subsalicylate
bis′-muth sub-sal-ih′-sah-late
(Bismed[CAN], Colo-Fresh, Devrom, Kaopectate, Pepto-Bismol)

CATEGORY AND SCHEDULE
Pregnancy Risk Category: C
OTC

MECHANISM OF ACTION
An antinauseant and antiulcer agent that absorbs water and toxins in the large intestine and forms a protective coating in the intestinal mucosa. Also possesses antisecretory and antimicrobial effects. ***Therapeutic Effect:*** Prevents diarrhea. Helps treat *Helicobacter-pylori*-associated peptic ulcer disease.

AVAILABILITY
Caplet (Devrom): 200 mg.
Liquid (Kaopectate, Pepto-Bismol): 262 mg/15 ml, 525 mg/15 ml.
Tablet (Colo-Fresh): 324 mg.
Tablets (Chewable [Devrom]): *(Devrom):* 200 mg.
Tablets (Chewable [Pepto-Bismol]): 262 mg.

INDICATIONS AND DOSAGES
▸ **Diarrhea, Gastric Distress**
PO
Adults, Elderly. 2 tablets (30 ml) q30–60min. Maximum: 8 doses in 24 hr.
Children 9–12 yr. 1 tablet or 15 ml q30–60min. Maximum: 8 doses in 24 hr.
Children 6–8 yr. Two-thirds of a tablet or 10 ml q30–60min. Maximum: 8 doses in 24 hr.
Children 3–5 yr. One-third of a tablet or 5 ml q30–60min. Maximum: 8 doses in 24 hr.

▸ ***H. Pylori*–Associated Duodenal Ulcer, Gastritis**
PO
Adults, Elderly. 525 mg 4 times a day, with 500 mg amoxicillin and 500 mg metronidazole, 3 times a day after meals, for 7–14 days.

▸ **Chronic Infant Diarrhea**
PO
Children 2–24 mo. 2.5 ml q4h.

OFF-LABEL USES

Prevention of traveler's diarrhea

CONTRAINDICATIONS

Bleeding ulcers, gout, hemophilia, hemorrhagic states, renal impairment

INTERACTIONS

Drug

Anticoagulants, heparin, thrombolytics: May increase the risk of bleeding.
Aspirin, other salicylates: May increase the risk of salicylate toxicity.
Insulin, oral antidiabetics: Large dose may increase the effects of insulin and oral antidiabetics.
Tetracyclines: May decrease the absorption of tetracyclines.

Herbal

None known.

Food

None known.

Drug interactions of concern to dentistry

- Salicylate toxicity: other salicylates
- Decreased absorption of tetracyclines
- Suspected reduction in antihypertensives and vasodilator effects of ACE inhibitors; monitor blood pressure if used concurrently

DIAGNOSTIC TEST EFFECTS

May alter serum alkaline phosphatase, AST (SGOT), ALT (SGPT), and uric acid levels. May decrease serum potassium level. May prolong PT.

SIDE EFFECTS

Frequent
Grayish black stools
Rare
Constipation

SERIOUS REACTIONS

! Debilitated patients and infants may develop impaction.

DENTAL CONSIDERATIONS

General:

- Avoid prescribing aspirin-containing products for analgesia.

bisoprolol fumarate

bis-ope′-pro-lal
(Bicor[AUS], Zebeta)
Do not confuse Zebeta with DiaBeta.

CATEGORY AND SCHEDULE

Pregnancy Risk Category: C (D if used in second or third trimester)

MECHANISM OF ACTION

An antihypertensive that blocks beta$_1$-adrenergic receptors in cardiac tissue. ***Therapeutic Effect:*** Slows sinus heart rate and decreases BP.

PHARMACOKINETICS

Well absorbed from the GI tract. Protein binding: 26%–33%. Metabolized in the liver. Primarily excreted in urine. Not removed by hemodialysis. ***Half-life:*** 9–12 hr (increased in impaired renal function).

AVAILABILITY

Tablets: 5 mg, 10 mg.

INDICATIONS AND DOSAGES

Hypertension

PO

Adults. Initially, 5 mg/day. May increase up to 20 mg/day.

Elderly. Initially, 2.5–5 mg/day. May increase by 2.5–5 mg/day. Maximum: 20 mg/day.

Dosage in Hepatic Impairment

For adults and elderly patients with cirrhosis or hepatitis whose creatinine clearance is less than 40 ml/minute, initially give 2.5 mg.

OFF-LABEL USES

Angina pectoris, premature ventricular contractions, supraventricular arrhythmias

CONTRAINDICATIONS

Cardiogenic shock, overt cardiac failure, second- or third-degree heart block

INTERACTIONS

Drug

Cimetidine: May increase bisoprolol blood concentration.
Diuretics, other antihypertensives: May increase the hypotensive effect of bisoprolol.
Insulin, oral hypoglycemics: May mask symptoms of hypoglycemia and prolong the hypoglycemic effect of these drugs.
NSAIDs: May decrease antihypertensive effect.
Sympathomimetics, xanthines: May mutually inhibit effects.

Herbal

None known.

Food

None known.

Drug interactions of concern to dentistry

- Decreased antihypertensive effects: NSAIDs, indomethacin, sympathomimetics
- May slow metabolism of lidocaine
- Decreased β-blocking effects (or decreased β-adrenergic effects) of epinephrine, levonordefrin, isoproterenol, and other sympathomimetics

DIAGNOSTIC TEST EFFECTS

May increase antinuclear antibody titer and BUN, serum lipoprotein, creatinine, potassium, uric acid, and triglyceride levels.

SIDE EFFECTS

Frequent

Hypotension manifested as dizziness, nausea, diaphoresis, headache, cold extremities, fatigue, constipation or diarrhea

Occasional

Insomnia, flatulence, urinary frequency, impotence or decreased libido

Rare

Rash, arthralgia, myalgia, confusion (especially in the elderly), altered taste

SERIOUS REACTIONS

! Overdose may produce profound bradycardia and hypotension.
! Abrupt withdrawal may result in diaphoresis, palpitations, headache, and tremulousness.
! Bisoprolol administration may precipitate CHF and MI in patients with heart disease; thyroid storm in those with thyrotoxicosis; and peripheral ischemia in those with existing peripheral vascular disease.
! Hypoglycemia may occur in patients with previously controlled diabetes.
! Thrombocytopenia, including unusual bruising and bleeding, occurs rarely.

DENTAL CONSIDERATIONS

General:

- Monitor vital signs at every appointment because of cardiovascular side effects.
- After supine positioning, have patient sit upright for at least 2 min to avoid orthostatic hypotension.

- Patients on chronic drug therapy may rarely have symptoms of blood dyscrasias, which can include infection, bleeding, and poor healing.
- Assess salivary flow as a factor in caries, periodontal disease, and candidiasis.
- Stress from dental procedures may compromise cardiovascular function; determine patient risk.
- Short appointments and a stress reduction protocol may be required for anxious patients.
- Use vasoconstrictors with caution, in low doses, and with careful aspiration. Avoid use of gingival retraction cord with epinephrine.

Consultations:

- In a patient with symptoms of blood dyscrasias, request a medical consultation for blood studies and postpone dental treatment until normal values are reestablished.
- Medical consultation may be required to assess disease control and patient's ability to tolerate stress.
- Take precautions if general anesthesia is required for dental surgery.

Teach Patient/Family:

- *When chronic dry mouth occurs, advise patient:*
  - To avoid mouth rinses with high alcohol content because of drying effects
  - To use daily home fluoride products for anticaries effect
  - To use sugarless gum, frequent sips of water, or saliva substitutes

bitolterol

bye-tole'-ter-ol
(Tornalate)

CATEGORY AND SCHEDULE

Pregnancy Risk Category: C

MECHANISM OF ACTION

An antiadrenergic, sympatholytic agent that stimulates beta2-adrenergic receptors in lungs.
Therapeutic Effect: Relaxes bronchial smooth muscle, relieves bronchospasm, reduces airway resistance.

PHARMACOKINETICS

Onset of action is rapid with duration of 4–8 hrs. Rapidly absorbed following aerosol administration. Primarily distributed to lungs. Metabolized in liver. Excreted in urine and feces.
Half-life: 3 hrs.

AVAILABILITY

Aerosol for oral inhalation: 0.8% (Tornalate).
Solution for oral inhalation: 0.2% (Tornalate).

INDICATIONS AND DOSAGES

▸ **Brochospasm**

INHALATION

Adults, Elderly, Children 12 yrs and older. Use 2 inhalations, separated by 1–3 minute interval. A third inhalation may be required.

▸ **Prevention of Bronchospasm**

INHALATION

Adults, Elderly, Children 12 yrs and older. Use 2 inhalations q8h.
Do not exceed 3 inhalations q6h, or 2 inhalations q4h.

OFF-LABEL USES

Chronic obstructive pulmonary disease

CONTRAINDICATIONS

History of hypersensitivity to sympathomimetics, bitolterol, or any of its components.

INTERACTIONS

Drug

Beta-blockers: May decrease effects of beta blockers.

B

Digoxin: May increase risk of arrhythmias.
MAOIs, tricyclic antidepressants, sympathomimetic agents, inhaled anesthetics: May increase the risk of toxicity.
Aminophylline: May increase risk of cardiotoxicity.

Herbal
None known.

Food
None known.

Drug interactions of concern to dentistry
• Significant reduction of effects: β-adrenergic blockers
• Potentiation of CV effects: MAOIs, tricyclic antidepressants, methylxanthine

DIAGNOSTIC TEST EFFECTS
May decrease potassium.

IV INCOMPATIBILITIES
Phenytoin, propofol (Diprivan)

IV COMPATIBILITIES
Amiodarone (Cordarone), atracurium (Tacrium), calcium chloride, calcium gluconate, digoxin, dopamine (Intropin), esmolol (Brevibloc), famotidine (Pepcid), insulin, isoproterenol, lidocaine, potassium, quinidine, ranitidine (Zantac), sodium bicarbonate, theophylline, verapamil

SIDE EFFECTS
Frequent
Tremor
Occasional
Cough, dry or irritated mouth/throat, headache, nausea, vomiting
Rare
Dizziness, vertigo, palpitations, insomnia

SERIOUS REACTIONS
! Although tolerance to the bronchodilating effect has not been observed, prolonged or too frequent use may lead to tolerance.
! Severe paradoxical bronchoconstriction may occur with excessive use.

DENTAL CONSIDERATIONS
General:
• Assess salivary flow as a factor in caries, periodontal disease, and candidiasis.
• Consider semisupine chair position for patients with respiratory disease.
• Acute asthmatic episodes may be precipitated in the dental office. A rapid-acting sympathomimetic inhalant (rescue inhaler) should be available for emergency use. Many patients may already have a prescribed rescue inhaler they normally use for acute asthmatic events.

Consultations:
• Medical consultation may be required to assess disease control and patient's ability to tolerate stress.

Teach Patient/Family:
• Importance of gargling, rinsing mouth with water, and expectorating after each aerosol dose
• *When chronic dry mouth occurs advise patient:*
  • To avoid mouth rinses with high alcohol content due to drying effects
  • To use daily home fluoride products for anticaries effect
  • To use sugarless gum, frequent sips of water or saliva substitutes

bivalirudin
bye-va-leer′-u-din
(Angiomax)

CATEGORY AND SCHEDULE
Pregnancy Risk Category: B

MECHANISM OF ACTION
An anticoagulant that specifically and reversibly inhibits thrombin by binding to its receptor sites.

Therapeutic Effect: Decreases acute ischemic complications in patients with unstable angina pectoris.

PHARMACOKINETICS

Route	Onset	Peak	Duration
IV	Immediate	N/A	1 hr

Primarily eliminated by kidneys. Twenty-five percent removed by hemodialysis. ***Half-life:*** 25 min (increased in moderate to severe renal impairment).

AVAILABILITY

Injection, Powder for Reconstitution: 250 mg.

INDICATIONS AND DOSAGES

▸ Anticoagulant in Patients with Unstable Angina who are Undergoing Percutaneous Transluminal Coronary Angioplasty (PTCA) in Conjunction with Aspirin

IV

Adults, Elderly. 1 mg/kg as IV bolus followed by 4-hr IV infusion at rate of 2.5 mg/ kg/hr. After initial 4-hr infusion is completed, give additional IV infusion at rate of 0.2 mg/ kg/hr for 20 hr or less, if necessary.

▸ Dosage in Renal Impairment

GFR	Dosage Reduced by
30–59 ml/min	20%
10–29 ml/min	60%
Dialysis	90%

CONTRAINDICATIONS

Active major bleeding

INTERACTIONS

Drug

Platelet aggregation inhibitors other than aspirin, thrombolytics, warfarin: May increase the risk of bleeding complications.

Herbal

Ginkgo biloba: May increase the risk of bleeding.

Food

None known.

Drug interactions of concern to dentistry

- Increased risk of bleeding: anticoagulants, antiplatelet agents, thrombolytics, ginkgo biloba (herb)

DIAGNOSTIC TEST EFFECTS

Prolongs aPTT and PT.

IV INCOMPATIBILITIES

Do not mix with other medications.

SIDE EFFECTS

Frequent (42%)

Back pain

Occasional (15%–12%)

Nausea, headache, hypotension, generalized pain

Rare (8%–4%)

Injection site pain, insomnia, hypertension, anxiety, vomiting, pelvic or abdominal pain, bradycardia, nervousness, dyspepsia, fever, urine retention

SERIOUS REACTIONS

! A hemorrhagic event occurs rarely and is characterized by a fall in BP or Hct.

DENTAL CONSIDERATIONS

General:

- Intended for use in hospitals or emergency rooms.
- Patients are at risk of bleeding, check for oral signs.
- Provide palliative dental care for dental emergencies only.

Consultations:

- Medical consultation should include routine blood counts including platelet counts and bleeding time.

B

• In a patient with symptoms of blood dyscrasias, request a medical consultation for blood studies and postpone treatment until normal values are reestablished.

Teach Patient/Family:

• To use soft tooth brush to reduce risk of bleeding
• Importance of good oral hygiene to prevent soft tissue inflammation
• To report oral lesions, soreness, or bleeding to dentist
• To prevent trauma when using oral hygiene aids
• Importance of updating health and medication history if physician makes any changes in evaluation or drug regimens; include OTC, herbal, and nonherbal remedies in the update

bleomycin sulfate

blee-oh-my′-sin
(Blenamax[AUS], Blenoxane)

CATEGORY AND SCHEDULE

Pregnancy Risk Category: D

MECHANISM OF ACTION

A glycopeptide antibiotic whose mechanism of action is unknown. Is most effective in the G_2 phase of cell division. ***Therapeutic Effect:*** Appears to inhibit DNA synthesis and, to a lesser extent, RNA and protein synthesis.

AVAILABILITY

Powder for Injection: 15 units, 30 units.

INDICATIONS AND DOSAGES

▸ **As Monotherapy to Treat Testicular Carcinoma; Lymphomas (including Hodgkin's disease, choriocarcinoma, reticulum cell sarcoma, and lymphosarcoma); and Squamous Cell Carcinomas of the Head and Neck (including mouth, tongue, tonsil, nasopharynx, oropharynx, sinus, palate, lip, buccal mucosa, gingiva, epiglottis, and larynx)**

IV, IM, Subcutaneous
Adults, Elderly. 10–20 units/m^2 (0.25–0.5 units/kg) 1–2 times/wk.
IV (continuous)
Adults, Elderly. 15 units/m^2 over 24 hr for 4 days.

▸ **In Combination Therapy to Treat Testicular Carcinoma; Lymphomas (including Hodgkin's disease, choriocarcinoma, reticulum cell sarcoma, and lymphosarcoma); and Squamous Cell Carcinomas of the Head and Neck (including mouth, tongue, tonsil, nasopharynx, oropharynx, sinus, palate, lip, buccal mucosa, gingiva, epiglottis, and larynx)**

IV, IM
Adults, Elderly. 3–4 units/m^2.
As a sclerosing agent to treat malignant pleural effusions and prevent recurrent pleural effusions.
INTRAPLEURAL
Adults, Elderly. 60–240 units as a single injection.

OFF-LABEL USES

Treatment of mycosis fungoides, osteosarcoma, ovarian tumors, renal carcinoma, soft-tissue sarcoma

CONTRAINDICATIONS

Previous allergic reaction

INTERACTIONS

Drug

Cisplatin: May decrease bleomycin clearance and increase the risk of bleomycin toxicity (from cisplatin-induced renal impairment).
Live-virus vaccines: May potentiate virus replication, increase vaccine

side effects, and decrease the patient's antibody response to the vaccine.
Other antineoplastics: May increase the risk of bleomycin toxicity.

Herbal

None known.

Food

None known.

Drug interactions of concern to dentistry

- None reported

DIAGNOSTIC TEST EFFECTS

None known.

IV INCOMPATIBILITIES

None known by Y-site administration.

IV COMPATIBILITIES

Cefepime (Maxipime), dacarbazine (DTIC), dexamethasone (Decadron), diphenhydramine (Benadryl), fludarabine (Fludara), gemcitabine (Gemzar), ondansetron (Zofran), paclitaxel (Taxol), piperacillin and tazobactam (Zosyn), vinblastine (Velban), vinorelbine (Navelbine)

SIDE EFFECTS

Frequent

Anorexia, weight loss, erythematous skin swelling, urticaria, rash, striae, vesiculation, hyperpigmentation (particularly at areas of pressure, skin folds, cuticles, IM injection sites, and scars), stomatitis (usually evident 1 to 3 weeks after initial therapy); may also be accompanied by decreased skin sensitivity followed by skin hypersensitivity, nausea, vomiting, alopecia, and—with parenteral form—fever or chills (typically occurring a few hours after large single dose and lasting 4–12 hrs).

SERIOUS REACTIONS

! Interstitial pneumonitis occurs in 10% of patients and occasionally progresses to pulmonary fibrosis. This condition appears to be dose- or age-related, occurring more often in patients receiving a total dose greater than 400 units and those older than 70 years.

! Nephrotoxicity and hepatotoxicity occur infrequently.

DENTAL CONSIDERATIONS

General:

- Monitor vital signs at every appointment due to cardiovascular side effects.
- Examine for oral manifestation of opportunistic infection.
- This drug may be used in the hospital or on an outpatient basis. Confirm the patient's disease and treatment status.
- Chlorhexidine mouth rinse prior to and during chemotherapy may reduce severity of mucositis.
- Patient on chronic drug therapy may rarely present with symptoms of blood dyscrasias, which can include infection, bleeding, and poor healing. If dyscrasia is present, caution patient to prevent oral tissue trauma when using oral hygiene aids.
- Palliative medication may be required for management of oral side effects.
- Patients may have received other chemotherapy or radiation; confirm medical and drug history.
- Patients may be taking a prophylactic antiinfective.
- Place on frequent recall due to oral side effects.

Consultations:

- Consult physician; prophylactic or therapeutic antiinfectives may be indicated if surgery or periodontal treatment is required.

• Medical consultation may be required to assess immunologic status during cancer chemotherapy and determine safety risk, if any, posed by the required dental treatment.
• Medical consultation may be required to assess disease control and patient's ability to tolerate stress.

Teach Patient/Family:
• To be aware of oral side effects
• Importance of good oral hygiene to prevent soft tissue inflammation
• To report oral lesions, soreness, or bleeding to dentist
• To prevent trauma when using oral hygiene aids
• Importance of updating health and medication history if physician makes any changes in evaluation or drug regimens; include OTC, herbal, and nonherbal remedies in the update

bosentan

bo′-sen-tan
(Tracleer)
Do not confuse with Tricor.

CATEGORY AND SCHEDULE

Pregnancy Risk Category: X

MECHANISM OF ACTION

An endothelin receptor antagonist that blocks endothelin-1, the neurohormone that constricts pulmonary arteries. ***Therapeutic Effect:*** Improves exercise ability and slows clinical worsening of pulmonary arterial hypertension (PAH).

PHARMACOKINETICS

Highly bound to plasma proteins, mainly albumin. Metabolized in the liver. Eliminated by biliary excretion. ***Half-life:*** Approximately 5 hr.

AVAILABILITY

Tablets: 62.5 mg, 125 mg.

INDICATIONS AND DOSAGES

▸ PAH in those with World Health Organization Class III or IV Symptoms

PO

Adults, Elderly. 62.5 mg twice a day for 4 wk; then increase to maintenance dosage of 125 mg twice a day.
Children weighing less than 40 kg. 62.5 mg twice a day.

CONTRAINDICATIONS

Administration with cyclosporine or glyburide, pregnancy

INTERACTIONS

Drug

Atorvastatin, glyburide, hormonal contraceptives (including oral, injectable, and implantable), lovastatin, simvastatin, warfarin: May decrease the plasma concentrations of these drugs.
Cyclosporine, ketoconazole: May increase plasma concentration of bosentan.

Herbal

None known.

Food

None known.

Drug interactions of concern to dentistry

• Increased plasma concentrations: ketoconazole and possible other drugs that inhibit or induce CYP450 enzymes involved with metabolism
• See contraindications for other drugs

DIAGNOSTIC TEST EFFECTS

May increase serum bilirubin, AST (SGOT), and ALT (SGPT) levels. May decrease blood Hgb and Hct levels.

SIDE EFFECTS

Occasional

Headache, nasopharyngitis, flushing

Rare

Dyspepsia (heartburn, epigastric distress), fatigue, pruritus, hypotension

SERIOUS REACTIONS

! Abnormal hepatic function, lower extremity edema, and palpitations occur rarely.

DENTAL CONSIDERATIONS

General:

- Acute pulmonary arterial hypertension rarely occurs and is a major medical problem. Patients are at high risk.
- Chronic pulmonary arterial hypertension also occurs. Patients may be taking a variety of antihypertensive medications. It is advisable to consult with the physician of record to determine quality of disease control, patient's ability to tolerate stress, and, with this particular drug, liver function.

Teach Patient/Family:

- Importance of good oral hygiene to prevent tissue inflammation and dental caries
- Importance of updating health and drug history if physician makes any changes in evaluation or drug regimens

brimonidine

bry-mo′-nih-deen

(Alphagan P)

Do not confuse with bromocriptine.

CATEGORY AND SCHEDULE

Pregnancy Risk Category: B

MECHANISM OF ACTION

An ophthalmic agent that is a selective alpha$_2$-adrenergic agonist. ***Therapeutic Effect:*** Reduces intraocular pressure (IOP).

PHARMACOKINETICS

Plasma concentrations peak within 0.5 to 2.5 hours after ocular administration. Distributed into aqueous humor. Metabolized in liver. Primarily excreted in urine. ***Half-life:*** 3 hrs.

AVAILABILITY

Ophthalmic Solution: 0.15% (Alphagan P) [contains Purite 0.005% as preservative].

INDICATIONS AND DOSAGES

▸ **Glaucoma, Ocular Hypertension**

OPHTHALMIC

Adults, Elderly, Children 2 yrs and older: 1 drop in affected eye(s) 3 times/day.

CONTRAINDICATIONS

Concurrent use of monoamine oxidase (MAO) inhibitor therapy, hypersensitivity to brimonidine tartrate or any other component of the formulation

INTERACTIONS

Drug

Alcohol, CNS depressants: May increase the effect of brimonidine.

Alpha-agonists: May decrease pulse and blood pressure

Beta-blockers (ophthalmic and systemic), other antihypertensives, cardiac glycosides: May cause adverse effects.

Clonidine, tricyclic antidepressants: May blunt the hypotensive effect of these drugs.

MAOIs: May increase risk of hypertensive urgency or emergency.

B

Herbal
None known.
Food
None known.
Drug interactions of concern to dentistry
• Drug interactions have not been studied; however, the following possibilities exist:
  • Increased CNS depression: opioids, sedatives, alcohol, and general anesthetics
  • Possible risk of interference with lowering intraocular pressure: anticholinergic drugs or drugs with anticholinergic actions; tricyclic antidepressants

DIAGNOSTIC TEST EFFECTS
None known.

SIDE EFFECTS
Occasional
Allergic conjunctivitis, conjunctival hyperemia, eye pruritus, burning sensation, conjunctival folliculosis, oral dryness, visual disturbances

SERIOUS REACTIONS
! Bradycardia, hypotension, iritis, miosis, skin reactions, including erythema, eyelid, pruritus, rash, and vasodilation, and tachycardia have been reported.

DENTAL CONSIDERATIONS
General:
• Assess salivary flow as factor in caries, periodontal disease, and candidiasis.
• Avoid dental light in patient's eyes; offer dark glasses for patient comfort.
• Question patient about compliance with prescribed drug regimen for glaucoma.
• Avoid drugs with anticholinergic activity, such as antihistamines, opioids, benzodiazepines, propantheline, atropine, and scopolamine.
• Monitor vital signs at every appointment because of cardiovascular side effects.

Consultations:
• Consultation with physician may be necessary if sedation or general anesthesia is required.

Teach Patient/Family:
• Importance of updating health and drug history if physician makes any changes in evaluation or drug regimens
• *When chronic dry mouth occurs, advise patient:*
  • To avoid mouth rinses with high alcohol content because of drying effects
  • To use daily home fluoride products for anticaries effect
  • To use sugarless gum, frequent sips of water, or saliva substitutes

brinzolamide
brin-zol′-a-mide
(Azopt)

CATEGORY AND SCHEDULE
Pregnancy Risk Category: C

MECHANISM OF ACTION
An ophthalmic agent that inhibits carbonic anhydrase. Decreases aqueous humor secretion.
Therapeutic Effect: Reduces intraocular pressure (IOP).

PHARMACOKINETICS
Systemically absorbed to some degree. Protein binding: 60%. Distributed extensively in red blood cells. Site of metabolism has not been established. Metabolized to active and inactive metabolites. Primarily excreted unchanged in urine.

AVAILABILITY
Ophthalmic suspension: 1% (Azopt).

INDICATIONS AND DOSAGES
▸ Glaucoma, Ocular Hypertension
OPHTHALMIC
Adults, Elderly. Instill 1 drop in affected eye(s) 3 times/day.

CONTRAINDICATIONS
Hypersensitivity to brinzolamide or any other component of the formulation

INTERACTIONS
Drug
None known.
Herbal
None known.
Food
None known.
Drug interactions of concern to dentistry
• Avoid drugs that can exacerbate glaucoma (e.g., anticholinergics)

DIAGNOSTIC TEST EFFECTS
None known.

SIDE EFFECTS
Occasional
Blurred vision, bitter taste, dry eye, ocular discharge, ocular discomfort and pain, ocular pruritus, headache, rhinitis
Rare
Allergic reactions, alopecia, chest pain, conjunctivitis, diarrhea, diplopia, dizziness, dry mouth, dyspnea, dyspepsia, eye fatigue, hypertonia, keratoconjunctivitis, keratopathy, kidney pain, lid margin crusting or sticky sensation, nausea, pharyngitis, tearing, urticaria

SERIOUS REACTIONS
! Electrolyte imbalance, development of an acidotic state, and possible CNS effects may occur.

DENTAL CONSIDERATIONS
General:
• Avoid dental light in patient's eyes; offer dark glasses for patient comfort.
• Question patient about compliance with prescribed drug regimen for glaucoma.
Consultations:
• Medical consult may be required to assess disease control.

bromocriptine mesylate
broe-moe-krip′-teen
(Apo-Bromocriptine[CAN], Bromohexal[AUS], Kripton[AUS], Parlodel)
Do not confuse bromocriptine with benztropine, or Parlodel with pindolol.

CATEGORY AND SCHEDULE
Pregnancy Risk Category: C

MECHANISM OF ACTION
A dopamine agonist that directly stimulates dopamine receptors in the corpus striatum and inhibits prolactin secretion. Also suppresses secretion of growth hormone.
Therapeutic Effect: Improves symptoms of parkinsonism, suppresses galactorrhea, and reduces serum growth hormone concentrations in acromegaly.

PHARMACOKINETICS
Indication	Onset	Peak	Duration
Prolactin lowering	2 hr	8 hr	24 hr
Antiparkinson	0.5–1.5 hr	2 hr	N/A
Growth hormone suppressant	1–2 hr	4–8 wk	4–8 hr

Minimally absorbed from the GI tract. Protein binding: 90%–96%. Metabolized in the liver. Excreted in feces by biliary secretion. ***Half-life:*** 15 hr.

AVAILABILITY

Capsules: 5 mg.
Tablets: 2.5 mg.

INDICATIONS AND DOSAGES

▸ Hyperprolactinemia

PO

Adults, Elderly. Initially, 1.25–2.5 mg/day. May increase by 2.5 mg/day at 3-to 7-day intervals. Range: 2.5 mg 2-3 times a day.

▸ Parkinson's Disease

PO

Adults, Elderly. Initially, 1.25 mg twice a day. May increase by 2.5 mg/day every 14–28 days. Range: 30–90 mg/day.

▸ Acromegaly

PO

Adults, Elderly. Initially, 1.25–2.5 mg. May increase at 3–7 day intervals. Usual dose 20–30 mg/day.

OFF-LABEL USES

Treatment of cocaine addiction, hyperprolactinemia associated with pituitary adenomas, neuroleptic malignant syndrome

CONTRAINDICATIONS

Hypersensitivity to ergot alkaloids, peripheral vascular disease, pregnancy, severe ischemic heart disease, uncontrolled hypertension

INTERACTIONS

Drug

Alcohol: May produce a disulfiram-like reaction (chest pain, confusion, flushed face, nausea, vomiting).
Erythromycin, ritonavir: May increase bromocriptine blood concentration and risk of toxicity.
Estrogens, progestins: May decrease the effects of bromocriptine.
Haloperidol, MAOIs, phenothiazines, risperidone: May decrease bromocriptine's prolactin-lowering effect.
Hypotension-producing medications: May increase hypotension.
Levodopa: May increase the effects of bromocriptine.

Herbal

None known.

Food

None known.

Drug interactions of concern to dentistry

- Decreased action: phenothiazines, loxapine, haloperidol, droperidol, amitriptyline
- Increased plasma levels: erythromycin

DIAGNOSTIC TEST EFFECTS

May increase plasma growth hormone concentration.

SIDE EFFECTS

Frequent

Nausea (49%), headache (19%), dizziness (17%)

Occasional (7%–3%)

Fatigue, lightheadedness, vomiting, abdominal cramps, diarrhea, constipation, nasal congestion, somnolence, dry mouth

Rare

Muscle cramps, urinary hesitancy

SERIOUS REACTIONS

! Visual or auditory hallucinations have been noted in patients with Parkinson's disease.
! Long-term, high-dose therapy may produce continuing rhinorrhea, syncope, GI hemorrhage, peptic ulcer, and severe abdominal pain.

DENTAL CONSIDERATIONS

General:

- Monitor vital signs at every appointment because of cardiovascular side effects.
- After supine positioning, have patient sit upright for at least 2 min to avoid orthostatic hypotension.
- Assess salivary flow as a factor in caries, periodontal disease, and candidiasis.
- Short appointments may be required because of disease effects on musculature.

Consultations:

- Medical consultation may be required to assess disease control.

Teach Patient/Family:

- To avoid mouth rinses with high alcohol content because of drying effects

brompheniramine

brome-fen-ir′-a-meen

(BroveX, BroveX CT, Codimal A, Colhist, Dimetane, Dimetane Extentabs, Dimetapp, Lodrane 12 Hour, Nasahist B, ND Stat)

CATEGORY AND SCHEDULE

Pregnancy Risk Category: B

OTC (tablets, elixir)

MECHANISM OF ACTION

An alklamine that competes with histamine at histaminic receptor sites. Inhibits central acetylcholine. ***Therapeutic Effect:*** Results in anticholinergic, antipruritic, antitussive, antiemetic effects. Produces antidyskinetic, sedative effect.

PHARMACOKINETICS

Rapidly absorbed after PO administration. Widely distributed. Metabolized in liver. Primarily excreted in urine. ***Half-life:*** 25 hrs.

AVAILABILITY

Tablets: 4 mg (Dimetane).
Tablets, chewable (extended-release): 12 mg (BroveX CT).
Tablets (extended-release): 6 mg (Lodrane 12 Hour).
Tablets (timed-release): 8 mg, 12 mg (Dimetane Extentabs).
Elixir: 2 mg/ 5 ml (Dimetapp).
Oral Suspension: 12 mg/5 ml (BroveX).

INDICATIONS AND DOSAGES

▸ Allergic Rhinitis, Anaphylaxis, Urticarial Transfusion Reactions, Urticaria

PO

Adults, Elderly, Children 12 yrs and older. 4 mg q4–6h or 8–12 mg extended/timed-release q12h.
Children younger than 12 yrs. 1–2 mg q4–6h.

▸ Amelioration of Allergic Reactions to Blood or Plasma, Anaphylaxis as an Adjunct to Epinephrine and other Standard Measures after the Acute Symptoms Have Been Controlled, Other Uncomplicated Allergic Conditions of the Immediate Type When Oral Therapy Is Impossible or Contraindicated

IM/IV/SC

Adults, Elderly, Children 12 yrs and older. 5–20 mg/day in 2 divided doses. Maximum: 40 mg/day.
Children younger than 12 yrs. 0.125 mg/kg/day or 3.75 mg/m^2 in 3–4 divided doses.

CONTRAINDICATIONS

Concurrent MAOI therapy, focal CNS lesions, newborn or premature infants, hypersensitivity to brompheniramine or related drugs

INTERACTIONS

Drug

Anticholinergics: May increase anticholinergic effects.
MAOIs: May increase anticholinergic and CNS depressant effects.
Procarbazine: May increase CNS depressant effects.

Herbal

None known.

Food

None known.

Drug interactions of concern to dentistry

- Increased CNS depression: alcohol, all CNS depressants
- Additive photosensitization: tetracyclines
- Increased drying effect: anticholinergics
- Hypotension: general anesthetics

DIAGNOSTIC TEST EFFECTS

May suppress wheal and flare reactions to antigen skin testing unless antihistamines are discontinued 4 days before testing.

SIDE EFFECTS

Frequent

Drowsiness, dizziness, dry mouth, nose, or throat, urinary retention, thickening of bronchial secretions
Elderly: Sedation, dizziness, hypotension

Occasional

Epigastric distress, flushing, blurred vision, tinnitus, paresthesia, sweating, chills

SERIOUS REACTIONS

! Children may experience dominant paradoxical reactions, including restlessness, insomnia, euphoria, nervousness, and tremors.
! Overdosage in children may result in hallucinations, seizures, and death.
! Hypersensitivity reaction, such as eczema, pruritus, rash, cardiac disturbances, and photosensitivity, may occur.

DENTAL CONSIDERATIONS

General:

- Assess salivary flow as a factor in caries, periodontal disease, and candidiasis.
- Consider semisupine chair position for patients with respiratory disease.
- Determine why the patient is taking the drug.

Teach Patient/Family:

- Importance of good oral hygiene to prevent soft tissue inflammation
- To avoid mouth rinses with high alcohol content because of drying effects

buclizine hydrochloride

bew'-klih-zeen
(Bucladin-S)

CATEGORY AND SCHEDULE

Pregnancy Risk Category: C

MECHANISM OF ACTION

A centrally acting agent that suppresses nausea and vomiting. Buclizine is an anticholinergic that reduces labyrinth excitability and diminishes vestibular stimulation of labyrinth, affecting chemoreceptor trigger zone (CTZ). Possesses anticholinergic activity. ***Therapeutic Effect:*** Reduces nausea, vomiting, vertigo.

PHARMACOKINETICS

None reported.

AVAILABILITY

Tablets (softabs): 50 mg (Bucladin-S).

INDICATIONS AND DOSAGES

▸ Motion Sickness

PO

Adults, Elderly, Children 12 yrs and older. 50 mg 30 minutes before travel. Dose may be repeated every 4–6 hours as needed. Maximum: 150 mg/day.

CONTRAINDICATIONS

Early pregnancy, hypersensitivity to buclizine or other components of the formulation including tartrazine

INTERACTIONS

Drug

Alcohol, central nervous system (CNS) depression-producing medications: May increase CNS depressant effect.
Apomorphine: May decrease the emetic response of apomorphine.
Other anticholinergics: May potentiate anticholinergic effects.

Herbal

None known.

Food

None known.

Drug interactions of concern to dentistry

- Increased risk of drowsiness: CNS depressants and alcohol

DIAGNOSTIC TEST EFFECTS

May produce false-negative results using allergen extracts for skin tests.

SIDE EFFECTS

Frequent
Drowsiness
Occasional
Dryness of mouth, headache, jitteriness

SERIOUS REACTIONS

! Children may experience dominant paradoxical reaction, including restlessness, insomnia, euphoria, nervousness, and tremors.
! Overdosage in children may result in hallucinations, convulsions, and death.
! Hypersensitivity reaction, marked by eczema, pruritus, rash, cardiac disturbances, and photosensitivity, may occur.
! Overdosage may vary from CNS depression, such as sedation, apnea, cardiovascular collapse, or death, to severe paradoxical reaction, including hallucinations, tremor, or seizures.

DENTAL CONSIDERATIONS

General:

- Symptoms may preclude elective dental treatment.
- Assess salivary flow as a factor in caries, periodontal disease, and candidiasis.
- Consider semisupine chair position for patient comfort because of GI effects of disease.

Teach Patient/Family:

- Importance of good oral hygiene to prevent soft tissue inflammation.
- *When chronic dry mouth occurs advise patient:*
  - To avoid mouth rinses with high alcohol content due to drying effects
  - To use daily home fluoride products for anticaries effect
  - To use sugarless gum, frequent sips of water or saliva substitutes

budesonide

bu-dess′-ah-nide
(Burinex[AUS], Entocort EC, Pulmicort Respules, Pulmicort Turbuhaler, Rhinocort Aqua, Rhinocort Aqueous[AUS], Rhinocort Hayfever[AUS])

CATEGORY AND SCHEDULE

Pregnancy Risk Category: B

B

MECHANISM OF ACTION

A glucocorticoid that inhibits the accumulation of inflammatory cells and decreases and prevents tissues from responding to the inflammatory process. ***Therapeutic Effect:*** Relieves symptoms of allergic rhinitis or Crohn's disease.

PHARMACOKINETICS

Minimally absorbed from nasal tissue; moderately absorbed from inhalation. Protein binding: 88%. Primarily metabolized in the liver. ***Half-life:*** 2–3 hr.

AVAILABILITY

Capsules (Entocort EC): 3 mg.
Powder for oral inhalation (Pulmicort Turbuhaler): 200 mcg per inhalation.
Suspension for oral inhalation (Pulmicort Respules): 0.25 mg/2 ml; 0.5 mg/2 mg.
Nasal spray (Rhinocort Aqua): 32 mcg/spray.

INDICATIONS AND DOSAGES

▸ Rhinitis

INTRANASAL (RHINOCORT AQUA)

Adults, Elderly, Children 6 yr and older. 1 spray in each nostril once a day. Maximum: 8 sprays/day for adults and children 12 yr and older; 4 sprays/day for children younger than 12 yr.

▸ Bronchial Asthma

NEBULIZATION

Children 6 mo–8 yr. 0.25–1 mg/day titrated to lowest effective dosage.

INHALATION

Adults, Elderly, Children 6 yr and older. Initially, 200–400 mcg twice a day. Maximum: Adults: 800 mcg twice a day. Children: 400 mcg twice a day.

▸ Crohn's Disease

PO

Adults, Elderly. 9 mg once a day for up to 8 wk.

OFF-LABEL USES

Treatment of vasomotor rhinitis

CONTRAINDICATIONS

Hypersensitivity to any corticosteroid or its components, persistently positive sputum cultures for *Candida albicans*, primary treatment of status asthmaticus, systemic fungal infections, untreated localized infection involving nasal mucosa

INTERACTIONS

Drug

None known.

Herbal

None known.

Food

None known.

Drug interactions of concern to dentistry

- None reported

DIAGNOSTIC TEST EFFECTS

None known.

SIDE EFFECTS

Frequent (> 3%)

Nasal: Mild nasopharyngeal irritation, burning, stinging, or dryness; headache; cough
Inhalation: Flu-like symptoms, headache, pharyngitis

Occasional (3%–1%)

Nasal: Dry mouth, dyspepsia, rebound congestion, rhinorrhea, loss of taste
Inhalation: Back pain, vomiting, altered taste, voice changes, abdominal pain, nausea, dyspepsia

SERIOUS REACTIONS

! An acute hypersensitivity reaction marked by urticaria, angioedema, and severe bronchospasm, occurs rarely.

DENTAL CONSIDERATIONS

General:

- Evaluate respiration characteristics and rate.
- Assess salivary flow as a factor in caries, periodontal disease, and candidiasis.
- Midday appointments are suggested with stress reduction protocol for anxious patients.
- Place on frequent recall because of oral side effects.
- Acute asthmatic episodes may be precipitated in the dental office. Rapid-acting sympathomimetic inhalants should be available for emergency use. Budesonide is not a rapid-acting drug and is not intended for use in acute asthmatic attacks.

Consultations:

- Medical consultation may be required to assess disease control.

Teach Patient/Family:

- Importance of good oral hygiene to prevent soft tissue inflammation
- That gargling and rinsing with water after each dose helps prevent fungal infection
- *When chronic dry mouth occurs, advise patient:*
  - To avoid mouth rinses with high alcohol content because of drying effects
  - To use daily home fluoride products for anticaries effect
  - To use sugarless gum, frequent sips of water, or artificial saliva substitutes

bumetanide

byoo-met′-a-nide
(Bumex, Burinex[CAN])

CATEGORY AND SCHEDULE

Pregnancy Risk Category: C (D if used in pregnancy-induced hypertension)

MECHANISM OF ACTION

A loop diuretic that enhances excretion of sodium, chloride, and to lesser degree, potassium, by direct action at the ascending limb of the loop of Henle and in the proximal tubule. ***Therapeutic Effect:*** Produces diuresis.

PHARMACOKINETICS

Route	Onset	Peak	Duration
PO	30–60 min	60–120 min	4–6 hr
IV	Rapid	15–30 min	2–3 hr
IM	40 min	60–120 min	4–6 hr

Completely absorbed from the GI tract (absorption decreased in CHF and nephrotic syndrome). Protein binding: 94%–96%. Partially metabolized in the liver. Primarily excreted in urine. Not removed by hemodialysis. ***Half-life:*** 1–1.5 hr.

AVAILABILITY

Tablets: 0.5 mg, 1 mg, 2 mg.
Injection: 0.25 mg/ml.

INDICATIONS AND DOSAGES

▸ **Edema**

PO

Adults, Children older than 18 yr. 0.5–2 mg as a single dose in the morning. May repeat at q4–5hr.
Elderly. 0.5 mg/day, increased as needed.

IV, IM

Adults, Elderly. 0.5–2 mg/dose; may repeat in 2–3 hr. Or 0.5–1 mg/hr by continuous IV infusion.

▸ **Hypertension**

PO

Adults, Elderly. Initially, 0.5 mg/day. Range: 1–4 mg/day. Maximum: 5 mg/day. Larger doses may be given 2–3 doses/day.

▸ **Usual Pediatric Dosage**

PO, IV, IM

Children. 0.015–0.1 mg/kg/dose q6–24h.

B

OFF-LABEL USES
Treatment of hypercalcemia, hypertension

CONTRAINDICATIONS
Anuria, hepatic coma, severe electrolyte depletion

INTERACTIONS
Drug
Amphotericin B, nephrotoxic and ototoxic medications: May increase the risk of nephrotoxicity and ototoxicity.
Anticoagulants, heparin: May decrease the effects of these drugs.
Lithium: May increase the risk of lithium toxicity.
Other hypokalemia-causing medications: May increase the risk of hypokalemia.
Herbal
None known.
Food
None known.
Drug interactions of concern to dentistry
- Decreased diuretic effect: NSAIDs, indomethacin
- Masked ototoxicity: phenothiazines
- Increased electrolyte imbalance: nondepolarizing skeletal muscle relaxants, corticosteroids

DIAGNOSTIC TEST EFFECTS
May increase blood glucose, BUN, serum uric acid, and urinary phosphate levels. May decrease serum calcium, chloride, magnesium, potassium, and sodium levels.

IV INCOMPATIBILITIES
Midazolam (Versed)
IV COMPATIBILITIES
Aztreonam (Azactam), cefepime (Maxipime), diltiazem (Cardizem), dobutamine (Dobutrex), furosemide (Lasix), lorazepam (Ativan), milrinone (Primacor), morphine, piperacillin and tazobactam (Zosyn), propofol (Diprivan)

SIDE EFFECTS
Expected
Increased urinary frequency and urine volume
Frequent
Orthostatic hypotension, dizziness
Occasional
Blurred vision, diarrhea, headache, anorexia, premature ejaculation, impotence, dyspepsia
Rare
Rash, urticaria, pruritus, asthenia, muscle cramps, nipple tenderness

SERIOUS REACTIONS
! Vigorous diuresis may lead to profound water and electrolyte depletion, resulting in hypokalemia, hyponatremia, dehydration, coma, and circulatory collapse.
! Ototoxicity — manifested as deafness, vertigo, or tinnitus — may occur, especially in patients with severe renal impairment and those taking other ototoxic drugs.
! Blood dyscrasias and acute hypotensive episodes have been reported.

DENTAL CONSIDERATIONS
General:
- Monitor vital signs at every appointment because of cardiovascular side effects.
- Patients on chronic drug therapy may rarely have symptoms of blood dyscrasias, which can include infection, bleeding, and poor healing.
- After supine positioning, have patient sit upright for at least 2 min to avoid orthostatic hypotension.
- Assess salivary flow as a factor in caries, periodontal disease, and candidiasis.
- Limit use of sodium-containing products, such as saline IV fluids, for patients with a dietary salt restriction.

• Patients on high-potency diuretics should be monitored for serum K^+ levels.

Consultations:

• In a patient with symptoms of blood dyscrasias, request a medical consultation for blood studies and postpone dental treatment until normal values are reestablished.

• Medical consultation may be required to assess disease control.

Teach Patient/Family:

• Importance of good oral hygiene to prevent soft tissue inflammation

• Caution to prevent injury when using oral hygiene aids

• *When chronic dry mouth occurs, advise patient:*

  • To avoid mouth rinses with high alcohol content because of drying effects

  • To use daily home fluoride products for anticaries effect

  • To use sugarless gum, frequent sips of water, or saliva substitutes

bupivacaine

byoo-piv′-a-caine
(Marcaine, Marcaine Spinal, Sensorcaine, Sensorcaine-MPF)

CATEGORY AND SCHEDULE

Pregnancy Risk Category: C

MECHANISM OF ACTION

An amide-type anesthetic that stabilizes neuronal membranes and prevents initiation and transmission of nerve impulses, thereby effecting local anesthetic actions. ***Therapeutic Effect:*** Produces local analgesia.

PHARMACOKINETICS

Onset of action occurs within 4–10 minutes depending on route of administration. Duration is 1.5–8.5 hrs. Well absorbed. Protein binding: 95%. Metabolized in liver. Excreted in urine. ***Half-life:*** 1.5–5.5 hrs (Adults), 8.1 hrs. (Neonates)

AVAILABILITY

Injection: 0.25% (Marcaine, Sensorcaine-MPF, 0.5% (Marcaine, Sensorcaine-MPF, 0.75% (Marcaine, Marcaine Spinal, Sensorcaine-MPF).

INDICATIONS AND DOSAGES

Dose varies with procedure, depth of anesthesia, vascularity of tissues, duration of anesthesia and condition of patient.

▸ Analgesic, Epidural (partial to moderate motor blockade)

IV

Adults, Elderly. 10–20 ml (25–50 mg) of a 0.25% solution. Repeat once q3h as needed.

Children more than 10 kg.
1–2.5 mg/kg single dose as a 0.125% or 0.25% solution or 0.2–0.4 mg/kg/hr continuous infusion as a 0.1%, 0.125%, or 0.25% solution. Maximum: 0.4 mg/kg/hr.

Children less than 10 kg.
1–1.25 mg/kg single dose as a 0.125% or 0.25% solution or 0.1–0.2 mg/kg/hr continuous infusion as a 0.1%, 0.125%, or 0.25% solution. Maximum: 0.2 mg/kg/hr.

▸ Analgesic, Epidural (moderate to complete motor blockade)

IV

Adults, Elderly. 10–20 ml (50–100 mg) as a 0.5% solution. Repeat once q3h as needed.

Children more than 10 kg.
1–2.5 mg/kg single dose as a 0.125% or 0.25% solution or 0.2–0.4 mg/kg/hr continuous infusion as a 0.1%, 0.125%, or 0.25% solution. Maximum: 0.4 mg/kg/hr.

Children less than 10 kg.
1–1.25 mg/kg single dose as a

0.125% or 0.25% solution or 0.1–0.2 mg/kg/hr continuous infusion as a 0.1%, 0.125%, or 0.25% solution. Maximum: 0.2 mg/kg/hr.

▸ **Analgesic, Epidural (complete motor blockade)**

IV

Adults. 10–20 ml (75–150 mg) as a 0.75% solution. Repeat once q3h as needed.

Children more than 10 kg. 1–2.5 mg/kg single dose as a 0.125% or 0.25% solution or 0.2–0.4 mg/kg/hr continuous infusion as a 0.1%, 0.125%, or 0.25% solution. Maximum: 0.4 mg/kg/hr.

Children less than 10 kg. 1–1.25 mg/kg single dose as a 0.125% or 0.25% solution or 0.1–0.2 mg/kg/hr continuous infusion as a 0.1%, 0.125%, or 0.25% solution. Maximum: 0.2 mg/kg/hr.

▸ **Analgesic, Intrapleural**

IV

Adults, Elderly. 10–30 ml bolus of 0.25%, 0.375%, or 0.5% q4–8h or 0.375% solution with epinephrine continuous infusion at 6 ml/hr after 20 ml loading dose.

▸ **Analgesic, Caudal (moderate to complete blockade)**

IV

Adults, Elderly. 15–30 mL of 0.5% solution (75–150 mg) OR 0.25% solution (37.5–75 mg), repeated once every 3 hr as needed

Children more than 10 kg. 1–2.5 mg/kg single dose as a 0.125% or 0.25% solution or 0.2–0.4 mg/kg/hr continuous infusion as a 0.1%, 0.125%, or 0.25% solution. Maximum: 0.4 mg/kg/hr.

Children less than 10 kg. 1–1.25 mg/kg single dose as a 0.125% or 0.25% solution or 0.1–0.2 mg/kg/hr continuous infusion as a 0.1%, 0.125%, or 0.25% solution. Maximum: 0.2 mg/kg/hr.

▸ **Analgesic, Dental**

IV

Adults, Elderly. 1.8–3.6 ml of 0.5% solution (9–18 mg) with epinephrine. A second dose of 9 mg may be administered. Maximum: 90 mg total dose.

▸ **Analgesic, Peripheral Nerve Block (moderate to complete motor blockade)**

IV

Adults, Elderly. 5–37.5 ml (25–175 mg) of 0.5% solution or 5–70 ml (12.5–175 mg) of 0.25% solution. Repeat q3h as needed. Maximum: up to 400 mg/day.

Children 12 years and older. 0.3–2.5 mg/kg as a 0.25% or 0.5% solution. Maximum: 1 ml/kg of 0.25% solution or 0.5 ml/kg of 0.5% solution.

▸ **Analgesic, Retrobulbar (complete motor blockade)**

IV

Adults, Elderly. 2–4 ml (15–30 mg) of 0.75% solution.

▸ **Analgesic, Sympathetic blockade**

IV

Adults, Elderly. 20–50 ml (50–125 mg) of 0.25% (no epinephrine) solution. Repeat once q3h as needed.

▸ **Analgesic, Hyperbaric Spinal (obstetrical, normal vaginal delivery)**

IV

Adults, Elderly. 0.8 ml (6 mg) bupivacaine in dextrose as 0.75% solution

▸ **Analgesic, Hyperbaric Spinal (obstetrical, cesarean section)**

IV

Adults, Elderly. 1–1.4 ml (7.5–10.5 mg) bupivacaine in dextrose as 0.75% solution.

▸ **Anesthesia, Hyperbaric Spinal (surgical, lower extremity and**

B

perineal procedures)
IV
Adults, Elderly. 1 ml (7.5 mg) bupivacaine in dextrose as 0.75% solution
Children 12 years and older. 0.3–0.6 mg/kg bupivacaine in dextrose as a 0.75% solution

▸ **Anesthesia, Spinal (surgical, lower abdominal procedures)**
IV
Adults, Elderly. 1.6 ml (12 mg) bupivacaine in dextrose as 0.75% solution.
Children 12 years and older. 0.3–0.6 mg/kg bupivacaine in dextrose as a 0.75% solution

▸ **Anesthesia, Spinal (surgical, hyperbaric, upper abdominal procedures)**
IV
Adults, Elderly. 2 ml (15 mg) bupivacaine in dextrose administered in horizontal position
Children 12 years and older. 0.3–0.6 mg/kg bupivacaine in dextrose as a 0.75% solution

▸ **Analgesic, Local Infiltration**
IV
Adults, Elderly. 0.25% solution. Maximum: 225 mg with epinephrine or 175 mg without epinephrine.
Children 12 years and older. 0.5–2.5 mg/kg as a 0.25% or 0.5% solution. Maximum: 1 ml/kg of 0.25% solution or 0.5 ml/kg of 0.5% solution.

CONTRAINDICATIONS

Local infection at the site of proposed lumbar puncture (spinal anesthesia), obstetrical paracervical block anesthesia, septicemia (spinal anesthesia), severe hemorrhage, severe hypotension or shock, arrhythmias such as complete heart block, which severely restrict cardiac output (spinal anesthesia), sulfite allergy (epinephrine containing solutions only), hypersensitivity to bupivacaine products or to other amide-type anesthetics

INTERACTIONS

Drug

Angiotensin converting enzyme inhibitors: May increase risk of bradycardia and hypotension, as well as loss of consciousness.
Beta-blockers, ergot-type oxytocics, MAO inhibitors, TCAs, phenothiazines, vasopressors: May increase the risk of bupivacaine toxicity.
Cisatracurium, rapacuronium: May increase neuromuscular blocking action.
Hyaluronidase: May increase incidence of systemic reaction to bupivacaine.
Propofol: May increase hypnotic effect of propofol.
Ropivacaine: May prolong effect of intrathecal bupivacaine.
Verapamil: May increase risk of heart block.

Herbal

St. John's Wort: May increase risk of cardiovascular collapse and/or delay emergence from anesthesia.

Food

None known.

Drug interactions of concern to dentistry

- CNS depressants: may see increased risk of CNS depression with all CNS depressants, especially in children and when larger doses are used
- Avoid placing dental cartridges in disinfectant solutions with heavy metals or surface-active agents; may see release of metal ions into local anesthetic solutions, with tissue irritation following injection

B

• Avoid excessive exposure of dental cartridges to light or heat; it hastens deterioration of vasoconstrictor; color change in local anesthetic solution indicates breakdown of vasoconstrictor
• Risk of cardiovascular side effects: rapid intravascular administration of local anesthetic containing vasoconstrictor, either alone or in patients taking tricyclic antidepressants, MAOIs, digitalis drugs, cocaine, phenothiazines, β-blockers, and in the presence of halogenated hydrocarbon general anesthetics; always use the smallest effective vasoconstrictor dose and careful aspiration technique
• Avoid use of vasoconstrictors in patients with uncontrolled hyperthyroidism, diabetes, angina, or hypertension; refer these patients for medical treatment before elective dental procedures

DIAGNOSTIC TEST EFFECTS
None known.

IV INCOMPATIBILITIES
None known.

IV COMPATIBILITIES
Fentanyl, hydromorphone (Dilaudid), morphine

SIDE EFFECTS
Occasional
Hypotension, bradycardia, palpitations, respiratory depression, dizziness, headache, vomiting, nausea, restlessness, weakness, blurred vision, tinnitus, apnea

SERIOUS REACTIONS
! Arterial hypotension, bradycardia, ventricular arrhythmias, central nervous system (CNS) depression and excitation, convulsions, respiratory arrest, tinnitus have been reported.

! Solutions with epinephrine contain metabisulfite, a sulfite that may cause allergic-type reactions, including anaphylaxis.

DENTAL CONSIDERATIONS
General:
• Monitor vital signs at every appointment because of cardiovascular and respiratory side effects.
• Lubricate dry lips before injection or dental treatment as required.

Teach Patient/Family:
• To use care to prevent injury while numbness exists; do not chew gum or eat following dental anesthesia
• That numbness with this drug is expected to last for a considerable period
• To report any signs of infection, muscle pain, or fever to dentist when oral sensations return
• To report any unusual soft tissue reactions

buprenorphine hydrochloride
byoo-pre-nor′-feen

SCHEDULE V
(Buprenex, Subutex, Temgesic[CAN])

CATEGORY AND SCHEDULE
Pregnancy Risk Category: C
Controlled Substance: Schedule V (opioid agonist), III (tablet)

MECHANISM OF ACTION
An opioid agonist-antagonist that binds with opioid receptors in the CNS. ***Therapeutic Effect:*** Alters the perception of and emotional response to pain; blocks

the effects of heroin and produces minimal opioid withdrawal symptoms.

AVAILABILITY

Tablets (Sublingual): 2 mg, 8 mg.
Injection: 0.3 mg/ml.

INDICATIONS AND DOSAGES

▸ Analgesia

IV, IM
Adults, Children older than 12 yr. 0.3 mg q6–8h as needed. May repeat once in 30–60 min. Range: 0.15–0.6 mg q4–8h as needed.
Children 2–12 yr. 2-6 mcg/kg q4–6h as needed.
Elderly. 0.15 mg q6h as needed.

▸ Opioid Dependence

SUBLINGUAL
Adults, Elderly, Children older than 16 yr. Initially, 12–16 mg/day, beginning at least 4 hr after last use of heroin or short-acting opioid. Maintenance: 16 mg/day. Range: 4–24 mg/day. Patients should be switched to buprenorphine and naloxone combination, is preferred for maintenance treatment.

CONTRAINDICATIONS

Hypersensitivity to buprenorphine; hypersensitivity to naloxone for those receiving the fixed combination product containing naloxone (Suboxone)

INTERACTIONS

Drug

CNS depressants, MAOIs: May increase CNS or respiratory depression and hypotension.
Other opioid analgesics: May decrease the effects of other opioid analgesics.

Herbal

Kava kava, St. John's wort, valerian: May increase CNS depression.

Food

None known.

Drug interactions of concern to dentistry

- Increased risk of respiratory and cardiovascular collapse: benzodiazepines
- Increased CNS depression: all CNS depressants, concomitant use of other opioids

DIAGNOSTIC TEST EFFECTS

May increase serum amylase and lipase levels.

SIDE EFFECTS

Frequent

Tablet: Headache, pain, insomnia, anxiety, depression, nausea, abdominal pain, constipation, back pain, weakness, rhinitis, withdrawal syndrome, infection, diaphoresis
Injection (> 10%): Sedation

Occasional

Injection: Hypotension, respiratory depression, dizziness, headache, vomiting, nausea, vertigo

SERIOUS REACTIONS

! Overdose results in cold and clammy skin, weakness, confusion, severe respiratory depression, cyanosis, pinpoint pupils, and extreme somnolence progressing to seizures, stupor, and coma.

DENTAL CONSIDERATIONS

General:

- Patients taking this drug for opioid dependence; avoid the use of any drug with abuse potential.
- Consider aspirin, acetaminophen, or NSAIDs for the management of dental-related pain.

- Monitor vital signs at every appointment because of cardiovascular side effects.
- After supine positioning, have patient sit upright for at least 2 minutes to avoid orthostatic hypotension.
- Assess salivary flow as a factor in caries, periodontal disease, and candidiasis.
- Consider semisupine chair position for patient comfort if GI or respiratory side effects occur.
- Take precautions if dental surgery is anticipated and general anesthesia is required.
- If opioid or sedative drugs are required for patient management and comfort, advise current drug abuse care facility or aftercare program as appropriate.

Consultations:

- Consultations may be difficult to obtain where treatment confidentiality of drug dependence is followed.
- Medical consultation may be required to assess disease control.

Teach Patient/Family:

- Importance of good oral hygiene to prevent soft tissue inflammation.
- *When chronic dry mouth occurs, advise patient:*
  - To avoid mouth rinses with high alcohol content because of drying effects
  - To use daily home fluoride products for anticaries effect
  - To use sugarless gum, frequent sips of water, or saliva substitutes

bupropion

byoo-proe′-pee-on
(Wellbutrin, Wellbutrin SR, Wellbutrin XL, Zyban, Zyban sustained release[AUS])
Do not confuse bupropion with buspirone, Wellbutrin with Wellcovorin or Wellferon, or Zyban with Zagam.

CATEGORY AND SCHEDULE

Pregnancy Risk Category: B

MECHANISM OF ACTION

An aminoketone that blocks the reuptake of neurotransmitters, including serotonin and norepinephrine at CNS presynaptic membranes, increasing their availability at postsynaptic receptor sites. Also reduces the firing rate of noradrenergic neurons. ***Therapeutic Effect:*** Relieves depression and nicotine withdrawal symptoms.

PHARMACOKINETICS

Rapidly absorbed from the GI tract. Protein binding: 84%. Crosses the blood-brain barrier. Undergoes extensive first-pass metabolism in the liver to active metabolite. Primarily excreted in urine. ***Half-life:*** 14 hr.

AVAILABILITY

Tablets (Wellbutrin): 75 mg, 100 mg.
Tablets (Extended-Release [Wellbutrin XL]): 150 mg, 300 mg.
Tablets (Sustained-Release [Wellbutrin SR]): 100 mg, 150 mg, 200 mg.
Tablets (Sustained-Release [Zyban]): 150 mg.

INDICATIONS AND DOSAGES

▸ **Depression**

PO (Immediate-Release)

Adults. Initially, 100 mg twice a day. May increase to 100 mg 3 times a day no sooner than 3 days after beginning therapy. Maximum: 450 mg/day.
Elderly. 37.5 mg twice a day. May increase by 37.5 mg q3–4 days. Maintenance: Lowest effective dosage.
PO (Sustained-Release)
Adults. Initially, 150 mg/day as a single dose in the morning. May increase to 150 mg twice a day as early as day 4 after beginning therapy. Maximum: 400 mg/day.
Elderly. 50–100 mg/day. May increase by 50–100 mg/day q3–4 days. Maintenance: Lowest effective dosage.
PO (Extended-Release)
Adults. 150 mg once a day. May increase to 300 mg once a day. Maximum: 450 mg a day.

▸ **Smoking Cessation**

PO
Adults. Initially, 150 mg a day for 3 days; then 150 mg twice a day for 7–12 wk.

OFF-LABEL USES

Treatment of attention deficit hyperactivity disorder in adults and children

CONTRAINDICATIONS

Current or prior diagnosis of anorexia nervosa or bulimia, seizure disorder, use within 14 days of MAOIs.

INTERACTIONS

Drug

Alcohol, lithium, ritonavir, trazodone, tricyclic antidepressants: May increase the risk of seizures.
MAOIs: May increase the risk of neuroleptic malignant syndrome and acute bupropion toxicity.

Herbal

None known.

Food

None known.

Drug interactions of concern to dentistry

- Increased adverse reactions (seizures): tricyclic antidepressants, phenothiazines, benzodiazepines, alcohol, haloperidol, and trazodone
- Decreased serum levels with carbamazepine
- Inhibits CYP2D6 isoenzymes; use with caution; other drugs metabolized by this enzyme

DIAGNOSTIC TEST EFFECTS

May decrease serum WBC count.

SIDE EFFECTS

Frequent (32%–18%)
Constipation, weight gain or loss, nausea, vomiting, anorexia, dry mouth, headache, diaphoresis, tremor, sedation, insomnia, dizziness, agitation
Occasional (10%–5%)
Diarrhea, akinesia, blurred vision, tachycardia, confusion, hostility, fatigue

SERIOUS REACTIONS

! The risk of seizures increases in patients taking more than 150 mg/dose of bupropion, in patients with a history of bulimia or seizure disorders, and in patients discontinuing drugs that may lower the seizure threshold.

DENTAL CONSIDERATIONS

General:

- Assess salivary flow as a factor in caries, periodontal disease, and candidiasis.
- Short appointments and a stress reduction protocol may be required for anxious patients.

B

- See nicotine dose forms for additional smoking cessation considerations.

Consultations:

- Medical consultation may be required to assess disease control and patient's ability to tolerate stress.
- Physician should be informed if significant xerostomic side effects occur (e.g., increased caries, sore tongue, problems eating or swallowing, difficulty wearing prosthesis) so that a medication change can be considered.

Teach Patient/Family:

- *When chronic dry mouth occurs, advise patient:*
  - To avoid mouth rinses with high alcohol content because of drying effects
  - To use daily home fluoride products for anticaries effect
  - To use sugarless gum, frequent sips of water, or saliva substitutes

buspirone hydrochloride

byoo-spir′-own
(BuSpar, Buspirex[CAN], Bustab[CAN])
Do not confuse buspirone with bupropion.

CATEGORY AND SCHEDULE

Pregnancy Risk Category: B

MECHANISM OF ACTION

Although its exact mechanism of action is unknown, this nonbarbiturate is thought to bind to serotonin and dopamine receptors in the CNS. The drug may also increase norepinephrine metabolism in the locus ceruleus. ***Therapeutic Effect:*** Produces anxiolytic effect.

PHARMACOKINETICS

Rapidly and completely absorbed from the GI tract. Protein binding: 95%. Undergoes extensive first-pass metabolism. Metabolized in the liver to active metabolite. Primarily excreted in urine. Not removed by hemodialysis. ***Half-life:*** 2–3 hr.

AVAILABILITY

Tablets: 5 mg, 7.5 mg, 10 mg, 15 mg, 30 mg.

INDICATIONS AND DOSAGES

▸ Short-Term Management (up to 4 weeks) of Anxiety Disorders

PO

Adults. 5 mg 2–3 times a day or 7.5 mg twice a day. May increase by 5 mg/day every 2–4 days. Maintenance: 15–30 mg/day in 2-3 divided doses. Maximum: 60 mg/day.

Elderly. Initially, 5 mg twice a day. May increase by 5 mg/day every 2-3 days. Maximum: 60 mg/day.

Children. Initially, 5 mg/day. May increase by 5 mg/day at weekly intervals. Maximum: 60 mg/day.

OFF-LABEL USES

Management of panic attack, premenstrual syndrome (aches, pain, fatigue, irritability)

CONTRAINDICATIONS

Concurrent use of MAOIs, severe hepatic or renal impairment

INTERACTIONS

Drug

Alcohol, other CNS depressants: Potentiates effects of buspirone and may increase sedation.

Erythromycin, itraconazole: May increase buspirone blood concentration and risk of toxicity.

MAOIs: May increase BP.

Herbal

Kava kava: May increase sedation.

Food

Grapefruit, grapefruit juice: May increase buspirone blood concentration and risk of toxicity.

Drug interactions of concern to dentistry

- Increased sedation: alcohol, all CNS depressants
- Increased plasma levels: fluconazole, ketoconazole, itraconazole, miconazole, erythromycin, clarithromycin, troleandomycin

DIAGNOSTIC TEST EFFECTS

None known.

SIDE EFFECTS

Frequent (12%–6%)

Dizziness, somnolence, nausea, headache

Occasional (5%–2%)

Nervousness, fatigue, insomnia, dry mouth, lightheadedness, mood swings, blurred vision, poor concentration, diarrhea, paraesthesia

Rare

Muscle pain and stiffness, nightmares, chest pain, involuntary movements

SERIOUS REACTIONS

! Buspirone does not appear to cause drug tolerance, psychological or physical dependence, or withdrawal syndrome.

! Overdose may produce severe nausea, vomiting, dizziness, drowsiness, abdominal distention, and excessive pupil contraction.

DENTAL CONSIDERATIONS

General:

- Monitor vital signs at every appointment because of cardiovascular side effects.
- Assess salivary flow as a factor in caries, periodontal disease, and candidiasis.
- Short appointments and a stress reduction protocol may be required for anxious patients.
- Determine why the patient is taking the drug.

Consultations:

- Medical consultation may be required to assess disease control.

Teach Patient/Family:

- *When chronic dry mouth occurs, advise patient:*
  - To avoid mouth rinses with high alcohol content because of drying effects
  - To use daily home fluoride products for anticaries effect
  - To use sugarless gum, frequent sips of water, or saliva substitutes

busulfan

bew-sull′-fan

(Busulfex, Myleran)

Do not confuse Myleran with Alkeran, Leukeran, or Mylicon.

CATEGORY AND SCHEDULE

Pregnancy Risk Category: D

MECHANISM OF ACTION

An alkylating agent that interferes with DNA replication and RNA synthesis. Cell cycle-phase nonspecific. ***Therapeutic Effect:*** Disrupts nucleic acid function and causes myelosuppression.

PHARMACOKINETICS

Completely absorbed from the GI tract. Protein binding: 33%. Metabolized in the liver. Primarily excreted in urine. Minimally removed by hemodialysis. ***Half-life:*** 2.5 hr.

B

AVAILABILITY

Tablets (Myleran): 2 mg.
Injection solution (Busulfan): 60-mg ampule.

INDICATIONS AND DOSAGES

Remission Induction in Chronic Myelogenous Leukemia (CML)

PO
Adults, Elderly. 4–8 mg/day up to 12 mg/day. Maintenance: 1–4 mg/day to 2 mg/wk. Continue until WBC count is 10,000–20,000/mm^3, resume when WBC count reaches 50,000/mm^3.
Children. 0.06–0.12 mg/kg/day. Maintenance: Titrate to maintain leukocyte count above 40,000/mm^3, reduce dose by 50% if count is 30,000–40,000/mm^3, and discontinue if the count is 20,000/mm^3 or less

Marrow Ablative Conditioning for Bone Marrow Transplantation

IV
Adults, Elderly, Children weighing more than 12 kg. 0.8 mg/kg/dose q6h for total of 16 doses. (Use IBW or ABW, whichever is lower)
Children weighing 12 kg or less. 1.1 mg/kg/dose (IBW) q6h for 16 doses.
PO
Adults, Elderly, Children. 1 mg/kg/dose (IBW) q6h for 16 doses.

OFF-LABEL USES

Treatment of acute myelocytic leukemia

CONTRAINDICATIONS

Disease resistance to previous therapy with this drug

INTERACTIONS

Drug

Antigout medications: May decrease the effects of these drugs.
Bone marrow depressants: May increase the risk of myelosuppression.
Fosphenytoin, phenytoin: May decrease plasma concentrations of busulfan.
Live-virus vaccines: May potentiate virus replication, increase vaccine side effects, and decrease the patient's antibody response to the vaccine.

Herbal

None known.

Food

None known.

Drug interactions of concern to dentistry

- Acetaminophen may reduce clearance if given within 72 hr before busulfan administration

DIAGNOSTIC TEST EFFECTS

May decrease serum magnesium, potassium, phosphates, and sodium levels. May increase blood glucose, BUN, and serum calcium, alkaline phosphatase, bilirubin, creatinine, and ALT levels.

IV INCOMPATIBILITIES

Don't mix busulfan with any other medications.

SIDE EFFECTS

Expected (98%-72%)
Nausea, stomatitis, vomiting, anorexia, insomnia, diarrhea, fever, abdominal pain, anxiety
Frequent (69%-44%)
Headache, rash, asthenia, infection, chills, tachycardia, dyspepsia
Occasional (38%-16%)
Constipation, dizziness, edema, pruritus, cough, dry mouth, depression, abdominal enlargement, pharyngitis, hiccups, back pain, alopecia, myalgia
Rare (13%-5%)
Injection site pain, arthralgia, confusion, hypotension, lethargy

SERIOUS REACTIONS

! Busulfan's major adverse effect is myelosuppression resulting in hematologic toxicity, as evidenced by anemia, severe leukopenia, and severe thrombocytopenia.
! Very high busulfan dosages may produce blurred vision, muscle twitching, and tonic-clonic seizures.
! Long-term therapy (more than 4 years) may produce pulmonary syndrome ("busulfan lung"), characterized by persistent cough, congestion, crackles, and dyspnea.
! Hyperuricemia may produce uric acid nephropathy, renal calculi, and acute renal failure.

DENTAL CONSIDERATIONS

General:

• Patients taking opioids for acute or chronic pain should be given alternative analgesics for dental pain.
• Consider semisupine chair position for patient comfort if GI side effects occur.
• Chlorhexidine mouth rinse (nonalcoholic) before and during chemotherapy may reduce severity of mucositis.
• Patients on chronic drug therapy may rarely have symptoms of blood dyscrasias, which can include infection, bleeding, and poor healing.
• Palliative medication may be required for management of oral side effects.
• Apply lubricant to dry lips for patient comfort before dental procedures.
• Assess salivary flow as factor in caries, periodontal disease, and candidiasis.
• Patients in active chemotherapy treatment should have adequate white blood cell (WBC) count before completing dental procedures that may produce a wound. Consultation with the oncologist may be required to determine WBC counts before treatment.

Consultations:

• Medical consultation may be required to assess disease control and patient's ability to tolerate stress.
• In a patient with symptoms of blood dyscrasias, request a medical consultation for blood studies and postpone dental treatment until normal values are reestablished.
• Consult oncologist; prophylactic or therapeutic antibiotics may be indicated to prevent or treat infection if surgery or deep scaling is planned.

Teach Patient/Family:

• Importance of good oral hygiene to prevent soft tissue inflammation
• To prevent trauma when using oral hygiene aids
• To report oral lesions, soreness, or bleeding to dentist
• That secondary oral infection may occur; must see dentist immediately if infection occurs
• Importance of updating medical/drug record if physician makes any changes in evaluation or drug regimen
• *When chronic dry mouth occurs, advise patient:*
  • To avoid mouth rinses with high alcohol content because of drying effects
  • To use daily home fluoride products for anticaries effect
  • To use sugarless gum, frequent sips of water, or artificial saliva substitutes

B

butabarbital sodium

byoo-tah-**bar**-bi-tal
(Butisol)

CATEGORY AND SCHEDULE

Pregnancy Risk Category: D
Controlled Substance: Schedule III

MECHANISM OF ACTION

A barbiturate and nonselective CNS depressant that binds at GABA receptor complex, enhancing GABA activity. ***Therapeutic Effect:*** Produces hypnotic effect due to CNS depression.

PHARMACOKINETICS

Widely distributed. Metabolized in liver. Minimally excreted unchanged in urine. ***Half-life:*** 34–100 hr.

AVAILABILITY

Tablets: 30 mg, 50 mg (Butisol).
Elixir: 30 mg/5 ml (Butisol).

INDICATIONS AND DOSAGES

▸ Insomnia, Short-Term

PO
Adults. 50–100 mg at bedtime.

▸ Preoperative Sedation

PO
Adults. 50–100 mg, 60–90 min before surgery.
Children. 2–6 mg/kg. Maximum: 100 mg.

▸ Sedation, Daytime

PO
Adults. 15–30 mg 3–4 times/day.

CONTRAINDICATIONS

Porphyria, barbiturate sensitivity

INTERACTIONS

Drug

Alcohol, CNS depressants: May increase the effects of butabarbital.
Doxycycline, estradiol, glucocorticoids, griseofulvin, metronidazole, oral anticoagulants, quinidine, tricyclic antidepressants: May decrease the effects of doxycycline, estradiol, glucocorticoids, griseofulvin, metronidazole, oral anticoagulants, quinidine, tricyclic antidepressants.
MAOIs: May prolong the effects of butabarbital.
Valproic acid: Decreases the metabolism and increases the concentration and risk of toxicity of butabarbital.

Herbal

None known.

Food

None known.

Drug interactions of concern to dentistry

- Nephrotoxicity and/or hepatotoxicity: halogenated hydrocarbon anesthetics
- Increased CNS depression: alcohol and all other CNS depressants
- Increased metabolism of: oral anticoagulants, glucocorticoids, carbamazepine, tricyclic antidepressants

DIAGNOSTIC TEST EFFECTS

None known.

SIDE EFFECTS

Occasional

Somnolence

Rare

Confusion, dizziness, agitation, nausea, vomiting, constipation, headache, hypotension, acnes

SERIOUS REACTIONS

! Skin eruptions appear as hypersensitivity reaction.
! Blood dyscrasias, liver disease, and hypocalcemia occur rarely.

DENTAL CONSIDERATIONS

General:

- Determine why patient is taking the drug.

- Monitor vital signs at every appointment due to cardiovascular side effects.
- Patient on chronic drug therapy may rarely present with symptoms of blood dyscrasias, which can include infection, bleeding and poor healing. If dyscrasia is present, caution patient to prevent oral tissue trauma when using oral hygiene aids.
- *When used for sedation in dentistry:*
  - Have responsible person drive patient to and from dental office when drug used for conscious sedation.
  - After supine positioning, have patient sit upright for at least 2 min before standing to avoid orthostatic hypotension.
  - Geriatric patients are more susceptible to drug effects, use lower dose.
  - Barbiturates induce certain liver enzymes that can alter the metabolism of other drugs (see drug interactions).

Consultations:

- In a patient with symptoms of blood dyscrasias, request a medical consultation for blood studies and postpone treatment until normal values are reestablished.

Teach Patient/Family:

- To avoid driving or other activities requiring mental alertness
- To avoid alcohol ingestion or CNS depressants; serious CNS depression may result
- To avoid OTC preparations that contain CNS depressants (antihistamine, cold remedies)
- Importance of updating health and medication history if physician makes any changes in evaluation or drug regimens; include OTC, herbal, and nonherbal remedies in the update

butenafine

byoo-ten′-a-feen
(Mentax)

CATEGORY AND SCHEDULE

Pregnancy Risk Category: B

MECHANISM OF ACTION

An antifungal agent that locks biosynthesis of ergosterol, essential for fungal cell membrane. Fungicidal. ***Therapeutic Effect:*** Relieves athlete's foot.

PHARMACOKINETICS

Total amount absorbed into systemic circulation has not been determined. Metabolized in liver. Excreted in urine. ***Half-life:*** 35 hrs.

AVAILABILITY

Cream: 1% (Mentax).

INDICATIONS AND DOSAGES

▸ Tinea Pedis, Tinea Corporis, Tinea Cruris, Tinea Versicolor

TOPICAL

Adults, Elderly, Children 12 yrs and older. Apply to affected area and immediate surrounding skin daily for 4 wks.

OFF-LABEL USES

Onychomycosis, seborrheic dermatitis

CONTRAINDICATIONS

Hypersensitivity to butenafine or any component of the formulation

INTERACTIONS

Drug

None known.

Herbal

None known.

Food

None known.

B

Drug interactions of concern to dentistry
- None reported

DIAGNOSTIC TEST EFFECTS
None known.

SIDE EFFECTS
Occasional (2%)
Contact dermatitis, burning/stinging, worsening of the condition
Rare (< 2%)
Erythema, irritation, pruritus

SERIOUS REACTIONS
! None known.

butoconazole
byoo-toe-ko′-na-zole
(Gynazole-1, Femstat One[CAN])Mycelex-32%

CATEGORY AND SCHEDULE
Pregnancy Risk Category: C

MECHANISM OF ACTION
An antifungal similar to imidazole derivatives that inhibits the steroid synthesis, a vital component of fungal cell formation, thereby damaging the fungal cell membrane.
Therapeutic Effect: Fungistatic.

PHARMACOKINETICS
Not known.

AVAILABILITY
Cream: 2% (Mycelex-3, OTC)
Cream: 2% (Gynazole-1, prefilled applicator)

INDICATIONS AND DOSAGES
▸ Treatment of Candidiasis
TOPICAL
Adults, Elderly. Insert 1 applicatorful intravaginally at bedtime for up to 3 or 6 days.

CONTRAINDICATIONS
Hypersensitivity to butoconazole or any of its components

INTERACTIONS
Drug
Not known.
Herbal
Not known.
Food
Not known.

SIDE EFFECTS
Occasional
Vaginal itching, burning, irritation

SERIOUS REACTIONS
! Soreness, swelling, pelvic pain, or cramping rarely occurs.

DENTAL CONSIDERATIONS
General:
- Examine oral mucous membranes for signs of yeast infection.
- Broad-spectrum antibiotics for dental infections may cause vaginal yeast infection.

butorphanol tartrate
byoo-tor′-fa-nole

SCHEDULE IV
(Stadol, Stadol NS)
Do not confuse butorphanol with butabarbital or Stadol with Haldol.

CATEGORY AND SCHEDULE
Pregnancy Risk Category: C, D if used for prolonged time, high dose at term
Controlled Substance: Schedule IV

MECHANISM OF ACTION
An opioid that binds to opiate receptor sites in the CNS.

Reduces intensity of pain stimuli incoming from sensory nerve endings. ***Therapeutic Effect:*** Alters pain perception and emotional response to pain.

PHARMACOKINETICS

Route	Onset	Peak	Duration
IM	10–30 min	30–60 min	3–4 hr
IV	less than 1 min	30 min	2–4 hr
Nasal	15 min	1–2 hr	4–5 hr

Rapidly absorbed after IM injection. Protein binding: 80%. Extensively metabolized in the liver. Primarily excreted in urine. ***Half-life:*** 2.5–4 hr.

AVAILABILITY

Injection: 1 mg/ml, 2 mg/ml.
Nasal Spray: 10 mg/ml.

INDICATIONS AND DOSAGES

▸ Analgesia

IV
Adults. 0.5–2 mg q3–4h as needed.
Elderly. 1 mg q4–6h as needed.
IM
Adults. 1–4 mg q3–4h as needed.
Elderly. 1 mg q4–6h as needed.

▸ Migraine

NASAL
Adults. 1 mg or 1 spray in one nostril. May repeat in 60–90 min. May repeat 2-dose sequence q3–4h as needed. Alternatively, 2 mg or 1 spray each nostril if patient remains recumbent, may repeat in 3–4 hrs.

CONTRAINDICATIONS

CNS disease that affects respirations, physical dependence on other opioid analgesics, preexisting respiratory depression, pulmonary disease

INTERACTIONS

Drug

Alcohol, CNS depressants: May increase CNS or respiratory depression and hypotension.
Buprenorphine: Effects may be decreased with buprenorphine.
MAOIs: May produce severe, fatal reaction unless dose is reduced by one-fourth.

Herbal

None known.

Food

None known.

Drug interactions of concern to dentistry

- Increased CNS depression: alcohol and all CNS depressants
- Decreased effects of: buprenorphine
- Use caution or avoid use in patients taking MAOIs
- Avoid use in narcotic-dependent persons
- Possible decrease in effects: drugs that induce CYP3A4 isoenzymes (phenobarbital, carbamazepine)
- Possible increase in effects: drugs that inhibit CYP3A4 isoenzymes (ketoconazole, itraconazole, erythromycin, protease inhibitors)

DIAGNOSTIC TEST EFFECTS

None known.

IV INCOMPATIBILITIES

Amphotericin B complex (Abelcet, AmBisome, Amphotec)

IV COMPATIBILITIES

Atropine, diphenhydramine (Benadryl), droperidol (Inapsine), hydroxyzine (Vistaril), morphine, promethazine (Phenergan), propofol (Diprivan)

SIDE EFFECTS

Frequent

Parenteral: Somnolence (43%), dizziness (19%)

Nasal: Nasal congestion (13%), insomnia (11%)

Occasional

Parenteral (3%–9%): Confusion, diaphoresis, clammy skin, lethargy, headache, nausea, vomiting, dry mouth

Nasal (3%–9%): Vasodilation, constipation, unpleasant taste, dyspnea, epistaxis, nasal irritation, upper respiratory tract infection, tinnitus

Rare

Parenteral: Hypotension, pruritus, blurred vision, sensation of heat, CNS stimulation, insomnia

Nasal: Hypertension, tremor, ear pain, paresthesia, depression, sinusitis

SERIOUS REACTIONS

! Abrupt withdrawal after prolonged use may produce symptoms of narcotic withdrawal, such as abdominal cramping, rhinorrhea, lacrimation, anxiety, increased temperature, and piloerection or goose bumps.

! Overdose results in severe respiratory depression, skeletal muscle flaccidity, cyanosis, and extreme somnolence progressing to seizures, stupor, and coma.

! Tolerance to analgesic effect and physical dependence may occur with chronic use.

DENTAL CONSIDERATIONS

General:

- Monitor vital signs at every appointment due to cardiovascular side effects.
- This is an acute-use drug, it is doubtful that patients will undergo dental treatment during severe migraine attacks.
- After supine positioning, have patient sit upright for at least 2 min before standing to avoid orthostatic hypotension.
- Psychologic and physical dependence may occur with chronic administration.
- Determine why patient is taking the drug.
- If additional analgesia is required for dental pain, consider alternative analgesics (NSAIDs) in patients taking narcotics for acute or chronic pain.

Teach Patient/Family:

- To avoid driving or other activities requiring mental alertness
- To avoid alcohol ingestion or CNS depressants; serious CNS depression may result
- To avoid OTC preparations that contain CNS depressants (antihistamine, cold remedies)
- Importance of updating health and medication history if physician makes any changes in evaluation or drug regimens; include OTC, herbal, and nonherbal remedies in the update

cabergoline

cab-err-go′-leen
(Dostinex)

CATEGORY AND SCHEDULE

Pregnancy Risk Category: B

MECHANISM OF ACTION

Agonist at dopamine D2 receptors suppressing prolactin secretion. ***Therapeutic effects:*** Shrinks prolactinomas, restores gonadal function.

PHARMACOKINETICS

Cabergoline is administered orally and undergoes significant first-pass metabolism following systemic absorption. Extensively metabolized in the liver. Elimination is primarily in the feces. ***Half-life:*** 80 hrs.

AVAILABILITY

Tablet: 0.5 mg

INDICATIONS AND DOSAGES

▸ **Hyperprolactemia (Idiopathic or Primary Pituitary Adenomas)**

PO

Adults, elderly. 0.25 mg 2 times per week, titrate by 0.25 mg/dose no more than every 4 weeks up to 1 mg 2 times per week

PV

Adults. 0.5 mg 2 to five times per week

▸ **Parkinson's Disease**

PO

Adults. 0.5 mg/day and titrate to response. Mean effective dose is 3 mg/day and ranges from 0.5 – 6 mg/day.

▸ **Restless Legs Syndrome (RLS)**

PO

Adults. 0.5 mg once daily at bedtime, slowly titrate until symptoms resolve or drug-intolerance limits further adjustment. Mean effective dose is 2 mg/day and ranges from 1–4 mg/day.

OFF-LABEL USES

Parkinson's disease, restless legs syndrome (RLS)

CONTRAINDICATIONS

Hypersensitivity to cabergoline, ergot alkaloids or any one of its components.
Uncontrolled hypertension.

INTERACTIONS

Drug

Antihypertensives: May increase hypotensive effect.
Cimetidine, haloperidol, loxapine, MAOIs, methyldopa, metoclopramide, molindone, olanzapine, phenothiazines, pimozide, reserpine, risperidone, thiothixene, tricyclic antidepressants: Antagonizes the prolactin-lowering effect of cabergoline.
Antipsychotics, phenothiazine-type antiemetics: Cabergoline may diminish the effects of these dopamine agonists.
Levodopa: Additive neurologic effects are possible.
Ergot alkaloids: May lead to ergot toxicity.
Anti-retroviral drugs: May lead to ergot toxicity.
Imatinib: May increase the risk of ergot-related side effects.

Herbal

None known.

Food

None known.

Drug interactions of concern to dentistry

- None reported

C

DIAGNOSTIC TEST EFFECTS

None known.

SIDE EFFECTS

Frequent

Nausea, orthostatic hypotension, confusion, dyskinesia, hallucinations, peripheral edema

Occasional

Headache, vertigo, dizziness, dyspepsia, postural hypotension, constipation, asthenia, fatigue, abdominal pain, drowsiness

Rare

Vomiting, dry mouth, diarrhea, flatulence, anxiety, depression, dysmenorrheal, dyspepsia, mastalgia, paresthesias, vertigo, visual impairment, pleuropulmonary changes, pleural effusion, pulmonary fibrosis, heart failure, peptic ulcer

SERIOUS REACTIONS

! Overdosage may produce nasal congestion, syncope, or hallucinations.

DENTAL CONSIDERATIONS

General:

- Determine why patient is taking the drug.
- Monitor vital signs at every appointment due to cardiovascular side effects.
- After supine positioning, have patient sit upright for at least 2 min before standing to avoid orthostatic hypotension.
- Use precaution if sedation or general anesthesia is required; risk of hypotensive episode.
- Assess salivary flow as a factor in caries, periodontal disease, and candidiasis.
- Consider semisupine chair position for patient comfort if GI side effects occur.

Consultations:

- Medical consultation may be required to assess disease control.

Teach Patient/Family:

- *When chronic dry mouth occurs advise patient:*
  - To avoid mouth rinses with high alcohol content due to drying effects
  - To use daily home fluoride products for anticaries effect
  - To use sugarless gum, frequent sips of water or saliva substitutes
- Importance of updating health and medication history if physician makes any changes in evaluation or drug regimens; include OTC, herbal, and nonherbal remedies in the update

calcitonin

kal-si-toe′-nin

(Calcimar, Caltine[CAN], Cibacalcin, Miacalcin)

Do not confuse calcitonin with calcitriol.

CATEGORY AND SCHEDULE

Pregnancy Risk Category: C

MECHANISM OF ACTION

A synthetic hormone that decreases osteoclast activity in bones, decreases tubular reabsorption of sodium and calcium in the kidneys, and increases absorption of calcium in the GI tract. ***Therapeutic Effect:*** Regulates serum calcium concentrations.

PHARMACOKINETICS

Injection form rapidly metabolized (primarily in kidneys); primarily excreted in urine. Nasal form rapidly absorbed. ***Half-life:*** 70–90 min (injection); 43 min (nasal).

AVAILABILITY

Injection: 200 international units/ml (calcitonin-salmon), 500 mg (calcitonin-human).

Nasal Spray: 200 international units/activation (calcitonin-salmon).

INDICATIONS AND DOSAGES

▸ Skin Testing Before Treatment in Patients with Suspected Sensitivity to Calcitonin-Salmon

INTRACUTANEOUS

Adults, Elderly. Prepare a 10-international units/ml dilution; withdraw 0.05 ml from a 200-international units/ml vial in a tuberculin syringe; fill up to 1 ml with 0.9% NaCl. Take 0.1 ml and inject intracutaneously on inner aspect of forearm. Observe after 15 min; a positive response is the appearance of more than mild erythema or wheal.

▸ Paget's Disease

IM, SUBCUTANEOUS

Adults, Elderly. Initially, 100 international units/day. Maintenance: 50 international units/day or 50–100 international units every 1–3 days.

INTRANASAL

Adults, Elderly. 200–400 international units/day.

▸ Osteoporosis Imperfecta

IM, SUBCUTANEOUS

Adults. 2 international units/kg 3 times a week.

▸ Postmenopausal Osteoporosis

IM, SUBCUTANEOUS

Adults, Elderly. 100 international units/day with adequate calcium and vitamin D intake.

INTRANASAL

Adults, Elderly. 200 international units/day as a single spray, alternating nostrils daily.

▸ Hypercalcemia

IM, SUBCUTANEOUS

Adults, Elderly. Initially, 4 international units/kg q12h; may increase to 8 international units/kg q12h if no response in 2 days; may further increase to 8 international units/kg q6h if no response in another 2 days.

OFF-LABEL USES

Treatment of secondary osteoporosis due to drug therapy or hormone disturbance

CONTRAINDICATIONS

Hypersensitivity to gelatin desserts or salmon protein

INTERACTIONS

Drug

None known.

Herbal

None known.

Food

None known.

Drug interactions of concern to dentistry

- Supplemental calcium and vitamin D may already be used; do not use additional amounts

DIAGNOSTIC TEST EFFECTS

None known.

SIDE EFFECTS

Frequent

IM, Subcutaneous (10%): Nausea (may occur 30 min after injection, usually diminishes with continued therapy), inflammation at injection site

Nasal (12%–10%): Rhinitis, nasal irritation, redness, sores

Occasional

IM, Subcutaneous (5%–2%): Flushing of face or hands

Nasal (5%–3%): Back pain, arthralgia, epistaxis, headache

Rare

IM, Subcutaneous: Epigastric discomfort, dry mouth, diarrhea, flatulence

Nasal: Itching of earlobes, edema of feet, rash, diaphoresis

SERIOUS REACTIONS

! Patients with a protein allergy may develop a hypersensitivity reaction.

C

DENTAL CONSIDERATIONS

General:

- Consider semisupine chair position for patient comfort because of effects of disease or if GI side effects occur.
- Assess salivary flow as factor in caries, periodontal disease, and candidiasis.

Teach Patient/Family:

- Importance of good oral hygiene to prevent soft tissue inflammation
- *When chronic dry mouth occurs, advise patient:*
  - To avoid mouth rinses with high alcohol content because of drying effects
  - To use daily home fluoride products for anticaries effect
  - To use sugarless gum, frequent sips of water, or saliva substitutes

candesartan cilexetil

kan-de-sar′-tan
(Atacand)

CATEGORY AND SCHEDULE

Pregnancy Risk Category: C (D if used in second or third trimester)

MECHANISM OF ACTION

An angiotensin II receptor, type AT_1, antagonist that blocks the vasoconstrictor and aldosterone-secreting effects of angiotensin II, inhibiting the binding of angiotensin II to the AT_1 receptors. ***Therapeutic Effect:*** Causes vasodilation, decreases peripheral resistance, and decreases BP.

PHARMACOKINETICS

Route	Onset	Peak	Duration
PO	2–3 hr	6–8 hr	Greater than 24 hr

Rapidly, completely absorbed. Protein binding: greater than 99%. Undergoes minor hepatic metabolism to inactive metabolite. Excreted unchanged in urine and in the feces through the biliary system. Not removed by hemodialysis.
Half-life: 9 hr.

AVAILABILITY

Tablets: 4 mg, 8 mg, 16 mg, 32 mg.

INDICATIONS AND DOSAGES

▶ Hypertension Alone or in Combination with Other Antihypertensives

PO

Adults, Elderly, Patients with mildly impaired liver or renal function. Initially, 16 mg once a day in those who are not volume depleted. Can be given once or twice a day with total daily doses of 8–32 mg. Give lower dosage in those treated with diuretics or with severely impaired renal function.

OFF-LABEL USES

Treatment of heart failure

CONTRAINDICATIONS

Hypersensitivity to candesartan

INTERACTIONS

Drug

None known.

Herbal

None known.

Food

None known.

Drug interactions of concern to dentistry

- Potential for increased hypotensive effects with other hypotensive and sedative drugs

DIAGNOSTIC TEST EFFECTS

May increase BUN, serum alkaline phosphatase, serum bilirubin, serum creatinine, AST (SGOT), and ALT(SGPT) levels. May decrease blood Hgb and Hct levels.

SIDE EFFECTS

Occasional (6%–3%)
Upper respiratory tract infection, dizziness, back and leg pain
Rare (2%–1%)
Pharyngitis, rhinitis, headache, fatigue, diarrhea, nausea, dry cough, peripheral edema

SERIOUS REACTIONS

! Overdosage may manifest as hypotension and tachycardia. Bradycardia occurs less often. Institute supportive measures.

DENTAL CONSIDERATIONS

General:

- Monitor vital signs at every appointment in patients with history of hypertension.
- Evaluate respiration characteristics and rate.
- Consider semisupine chair position for patient comfort if GI side effects occur.
- Limit use of sodium-containing products, such as saline IV fluids, for those patients with a dietary salt restriction.
- Stress from dental procedures may compromise cardiovascular function; determine patient risk.
- Short appointments and a stress reduction protocol may be required for anxious patients.
- Use precaution if sedation or general anesthesia is required; risk of hypotensive episode.

Consultations:

- Medical consultation may be required to assess disease control and patient's ability to tolerate stress.

Teach Patient/Family:

- Importance of updating health and drug history if physician makes any changes in evaluation or drug regimens

capecitabine

cap-eh-site′-ah-bean
(Xeloda)
Do not confuse Xeloda with Xenical.

CATEGORY AND SCHEDULE

Pregnancy Risk Category: D

MECHANISM OF ACTION

An antimetabolite that is enzymatically converted to 5-fluorouracil. Inhibits enzymes necessary for synthesis of essential cellular components. ***Therapeutic Effect:*** Interferes with DNA synthesis, RNA processing, and protein synthesis.

PHARMACOKINETICS

Readily absorbed from the GI tract. Protein binding: less than 60%. Metabolized in the liver. Primarily excreted in urine. ***Half-life:*** 45 min.

AVAILABILITY

Tablets: 150 mg, 500 mg.

C

INDICATIONS AND DOSAGES

▸ **Metastatic Breast Cancer, Colon Cancer**

PO

Adults, Elderly. Initially, 2,500 mg/m^2/day in 2 equally divided doses approximately q12h for 2 wk. Follow with a 1-wk rest period; given in 3-wk cycles.

CONTRAINDICATIONS

Severe renal impairment

INTERACTIONS

Drug

Warfarin: May alter the effects of warfarin.

Herbal

None known.

Food

None known.

Drug interactions of concern to dentistry

• Dental drug interactions not reported; however, patients taking this drug with coumarin oral anticoagulants have altered coagulation parameters, bleeding, or both; INR or PT should be physician monitored

DIAGNOSTIC TEST EFFECTS

May increase serum alkaline phosphatase, bilirubin, AST (SGOT), and ALT (SGPT) levels. May decrease blood Hct, Hgb level, and WBC count.

SIDE EFFECTS

Frequent (> 5%)

Diarrhea (sometimes severe), nausea, vomiting, stomatitis, hand-and-foot syndrome (painful palmar-plantar swelling with paresthesia, erythema, and blistering), fatigue, anorexia, dermatitis

Occasional (< 5%)

Constipation, dyspepsia, nail disorder, headache, dizziness, insomnia, edema, myalgia

SERIOUS REACTIONS

! Serious reactions may include myelosuppression (evidenced by neutropenia, thrombocytopenia, and anemia), cardiovascular toxicity (marked by angina, cardiomyopathy, and deep vein thrombosis), respiratory toxicity (marked by dyspnea, epistaxis, and pneumonia), and lymphedema.

DENTAL CONSIDERATIONS

General:

• Monitor vital signs at every appointment because of cardiovascular side effects.

• Patients on chronic drug therapy may have symptoms of blood dyscrasias, which can include infection, bleeding, and poor healing.

• Patients taking opioids for acute or chronic pain should be given alternative analgesics for dental pain.

• Short appointments and a stress reduction protocol may be required for anxious patients.

• Consider semisupine chair position for patient comfort if GI side effects occur.

• Question patient about tolerance of NSAIDs or aspirin related to GI side effects of drug.

• Consider local hemostasis measures to control and prevent excessive bleeding.

• Examine for oral manifestation of opportunistic infection.

• Be aware of oral side effects and potential sequelae.

• Palliative medication may be required for management of oral side effects.

- Avoid dental light in patient's eyes; offer dark glasses for patient comfort.
- Prophylactic or therapeutic antibiotics may be indicated to prevent or treat infection if surgery or periodontal debridement is required.

Consultations:
- In a patient with symptoms of blood dyscrasias, request a medical consultation for blood studies and postpone treatment until normal values are reestablished.
- Medical consultation may be required to assess disease control and patient's ability to receive dental treatment.
- Consultation with physician may be necessary if sedation or general anesthesia is required.

Teach Patient/Family:
- To prevent trauma when using oral hygiene aids
- That secondary oral infection may occur; need to see dentist immediately if infection occurs
- Importance of good oral hygiene to prevent soft tissue inflammation
- To report oral lesions, soreness, or bleeding to dentist
- Importance of updating health and drug history if physician makes any changes in evaluation or drug regimens

capsaicin
cap-say′-sin
(Zostrix)
Do not confuse with Zovirax.

CATEGORY AND SCHEDULE
Pregnancy Risk Category: C
OTC

MECHANISM OF ACTION
A topical analgesic that depletes and prevents reaccumulation of the chemomediator of pain impulses (substance P) from peripheral sensory neurons to CNS.
Therapeutic Effect: Relieves pain.

PHARMACOKINETICS
None reported.

AVAILABILITY
Cream: 0.025%, 0.075% (Zostrix).

INDICATIONS AND DOSAGES
▸ **Treatment of Neuralgia, Osteoarthritis, Rheumatoid Arthritis**
TOPICAL
Adults, Elderly, Children older than 2 yrs. Apply directly to affected area 3–4 times/day. Continue for 14 to 28 days for optimal clinical response.

OFF-LABEL USES
Treatment of neurogenic pain

CONTRAINDICATIONS
Hypersensitivity to capsaicin or any component of the formulation

INTERACTIONS
Drug
Anticoagulants, antiplatelet agents, low molecular weight heparins, thrombolytic agents: May increase risk of bleeding.
Herbal
None known.
Food
None known.
Drug interactions of concern to dentistry
- None reported

DIAGNOSTIC TEST EFFECTS
None known.

C

SIDE EFFECTS

Frequent

Burning, stinging, erythema at site of application

SERIOUS REACTIONS

! None known.

DENTAL CONSIDERATIONS

General:

- Determine why the patient is taking the drug.
- Consider location of lesions and alter dental procedures accordingly.

Teach Patient/Family:

- To wash hands thoroughly after use and avoid contact with mouth or eyes

captopril

cap′-toe-pril

(Acenorm[AUS], Capoten, Captohexal[AUS], Novo-Captoril[CAN], Topace[AUS])

Do not confuse captopril with Capitrol.

CATEGORY AND SCHEDULE

Pregnancy Risk Category: C (D if used in second or third trimester)

MECHANISM OF ACTION

An ACE inhibitor that suppresses the renin-angiotensin-aldosterone system and prevents conversion of angiotensin I to angiotensin II, a potent vasoconstrictor; may also inhibit angiotensin II at local vascular and renal sites. Decreases plasma angiotensin II, increases plasma renin activity, and decreases aldosterone secretion. ***Therapeutic Effect:*** Reduces peripheral arterial resistance, pulmonary capillary wedge pressure; improves cardiac output and exercise tolerance.

PHARMACOKINETICS

Route	Onset	Peak	Duration
PO	0.25 hr	0.5–1.5 hr	Dose-related

Rapidly, well absorbed from the GI tract (absorption is decreased in the presence of food). Protein binding: 25%–30%. Metabolized in the liver. Primarily excreted in urine. Removed by hemodialysis. ***Half-life:*** less than 3 hr (increased in those with impaired renal function).

AVAILABILITY

Tablets: 12.5 mg, 25 mg, 50 mg, 100 mg.

INDICATIONS AND DOSAGES

▸ **Hypertension**

PO

Adults, Elderly. Initially, 12.5–25 mg 2–3 times a day. After 1–2 wk, may increase to 50 mg 2–3 times a day. Diuretic may be added if no response in additional 1–2 wk. If taken in combination with diuretic, may increase to 100–150 mg 2–3 times a day after 1–2 wk. Maintenance: 25–150 mg 2–3 times a day. Maximum: 450 mg/day.

▸ **CHF**

PO

Adults, Elderly. Initially, 6.25–25 mg 3 times a day. Increase to 50 mg 3 times a day. After at least 2 wk, may increase to 50–100 mg 3 times a day. Maximum: 450 mg/day.

▸ **Post-Myocardial Infarction, Impaired Liver Function**

PO

Adults, Elderly. 6.25 mg a day, then 12.5 mg 3 times a day. Increase to 25 mg 3 times a day over several days up to 50 mg 3 times a day over several weeks.

▸ Diabetic Nephropathy Prevention of Kidney Failure
PO
Adults, Elderly. 25 mg 3 times a day.
Children. Initially 0.3–0.5 mg/kg/dose titrated up to a maximum of 6 mg/kg/day in 2–4 divided doses.
Neonates. Initially, 0.05–0.1 mg/kg/dose q8–24h titrated up to 0.5 mg/kg/dose given q6–24h.

▸ Dosage in Renal Impairment
Creatinine clearance 10–50 ml/min. 75% of normal dosage.
Creatinine clearance less than 10 ml/min. 50% of normal dosage.

OFF-LABEL USES
Diagnosis of anatomic renal artery stenosis, hypertensive crisis, rheumatoid arthritis

CONTRAINDICATIONS
History of angioedema from previous treatment with ACE inhibitors

INTERACTIONS
Drug
Alcohol, antihypertensives, diuretics: May increase the effects of captopril.
Lithium: May increase lithium blood concentration and risk of lithium toxicity.
NSAIDs: May decrease the effects of captopril.
Potassium-sparing diuretics, potassium supplements: May cause hyperkalemia.
Herbal
None known.
Food
All food: Food significantly reduces drug absorption by 30% to 40%.
Drug interactions of concern to dentistry
- Increased hypotension: alcohol, phenothiazines
- Decreased hypotensive effects: indomethacin and possibly other NSAIDs, sympathomimetics
- Suspected reduction in the antihypertensive and vasodilator effects by salicylates; monitor blood pressure if used concurrently

DIAGNOSTIC TEST EFFECTS
May increase BUN, serum alkaline phosphatase, serum bilirubin, serum creatinine, serum potassium, AST (SGOT), and ALT(SGPT) levels. May decrease serum sodium levels. May cause positive antinuclear antibody titer.

SIDE EFFECTS
Frequent (7%–4%)
Rash
Occasional (4%–2%)
Pruritus, dysgeusia (altered taste)
Rare (< 2%–0.5%)
Headache, cough, insomnia, dizziness, fatigue, paraesthesia, malaise, nausea, diarrhea or constipation, dry mouth, tachycardia

SERIOUS REACTIONS
! Excessive hypotension (“first-dose syncope”) may occur in patients with CHF and in those who are severely salt and volume depleted.
! Angioedema (swelling of face and lips) and hyperkalemia occur rarely.
! Agranulocytosis and neutropenia may be noted in those with collagen vascular disease, including scleroderma and systemic lupus erythematosus, and impaired renal function.
! Nephrotic syndrome may be noted in those with history of renal disease.

DENTAL CONSIDERATIONS
General:
- Monitor vital signs at every appointment because of cardiovascular side effects.

• After supine positioning, have patient sit upright for at least 2 min before standing to avoid orthostatic hypotension.
• Patients on chronic drug therapy may rarely have symptoms of blood dyscrasias, which can include infection, bleeding, and poor healing.
• Assess salivary flow as a factor in caries, periodontal disease, and candidiasis.
• Limit use of sodium-containing products, such as saline IV fluids, for patients with a dietary salt restriction.
• Stress from dental procedures may compromise cardiovascular function; determine patient risk.
• Short appointments and a stress reduction protocol may be required for anxious patients.

Consultations:
• Medical consultation may be required to assess patient's ability to tolerate stress.
• In a patient with symptoms of blood dyscrasias, request a medical consultation for blood studies and postpone dental treatment until normal values are reestablished.
• Take precautions if dental surgery is anticipated and sedation or general anesthesia is required; risk of hypotensive episode.

Teach Patient/Family:
• Importance of good oral hygiene to prevent soft tissue inflammation
• Caution to prevent injury when using oral hygiene aids
• *When chronic dry mouth occurs, advise patient:*
  • To avoid mouth rinses with high alcohol content because of drying effects
  • To use daily home fluoride products for anticaries effect
  • To use sugarless gum, frequent sips of water, or saliva substitutes

carbachol

kar′-ba-kole
(Caroptic, Isopto Carbachol, Miostat)

CATEGORY AND SCHEDULE

Pregnancy Risk Category: C

MECHANISM OF ACTION

A direct-acting parasympathomimetic agent that stimulates cholinergic receptors resulting in muscarinic and nicotinic effects. Indirectly promotes release of acetylcholine. ***Therapeutic Effect:*** Produces contraction of the iris sphincter muscle, resulting in miosis, and reduction in intraocular pressure associated with decreased resistance to aqueous humor outflow.

PHARMACOKINETICS

None reported.

AVAILABILITY

Intraocular Solution: 0.01% (Miostat).
Ophthalmic Solution: 0.75% (Isopto Carbachol), 1.5% (Isopto Carbachol), 3% (Carboptic, Isopto Carbachol).

INDICATIONS AND DOSAGES

▸ **Glaucoma**
OPHTHALMIC
Adults, Elderly. Instill 1–2 drops of 0.75–3% solution in affected eye(s) up to 3 times/day.

▸ **Miosis, Ophthalmic Surgery**
OPHTHALMIC
Adults, Elderly. Instill 0.5 ml of 0.01% solution into anterior chamber before or after securing sutures.

OFF-LABEL USES

Postoperative intraocular pressure

CONTRAINDICATIONS
Acute iritis, hypersensitivity to carbachol or any component of the formulation

INTERACTIONS
Drug
None known.
Herbal
None known.
Food
None known.
Drug interactions of concern to dentistry
• None reported

DIAGNOSTIC TEST EFFECTS
None known.

SIDE EFFECTS
Occasional
Blurred vision, burning/irritation of eye, decreased night vision, headache.

SERIOUS REACTIONS
! Retinal detachment has been reported.
! Systemic absorption which includes arrhythmia, hypotension, syncope, asthma occurs rarely.

DENTAL CONSIDERATIONS
General:
• Determine why patient is taking the drug.
• Avoid drugs with anticholinergic activity, such as antihistamines, opioids, benzodiazepines, propantheline, atropine, and scopolamine.
• Avoid dental light in patient's eyes; offer dark glasses for patient comfort.
• Protect patient's eyes from accidental spatter during dental treatment.
• Question glaucoma patient about compliance with prescribed drug regimen.

Consultations:
• Medical consultation may be required to assess disease control.

Teach Patient/Family:
• Importance of updating health and medication history if physician makes any changes in evaluation or drug regimens; include OTC, herbal, and nonherbal remedies in the update

carbamazepine
kar-ba-maz′-e-peen
(Apo-Carbamazepine[CAN], Carbatrol, Epitol, Equetro, Tegretol, Tegretol CR[AUS], Tegretol XR, Teril[AUS])
Do not confuse Tegretol with Cartrol, Toradol, or Trental.

CATEGORY AND SCHEDULE
Pregnancy Risk Category: D

MECHANISM OF ACTION
An iminostilbene derivative that decreases sodium and calcium ion influx into neuronal membranes, reducing post-tetanic potentiation at synapses. ***Therapeutic Effect:*** Reduces seizure activity.

PHARMACOKINETICS
Slowly and completely absorbed from the GI tract. Protein binding: 75%. Metabolized in the liver to active metabolite. Primarily excreted in urine. Not removed by hemodialysis. ***Half-life:*** 25–65 hr (decreased with chronic use).

AVAILABILITY
Capsules (Extended-Release [Carbatrol]): 100 mg, 200 mg, 400 mg.

C

Capsules (Extended-Release [Equetro]): 100 mg, 200 mg, 300 mg.
Suspension (Tegretol): 100 mg/5 ml.
Tablets (Epitol, Tegretol): 200 mg.
Tablets (Chewable [Tegretol]): 100 mg.
Tablets (Extended-Release [Tegretol XR]): 100 mg, 200 mg, 400 mg.

INDICATIONS AND DOSAGES

▸ Seizure Control

PO

Adults, Children older than 12 yr. Initially, 200 mg twice a day. May increase dosage by 200 mg/day at weekly intervals. Range: 400–1200 mg/day in 2–4 divided doses. Maximum: 1.6–2.4 g/day.
Children 6–12 yr. Initially, 100 mg twice a day. May increase by 100 mg/day at weekly intervals. Range: 20–30 mg/kg/day. Maxiumum: 1000 mg/day.
Children younger than 6 yr. Initially 5 mg/kg/day. May increase at weekly intervals to 10 mg/kg/day up to 20 mg/kg/day.
Elderly. Initially 100 mg 1–2 times a day. May increase by 100 mg/day at weekly intervals. Usual dose 400–1000 mg/day.

▸ Trigeminal Neuralgia, Diabetic Neuropathy

PO

Adults. Initially, 100 mg twice a day. May increase by 100 mg twice a day up to 400–800 mg/day. Maxiumum: 1200 mg/day.
Elderly. Initially 100 mg 1–2 times a day. May increase by 100 mg/day at weekly intervals. Usual dose 400–1000 mg/day.

OFF-LABEL USES

Treatment of alcohol withdrawal, bipolar disorder, diabetes insipidus, neurogenic pain, psychotic disorders

CONTRAINDICATIONS

Concomitant use of MAOIs, history of myelosuppression, hypersensitivity to tricyclic antidepressants

INTERACTIONS

Drug

Anticoagulants, clarithromycin, diltiazem, erythromycin, estrogens, propoxyphene, quinidine, steroids: May decrease the effects of these drugs.
Antipsychotics, haloperidol, tricyclic antidepressants: May increase CNS depressant effects.
Cimetidine: May increase carbamazepine blood concentration and risk of toxicity.
Isoniazid: May increase metabolism of isoniazid; may increase carbamazepine blood concentration and risk of toxicity.
MAOIs: May cause seizures and hypertensive crisis.
Other anticonvulsants, barbiturates, benzodiazepines, valproic acid: May increase the metabolism of these drugs.
Verapamil: May increase the toxicity of carbamazepine.

Herbal

None known.

Food

Grapefruit, grapefruit juice: May increase the absorption and blood concentration of carbamazepine.

Drug interactions of concern to dentistry

- Decreased metabolism: erythromycin, clarithromycin, propoxyphene, troleandomycin, metronidazole, ketoconazole, fluconazole, itraconazole, or any drug that inhibits CYP450 3A4 enzymes
- Increased serum levels: tricyclic antidepressants, fluoxetine, fluvoxamine, nefazodone, ketoconazole, itraconazole

• Increased CNS depression: haloperidol, phenothiazines
• Decreased half-life: doxycycline
• Potential hepatotoxicity: chronic high doses of carbamazepine with acetaminophen
• Decreased effects of phenobarbital, corticosteroids, benzodiazepines, doxycycline, sertraline

DIAGNOSTIC TEST EFFECTS

May increase BUN and blood glucose levels and serum alkaline phosphatase, bilirubin, AST (SGOT), ALT (SGPT), protein, cholesterol, HDL, and triglyceride levels. May decrease serum calcium and thyroid hormone (T_3, T_4, T_4 index) levels. Therapeutic serum level is 4–12 mcg/ml; toxic serum level is greater than 12 mcg/ml.

SIDE EFFECTS

Frequent

Drowsiness, dizziness, nausea, vomiting

Occasional

Visual abnormalities (spots before eyes, difficulty focusing, blurred vision), dry mouth or pharynx, tongue irritation, headache, fluid retention, diaphoresis, constipation or diarrhea, behavioral changes in children

SERIOUS REACTIONS

! Toxic reactions may include blood dyscrasias (such as aplastic anemia, agranulocytosis, thrombocytopenia, leukopenia, leukocytosis, and eosinophilia), cardiovascular disturbances (such as CHF, hypotension or hypertension, thrombophlebitis and arrhythmias), and dermatologic effects (such as rash, urticaria, pruritus, and photosensitivity).
! Abrupt withdrawal may precipitate status epilepticus.

DENTAL CONSIDERATIONS

General:

• Monitor vital signs at every appointment because of cardiovascular side effects.
• Patients on chronic drug therapy may rarely have symptoms of blood dyscrasias, which can include infection, bleeding, and poor healing.
• Assess salivary flow as a factor in caries, periodontal disease, and candidiasis.
• Short appointments and a stress reduction protocol may be required for anxious patients.
• Talk with patient about type of epilepsy, seizure frequency, and quality of seizure control.

Consultations:

• In a patient with symptoms of blood dyscrasias, request a medical consultation for blood studies and postpone dental treatment until normal values are reestablished.
• Medical consultation may be required to assess disease control and patient's ability to tolerate stress.

Teach Patient/Family:

• Importance of good oral hygiene to prevent soft tissue inflammation
• Caution to prevent injury when using oral hygiene aids
• Caution patients about driving or performing other tasks requiring alertness.
• *When chronic dry mouth occurs, advise patient:*
  • To avoid mouth rinses with high alcohol content because of drying effects
  • To use daily home fluoride products for anticaries effect
  • To use sugarless gum, frequent sips of water, or saliva substitutes

C

carbamide peroxide

(Auro Ear Drops, Debrox, E•R•O Ear, GlyOxide, Mollifene Ear Wax Removing, Murine Ear Drops, Orajel Perioseptic, Proxigel) (gel, solution)

CATEGORY AND SCHEDULE

Pregnancy Risk Category: C

MECHANISM OF ACTION

A cerumenolytic that releases oxygen on contact with moist mouth tissues to provide cleansing effects, reduce inflammation, relieve pain, and inhibit odor-forming bacteria. In the ear, oxygen is released and hydrogen peroxide is reduced to water, which enables the chemical reaction. ***Therapeutic Effect:*** Relieves inflammation of gums and lips. Emulsifies and disperses ear wax.

PHARMACOKINETICS

Not known.

AVAILABILITY

Gel, oral: 10% (Proxigel).
Solution, oral: 10% (Gly-Oxide), 15% (Orajel Perioseptic).
Solution, otic: 6.5% (Auro Ear Drops, Debrox, E•R•O Ear, Mollifene Ear Wax Removing, Murine Ear Drops)

INDICATIONS AND DOSAGES

▸ **Earwax Removal**

TOPICAL, SOLUTION

Adults, Elderly, Children 12 yrs or older. Tilt head and administer 5–10 drops twice a day for up to 4 days.
Children 12 years or younger. Tilt head and administer 1–5 drops twice a day for up to 4 days.

▸ **Oral Lesions**

TOPICAL, GEL

Adults, Elderly, Children. Apply to affected area 4 times a day.

TOPICAL, SOLUTION

Adults, Elderly, Children. Apply several drops undiluted on affected area 4 times a day after meals and at bedtime.

OFF-LABEL USES

Dental whitener

CONTRAINDICATIONS

Dizziness, ear discharge or drainage, ear injury, ear pain, irritation, or rash, hypersensitivity to carbamide peroxide or any one of its components

INTERACTIONS

Drug

None known.

Herbal

None known.

Food

None known.

Drug interactions of concern to dentistry

- None reported

DIAGNOSTIC TEST EFFECTS

Not known.

SIDE EFFECTS

Occasional

Oral: Gingival sensitivity

SERIOUS REACTIONS

! Opportunistic infections caused by organisms like Candida albicans is possible with prolonged use.

DENTAL CONSIDERATIONS

General:

- For oral ulcers, perform an oral exam to rule out possible local contributing factors such as broken tooth or filling or ill-fitting dentures.

• Question patient about symptom history; onset, duration, and frequency.
• This drug is the principal ingredient in tooth bleaching or whiting agents; avoid excessive use.

Teach Patient/Family:

• Caution patient that if symptoms do not abate or worsen within 7 days to see the dentist

carbinoxamine maleate

kar-bi-**nox**-a-meen
(Carboxine, Histex CT, Histex I/E, Histex PD, Histex Pd 12, Palgic, Pediatex, Pediox)

CATEGORY AND SCHEDULE

Pregnancy Risk Category: C

MECHANISM OF ACTION

An antihistamine that exhibits H_1 receptor blocking action.
Therapeutic Effect: Prevents allergic responses mediated by histamine, such as rhinitis.

PHARMACOKINETICS

Virtually no intact drug is excreted in urine. ***Half-life:*** 1–20 hr.

AVAILABILITY

Capsules: 10 mg (Histex I/E).
Liquid: 1.75 mg/5 ml (Carboxine), 2 mg/5 ml (Histex PD), 4 mg/5 ml (Histex PD, Palgic, Pediox).
Suspension (Maleate-Tannate [Histex Pd 12]): 2–6 mg/5 ml.
Tablets (Palgic): 4 mg.
Tablets (Extended-Release [Histex CT]): 8 mg.

INDICATIONS AND DOSAGES

▸ Allergic Rhinitis

PO

Adults, Children 6 yr and Older. 1 tsp 4 times/day.
Children 18 mo–6 yr. 1/2 tsp 4 times/day.
Children 9–18 mo. 1/4–1/2 tsp 4 times/day.

CONTRAINDICATIONS

Hypersensitivity or idiosyncrasy to any ingredients, patients taking MAOIs

INTERACTIONS

Drug

Alcohol, other CNS depressants: May increase CNS depressant effects.
Anticholinergics: May increase anticholinergic effects.
MAOIs: May increase the anticholinergic and CNS depressant effects of carbinoxamine.

Herbal

None known.

Food

None known.

Drug interactions of concern to dentistry

• Increased sedation: alcohol and all CNS depressants
• Prolonged sedative and anticholinergic effects: MAOIs

DIAGNOSTIC TEST EFFECTS

None known.

SIDE EFFECTS

Frequent

Somnolence, dizziness, muscle weakness, hypotension, urine retention, thickening of bronchial secretions, dry mouth, nose, throat, or lips; in elderly, sedation, dizziness, hypotension

Occasional

Epigastric distress, vomiting, headache

C

Rare
Excitability in children

SERIOUS REACTIONS

! Overdose symptoms may vary from CNS depression, including sedation, apnea, hypotension, cardiovascular collapse, and death, to severe paradoxical reactions, such as hallucinations, tremor, and seizures.

DENTAL CONSIDERATIONS

General:

- Assess salivary flow as a factor in caries, periodontal disease, and candidiasis.
- Determine why patient is taking the drug.

Teach Patient/Family:

- Importance of good oral hygiene to prevent soft tissue inflammation
- To prevent trauma when using oral hygiene aids
- *When chronic dry mouth occurs advise patient:*
  - To avoid mouth rinses with high alcohol content due to drying effects
  - To use daily home fluoride products for anticaries effect
  - To use sugarless gum, frequent sips of water or saliva substitutes

carboplatin

car-bow-play'-tin
(Paraplatin)
Do not confuse carboplatin with Cisplatin or Platinol.

CATEGORY AND SCHEDULE

Pregnancy Risk Category: D

MECHANISM OF ACTION

A platinum coordination complex that inhibits DNA synthesis by cross-linking with DNA strands, preventing cell division. Cell cycle-phase nonspecific. ***Therapeutic Effect:*** Interferes with DNA function.

PHARMACOKINETICS

Protein binding: Low. Hydrolyzed in solution to active form. Primarily excreted in urine. ***Half-life:*** 2.6–5.9 hr.

AVAILABILITY

Powder for Injection: 50 mg, 150 mg, 450 mg.
Injection Solution: 10 mg/ml.

INDICATIONS AND DOSAGES

▸ Ovarian Carcinoma (Monotherapy)
IV
Adults. 360 mg/m^2 on day 1, every 4 wk. Don't repeat dose until neutrophil and platelet counts are within acceptable levels. Adjust drug dosage in previously treated patients based on lowest post-treatment platelet or neutrophil count. Increase dosage only once to no more than 125% of starting dose.

▸ Ovarian Carcinoma (Combination Therapy)
IV
Adults. 300 mg/m^2 (with cyclophosphamide) on day 1, every 4 wk. Don't repeat dose until neutrophil and platelet counts are within acceptable levels.
Children. 300–600 mg/m^2 every 4 wk for solid tumor, or 175 mg/m^2 every 4 wk for brain tumor.

▸ Dosage in Renal Impairment
Initial dosage is based on creatinine clearance; subsequent dosages are based on the patient's tolerance and degree of myelosuppression.

Creatinine Clearance	Dosage Day 1
60 ml/min or greater	360 mg/m^2
41–59 ml/min	250 mg/m^2
16–40 ml/min	200 mg/m^2

OFF-LABEL USES
Treatment of bony and soft tissue sarcomas; germ cell tumors; neuroblastoma; pediatric brain tumor; small-cell lung cancer; solid tumors of the bladder, cervix, and testes; squamous cell carcinoma of the esophagus

CONTRAINDICATIONS
History of severe allergic reaction to cisplatin, platinum compounds, or mannitol; severe bleeding, severe myelosuppression

INTERACTIONS
Drug
Bone marrow depressants: May increase myelosuppression.
Live-virus vaccines: May potentiate virus replication, increase vaccine side effects, and decrease the patient's antibody response to the vaccine.
Nephrotoxic, ototoxic medications: May increase the risk of nephrotoxicity.
Herbal
None known.
Food
None known.
Drug interactions of concern to dentistry
- None reported

DIAGNOSTIC TEST EFFECTS
May decrease serum electrolyte levels, including calcium, magnesium, potassium, and sodium. High dosages (more than 4 times the recommended dosage) may elevate BUN and serum alkaline phosphatase, bilirubin, creatinine, and AST SGOT levels.

IV INCOMPATIBILITIES
Amphotericin B complex (Abelcet, AmBisome, Amphotec)
IV COMPATIBILITIES
Etoposide (VePesid), granisetron (Kytril), ondansetron (Zofran), paclitaxel (Taxol)

SIDE EFFECTS
Frequent
Nausea (75%–80%), vomiting (65%)
Occasional
Generalized pain (17%), diarrhea or constipation (6%), peripheral neuropathy (4%)
Rare (3%–2%)
Alopecia, asthenia, hypersensitivity reaction (erythema, pruritus, rash, urticaria)

SERIOUS REACTIONS
! Myelosuppression may be severe, resulting in anemia, infection, (sepsis, pneumonia), and bleeding.
! Prolonged treatment may result in peripheral neurotoxicity.

DENTAL CONSIDERATIONS
General:
- Determine why patient is taking the drug.
- If additional analgesia is required for dental pain, consider alternative analgesics (NSAIDs) in patients taking narcotics for acute or chronic pain.
- Examine for oral manifestation of opportunistic infection.
- Avoid prescribing aspirin-containing products.
- This drug may be used in the hospital or on an outpatient basis. Confirm the patient's disease and treatment status.

• Patient on chronic drug therapy may rarely present with symptoms of blood dyscrasias, which can include infection, bleeding, and poor healing. If dyscrasia is present, caution patient to prevent oral tissue trauma when using oral hygiene aids.
• Short appointments and a stress reduction protocol may be required for anxious patients.
• Patients may have received other chemotherapy or radiation; confirm medical and drug history.
• Patients may be at risk of bleeding, check for oral signs.
• Patients may be at risk of infection.
• Patients may be taking prophylactic antiinfectives.
• Oral infections should be eliminated and/or treated aggressively.

Consultations:

• Medical consultation should include routine blood counts including platelet counts and bleeding time.
• Consult physician; prophylactic or therapeutic antiinfectives may be indicated if surgery or periodontal treatment is required.
• Medical consultation may be required to assess immunologic status during cancer chemotherapy and determine safety risk, if any, posed by the required dental treatment.
• Medical consultation may be required to assess disease control and patient's ability to tolerate stress.

Teach Patient/Family:

• Secondary oral infection may occur; need to see dentist immediately if infection occurs
• Importance of good oral hygiene to prevent soft tissue inflammation
• To report oral lesions, soreness, or bleeding to dentist
• To prevent trauma when using oral hygiene aids
• Importance of updating health and medication history if physician makes any changes in evaluation or drug regimens; include OTC, herbal, and nonherbal remedies in the update

carisoprodol

kar-i-so-pro′-dol
(Soma)

CATEGORY AND SCHEDULE

Pregnancy Risk Category: C

MECHANISM OF ACTION

A centrally acting skeletal muscle relaxant whose exact mechanism is unknown. Effects may be due to its CNS depressant actions.
Therapeutic Effect: Relieves muscle spasms and pain.

AVAILABILITY

Tablets: 350 mg.

INDICATIONS AND DOSAGES

▸ Adjunct to Rest, Physical Therapy, Analgesics, and Other Measures for Relief of Discomfort from Acute, Painful Musculoskeletal Conditions

PO

Adults, Elderly. 350 mg 4 times a day.

CONTRAINDICATIONS

Acute intermittent porphyria, sensitivity to meprobamate

INTERACTIONS

Drug

Alcohol, other CNS depressants: May increase CNS depression.

Herbal

None known.

Food
None known.

Drug interactions of concern to dentistry
• Increased CNS depression: alcohol, all CNS depressants

DIAGNOSTIC TEST EFFECTS
None known.

SIDE EFFECTS
Frequent (> 10%)
Somnolence
Occasional (10%–1%)
Tachycardia, facial flushing, dizziness, headache, lightheadedness, dermatitis, nausea, vomiting, abdominal cramps, dyspnea

SERIOUS REACTIONS
! Overdose may cause CNS and respiratory depression, shock, and coma.

DENTAL CONSIDERATIONS
General:
• When used in dentistry, may be more effective when used in combination with aspirin or NSAIDs.
Teach Patient/Family:
• To use electric toothbrush if patient has difficulty holding conventional devices

carmustine
car-muss′-teen
(BiCNU, Gliadel)

CATEGORY AND SCHEDULE
Pregnancy Risk Category: D

MECHANISM OF ACTION
An alkylating agent and nitrosourea that inhibits DNA and RNA synthesis by cross-linking with DNA and RNA strands, preventing cell division. Cell cycle-phase nonspecific. ***Therapeutic Effect:*** Interferes with DNA and RNA function.

AVAILABILITY
Powder for Injection (BiCNu): 100 mg.
Wafer (Gliadel): 7.7 mg.

INDICATIONS AND DOSAGES
▸ **Disseminated Hodgkin's Disease, Non-Hodgkin's Lymphoma, Multiple Myeloma, and Primary and Metastatic Brain Tumors in Previously Untreated Patients (Monotherapy)**
IV (BiCNu)
Adults, Elderly. 150–200 mg/m^2 as a single dose or 75–100 mg/m^2 on 2 successive days.
Children. 200–250 mg/m^2 every 4–6 wk as a single dose.
! Implantation (Gliadel)
Adults, Elderly, Children. Up to 8 wafers may be placed in resection cavity.

OFF-LABEL USES
Treatment of hepatic or GI carcinoma, malignant melanoma, mycosis fungoides

CONTRAINDICATIONS
None known.

INTERACTIONS
Drug
Bone marrow depressants, cimetidine: May enhance carmustine's myelosuppressive effect.

Hepatotoxic, nephrotoxic medications: May increase the risk of hepatotoxicity or nephrotoxicity.
Live-virus vaccines: May potentiate virus replication, increase vaccine side effects, and decrease the patient's antibody response to the vaccine.

Herbal
None known.

Food
None known.

Drug interactions of concern to dentistry
- None reported

DIAGNOSTIC TEST EFFECTS
May increase BUN, and serum alkaline phosphatase, bilirubin, AST (SGOT), and ALT (SGPT) levels.

IV INCOMPATIBILITIES
Allopurinol (Aloprim)

SIDE EFFECTS
Frequent
Nausea and vomiting within minutes to 2 hr after administration (may last up to 6 hr)

Occasional
Diarrhea, esophagitis, anorexia, dysphagia

Rare
Thrombophlebitis

SERIOUS REACTIONS
! Hematologic toxicity due to myelosuppression occurs frequently. Thrombocytopenia occurs about 4 weeks after carmustine treatment begins and lasts 1 to 2 weeks.
! Leukopenia is evident 5 to 6 weeks after treatment begins and lasts 1 to 2 weeks. Anemia occurs less frequently and is less severe.
! Mild, reversible hepatotoxicity also occurs frequently.
! Prolonged high-dose carmustine therapy may produce impaired renal function and pulmonary toxicity (pulmonary infiltrate or fibrosis).

DENTAL CONSIDERATIONS
General:
- Determine why patient is taking the drug.
- If additional analgesia is required for dental pain, consider alternative analgesics (NSAIDs) in patients taking narcotics for acute or chronic pain.
- Avoid products that affect platelet function, such as aspirin and NSAIDs.
- This drug may be used in the hospital or on an outpatient basis. Confirm the patient's disease and treatment status.
- Consider semisupine chair position for patient comfort if GI side effects occur.
- Patient on chronic drug therapy may rarely present with symptoms of blood dyscrasias, which can include infection, bleeding and poor healing. If dyscrasia is present, caution patient to prevent oral tissue trauma when using oral hygiene aids.
- Examine for oral manifestation of opportunistic infection.
- Consider local hemostasis measures to prevent excessive bleeding.
- Monitor vital signs at every appointment due to cardiovascular side effects.
- Caution: use of potentially hepatotoxic drugs.

Consultations:
- Medical consultation should include routine blood counts including platelet counts and bleeding time.
- Consult physician; prophylactic or therapeutic antiinfectives may be indicated if surgery or periodontal treatment is required.

• In a patient with symptoms of blood dyscrasias, request a medical consultation for blood studies and postpone treatment until normal values are reestablished.
• Medical consultation may be required to assess disease control and patient's ability to tolerate stress.

Teach Patient/Family:

• Importance of good oral hygiene to prevent soft tissue inflammation
• To prevent trauma when using oral hygiene aids
• Importance of updating health and medication history if physician makes any changes in evaluation or drug regimens; include OTC, herbal, and nonherbal remedies in the update
• To report oral lesions, soreness, or bleeding to dentist

carteolol

kar-tee′-oh-lole
(Cartrol, Ocupress)
Do not confuse with carvedilol.

CATEGORY AND SCHEDULE

Pregnancy Risk Category: C/D if after first trimester

MECHANISM OF ACTION

An antihypertensive that blocks beta1-adrenergic receptor at normal doses and beta2-adrenergic receptors at large doses. Predominantly blocks beta1-adrenergic receptors in cardiac tissue. Reduces aqueous humor production. ***Therapeutic Effect:*** Slows sinus heart rate, decreases cardiac output, decreases blood pressure (B/P), increases airway resistance, decreases intraocular pressure.

PHARMACOKINETICS

Well absorbed from the gastrointestinal (GI) tract. Protein binding: unknown. Minimally metabolized in liver. Primarily excreted unchanged in urine. Not removed by hemodialysis. ***Half-life:*** 6 hrs (increased in decreased renal function).

AVAILABILITY

Ophthalmic solution: 1% (Ocupress).
Tablets: 2.5 mg, 5 mg (Cartrol).

INDICATIONS AND DOSAGES

▸ **Hypertension**

PO

Adults, Elderly. Initially, 2.5 mg/day as single dose either alone or in combination with diuretic. May increase gradually to 5–10 mg/day as a single dose. Maintenance: 2.5–5 mg/day.

▸ **Dosage in Renal Impairment**

Creatinine Clearance	Dosage Interval
>60 ml/min	24 hrs
20–60 ml/min	48 hrs
<20 ml/min	72 hrs

▸ **Open-Angle Glaucoma, Ocular Hypertension**

OPHTHALMIC

Adults, Elderly. 1 drop 2 times/day.

OFF-LABEL USES

Combination with miotics decreases IOP in acute/chronic angle closure glaucoma, treatment of secondary glaucoma, malignant glaucoma, angle closure glaucoma during/after iridectomy

CONTRAINDICATIONS

Bronchial asthma, COPD, bronchospasm, overt cardiac failure, cardiogenic shock, heart block greater than first degree, persistently severe bradycardia

INTERACTIONS

Drug

Cimetidine: May increase carteolol concentrations.
Diuretics, other hypotensives: May increase hypotensive effect.
Insulin, oral hypoglycemics: May mask symptoms of hypoglycemia and prolong hypoglycemic effect of these drugs.
MAOIs: May produce hypertension.
NSAIDs: May decrease antihypertensive effects.
Sympathomimetics, xanthines: May mutually inhibit effects of carteolol.

Herbal

None known.

Food

None known.

Drug interactions of concern to dentistry

- Decreased hypotensive effect: indomethacin, NSAIDs
- Increased hypotension, myocardial depression: hydrocarbon inhalation anesthetics
- Hypertension, bradycardia: sympathomimetics (epinephrine, ephedrine)
- Bradycardia: fluoxetine, paroxetine

DIAGNOSTIC TEST EFFECTS

May increase serum ANA titer, BUN, serum LDH, lipoprotein, alkaline phosphatase, bilirubin, creatinine, potassium, triglyceride, uric acid, SGOT (AST), and SGPT (ALT) levels.

SIDE EFFECTS

Frequent

Oral: Hypotension manifested as dizziness, nausea, diaphoresis, headache, cold extremities, fatigue, constipation/diarrhea
Ophthalmic: Redness of eye or inside of eyelids, decreased night vision

Occasional

Oral: Insomnia, flatulence, urinary frequency, impotence or decreased libido
Ophthalmic: Blepharoconjunctivitis, edema, droopy eyelid, staining of cornea, blurred vision, brow ache, increased light sensitivity, burning, stinging

Rare

Rash, arthralgia, myalgia, confusion (especially elderly), taste disturbances

SERIOUS REACTIONS

! Abrupt withdrawal (particularly in those with coronary artery disease) may produce angina or precipitate MI.
! May precipitate thyroid crisis in those with thyrotoxicosis.
! Beta-blockers may mask signs and symptoms of acute hypoglycemia (tachycardia, B/P changes) in diabetic patients.

DENTAL CONSIDERATIONS

General:

- Monitor vital signs at every appointment because of cardiovascular side effects.
- After supine positioning, have patient sit upright for at least 2 min before standing to avoid orthostatic hypotension.
- Assess salivary flow as a factor in caries, periodontal disease, and candidiasis.
- Patients on chronic drug therapy may rarely have symptoms of blood dyscrasias, which can include infection, bleeding, and poor healing.
- Limit use of sodium-containing products, such as saline IV fluids, for those patients with a dietary salt restriction.

- Stress from dental procedures may compromise cardiovascular function; determine patient risk.
- Short appointments and a stress reduction protocol may be required for anxious patients.

Consultations:

- In a patient with symptoms of blood dyscrasias, request a medical consultation for blood studies and postpone dental treatment until normal values are reestablished.
- Medical consultation may be required to assess disease control and patient's ability to tolerate stress.

Teach Patient/Family:

- To report oral lesions, soreness, or bleeding to dentist
- *When chronic dry mouth occurs, advise patient:*
  - To avoid mouth rinses with high alcohol content because of drying effects
  - Of need for daily home fluoride to prevent caries
  - To use sugarless gum, frequent sips of water, or saliva substitutes

caspofungin acetate

cas-poe-fun′-gin
(Cancidas)

CATEGORY AND SCHEDULE

Pregnancy Risk Category: C

MECHANISM OF ACTION

An antifungal that inhibits the synthesis of glucan, a vital component of fungal cell formation, thereby damaging the fungal cell membrane. ***Therapeutic Effect:*** Fungistatic.

PHARMACOKINETICS

Distributed in tissue. Extensively bound to albumin. Protein binding: 97%. Slowly metabolized in liver to active metabolite. Excreted primarily in urine and to a lesser extent in feces. Not removed by hemodialysis. ***Half-life:*** 40–50 hr.

AVAILABILITY

Powder for Injection: 50-mg, 70-mg vials.

INDICATIONS AND DOSAGES

▸ Aspergillosis

IV

Adults, Elderly, Children older than 12 yr. Give single 70-mg loading dose on day 1, followed by 50 mg/day thereafter. For patients with moderate hepatic insufficiency, daily dose reduced to 35 mg.

▸ Invasive Candidiasis

IV

Adults, Elderly. Initially, 70 mg followed by 50 mg daily.

▸ Esophageal Candidiasis

IV

Adult, Elderly. 50 mg a day.

CONTRAINDICATIONS

None known.

INTERACTIONS

Drug

Carbamazepine, cyclosporine, dexamethasone, efavirenz, nelfinavir, nevirapine, phenytoin, rifampin: May increase blood concentration of caspofungin.
Tacrolimus: May decrease the effect of tacrolimus.

Herbal

None known.

Food

None known.

Drug interactions of concern to dentistry
- Reduction in concentration: dexamethasone, carbamazepine

DIAGNOSTIC TEST EFFECTS
May increase PT, as well as serum alkaline phosphatase, serum bilirubin, serum creatinine, LDH, AST(SGOT), ALT(SGPT), serum uric acid, urine pH, urine protein, urine RBC, and urine WBC levels. May decrease Hgb, Hct, platelet count, and serum albumin, serum bicarbonate, serum protein, and serum potassium levels.

IV INCOMPATIBILITIES
Don't mix caspofungin with any other medication or use dextrose as a diluent.

SIDE EFFECTS
Frequent (26%)
Fever
Occasional (11%–4%)
Headache, nausea, phlebitis
Rare (3% or less)
Paresthesia, vomiting, diarrhea, abdominal pain, myalgia, chills, tremor, insomnia

SERIOUS REACTIONS
! Hypersensitivity reactions (characterized by rash, facial swelling, pruritus, and a sensation of warmth) may occur.

DENTAL CONSIDERATIONS
General:
- For selected infections in the hospital setting.
- Provide palliative dental care for dental emergencies only.
- Patient on chronic drug therapy may rarely present with symptoms of blood dyscrasias, which can include infection, bleeding, and poor healing. If dyscrasia is present, caution patient to prevent oral tissue trauma when using oral hygiene aids.

Consultations:
- In a patient with symptoms of blood dyscrasias, request a medical consultation for blood studies and postpone treatment until normal values are reestablished.
- Medical consultation may be required to assess disease control and patient's ability to tolerate stress.
- Medical consultation should include partial prothrombin time, prothrombin time, or INR.

Teach Patient/Family:
- Importance of good oral hygiene to prevent soft tissue inflammation
- To report oral lesions, soreness, or bleeding to dentist
- To prevent trauma when using oral hygiene aids

cefaclor
sef′-a-klor
(Apo-Cefaclor[CAN], Ceclor, Ceclor CD, Cefkor[AUS], Cefkor CD[AUS], Keflor[AUS])

CATEGORY AND SCHEDULE
Pregnancy Risk Category: B

MECHANISM OF ACTION
A second-generation cephalosporin that binds to bacterial cell membranes and inhibits cell wall synthesis.
Therapeutic Effect: Bactericidal.

PHARMACOKINETICS
Well absorbed from the GI tract. Protein binding: 25%. Widely distributed. Primarily excreted unchanged in urine. Moderately removed by hemodialysis.
Half-life: 0.6–0.9 hr (increased in impaired renal function).

AVAILABILITY

Capsules (Ceclor): 250 mg, 500 mg.
Oral Suspension (Ceclor): 125 mg/5 ml, 187 mg/5 ml, 250 mg/5 ml, 375 mg/5 ml.
Tablets (Extended-release [Ceclor CD]): 375 mg, 500 mg.
Tablets (Chewable [Raniclor]): 125 mg, 187 mg, 250 mg, 375 mg.

INDICATIONS AND DOSAGES

▸ Bronchitis

PO (Extended-Release)
Adults, Elderly. 500 mg q12h for 7 days.

▸ Lower Respiratory Tract Infections

PO
Adults, Elderly. 250–500 mg q8h.

▸ Otitis Media

PO
Children. 20–40 mg/kg/day in 2–3 divided doses.
Maximum: 1 g/day.

▸ Pharyngitis, Skin/Skin Structure Infections, Tonsillitis

PO (Extended-Release)
Adults, Elderly. 375 mg q12h.
PO (Regular-Release)
Adults, Elderly. 250–500 mg q8h.
Children. 20–40 mg/kg/day in 2–3 divided doses. Maxiumum: 1 g/day.

▸ Urinary Tract Infections

PO
Adults, Elderly. 250–500 mg q8h.
Children. 20–40 mg/kg/day in 2–3 divided doses q8h.
Maximum: 1 g/day.
PO (Extended-Release)
Adults, Children older than 16 yr. 375–500 mg q12h.

▸ Otitis Media

PO
Children older than 1 mo.
40 mg/kg/day in divided doses q8h.
Maximum: 1 g/day.

▸ Dosage in Renal Impairment

Decreased dosage may be necessary in patients with creatinine clearance less than 40 ml/min.

CONTRAINDICATIONS

History of anaphylactic reaction to penicillins or hypersensitivity to cephalosporins

INTERACTIONS

Drug

Probenecid: May increase cefaclor blood concentration.

Herbal

None known.

Food

None known.

Drug interactions of concern to dentistry

- Decreased bactericidal effects: tetracyclines, erythromycins
- Increased and prolonged serum levels: probenecid
- Oral contraceptives: advise patient of a potential risk for decreased contraceptive action, to maintain compliance with oral contraceptive use while using antibiotics, and to consider the use of additional nonhormonal contraception

DIAGNOSTIC TEST EFFECTS

May increase BUN level and serum alkaline phosphatase, bilirubin, creatinine, LDH, AST (SGOT), and ALT (SGPT) levels. May cause a positive direct or indirect Coombs' test.

SIDE EFFECTS

Frequent

Oral candidiasis, mild diarrhea, mild abdominal cramping, vaginal candidiasis

Occasional

Nausea, serum sickness-like reaction (marked by fever and joint pain; usually occurs after the second course of therapy and resolves after the drug is discontinued)

Rare

Allergic reaction (pruritus, rash, and urticaria)

SERIOUS REACTIONS

! Antibiotic-associated colitis and other superinfections may result from altered bacterial balance.

! Nephrotoxicity may occur, especially in patients with pre-existing renal disease.

! Patients with a history of allergies, especially to penicillin, are at increased risk for developing a severe hypersensitivity reaction, marked by severe pruritus, angioedema, bronchospasm, and anaphylaxis.

DENTAL CONSIDERATIONS

General:

- Take precautions regarding allergy to medication.
- Determine why the patient is taking the drug.

Consultations:

- Medical consultation may be required to assess disease control.

Teach Patient/Family:

- Importance of good oral hygiene to prevent soft tissue inflammation
- To avoid mouth rinses with high alcohol content because of drying effects and possible drug–drug reaction
- *When used for dental infection, advise patient:*
  - To report sore throat, oral burning sensation, fever, and fatigue, any of which could indicate superinfection
  - To take at prescribed intervals and complete dosage regimen
  - To immediately notify the dentist if signs or symptoms of infection increase

cefadroxil

sef-a-drox′-ill

(Duricef)

CATEGORY AND SCHEDULE

Pregnancy Risk Category: B

MECHANISM OF ACTION

A first-generation cephalosporin that binds to bacterial cell membranes and inhibits cell wall synthesis. ***Therapeutic Effect:*** Bactericidal.

PHARMACOKINETICS

Well absorbed from the GI tract. Protein binding: 15%–20%. Widely distributed. Primarily excreted unchanged in urine. Removed by hemodialysis. ***Half-life:*** 1.2–1.5 hr (increased in impaired renal function).

AVAILABILITY

Capsules: 500 mg.

Oral Suspension: 250 mg/5 ml, 500 mg/5 ml.

Tablets: 1,000 mg.

INDICATIONS AND DOSAGES

▶ **UTIs**

PO

Adults, Elderly. 1–2 g/day as a single dose or in 2 divided doses.

Children. 30 mg/kg/day in 2 divided doses. Maximum: 2 g/day.

▶ **Skin and Skin-Structure Infections, Group A Beta-Hemolytic Streptococcal Pharyngitis, Tonsillitis**

PO

Adults, Elderly. 1–2 g in 2 divided doses.

Children. 30 mg/kg/day in 2 divided doses. Maximum: 2 g/day.

Impetigo

PO

Children. 30 mg/kg/day as a single or in 2 divided doses. Maximum: 2 g/day.

Dosage in Renal Impairment

After an initial 1-g dose, dosage and frequency are modified on the basis of creatinine clearance and the severity of the infection.

Creatinine Clearance	Dosage Interval
25–50 ml/min	500 mg q12h
10–25 ml/min	500 mg q24h
0–10 ml/min	500 mg q36h

CONTRAINDICATIONS

History of anaphylactic reaction to penicillins or hypersensitivity to cephalosporins

INTERACTIONS

Drug

Probenecid: Increases cefadroxil blood concentration.

Herbal

None known.

Food

None known.

Drug interactions of concern to dentistry

- Decreased bactericidal effects: tetracyclines, erythromycins
- Increased and prolonged serum levels: probenecid
- Oral contraceptives: advise patient of a potential risk for decreased contraceptive action, to maintain compliance with oral contraceptive use while using antibiotics, and to consider the use of additional nonhormonal contraception

DIAGNOSTIC TEST EFFECTS

May increase BUN level and serum alkaline phosphatase, bilirubin, creatinine, LDH, AST (SGOT), and ALT (SGPT) levels. May cause a positive direct or indirect Coombs' test.

SIDE EFFECTS

Frequent

Oral candidiasis, mild diarrhea, mild abdominal cramping, vaginal candidiasis

Occasional

Nausea, unusual bruising or bleeding, serum sickness-like reaction (marked by fever and joint pain; usually occurs after the second course of therapy and resolves after the drug is discontinued)

Rare

Allergic reaction (rash, pruritus, urticaria), thrombophlebitis (pain, redness, swelling at injection site)

SERIOUS REACTIONS

! Antibiotic-associated colitis and other superinfections may result from altered bacterial balance.

! Nephrotoxicity may occur, especially in patients with pre-existing renal disease.

! Patients with a history of allergies, especially to penicillin, are at increased risk for developing a severe hypersensitivity reaction, marked by severe pruritus, angioedema, bronchospasm, and anaphylaxis.

DENTAL CONSIDERATIONS

General:

- Take precautions regarding allergy to medication.
- Determine why the patient is taking the drug.

Consultations:

- Medical consultation may be required to assess disease control.

Teach Patient/Family:
- Importance of good oral hygiene to prevent soft tissue inflammation
- To avoid mouth rinses with high alcohol content because of drying effects and possible drug–drug reaction
- *When used for dental infection, advise patient:*
  - To report sore throat, oral burning sensation, fever, and fatigue, any of which could indicate superinfection
  - To take at prescribed intervals and complete dosage regimen
  - To immediately notify the dentist if signs or symptoms of infection increase

cefazolin sodium

sef-a′-zoe-lin
(Ancef, Kefzol)
Do not confuse cefazolin with cefprozil or Cefzil.

CATEGORY AND SCHEDULE

Pregnancy Risk Category: B

MECHANISM OF ACTION

A first-generation cephalosporin that binds to bacterial cell membranes and inhibits cell wall synthesis.
Therapeutic Effect: Bactericidal.

PHARMACOKINETICS

Widely distributed. Protein binding: 85%. Primarily excreted unchanged in urine. Moderately removed by hemodialysis. ***Half-life:*** 1.4–1.8 hr (increased in impaired renal function).

AVAILABILITY

Injection: 500 mg, 1 g.
Ready-to-Hang Infusion: 1 g/50 ml, 2 g/100 ml.

INDICATIONS AND DOSAGES

▸ Uncomplicated UTIs
IV, IM
Adults, Elderly. 1 g q12h.

▸ Mild to Moderate Infections
IV, IM
Adults, Elderly. 250–500 mg q8–12h.

▸ Severe infections
IV, IM
Adults, Elderly. 0.5–1 g q6–8h.

▸ Life-Threatening Infections
IV, IM
Adults, Elderly. 1–1.5 g q6h.
Maximum: 12 g/day.

▸ Perioperative Prophylaxis
IV, IM
Adults, Elderly. 1 g 30–60 min before surgery, 0.5–1 g during surgery, and q6–8h for up to 24 hrs postoperatively.

▸ Usual Pediatric Dosage
Children. 50–100 mg/kg/day in divided doses q8h. Maximum: 6 g/day.
Neonates older than 7 days. 40–60 mg/kg/day in divided doses q8–12h.
Neonates 7 days and younger. 40 mg/kg/day in divided doses q12h.

▸ Dosage in Renal Impairment
Dosing frequency is modified on the basis of creatinine clearance.

Creatinine Clearance	Dosage Interval
10–30 ml/min	Usual dose q12h
less than 10 ml/min	Usual dose q24h

CONTRAINDICATIONS

History of anaphylactic reaction to penicillins or hypersensitivity to cephalosporins

INTERACTIONS

Drug

Probenecid: Increases cefazolin blood concentration.

Herbal
None known.
Food
None known.
Drug interactions of concern to dentistry
• Decreased bactericidal effects: tetracyclines, erythromycins
• Increased and prolonged serum levels: probenecid
• Oral contraceptives: advise patient of a potential risk for decreased contraceptive action, to maintain compliance with oral contraceptive use while using antibiotics, and to consider the use of additional nonhormonal contraception

DIAGNOSTIC TEST EFFECTS

May increase BUN level and serum alkaline phosphatase, bilirubin, creatinine, LDH, AST (SGOT), and ALT (SGPT) levels. May cause a positive direct or indirect Coombs' test

IV INCOMPATIBILITIES

Amikacin (Amikin), amiodarone (Cordarone), hydromorphone (Dilaudid)

IV COMPATIBILITIES

Calcium gluconate, diltiazem (Cardizem), famotidine (Pepcid), heparin, insulin (regular), lidocaine, magnesium sulfate, midazolam (Versed), morphine, multivitamins, potassium chloride, propofol (Diprivan), vecuronium (Norcuron)

SIDE EFFECTS

Frequent
Discomfort with IM administration, oral candidiasis, mild diarrhea, mild abdominal cramping, vaginal candidiasis
Occasional
Nausea, serum sickness-like reaction (marked by fever and joint pain; usually occurs after the second course of therapy and resolves after the drug is discontinued)
Rare
Allergic reaction (rash, pruritus, urticaria), thrombophlebitis (pain, redness, swelling at injection site)

SERIOUS REACTIONS

! Antibiotic-associated colitis and other superinfections may result from altered bacterial balance.
! Nephrotoxicity may occur, especially in patients with pre-existing renal disease.
! Patients with a history of allergies, especially to penicillin, are at increased risk for developing a severe hypersensitivity reaction, marked by severe pruritus, angioedema, bronchospasm, and anaphylaxis.

DENTAL CONSIDERATIONS

General:
• Take precautions regarding allergy to medication.
• Determine why the patient is taking the drug.
Consultations:
• Medical consultation may be required to assess disease control.
Teach Patient/Family:
• Importance of good oral hygiene to prevent soft tissue inflammation
• To avoid mouth rinses with high alcohol content because of drying effects and possible drug–drug reaction
• *When used for dental infection, advise patient:*
  • To report sore throat, oral burning sensation, fever, and fatigue, any of which could indicate superinfection
  • To take at prescribed intervals and complete dosage regimen
  • To immediately notify the dentist if signs or symptoms of infection increase

C

cefdinir

sef′-di-neer
(Omnicef)

CATEGORY AND SCHEDULE

Pregnancy Risk Category: B

MECHANISM OF ACTION

A third-generation cephalosporin that binds to bacterial cell membranes and inhibits cell wall synthesis. ***Therapeutic Effect:*** Bactericidal.

PHARMACOKINETICS

Moderately absorbed from the GI tract. Protein binding: 60%–70%. Widely distributed. Not appreciably metabolized. Primarily excreted unchanged in urine. Minimally removed by hemodialysis. ***Half-life:*** 1–2 hr (increased in impaired renal function).

AVAILABILITY

Capsules: 300 mg.
Oral Suspension: 125 mg/5 ml, 250 mg/5 ml.

INDICATIONS AND DOSAGES

▸ Community-Acquired Pneumonia
PO
Adults, Elderly, Children 13 yr and older. 300 mg q12h for 10 days.

▸ Acute Exacerbation of Chronic bronchitis
PO
Adults, Elderly. 300 mg q12h for 5–10 days.

▸ Acute Maxillary Sinusitis
PO
Adults, Elderly, Children 13 yr and older. 300 mg q12h or 600 mg q24h for 10 days.
Children 6 mo–12 yr. 7 mg/kg q12h or 14 mg/kg q24h for 10 days.

▸ Pharyngitis or Tonsillitis
PO
Adults, Elderly, Children 13 yr and older. 300 mg q12h for 5–10 days or 600 mg q24h for 10 days.
Children 6 mos-12 yrs. 7 mg/kg q12h for 5–10 days or 14 mg/kg q24h for 10 days.

▸ Uncomplicated Skin or Skin-Structure Infections
PO
Adults, Elderly, Children 13 yr and older. 300 mg q12h for 10 days.
Children 6 mo–12 yr. 7 mg/kg q12h for 10 days.

▸ Acute Bacterial Otitis Media
PO (Capsules)
Children 6 mo–12 yr. 7 mg/kg q12h or 14 mg/kg q24h for 10 days.

▸ Usual Pediatric Dosage for Oral Suspension
Children weighing 81–95 lb (37–43 kg). 12.5 ml (2.5 tsp) q12h or 25 ml (5 tsp) q24h.
Children weighing 61–80 lb (28–36 kg). 10 ml (2 tsp) q12h or 20 ml (4 tsp) q24h.
Children weighing 41–60 lb (19–27 kg). 7.5 ml (1 tsp) q12h or 15 ml (3 tsp) q24h.
Children weighing 20–40 lb (9–18 kg). 5 ml (1 tsp) q12h or 10 ml (2 tsp) q24h.
Infants weighing less than 20 lb (9 kg). 2.5 ml (1/2 tsp) q12h or 5 ml (1 tsp) q24h.

▸ Dosage in Renal Impairment
For patients with creatinine clearance less than 30 ml/min, dosage is 300 mg/day as single daily dose. For hemodialysis patients, dosage is 300 mg or 7 mg/kg/dose every other day.

CONTRAINDICATIONS

History of anaphylactic reaction to penicillins or hypersensitivity to cephalosporins

INTERACTIONS

Drug

Antacids: Decrease cefdinir blood concentration.
Probenecid: Increases cefdinir blood concentration.

Herbal

None known.

Food

None known.

Drug interactions of concern to dentistry

- Absorption retarded by iron salts, magnesium, or aluminum antacids: take antiinfective dose at least 2 hr before antacids or iron preparations
- Increased plasma levels: probenecid
- Oral contraceptives: advise patient of a potential risk for decreased contraceptive action, to maintain compliance with oral contraceptive use while using antibiotics, and to consider the use of additional nonhormonal contraception

DIAGNOSTIC TEST EFFECTS

May increase serum alkaline phosphatase, bilirubin, LDH, AST (SGPT), and ALT (SGOT) levels. May produce a false-positive reaction for ketones in urine.

SIDE EFFECTS

Frequent

Oral candidiasis, mild diarrhea, mild abdominal cramping, vaginal candidiasis

Occasional

Nausea, serum sickness-like reaction (marked by fever and joint pain; usually occurs after the second course of therapy and resolves after the drug is discontinued)

Rare

Allergic reaction (rash, pruritus, urticaria)

SERIOUS REACTIONS

! Antibiotic-associated colitis and other superinfections may result from altered bacterial balance.
! Nephrotoxicity may occur, especially in patients with pre-existing renal disease.
! Patients with a history of allergies, especially to penicillin, are at increased risk for developing a severe hypersensitivity reaction, marked by severe pruritus, angioedema, bronchospasm, and anaphylaxis.

DENTAL CONSIDERATIONS

General:

- Use precaution regarding allergy to medication.
- Determine why patient is taking the drug.
- Examine for oral manifestation of opportunistic infection.

Consultations:

- Medical consultation may be required to assess disease control.

Teach Patient/Family:

- Importance of good oral hygiene to prevent soft tissue inflammation

cefditoren pivoxil

seff-di-tore′-en
(Spectracef)

CATEGORY AND SCHEDULE

Pregnancy Risk Category: B

MECHANISM OF ACTION

A third-generation cephalosporin that binds to bacterial cell membranes and inhibits cell wall synthesis.
Therapeutic Effect: Bactericidal.

C

PHARMACOKINETICS
Moderately absorbed from the GI tract. Protein binding: 88%. Not metabolized. Excreted in the urine. Minimally removed by hemodialysis. ***Half-life:*** 1.6 hr (half-life increased with impaired renal function).

AVAILABILITY
Tablets: 200 mg.

INDICATIONS AND DOSAGES
▶ Pharyngitis, Tonsillitis, Skin Infections
PO
Adults, Elderly, Children older than 12 yr. 200 mg twice a day for 10 days.

▶ Acute Exacerbation of Chronic Bronchitis
PO
Adults, Elderly, Children older than 12 yr. 400 mg twice a day for 10 days.

▶ Community-Acquired Pneumonia
PO
Adults, Elderly, Children older than 12 yr. 400 mg 2 twice a day for 14 days.

▶ Dosage in Renal Impairment
Dosage and frequency are modified on the basis of creatinine clearance.

Creatinine Clearance	Dosage
50–80 ml/min	No adjustment necessary.
30–49 ml/min	200 mg twice a day
less than 30 ml/min	200 mg once a day

CONTRAINDICATIONS
Carnitive deficiency, inborn errors of metabolism, known allergy to cephalosporins, hypersensitivity to milk protein

INTERACTIONS
Drug
Antacids containing magnesium or aluminum, H_2 receptor antagonists: May decrese the absorption of cefditoren.
Probenecid: May increase the absorption of cefditoren.
Herbal
None known.
Food
High-fat meals: Increase the cefditoren plasma concentration.
Drug interactions of concern to dentistry
- Reduced absorption: concurrent use with antacids, H_2-receptor antagonist
- Increased and prolonged serum levels: probenecid
- Does not alter pharmacokinetics of ethinyl estradiol

DIAGNOSTIC TEST EFFECTS
May cause a positive direct or indirect Coombs' test and a false-positive reaction to glycosuria.

SIDE EFFECTS
Occasional (11%)
Diarrhea
Rare (4%–1%)
Nausea, headache, abdominal pain, vaginal candidiasis, dyspepsia, vomiting

SERIOUS REACTIONS
! Antibiotic-associated colitis and other superinfections may occur.
! Patients with a history of allergies, especially to penicillin, are at increased risk for developing a severe hypersensitivity reaction, marked by severe pruritus, angioedema, bronchospasm, and anaphylaxis.

DENTAL CONSIDERATIONS

General:

• Precaution regarding allergy to medication.
• Assess salivary flow as a factor in caries, periodontal disease, and candidiasis.
• Determine why patient is taking the drug.
• Consider semisupine chair position for patient comfort if GI side effects occur.
• Consult with patient's physician if an acute dental infection occurs and another antiinfective is required.
• Examine for oral manifestation of opportunistic infection.
• Patients on chronic drug therapy may rarely have symptoms of blood dyscrasias, which can include infection, bleeding, and poor healing.

Consultations:

• Medical consultation may be required to assess disease control
• In a patient with symptoms of blood dyscrasias, request a medical consultation for blood studies and postpone treatment until normal values are reestablished.

Teach Patient/Family:

• Importance of good oral hygiene to prevent soft tissue inflammation and infection
• *When chronic dry mouth occurs, advise patient:*
  • To avoid mouth rinses with high alcohol content because of drying effects
  • To use daily home fluoride products for anticaries effect
  • To use sugarless gum, frequent sips of water, or saliva substitutes

C

cefepime

sef′-e-peem
(Maxipime)
Do not confuse cefepime with ceftidine.

CATEGORY AND SCHEDULE

Pregnancy Risk Category: B

MECHANISM OF ACTION

A fourth-generation cephalosporin that binds to bacterial cell membranes and inhibits cell wall synthesis. ***Therapeutic Effect:*** Bactericidal.

PHARMACOKINETICS

Well absorbed after IM administration. Protein binding: 20%. Widely distributed. Primarily excreted unchanged in urine. Removed by hemodialysis. ***Half-life:*** 2–2.3 hr (increased in impaired renal function, and in the elderly).

AVAILABILITY

Powder for Injection: 500 mg, 1 g, 2 g.

INDICATIONS AND DOSAGES

▸ Pneumonia

IV
Adults, Elderly. 1–2 g q12h for 7–10 days.
Children 2 mo and older. 50 mg/kg q12h. Maximum: 2 g/dose.

▸ Intra-Abdominal Infections

IV
Adults, Elderly. 2 g q12h for 10 days.

▸ Skin and Skin Structure Infections

IV
Adults, Elderly. 2 g q12h for 10 days.
Children 2 mo and older. 50 mg/kg q12h. Maximum: 2 g/dose.

C

▸ **UTIs**
IV
Adults, Elderly. 0.5–2 g q12h for 7–10 days.
Children 2 mo and older. 50 mg/kg q12h. Maximum: 2 g/dose.
▸ **Febrile Neutropenia**
IV
Adults, Elderly. 2 g q8h.
Children 2 mo and older. 50 mg/kg q8h. Maximum: 2 g/dose.
▸ **Dosage in Renal Impairment**
Dosage and frequency are modified on the basis of creatinine clearance and the severity of the infection.

Creatinine Clearance	Dose
30–60 ml/min	0.5–2 g q24h
11–29 ml/min	0.5–1 g q24h
10 ml/min or less	0.25–0.5 g q24h

CONTRAINDICATIONS
History of anaphylactic reaction to penicillins or hypersensitivity to cephalosporins

INTERACTIONS
Drug
Probenecid: May increase cefepime blood concentration.
Herbal
None known.
Food
None known.
Drug interactions of concern to dentistry
- Increased risk of nephrotoxicity, ototoxicity: aminoglycosides in high doses, furosemide

DIAGNOSTIC TEST EFFECTS
May increase serum alkaline phosphatase, bilirubin, LDH, AST (SGOT), and ALT (SGPT) levels. May cause a positive direct or indirect Coombs' test.

IV INCOMPATIBILITIES
Acyclovir (Zovirax), amphotericin (Fungizone), cimetidine (Tagamet), ciprofloxacin (Cipro), cisplatin (Platinol), dacarbazine (DTIC), daunorubicin (Cerubidine), diazepam (Valium), diphenhydramine (Benadryl), dobutamine (Dobutrex), dopamine (Intropin), doxorubicin (Adriamycin), droperidol (Inapsine), famotidine (Pepcid), ganciclovir (Cytovene), haloperidol (Haldol), magnesium, magnesium sulfate, mannitol, meperidine (Demerol), metoclopramide (Reglan), morphine, ofloxacin (Floxin), ondansetron (Zofran), vancomycin (Vancocin)
IV COMPATIBILITIES
Bumetanide (Bumex), calcium gluconate, furosemide (Lasix), hydromorphone (Dilaudid), lorazepam (Ativan), propofol (Diprivan)

SIDE EFFECTS
Frequent
Discomfort with IM administration, oral candidiasis, mild diarrhea, mild abdominal cramping, vaginal candidiasis
Occasional
Nausea, serum sickness-like reaction (marked by fever and joint pain; usually occurs after the second course of therapy and resolves after the drug is discontinued)
Rare
Allergic reaction (rash, pruritus, urticaria), thrombophlebitis (pain, redness, swelling at injection site)

SERIOUS REACTIONS
! Antibiotic-associated colitis manifested and other superinfections may result from altered bacterial balance.
! Nephrotoxicity may occur, especially in patients with pre-existing renal disease.
! Patients with a history of allergies, especially to penicillin, are at

increased risk for developing a severe hypersensitivity reaction, marked by severe pruritus, angioedema, bronchospasm, and anaphylaxis.

DENTAL CONSIDERATIONS

General:

- Precaution regarding allergy to medication.
- Determine why patient is taking the drug.
- Oral contraceptives: advise patient of a potential risk for decreased contraceptive action, to maintain compliance with oral contraceptive use while using antibiotics, and to consider the use of additional nonhormonal contraception

Consultation:

- Medical consultation may be required to assess disease control.

Teach Patient/Family:

- Importance of good oral hygiene to prevent soft tissue inflammation
- To report sore throat, oral burning sensation, fever, and fatigue, any of which could indicate presence of a superinfection

cefixime

sef-ix′-zeem

(Suprax)

Do not confuse Suprax with Sporanox, Surbex, or Surfak.

CATEGORY AND SCHEDULE

Pregnancy Risk Category: B

MECHANISM OF ACTION

A third-generation cephalosporin that binds to bacterial cell membranes and inhibits cell wall synthesis.
Therapeutic Effect: Bactericidal.

PHARMACOKINETICS

Moderately absorbed from the GI tract. Protein binding: 65%–70%. Widely distributed. Primarily excreted unchanged in urine. Minimally removed by hemodialysis. ***Half-life:*** 3–4 hr (increased in renal impairment).

AVAILABILITY

Oral Suspension: 100 mg/5 ml.
Tablets: 200 mg, 400 mg.

INDICATIONS AND DOSAGES

▸ Otitis Media, Acute Bronchitis, Acute Exacerbations of Chronic Bronchitis, Pharyngitis, Tonsillitis, and Uncomplicated UTIs

PO

Adults, Elderly, Children weighing more than 50 kg. 400 mg/day as a single dose or in 2 divided doses.
Children 6 mo–12 yr weighing less than 50 kg. 8 mg/kg/day as a single dose or in 2 divided doses.
Maximum: 400 mg.

▸ Uncomplicated Gonorrhea

PO

Adults. 400 mg as a single dose.

▸ Dosage in Renal Impairment

Dosage is modified on the basis of creatinine clearance.

Creatinine Clearance	% of Usual Dose
21–60 ml/min	75%
20 ml/min or less	50%

CONTRAINDICATIONS

History of anaphylactic reaction to penicillins, hypersensitivity to cephalosporins

INTERACTIONS

Drug

Probenecid: Increases serum concentration of cefixime.

C

Herbal
None known.
Food
None known.
Drug interactions of concern to dentistry
• Decreased bactericidal effects: tetracyclines, erythromycins
• Increased and prolonged serum levels: probenecid
• Oral contraceptives: advise patient of a potential risk for decreased contraceptive action, to maintain compliance with oral contraceptive use while using antibiotics, and to consider the use of additional nonhormonal contraception

DIAGNOSTIC TEST EFFECTS

May increase BUN and serum alkaline phosphatase, bilirubin, creatinine, AST (SGOT), and ALT (SGPT) levels. May increase LDH level. May cause a positive direct or indirect Coombs' test.

SIDE EFFECTS

Frequent
Oral candidiasis, mild diarrhea, mild abdominal cramping, vaginal candidiasis
Occasional
Nausea, serum sickness-like reaction (marked by arthralgia and fever; usually occurs after second course of therapy and resolves after drug is discontinued)
Rare
Allergic reaction (rash, pruritus, urticaria)

SERIOUS REACTIONS

! Antibiotic-associated colitis and other superinfections may result from altered bacterial balance.
! Nephrotoxicity may occur, especially in patients with pre-existing renal disease.
! Patients with a history of allergies, especially to penicillin, are at increased risk for developing a severe hypersensitivity reaction, marked by severe pruritus, angioedema, bronchospasm, and anaphylaxis.

DENTAL CONSIDERATIONS

General:
• Take precautions regarding allergy to medication.
• Determine why the patient is taking the drug.
Consultations:
• Medical consultation may be required to assess disease control.
Teach Patient/Family:
• Importance of good oral hygiene to prevent soft tissue inflammation
• To avoid mouth rinses with high alcohol content because of drying effects and possible drug–drug reaction
• *When used for dental infection, advise patient:*
  • To report sore throat, oral burning sensation, fever, and fatigue, any of which could indicate superinfection
  • To take at prescribed intervals and complete dosage regimen
  • To immediately notify the dentist if signs or symptoms of infection increase

cefonicid sodium

sef-on-**ih**-sid
(Monocid)
Do not confuse with cefoxitin.

CATEGORY AND SCHEDULE

Pregnancy Risk Category: B

C

MECHANISM OF ACTION
A second-generation cephalosporin that binds to bacterial cell membranes and inhibits cell wall synthesis. ***Therapeutic Effect:*** Bactericidal.

PHARMACOKINETICS
Protein binding: greater than 90%. Widely distributed. Not metabolized. Primarily excreted unchanged in urine. Not removed by hemodialysis. **Half-life:** 4.5 hr.

AVAILABILITY
Powder for Injection: 500 mg, 1 g (Monocid).

INDICATIONS AND DOSAGES
UTIs
IV, IM
Adults, elderly. 0.5 g q24h.
Mild to Moderate Infections
IV, IM
Adults, elderly. 1 g q24h.
Severe or Life-Threatening Infections
IV, IM
Adults, elderly. 2 g q24h.
Surgical Prophylaxis
IV
Adults, elderly. 1 g 60 min before surgery.
Dosage in Renal Impairment
Dosage and frequency are modified on the basis of creatinine clearance and the severity of infection.

Creatinine clearance	Dosage (mild to moderate infections)
60–79 ml/min	10 mg/kg q24h
59–40 ml/min	8 mg/kg q24h
39–20 ml/min	4 mg/kg q24h
19–10 ml/min	4 mg/kg q48h
9–5 ml/min	4 mg/kg q3–5 days
Less than 5 ml/min	3 mg/kg q3–5 days

CONTRAINDICATIONS
History of anaphylactic reaction to penicillins or hypersensitivity to cephalosporins

INTERACTIONS
Drug
Alcohol: May produce a disulfiram-like reaction (facial flushing, headache, nausea, sweating, tachycardia).
Heparin, other anticoagulants: May increase the risk of bleeding.
Herbal
None known.
Food
None known.
Drug interactions of concern to dentistry
- Increased or prolonged plasma levels: probenecid

DIAGNOSTIC TEST EFFECTS
May increase BUN level and serum alkaline phosphatase, creatinine, AST, and ALT levels. May prolong prothrombin time and produce a positive direct or indirect Coombs' test. Interferes with cross-matching procedures and hematologic tests.

SIDE EFFECTS
Frequent
Discomfort with IM administration, oral candidiasis, mild diarrhea, mild abdominal cramping, vaginal candidiasis
Occasional
Nausea, unusual bleeding or bruising, serum sickness-like reaction (marked by fever and joint pain)
Rare
Allergic reaction (rash, pruritus, urticaria), thrombophlebitis (pain, redness, swelling at injection site)

SERIOUS REACTIONS
Antibiotic-associated colitis and other superinfections may result from altered bacterial balance.

Nephrotoxicity may occur, especially in patients with preexisting renal disease.
Patients with a history of allergies, especially to penicillin, are at an increased risk for developing a severe hypersensitivity reaction, marked by severe pruritus, angioedema, bronchospasm, and anaphylaxis.

DENTAL CONSIDERATIONS

General:

- For selected infections in the hospital setting; provide palliative emergency dental care only.
- Caution: use in patients with a history of antibiotic-associated colitis.
- Determine why patient is taking the drug.
- Examine for oral manifestation of opportunistic infection.
- Caution regarding allergy to medication.

Consultations:

- CONIF
- Medical consultation may be required to assess disease control and patient's ability to tolerate stress.

Teach Patient/Family:

- Importance of good oral hygiene to prevent soft tissue inflammation
- To report sore throat, oral burning sensation, fever, or fatigue, any of which could indicate presence of a superinfection

cefoperazone

sef-oh-per′-a-zone
(Cefobid)
Do not confuse with ceftin, cefotetan, and cefamandole.

CATEGORY AND SCHEDULE

Pregnancy Risk Category: B

MECHANISM OF ACTION

A third-generation cephalosporin that binds to bacterial cell membranes. ***Therapeutic Effect:*** Inhibits synthesis of bacterial cell wall. Bactericidal.

PHARMACOKINETICS

Widely distributed, including cerebrospinal fluid (CSF). Protein binding: 82%–93%. Metabolized and excreted in kidney and urine. Removed by hemodialysis. **Half-life:** 1.6–2.4 hrs (half-life is increased with impaired renal function).

AVAILABILITY

Injection, premixed frozen: 1 g (Cefobid).
Powder for Injection: 1 g, 2 g (Cefobid).

INDICATIONS AND DOSAGES

▸ Mild to Moderate Infections

IM/IV
Adults, Elderly. 2–4 g/day in 2 divided doses q12h.

▸ Severe or Life-Threatening Infections

IM/IV
Adults, Elderly. Total daily dose and/or frequency may be increased to 6–12 g/day divided into 2, 3, or 4 equal doses of 1.5–4 g per dose.
Dosage in renal and/or hepatic impairment
Do not exceed 4 g/day in those with liver disease and/or biliary obstruction. Modification of dose usually not necessary in those with renal impairment. Dose should not exceed 1–2 g/day in those with both hepatic and substantial renal impairment.

OFF-LABEL USES

Treatment of Lyme disease

C

CONTRAINDICATIONS
Anaphylactic reaction to penicillins, history of hypersensitivity to cephalosporins or any one of its components.

INTERACTIONS
Drug
Alcohol: A disulfiram-like reaction (facial flushing, headache, nausea, sweating, tachycardia) may occur when alcohol is ingested during cefoperzone therapy.
Anticoagulants, heparin, thrombolytics: May increase the risk of bleeding with these drugs.
Probenecid: May increase serum concentrations of cefoperazone.
Herbal
None known.
Food
None known.
Drug interactions of concern to dentistry
- Avoid alcohol, risk of disulfiram-like reaction
- Increased risk of bleeding: drugs that interfere with platelet action

DIAGNOSTIC TEST EFFECTS
Positive direct/indirect Coombs' test may occur (interferes with hematologic tests, cross-matching procedures). Prothrombin times may be increased. May increase BUN, serum creatinine, SGOT (AST), SGPT (ALT), alkaline phosphatase concentrations.

IV INCOMPATIBILITIES
Amifostine (Ethyol), amikacin, gentamycin, kanamycin, labetolol (Cardene), meperidine (Demerol), neomycin, nicardipine (Cardene), ondansetron (Zofran), perphenazine (Trilafon), promethazine (Phenergan), sargramostim (Leukine), streptomycin, tobramycin, vinorelbine (Navelbine)

IV COMPATIBILITIES
Acyclovir (Zovirax), allopurinol (Aloprim), aztreonam (Azactam), cimetidine (Tagamet), clindamycin (Cleocin Phosphate), cyclosporine (Sandimmune), enalapril (Vasotec), esmolol(Brevibloc), famotidine (Pepcid), fenoldopam (Corlopam), fludarabine (Fludara), foscarnet (Foscavir), furosemide (Lasix), heparin (Hep-Lock), hydromorphone (Dilaudid), lidocaine (Xylocaine), magnesium, propofol (Diprivan), ranitidine (Zantac)

SIDE EFFECTS
Frequent
Discomfort with IM administration, oral candidiasis, mild diarrhea, mild abdominal cramping, vaginal candidiasis
Occasional
Nausea, unusual bruising/bleeding, serum sickness reaction
Rare
Allergic reaction, rash, pruritus, urticaria, thrombophlebitis (pain, redness, swelling at injection site)

SERIOUS REACTIONS
! Antibiotic-associated colitis manifested as severe abdominal pain and tenderness, fever, and watery and severe diarrhea, and other superinfections may result from altered bacterial balance.
! Nephrotoxicity may occur, especially in patients with preexisting renal disease. Severe hypersensitivity reaction including severe pruritus, angioedema, bronchospasm, and anaphylaxis, particularly in patients with a history of allergies, especially to penicillins, may occur.

DENTAL CONSIDERATIONS
General:
- For selected infections in the hospital setting; provide

C

palliative emergency dental treatment only.
- Caution: use in patients with a history of antibiotic-associated colitis.
- Caution: may interfere with prothrombin levels.
- Examine for oral manifestation of opportunistic infection.
- Determine why patient is taking the drug.
- Caution regarding allergy to medication.

Consultations:
- CONIF
- Medical consultation may be required to assess disease control and patient's ability to tolerate stress.
- Medical consultation should include partial prothrombin time, prothrombin time, or INR.

Teach Patient/Family:
- Importance of good oral hygiene to prevent soft tissue inflammation
- To report sore throat, oral burning sensation, fever, or fatigue, any of which could indicate presence of a superinfection

cefotaxime sodium

sef-oh-taks′-eem
(Claforan)
Do not confuse cefotaxime with cefoxitin, ceftizoxime, or cefuroxime, or Claforan with Claritin.

CATEGORY AND SCHEDULE
Pregnancy Risk Category: B

MECHANISM OF ACTION
A third-generation cephalosporin that binds to bacterial cell membranes and inhibits cell wall synthesis. **Therapeutic Effect:** Bactericidal.

PHARMACOKINETICS
Widely distributed, including to CSF. Protein binding: 30%–50%. Partially metabolized in the liver to active metabolite. Primarily excreted in urine. Moderately removed by hemodialysis. ***Half-life:*** 1 hr (increased in impaired renal function).

AVAILABILITY
Powder for Injection: 500 mg, 1 g, 2 g.

INDICATIONS AND DOSAGES
▸ Uncomplicated Infections
IV, IM
Adults, Elderly. 1 g q12h.
▸ Mild to Moderate Infections
IV, IM
Adults, Elderly. 1–2 g q8h.
▸ Severe Infections
IV, IM
Adults, Elderly. 2 g q6–8h.
▸ Life-Threatening Infections
IV, IM
Adults, Elderly. 2 g q4h.
Children: 2 g q4h. Maximum: 12 g/day.
▸ Gonorrhea
IM
Adults. (Male): 1 g as a single dose. (Female): 0.5 g as a single dose.
▸ Perioperative Prophylaxis
IV, IM
Adults, Elderly. 1 g 30–90 min before surgery.
▸ Cesarean Section
IV
Adults. 1 g as soon as umbilical cord is clamped, then 1 g 6 and 12 hr after first dose.
▸ Usual Pediatric Dosage
Children weighing 50 kg or more. 1–2 g q6–8h.
Children 1 mo–12 yr weighing less than 50 kg. 100–200 mg/kg/day in divided doses q6–8h.

Dosage in Renal Impairment

For patients with creatinine clearance less than 20 ml/min give half of dose at usual dosing intervals.

OFF-LABEL USES

Treatment of Lyme disease

CONTRAINDICATIONS

History of anaphylactic reaction to penicillins or hypersensitivity to cephalosporins

INTERACTIONS

Drug

Probenecid: May increase cefotaxime blood concentration.

Herbal

None known.

Food

None known.

Drug interactions of concern to dentistry

- Increased or prolonged plasma levels: probenecid

DIAGNOSTIC TEST EFFECTS

May increase liver function test results and produce a positive direct or indirect Coombs' test

IV INCOMPATIBILITIES

Allopurinol (Aloprim), filgrastim (Neupogen), fluconazole (Diflucan), hetastarch (Hespan), pentamidine (Pentam IV), vancomycin (Vancocin)

IV COMPATIBILITIES

Diltiazem (Cardizem), famotidine (Pepcid), hydromorphone (Dilaudid), lorazepam (Ativan), magnesium sulfate, midazolam (Versed), morphine, propofol (Diprivan)

SIDE EFFECTS

Frequent

Discomfort with IM administration, oral candidiasis, mild diarrhea, mild abdominal cramping, vaginal candidiasis

Occasional

Nausea, serum sickness-like reaction (marked by fever and joint pain; usually occurs after the second course of therapy and resolves after the drug is discontinued)

Rare

Allergic reaction (rash, pruritus, urticaria), thrombophlebitis (pain, redness, swelling at injection site)

SERIOUS REACTIONS

! Antibiotic-associated colitis and other superinfections may result from altered bacterial balance.

! Nephrotoxicity may occur, especially in patients with pre-existing renal disease.

! Patients with a history of allergies, especially to penicillin, are at increased risk for developing a severe hypersensitivity reaction, marked by severe pruritus, angioedema, bronchospasm, and anaphylaxis.

DENTAL CONSIDERATIONS

General:

- For selected infections in the hospital setting; provide palliative emergency dental treatment only.
- Caution: use in patients with a history of antibiotic-associated colitis.
- Examine for oral manifestation of opportunistic infection.
- Determine why patient is taking the drug.
- Caution regarding allergy to medication.

Consultations:

- CONIF
- Medical consultation may be required to assess disease control and patient's ability to tolerate stress.

Teach Patient/Family:

- Importance of good oral hygiene to prevent soft tissue inflammation

• To report sore throat, oral burning sensation, fever, or fatigue, any of which could indicate presence of a superinfection

cefotetan disodium

sef′-oh-tee-tan
(Apatef[AUS], Cefotan)
Do not confuse cefotetan with cefoxitin or Ceftin.

CATEGORY AND SCHEDULE

Pregnancy Risk Category: B

MECHANISM OF ACTION

A second-generation cephalosporin that binds to bacterial cell membranes and inhibits cell wall synthesis. ***Therapeutic Effect:*** Bactericidal.

PHARMACOKINETICS

Protein binding: 78%–91%. Primarily excreted unchanged in urine. Minimally removed by hemodialysis. ***Half-life:*** 3–4.6 hr (increased in impaired renal function).

AVAILABILITY

Powder for Injection: 1 g, 2 g.

INDICATIONS AND DOSAGES

▸ UTIs
IV, IM
Adults, Elderly. 1–2 g in divided doses q12–24h.

▸ Mild to Moderate Infections
IV, IM
Adults, Elderly. 1–2 g q12h.

▸ Severe Infections
IV, IM
Adults, Elderly. 2 g q12h.

▸ Life-Threatening Infections
IV, IM
Adults, Elderly. 3 g q12h.

▸ Perioperative Prophylaxis
IV
Adults, Elderly. 1–2 g 30–60 min before surgery.

▸ Cesarean Section
IV
Adults. 1–2 g as soon as umbilical cord is clamped.

▸ Usual Pediatric Dosage
Children. 40–80 mg/kg/day in divided doses q12h. Maximum: 6 g/day.

▸ Dosage in Renal Impairment
Dosing frequency is modified on the basis of creatinine clearance and the severity of the infection.

Creatinine Clearance	Dosage Interval
10–30 ml/min	Usual dose q24h
less than 10 ml/min	Usual dose q48h

CONTRAINDICATIONS

History of anaphylactic reaction to penicillins or hypersensitivity to cephalosporins

INTERACTIONS

Drug

Alcohol: May produce a disulfiram-like reaction (facial flushing, headache, nausea, pruritus, tachycardia).
Heparin, other anticoagulants: May increase the risk of bleeding.

Herbal

None known.

Food

None known.

Drug interactions of concern to dentistry

• Avoid alcohol, risk of disulfiram-like reaction
• Increased or prolonged plasma levels: probenecid
• Increased risk of bleeding: drugs that interfere with platelet action

DIAGNOSTIC TEST EFFECTS

May increase BUN level and serum alkaline phosphatase, creatinine, AST (SGOT), and ALT (SGPT) levels. May prolong prothrombin time and produce a positive direct or indirect Coombs' test. Interferes with crossmatching procedures and hematologic tests.

IV INCOMPATIBILITIES

Vancomycin (Vancocin)

IV COMPATIBILITIES

Diltiazem (Cardizem), famotidine (Pepcid), heparin, insulin (regular), morphine, propofol (Diprivan)

SIDE EFFECTS

Frequent

Discomfort with IM administration, oral candidiasis, mild diarrhea, mild abdominal cramping, vaginal candidiasis

Occasional

Nausea, unusual bleeding or bruising, serum sickness-like reaction (marked by fever and joint pain; usually occurs after the second course of therapy and resolves after the drug is discontinued)

Rare

Allergic reaction (rash, pruritus, urticaria), thrombophlebitis (pain, redness, swelling at injection site)

SERIOUS REACTIONS

! Antibiotic-associated colitis and other superinfections may result from altered bacterial balance.

! Nephrotoxicity may occur, especially in patients with pre-existing renal disease.

! Patients with a history of allergies, especially to penicillin, are at increased risk for developing a severe hypersensitivity reaction, marked by severe pruritus, angioedema, bronchospasm, and anaphylaxis.

DENTAL CONSIDERATIONS

General:

- For selected infections in the hospital setting; provide palliative emergency dental treatment only
- Caution: use in patients with a history of antibiotic-associated colitis
- Caution: may interfere with prothrombin levels
- Examine for oral manifestation of opportunistic infection
- Determine why patient is taking the drug
- Caution regarding allergy to medication

Consultations:

- CONIF
- Medical consultation may be required to assess disease control and patient's ability to tolerate stress
- Medical consultation should include partial prothrombin time, prothrombin time, or INR

Teach Patient/Family:

- Importance of good oral hygiene to prevent soft tissue inflammation
- To report sore throat, oral burning sensation, fever, or fatigue, any of which could indicate presence of a superinfection

cefoxitin sodium

se-fox′-i-tin

(Mefoxin)

Do not confuse cefoxitin with cefotaxime, cefotetan, or Cytoxan.

CATEGORY AND SCHEDULE

Pregnancy Risk Category: B

MECHANISM OF ACTION

A second-generation cephalosporin that binds to bacterial cell membranes and inhibits cell

C

wall synthesis. ***Therapeutic Effect:*** Bactericidal.

AVAILABILITY

Powder for Injection: 1 g, 2 g.

INDICATIONS AND DOSAGES

▸ Mild to Moderate Infections

IV, IM

Adults, Elderly. 1–2 g q6–8h.

▸ Severe Infections

IV, IM

Adults, Elderly. 1 g q4h or 2 g q6–8h up to 2 g q4h.

▸ Uncomplicated Gonorrhea

IM

Adults. 2 g one time with 1 g probenecid.

▸ Perioperative Prophylaxis

IV, IM

Adults, Elderly. 2 g 30–60 min before surgery, then q6h for up to 24 hr after surgery.

Children older than 3 mo. 30–40 mg/kg 30–60 min before surgery, then q6h for up to 24 hr after surgery.

▸ Cesarean Section

IV

Adults. 2 g as soon as umbilical cord is clamped, then 2 g 4 and 8 hr after first dose, then q6h for up to 24 hr.

▸ Usual Pediatric Dosage

Children older than 3 mo.
80–160 mg/kg/day in 4–6 divided doses. Maximum: 12 g/day.

Neonates. 90–100 mg/kg/day in divided doses q6–8h.

▸ Dosage in Renal Impairment

After a loading dose of 1–2 g, dosage and frequency are modified on the basis of creatinine clearance and the severity of the infection.

Creatinine Clearance	Dosage
30–50 ml/min	1–2 g q8–12h
10–29 ml/min	1–2 g q12–24h
5–9 ml/min	500 mg–1 g q12–24h
less than 5 ml/min	500 mg–1 g q24–48h

CONTRAINDICATIONS

History of anaphylactic reaction to penicillins or hypersensitivity to cephalosporins

INTERACTIONS

Drug

Probenecid: Increases serum concentration of cefoxitin.

Herbal

None known.

Food

None known.

Drug interactions of concern to dentistry

- Increased or prolonged plasma levels: probenecid

DIAGNOSTIC TEST EFFECTS

May increase BUN level and serum alkaline phosphatase, creatinine, AST (SGOT), and ALT (SGPT) levels. May produce a positive direct or indirect Coombs' test. Interferes with crossmatching procedures and hematologic tests.

IV INCOMPATIBILITIES

Filgrastim (Neupogen), pentamidine (Pentam IV), vancomycin (Vancocin)

IV COMPATIBILITIES

Diltiazem (Cardizem), famotidine (Pepcid), heparin, hydromorphone (Dilaudid), magnesium sulfate, morphine, multivitamins, propofol (Diprivan)

SIDE EFFECTS

Frequent

Discomfort with IM administration, oral candidiasis, mild diarrhea, mild abdominal cramping, vaginal candidiasis

Occasional

Nausea, serum sickness-like reaction (marked by fever and joint pain; usually occurs after the second course of therapy and resolves after the drug is discontinued).

Rare
Allergic reaction (pruritus, rash, urticaria), thrombophlebitis (pain, redness, swelling at injection site)

SERIOUS REACTIONS

! Antibiotic-associated colitis and other superinfections may result from altered bacterial balance.
! Nephrotoxicity may occur, especially in patients with pre-existing renal disease.
! Patients with a history of allergies, especially to penicillin, are at increased risk for developing a severe hypersensitivity reaction, marked by severe pruritus, angioedema, bronchospasm, and anaphylaxis.

DENTAL CONSIDERATIONS

General:

- For selected infections in the hospital setting; provide palliative emergency dental treatment only.
- Caution: use in patients with a history of antibiotic-associated colitis.
- Examine for oral manifestation of opportunistic infection.
- Determine why patient is taking the drug.
- Caution regarding allergy to medication.

Consultations:

- Consult patient's physician if an acute dental infection occurs and another antiinfective is required.
- Medical consultation may be required to assess disease control and patient's ability to tolerate stress.

Teach Patient/Family:

- Importance of good oral hygiene to prevent soft tissue inflammation
- To report sore throat, oral burning sensation, fever, or fatigue, any of which could indicate presence of a superinfection

cefpodoxime proxetil

sef-pod′-ox-ime
(Vantin)
Do not confuse Vantin with Ventolin.

CATEGORY AND SCHEDULE

Pregnancy Risk Category: B

MECHANISM OF ACTION

A third-generation cephalosporin that binds to bacterial cell membranes and inhibits cell wall synthesis. ***Therapeutic Effect:*** Bactericidal.

PHARMACOKINETICS

Well absorbed from the GI tract (food increases absorption). Protein binding: 21%–40%. Widely distributed. Primarily excreted unchanged in urine. Partially removed by hemodialysis. ***Half-life:*** 2.3 hr (increased in impaired renal function and elderly patients).

AVAILABILITY

Oral Suspension: 50 mg/5 ml, 100 mg/5 ml.
Tablets: 100 mg, 200 mg.

INDICATIONS AND DOSAGES

▸ **Chronic Bronchitis, Pneumonia**
PO
Adults, Elderly, Children older than 13 yr. 200 mg q12h for 10–14 days.

▸ **Gonorrhea, Rectal Gonococcal Infection (Female Patients Only)**
PO
Adults, Children older than 13 yr. 200 mg as a single dose.

▸ **Skin and Skin-Structure Infections**
PO
Adults, Elderly, Children older than 13 yr. 400 mg q12h for 7–14 days.

C

▸ **Pharyngitis, Tonsillitis**
PO
Adults, Elderly, Children older than 13 yr. 100 mg q12h for 5–10 days.
Children 6 mo–13 yr. 5 mg/kg q12h for 5–10 days. Maximum: 100 mg/dose.

▸ **Acute Maxillary Sinusitis**
PO
Adults, Children older than 13 yr. 200 mg twice a day for 10 days.
Children 2 mos-13 yr. 5 mg/kg q12h for 10 days. Maximum: 400 mg/day.

▸ **UTIs**
PO
Adults, Elderly, Children older than 13 yr. 100 mg q12h for 7 days.

▸ **Acute Otitis Media**
PO
Children 6 mos-13 yr. 5 mg/kg q12h for 5 days. Maximum: 400 mg/dose.

▸ **Dosage in Renal Impairment**
For patients with creatinine clearance less than 30 ml/min, usual dose is given q24h. For patients on hemodialysis, usual dose is given 3 times/wk after dialysis.

CONTRAINDICATIONS

History of anaphylactic reaction to penicillins or hypersensitivity to cephalosporins

INTERACTIONS

Drug

Antacids, H_2 antagonists: May decrease cefpodoxime absorption.
Probenecid: May increase cefpodoxime blood concentration.

Herbal

None known.

Food

None known.

Drug interactions of concern to dentistry

- Decreased bactericidal effects: tetracyclines, erythromycins
- Increased and prolonged serum levels: probenecid
- Oral contraceptives: advise patient of a potential risk for decreased contraceptive action, to maintain compliance with oral contraceptive use while using antibiotics, and to consider the use of additional nonhormonal contraception

DIAGNOSTIC TEST EFFECTS

May increase BUN level and serum alkaline phosphatase, bilirubin, creatinine, LDH, AST (SGOT), and ALT (SGPT) levels. May produce a positive direct or indirect Coombs' test.

SIDE EFFECTS

Frequent

Oral candidiasis, mild diarrhea, mild abdominal cramping, vaginal candidiasis

Occasional

Nausea, serum sickness-like reaction (marked by fever and joint pain; usually occurs after the second course of therapy and resolves after the drug is discontinued)

Rare

Allergic reaction (pruritus, rash, urticaria)

SERIOUS REACTIONS

! Antibiotic-associated colitis and other superinfections may result from altered bacterial balance.

! Nephrotoxicity may occur, especially in patients with pre-existing renal disease.

! Patients with a history of allergies, especially to penicillin, are at increased risk for developing a severe hypersensitivity reaction, marked by severe pruritus, angioedema, bronchospasm, and anaphylaxis.

DENTAL CONSIDERATIONS

General:

- Take precautions regarding allergy to medication.
- Determine why the patient is taking the drug.

Consultations:

- Medical consultation may be required to assess disease control.

Teach Patient/Family:

- Importance of good oral hygiene to prevent soft tissue inflammation
- To avoid mouth rinses with high alcohol content because of drying effects and possible drug–drug reaction
- *When used for dental infection, advise patient:*
  - To report sore throat, oral burning sensation, fever, and fatigue, any of which could indicate superinfection
  - To take at prescribed intervals and complete dosage regimen
  - To immediately notify the dentist if signs or symptoms of infection increase

cefprozil

sef-pro′-zil

(Cefzil)

Do not confuse cefprozil with Cefazolin or Cefzil with Cefol, Ceftin, or Kefzol.

CATEGORY AND SCHEDULE

Pregnancy Risk Category: B

MECHANISM OF ACTION

A second-generation cephalosporin that binds to bacterial cell membranes and inhibits cell wall synthesis. ***Therapeutic Effect:*** Bactericidal.

PHARMACOKINETICS

Well absorbed from the GI tract. Protein binding: 36%–45%. Widely distributed. Primarily excreted unchanged in urine. Moderately removed by hemodialysis. ***Half-life:*** 1.3 hr (increased in impaired renal function).

AVAILABILITY

Oral Suspension: 125 mg/5 ml, 250 mg/5 ml.
Tablets: 250 mg, 500 mg.

INDICATIONS AND DOSAGES

▸ Pharyngitis, Tonsillitis

PO

Adults, Elderly. 500 mg q24h for 10 days.
Children 2–12 yr. 7.5 mg/kg q12h for 10 days.

▸ Acute Bacterial Exacerbation of Chronic Bronchitis, Secondary Bacterial Infection of Acute Bronchitis

PO

Adults, Elderly. 500 mg q12h for 10 days.

▸ Skin and Skin-Structure Infections

PO

Adults, Elderly. 250–500 mg q12h for 10 days.
Children. 20 mg/kg q24h for 10 days.

▸ Acute Sinusitis

PO

Adults, Elderly. 250–500 mg q12h for 10 days.
Children 6 mo–12 yr. 7.5–15 mg/kg q12h for 10 days.

▸ Otitis Media

PO

Children 6 mo–12 yr. 15 mg/kg q12h for 10 days. Maximum: 1 g/day.

▸ Dosage in Renal Impairment

Patients with creatinine clearance less than 30 ml/min receive 50% of usual dose at usual interval.

C

CONTRAINDICATIONS
History of anaphylactic reaction to penicillins or hypersensitivity to cephalosporins

INTERACTIONS
Drug
Probenecid: Increases serum concentration of cefprozil.
Herbal
None known.
Food
None known.
Drug interactions of concern to dentistry
- Decreased bactericidal effects: tetracyclines, erythromycins
- Increased and prolonged serum levels: probenecid
- Oral contraceptives: advise patient of a potential risk for decreased contraceptive action, to maintain compliance with oral contraceptive use while using antibiotics, and to consider the use of additional nonhormonal contraception

DIAGNOSTIC TEST EFFECTS
May increase liver function test results. May produce a positive direct or indirect Coombs' test. Interferes with crossmatching procedures and hematologic tests.

SIDE EFFECTS
Frequent
Oral candidiasis, mild diarrhea, mild abdominal cramping, vaginal candidiasis
Occasional
Nausea, serum sickness reaction (marked by fever and joint pain; usually occurs after the second course of therapy and resolves after the drug is discontinued)
Rare
Allergic reaction (pruritus, rash, urticaria)

SERIOUS REACTIONS
! Antibiotic-associated colitis and other superinfections may result from altered bacterial balance.
! Nephrotoxicity may occur, especially in patients with pre-existing renal disease.
! Patients with a history of allergies, especially to penicillin, are at increased risk for developing a severe hypersensitivity reaction, marked by severe pruritus, angioedema, bronchospasm, and anaphylaxis.

DENTAL CONSIDERATIONS
General:
- Take precautions regarding allergy to medication.
- Determine why the patient is taking the drug.
- Examine for evidence of oral manifestations of blood dyscrasia (infection, bleeding, poor healing) and superinfection.

Consultations:
- Medical consultation may be required to assess disease control.

Teach Patient/Family:
- Importance of good oral hygiene to prevent soft tissue inflammation
- To avoid mouth rinses with high alcohol content because of drying effects and possible drug–drug reaction
- *When used for dental infection, advise patient:*
  - To report sore throat, oral burning sensation, fever, and fatigue, any of which could indicate superinfection
  - To take at prescribed intervals and complete dosage regimen
  - To immediately notify the dentist if signs or symptoms of infection increase

ceftazidime

sef-taz′-i-deem
(Ceptaz, Fortaz, Fortum[AUS], Tazicef, Tazidime)
Do not confuse ceftazidime with ceftizoxime.

CATEGORY AND SCHEDULE

Pregnancy Risk Category: B

MECHANISM OF ACTION

A third-generation cephalosporin that binds to bacterial cell membranes and inhibits cell wall synthesis. ***Therapeutic Effect:*** Bactericidal.

PHARMACOKINETICS

Widely distributed (including to CSF). Protein binding: 5%–17%. Primarily excreted unchanged in urine. Removed by hemodialysis. ***Half-life:*** 2 hr (increased in impaired renal function).

AVAILABILITY

Powder for Injection (Fortaz, Tazicef, Tazidime): 500 mg, 1 g, 2 g.

INDICATIONS AND DOSAGES

▸ UTIs
IV, IM
Adults. 250–500 mg q8–12h.

▸ Mild to Moderate Infections
IV, IM
Adults. 1 g q8–12h.

▸ Uncomplicated Pneumonia, Skin and Skin-Structure Infections
IV, IM
Adults. 0.5–1 g q8h.

▸ Bone and Joint Infections
IV, IM
Adults. 2 g q12h.

▸ Meningitis, Serious Gynecologic and Intra-Abdominal Infections
IV, IM
Adults. 2 g q8h.

▸ Pseudomonal Pulmonary Infections in Patients with Cystic Fibrosis
IV
Adults. 30–50 mg/kg q8h. Maximum: 6 g/day.

▸ Usual Elderly Dosage
Elderly (normal renal function). 500 mg–1 g q12h.

▸ Usual Pediatric Dosage
Children 1 mo–12 yr. 100–150 mg/kg/day in divided doses q8h. Maximum: 6 g/day.
Neonates 0–4 wk. 100–150 mg/kg/day in divided doses q8–12h.

▸ Dosage in Renal Impairment
After an initial 1-g dose, dosage and frequency are modified on the basis of creatinine clearance and the severity of the infection.

Creatinine Clearance	Dosage
31–50 ml/min	1 g q12h
16–30 ml/min	1 g q24h
6–15 ml/min	500 mg q24h
less than 5 ml/min	500 mg q48h

CONTRAINDICATIONS

History of anaphylactic reaction to penicillins or hypersensitivity to cephalosporins

INTERACTIONS

Drug
None known.

Herbal
None known.

Food
None known.

Drug interactions of concern to dentistry
- None reported

DIAGNOSTIC TEST EFFECTS

May increase BUN level and serum alkaline phosphatase, creatinine, LDH, AST (SGOT), and ALT (SGPT) levels. May produce a positive direct or indirect Coombs' test. Interferes with crossmatching procedures and hematologic tests.

IV INCOMPATIBILITIES

Amphotericin B complex (AmBisome, Amphotec, Abelcet), doxorubicin liposomal (Doxil), fluconazole (Diflucan), idarubicin (Idamycin), midazolam (Versed), pentamidine (Pentam IV), vancomycin (Vancocin)

IV COMPATIBILITIES

Diltiazem (Cardizem), famotidine (Pepcid), heparin, hydromorphone (Dilaudid), morphine, propofol (Diprivan)

SIDE EFFECTS

Frequent

Discomfort with IM administration, oral candidiasis, mild diarrhea, mild abdominal cramping, vaginal candidiasis

Occasional

Nausea, serum sickness-like reaction (marked by fever and joint pain; usually occurs after the second course of therapy and resolves after the drug is discontinued)

Rare

Allergic reaction (pruritus, rash, urticaria), thrombophlebitis (pain, redness, swelling at injection site)

SERIOUS REACTIONS

! Antibiotic-associated colitis and other superinfections may result from altered bacterial balance.

! Nephrotoxicity may occur, especially in patients with pre-existing renal disease.

! Patients with a history of allergies, especially to penicillin, are at increased risk for developing a severe hypersensitivity reaction, marked by severe pruritus, angioedema, bronchospasm, and anaphylaxis.

DENTAL CONSIDERATIONS

General:

- For selected infections in the hospital setting; provide palliative emergency dental treatment only.
- Caution: use in patients with a history of antibiotic-associated colitis.
- Examine for oral manifestation of opportunistic infection.
- Determine why patient is taking the drug.
- Caution regarding allergy to medication.

Consultations:

- CONIF
- Medical consultation may be required to assess disease control and patient's ability to tolerate stress.

Teach Patient/Family:

- Importance of good oral hygiene to prevent soft tissue inflammation
- To report sore throat, oral burning sensation, fever, or fatigue, any of which could indicate presence of a superinfection

ceftibuten

cef′-te-bute-in

(Cedax)

CATEGORY AND SCHEDULE

Pregnancy Risk Category: B

MECHANISM OF ACTION

A third-generation cephalosporin that binds to bacterial cell membranes and inhibits cell wall synthesis. ***Therapeutic Effect:*** Bactericidal.

PHARMACOKINETICS

Rapidly absorbed from the gastrointestinal tract. Excreted primarily in urine. ***Half-life:*** 2–3h.

AVAILABILITY

Capsules: 400 mg.
Oral Suspension: 90 mg/5 ml.

INDICATIONS AND DOSAGES

▸ Chronic Bronchitis

PO

Adults, Elderly. 400 mg/day once a day for 10 days.

▸ Pharyngitis, Tonsillitis

PO

Adults, Elderly. 400 mg once a day for 10 days.

Children older than 6 mo. 9 mg/kg once a day for 10 days. Maximum: 400 mg/day.

▸ Otitis Media

PO

Children older than 6 mo. 9 mg/kg once a day for 10 days. Maximum: 400 mg/day.

▸ Dosage in Renal Impairment

Dosage is modified on the basis of creatinine clearance.

Creatinine Clearance	Dosage
50 ml/min and higher	400 mg or 9 mg/kg q24h
30–49 ml/min	200 mg or 4.5 mg/kg q24h
less than 30 ml/min	100 mg or 2.25 mg/kg q24h

CONTRAINDICATIONS

History of anaphylactic reaction to penicillins or hypersensitivity to cephalosporins

INTERACTIONS

Drug

Aminoglycosides: Increased risk of nephrotoxicity.
Probenecid: Increases serum ceftibuten level.

Herbal

None known.

Food

None known.

Drug interactions of concern to dentistry

- Decreased bactericidal effects: tetracyclines, erythromycins
- Increased and prolonged serum levels: probenecid
- Aminoglycosides increase nephrotoxic potential
- Oral contraceptives: advise patient of a potential risk for decreased contraceptive action, to maintain compliance with oral contraceptive use while using antibiotics, and to consider the use of additional nonhormonal contraception

DIAGNOSTIC TEST EFFECTS

May increase BUN level and serum alkaline phosphatase, bilirubin, creatinine, LDH, AST (SGOT), and ALT (SGPT) levels. May produce a positive direct or indirect Coombs' test.

SIDE EFFECTS

Frequent

Oral candidiasis, mild diarrhea (discharge, itching)

Occasional

Nausea, serum sickness-like reaction (marked by fever and joint pain; usually occurs after the second course of therapy and resolves after the drug is discontinued)

Rare

Allergic reaction (rash, pruritus, urticaria)

SERIOUS REACTIONS

! Antibiotic-associated colitis and other superinfections may result from altered bacterial balance.

! Nephrotoxicity may occur, especially in patients with pre-existing renal disease.

! Patients with a history of allergies, especially to penicillin, are at increased risk for developing a severe hypersensitivity reaction, marked by severe pruritus, angioedema, bronchospasm, and anaphylaxis.

DENTAL CONSIDERATIONS

General:

- Take precautions regarding allergy to medication.
- Assess salivary flow as factor in caries, periodontal disease, and candidiasis.
- Oral suspension contains sucrose; patient should rinse mouth after use.
- Determine why the patient is taking the drug.

Consultations:

- Medical consultation may be required to assess disease control.

Teach Patient/Family:

- Importance of good oral hygiene to prevent soft tissue inflammation
- *When used for dental infection, advise patient:*
  - To report sore throat, oral burning sensation, fever, and fatigue, any of which could indicate superinfection
  - To take at prescribed intervals and complete dosage regimen
  - To immediately notify the dentist if signs or symptoms of infection increase

ceftizoxime sodium

sef-ti-zox′-eem
(Cefizox)
Do not confuse ceftizoxime with cefotaxime or ceftazidime.

CATEGORY AND SCHEDULE

Pregnancy Risk Category: B

MECHANISM OF ACTION

A third-generation cephalosporin that binds to bacterial cell membranes and inhibits cell wall synthesis. ***Therapeutic Effect:*** Bactericidal.

PHARMACOKINETICS

Widely distributed (including to CSF). Protein binding: 30%. Primarily excreted unchanged in urine. Moderately removed by hemodialysis. ***Half-life:*** 1.7 hr (increased in impaired renal function).

AVAILABILITY

Powder for Injection: 500 mg, 1 g, 2 g.

INDICATIONS AND DOSAGES

▸ **Uncomplicated UTIs**
IV, IM
Adults, Elderly. 500 mg q12h.

▸ **Mild, Moderate, or Severe Infections of the Biliary, Respiratory, and GU Tracts; Skin, Bone, and Intra-Abdominal Infections; Meningitis; and Septicemia**
IV, IM
Adults, Elderly. 1–2 g q8–12h.

▸ **Life-Threatening Infections of the Biliary, Respiratory, and GU Tracts; Skin, Bone and Intra-Abdominal Infections; Meningitis; and Septicemia**
IV
Adults, Elderly. 3–4 g q8h, up to 2 g q4h.

▸ **Pelvic Inflammatory Disease (PID)**
IV
Adults. 2 g q4–8h.

▸ **Uncomplicated Gonorrhea**
IM
Adults. 1 g one time.

▸ **Usual Pediatric Dosage**
Children older than 6 mo: 50 mg/kg q6–8h.
Maximum: 12 g/day.

Dosage in Renal Impairment

After a loading dose of 0.5–1 g, dosage and frequency are modified on the basis of creatinine clearance and the severity of the infection.

Creatinine Clearance	Dosage
50–79 ml/min	0.5 g–1.5 g q8h
5–49 ml/min	0.25 g–1 g q12h
less than 5 ml/min	0.25–0.5 g q24h or 0.5 g–1 g q48h

CONTRAINDICATIONS

History of anaphylactic reaction to penicillins or hypersensitivity to cephalosporins

INTERACTIONS

Drug

Probenecid: Increases serum concentration of ceftizoxime.

Herbal

None known.

Food

None known.

Drug interactions of concern to dentistry

• Increased or prolonged plasma levels: probenecid

DIAGNOSTIC TEST EFFECTS

May increase BUN level and serum alkaline serum phosphatase, creatinine, AST (SGOT), and ALT (SGPT) levels. May produce a positive direct or indirect Coombs' test.

IV INCOMPATIBILITIES

Filgrastim (Neupogen)

IV COMPATIBILITIES

Hydromorphone (Dilaudid), morphine, propofol (Diprivan)

SIDE EFFECTS

Frequent

Discomfort with IM administration, oral candidiasis, mild diarrhea, mild abdominal cramping, vaginal candidiasis

Occasional

Nausea, serum sickness-like reaction (fever, joint pain; usually occurs after the second course of therapy and resolves after the drug is discontinued)

Rare

Allergic reaction (rash, pruritus, urticaria), thrombophlebitis (pain, redness, swelling at injection site)

SERIOUS REACTIONS

! Antibiotic-associated colitis manifested and other superinfections may result from altered bacterial balance.

! Nephrotoxicity may occur, especially in patients with pre-existing renal disease.

! Patients with a history of allergies, especially to penicillin, are at increased risk for developing a severe hypersensitivity reaction, marked by severe pruritus, angioedema, bronchospasm, and anaphylaxis.

DENTAL CONSIDERATIONS

General:

• For selected infections in the hospital setting; provide palliative emergency dental treatment only.

• Caution: use in patients with a history of antibiotic-associated colitis.

• Examine for oral manifestation of opportunistic infection.

• Determine why patient is taking the drug.

• Caution regarding allergy to medication.

Consultations:

• CONIF

• Medical consultation may be required to assess disease control and patient's ability to tolerate stress.

C

Teach Patient/Family:
- Importance of good oral hygiene to prevent soft tissue inflammation
- To report sore throat, oral burning sensation, fever, or fatigue, any of which could indicate presence of a superinfection

ceftriaxone sodium

sef-try-ax′-one
(Rocephin)

CATEGORY AND SCHEDULE

Pregnancy Risk Category: B

MECHANISM OF ACTION

A third-generation cephalosporin that binds to bacterial cell membranes and inhibits cell wall synthesis. ***Therapeutic Effect:*** Bactericidal.

PHARMACOKINETICS

Widely distributed (including to CSF). Protein binding: 83%–96%. Primarily excreted unchanged in urine. Not removed by hemodialysis. ***Half-life:*** 4.3–4.6 hr IV; 5.8–8.7 hr IM (increased in impaired renal function).

AVAILABILITY

Powder for Injection: 250 mg, 500 mg, 1 g, 2 g.

INDICATIONS AND DOSAGES

▸ **Mild to Moderate Infections**
IV, IM
Adults, Elderly. 1–2 g as a single dose or in 2 divided doses.

▸ **Serious Infections**
IV, IM
Adults, Elderly. Up to 4 g/day in 2 divided doses.
Children. 50–75 mg/kg/day in divided doses q12h. Maximum: 2 g/day.

▸ **Skin and Skin-Structure Infections**
IV, IM
Children. 50–75 mg/kg/day as a single dose or in 2 divided doses. Maximum: 2 g/day.

▸ **Meningitis**
IV
Children. Initially, 75 mg/kg, then 100 mg/kg/day as a single dose or in divided doses q12h. Maximum: 4 g/day.

▸ **Lyme Disease**
IV
Adults, Elderly. 2–4 g a day for 10–14 days.

▸ **Acute Bacterial Otitis Media**
IM
Children. 50 mg/kg once a day for 3 days. Maximum: 1 g/day.

▸ **Perioperative Prophylaxis**
IV, IM
Adults, Elderly. 1 g 0.5–2 hrs before surgery.

▸ **Uncomplicated Gonorrhea**
IM
Adults. 250 mg plus doxycycline one time.

▸ **Dosage in Renal Impairment**
Dosage modification is usually unnecessary, but liver and renal function test results should be monitored in those with both renal and liver impairment or severe renal impairment.

CONTRAINDICATIONS

History of anaphylactic reaction to penicillins or hypersensitivity to cephalosporins

INTERACTIONS

Drug
None known.
Herbal
None known.
Food
None known.

Drug interactions of concern to dentistry

- None reported

DIAGNOSTIC TEST EFFECTS

May increase BUN level and serum alkaline phosphatase, bilirubin, creatinine, AST (SGOT), and ALT (SGPT) levels. May produce a positive direct or indirect Coombs' test. Interferes with crossmatching procedures and hematologic tests.

IV INCOMPATIBILITIES

Aminophylline, amphotericin B complex (AmBisome, Amphotec, Abelcet), filgrastim (Neupogen), fluconazole (Diflucan), labetalol (Normodyne), pentamidine (Pentam IV), vancomycin (Vancocin)

IV COMPATIBILITIES

Diltiazem (Cardizem), heparin, lidocaine, morphine, propofol (Diprivan)

SIDE EFFECTS

Frequent

Discomfort with IM administration, oral candidiasis, mild diarrhea, mild abdominal cramping, vaginal candidiasis

Occasional

Nausea, serum sickness-like reaction (marked by fever and joint pain; usually occurs after the second course of therapy and resolves after the drug is discontinued)

Rare

Allergic reaction (rash, pruritus, urticaria), thrombophlebitis (pain, redness, swelling at injection site)

SERIOUS REACTIONS

! Antibiotic-associated colitis and other superinfections may result from altered bacterial balance.

! Nephrotoxicity may occur, especially in patients with pre-existing renal disease.

! Patients with a history of allergies, especially to penicillin, are at increased risk for developing a severe hypersensitivity reaction, marked by severe pruritus, angioedema, bronchospasm, and anaphylaxis.

DENTAL CONSIDERATIONS

General:

- For selected infections in the hospital setting; provide palliative emergency dental treatment only.
- Caution: use in patients with a history of antibiotic-associated colitis.
- Caution: may interfere with prothrombin levels.
- Examine for oral manifestation of opportunistic infection.
- Determine why patient is taking the drug.
- Caution regarding allergy to medication.

Consultations:

- CONIF
- Medical consultation may be required to assess disease control and patient's ability to tolerate stress.
- Medical consultation should include partial prothrombin time, prothrombin time, or INR.

Teach Patient/Family:

- Importance of good oral hygiene to prevent soft tissue inflammation
- To report sore throat, oral burning sensation, fever, or fatigue, any of which could indicate presence of a superinfection

C

cefuroxime axetil/ cefuroxime sodium

cef-yur-ox′-ime
(cefuroxime axetil) Ceftin, Zinnat[AUS](cefuroxime sodium) Kefurox, Zinacef
Do not confuse cefuroxime with cefotaxime or deferoxamine or Ceftin with Cefzil.

CATEGORY AND SCHEDULE

Pregnancy Risk Category: B

MECHANISM OF ACTION

A second-generation cephalosporin that binds to bacterial cell membranes and inhibits cell wall synthesis. ***Therapeutic Effect:*** Bactericidal.

PHARMACOKINETICS

Rapidly absorbed from the GI tract. Protein binding: 33%–50%. Widely distributed (including to CSF). Primarily excreted unchanged in urine. Moderately removed by hemodialysis. ***Half-life:*** 1.3 hr (increased in impaired renal function).

AVAILABILITY

Oral Suspension: 125 mg/5 ml, 250 mg/5 ml.
Tablets: 250 mg, 500 mg.
Powder for Injection: 750 mg, 1.5 g.

INDICATIONS AND DOSAGES

▸ Ampicillin-Resistant Influenza; Bacterial Meningitis; Early Lyme Disease; GU Tract, Gynecologic, Skin, and Bone Infections; Septicemia; Gonorrhea, and Other Gonococcal Infections

IV, IM
Adults, Elderly. 750 mg–1.5 g q8h.
Children. 75–100 mg/kg/day divided q8h. Maximum: 8 g/day.
Neonates. 50–100 mg/kg/day divided q12h.
PO
Adults, Elderly. 125–500 mg twice a day, depending on the infection.

▸ Pharyngitis, Tonsillitis

PO
Children 3 mo–12 yr. 125 mg (tablets) q12h or 20 mg/kg/day (suspension) in 2 divided doses.

▸ Acute Otitis Media, Acute Bacterial Maxillary Sinusitis, Impetigo

PO
Children 3 mo–12 yr. 250 mg (tablets) q12h or 30 mg/kg/day (suspension) in 2 divided doses.

▸ Bacterial Meningitis

IV
Children 3 mo–12 yr. 200–240 mg/kg/day in divided doses q6–8h.

▸ Perioperative Prophylaxis

IV
Adults, Elderly. 1.5 g 30–60 min before surgery and 750 mg q8h after surgery.

▸ Usual Neonatal Dosage

IV, IM
Neonates. 20–100 mg/kg/day in divided doses q12h.

▸ Dosage in Renal Impairment

Adult dosage and frequency are modified based on creatinine clearance and the severity of the infection.

Creatinine Clearance	Dosage
greater than 20 ml/min	750 mg–1 g q8h
10–20 ml/min	750 mg q12h
less than 10 ml/min	750 mg q24h

CONTRAINDICATIONS

History of anaphylactic reaction to penicillins or hypersensitivity to cephalosporins

INTERACTIONS

Drug

Probenecid: Increases serum concentration of cefuroxime.

Herbal

None known.

Food

None known.

Drug interactions of concern to dentistry

- Decreased bactericidal effects: tetracyclines, erythromycins
- Increased and prolonged serum levels: probenecid
- Oral contraceptives: advise patient of a potential risk for decreased contraceptive action, to maintain compliance with oral contraceptive use while using antibiotics, and to consider the use of additional nonhormonal contraception

DIAGNOSTIC TEST EFFECTS

May increase serum alkaline phosphatase, bilirubin, LDH, AST (SGOT), and ALT (SGPT) levels. May produce a positive direct or indirect Coombs' test. Interferes with crossmatching procedures, hematologic tests.

IV INCOMPATIBILITIES

Filgrastim (Neupogen), fluconazole (Diflucan), midazolam (Versed), vancomycin (Vancocin)

IV COMPATIBILITIES

Diltiazem (Cardizem), hydromorphone (Dilaudid), morphine, propofol (Diprivan)

SIDE EFFECTS

Frequent

Discomfort with IM administration, oral candidiasis, mild diarrhea, mild abdominal cramping, vaginal candidiasis

Occasional

Nausea, serum sickness-like reaction (marked by fever and joint pain; usually occurs after the second course of therapy and resolves after the drug is discontinued)

Rare

Allergic reaction (rash, pruritus, urticaria), thrombophlebitis (pain, redness, swelling at injection site)

SERIOUS REACTIONS

! Antibiotic-associated colitis and other superinfections may result from altered bacterial balance.

! Nephrotoxicity may occur, especially in patients with pre-existing renal disease.

! Patients with a history of allergies, especially to penicillin, are at increased risk for developing a severe hypersensitivity reaction, marked by severe pruritus, angioedema, bronchospasm, and anaphylaxis.

DENTAL CONSIDERATIONS

General:

- Take precautions regarding allergy to medication.
- Determine why the patient is taking the drug.

Consultations:

- Medical consultation may be required to assess disease control.

Teach Patient/Family:

- Importance of good oral hygiene to prevent soft tissue inflammation
- To avoid mouth rinses with high alcohol content because of drying effects and possible drug–drug reaction
- *When used for dental infection, advise patient:*
  - To report sore throat, oral burning sensation, fever, and fatigue, any of which could indicate superinfection

- To take at prescribed intervals and complete dosage regimen
- To immediately notify the dentist if signs or symptoms of infection increase

celecoxib

sel-eh-cox′-ib
(Celebrex, DisperDose, Panixine)
Do not confuse Celebrex with Cerebyx or Celexa.

CATEGORY AND SCHEDULE

Pregnancy Risk Category: C (D if used in third trimester or near delivery)

MECHANISM OF ACTION

An NSAID that inhibits cyclo-oxygenase-2, the enzyme responsible for prostaglandin synthesis. Mechanism of action in treating familial adenomatous polyposis is unknown. ***Therapeutic Effect:*** Reduces inflammation and relieves pain.

PHARMACOKINETICS

Widely distributed. Protein binding: 97%. Metabolized in the liver. Primarily eliminated in feces. ***Half-life:*** 11.2 hr.

AVAILABILITY

Capsules: 100 mg, 200 mg, 400 mg.

INDICATIONS AND DOSAGES

▸ Osteoarthritis

PO

Adults, Elderly. 200 mg/day as a single dose or 100 mg twice a day.

▸ Rheumatoid Arthritis

PO

Adults, Elderly. 100–200 mg twice a day.

▸ Acute Pain

PO

Adults, Elderly. Initially, 400 mg with additional 200 mg on day 1, if needed. Maintenance: 200 mg twice a day as needed.

▸ Familial Adenomatous Polyposis

PO

Adults, Elderly. 400 mg twice daily (with food).

CONTRAINDICATIONS

Hypersensitivity to aspirin, NSAIDs, or sulfonamides

INTERACTIONS

Drug

Fluconazole: May increase celecoxib blood level.
Lithium: May increase lithium blood levels.
Warfarin: May increase the risk of bleeding.

Herbal

None known.

Food

None known.

Drug interactions of concern to dentistry

- Increased plasma levels: fluconazole
- Increased risk of GI bleeding: long-duration NSAIDs, aspirin (except low doses), oral glucocorticoids, alcoholism, smoking, older age, generally poor health
- Increased plasma levels of lithium
- Possible risk of increased INR in elderly patients taking warfarin
- Possible reduction in blood pressure control: ACE inhibitors
- First-time users of SSRIs also taking NSAIDs may have a higher risk of GI side effects; until more data are available, it may be advisable to avoid use of NSAIDs in these patients (*Br J Clin Pharmacol* 55:591–595, 2003)

DIAGNOSTIC TEST EFFECTS
May increase AST (SGOT) and ALT (SGPT) levels.

SIDE EFFECTS
Frequent (> 5%)
Diarrhea, dyspepsia, headache, upper respiratory tract infection
Occasional (5%–1%)
Abdominal pain, flatulence, nausea, back pain, peripheral edema, dizziness, rash

SERIOUS REACTIONS
! None known.

DENTAL CONSIDERATIONS
General:
- Patients on chronic drug therapy may rarely have symptoms of blood dyscrasias, which can include infection, bleeding, and poor healing.
- Assess salivary flow as a factor in caries, periodontal disease, and candidiasis.
- Consider semisupine chair position for patient comfort because of effects of disease and GI side effects of drug.

Teach Patient/Family:
- Importance of good oral hygiene to prevent soft tissue inflammation
- Importance of updating health and drug history if physician makes any changes in evaluation or drug regimens
- Use of electric toothbrush if patient has difficulty holding conventional devices
- *When chronic dry mouth occurs, advise patient:*
  - To avoid mouth rinses with high alcohol content because of drying effects
  - To use daily home fluoride products for anticaries effect
  - To use sugarless gum, frequent sips of water, or saliva substitutes

cephalexin
sef-a-lex′-in
(Apo-Cephalex[CAN], Biocef, Ceporex[AUS], Ibilex[AUS], Keflex, Keftab, Novolexin[CAN])

CATEGORY AND SCHEDULE
Pregnancy Risk Category: B

MECHANISM OF ACTION
A first-generation cephalosporin that binds to bacterial cell membranes and inhibits cell wall synthesis. ***Therapeutic Effect:*** Bactericidal.

PHARMACOKINETICS
Rapidly absorbed from the GI tract. Protein binding: 10%–15%. Widely distributed. Primarily excreted unchanged in urine. Moderately removed by hemodialysis. ***Half-life:*** 0.9–1.2 hr (increased in impaired renal function).

AVAILABILITY
Capsules (Biocef): 500 mg.
Capsules (Keflex): 250 mg, 500 mg.
Powder for Oral Suspension (Biocef): 125 mg/5 ml, 250 mg/5 ml.
Tablets: 250 mg, 500 mg.
Tablets (Keftab): 500 mg.

INDICATIONS AND DOSAGES
▸ Bone Infections, Prophylaxis of Rheumatic Fever, Follow-up to Parenteral Therapy
PO
Adults, Elderly. 250–500 mg q6h up to 4 g/day.
▸ Streptococcal Pharyngitis, Skin and Skin-Structure Infections, Uncomplicated Cystitis
PO
Adults, Elderly. 500 mg q12h.
▸ Usual Pediatric Dosage
Children. 25–100 mg/kg/day in 2–4 divided doses.

C

Otitis Media
PO
Children. 75–100 mg/kg/day in 4 divided doses.

Dosage in Renal Impairment
After usual initial dose, dosing frequency is modified on the basis of creatinine clearance and the severity of the infection.

Creatinine Clearance	Dosage Interval
10–40 ml/min	Usual dose q8–12h
less than 10 ml/min	Usual dose q12–24h

CONTRAINDICATIONS
History of anaphylactic reaction to penicillins or hypersensitivity to cephalosporins

INTERACTIONS
Drug
Probenecid: Increases serum concentration of cephalexin.
Herbal
None known.
Food
None known.
Drug interactions of concern to dentistry
- Decreased bactericidal effects: tetracyclines, erythromycins
- Increased and prolonged serum levels: probenecid
- Oral contraceptives: advise patient of a potential risk for decreased contraceptive action, to maintain compliance with oral contraceptive use while using antibiotics, and to consider the use of additional nonhormonal contraception

DIAGNOSTIC TEST EFFECTS
May increase serum alkaline phosphatase, AST (SGOT), and ALT (SGPT) levels. May produce a positive direct or indirect Coombs' test. Interferes with crossmatching procedures and hematologic tests.

SIDE EFFECTS
Frequent
Oral candidiasis, mild diarrhea, mild abdominal cramping, vaginal candidiasis
Occasional
Nausea, serum sickness-like reaction (marked by fever and joint pain; ususally occurs after the second course of therapy and resolves after the drug is discontinued)
Rare
Allergic reaction (rash, pruritus, urticaria)

SERIOUS REACTIONS
! Antibiotic-associated colitis and other superinfections may result from altered bacterial balance.
! Nephrotoxicity may occur, especially in patients with pre-existing renal disease.
! Patients with a history of allergies, especially to penicillin, are at increased risk for developing a severe hypersensitivity reaction, marked by severe pruritus, angioedema, bronchospasm, and anaphylaxis.

DENTAL CONSIDERATIONS
General:
- Take precautions regarding allergy to medication.
- Determine why the patient is taking the drug.

Consultations:
- Medical consultation may be required to assess disease control.

Teach Patient/Family:
- Importance of good oral hygiene to prevent soft tissue inflammation

- To avoid mouth rinses with high alcohol content because of drying effects and possible drug–drug reaction
- *When used for dental infection, advise patient:*
  - To report sore throat, oral burning sensation, fever, and fatigue, any of which could indicate superinfection
  - To take at prescribed intervals and complete dosage regimen
  - To immediately notify the dentist if signs or symptoms of infection increase

cephradine

sef′-ra-deen
(Velosef)

CATEGORY AND SCHEDULE

Pregnancy Risk Category: B

MECHANISM OF ACTION

A first-generation cephalosporin that binds to bacterial cell membranes. Inhibits synthesis of bacterial cell wall. ***Therapeutic Effect:*** Bactericidal.

PHARMACOKINETICS

Well absorbed from the gastrointestinal (GI) tract. Protein binding: 18%–20%. Widely distributed. Primarily excreted unchanged in urine. Removed by hemodialysis. **Half-life:** 1–2 hrs (half-life is increased with impaired renal function).

AVAILABILITY

Capsules: 250 mg, 500 mg (Velosef).
Oral Suspension: 125 mg/5 ml, 250 mg/5ml (Velosef).

INDICATIONS AND DOSAGES

▸ Mild, Moderate, or Severe Infections of the Respiratory, and Genitourinary (GU) Tracts; Bone, Joint, and Skin Infections; Prostatitis; Otitis Media

PO
Adults, Elderly. 250–500 mg q6h. Maximum: 8 g/day.
Children older than 9 mo. 25–50 mg/kg/day in divided doses q6–12h. Maximum: 4 g/day.
Dosage in renal impairment
Dosage and frequency are based on the degree of renal impairment and the severity of infection. After initial 1-g dose:

Creatinine Clearance	Dosage Interval
10–50 ml/min	250 mg q6h
0–10 ml/min	125 mg q6h

CONTRAINDICATIONS

History of hypersensitivity to penicillins and cephalosporins

INTERACTIONS

Drug

Diuretics: Increases risk of nephrotoxicity.
Probenecid: Increases cephradine blood concentration.

Herbal

None known.

Food

Food: Delays absorption and reduces peak levels when administered immediately before oral cephradine.

Drug interactions of concern to dentistry

- Decreased bactericidal effects: tetracyclines, erythromycins
- Increased and prolonged serum levels: probenecid
- Oral contraceptives: advise patient of a potential risk for decreased contraceptive action, to maintain

C

compliance with oral contraceptive use while using antibiotics, and to consider the use of additional nonhormonal contraception

DIAGNOSTIC TEST EFFECTS

Positive direct or indirect Coombs' test. False-positive serum or urine creatinine with Jaffé reaction, urinary proteins and steroids, and glucose test using cupric sulfate (Benedict's solution, Clinitest, Fehling's solution).

SIDE EFFECTS

Frequent
Diarrhea, mild abdominal cramping, vaginal candidiasis (discharge, itching)
Occasional
Nausea, headache, unusual bruising or bleeding, serum sickness reaction (fever, joint pain)
Rare
Allergic reaction (rash, pruritus, urticaria)

SERIOUS REACTIONS

! Antibiotic-associated colitis as evidenced by severe abdominal pain and tenderness, fever, and watery and severe diarrhea, and other superinfections may result from altered bacterial balance.
! Nephrotoxicity may occur, especially in patients with preexisting renal disease.
! Severe hypersensitivity reaction including severe pruritus, angioedema, bronchospasm, and anaphylaxis, particularly in patients with history of allergies, especially penicillin, may occur.

DENTAL CONSIDERATIONS

General:
- Take precautions regarding allergy to medication.
- Determine why the patient is taking the drug.

Consultations:
- Medical consultation may be required to assess disease control.

Teach Patient/Family:
- Importance of good oral hygiene to prevent soft tissue inflammation
- To avoid mouth rinses with high alcohol content because of drying effects and possible drug–drug reaction
- *When used for dental infection, advise patient:*
  - To report sore throat, oral burning sensation, fever, and fatigue, any of which could indicate superinfection
  - To take at prescribed intervals and complete dosage regimen
  - To immediately notify the dentist if signs or symptoms of infection increase

cetirizine

si-tear′-a-zeen
(Reactine[CAN], Zyrtec)
Do not confuse Zyrtec with Zantac or Zyprexa.

CATEGORY AND SCHEDULE

Pregnancy Risk Category: B

MECHANISM OF ACTION

A second-generation piperazine that competes with histamine for H_1-receptor sites on effector cells in the GI tract, blood vessels, and respiratory tract. ***Therapeutic Effect:*** Prevents allergic response, produces mild bronchodilation, blocks histamine-induced bronchitis.

PHARMACOKINETICS

Route	Onset	Peak	Duration
PO	less than 1 hr	4–8 hr	less than 24 hr

Rapidly and almost completely absorbed from the GI tract (absorption not affected by food). Protein binding: 93%. Undergoes low first-pass metabolism; not extensively metabolized. Primarily excreted in urine (more than 80% as unchanged drug). ***Half-life:*** 6.5–10 hr.

AVAILABILITY

Syrup: 5 mg/5 ml.
Tablets: 5 mg, 10 mg.
Tablets (Chewable): 5 mg, 10 mg.

INDICATIONS AND DOSAGES

▸ Allergic Rhinitis, Urticaria

PO

Adults, Elderly, Children older than 5 yr. Initially, 5–10 mg/day as a single or in 2 divided doses.
Children 2–5 yr. 2.5 mg/day. May increase up to 5 mg/day as a single or in 2 divided doses.
Children 12–23 mo. Initially, 2.5 mg/day. May increase up to 5 mg/day in 2 divided doses.
Children 6–11 mo. 2.5 mg once a day.

▸ Dosage in Renal or Hepatic impairment

For adult and elderly patients with renal impairment (creatinine clearance of 11–31 ml/min), those receiving hemodialysis (creatinine clearance of < 7 ml/min), and those with hepatic impairment, dosage is decreased to 5 mg once a day.

OFF-LABEL USES

Treatment of bronchial asthma

CONTRAINDICATIONS

Hypersensitivity to cetirizine or hydroxyzine

INTERACTIONS

Drug

Alcohol, other CNS depressants: May increase CNS depression.

Herbal

None known.

Food

None known.

Drug interactions of concern to dentistry

- No drug interactions reported, but should be similar to other antihistamines; anticipate increased sedation with other CNS depressants and increased anticholinergic effects with anticholinergic drugs

DIAGNOSTIC TEST EFFECTS

May suppress wheal and flare reactions to antigen skin testing, unless drug is discontinued 4 days before testing.

SIDE EFFECTS

Occasional (10%–2%)

Pharyngitis; dry mucous membranes, nose, or throat; nausea and vomiting; abdominal pain; headache; dizziness; fatigue; thickening of mucus; somnolence; photosensitivity; urine retention

SERIOUS REACTIONS

! Children may experience paradoxical reactions, including restlessness, insomnia, euphoria, nervousness, and tremor.

! Dizziness, sedation, and confusion are more likely to occur in elderly patients.

DENTAL CONSIDERATIONS

General:

- Assess salivary flow as factor in caries, periodontal disease, and candidiasis.

Teach Patient/Family:

- *When chronic dry mouth occurs, advise patient:*
  - To avoid mouth rinses with high alcohol content because of drying effects

C

• To use daily home fluoride products for anticaries effect
• To use sugarless gum, frequent sips of water, or saliva substitutes

cetuximab

ceh-tux′-ih-mab
(Erbitux)

CATEGORY AND SCHEDULE

Pregnancy Risk Category: C

MECHANISM OF ACTION

A monoclonal antibody that binds to the epidermal growth factor receptor (EGFR), a glycoprotein on normal and tumor cells, thus inhibiting cell growth and inducing apoptosis.
Therapeutic Effect: Inhibits the growth and survival of tumor cells that overexpress EGFR.

PHARMACOKINETICS

Reaches steady state levels by the third weekly infusion. Clearance decreases as dose increases.
Half-life: 114 hr (range, 75–188 hr).

AVAILABILITY

Injection: 2 mg/ml.

INDICATIONS AND DOSAGES

▸ **Metastatic Colorectal Carcinoma**

IV

Adults, Elderly. Initially, 400 mg/m^2 as a loading dose. Maintenance: 250 mg/m^2 infused over 60 minutes weekly.

CONTRAINDICATIONS

None known.

INTERACTIONS

Drug

None known.

Herbal

None known.

Food

None known.

Drug interactions of concern to dentistry

• Dental drug interactions have not been studied

DIAGNOSTIC TEST EFFECTS

May decrease WBC count, hematocrit, and hemoglobin level.

IV COMPATIBILITIES

Irinotecan (Camptosar)

SIDE EFFECTS

Frequent (90%–25%)

Acneiform rash, malaise, fever, nausea, diarrhea, constipation, headache, abdominal pain, anorexia, vomiting

Occasional (16%–10%)

Nail disorder, back pain, stomatitis, peripheral edema, pruritus, cough, insomnia

Rare (9%–5%)

Weight loss, depression, dyspepsia, conjunctivitis, alopecia

SERIOUS REACTIONS

! Anemia occurs in 10% of patients.
! A severe infusion reaction, characterized by rapid onset of airway obstruction, a precipitous drop in blood pressure, and severe urticaria, occurs rarely.
! Dermatologic toxicity, pulmonary embolus, leukopenia, and renal failure occur rarely.

DENTAL CONSIDERATIONS

General:

• Monitor vital signs at every appointment due to cardiovascular side effects.
• If additional analgesia is required for dental pain, consider alternative analgesics (NSAIDs) in patients

taking narcotics for acute or chronic pain.
- Examine for oral manifestation of opportunistic infection.
- Consider semisupine chair position for patient comfort because of GI effects of disease.
- Patient on chronic drug therapy may rarely present with symptoms of blood dyscrasias, which can include infection, bleeding and poor healing. If dyscrasia is present, caution patient to prevent oral tissue trauma when using oral hygiene aids.
- Advise patient if dental drugs prescribed have a potential for photosensitivity.
- Patients may be taking a prophylactic antiinfective.
- Caution in the use of drugs that may cause diarrhea or constipation.
- Patients may have received other chemotherapy or radiation; confirm medical and drug history.

Consultations:
- Consult physician; prophylactic or therapeutic antiinfectives may be indicated if surgery or periodontal treatment is required.
- Medical consultation may be required to assess immunologic status during cancer chemotherapy and determine safety risk, if any, posed by the required dental treatment.
- Medical consultation may be required to assess disease control and patient's ability to tolerate stress.
- Medical consultation should include routine blood counts including platelet counts and bleeding time.

Teach Patient/Family:
- Importance of good oral hygiene to prevent soft tissue inflammation
- To report oral lesions, soreness, or bleeding to dentist
- To prevent trauma when using oral hygiene aids
- Importance of updating health and medication history if physician makes any changes in evaluation or drug regimens; include OTC, herbal, and nonherbal remedies in the update

cevimeline

sev-im′-el-ine
(Evoxac)
Do not confuse Evoxac with Eurax.

CATEGORY AND SCHEDULE
Pregnancy Risk Category: C

MECHANISM OF ACTION
A cholinergic agonist that binds to muscarinic receptors of effector cells, thereby increasing secretion of exocrine glands, such as salivary glands. ***Therapeutic Effect:*** Relieves dry mouth.

AVAILABILITY
Capsules: 30 mg.

INDICATIONS AND DOSAGES
▸ **Dry Mouth**
PO
Adults. 30 mg 3 times a day.

CONTRAINDICATIONS
Acute iritis, angle-closure glaucoma, uncontrolled asthma

INTERACTIONS
Drug
Amiodarone, diltiazem, erythromycin, fluoxetine, itraconazole, ketoconazole, paroxetine, quinidine, ritonavir, verapamil: May increase the effects of cevimeline.

C

Atropine, phenothiazines, tricyclic antidepressants: May decrease the effects of cevimeline.
Beta blockers: May increase the risk of conduction disturbances.

Herbal

None known.

Food

All foods: Decreases the absorption rate of cevimeline.

Drug interactions of concern to dentistry

- Use with caution in patients taking β-adrenergic blockers: possible conduction disturbances.
- There are no specific data on dental drug interactions; however, use caution with other cholinergic agonists.
- There is always the possibility that a cholinergic antagonist could interfere with this drug's action.
- Although there are no supporting data, use with caution in patients taking drugs that inhibit cytochrome P-450 (CYP3A3/4 and CYP2D6 isoenzymes).

DIAGNOSTIC TEST EFFECTS

None known.

SIDE EFFECTS

Frequent (19%–11%)

Diaphoresis, headache, nausea, sinusitis, rhinitis, upper respiratory tract infection, diarrhea

Occasional (10%–3%)

Dyspepsia, abdominal pain, cough, UTI, vomiting, back pain, rash, dizziness, fatigue

Rare (2%–1%)

Skeletal pain, insomnia, hot flashes, excessive salivation, rigors, anxiety

SERIOUS REACTIONS

! Cevimeline use may result in decreased visual acuity, especially at night, and impaired depth perception.

DENTAL CONSIDERATIONS

General:

- Assess salivary flow as a factor in caries, periodontal disease, and candidiasis.
- Place on frequent recall to assess effectiveness.
- Consider semisupine chair position for patient comfort if GI side effects occur.

Consultations:

- Medical consultation may be required to assess disease control.
- Medical consultation may be necessary before prescribing for those patients with cardiovascular or respiratory disease.

Teach Patient/Family:

- That this drug may cause visual disturbances, especially with night driving, which may impair driving safety
- That the patient should drink extra fluids (water) to compensate for excessive sweating
- *When chronic dry mouth occurs, advise patient:*
    - To avoid mouth rinses with high alcohol content because of drying effects
    - Of need for daily home fluoride to prevent caries
    - To use sugarless gum, frequent sips of water, or saliva substitutes

chloral hydrate

klor-al hye′-drate
Schedule IV
(Aquachloral Supprettes, PMS-Chloral Hydrate[CAN], Somnote)

CATEGORY AND SCHEDULE

Pregnancy Risk Category: C

MECHANISM OF ACTION

A nonbarbiturate chloral derivative that produces CNS depression. ***Therapeutic Effect:*** Induces quiet, deep sleep, with only a slight decrease in respiratory rate and BP.

AVAILABILITY

Capsules (Somnote): 500 mg.
Syrup: 500 mg/5 ml.
Suppositories (Aquachloral Supprettes): 324 mg, 648 mg.

INDICATIONS AND DOSAGES

▸ Premedication for Dental or Medical Procedures

PO, Rectal
Adults. 0.5–1 g.
Children. 75 mg/kg up to 1 g total.

▸ Premedication for EEG

PO, Rectal
Adults. 0.5–1.5 g.
Children. 25–50 mg/kg/dose 30–60 min prior to EEG. May repeat in 30 min. Maximum: 1 g for infants, 2 g for children.

CONTRAINDICATIONS

Gastritis, marked hepatic or renal impairment, severe cardiac disease

INTERACTIONS

Drug

Alcohol, other CNS depressants: May increase the effects of chloral hydrate.
Furosemide (IV): May alter BP and cause diaphoresis if given within 24 hours after chloral hydrate,
Warfarin: May increase the effect of warfarin.

Herbal

None known.

Food

None known.

Drug interactions of concern to dentistry

• Increased action of both drugs: alcohol, all CNS depressants, including nitrous oxide

DIAGNOSTIC TEST EFFECTS

None known.

SIDE EFFECTS

Occasional

Gastric irritation (nausea, vomiting, flatulence, diarrhea), rash, sleepwalking

Rare

Headache, paradoxical CNS hyperactivity or nervousness in children, excitement or restlessness in the elderly (particularly in patients with pain).

SERIOUS REACTIONS

! Overdose may produce somnolence, confusion, slurred speech, severe incoordination, respiratory depression, and coma.

DENTAL CONSIDERATIONS

General:

• Consider semisupine chair position for patient comfort because of GI side effects of drug.
• Administer syrup in juice or beverage to mask taste and reduce GI upset.
• Contraindicated for use in patients with GI ulcerative disease.
• Have someone drive patient to and from dental office when drug used for conscious sedation.
• Geriatric patients are more susceptible to drug effects; use lower dose.
• Psychologic and physical dependence may occur with chronic administration.

C

chlordiazepoxide

klor-dye-az-e-pox′-ide
Schedule IV
(Apo-Chlordiazepoxide[CAN], Librium, Novopoxide[CAN])
Do not confuse Librium with Librax.

CATEGORY AND SCHEDULE

Pregnancy Risk Category: D

MECHANISM OF ACTION

A benzodiazepine that enhances the action of the inhibitory neurotransmitter gamma-aminobutyric acid in the CNS. ***Therapeutic Effect:*** Produces anxiolytic effect.

AVAILABILITY

Capsules: 5 mg, 10 mg, 25 mg.
Injection Powder for Reconstitution. 100 mg.

INDICATIONS AND DOSAGES

▸ Alcohol Withdrawal Symptoms

PO
Adults, Elderly. 50–100 mg. May repeat q2–4h. Maximum: 300 mg/24 hr.

▸ Anxiety

PO
Adults. 15–100 mg/day in 3–4 divided doses.
Elderly. 5 mg 2–4 times a day.
IV, IM
Adults. Initially, 50–100 mg, then 25–50 mg 3–4 times a day as needed.

OFF-LABEL USES

Treatment of panic disorder, tension headache, tremors

CONTRAINDICATIONS

Acute alcohol intoxication, acute angle-closure glaucoma

INTERACTIONS

Drug

Alcohol, other CNS depressants: May increase CNS depression.

Herbal

Kava kava, valerian: May increase CNS depression.

Food

None known.

Drug interactions of concern to dentistry

- Delayed elimination: erythromycin
- Increased CNS depression: CNS depressants, alcohol, disulfiram, nefazodone
- Increased serum levels and prolonged effects of benzodiazepines: ketoconazole, itraconazole, fluconazole, miconazole (systemic), cimetidine, fluvoxamine, omeprazole, rifabutin, rifampin
- Contraindicated with ritonavir, indinavir, saquinavir
- Possible increase in CNS side effects: kava (herb)
- Decreased plasma levels: St. John's wort (herb)

DIAGNOSTIC TEST EFFECTS

None known. Therapeutic serum drug level is 1–3 mcg/ml; toxic serum drug level is greater than 5 mcg/ml.

SIDE EFFECTS

Frequent

Pain at IM injection site; somnolence, ataxia, dizziness, confusion with oral dose (particularly in elderly or debilitated patients)

Occasional

Rash, peripheral edema, GI disturbances

Rare

Paradoxical CNS reactions, such as hyperactivity or nervousness in children and excitement or restlessness in the elderly (generally noted during first 2 weeks of therapy, particularly in presence of uncontrolled pain)

SERIOUS REACTIONS

! IV administration may produce pain, swelling, thrombophlebitis, and carpal tunnel syndrome.
! Abrupt or too-rapid withdrawal may result in pronounced restlessness, irritability, insomnia, hand tremors, abdominal or muscle cramps, diaphoresis, vomiting, and seizures.
! Overdose results in somnolence, confusion, diminished reflexes, and coma.

DENTAL CONSIDERATIONS

General:

- After supine positioning, have patient sit upright for at least 2 min to avoid orthostatic hypotension.
- Assess salivary flow as a factor in caries, periodontal disease, and candidiasis.
- Psychologic and physical dependence may occur with chronic administration.
- Geriatric patients are more susceptible to drug effects; use lower dose.
- Have someone drive patient to and from dental office if used for conscious sedation.

Consultations:

- Medical consultation may be required to assess disease control.

Teach Patient/Family:

- Importance of good oral hygiene to prevent soft tissue inflammation
- To avoid mouth rinses with high alcohol content because of drying effects

chlorhexidine gluconate

klor-**hex**-i-deen
(Chlorhexidine Mouthwash[AUS], Chlorhexidine Obstetric Lotion[AUS], Chlorohex Gel[AUS], Chlorohex Gel Forte[AUS], Chlorohex Mouth Rinse[AUS], Peridex, PerioChip, PerioGard, Perisol)

CATEGORY AND SCHEDULE

Pregnancy Risk Category: C

MECHANISM OF ACTION

An antiseptic and antimicrobial agent that is active against a broad spectrum of microbes. The chlorhexidine molecule, due to its positive charge, reacts with the microbial cell surface, destroys the integrity of the cell membrane, penetrates into the cell, precipitates the cytoplasm, and the cell dies. ***Therapeutic Effect:*** Causes cell death.

PHARMACOKINETICS

Initially, the chlorhexidine gluconate dental chip releases approximately 40% of the drug within the first 24 hr, then releases the remainder in an almost linear fashion for 7–10 days. Approximately 30% of the active ingredient, chlorhexidine gluconate, is retained in the oral cavity following oral rinsing. This retained drug is slowly released into the oral fluids. Poorly absorbed from the GI track. Primarily excreted in feces.
Half-life: Unknown.

AVAILABILITY

Oral liquid (Peridex, PerioGard): 0.12%.
Oral insert (PerioChip): 2.5 mg.
Topical liquid (Peridex, Perisol): 0.12%, 0.5%, 2%, 4%.

C

INDICATIONS AND DOSAGES

▸ **Gingivitis**

ORAL RINSE

Adults, Elderly. Swish and spit for 30 sec twice daily.

▸ **Periodontitis**

ORAL INSERT

Adults, Elderly. One chip is inserted into a periodontal pocket; insert a new chip q3mo; maximum of 8 chips per dental visit.

UNLABELED USES

Treatment of acute necrotizing ulcerative gingivitis, aphthous stomatitis, dental caries (prophylaxis), dental plaque (prophylaxis), denture stomatitis, mouth infection, necrotizing ulcerative periodontitis, nosocomial respiratory tract (prophylaxis)

CONTRAINDICATIONS

Hypersensitivity to chlorhexidine gluconate or any component of the formulation

INTERACTIONS

Drug

None known.

Herbal

None known.

Food

None known.

Drug interactions of concern to dentistry

- None reported

DIAGNOSTIC TEST EFFECTS

None known.

SIDE EFFECTS

Occasional

Altered taste, staining of tooth, toothache

SERIOUS REACTIONS

Anaphylaxis has been reported.

Drug interactions of concern to dentistry

Disulfiram-like effects resulting from alcohol content: Antabuse, metronidazole

DENTAL CONSIDERATIONS

General:

- Perform dental examination and prophylaxis/scaling/root planing before starting rinse.
- Place on frequent recall because of oral side effects.
- Use discretion when prescribing to patients with anterior facial restorations with rough surfaces or margins.

Teach Patient/Family:

- Instruct patient to eat, brush, and floss before using rinse
- Do not rinse with water after using chlorhexidine
- Not to dilute solution; not to swallow solution
- Inform patient of oral side effects

DENTAL CONSIDERATIONS

General:

- Do not brush or use dental floss at site of chip placement.

Teach Patient/Family:

- To notify dentist immediately if chip is dislodged or if pain, swelling, or other symptoms occur

chloroquine/chloroquine phosphate

klor′-oh-kwin

(Aralen hydrochloride, Aralen[CAN]) (Aralen phosphate)

CATEGORY AND SCHEDULE

Pregnancy Risk Category: C

C

MECHANISM OF ACTION

An amebecide that concentrates in parasite acid vesicles and may interfere with parasite protein synthesis. ***Therapeutic Effect:*** Increases pH and inhibits parasite growth.

PHARMACOKINETICS

Rate of absorption is variable. Chloroquine is almost completely absorbed from the gastrointestinal (GI) tract. Protein binding: 50%–65%. Widely distributed into body tissues such as eyes, heart, kidneys, liver, and lungs. Partially metabolized to active de-ethylated metabolites (principle metabolite is desethylchloroquine). Excreted in urine. Removed by hemodialysis. ***Half-life:*** 1–2 mos.

AVAILABILITY

Tablets: 250 mg, 500 mg (Aralen).

INDICATIONS AND DOSAGES

▸ Chloroquine Phosphate

Treatment of malaria (acute attack): Dose (mg base)

Dose	Time	Adults	Children
Initial	Day 1	600 mg	10 mg/kg
Second	6 hrs later	300 mg	5 mg/kg
Third	Day 2	300 mg	5 mg/kg
Fourth	Day 3	300 mg	5 mg/kg

▸ Suppression of Malaria

PO

Adults. 300 mg (base)/wk on same day each week beginning 2 wks before exposure; continue for 6–8 wks after leaving endemic area.
Children. 5 mg (base)/kg/wk.

▸ Malaria Prophylaxis

PO

Adults. 600 mg base initially given in 2 divided doses 6 hrs apart.
Children. 10 mg base/kg.

▸ Amebiasis

PO

Adults. 1 g (600 mg base) daily for 2 days; then, 500 mg (300 mg base)/day for at least 2–3 wks.

▸ Chloroquine HCL

Treatment of malaria

IM

Adults. Initially, 160–200 mg base (4–5 ml), repeat in 6 hrs. Maximum: 800 mg base in first 24 hrs. Begin oral therapy as soon as possible and continue for 3 days until approximately 1.5 g base given.
Children. Initially, 5 mg base/kg, repeat in 6 hrs. Do not exceed 10 mg base/kg/24 hrs.

▸ Amebiasis

IM

Adults. 160–200 mg base (4–5 ml) daily for 10–12 days. Change to oral therapy as soon as possible.

OFF-LABEL USES

Treatment of sarcoid-associated hypercalcemia, juvenile arthritis, rheumatoid arthritis, systemic lupus erythematosus, solar urticaria, chronic cutaneous vasculitis

CONTRAINDICATIONS

Hypersensitivity to 4-aminoquinoline compounds, retinal or visual field changes

INTERACTIONS

Drug

Alcohol: May increase GI irritation.
Penicillamine: May increase concentration of penicillamine and increase risk of hematologic, renal or severe skin reaction.
Ampicillin: May reduce the absorption of ampicillin. Separate administration by 2 hours.
Antacids and kaolin: May be decreased due to GI binding with kaolin or magnesium trisilicate.

C

Cimetidine: May increase levels of chloroquine.
Cyclosporine: May increase cyclosporine concentrations.
CYP2D6 inhibitors (chlorpromazine, delavirdine, fluoxetine, miconazole, paroxetine, pergolide, quinidine, quinine, ritonavir, ropinirole): May increase the levels and effects of chloroquine.
CYP2D6 substrates (amphetamines, selected beta-blockers, dextromethorphan, fluoxetine, lidocaine, mirtazapine, nefazodone, paroxetine, risperidone, ritonavir, thioridazine, tricyclic antidepressants, venlafaxine): May increase the levels and effects of CYP2D6 substrates.
CYP2D6 prodrug substrates: Chloroquine may decrease the levels and effects of CYP2D6 prodrug substrates.
CYP3A4 inducers (aminoglutethimide, carbamazepine, nafcillin, nevirapine, phenobarbital, phenytoin, and rifamycins): CYP3A4 inducers may decrease the levels and effects of chloroquine.
CYP3A4 inhibitors (azole antifungals, ciprofloxacin, clarithromycin, diclofenac, doxycycline, erythromycin, imatinib, isoniazid, nefazodone, nicardipine, propofol, protease inhibitors, quinidine, and verapamil): May increase the levels and effects of chloroquine.
Praziquantel: May decrease praziquantel concentrations.

Herbal
None known.

Food
None known.

Drug interactions of concern to dentistry
- Hepatotoxicity: alcohol, hepatotoxic drugs

DIAGNOSTIC TEST EFFECTS
Acute decrease in Hct, Hgb, RBC count may occur.

SIDE EFFECTS
Frequent
Discomfort with IM administration, mild transient headache, anorexia, nausea, vomiting
Occasional
Visual disturbances (blurring, difficulty focusing); nervousness, fatigue, pruritus esp. of palms, soles, scalp; bleaching of hair, irritability, personality changes, diarrhea, skin eruptions
Rare
Phlebitis or thrombophlebitis at IV injection site, abdominal cramps, headache, hypotension

SERIOUS REACTIONS
! Ocular toxicity and ototoxicity have been reported.
! Prolonged therapy: peripheral neuritis and neuromyopathy, hypotension, ECG changes, agranulocytosis, aplastic anemia, thrombocytopenia, convulsions, psychosis.
! Overdosage includes symptoms of headache, vomiting, visual disturbance, drowsiness, convulsions, hypokalemia followed by cardiovascular collapse, and death.

DENTAL CONSIDERATIONS
General:
- Patients on chronic drug therapy may rarely have symptoms of blood dyscrasias, which can include infection, bleeding, and poor healing.
- Avoid dental light in patient's eyes; offer dark glasses for patient comfort.
- Determine why the patient is taking the drug.

Consultations:

- In a patient with symptoms of blood dyscrasias, request a medical consultation for blood studies and postpone dental treatment until normal values are reestablished.

Teach Patient/Family:

- Importance of good oral hygiene to prevent soft tissue inflammation
- To avoid mouth rinses with high alcohol content because of drying effects

chlorothiazide

klor-oh-thye′-a-zide
(Diuril, Diuril Sodium)

CATEGORY AND SCHEDULE

Pregnancy Risk Category: C

MECHANISM OF ACTION

A sulfonamide derivative that acts as a thiazide diuretic and antihypertensive. As a diuretic blocks reabsorption of water, the electrolytes sodium and potassium at cortical diluting segment of distal tubule. As an antihypertensive reduces plasma, extracellular fluid volume, decreases peripheral vascular resistance (PVR) by direct effect on blood vessels. ***Therapeutic Effect:*** Promotes diuresis, reduces blood pressure (B/P).

PHARMACOKINETICS

Poorly absorbed from the gastrointestinal (GI) tract. Not metabolized. Primarily excreted unchanged in urine. Not removed by hemodialysis. ***Half-life:*** 45–120 min.

AVAILABILITY

Powder for injection, lyophilized: 0.5 g.
Oral suspension: 250 mg/5 ml (Diuril).
Tablets: 250 mg, 500 mg (Diuril).

INDICATIONS AND DOSAGES

▸ Edema, Hypertension

PO

Adults. 0.5–1 g 1–2 times/day. May give every other day or 3–5 days/wk.
Children 12 years and older. 10–20 mg/kg/dose in divided doses q8–12h. Maximum: 2g/day.
Children 2–12 yrs. 1 g/day.
Children 6 mos-2 yrs. 10–20 mg/kg/day in divided doses q12–24h. Maximum: 375 mg/day.
Children younger than 6 mos. 20–30 mg/kg/day in divided doses q12h. Maximum: 375 mg/day.

▸ Hypertension

IV

Adults. 0.5–1 g in divided doses q12–24h.

OFF-LABEL USES

Treatment of diabetes insipidus, prevention of calcium-containing renal stones

CONTRAINDICATIONS

Anuria, history of hypersensitivity to sulfonamides or thiazide diuretics, renal decompensation

INTERACTIONS

Drug

Cholestyramine, colestipol: May decrease the absorption and effects of chlorothiazide.
Digoxin: May increase the risk of toxicity of digoxin caused by hypokalemia.
Lithium: May increase the risk of toxicity of lithium.
NSAIDs: May decrease the absorption and effects of chlorothiazide.
Probenecid: May increase concentrations of chlorothiazide.

Herbal

Ginkgo biloba: May increase blood pressure.
Licorice: May increase risk of hypokalemia and decrease effectiveness of chlorothiazide.
Ma Huang: May decrease hypotensive effect of chlorothiazide.
Yohimbe: May decrease effects of chlorothiazide.

Food

None known.

Drug interactions of concern to dentistry

- Increased photosensitization: tetracyclines
- Decreased hypotensive response, nephrotoxicity: indomethacin and other NSAIDs

DIAGNOSTIC TEST EFFECTS

None known.

SIDE EFFECTS

Expected

Increase in urine frequency and volume

Frequent

Potassium depletion

Occasional

Postural hypotension, headache, gastrointestinal (GI) disturbances, photosensitivity reaction, muscle spasms, alopecia, rash, urticaria

SERIOUS REACTIONS

! Vigorous diuresis may lead to profound water loss and electrolyte depletion, resulting in hypokalemia, hyponatremia, and dehydration.
! Acute hypotensive episodes may occur.
! Hyperglycemia may be noted during prolonged therapy.
! GI upset, pancreatitis, dizziness, paresthesias, headache, blood dyscrasias, pulmonary edema, allergic pneumonitis, and dermatologic reactions occur rarely.
! Overdosage can lead to lethargy and coma without changes in electrolytes or hydration.

DENTAL CONSIDERATIONS

General:

- Monitor vital signs at every appointment because of cardiovascular side effects.
- After supine positioning, have patient sit upright for at least 2 min before standing to avoid orthostatic hypotension.
- Patients on chronic drug therapy may rarely have symptoms of blood dyscrasias, which can include infection, bleeding, and poor healing.
- Assess salivary flow as a factor in caries, periodontal disease, and candidiasis.
- Limit use of sodium-containing products, such as saline IV fluids, for patients with a dietary salt restriction.
- Stress from dental procedures may compromise cardiovascular function; determine patient risk.
- Short appointments and a stress reduction protocol may be required for anxious patients.
- Patients taking diuretics should be monitored for serum K^+ levels.

Consultations:

- In a patient with symptoms of blood dyscrasias, request a medical consultation for blood studies and postpone dental treatment until normal values are reestablished.
- Medical consultation may be required to assess disease control and patient's ability to tolerate stress.
- Physician should be informed if significant xerostomic side effects occur (increased caries, sore tongue, problems eating or swallowing, difficulty wearing prosthesis) so that a medication change can be considered.

Teach Patient/Family:
- Importance of good oral hygiene to prevent soft tissue inflammation
- Caution to prevent injury when using oral hygiene aids
- *When chronic dry mouth occurs, advise patient:*
  - To avoid mouth rinses with high alcohol content because of drying effects
  - To use daily home fluoride products for anticaries effect
  - To use sugarless gum, frequent sips of water, or saliva substitutes

chlorpheniramine

klor-fen-ir′-a-meen
(Aller-Chlor, Chlor-Trimeton, Chlor-Trimeton Allergy, Chlor-Trimeton Allergy 12 Hour, Chlor-Trimeton Allergy 8 Hour, Chlor-Tripolon[CAN], Chlorate, Chlorphen, Diabetic Tussin Allergy Relief)
Do not confuse with chlorpromazine or chlorpropamide.

CATEGORY AND SCHEDULE

Pregnancy Risk Category: C
OTC (tablets, syrup)

MECHANISM OF ACTION

A propylamine derivative antihistamine that competes with histamine for histamine receptor sites on cells in the blood vessels, gastrointestinal (GI) tract, and respiratory tract. ***Therapeutic Effect:*** Inhibits symptoms associated with seasonal allergic rhinitis such as increased mucus production and sneezing.

PHARMACOKINETICS

Well absorbed after PO and parenteral administration. Food delays absorption. Widely distributed. Metabolized in liver. Primarily excreted in urine. Not removed by dialysis. ***Half-life:*** 20 hrs.

AVAILABILITY

Injection: 10 mg/ml, 100 mg/ml.
Syrup: 2 mg/5 ml (Aller-Chlor, Diabetic Tussin Allergy Relief [sugar free]).
Tablets: 4 mg (Aller-Chlor, Chlor-Trimeton, Chlorate, Chlorphen).
Tablets (sustained-release): 8 mg (Chlor-Trimeton Allergy 8 Hour), 12 mg (Chlor-Trimeton Allergy 12 Hour).

INDICATIONS AND DOSAGES

▸ **Allergic Rhinitis, Common Cold**

PO

Adults, Elderly. 4 mg q6–8h or 8–12 mg (sustained-release) q8–12h. Maximum: 24 mg/day.
Children 12 yrs and older. 4 mg q6–8h or 8 mg (sustained-release) q12h. Maximum: 24 mg/day.
Children 6–11 yrs. 2 mg q4–6h. Maximum: 12 mg/day.

IM/IV/SC

Adults, Elderly. 5–40 mg as a single dose. Maximum: 40 mg/day.

SC

Children 6 yrs and older. 87.5 mcg/kg or 2.5 mg/m^2 4 times/day.

CONTRAINDICATIONS

Hypersensitivity to chlorpheniramine or its components

INTERACTIONS

Drug

Alcohol, central nervous system (CNS) depressants: May increase CNS depressant effects.

Anticholinergics: May increase anticholinergic effects.
MAOIs: May increase anticholinergic and CNS depressant effects.
Phenytoin, fosphenytoin: May increase the risk of phenytoin toxicity.
Procarbazine: May increase CNS depressant effects.

Herbal
None known.

Food
None known.

Drug interactions of concern to dentistry
- Increased CNS depression: alcohol, all CNS depressants
- Increased anticholinergic effect: other anticholinergics, phenothiazines, tricyclic antidepressants

DIAGNOSTIC TEST EFFECTS
None known.

IV INCOMPATIBILITIES
Calcium, iodipamide, kanamycin (Kantrex), norepinephrine (Levophed), pentobarbital (Nembutal)

IV COMPATIBILITIES
Amikacin (Amikin), corticotropin, cortisone, hyaluronidase (Wydase), penicillin G

SIDE EFFECTS
Frequent
Drowsiness, dizziness, muscular weakness, hypotension, dry mouth, nose, throat, and lips, urinary retention, thickening of bronchial secretions
Elderly: Sedation, dizziness, hypotension

Occasional
Epigastric distress, flushing, visual or hearing disturbances, paresthesia, diaphoresis, chills

SERIOUS REACTIONS
! Children may experience dominant paradoxical reactions, including restlessness, insomnia, euphoria, nervousness, and tremors.
! Overdosage in children may result in hallucinations, seizures, and death.
! Hypersensitivity reaction, such as eczema, pruritus, rash, cardiac disturbances, and photosensitivity, may occur.
! Overdosage may vary from CNS depression, including sedation, apnea, hypotension, cardiovascular collapse, or death to severe paradoxical reaction, such as hallucinations, tremor, and seizures.

DENTAL CONSIDERATIONS
General:
- Assess salivary flow as a factor in caries, periodontal disease, and candidiasis.
- Consider semisupine chair position for patients with respiratory disease.
- Determine why the patient is taking the drug.

Teach Patient/Family:
- Importance of good oral hygiene to prevent soft tissue inflammation
- Caution to prevent injury when using oral hygiene aids
- *When chronic dry mouth occurs, advise patient:*
  - To avoid mouth rinses with high alcohol content because of drying effects
  - To use daily home fluoride products for anticaries effect
  - To use sugarless gum, frequent sips of water, or saliva substitutes

chlorpromazine

klor-proe′-ma-zeen
(Chlorpromanyl[CAN], Largactil[CAN], Thorazine)
Do not confuse chlorpromazine with chlorpropamide, clomipramine, or prochlorperazine, or Thorazine with thiamide or thioridazine.

CATEGORY AND SCHEDULE

Pregnancy Risk Category: C

MECHANISM OF ACTION

A phenothiazine that blocks dopamine neurotransmission at postsynaptic dopamine receptor sites. Possesses strong anticholinergic, sedative, and antiemetic effects; moderate extrapyramidal effects; and slight antihistamine action.
Therapeutic Effect: Relieves nausea and vomiting; improves psychotic conditions; controls intractable hiccups and porphyria.

PHARMACOKINETICS

Rapidly absorbed after oral or IM administration. Protein binding: 92%–97%. Metabolized in the liver. Excreted in urine. ***Half-life:*** 6 hr.

AVAILABILITY

Oral Concentrate: 30 mg/ml, 100 mg/ml.
Syrup: 10 mg/5 ml.
Tablets: 10 mg, 25 mg, 50 mg, 100 mg, 200 mg.
Capsules (Sustained-Release): 30 mg, 75 mg, 150 mg.
Injection (Thorazine): 25 mg/ml.
Suppositories: 25 mg, 100 mg.

INDICATIONS AND DOSAGES

▸ Severe Nausea or Vomiting
PO
Adults, Elderly. 10–25 mg q4–6h.
Children. 0.5–1 mg/kg q4–6h.
IV, IM
Adults, Elderly. 25–50 mg q4–6h.
Children. 0.5–1 mg/kg q6–8h.
RECTAL
Adults, Elderly. 50–100 mg q6–8h.
Children. 1 mg/kg q6–8h.

▸ Psychotic Disorders
PO
Adults, Elderly. 30–800 mg/day in 1–4 divided doses.
Children older than 6 mo. 0.5–1 mg/kg q4–6h.
IV, IM
Adults, Elderly. Initially, 25 mg; may repeat in 1–4 hr. May gradually increase to 400 mg q4–6h. Maximum: 300–800 mg/day.
Children older than 6 mo. 0.5–1 mg/kg q6–8h. Maximum: 75 mg/day for children 5–12 yr; 40 mg/day for children younger than 5 yr.

▸ Intractable Hiccups
PO, IV, IM
Adults. 25–50 mg 3 times a day.

▸ Porphyria
PO
Adults. 25–50 mg 3–4 times a day.
IM
Adults, Elderly. 25 mg 3–4 times a day.

OFF-LABEL USES

Treatment of choreiform movement of Huntington's disease

CONTRAINDICATIONS

Comatose states, myelosuppression, severe cardiovascular disease, severe CNS depression, subcortical brain damage

INTERACTIONS

Drug

Alcohol, other CNS depressants: May increase respiratory depression and the hypotensive effects of chlorpromazine.

Antithyroid agents: May increase the risk of agranulocytosis.
Extrapyramidal symptom-producing medications: Increased risk of extrapyramidal symptoms.
Hypotensives: May increase hypotension.
Levodopa: May decrease the effects of levodopa.
Lithium: May decrease the absorption of chlorpromazine and produce adverse neurologic effects.
MAOIs, tricyclic antidepressants: May increase the anticholinergic and sedative effects of chlorpromazine.

Herbal
None known.

Food
None known.

Drug interactions of concern to dentistry
- Increased sedation: other CNS depressants, alcohol, barbiturate anesthetics, opioid analgesics
- Hypotension, tachycardia: epinephrine (systemic)
- Increased extrapyramidal effects: related drugs, such as haloperidol, droperidol, and metoclopramide
- Additive photosensitization: tetracyclines
- Increased anticholinergic effects: anticholinergics

DIAGNOSTIC TEST EFFECTS
May produce false-positive pregnancy and phenylketonuria (PKU) test results. May cause ECG changes, including Q- and T-wave disturbances. Therapeutic serum level is 50–300 mcg/ml; toxic serum level is greater than 750 mcg/ml.

SIDE EFFECTS
Frequent
Somnolence, blurred vision, hypotension, color vision or night vision disturbances, dizziness, decreased sweating, constipation, dry mouth, nasal congestion

Occasional
Urinary retention, photosensitivity, rash, decreased sexual function, swelling or pain in breasts, weight gain, nausea, vomiting, abdominal pain, tremors

SERIOUS REACTIONS
! Extrapyramidal symptoms appear to be dose related and are divided into three categories: akathisia (including inability to sit still, tapping of feet), parkinsonian symptoms (such as masklike face, tremors, shuffling gait, hypersalivation), and acute dystonias (including torticollis, opisthotonos, and oculogyric crisis). A dystonic reaction may also produce diaphoresis and pallor.
! Tardive dyskinesia, including tongue protrusion, puffing of the cheeks, and puckering of the mouth is a rare reaction that may be irreversible.
! Abrupt discontinuation after long-term therapy may precipitate nausea, vomiting, gastritis, dizziness, and tremors.
! Blood dyscrasias, particularly agranulocytosis and mild leukopenia, may occur.
! Chlorpromazine may lower the seizure threshold.

DENTAL CONSIDERATIONS
General:
- Monitor vital signs at every appointment because of cardiovascular side effects.
- Patients on chronic drug therapy may rarely have symptoms of blood dyscrasias, which can include infection, bleeding, and poor healing.
- After supine positioning, have patient sit upright for at least 2 min before standing to avoid orthostatic hypotension.

- Assess salivary flow as a factor in caries, periodontal disease, and candidiasis.
- Avoid dental light in patient's eyes; offer dark glasses for patient comfort.
- Assess for presence of extrapyramidal motor symptoms, such as tardive dyskinesia and akathisia. Extrapyramidal motor activity may complicate dental treatment.
- Geriatric patients are more susceptible to drug effects; use a lower dose.

Consultations:

- In a patient with symptoms of blood dyscrasias, request a medical consultation for blood studies and postpone dental treatment until normal values are reestablished.
- Take precautions if dental surgery is anticipated and anesthesia is required.
- If signs of tardive dyskinesia or akathisia are present, refer to physician.
- Physician should be informed if significant xerostomic side effects occur (increased caries, sore tongue, problems eating or swallowing, difficulty wearing prosthesis) so that a medication change can be considered.

Teach Patient/Family:

- Importance of good oral hygiene to prevent soft tissue inflammation
- Caution to prevent injury when using oral hygiene aids
- To use electric toothbrush if patient has difficulty holding conventional devices
- *When chronic dry mouth occurs, advise patient:*
  - To avoid mouth rinses with high alcohol content because of drying effects
  - To use daily home fluoride products for anticaries effect
  - To use sugarless gum, frequent sips of water, or saliva substitutes

chlorpropamide

klor-pro′-pa-mide
(Apo-Chlorpropamide[CAN], Diabinese)
Do not confuse with chlorpromazine.

CATEGORY AND SCHEDULE

Pregnancy Risk Category: C

MECHANISM OF ACTION

A first-generation sulfonylurea that promotes release of insulin from beta cells of pancreas. ***Therapeutic Effect:*** Lowers blood glucose concentration.

PHARMACOKINETICS

Rapidly absorbed from the gastrointestinal (GI) tract. Protein binding: 60%–90%. Extensively metabolized in liver. Excreted primarily urine. Removed by hemodialysis. ***Half-life:*** 30–42 hrs.

AVAILABILITY

Tablets: 100 mg, 250 mg (Diabenese).

INDICATIONS AND DOSAGES

▸ Diabetes Mellitus, Combination Therapy

PO

Adults. Initially, 250 mg once a day. Maintenance: 250–500 mg once a day. Maximum: 750 mg/day.
Elderly. Initially, 100–125 mg once a day. Maintenance: 100–250 mg once a day. Increase or decrease by 50–125 mg a day for 3–5 day intervals.

▸ Renal Function Impairment

Not recommended.

OFF-LABEL USES

Neurogenic diabetes insipidus

C

CONTRAINDICATIONS
Diabetic complications, such as ketosis, acidosis, and diabetic coma, severe liver or renal impairment, sole therapy for type 1 diabetes mellitus, or hypersensitivity to sulfonylureas

INTERACTIONS
Drug
Alcohol: Disulfiram-like reactions may occur. Symptoms of low blood sugar including sweating, shaking, weakness, drowsiness, and trouble concentrating will occur.
Beta-blockers, MAOIs, NSAIDs, salicylates: May increase hypoglycemic effect.
Fluoroquinolone antibiotics: May increase the risk of hypoglycemia.
Glucocorticoids, thiazide diuretics: May increase blood glucose.
Oral contraceptives: May increase blood glucose.
Herbal
Bitter melon: May increase the risk of hypoglycemia.
St. John's Wort: May increase the risk of hypoglycemia.
Food
None known.
Drug interactions of concern to dentistry
- Increased hypoglycemic effects: salicylates, NSAIDs, ketoconazole, miconazole
- Decreased action: corticosteroids, sympathomimetics
- Disulfiram-like reaction: alcohol

DIAGNOSTIC TEST EFFECTS
None known.

SIDE EFFECTS
Frequent
Headache, upper respiratory tract infection
Occasional
Sinusitis, myalgia (muscle aches), pharyngitis, aggravated diabetes mellitus

SERIOUS REACTIONS
! Possible increased risk of cardiovascular mortality with this class of drugs.
! Overdosage can cause severe hypoglycemia prolonged by extended half-life.

DENTAL CONSIDERATIONS
General:
- Patients on chronic drug therapy may rarely have symptoms of blood dyscrasias, which can include infection, bleeding, and poor healing.
- Short appointments and a stress reduction protocol may be required for anxious patients.
- Question patient about self-monitoring of drug's antidiabetic effect, including blood glucose values or finger-stick records.
- Ensure that patient is following prescribed diet and regularly takes medication.
- Determine if medication controls disease. Patients with diabetes may be more susceptible to infection and have delayed wound healing.
- Avoid prescribing aspirin-containing products.

Consultations:
- In a patient with symptoms of blood dyscrasias, request a medical consultation for blood studies and postpone dental treatment until normal values are reestablished.
- Medical consultation may be required to assess disease control.
- Medical consultation may include data from patient's blood glucose monitoring, including glycosylated hemoglobin or HbA_{1c} testing.

Teach Patient/Family:
- Importance of good oral hygiene to prevent soft tissue inflammation
- Caution to prevent injury when using oral hygiene aids
- To avoid mouth rinses with high alcohol content because of drying effects

chlorthalidone

klor-thal′-i-doan
(Apo-Chlorthalidone[CAN], Hygroton[AUS], Thalitone)

CATEGORY AND SCHEDULE

Pregnancy Risk Category: B (D if used in pregnancy-induced hypertension)

MECHANISM OF ACTION

A thiazide diuretic that blocks reabsorption of sodium, potassium, and water at the distal convoluted tubule; also decreases plasma and extracellular fluid volume and peripheral vascular resistance. ***Therapeutic Effect:*** Produces diuresis; lowers BP.

PHARMACOKINETICS

Route	Onset	Peak	Duration
PO (diuretic)	2 hr	2–6 hr	Up to 36 hr

Rapidly absorbed from the GI tract. Excreted unchanged in urine. ***Half-life:*** 35–50 hr. Onset of antihypertensive effect: 3–4 days; optimal therapeutic effect: 3–4 wk.

AVAILABILITY

Tablets: 15 mg, 25 mg, 50 mg, 100 mg.

INDICATIONS AND DOSAGES

▸ Hypertension, Edema

PO

Adults. 25–100 mg/day or 100 mg 3 times a week.

Elderly. Initially, 12.5–25 mg/day or every other day.

CONTRAINDICATIONS

Anuria, history of hypersensitivity to sulfonamides or thiazide diuretics, renal decompensation

INTERACTIONS

Drug

Cholestyramine, colestipol: May decrease the absorption and effects of chlorthalidone.

Digoxin: May increase the risk of digoxin toxicity associated with chlorthalidone-induced hyperkalemia.

Lithium: May increase the risk of lithium toxicity.

Herbal

None known.

Food

None known.

Drug interactions of concern to dentistry
- Increased photosensitization: tetracyclines
- Decreased hypotensive response, nephrotoxicity: NSAIDs, indomethacin

DIAGNOSTIC TEST EFFECTS

May increase blood glucose and serum cholesterol, LDL, bilirubin, calcium, creatinine, uric acid, and triglyceride levels. May decrease urinary calcium and serum magnesium, potassium, and sodium levels.

SIDE EFFECTS

Expected

Increase in urinary frequency and urine volume

C

Frequent
Potassium depletion (rarely produces symptoms)
Occasional
Anorexia, impotence, diarrhea, orthostatic hypotension, GI disturbances, photosensitivity
Rare
Rash

SERIOUS REACTIONS

! Vigorous diuresis may lead to profound water and electrolyte depletion, resulting in hypokalemia, hyponatremia, and dehydration.
! Acute hypotensive episodes may occur.
! Hyperglycemia may occur during prolonged therapy.
! Overdose can lead to lethargy and coma without changes in electrolytes or hydration.

DENTAL CONSIDERATIONS

General:
- Monitor vital signs at every appointment because of cardiovascular side effects.
- After supine positioning, have patient sit upright for at least 2 min before standing to avoid orthostatic hypotension.
- Patients on chronic drug therapy may rarely have symptoms of blood dyscrasias, which can include infection, bleeding, and poor healing.
- Assess salivary flow as a factor in caries, periodontal disease, and candidiasis.
- Limit use of sodium-containing products, such as saline IV fluids, for those patients with a dietary salt restriction.
- Short appointments and a stress reduction protocol may be required for anxious patients.
- Stress from dental procedures may compromise cardiovascular function; determine patient risk.

Consultations:
- In a patient with symptoms of blood dyscrasias, request a medical consultation for blood studies and postpone dental treatment until normal values are reestablished.
- Medical consultation may be required to assess disease control and patient's ability to tolerate stress.

Teach Patient/Family:
- Importance of good oral hygiene to prevent soft tissue inflammation
- Caution to prevent injury when using oral hygiene aids
- *When chronic dry mouth occurs, advise patient:*
  - To avoid mouth rinses with high alcohol content because of drying effects
  - To use daily home fluoride products for anticaries effect
  - To use sugarless gum, frequent sips of water, or saliva substitutes

chlorzoxazone

klor-zox′-a-zone
(Parafon Forte DSC, Remular, Remular-S)
Do not confuse with chlorthalidone.

CATEGORY AND SCHEDULE

Pregnancy Risk Category: C

MECHANISM OF ACTION

A skeletal muscle relaxant that inhibits transmission of reflexes at the spinal cord level. ***Therapeutic Effect:*** Relieves muscle spasticity.

PHARMACOKINETICS
Readily absorbed from the gastrointestinal (GI) tract. Metabolized in liver. Primarily excreted in urine. ***Half-life:*** 1.1 hrs.

AVAILABILITY
Caplets: 500 mg (Parafon Forte DSC).
Tablets: 250 mg.

INDICATIONS AND DOSAGES
▸ Musculoskeletal Pain
PO
Adults, Elderly. 250–500 mg 3–4 times/day. Maximum: 750 mg 3–4 day.
Children. 20 mg/kg/day in 3–4 divided doses.

CONTRAINDICATIONS
Hypersensitivity to chlorzoxazone or any one of its components.

INTERACTIONS
Drug
Alcohol, central nervous system (CNS) depressants: May increase CNS depression.
Herbal
Garlic: May decrease the effectiveness of chlorzoxazone.
Kava: May increase CNS depression.
St. John's Wort: May decrease the effectiveness of chlorzoxazone.
Food
None known.
Drug interactions of concern to dentistry
- Increased CNS depression: alcohol, narcotics, barbiturates, sedatives, hypnotics

DIAGNOSTIC TEST EFFECTS
False-positive for serum aprobarbital when using Toxi-Lab Screen.

SIDE EFFECTS
Frequent
Drowsiness, fever, headache
Occasional
Nausea, vomiting, stomach cramps, rash

SERIOUS REACTIONS
! Overdosage results in nausea, vomiting, diarrhea, and hypotension.

DENTAL CONSIDERATIONS
General:
- Determine why the patient is taking the drug.
- Consider semisupine chair position if back is involved.
- When used for dental-related problems, consider aspirin or NSAIDs to improve response.

cholestyramine resin
koe-less-tir′-a-meen
(Novo-Cholamine[CAN], Prevalite, Questran[CAN], Questran Lite[AUS])
Do not confuse Questran with Quarzan.

CATEGORY AND SCHEDULE
Pregnancy Risk Category: B

MECHANISM OF ACTION
An antihyperlipoproteinemic that binds with bile acids in the intestine, forming an insoluble complex. Binding results in partial removal of bile acid from enterohepatic circulation. ***Therapeutic Effect:*** Removes LDL cholesterol from plasma.

PHARMACOKINETICS
Not absorbed from the GI tract. Decreases in serum LDL apparent

in 5 to 7 days and in serum cholesterol in 1 mo. Serum cholesterol returns to baseline levels about 1 mo after drug is discontinued.

AVAILABILITY

Powder for Oral Suspension: 4 g.

INDICATIONS AND DOSAGES

▸ Primary Hypercholesterolemia

PO

Adults, Elderly. 3–4 g 3–4 times a day. Maximum: 16–32 g/day in 2–4 divided doses.
Children older than 10 yr. 2 g/day. Maximum: 8 g/day in 2 or more divided doses.
Children 10 yr and younger. Initially, 2 g/day. Range: 1–4 g/day.

▸ Pruritis

PO

Adults, Elderly. 4 g 1–2 times a day. Maintenance: Up to 24 g/day in divided doses.

OFF-LABEL USES

Treatment of diarrhea (due to bile acids), hyperoxaluria

CONTRAINDICATIONS

Complete biliary obstruction, hypersensitivity to cholestyramine or tartrazine (frequently seen in aspirin hypersensitivity)

INTERACTIONS

Drug

Anticoagulants: May increase effects of these drugs by decreasing level of vitamin K.
Digoxin, folic acid, penicillins, propranolol, tetracyclines, thiazides, thyroid hormones, other medications: May bind and decrease absorption of these drugs.
Oral vancomycin: Binds and decreases the effects of oral vancomycin.
Warfarin: May decrease warfarin absorption.

Herbal

None known.

Food

None known.

Drug interactions of concern to dentistry

- Decreased absorption of tetracyclines, cephalexin, phenobarbital, corticosteroids, clindamycin, penicillins; administer doses several hours apart

DIAGNOSTIC TEST EFFECTS

May increase serum alkaline phosphatase, serum magnesium, AST (SGOT), and ALT (SGPT) levels. May decrease serum calcium, potassium, and sodium levels. May prolong prothrombin time.

SIDE EFFECTS

Frequent

Constipation (may lead to fecal impaction), nausea, vomiting, abdominal pain, indigestion

Occasional

Diarrhea, belching, bloating, headache, dizziness

Rare

Gallstones, peptic ulcer disease, malabsorption syndrome

SERIOUS REACTIONS

! GI tract obstruction, hyperchloremic acidosis, and osteoporosis secondary to calcium excretion may occur.
! High dosage may interfere with fat absorption, resulting in steatorrhea.

DENTAL CONSIDERATIONS

General:

- Consider semisupine chair position for patient comfort because of GI side effects of disease.

ciclopirox

sye-kloe-peer′-ox
(Loprox, Penlac)
Do not confuse with ciprofloxacin.

CATEGORY AND SCHEDULE

Pregnancy Risk Category: B

MECHANISM OF ACTION

An antifungal that inhibits the transport of essential elements in the fungal cell, thereby interfering with biosynthesis in fungi. ***Therapeutic Effect:*** Results in fungal cell death.

PHARMACOKINETICS

Absorbed through intact skin. Distributed to epidermis, dermis, including hair, hair follicles, and sebaceous glands. Protein binding: 98%. Primarily excreted in urine and to a lesser extent in feces. ***Half-life:*** 1.7 hrs.

AVAILABILITY

Cream: 0.77% (Loprox).
Gel: 0.77% (Loprox).
Lotion: 0.77% (Loprox TS).
Shampoo: 0.77% (Loprox).
Topical Solution, nail lacquer: 8% (Penlac).

INDICATIONS AND DOSAGES

▸ Tinea Pedis

TOPICAL
Adults, Elderly, Children 10 yrs and older. Apply 2 times a day until signs and symptoms significantly improve.

▸ Tinea Cruris, Tinea Corporis

TOPICAL
Adults, Elderly, Children 10 yrs and older. Apply 2 times a day until signs and symptoms significantly improve.

▸ Onychomycosis

TOPICAL (solution)
Adults, Elderly, Children 10 yrs and older. Apply to the affected area (nails) daily. Remove with alcohol every 7 days.

▸ Seborrheic Dermatitis

SHAMPOO
Adults, Elderly, Children 10 yrs and older. Apply to affected scalp areas 2 times a day, in the morning and evening for 4 weeks.

CONTRAINDICATIONS

Hypersensitivity to ciclopirox or any one of its components

INTERACTIONS

Drug
Not known.

Herbal
Not known.

Food
Not known.

Drug interactions of concern to dentistry

- None reported

DIAGNOSTIC TEST EFFECTS

None known.

SIDE EFFECTS

Rare
Topical: Irritation, burning, redness, pain at the site of application

SERIOUS REACTIONS

! None known.

C

cimetidine

sye-met′-i-deen
(Apo-Cimetidine[CAN], Cimehexal[AUS], Magicul[AUS], Novocimetine[CAN], Peptol[CAN], Sigmetadine[AUS], Tagamet, Tagamet HB)
Do not confuse cimetidine with simethicone.

CATEGORY AND SCHEDULE

Pregnancy Risk Category: B
OTC (100 mg tablets)

MECHANISM OF ACTION

An antiulcer agent and gastric acid secretion inhibitor that inhibits histamine action at histamine 2 receptor sites of parietal cells. ***Therapeutic Effect:*** Inhibits gastric acid secretion during fasting, at night, or when stimulated by food, caffeine, or insulin.

PHARMACOKINETICS

Well absorbed from the GI tract. Protein binding: 15%–20%. Widely distributed. Metabolized in the liver. Primarily excreted in urine. Not removed by hemodialysis. ***Half-life:*** 2 hr; increased with impaired renal function.

AVAILABILITY

Tablets (Tagamet HB): 100 mg, 200 mg.
Tablets (Tagamet): 200 mg, 300 mg, 400 mg, 800 mg.
Liquid (Tagamet): 300 mg/5 ml.
Liquid (Tagamet HB): 200 mg/20 ml.
Injection (Tagamet): 150 mg/ml.

INDICATIONS AND DOSAGES

▸ Active Ulcer
PO
Adults, Elderly. 300 mg 4 times a day or 400 mg twice a day or 800 mg at bedtime.
IV, IM
Adults, Elderly. 300 mg q6h or 150 mg as single dose followed by 37.5 mg/hr continuous infusion.

▸ Prevention of Duodenal Ulcer
PO
Adults, Elderly. 400–800 mg at bedtime.

▸ Gastric Hypersecretory Secretions
PO, IV, IM
Adults, Elderly. 300–600 mg q6h. Maximum: 2,400 mg/day.
Children. 20–40 mg/kg/day in divided doses q6h.
Infants. 10–20 mg/kg/day in divided doses q6–12h.
Neonates. 5–10 mg/kg/day in divided doses q8–12h.

▸ Gastrointestinal Reflux Disease
PO
Adults, Elderly. 800 mg twice a day or 400 mg 4 times a day for 12 wks.

▸ OTC use
PO
Adults, Elderly. 100 mg up to 30 min before meals. Maximum: 2 doses/day.

▸ Prevention of Upper GI Bleeding
IV Infusion
Adults, Elderly. 50 mg/hr.

▸ Dosage in Renal Impairment
Dosage is based on a 300-mg dose in adults. Dosage interval is modified on the basis of creatinine clearance.

Creatinine Clearance	Dosage Interval
greater than 40 ml/min	q6h
20–40 ml/min	q8h or decrease dose by 25%
less than 20 ml/min	q12h or decrease dose by 50%

Give after hemodialysis and q12h between dialysis sessions.

OFF-LABEL USES
Prevention of aspiration pneumonia; treatment of acute urticaria, chronic warts, upper GI bleeding

CONTRAINDICATIONS
Hypersensitivity to other H_2-antagonists

INTERACTIONS
Drug
Antacids: May decrease the absorption of cimetidine.
Calcium channel blockers, cyclosporine, lidocaine, metoprolol, metronidazole, oral anticoagulants, oral antidiabetics, phenytoin, propranolol, theophylline, tricyclic antidepressants: May decrease the metabolism and increase the blood concentrations of these drugs.
Ketoconazole: May decrease the absorption of ketoconazole.
Herbal
None known.
Food
None known.
Drug interactions of concern to dentistry
- GI ulceration, bleeding: aspirin, NSAIDs
- Decreased absorption: sodium bicarbonate, anticholinergics
- Decreased absorption of fluconazole, ketoconazole, tetracycline (take doses 2 hr apart), ferrous salts
- Increased blood levels of metronidazole, alcohol, lidocaine, narcotic analgesics, benzodiazepines, carbamazepine

DIAGNOSTIC TEST EFFECTS
Interferes with skin tests using allergen extracts. May increase prolactin, serum creatinine, and transaminase levels. May decrease parathyroid hormone concentration.

IV INCOMPATIBILITIES
Allopurinol (Aloprim), amphotericin B complex (AmBisome, Amphotec, Abelcet), cefepime (Maxipime)
IV COMPATIBILITIES
Aminophylline, diltiazem (Cardizem), furosemide (Lasix), heparin, hydromorphone (Dilaudid), insulin (regular), lidocaine, lorazepam (Ativan), midazolam (Versed), morphine, potassium chloride, propofol (Diprivan)

SIDE EFFECTS
Occasional (4%–2%)
Headache
Elderly and severely ill patients, patients with impaired renal function: Confusion, agitation, psychosis, depression, anxiety, disorientation, hallucinations. Effects reverse 3 to 4 days after discontinuance.
Rare (less than 2%)
Diarrhea, dizziness, somnolence, nausea, vomiting, gynecomastia, rash, impotence

SERIOUS REACTIONS
! Rapid IV administration may produce cardiac arrhythmias and hypotension.

DENTAL CONSIDERATIONS
General:
- Monitor vital signs at every appointment because of cardiovascular side effects.
- Consider semisupine chair position for patient comfort because of GI side effects of disease.
- Avoid prescribing aspirin- or NSAID-containing products in patients with active upper GI disease; risk of irritation and ulceration exists.
- Sodium bicarbonate products can be used 1 hr before or 1 hr after cimetidine dose.

C

Teach Patient/Family:
- Importance of good oral hygiene to prevent soft tissue inflammation
- Caution to prevent injury when using oral hygiene aids

ciprofloxacin hydrochloride

sip-ro-floks′-a-sin hye-droe-klor′-ide
(C-Flox[AUS], Ciloquin[AUS], Ciloxan, Cipro, Ciproxin[AUS])
Do not confuse ciprofloxacin or Ciproxin with Ciloxan, cinoxacin, or Cytoxan.

CATEGORY AND SCHEDULE

Pregnancy Risk Category: C

MECHANISM OF ACTION

A fluoroquinolone that inhibits the enzyme DNA gyrase in susceptible bacteria, interfering with bacterial cell replication. ***Therapeutic Effect:*** Bactericidal.

PHARMACOKINETICS

Well absorbed from the GI tract (food delays absorption). Protein binding: 20%–40%. Widely distributed (including to CSF). Metabolized in the liver to active metabolite. Primarily excreted in urine. Minimal removal by hemodialysis. ***Half-life:*** 4–6 hr (increased in impaired renal function and the elderly).

AVAILABILITY

Tablets (Cipro): 100 mg, 250 mg, 500 mg, 750 mg.
Tablets (Extended-Release [Cipro XR]): 500 mg, 1000 mg.
Infusion: 200 mg/100 ml, 400 mg/200 ml.
Ophthalmic Ointment (Ciloxan): 0.3%.
Ophthalmic Suspension (Ciloxan): 0.3%.

INDICATIONS AND DOSAGES

▸ **Mild to Moderate UTIs**
PO
Adults, Elderly. 250 mg q12h.
IV
Adults, Elderly. 200 mg q12h.

▸ **Complicated UTIs, Mild to Moderate Respiratory Tract, Bone, Joint, Skin and Skin-Structure Infections; Infectious Diarrhea**
PO
Adults, Elderly. 500 mg q12h.
IV
Adults, Elderly. 400 mg q12h.

▸ **Severe, Complicated Infections**
PO
Adults, Elderly. 750 mg q12h.
IV
Adults, Elderly. 400 mg q12h.

▸ **Prostatitis**
PO
Adults, Elderly. 500 mg q12h for 28 days.

▸ **Uncomplicated Bladder Infection**
PO
Adults. 100 mg twice a day for 3 days.

▸ **Acute Sinusitis**
PO
Adults. 500 mg q12h.

▸ **Uncomplicated Gonorrhea**
PO
Adults. 250 mg as a single dose.

▸ **Cystic Fibrosis**
IV
Children. 30 mg/kg/day in 2–3 divided doses. Maximum: 1.2 g/day.
PO
Children. 40 mg/kg/day. Maximum: 2 g/day.

▸ **Corneal Ulcer**
OPHTHALMIC
Adults, Elderly. 2 drops q15min for 6 hr, then 2 drops q30min for the

remainder of first day, 2 drops q1h on second day, and 2 drops q4h on days 3–14.

▸ **Conjunctivitis**

OPHTHALMIC

Adults, Elderly. 1–2 drops q2h for 2 days, then 2 drops q4h for next 5 days.

▸ **Dosage in Renal Impairment**

Dosage and frequency are modified on the basis of creatinine clearance and the severity of the infection.

Creatinine Clearance	Dosage Interval
less than 30 ml/min	Usual dose q18–24h

▸ **Hemodialysis**

Adults, Elderly. 250–500 mg q24h (after dialysis).

▸ **Peritoneal Dialysis**

Adults, Elderly. 250–500 mg q24h (after dialysis).

OFF-LABEL USES

Treatment of chancroid

CONTRAINDICATIONS

Hypersensitivity to ciprofloxacin or other quinolones; for ophthalmic administration: vaccinia, varicella, epithelial herpes simplex, keratitis, mycobacterial infection, fungal disease of ocular structure, use after uncomplicated removal of a foreign body.

INTERACTIONS

Drug

Antacids, iron preparations, sucralfate: May decrease ciprofloxacin absorption.

Caffeine, oral anticoagulants: May increase the effects of these drugs.

Theophylline: Decreases clearance and may increase blood concentration and risk of toxicity of theophylline.

Herbal

None known.

Food

None known.

Drug interactions of concern to dentistry

- Decreased absorption: divalent, trivalent antacids, iron and zinc salts, calcium fortified juices
- Increased serum levels: probenecid
- Increased risk of bleeding with warfarin (monitor)
- Serious adverse effects with theophylline, caffeine

DIAGNOSTIC TEST EFFECTS

May increase BUN and serum alkaline phosphatase, bilirubin, creatinine, LDH, AST (SGOT), and ALT (SGPT) levels.

IV INCOMPATIBILITIES

Aminophylline, ampicillin and sulbactam (Unasyn), cefepime (Maxipime), dexamethasone (Decadron), furosemide (Lasix), heparin, hydrocortisone (Solu-Cortef), methylprednisolone (Solu-Medrol), phenytoin (Dilantin), sodium bicarbonate

IV COMPATIBILITIES

Calcium gluconate, diltiazem (Cardizem), dobutamine (Dobutrex), dopamine (Intropin), lidocaine, lorazepam (Ativan), magnesium, midazolam (Versed), potassium chloride

SIDE EFFECTS

Frequent (5%–2%)

Nausea, diarrhea, dyspepsia, vomiting, constipation, flatulence, confusion, crystalluria

Ophthalmic: Burning, crusting in corner of eye

C

Occasional (< 2%)
Abdominal pain or discomfort, headache, rash
Ophthalmic: Bad taste, sensation of something in eye, eyelid redness or itching
Rare (< 1%)
Dizziness, confusion, tremors, hallucinations, hypersensitivity reaction, insomnia, dry mouth, paresthesia

SERIOUS REACTIONS

! Superinfection (especially enterococcal or fungal), nephropathy, cardiopulmonary arrest, chest pain, and cerebral thrombosis may occur.
! Hypersensitivity reactions, including photosensitivity (as evidenced by rash, pruritus, blisters, edema, and burning skin), have occurred in patients receiving fluoroquinolones.
! Arthropathy may occur if the drug is given to children younger than 18 years.
! Sensitization to the ophthalmic form of the drug may contraindicate later systemic use of ciprofloxacin.

DENTAL CONSIDERATIONS

General:
- Determine why the patient is taking the drug.
- Avoid dental light in patient's eyes; offer dark glasses for patient comfort.
- Minimize exposure to sunlight and wear sunscreen if sun exposure is planned.
- Ruptures of the shoulder, hand, and Achilles tendon requiring surgical repair or resulting in prolonged disability have been reported with this drug.

Consultations:
- Consult with patient's physician if an acute dental infection occurs and another antiinfective is required.

Teach Patient/Family:
- To discontinue treatment and inform dentist immediately if patient experiences pain or inflammation of a tendon, and to rest and refrain from exercise

Drug interactions of concern to dentistry
- Specific studies have not been conducted with topical ciprofloxacin. See systemic drug for interactions.

DENTAL CONSIDERATIONS

General:
- Protect patient's eyes from accidental spatter during dental treatment.
- Avoid dental light in patient's eyes; offer dark glasses for patient comfort.

cisplatin

sis-plah′-tin
(Platinol-AQ)
Do not confuse cisplatin with carboplatin, or Platinol with Paraplatin or Patanol.

CATEGORY AND SCHEDULE

Pregnancy Risk Category: D

MECHANISM OF ACTION

A platinum coordination complex that inhibits DNA and to a lesser extent, RNA, protein synthesis by cross-linking with DNA strands, preventing cell division. Cell cycle-phase nonspecific. ***Therapeutic Effect:*** Interferes with DNA function.

PHARMACOKINETICS

Widely distributed. Protein binding: greater than 90%. Undergoes rapid nonenzymatic conversion to inactive metabolite. Excreted in urine. Removed by hemodialysis. ***Half-life:*** 58–73 hr (increased with impaired renal function).

AVAILABILITY

Injection: 10-mg (CAN) 50-mg, 100-mg vials.

INDICATIONS AND DOSAGES

▸ Advanced Bladder Carcinoma, Metastatic Ovarian Tumors, Metastatic Testicular Tumors

IV

Adults, Elderly, Children.

For intermittent dosage schedule, 37–75 mg/m^2 once every 2–3 wk or 50–100 mg/m^2 over 4–8 hr once every 21–28 days. For daily dosage schedule, 15–20 mg/m^2/day for 5 days every 3–4 wk.

▸ Dosage in Renal Impairment

Dosage is modified on the basis of creatinine clearance.

Creatinine Clearance	% of Dose
10–50 ml/min	75%
less than 10 ml/min	50%

OFF-LABEL USES

Breast, cervical, endometrial, gastric, head and neck, lung, and prostate carcinomas; germ cell tumors; neuroblastoma; osteosarcoma

CONTRAINDICATIONS

Hearing impairment, myelosuppression, pregnancy

INTERACTIONS

Drug

Antigout medications: May decrease the effects of these drugs.
Bone marrow depressants: May increase myelosuppression.
Live-virus vaccines: May potentiate virus replication, increase vaccine side effects, and decrease the patient's antibody response to the vaccine.
Nephrotoxic, ototoxic medications: May increase the risk of nephrotoxicity or ototoxicity.

Herbal

None known.

Food

None known.

Drug interactions of concern to dentistry

- Risk of masking ototoxicity: antihistamines

DIAGNOSTIC TEST EFFECTS

May increase BUN and serum creatinine, uric acid, and AST (SGOT) levels. May decrease creatinine clearance and serum calcium, magnesium, phosphate, potassium, and sodium levels. May cause a positive Coombs' test result.

IV INCOMPATIBILITIES

Amifostine (Ethyol), amphotericin B complex (Abelcet, AmBisome, Amphotec), cefepime (Maxipime), piperacillin and tazobactam (Zosyn), thiotepa

IV COMPATIBILITIES

Etoposide (VePesid), granisetron (Kytril), heparin, hydromorphone (Dilaudid), lorazepam (Ativan), magnesium sulfate, mannitol, morphine, ondansetron (Zofran)

SIDE EFFECTS

Frequent

Nausea, vomiting (generally beginning 1–4 hr after administration and lasting up to 24 hr); myelosuppression (affecting 25%–30% of patients with recovery generally occurring in 18–23 days).

C

Occasional
Peripheral neuropathy (with prolonged therapy [4–7 mo]). Pain or redness at injection site, loss of taste or appetite
Rare
Hemolytic anemia, blurred vision, stomatitis

SERIOUS REACTIONS

! An anaphylactic reaction manifested as angioedema, wheezing, tachycardia, and hypotension, may occur in the first few minutes of IV administration in patients previously exposed to cisplatin.
! Nephrotoxicity occurs in 28%–36% of patients treated with a single dose of cisplatin, usually during the second week of therapy.
! Ototoxicity, including tinnitus and hearing loss, occurs in 31% of patients treated with a single dose of cisplatin. It may be more severe in children and may become more frequent or severe with repeated doses.

DENTAL CONSIDERATIONS

General:
- Determine why patient is taking the drug.
- If additional analgesia is required for dental pain, consider alternative analgesics (NSAIDs) in patients taking narcotics for acute or chronic pain.
- Examine for oral manifestation of opportunistic infection.
- Avoid prescribing aspirin-containing products.
- This drug may be used in the hospital or on an outpatient basis. Confirm the patient's disease and treatment status.
- Chlorhexidine mouth rinse prior to and during chemotherapy may reduce severity of mucositis.
- Patient on chronic drug therapy may rarely present with symptoms of blood dyscrasias, which can include infection, bleeding and poor healing. If dyscrasia is present, caution patient to prevent oral tissue trauma when using oral hygiene aids.
- Palliative medication may be required for management of oral side effects.
- Short appointments and a stress reduction protocol may be required for anxious patients.
- Patients may have received other chemotherapy or radiation; confirm medical and drug history.
- Patients may be at risk of bleeding, check for oral signs.
- Oral infections should be eliminated and/or treated aggressively.
- Patients may be at risk of infection.

Consultations:
- Medical consultation should include routine blood counts including platelet counts and bleeding time.
- Consult physician; prophylactic or therapeutic antiinfectives may be indicated if surgery or periodontal treatment is required.
- Medical consultation may be required to assess immunologic status during cancer chemotherapy and determine safety risk, if any, posed by the required dental treatment.
- Medical consultation may be required to assess disease control and patient's ability to tolerate stress.

Teach Patient/Family:
- Secondary oral infection may occur; need to see dentist immediately if infection occurs
- To be aware of oral side effects
- Importance of good oral hygiene to prevent soft tissue inflammation
- To report oral lesions, soreness, or bleeding to dentist
- To prevent trauma when using oral hygiene aids

• Importance of updating health and medication history if physician makes any changes in evaluation or drug regimens; include OTC, herbal, and nonherbal remedies in the update

clarithromycin

clare-i-thro-mye′-sin
(Biaxin, Biaxin XL, Klacid[AUS])

CATEGORY AND SCHEDULE

Pregnancy Risk Category: C

MECHANISM OF ACTION

A macrolide that binds to ribosomal receptor sites of susceptible organisms, inhibiting protein synthesis of the bacterial cell wall. ***Therapeutic Effect:*** Bacteriostatic; may be bactericidal with high dosages or very susceptible microorganisms.

PHARMACOKINETICS

Well absorbed from the GI tract. Protein binding: 65%–75%. Widely distributed. Metabolized in the liver to active metabolite. Primarily excreted in urine. Not removed by hemodialysis. ***Half-life:*** 3–7 hr; metabolite 5–7 hr (increased in impaired renal function).

AVAILABILITY

Oral Suspension: 125 mg/5 ml, 250 mg/5 ml.
Tablets: 250 mg, 500 mg.
Tablets (Extended-Release): 500 mg.

INDICATIONS AND DOSAGES

▸ Bronchitis
PO
Adults, Elderly. 500 mg q12h for 7–14 days.

▸ Skin, Soft Tissue Infections
PO
Adults, Elderly. 250 mg q12h for 7–14 days.
Children. 7.5 mg/kg q12h for 10 days.

▸ MAC Prophylaxis
PO
Adults, Elderly. 500 mg 2 times/day.
Children. 7.5 mg/kg q12h. Maximum: 500 mg 2 times/day.

▸ MAC Treatment
PO
Adults, Elderly. 500 mg 2 times/day in combination.
Children. 7.5 mg/kg q12h in combination. Maximum: 500 mg 2 times/day.

▸ Pharyngitis, Tonsillitis
PO
Adults, Elderly. 250 mg q12h for 10 days.
Children. 7.5 mg/kg q12h for 10 days.

▸ Pneumonia
PO
Adults, Elderly. 250 mg q12h for 7–14 days.
Children. 7.5 mg/kg q12h.

▸ Maxillary Sinusitis
PO
Adults, Elderly. 500 mg q12h for 14 days.
Children. 7.5 mg/kg q12h. Maximum: 500 mg 2 times/day.

▸ H. pylori
PO
Adults, Elderly. 500 mg q12h for 10–14 days in combination.

▸ Acute Otitis Media
PO
Children. 7.5 mg/kg q12h for 10 days.

▸ Dosage in Renal Impairment
For patients with creatinine clearance less than 30 ml/min, reduce dose by 50% and administer once or twice a day.

C

CONTRAINDICATIONS

Hypersensitivity to clarithromycin or other macrolide antibiotics

INTERACTIONS

Drug

Carbamazepine, digoxin, theophylline: May increase blood concentration and toxicity of these drugs.
Rifampin: May decrease clarithromycin blood concentration.
Warfarin: May increase warfarin effects.
Zidovudine: May decrease blood concentration of zidovudine.

Herbal

None known.

Food

None known.

Drug interactions of concern to dentistry

- Decreased effect: anticholinergic drugs
- Increased effects of cyclosporine, warfarin, cilostazol, tacrolimus, pimozide, methylprednisolone, fluconazole, buspirone
- Decreased action of clindamycin, penicillins, lincomycin, rifabutin, rifampin, zidovudine
- Increased serum levels of carbamazepine, theophylline, digoxin
- Contraindicated with indinavir
- Suspected risk of increased CNS depression with alprazolam, diazepam, midazolam, triazolam
- Oral contraceptives: advise patient of a potential risk for decreased contraceptive action, to maintain compliance with oral contraceptive use while using antibiotics, and to consider the use of additional nonhormonal contraception
- Suspected increase in plasma levels of repaglinide
- Risk of severe myopathy or rhabdomyolysis: atorvastatin, fluvastatin, lovastatin, pravastatin

DIAGNOSTIC TEST EFFECTS

May (rarely) increase BUN, AST (SGOT), and ALT (SGPT) levels.

SIDE EFFECTS

Occasional (6%–3%)
Diarrhea, nausea, altered taste, abdominal pain
Rare (2%–1%)
Headache, dyspepsia

SERIOUS REACTIONS

! Antibiotic-associated colitis and other superinfections may result from altered bacterial balance.
! Hepatotoxicity and thrombocytopenia occur rarely.

DENTAL CONSIDERATIONS

General:

- Determine why the patient is taking the drug.
- May prove to be an alternative drug of choice for mild infections caused by a susceptible organism in patients who are allergic to penicillin.

Teach Patient/Family:

- Importance of good oral hygiene to prevent soft tissue inflammation
- *When used for dental infection, advise patient:*
  - To report sore throat, oral burning sensation, fever, and fatigue, any of which could indicate superinfection
  - To take at prescribed intervals and complete dosage regimen
  - To immediately notify the dentist if signs or symptoms of infection increase

clemastine fumarate

klem′-as-teen
(Dayhistol Allergy, Tavist Allergy)

CATEGORY AND SCHEDULE

Pregnancy Risk Category: B

MECHANISM OF ACTION

An ethanolamine that competes with histamine on effector cells in the GI tract, blood vessels, and respiratory tract. ***Therapeutic Effect:*** Relieves allergy symptoms, including urticaria, rhinitis, and pruritus.

PHARMACOKINETICS

Route	Onset	Peak	Duration
PO	15–60 min	5–7 hr	10–12 hr

Well absorbed from the GI tract. Metabolized in the liver. Excreted primarily in urine.

AVAILABILITY

Syrup (Dayhist, Tavist): 0.67 mg/5 ml.
Tablets (Dayhist, Tavist): 1.34 mg, 2.68 mg.

INDICATIONS AND DOSAGES

▸ **Allergic Rhinitis, Urticaria**

PO

Adults, Children older than 11 yr. 1.34 mg twice a day up to 2.68 mg 3 times a day. Maximum: 8.04 mg/day.
Children 6–11 yr. 0.67–1.34 mg twice a day. Maximum: 4.02 mg/day.
Children younger than 6 yr. 0.05 mg/kg/day divided into 2–3 doses per day. Maximum: 1.34 mg/day.
Elderly. 1.34 mg 1–2 times a day.

CONTRAINDICATIONS

Angle-closure glaucoma, hypersensitivity to clemastine, use within 14 days of MAOIs

INTERACTIONS

Drug

Alcohol, other CNS depressants: May increase CNS depression.
MAOIs: May increase the anticholinergic and CNS depressant effects of clemastine.

Herbal

None known.

Food

None known.

Drug interactions of concern to dentistry

- Increased CNS depression: all CNS depressants, alcohol
- Increased anticholinergic effect of anticholinergics, phenothiazines, tricyclic antidepressants

DIAGNOSTIC TEST EFFECTS

May suppress wheal and flare reactions to antigen skin testing unless drug is discontinued 4 days before testing.

SIDE EFFECTS

Frequent

Somnolence, dizziness, urine retention, thickening of bronchial secretions, dry mouth, nose, or throat; in elderly, sedation, dizziness, hypotension

Occasional

Epigastric distress, flushing, blurred vision, tinnitus, paresthesia, diaphoresis, chills

SERIOUS REACTIONS

! A hypersensitivity reaction, marked by eczema, pruritus, rash, cardiac disturbances, angioedema, and photosensitivity, may occur.

C

! Overdose symptoms may vary from CNS depression, including sedation, apnea, cardiovascular collapse, and death to severe paradoxical reaction, such as hallucinations, tremor, and seizures.
! Children may experience paradoxical reactions, such as restlessness, insomnia, euphoria, nervousness, and tremors.
! Overdose in children may result in hallucinations, seizures, and death.

DENTAL CONSIDERATIONS

General:

- Assess salivary flow as a factor in caries, periodontal disease, and candidiasis.
- Determine why the patient is taking the drug.

Teach Patient/Family:

- Importance of good oral hygiene to prevent soft tissue inflammation
- Caution to prevent injury when using oral hygiene aids
- *When chronic dry mouth occurs, advise patient:*
  - To avoid mouth rinses with high alcohol content because of drying effects
  - To use daily home fluoride products for anticaries effect
  - To use sugarless gum, frequent sips of water, or saliva substitutes

clindamycin

klin-da-mye′-sin
(Cleocin, Cleocin HCl[AUS], Clindesse, Dalacin[CAN], Dalacin C[AUS])

CATEGORY AND SCHEDULE

Pregnancy Risk Category: B

MECHANISM OF ACTION

A lincosamide antibiotic that inhibits protein synthesis of the bacterial cell wall by binding to bacterial ribosomal receptor sites. Topically, it decreases fatty acid concentration on the skin. ***Therapeutic Effect:*** Bacteriostatic. Prevents outbreaks of acne vulgaris.

PHARMACOKINETICS

Rapidly absorbed from the GI tract. Protein binding: 92%–94%. Widely distributed. Metabolized in the liver to some active metabolites. Primarily excreted in urine. Not removed by hemodialysis. ***Half-life:*** 2.4–3 hr (increased in impaired renal function and premature infants).

AVAILABILITY

Capsules: 75 mg, 150 mg, 300 mg.
Oral Solution: 75 mg/5 ml.
Injection: 150 mg/ml.
Topical Gel: 1%.
Topical Solution: 1%.
Vaginal Cream (Clindesse): 2%.
Vaginal Suppository: 100 mg.

INDICATIONS AND DOSAGES

▸ **Chronic Bone and Joint, Respiratory Tract, Skin and Soft Tissue, Intra-Abdominal, and Female GU Infections; Endocarditis; Septicemia**

PO
Adults, Elderly. 150–450 mg/dose q6–8h.
Children. 10–30 mg/kg/day in 3–4 divided doses. Maximum: 1.8 g/day.
IV, IM
Adults, Elderly. 1.2–1.8 g/day in 2–4 divided doses.
Children. 25–40 mg/kg/day in 3–4 divided doses. Maximum: 4.8 g/day.

▸ **Bacterial Vaginosis**
PO
Adults, Elderly. 300 mg twice a day for 7 days.
INTRAVAGINAL
Adults. One applicatorful at bedtime for 3–7 days or 1 suppository at bedtime for 3 days.
▸ **Acne Vulgaris**
TOPICAL
Adults. Apply thin layer to affected area twice a day.

OFF-LABEL USES

Treatment of malaria, otitis media, *Pneumocystis carinii* pneumonia, toxoplasmosis

CONTRAINDICATIONS

History of antibiotic-associated colitis, regional enteritis, or ulcerative colitis; hypersensitivity to clindamycin or lincomycin; known allergy to tartrazine dye

INTERACTIONS

Drug

Adsorbent antidiarrheals: May delay absorption of clindamycin.
Chloramphenicol, erythromycin: May antagonize the effects of clindamycin.
Neuromuscular blockers: May increase the effects of these drugs.

Herbal

None known.

Food

None known.

Drug interactions of concern to dentistry

- Decreased action: erythromycin, absorbent antidiarrheals
- Increased effects of nondepolarizing muscle relaxants, hydrocarbon inhalation anesthetics
- Avoid antiperistaltic drugs if diarrhea occurs
- Possible reduced blood levels of cyclosporine
- Oral contraceptives: advise patient of a potential risk for decreased contraceptive action, to maintain compliance with oral contraceptive use while using antibiotics, and to consider the use of additional nonhormonal contraception

DIAGNOSTIC TEST EFFECTS

May increase serum alkaline phosphatase, AST (SGOT), and ALT (SGPT) levels.

IV INCOMPATIBILITIES

Allopurinol (Aloprim), filgrastim (Neupogen), fluconazole (Diflucan), idarubicin (Idamycin)

IV COMPATIBILITIES

Amiodarone (Cordarone), diltiazem (Cardizem), heparin, hydromorphone (Dilaudid), magnesium sulfate, midazolam (Versed), morphine, multivitamins, propofol (Diprivan)

SIDE EFFECTS

Frequent

Systemic: Abdominal pain, nausea, vomiting, diarrhea
Topical: Dry scaly skin
Vaginal: Vaginitis, pruritus

Occasional

Systemic: Phlebitis or thrombophlebitis with IV administration, pain and induration at IM injection site, allergic reaction, urticaria, pruritus
Topical: Contact dermatitis, abdominal pain, mild diarrhea, burning or stinging
Vaginal: Headache, dizziness, nausea, vomiting, abdominal pain

Rare

Vaginal: Hypersensitivity reaction

SERIOUS REACTIONS

! Antibiotic-associated colitis and other superinfections may occur

during and several weeks after clindamycin therapy (including the topical form).
! Blood dyscrasias (leukopenia, thrombocytopenia) and nephrotoxicity (proteinuria, azotemia, oliguria) occur rarely.

DENTAL CONSIDERATIONS

General:
- Determine why the patient is taking the drug.

Consultations:
- Medical consultation may be required to assess disease control.

Teach Patient/Family:
- Importance of good oral hygiene to prevent soft tissue inflammation
- Caution to prevent injury when using oral hygiene aids
- *When used for dental infection, advise patient:*
  - To report sore throat, oral burning sensation, fever, and fatigue, any of which could indicate superinfection
  - To take at prescribed intervals and complete dosage regimen
  - To immediately notify the dentist if signs or symptoms of infection increase

clobetasol

klo-bet′-a-sol
(Alti-Clobetasol[CAN], Cormax, Dermovate[CAN], Gen-Clobetasol[CAN], Olux, Novo-Clobetasol[CAN], Temovate)

CATEGORY AND SCHEDULE

Pregnancy Risk Category: C

MECHANISM OF ACTION

A corticosteroid that inhibits accumulation of inflammatory cells at inflammation sites, phagocytosis, lysosomal enzyme release and synthesis or release of mediators of inflammation. ***Therapeutic Effect:*** Decreases or prevents tissue response to inflammatory process.

PHARMACOKINETICS

May be absorbed from intact skin. Metabolized in liver. Excreted in the urine.

AVAILABILITY

Cream: 0.05% (Cormax, Temovate).
Cream, in emollient base: 0.05% (Temovate).
Foam: 0.05% (Olux).
Gel: 0.05% (Temovate).
Ointment: 0.05% (Cormax, Temovate).
Topical Solution: 0.05% (Cormax, Temovate).

INDICATIONS AND DOSAGES

▸ **Anti-Inflammatory, Corticosteroid Replacement Therapy**

TOPICAL
Adults, Elderly, Children older than 12 yrs and older. Apply 2 times/day for 2 weeks.

FOAM
Adults, Elderly, Children older than 12 yrs and older. Apply 2 times/day for 2 wks.

CONTRAINDICATIONS

Hypersensitivity to clobetasol or other corticosteroids.

INTERACTIONS

Drug
None known.
Herbal
None known.
Food
None known.

Drug interactions of concern to dentistry

- None reported

DIAGNOSTIC TEST EFFECTS

None known.

SIDE EFFECTS

Frequent

Local irritation, dry skin, itching, redness

Occasional

Allergic contact dermatitis

Rare

Cushing's syndrome, numbness of fingers, skin atrophy

SERIOUS REACTIONS

! Overdosage can occur from topically applied clobetasol propionate absorbed in sufficient amounts to produce systemic effects producing reversible adrenal suppression, manifestations of Cushing's syndrome, hyperglycemia, and glucosuria in some patients.

CLOBETASOL PROPIONATE (TOPICAL FOAM)

DENTAL CONSIDERATIONS

General:

- Determine why patient is taking the drug.
- Avoid use of systemic corticosteroids unless a consultation is made.

CLOBETASOL PROPIONATE

DENTAL CONSIDERATIONS

General:

- Place on frequent recall to evaluate healing response.
- Topical adrenocorticosteroids are not indicated for treating plaque-related gingivitis, which should be treated by removal of local irritants and improved oral hygiene.

Teach Patient/Family:

- Importance of good oral hygiene to prevent soft tissue inflammation
- That use on oral herpetic ulcerations is contraindicated
- To apply at bedtime or after meals for maximum effect
- To apply with cotton-tipped applicator by pressing, not rubbing, paste on lesion
- When used for oral lesions, patient should return for oral evaluation if response of oral tissues has not occurred in 7–14 days

clocortolone

klo-kort′-o-lone

(Cloderm, Cloderm[CAN])

CATEGORY AND SCHEDULE

Pregnancy Risk Category: C

MECHANISM OF ACTION

A topical corticosteroid that inhibits accumulation of inflammatory cells at inflammation sites, suppresses mitotic activity, and cause vasoconstriction. ***Therapeutic Effect:*** Decreases or prevents tissue response to inflammatory process.

PHARMACOKINETICS

Absorption is variable and dependent upon many factors including integrity of skin, dose, vehicle used, and use of occlusive dressings. Small amounts may be absorbed from the skin. Metabolized in liver. Excreted in the urine and feces.

AVAILABILITY

Cream: 0.1%.

INDICATIONS AND DOSAGES

▸ **Dermatoses**

TOPICAL

Adults, Elderly, Children 12 yrs and older. Apply 1–4 times/day.

C

CONTRAINDICATIONS
Hypersensitivity to clocortolone pivalate or other corticosteroids; viral, fungal, or tubercular skin lesions

INTERACTIONS
Drug
None known.
Herbal
None known.
Food
None known.

DIAGNOSTIC TEST EFFECTS
None known.

SIDE EFFECTS
Occasional
Local irritation, burning, itching, redness
Allergic contact dermatitis
Rare
Hypertrichosis, hypopigmentation, maceration of skin, miliaria, perioral dermatitis, skin atrophy, striae

SERIOUS REACTIONS
! Overdosage can occur from topically applied clocortolone pivalate absorbed in sufficient amounts to produce systemic effects in some patients.

DENTAL CONSIDERATIONS
General:
- Determine why the patient is taking the drug.
- Place on frequent recall to evaluate healing response if used on a chronic basis.
- Apply lubricant to dry lips for patient comfort before dental procedures.

clofazimine
kloe-faz′-i-meen
(Lamprene)

CATEGORY AND SCHEDULE
Pregnancy Risk Category: C

MECHANISM OF ACTION
An antibiotic that binds to mycobacterial DNA. ***Therapeutic Effect:*** Inhibits mycobacterial growth and produces anti-inflammatory action.

AVAILABILITY
Capsules: 50 mg.

INDICATIONS AND DOSAGES
▸ **Leprosy**
PO
Adults, Elderly. 100 mg/day in combination with dapsone and rifampin for 3 yr then 100 mg/day as monotherapy.
Children. 1 mg/kg/day in combination with dapsone and rifampin.
▸ **Erythema Nodosum**
PO
Adults, Elderly. 100–200 mg/day for up to 3 mo, then 100 mg/day.

CONTRAINDICATIONS
None significant.

INTERACTIONS
Drug
Dapsone: May decrease the effects of clofazimine.
Herbal
None significant.
Food
All foods: May increase the absorption of clofazimine.

DIAGNOSTIC TEST EFFECTS
May increase blood glucose levels.

SIDE EFFECTS

Frequent (> 10%)

Dry skin, abdominal pain, nausea, vomiting, diarrhea, skin discoloration (pink to brownish-black)

Occasional (10%–1%)

Rash; pruritus; eye irritation; discoloration of sputum; sweat and urine

SERIOUS REACTIONS

! None significant.

Drug interactions of concern to dentistry

- None reported

DENTAL CONSIDERATIONS

General:

- Develop awareness of the patient's disease.

Teach Patient/Family:

- Importance of good oral hygiene to prevent soft tissue inflammation
- To avoid mouth rinses with high alcohol content because of drying effects

clofibrate

kloe-**fye**-brate

(Abitrate, Atromid-S, Claripex[CAN], Novofibrate[CAN])

CATEGORY AND SCHEDULE

Pregnancy Risk Category: C

MECHANISM OF ACTION

An antihyperlipidemic that enhances synthesis of lipoprotein lipase and reduces triglyceride-rich lipoproteins and VLDLs. ***Therapeutic Effect:*** Increases very-low-density lipoprotein (VLDL) catabolism and reduces total plasma triglyceride levels.

PHARMACOKINETICS

Well absorbed from the GI tract. Protein binding: 95%–97%. Metabolized in liver. Excreted primarily in urine, lesser amount in feces. ***Half-life:*** 14–35 hr.

AVAILABILITY

Capsules (Atromid-S): 500 mg.

INDICATIONS AND DOSAGES

Hypercholesterolemia

PO

Adults, Elderly. 2 g/day in divided doses. Some patients may respond to a lower dosage.

CONTRAINDICATIONS

Hypersensitivity to clofibrate, severe renal or hepatic dysfunction, pregnancy, nursing women, rhabdomyolysis, severe hyperkalemia, primary biliary cirrhosis

INTERACTIONS

Drug

- **Anticoagulants:** Potentiates effects of these drugs.
- **Bile acid sequestrants:** May impede clofibrate absorption.
- **Cyclosporine:** Increases risk of nephrotoxicity.
- **Hydroxymethylglutaryl-CoA reductase (HMG-CoA) inhibitors:** Increases risk of acute renal failure, rhabdomyolysis, severe myopathy.

Herbal

None known.

Food

None known.

Drug interactions of concern to dentistry

- None reported

DIAGNOSTIC TESTS

May increase AST and ALT levels.

C

clomiphene

kloe′-mi-feen
(Clomhexal[AUS], Clomid, Clomid[CAN], Milophene, Milophene[CAN], Serophene, Serophene[CAN])
Do not confuse with chlomipramine.

CATEGORY AND SCHEDULE

Pregnancy Risk Category: X

MECHANISM OF ACTION

An ovulation stimulator that promotes release of pituitary gonadotropins. ***Therapeutic Effect:*** Stimulates ovulation.

PHARMACOKINETICS

Readily absorbed. Time to peak occurs within 6.5 hrs. Undergoes enterohepatic recirculation. Primarily excreted in feces. ***Half-life:*** 5–7 days.

AVAILABILITY

Tablets: 50 mg (Clomid, Milophene, Serophene).

INDICATIONS AND DOSAGES

▸ Ovulatory Failure, Females

PO

Adults. 50 mg/day for 5 days (first course); start the regimen on the fifth day of cycle. Increase dose only if unresponsive to cyclic 50 mg. Maximum: 100 mg/day for 5 days.

OFF-LABEL USES

Infertility in males

CONTRAINDICATIONS

Liver dysfunction, abnormal uterine bleeding, enlargement or development of ovarian cyst, uncontrolled thyroid or adrenal dysfunction in the presence of an organic intracranial lesion such

SIDE EFFECTS

Frequent

Nausea, vomiting, loose stools, dyspepsia, flatulence, abdominal distress

Occasional

Headache, dizziness, fatigue

Rare

Muscle cramping, aching, weakness; skin rash, urticaria, pruritus; dry brittle hair, alopecia

SERIOUS REACTIONS

! May increase excretion of cholesterol into bile, leading to cholelithiasis.
! Various cardiac arrhythmias have been reported.
! Anemia and, more frequently, leukopenia have been reported.

DENTAL CONSIDERATIONS

General:

- Consider semisupine chair position for patient comfort if GI side effects occur.
- Patients on chronic drug therapy may rarely have symptoms of blood dyscrasias, which can include infection, bleeding, and poor healing.

Consultations:

- In a patient with symptoms of blood dyscrasias, request a medical consultation for blood studies and postpone treatment until normal values are reestablished.

Teach Patient/Family:

- Importance of good oral hygiene to prevent soft tissue inflammation

as pituitary tumor, pregnancy, hypersensitivity to clomipehene

INTERACTIONS

Drug

Danazol: May decrease the response of clomiphene.
Estradiol: May decrease estradiol.

Herbal

None known.

Food

None known.

Drug interactions of concern to dentistry

• None reported

DIAGNOSTIC TEST EFFECTS

Altered levels of thyroid function tests.

SIDE EFFECTS

Frequent (13%–10%)
Hot flashes, ovarian enlargement
Occasional (5%–2%)
Abdominal/pelvic discomfort, bloating, nausea, vomiting, breast discomfort (females)
Rare (< 1%)
Vision disturbances, abnormal menstrual flow, breast enlargement (males), headache, mental depression, ovarian cyst formation, thromboembolism, uterine fibroid enlargement

SERIOUS REACTIONS

! Thrombophlebitis, alopecia, and polyuria occurs rarely.

DENTAL CONSIDERATIONS

General:

• Consider semisupine chair position for patient comfort if GI side effects occur.
• Avoid dental light in patient's eyes; offer dark glasses for patient comfort.
• Be aware that patient may be in early stage of pregnancy.

clomipramine hydrochloride

klom-ip′-ra-meen
(Anafranil, Apo-Clomipramine[CAN], Clopram[AUS], Novo-Clopamine[CAN], Placil[AUS])
Do not confuse clomipramine with chlorpromazine, clomiphene, or imipramine, or Anafranil with alfentanil, enalapril, or nafarelin.

CATEGORY AND SCHEDULE

Pregnancy Risk Category: C

MECHANISM OF ACTION

A tricyclic antidepressant that blocks the reuptake of neurotransmitters, such as norepinephrine and serotonin, at CNS presynaptic membranes, increasing their availability at postsynaptic receptor sites. ***Therapeutic Effect:*** Reduces obsessive-compulsive behavior.

PHARMACOKINETICS

Well absorbed from GI tract. Protein binding: 97%. Principally bound to albumin. Distributed into cerebrospinal fluid. Metabolized in the liver. Undergoes extensive first-pass effect. Excreted in urine and feces. ***Half-life:*** 19–37 hr.

AVAILABILITY

Capsules: 25 mg, 50 mg, 75 mg.

INDICATIONS AND DOSAGES

▸ **Obsessive-Compulsive Disorder**

PO

Adults, Elderly. Initially, 25 mg/day. May gradually increase to 100 mg/day in the first 2 wk. Maximum: 250 mg/day.
Children 10 yr and older. Initially, 25 mg/day. May gradually increase up to maximum of 200 mg/day.

C

OFF-LABEL USES

Treatment of bulimia nervosa, cataplexy associated with narcolepsy, mental depression, neurogenic pain, panic disorder, ejaculatory disorders, pervasive developmental disorder

CONTRAINDICATIONS

Acute recovery period after MI, use within 14 days of MAOIs

INTERACTIONS

Drug

Alcohol, other CNS depressants: May increase CNS and respiratory depression and the hypotensive effects of clomipramine.
Antithyroid agents: May increase the risk of agranulocytosis.
Cimetidine: May increase clomipramine blood concentration and risk of toxicity.
Clonidine, guanadrel: May decrease the effects of these drugs.
MAOIs: May increase the risk of neuroleptic malignant syndrome, seizures, hyperpyresis, and hypertensive crisis.
Phenothiazines: May increase the anticholinergic and sedative effects of clomipramine.
Sympathomimetics: May increase the risk of cardiac effects.

Herbal

St. John's wort: May increase the risk of serotonin syndrome.

Food

None known.

Drug interactions of concern to dentistry

- Increased anticholinergic effects: muscarinic blockers, antihistamines, phenothiazines
- Increased effects of direct-acting sympathomimetics (epinephrine, levonordefrin)
- Potential risk of CNS depression: alcohol, barbiturates, benzodiazepines, and other CNS depressants
- Decreased antihypertensive effects: clonidine, guanadrel, guanethidine
- Use with caution, possible reduced metabolism: drugs metabolized by CYP450 2D6 isoenzymes
- Avoid concurrent use with St. John's wort (herb)

DIAGNOSTIC TEST EFFECTS

May alter the blood glucose level and EKG readings.

SIDE EFFECTS

Frequent

Somnolence, fatigue, dry mouth, blurred vision, constipation, sexual dysfunction (42%), ejaculatory failure (20%), impotence, weight gain (18%), delayed micturition, orthostatic hypotension, diaphoresis, impaired concentration, increased appetite, urine retention

Occasional

GI disturbances (such as nausea, GI distress, and metallic taste), asthenia, aggressiveness, muscle weakness

Rare

Paradoxical reactions (agitation, restlessness, nightmares, insomnia), extrapyramidal symptoms, (particularly fine hand tremor), laryngitis, seizures

SERIOUS REACTIONS

! Overdose may produce seizures; cardiovascular effects, such as severe orthostatic hypotension, dizziness, tachycardia, palpitations, and arrhythmias; and altered temperature regulation, including hyperpyrexia or hypothermia.

! Abrupt discontinuation after prolonged therapy may produce headache, malaise, nausea, vomiting, and vivid dreams.

! Anemia and agranulocytosis have been noted.

DENTAL CONSIDERATIONS

General:

• Take vital signs at every appointment because of cardiovascular side effects.
• Assess salivary flow as a factor in caries, periodontal disease, and candidiasis.
• Patients on chronic drug therapy may rarely have symptoms of blood dyscrasias, which can include infection, bleeding, and poor healing.
• After supine positioning, have patient sit upright for at least 2 min before standing to avoid orthostatic hypotension.
• Use vasoconstrictor with caution, in low doses, and with careful aspiration. Avoid use of gingival retraction cord with epinephrine.
• Place on frequent recall because of oral side effects.
• A stress reduction protocol may be required.

Consultations:

• In a patient with symptoms of blood dyscrasias, request a medical consultation for blood studies and postpone dental treatment until normal values are reestablished.
• Physician should be informed if significant xerostomic side effects occur (e.g., increased caries, sore tongue, problems eating or swallowing, difficulty wearing prosthesis) so that a medication change can be considered.
• Medical consultation may be required to assess disease control.

Teach Patient/Family:

• Importance of good oral hygiene to prevent soft tissue inflammation
• Caution to prevent injury when using oral hygiene aids
• *When chronic dry mouth occurs, advise patient:*
  • To avoid mouth rinses with high alcohol content because of drying effects
  • To use daily home fluoride products for anticaries effect
  • To use sugarless gum, frequent sips of water, or saliva substitutes

clonazepam

kloe-na′-zi-pam
Schedule IV
(Apo-Clonazepam[CAN], Clonapam[CAN], Klonopin, Paxam[AUS], Rivotril[CAN])
Do not confuse clonazepam with clonidine or lorazepam.

CATEGORY AND SCHEDULE

Pregnancy Risk Category: D

MECHANISM OF ACTION

A benzodiazepine that depresses all levels of the CNS; inhibits nerve impulse transmission in the motor cortex and suppresses abnormal discharge in petit mal seizures.
Therapeutic Effect: Produces anxiolytic and anticonvulsant effects.

PHARMACOKINETICS

Well absorbed from the GI tract. Protein binding: 85%. Metabolized in the liver. Excreted in urine. Not removed by hemodialysis. ***Half-life:*** 18–50 hr.

AVAILABILITY

Tablets: 0.5 mg, 1 mg, 2 mg.
Tablets (Disintegrating): 0.125 mg, 0.25 mg, 0.5 mg, 1 mg, 2 mg.

INDICATIONS AND DOSAGES

▸ Adjunctive Treatment of Lennox-Gastaut Syndrome (petit mal variant) and Akinetic, Myoclonic, and Absence (petit mal) Seizures

PO

Adults, Elderly, Children 10 yrs and older. 1.5 mg/day; may be increased in 0.5- to 1-mg increments every 3 days until seizures are controlled. Don't exceed maintenance dosage of 20 mg/day.

Infants, Children younger than 10 yr or weighing less than 30 kg. 0.01–0.03 mg/kg/day in 2–3 divided doses; may be increased by up to 0.5 mg every 3 days until seizures are controlled. Don't exceed maintenance dosage of 0.2 mg/kg/day.

▸ Panic Disorder

PO

Adults, Elderly. Initially, 0.25 mg twice a day; increased in increments of 0.125–0.25 mg twice a day every 3 days. Maximum: 4 mg/day.

OFF-LABEL USES

Adjunctive treatment of seizures; treatment of simple, complex partial, and tonic-clonic seizures

CONTRAINDICATIONS

Narrow-angle glaucoma, significant hepatic disease

INTERACTIONS

Drug

Alcohol, other CNS depressants: May increase CNS depressant effect.

Herbal

Kava kava: May increase sedation.

Food

None known.

Drug interactions of concern to dentistry

- Increased sedation: alcohol, all CNS depressants, indinavir, kava (herb)
- Risk of increased serum levels: drugs that inhibit CYP3A4 isoenzymes, ketoconazole, itraconazole, fluconazole, protease inhibitor, nefazodone
- Risk of decreased effect: St. John's wort (herb)

DIAGNOSTIC TEST EFFECTS

None known.

SIDE EFFECTS

Frequent

Mild, transient drowsiness; ataxia; behavioral disturbances (aggression, irritability, agitation), especially in children

Occasional

Rash, ankle or facial edema, nocturia, dysuria, change in appetite or weight, dry mouth, sore gums, nausea, blurred vision

Rare

Paradoxical CNS reactions, including hyperactivity or nervousness in children and excitement or restlessness in the elderly (particularly in the presence of uncontrolled pain).

SERIOUS REACTIONS

! Abrupt withdrawal may result in pronounced restlessness, irritability, insomnia, hand tremors, abdominal or muscle cramps, diaphoresis, vomiting, and status epilepticus.

! Overdose results in somnolence, confusion, diminished reflexes, and coma.

DENTAL CONSIDERATIONS

General:

- Patients on chronic drug therapy may rarely have symptoms of blood dyscrasias, which can include infection, bleeding, and poor healing.

- Assess salivary flow as a factor in caries, periodontal disease, and candidiasis.
- Psychologic and physical dependence may occur with chronic administration.
- Geriatric patients are more susceptible to drug effects; use lower dose.
- Ask about type of epilepsy, seizure frequency, and quality of seizure control.

Consultations:

- Medical consultation may be required to assess disease control.
- In a patient with symptoms of blood dyscrasias, request a medical consultation for blood studies and postpone dental treatment until normal values are reestablished.

Teach Patient/Family:

Importance of good oral hygiene to prevent soft tissue inflammation

Caution to prevent injury when using oral hygiene aids

- *When chronic dry mouth occurs, advise patient:*
  - To avoid mouth rinses with high alcohol content because of drying effects
  - To use daily home fluoride products for anticaries effect
  - To use sugarless gum, frequent sips of water, or saliva substitutes

clonidine

klon′-ih-deen

(Catapres, Catapres TTS, Dixarit[CAN], Duraclon)

Do not confuse clonidine with clomiphene, Klonopin, or quinidine, or Catapres with Cetapred.

CATEGORY AND SCHEDULE

Pregnancy Risk Category: C

MECHANISM OF ACTION

An antiadrenergic, sympatholytic agent that prevents pain signal transmission to the brain and produces analgesia at pre- and post-alpha-adrenergic receptors in the spinal cord. ***Therapeutic Effect:*** Reduces peripheral resistance; decreases BP and heart rate.

PHARMACOKINETICS

Route	Onset	Peak	Duration
PO	0.5–1 hr	2–4 hr	Up to 8 hr

Well absorbed from the GI tract. Transdermal best absorbed from the chest and upper arm; least absorbed from the thigh. Protein binding: 20%–40%. Metabolized in the liver. Primarily excreted in urine. Minimally removed by hemodialysis. ***Half-life:*** 12–16 hr (increased with impaired renal function).

AVAILABILITY

Tablets (Catapres): 0.1 mg, 0.2 mg, 0.3 mg.
Transdermal Patch (Catapres TTS): 2.5 mg (release at 0.1 mg/24 hr), 5 mg (release at 0.2 mg/24 hr), 7.5 mg (release at 0.3 mg/24 hr).
Injection (Duraclon): 100 mcg/ml, 500 mcg/ml.

INDICATIONS AND DOSAGES

▸ **Hypertension**

PO

Adults. Initially, 0.1 mg twice a day. Increase by 0.1–0.2 mg q2–4 days. Maintenance: 0.2–1.2 mg/day in 2–4 divided doses up to maximum of 2.4 mg/day.
Elderly. Initially, 0.1 mg at bedtime. May increase gradually.
Children. 5–25 mcg/kg/day in divided doses q6h. Increase at 5- to 7-day intervals. Maximum: 0.9 mg/day.

TRANSDERMAL
Adults, Elderly. System delivering 0.1 mg/24 hr up to 0.6 mg/24 hr q7 days.

▸ **Attention Deficit Hyperactivity Disorder (ADHD)**

PO
Children. Initially 0.05 mg/day. May increase by 0.05 mg/day q3–7 days. Maximum: 0.3–0.4 mg/day.

▸ **Severe Pain**

EPIDURAL
Adults, Elderly. 30–40 mcg/hr.
Children. Initially, 0.5 mcg/kg/hr, not to exceed adult dose.

OFF-LABEL USES

ADHD, diagnosis of pheochromocytoma, opioid withdrawal, prevention of migraine headaches, treatment of dysmenorrhea, menopausal flushing

CONTRAINDICATIONS

Epidural contraindicated in those patients with bleeding diathesis or infection at the injection site, and in those receiving anticoagulation therapy

INTERACTIONS

Drug

Beta blockers: Discontinuing these drugs may increase risk of clonidine-withdrawal hypertensive crisis.
Tricyclic antidepressants: May decrease effect of clonidine.

Herbal

None known.

Food

None known.

Drug interactions of concern to dentistry

- Increased CNS depression: alcohol, all CNS depressants
- Decreased hypotensive effects: NSAIDs, especially indomethacin, sympathomimetics, tricyclic anti-depressants

DIAGNOSTIC TEST EFFECTS

None known.

IV INCOMPATIBILITIES

None known.

IV COMPATIBILITIES

Bupivacaine (Marcaine, Sensorcaine), fentanyl (Sublimaze), heparin, ketamine (Ketalar), lidocaine, lorazepam (Ativan)

SIDE EFFECTS

Frequent

Dry mouth (40%), somnolence (33%), dizziness (16%), sedation, constipation (10%)

Occasional (5%–1%)

Tablets, injection: Depression, swelling of feet, loss of appetite, decreased sexual ability, itching eyes, dizziness, nausea, vomiting, nervousness
Transdermal: Itching, reddening or darkening of skin

Rare (less than 1%)

Nightmares, vivid dreams, cold feeling in fingers and toes

SERIOUS REACTIONS

! Overdose produces profound hypotension, irritability, bradycardia, respiratory depression, hypothermia, miosis (pupillary constriction), arrhythmias, and apnea.
! Abrupt withdrawal may result in rebound hypertension associated with nervousness, agitation, anxiety, insomnia, hand tingling, tremor, flushing, and diaphoresis.

DENTAL CONSIDERATIONS

General:

- Monitor vital signs at every appointment because of cardiovascular side effects.

• After supine positioning, have patient sit upright for at least 2 min before standing to avoid orthostatic hypotension.
• Limit use of sodium-containing products, such as saline IV fluids, for patients with a dietary salt restriction.
• Assess salivary flow as a factor in caries, periodontal disease, and candidiasis.
• Stress from dental procedures may compromise cardiovascular function; determine patient risk.
• Short appointments and a stress reduction protocol may be required for anxious patients.
• Consider drug in diagnosis of taste alterations.

Consultations:
• Medical consultation may be required to assess disease control.

Teach Patient/Family:
• *When chronic dry mouth occurs, advise patient:*
  • To avoid mouth rinses with high alcohol content because of drying effects
  • To use daily home fluoride products for anticaries effect
  • To use sugarless gum, frequent sips of water, or saliva substitutes

clopidogrel

clo-pid′-o-grill
(Iscover[AUS], Plavix)
Do not confuse Plavix with Paxil.

CATEGORY AND SCHEDULE

Pregnancy Risk Category: B

MECHANISM OF ACTION

A thienopyridine derivative that inhibits binding of the enzyme adenosine phosphate (ADP) to its platelet receptor and subsequent ADP-mediated activation of a glycoprotein complex. ***Therapeutic Effect:*** Inhibits platelet aggregation.

PHARMACOKINETICS

Route	Onset	Peak	Duration
PO	1 hr	2 hr	N/A

Rapidly absorbed. Protein binding: 98%. Extensively metabolized by the liver. Eliminated equally in the urine and feces. ***Half-life:*** 8 hr.

AVAILABILITY

Tablets: 75 mg.

INDICATIONS AND DOSAGES

▸ Myocardial Infarction (MI), Stroke Reduction
PO
Adults, Elderly. 75 mg once a day.

▸ Acute Coronary Syndrome
PO
Adults, Elderly. Initially, 300 mg loading dose, then 75 mg once a day (in combination with aspirin).

CONTRAINDICATIONS

Active bleeding, coagulation disorders, severe hepatic disease

INTERACTIONS

Drug
Fluvastatin, other NSAIDs, phenytoin, tamoxifen, tolbutamide, torsemide, warfarin: May interfere with metabolism of these drugs.

Herbal
Ginger, ginkgo biloba: May increase the risk of bleeding.

Food
None known.

Drug interactions of concern to dentistry

- Caution in use with NSAIDs

DIAGNOSTIC TEST EFFECTS

Prolongs bleeding time.

SIDE EFFECTS

Frequent (15%)
Skin disorders
Occasional (8%–6%)
Upper respiratory tract infection, chest pain, flulike symptoms, headache, dizziness, arthralgia
Rare (5%–3%)
Fatigue, edema, hypertension, abdominal pain, dyspepsia, diarrhea, nausea, epistaxis, dyspnea, rhinitis

SERIOUS REACTIONS

! None known.

DENTAL CONSIDERATIONS

General:

- Effects on platelet aggregation return to normal in 5–7 days.
- Patients on chronic drug therapy may rarely have symptoms of blood dyscrasias, which can include infection, bleeding, and poor healing.
- Consider local hemostasis measures to prevent excessive bleeding.
- Question patient about concurrent aspirin use.
- Monitor vital signs at every appointment because of cardiovascular disease.
- Consider semisupine chair position for patient comfort if GI side effects occur.

Consultations:

- Medical consultation may be required to assess disease control and patient's ability to tolerate stress.
- Consultation should include data on bleeding time.
- In a patient with symptoms of blood dyscrasias, request a medical consultation for blood studies and postpone treatment until normal values are reestablished.

Teach Patient/Family:

- Importance of updating health and drug history if physician makes any changes in evaluation or drug regimens
- Caution to prevent trauma when using oral hygiene aids
- To report any unusual or prolonged bleeding episodes after dental treatment

clorazepate dipotassium

klor-az′-e-pate
Schedule IV
(Novoclopate[CAN], Tranxene, Tranxene SD, Tranxene SD Half-Strength, T-Tab)
Do not confuse clorazepate with clofibrate.

CATEGORY AND SCHEDULE

Pregnancy Risk Category: D

MECHANISM OF ACTION

A benzodiazepine that depresses all levels of the CNS, including limbic and reticular formation, by binding to benzodiazepine receptor sites on the gamma-aminobutyric acid (GABA) receptor complex. Modulates GABA, a major inhibitory neurotransmitter in the brain. ***Therapeutic Effect:*** Produces anxiolytic effect, suppresses seizure activity.

AVAILABILITY

Tablets (Tranxene, T-Tab): 3.75 mg, 7.5 mg, 15 mg.
Tablets (Extended Release [Tranxene SD]): 22.5 mg.

Tablets (Extended-Release [Tranxene SD Half-Strength]): 11.25 mg.

INDICATIONS AND DOSAGES

▸ Anxiety

PO (Regular-Release)

Adults, Elderly. 7.5–15 mg 2–4 times a day.

PO (Sustained-Release)

Adults, Elderly. 11.25 mg or 22.5 mg once a day at bedtime.

▸ Anticonvulsant

PO

Adults, Elderly, Children older than 12 yr. Initially, 7.5 mg 2–3 times a day. May increase by 7.5 mg at weekly intervals. Maximum: 90 mg/day.

Children 9–12 yr. Initially, 3.75–7.5 mg twice a day. May increase by 2.75 mg at weekly intervals. Maximum: 60 mg/day.

▸ Alcohol Withdrawal

PO

Adults, Elderly. Initially, 30 mg, then 15 mg 2–4 times a day on first day. Gradually decrease dosage over subsequent days. Maximum: 90 mg/day.

CONTRAINDICATIONS

Acute narrow-angle glaucoma

INTERACTIONS

Drug

Alcohol, other CNS depressants: May increase CNS depressant effects.

Herbal

Kava kava, valerian: May increase CNS depression.

Food

None known.

Drug interactions of concern to dentistry

- Increased effects: CNS depressants, alcohol, opioid analgesics, general anesthetics, indinavir
- Increased serum levels and prolonged effect of benzodiazepines: fluconazole, ketoconazole, itraconazole, miconazole (systemic)
- Possible increase in CNS side effects: kava (herb)
- Contraindicated with saquinavir

DIAGNOSTIC TEST EFFECTS

None known. Therapeutic serum drug level is 0.12–1.5 mcg/ml; toxic serum drug level is greater than 5 mcg/ml.

SIDE EFFECTS

Frequent

Somnolence

Occasional

Dizziness, GI disturbances, nervousness, blurred vision, dry mouth, headache, confusion, ataxia, rash, irritability, slurred speech

Rare

Paradoxical CNS reactions, such as hyperactivity or nervousness in children and excitement or restlessness in the elderly or debilitated (generally noted during first 2 weeks of therapy, particularly in presence of uncontrolled pain)

SERIOUS REACTIONS

! Abrupt or too-rapid withdrawal may result in pronounced restlessness, irritability, insomnia, hand tremors, abdominal or muscle cramps, diaphoresis, vomiting, and seizures.

! Overdose results in somnolence, confusion, diminished reflexes, and coma.

DENTAL CONSIDERATIONS

General:

- Monitor vital signs at every appointment because of cardiovascular side effects.

• Assess salivary flow as a factor in caries, periodontal disease, and candidiasis.
• After supine positioning, have patient sit upright for at least 2 min to avoid orthostatic hypotension.
• Psychologic and physical dependence may occur with chronic administration.
• Geriatric patients are more susceptible to drug effects; use a lower dose.
• Short appointments and a stress reduction protocol may be required for anxious patients.
• Seizure: ask about type of epilepsy, seizure frequency and quality of seizure control.

Consultations:
• Medical consultation may be required to assess disease control and the patient's ability to tolerate stress.

Teach Patient/Family:
• *When chronic dry mouth occurs, advise patient:*
  • To avoid mouth rinses with high alcohol content because of drying effects
  • To use daily home fluoride products for anticaries effect
  • To use sugarless gum, frequent sips of water, or saliva substitutes

clotrimazole

kloe-try-mah-zole
(Canesten[CAN], Clotrimaderm[CAN], Mycelex, Mycelex OTC, Lotrimin, Gyne-Lotrimin, Trivagizole 3)

CATEGORY AND SCHEDULE

Pregnancy Risk Category: B (topical), C (troches)

MECHANISM OF ACTION

An antifungal that binds with phospholipids in fungal cell membrane. The altered cell membrane permeability. ***Therapeutic Effect:*** Inhibits yeast growth.

PHARMACOKINETICS

Poorly, erratically absorbed from GI tract. Bound to oral mucosa. Absorbed portion metabolized in liver. Eliminated in feces. Topical: Minimal systemic absorption (highest concentration in stratum corneum). Intravaginal: Small amount systemically absorbed. ***Half-life:*** 3.5–5 hrs.

AVAILABILITY

Combination pack: Vaginal tablet 100 mg and vaginal cream 1% (Mycelex-7).
Lotion: 1% (Lotrimin).
Topical Cream: 1% (Lotrimin, Lotrimin AF, Mycelex, Mycelex OTC).
Topical Solution: 1% (Lotrimin, Lotrimin AF, Mycelex, Mycelex OTC).
Troches: 10 mg (Mycelex).
Vaginal Cream: 1% (Gyne-Lotrimin, Mycelex-7), 2% (Gyne-Lotrimin 3, Mycelex-3, Trivagizole 3).
Vaginal Tablets: 100 mg, 500 mg (Gyne-Lotrimin, Mycelex-7).

INDICATIONS AND DOSAGES

▸ **Oropharyngeal Candidiasis Treatment**
PO
Adults, Elderly. 10 mg 5 times/day for 14 days.

▸ **Oropharyngeal Candidiasis Prophylaxis**
PO
Adults, Elderly. 10 mg 3 times/day.

▸ **Dermatophytosis, Cutaneous Candidiasis**
TOPICAL
Adults, Elderly. 2 times/day. Therapeutic effect may take up to 8 wks.

▸ **Vulvovaginal Candidiasis**
VAGINAL (Tablets)
Adults, Elderly. 1 tablet (100 mg) at bedtime for 7 days; 2 tablets (200 mg) at bedtime for 3 days; or 500 mg tablet one time.
Vaginal (Cream)
Adults, Elderly. 1 applicatorful at bedtime for 7–14 days.

OFF-LABEL USES
Topical: Treatment of paronychia, tinea barbae, tinea capitas.

CONTRAINDICATIONS
Hypersensitivity to clotrimazole or any component of the formulation, children 3 yrs

INTERACTIONS
Drug
Benzodiazepines: May increase benzodiazepine serum concentrations and increase risk of toxicity.
Ergot derivatives: May increase risk of ergotism (nausea, vomiting, vasospastic ischemia).
Fentanyl: May increase or prolong opioid effects (CNS depression).
Tacrolimus: May increase risk of tacrolimus toxicity.
Trimetrexate: May increase risk of trimetrexate toxicity.
Herbal
None known.
Food
None known.
Drug interactions of concern to dentistry
• None reported

DIAGNOSTIC TEST EFFECTS
May increase SGOT (AST).

SIDE EFFECTS
Frequent
Oral: Nausea, vomiting, diarrhea, abdominal pain
Occasional
Topical: Itching, burning, stinging, erythema, urticaria
Vaginal: Mild burning (tablets/cream); irritation, cystitis (cream)
Rare
Vaginal: Itching, rash, lower abdominal cramping, headache

SERIOUS REACTIONS
! None reported.

DENTAL CONSIDERATIONS
General:
• Determine why the patient is taking the drug.
• Examine oral mucous membranes for signs of fungal infection.
Teach Patient/Family:
• If used for oral infection: to soak full or partial dentures in an antifungal solution overnight until lesions are absent; prolonged infections may require fabrication of new prosthesis
• To dispose of toothbrush used during oral infection after oral lesions are absent to prevent reinoculation
• That long-term therapy may be necessary to clear infection; to complete entire course of medication

clozapine
klo′-za-peen
(Clopine[AUS], Clozaril, FazaClo)
Do not confuse clozapine with Cloxapen or clofazimine, or Clozaril with Clinoril or Colazal.

CATEGORY AND SCHEDULE
Pregnancy Risk Category: B

MECHANISM OF ACTION

A dibenzodiazepine derivative that interferes with the binding of dopamine at dopamine receptor sites; binds primarily at nondopamine receptor sites.
Therapeutic Effect: Diminishes schizophrenic behavior.

PHARMACOKINETICS

Absorbed rapidly and almost completely. Distributed rapidly and extensively. Crosses the blood-brain barrier. Protein binding: 95%. Metabolized in the liver. Excreted in urine and feces.
Half-life: 8 hr.

AVAILABILITY

Tablets (Clozaril): 12.5 mg, 25 mg, 100 mg.
Tablets (Orally-Disintegrating [FazaClo]): 25 mg, 100 mg.

INDICATIONS AND DOSAGES

▸ Schizophrenic Disorders, Reduce Suicidal Behavior

PO
Adults. Initially, 25 mg once or twice a day. May increase by 25–50 mg/day over 2 wk until dosage of 300–450 mg/day isachieved. May further increase by 50–100 mg/day no more than once or twice a week, Range: 200–600 mg/day. Maximum: 900 mg/day.
Elderly. Initially, 25 mg/day. May increase by 25 mg/day. Maximum: 450 mg/day.

CONTRAINDICATIONS

Coma, concurrent use of other drugs that may suppress bone marrow function, history of clozapine-induced agranulocytosis or severe granulocytopenia, myeloproliferative disorders, severe CNS depression

INTERACTIONS

Drug

Alcohol, other CNS depressants: May increase CNS depressant effects.
Bone marrow depressants: May increase myelosuppression.
Lithium: May increase the risk of confusion, dyskinesia, and seizures.
Phenobarbital: Decreases clozapine blood concentration.

Herbal

None known.

Food

None known.

Drug interactions of concern to dentistry

- Increased anticholinergic effects: anticholinergics
- Increased CNS depression: alcohol, all CNS depressant drugs
- Increased serum concentration, leukocytosis: erythromycin base
- Possible decreased effects: carbamazepine
- Increased plasma levels: ciprofloxacin

DIAGNOSTIC TEST EFFECTS

May increase serum glucose levels.

SIDE EFFECTS

Frequent

Somnolence (39%), salivation (31%), tachycardia (25%), dizziness (19%), constipation (14%)

Occasional

Hypotension (9%); headache (7%); tremor, syncope, diaphoresis, dry mouth (6%); nausea, visual disturbances (5%); nightmares, restlessness, akinesia, agitation, hypertension, abdominal discomfort or heartburn, weight gain (4%)

Rare

Rigidity, confusion, fatigue, insomnia, diarrhea, rash

SERIOUS REACTIONS

! Alert blood dyscrasias, particularly agranulocytosis and mild leukopenia, may occur.
! Seizures occur in about 3% of patients.
! Overdose produces CNS depression (including sedation, coma, and delirium), respiratory depression, and hypersalivation.

DENTAL CONSIDERATIONS

General:

- Monitor vital signs at every appointment because of cardiovascular and respiratory side effects.
- Patients on chronic drug therapy may rarely have symptoms of blood dyscrasias, which can include infection, bleeding, and poor healing.
- After supine positioning, have patient sit upright for at least 2 min before standing to avoid orthostatic hypotension.
- Assess salivary flow as a factor in caries, periodontal disease, and candidiasis.
- Determine why the patient is taking the drug.
- Place on frequent recall because of oral side effects.

Consultations:

- In a patient with symptoms of blood dyscrasias, request a medical consultation for blood studies and postpone dental treatment until normal values are reestablished.
- Medical consultation may be required to assess disease control and stress tolerance of patient.
- Physician should be informed if significant xerostomic side effects occur (e.g., increased caries, sore tongue, problems eating or swallowing, difficulty wearing prosthesis) so that a medication change can be considered.

Teach Patient/Family:

- Importance of good oral hygiene to prevent soft tissue inflammation
- Caution to prevent injury when using oral hygiene aids
- To use electric toothbrush if patient has difficulty holding conventional devices
- *When chronic dry mouth occurs, advise patient:*
  - To avoid mouth rinses with high alcohol content because of drying effects
  - To use daily home fluoride products for anticaries effect
  - To use sugarless gum, frequent sips of water, or saliva substitutes

cocaine hydrochloride

koe-kane′-
Schedule II
(Cocaine[CAN], Cocaine HCl)

CATEGORY AND SCHEDULE

Pregnancy Risk Category: C
Controlled substance: Schedule II

MECHANISM OF ACTION

A topical anesthetic that decreases membrane permeability, increases norepinephrine at postsynaptic receptor sites, producing intense vasoconstriction. ***Therapeutic Effect:*** Blocks conduction of nerve impulses.

PHARMACOKINETICS

Readily absorbed from all mucous membranes. Cocaine penetrates the CNS but is rapidly metabolized. Rapidly hydrolyzed in blood by serum cholinesterases. Metabolized in liver. Excreted in urine ***Half-life:*** 1–1.5 hrs.

AVAILABILITY

Powder, as hydrochloride: 5 g, 25 g (Cocaine HCl).
Topical solution, as hydrochloride: 40 mg/ml, 100 mg/ml (Cocaine HCl).

INDICATIONS AND DOSAGES

▸ **Anesthesia**

TOPICAL
Adults, Elderly, Children. 1–4% to mucous membranes. Maximum: 1–3 mg/kg (o4 400 mg). Dosage varies depending upon the area to be anesthetized, vascularity of the tissues, individual tolerance, and anesthetic technique. Administer lowest effective dose.

OFF-LABEL USES

Horner's syndrome (diagnosis)

CONTRAINDICATIONS

Hypersensitivity to cocaine or any component of the formulation.

INTERACTIONS

Drug

Alcohol: May increase heart rate and blood pressure.
Beta blockers: May decrease effects of beta-blockers.
Cholinesterase inhibitors: May increase effects and risk of toxicity.
Sympathomimetics: May increase CNS stimulation and risk of cardiovascular effects.
Tricyclic antidepressants, digoxin, methyldopa: May increase risk of arrhythmias.

Herbal

Hemp: May increase toxic effects of cocaine.
St. John's wort: May increase risk of cardiovascular collapse and/or delayed emergence from anesthesia.

Food

None known.

Drug interactions of concern to dentistry

- Sensitization to catecholamines, such as epinephrine; risk of serious cardiovascular events
- Avoid ester-type local anesthetics in patients with allergic reactions to cocaine

DIAGNOSTIC TEST EFFECTS

May give false-negative results of scintigraphy.

SIDE EFFECTS

Frequent

Loss of sense of smell and taste.

Occasional

Anxiety, central nervous system stimulation or depression.

SERIOUS REACTIONS

! Repeated nasal application may produce stuffy nose, and chronic rhinitis.
! Early signs of overdosage are increased blood pressure (B/P), increased pulse, irregular heartbeat, chills/fever, agitation, nervousness, confusion, inability to remain still, nausea, vomiting, abdominal pain, increased sweating, rapid breathing, and large pupils.
! Advanced signs of overdosage are arrhythmias, CNS hemorrhage, CHF, convulsions, delirium, hyperreflexia, loss of bladder/bowel control, and respiratory weakness.
! Late signs of overdosage are loss of reflexes, muscle paralysis, dilated pupils, LOC, cyanosis, pulmonary edema, cardiac and respiratory failure.

DENTAL CONSIDERATIONS

General:

- Acute-use drug for medical topical anesthesia.
- Abusers of cocaine may present with oral or nasal mucosal lesions

and dry mucous membranes, nervousness, and anxiety
- Caution drug interactions in chronic abusers of cocaine.
- Determine why patient is taking the drug.
- Monitor vital signs at every appointment due to cardiovascular side effects.
- Assess salivary flow as a factor in caries, periodontal disease, and candidiasis.
- If additional analgesia is required for dental pain, consider alternative analgesics (NSAIDs) in patients taking narcotics for acute or chronic pain.
- Use vasoconstrictor with caution, in low doses, and with careful aspiration. Avoid using gingival retraction cord containing epinephrine.
- Examine for oral manifestation of opportunistic infection.
- Psychologic and physical dependence may occur with chronic administration.
- Dental local anesthetics will not interfere with urine test for cocaine abuse.

Consultations:
- Notify recovery program director if controlled substances may be required for a patient in recovery from cocaine use.

Teach Patient/Family:
- *When chronic dry mouth occurs advise patient:*
  - To avoid mouth rinses with high alcohol content due to drying effects
  - To use daily home fluoride products for anticaries effect
  - To use sugarless gum, frequent sips of water or saliva substitutes.
  - To report oral lesions, soreness, or bleeding to dentist

codeine phosphate/ codeine sulfate

koe′-deen
Schedule II
(codeine phosphate)
Actacode[AUS], Codeine Phosphate Injection, Codeine Linctus[AUS](codeine sulfate) Contin[CAN]
Do not confuse codeine with Cardene or Lodine.

CATEGORY AND SCHEDULE

Pregnancy Risk Category: C (D if used for prolonged periods or at high dosages at term)
Controlled Substance: Schedule II (analgesic), III (fixed-combination form)

MECHANISM OF ACTION

An opioid agonist that binds to opioid receptors at many cites in the CNS, particularly in the medulla. This action inhibits the ascending pain pathways.
Therapeutic Effect: Alters the perception of and emotional response to pain, suppresses cough reflex.

AVAILABILITY

Tablets: 15 mg, 30 mg, 60 mg.
Oral Solution: 15 mg/5 ml.
Injection: 15 mg/ml, 30 mg/ml.

INDICATIONS AND DOSAGES

▸ Analgesia

PO, IM, SUBCUTANEOUS
Adults, Elderly. 30 mg q4–6h. Range: 15–60 mg.
Children. 0.5–1 mg/kg q4–6h. Maximum: 60 mg/dose.

▸ Cough

PO
Adults, Elderly, Children 12 yr and older. 10–20 mg q4–6h.

Children 6–11 yr. 5–10 mg q4–6h.
Children 2–5 yr. 2.5–5 mg q4–6h.

Dosage in Renal Impairment

Dosage is modified on the basis of creatinine clearance.

Creatinine Clearance	Dosage
10–50 ml/min	75% of usual dose
less than 10 ml/min	50% of usual dose

OFF-LABEL USES

Treatment of diarrhea

CONTRAINDICATIONS

None known.

INTERACTIONS

Drug

Alcohol, other CNS depressants: May increase CNS or respiratory depression, and hypotension.
MAOIs: May produce a severe, sometimes fatal reaction; plan to administer a test dose, which is one-quarter of usual codeine dose.

Herbal

None known.

Food

None known.

Drug interactions of concern to dentistry

- Increased sedation with other CNS depressants and alcohol
- Increased effects of anticholinergics

DIAGNOSTIC TEST EFFECTS

May increase serum amylase and lipase levels.

SIDE EFFECTS

Frequent

Constipation, somnolence, nausea, vomiting

Occasional

Paradoxical excitement, confusion, palpitations, facial flushing, decreased urination, blurred vision, dizziness, dry mouth, headache, hypotension (including orthostatic hypotension), decreased appetite, injection site redness, burning, or pain

Rare

Hallucinations, depression, abdominal pain, insomnia

SERIOUS REACTIONS

! Too-frequent use may result in paralytic ileus.
! Overdose may produce cold and clammy skin, confusion, seizures, decreased BP, restlessness, pinpoint pupils, bradycardia, respiratory depression, decreased LOC, and severe weakness.
! The patient who uses codeine repeatedly may develop a tolerance to the drug's analgesic effect, as well as physical dependence.

DENTAL CONSIDERATIONS

General:

- Monitor vital signs at every appointment because of cardiovascular and respiratory side effects.
- After supine positioning, have patient sit upright for at least 2 min to avoid orthostatic hypotension.
- Assess salivary flow as a factor in caries, periodontal disease, and candidiasis.
- Psychologic and physical dependence may occur with chronic administration.

Teach Patient/Family:

- *When chronic dry mouth occurs, advise patient:*
  - To avoid mouth rinses with high alcohol content because of drying effects
  - To use daily home fluoride products for anticaries effect
  - To use sugarless gum, frequent sips of water, or saliva substitutes

colchicine

kol′-chi-seen
(Colchicine, Colgout[AUS])

CATEGORY AND SCHEDULE

Pregnancy Risk Category: D

MECHANISM OF ACTION

An alkaloid that decreases leukocyte motility, phagocytosis, and lactic acid production. ***Therapeutic Effect:*** Decreases urate crystal deposits and reduces inflammatory process.

PHARMACOKINETICS

Rapidly absorbed from the GI tract. Highest concentration is in the liver, spleen, and kidney. Protein binding: 30%–50%. Reenters the intestinal tract by biliary secretion and is reabsorbed from the intestines. Partially metabolized in the liver. Eliminated primarily in feces.

AVAILABILITY

Tablets: 0.6 mg.
Injection: 1 mg.

INDICATIONS AND DOSAGES

▸ Acute Gouty Arthritis

PO

Adults, Elderly. 0.6–1.2 mg; then 0.6 mg q1–2h or 1–1.2 mg q2h, until pain is relieved or nausea, vomiting, or diarrhea occurs. Total dose: 4–8 mg.

IV

Adults, Elderly. Initially, 2 mg; then 0.5 mg q6h until satisfactory response. Maximum: 4 mg/wk or 4 mg/one course of treatment. If pain recurs, may give 1–2 mg/day for several days but no sooner than 7 days after a full course of IV therapy (total of 4 mg).

▸ Chronic Gouty Arthritis

PO

Adults, Elderly. 0.5–0.6 mg once weekly up to once a day, depending on number of attacks per year.

OFF-LABEL USES

To reduce frequency of recurrence of familial Mediterranean fever; treatment of acute calcium pyrophosphate deposition, amyloidosis, biliary cirrhosis, recurrent pericarditis, sarcoid arthritis

CONTRAINDICATIONS

Blood dyscrasias; severe cardiac, GI, hepatic, or renal disorders

INTERACTIONS

Drug

Bone marrow depressants: May increase the risk of blood dyscrasias.
NSAIDs: May increase the risk of bone marrow depression, neutropenia, and thrombocytopenia.

Herbal

None known.

Food

None known.

Drug interactions of concern to dentistry

- Increased risk of GI side effects: NSAIDs, alcohol
- Possible increased serum levels: erythromycin

DIAGNOSTIC TEST EFFECTS

May increase serum alkaline phosphatase and AST(SGOT) levels. May decrease platelet count.

IV INCOMPATIBILITIES

No information available via Y-site administration.

SIDE EFFECTS

Frequent

PO: Nausea, vomiting, abdominal discomfort

Occasional
PO: Anorexia
Rare
Hypersensitivity reaction, including angioedema
Parenteral: Nausea, vomiting, diarrhea, abdominal discomfort, pain or redness at injection site, neuritis in injected arm

SERIOUS REACTIONS

! Bone marrow depression, including aplastic anemia, agranulocytosis, and thrombocytopenia, may occur with long-term therapy.
! Overdose initially causes a burning feeling in the skin or throat, severe diarrhea, and abdominal pain. The patient then experiences fever, seizures, delirium, and renal impairment, marked by hematuria and oliguria. The third stage of overdose causes hair loss, leukocytosis, and stomatitis.

DENTAL CONSIDERATIONS

General:
- Consider drug in diagnosis of taste alteration.
- Patients on chronic drug therapy may rarely have symptoms of blood dyscrasias, which can include infection, bleeding, and poor healing.
- Avoid prescribing aspirin-containing products.

Consultations:
- Medical consultation may be required to assess disease control.
- In a patient with symptoms of blood dyscrasias, request a medical consultation for blood studies and postpone dental treatment until normal values are reestablished.

Teach Patient/Family:
- Importance of good oral hygiene to prevent soft tissue inflammation
- Caution to prevent injury when using oral hygiene aids
- To avoid mouth rinses with high alcohol content because of drying effects

colesevelam

koh-le-sev′-e-lam
(Welchol)

CATEGORY AND SCHEDULE

Pregnancy Risk Category: B

MECHANISM OF ACTION

A bile acid sequestrant and nonsystemic polymer that binds with bile acids in the intestines, preventing their reabsorption and removing them from the body. ***Therapeutic Effect:*** Decreases LDL cholesterol.

AVAILABILITY

Tablets: 625 mg.

INDICATIONS AND DOSAGES

▸ **To decrease LDL Cholesterol Level in Primary Hypercholesterolemia (Fredrickson type IIa)**
PO
Adults, Elderly. 3 tablets with meals twice a day or 6 tablets once a day with a meal. May increase daily dose to 7 tablets a day.

CONTRAINDICATIONS

Complete biliary obstruction, hypersensitivity to colesevelam

INTERACTIONS

Drug
Aspirin, clindamycin, digoxin, furosemide, glipizide, hydrocortisone, imipramine,

NSAIDs, phenytoin, propranolol, tetracyclines, thiazide diuretics, vitamins A, D, E, K: May decrease the absorption of these drugs.

Herbal

None known.

Food

None known.

Drug interactions of concern to dentistry

- None reported, but monitor if drugs with narrow therapeutic index are prescribed for dental conditions

DIAGNOSTIC TEST EFFECTS

None known.

SIDE EFFECTS

Frequent (12%–8%)

Flatulence, constipation, infection, dyspepsia (heartburn, epigastric distress)

SERIOUS REACTIONS

! GI tract obstruction may occur.

DENTAL CONSIDERATIONS

General:

- Consider semisupine chair position for patient comfort if GI side effects occur.
- Monitor vital signs at every appointment because of possibility of cardiovascular disease.

colestipol

koe-les′-ti-pole

(Colestid, Colestid[CAN])

CATEGORY AND SCHEDULE

Pregnancy Risk Category: C

MECHANISM OF ACTION

An antihyperlipoproteinemic that binds with bile acids in the intestine, forming an insoluble complex. Binding results in partial removal of bile acid from enterohepatic circulation. ***Therapeutic Effect:*** Removes low-density lipoproteins (LDL) and cholesterol from plasma.

PHARMACOKINETICS

Not absorbed from the gastrointestinal (GI) tract. Excreted in the feces.

AVAILABILITY

Granules: 5 g packet (Colestid).
Tablet: 1 g (Colestid).

INDICATIONS AND DOSAGES

▸ **Primary Hypercholesterolemia**

PO, granules

Adults, Elderly. Initially, 5 g 1–2 times/day. Range: 5–30 g/day once or in divided doses.

PO, tablets

Adults, Elderly. Initially, 2 g 1–2 times/day. Range: 2–16 g/day.

OFF-LABEL USES

Treatment of diarrhea (due to bile acids); hyperoxaluria

CONTRAINDICATIONS

Complete biliary obstruction, hypersensitivity to bile acid sequestering resins

INTERACTIONS

Drug

Anticoagulants: May increase effects of these drugs by decreasing vitamin K.

Digoxin, folic acid, penicillins, propranolol, tetracyclines, thiazides, thyroid hormones, and other medications: May bind and decrease absorption of these drugs.

Oral vancomycin: Binds and decreases the effects of oral vancomycin.

C

Warfarin: May decrease warfarin absorption.

Herbal

Vitamin A, vitamin E: May decrease vitamin A and E absorption.

Food

None known.

Drug interactions of concern to dentistry

- Decreased absorption of tetracyclines, cephalexin, phenobarbital, corticosteroids, clindamycin, penicillins; administer doses several hours apart

DIAGNOSTIC TEST EFFECTS

May decrease serum calcium, potassium, and sodium levels. May prolong prothrombin time.

SIDE EFFECTS

Frequent

Constipation (may lead to fecal impaction), nausea, vomiting, stomach pain, indigestion

Occasional

Diarrhea, belching, bloating, headache, dizziness

Rare

Gallstones, peptic ulcer, malabsorption syndrome

SERIOUS REACTIONS

! GI tract obstruction, hyperchloremic acidosis, and osteoporosis secondary to calcium excretion may occur.

! High dosage may interfere with fat absorption, resulting in steatorrhea.

DENTAL CONSIDERATIONS

General:

- Consider semisupine chair position for patient comfort because of GI side effects of disease.

cortisone acetate

kor′-ti-sone

(Cortate[AUS], Cortone[CAN])

Do not confuse cortisone with Cort-Dome.

CATEGORY AND SCHEDULE

Pregnancy Risk Category: C (D if used in the first trimester)

MECHANISM OF ACTION

An adrenocortical steroid that inhibits the accumulation of inflammatory cells at inflammation sites, phagocytosis, lysosomal enzyme release and synthesis, and release of mediators of inflammation.

Therapeutic Effect: Prevents or suppresses cell-mediated immune reactions. Decreases or prevents tissue response to inflammatory process.

AVAILABILITY

Tablets: 25 mg.

INDICATIONS AND DOSAGES

Dosage is dependent on the condition being treated and patient response.

▸ **Anti-Inflammation, Immunosuppression**

PO

Adults, Elderly. 25–300 mg/day in divided doses q12–24h.

Children. 2.5–10 mg/kg/day in divided doses q6–8h.

▸ **Physiologic Replacement**

PO

Adults, Elderly. 25–35 mg/day.

Children. 0.5–0.75 mg/kg/day in divided doses q8h.

CONTRAINDICATIONS

Hypersensitivity to corticosteroids, administration of live virus vaccine, peptic ulcers (except in life-threatening situations), systemic fungal infection

INTERACTIONS

Drug

Amphotericin: May increase hypokalemia.
Digoxin: May increase digoxin toxicity caused by hypokalemia.
Diuretics, insulin, oral hypoglycemics, potassium supplements: May decrease the effects of these drugs.
Hepatic enzyme inducers: May decrease the effects of cortisone.
Live-virus vaccines: May decrease the patient's antibody response to vaccine, increase vaccine side effects, and potentiate virus replication.

Herbal

None known.

Food

None known.

Drug interactions of concern to dentistry

- Decreased action: barbiturates, rifabutin, rifampin
- Increased GI side effects: alcohol, salicylates, NSAIDs
- Increased action: ketoconazole, macrolide antibiotics
- Hepatotoxicity: acetaminophen (chronic, high doses)

DIAGNOSTIC TEST EFFECTS

May increase blood glucose and serum lipid, amylase, and sodium levels. May decrease serum calcium, potassium, and thyroxine levels.

SIDE EFFECTS

Frequent

Insomnia, heartburn, anxiety, abdominal distention, increased diaphoresis, acne, mood swings, increased appetite, facial flushing, delayed wound healing, increased susceptibility to infection, diarrhea or constipation

Occasional

Headache, edema, change in skin color, frequent urination

Rare

Tachycardia, allergic reaction (such as rash and hives), psychological changes, hallucinations, depression

SERIOUS REACTIONS

! Long-term therapy may cause hypocalcemia, hypokalemia, muscle wasting in arms and legs, osteoporosis, spontaneous fractures, amenorrhea, cataracts, glaucoma, peptic ulcer disease, and CHF.
! Abrupt withdrawal following long-term therapy may cause anorexia, nausea, fever, headache, joint pain, rebound inflammation, fatigue, weakness, lethargy, dizziness, and orthostatic hypotension.

DENTAL CONSIDERATIONS

General:

- Monitor vital signs at every appointment because of cardiovascular side effects.
- Patients on chronic drug therapy may rarely have symptoms of blood dyscrasias, which can include infection, bleeding, and poor healing.
- Assess salivary flow as a factor in caries, periodontal disease, and candidiasis.
- Avoid prescribing aspirin-containing products.
- Symptoms of oral infections may be masked.
- Place on frequent recall to evaluate healing response.
- Prophylactic antibiotics may be indicated to prevent infection if surgery or deep scaling is planned.
- Determine dose and duration of steroid therapy for each patient to assess risk for stress tolerance and immunosuppression.
- Patients who have been or are currently on chronic steroid therapy (>2 wk) may require supplemental steroids for dental treatment.

• Determine why the patient is taking the drug.

Consultations:

• In a patient with symptoms of blood dyscrasias, request a medical consultation for blood studies and postpone dental treatment until normal values are reestablished.
• Medical consultation may be required to assess disease control and stress tolerance of patient.
• Consultation may be required to confirm steroid dose and duration of use.

Teach Patient/Family:

• Importance of good oral hygiene to prevent soft tissue inflammation
• Caution to prevent injury when using oral hygiene aids
• *When chronic dry mouth occurs, advise patient:*
  • To avoid mouth rinses with high alcohol content because of drying effects
  • To use daily home fluoride products for anticaries effect
  • To use sugarless gum, frequent sips of water, or saliva substitutes

cromolyn sodium

kroe′-moe-lin
(Apo-Cromolyn[CAN], Crolom, Gastrocom, Intal, Nasalcrom, Opticrom, Rynacrom[AUS])

CATEGORY AND SCHEDULE

Pregnancy Risk Category: B

MECHANISM OF ACTION

An antiasthmatic and antiallergic agent that prevents mast cell release of histamine, leukotrienes, and slow-reacting substances of anaphylaxis by inhibiting degranulation after contact with antigens. ***Therapeutic Effect:*** Helps prevent symptoms of asthma, allergic rhinitis, mastocytosis, and exercise-induced bronchospasm.

PHARMACOKINETICS

Minimal absorption after PO, inhalation, or nasal administration. Absorbed portion excreted in urine or by biliary system. ***Half-life:*** 80–90 min.

AVAILABILITY

Oral Concentrate (Gastrocrom): 100 mg/5ml.
Nasal Spray (Nasalcrom): 40 mg/ml.
Solution for Nebulization (Intal): 10 mg/ml.
Solution for Oral Inhalation (Intal): 800 mcg/inhalation.
Ophthalmic Solution (Crolom, Opticrom): 4%.

INDICATIONS AND DOSAGES

▶ Asthma

INHALATION (nebulization)
Adults, Elderly, Children older than 2 yr. 20 mg 3–4 times a day.
AEROSOL SPRAY
Adults, Elderly, Children 12 yrs and older. Initially, 2 sprays 4 times a day. Maintenance: 2–4 sprays 3–4 times a day.
Children 5–11 yr. Initially, 2 sprays 4 times a day, then 1–2 sprays 3–4 times a day.

▶ Prevention of Bronchospasm

INHALATION (nebulization)
Adults, Elderly, Children older than 2 yr. 20 mg within 1 hr before exercise or exposure to allergens.
AEROSOL SPRAY
Adults, Elderly, Children older than 5 yr. 2 sprays within 1 hr before exercise or exposure to allergens.

▸ **Food Allergy, Inflammatory Bowel Disease**
PO
Adults, Elderly, Children older than 12 yr. 200–400 mg 4 times a day.
Children 2–12 yr. 100–200 mg 4 times a day.
Maximum: 40 mg/kg/day.

▸ **Allergic Rhinitis**
INTRANASAL
Adults, Elderly, Children older than 6 yr. 1 spray each nostril 3–4 times a day. May increase up to 6 times a day.

▸ **Systemic Mastocytosis**
PO
Adults, Elderly, Children older than 12 yr. 200 mg 4 times a day.
Children 2–12 yr. 100 mg 4 times a day. Maximum: 40 mg/kg/day.
Children younger than 2 yr. 20 mg/kg/day in 4 divided doses. Maximum: 30 mg/kg/day (children 6 mo–2 yr).

▸ **Conjunctivitis**
OPHTHALMIC
Adults, Elderly, Children older than 4 yr. 1–2 drops in both eyes 4–6 times a day.

CONTRAINDICATIONS
Status asthmaticus

INTERACTIONS
Drug
None known.
Herbal
None known.
Food
None known.
Drug interactions of concern to dentistry
- None reported

DIAGNOSTIC TEST EFFECTS
None known.

SIDE EFFECTS
Frequent
PO: Headache, diarrhea
Inhalation: Cough, dry mouth and throat, stuffy nose, throat irritation, unpleasant taste
Nasal: Nasal burning, stinging, or irritation; increased sneezing
Ophthalmic: Eye burning or stinging
Occasional
PO: Rash, abdominal pain, arthralgia, nausea, insomnia
Inhalation: Bronchospasm, hoarseness, lacrimation
Nasal: Cough, headache, unpleasant taste, postnasal drip
Ophthalmic: Lacrimation and itching of eye
Rare
Inhalation: Dizziness, painful urination, arthralgia, myalgia, rash
Nasal: Epistaxis, rash
Ophthalmic: Chemosis or edema of conjunctiva, eye irritation

SERIOUS REACTIONS
! Anaphylaxis occurs rarely when cromolyn is given by the inhalation, nasal, or oral route.

DENTAL CONSIDERATIONS
General:
- Determine why patient is taking the drug.
- Protect patient's eyes from accidental spatter during dental treatment.
- Avoid dental light in patient's eyes; offer dark glasses for patient comfort.

DENTAL CONSIDERATIONS
General:
- Assess salivary flow as a factor in caries, periodontal disease, and candidiasis.
- Consider semisupine chair position for patients with respiratory disease.
- A stress reduction protocol may be required.

- Midday appointments and a stress reduction protocol may be required for anxious patients.
- Be aware that aspirin or sulfite preservatives in vasoconstrictor-containing products can exacerbate asthma.

Consultations:

- Consider drug in diagnosis of taste alteration and burning mouth syndrome.
- Medical consultation may be required to assess disease control and stress tolerance of patient.

Teach Patient/Family:

- For inhalation dosage forms, rinse mouth with water after each dose to prevent dryness
- *When chronic dry mouth occurs, advise patient:*
  - To avoid mouth rinses with high alcohol content because of drying effects
  - To use daily home fluoride products for anticaries effect
  - To use sugarless gum, frequent sips of water, or saliva substitutes

cyanocobalamin (vitamin B_{12})

sye-an-oh-koe-bal′-a-min
(Bedoz[CAN], Cytamen[AUS], Nascobal)

CATEGORY AND SCHEDULE

Pregnancy Risk Category: A (C if used in doses above recommended daily allowance)

MECHANISM OF ACTION

Acts as a coenzyme for various metabolic functions, including fat and carbohydrate metabolism and protein synthesis. ***Therapeutic Effect:*** Necessary for cell growth and replication, hematopoiesis, and myelin synthesis.

PHARMACOKINETICS

In the presence of calcium, absorbed systemically in lower half of ileum. Initially, bound to intrinsic factor; this complex passes down intestine, binding to receptor sites on ileal mucosa. Protein binding: High. Metabolized in the liver. Primarily eliminated unchanged in urine. ***Half-life:*** 6 days.

AVAILABILITY

Tablets: 50 mcg, 100 mcg, 250 mcg, 500 mcg, 1000 mcg, 5000 mcg.
Tablets (Extended-Release): 1500 mcg.
Injection: 1000 mcg/ml.
Nasal Gel (Nascobal):
500 mcg/0.1 ml.

INDICATIONS AND DOSAGES

▸ **Pernicious Anemia**

IM, SUBCUTANEOUS

Adults, Elderly. 100 mcg/day for 7 days, then every other day for 7 days, then every 3–4 days for 2–3 weeks. Maintenance: 100 mcg/month (oral 1000–2000 mcg/day).

Children. 30–50 mcg/day for 2 or more weeks. Maintenance: 100 mcg/month.

Neonates. 1000 mcg/day for 2 or more weeks. Maintenance: 50 mcg/month.

INTRANASAL

Adults, Elderly. 500 mcg once a week.

▸ **Uncomplicated Vitamin B_{12} Deficiency**

PO

Adults, Elderly. 1,000–2,000 mcg/day

IM, SUBCUTANEOUS

Adults, Elderly. 100 mcg/day for 5–10 days, followed by 100–200 mcg/mo.

▸ **Complicated Vitamin B_{12} Deficiency**
IM, SUBCUTANEOUS
Adults, Elderly. 1000 mcg (with IM or IV folic acid 15 mg) as a single dose, then 1000 mcg/day plus oral folic acid 5 mg/day for 7 days.

CONTRAINDICATIONS
Folic acid deficiency anemia, hereditary optic nerve atrophy, history of allergy to cobalamins

INTERACTIONS
Drug
Alcohol, colchicines: May decrease the absorption of cyanocobalamin.
Ascorbic acid: May destroy cyanocobalamin.
Folic acid (large doses): May decrease cyanocobalamin blood concentration.
Herbal
None known.
Food
None known.
Drug interactions of concern to dentistry
- Increased absorption: prednisone

DIAGNOSTIC TEST EFFECTS
None known.

SIDE EFFECTS
Occasional
Diarrhea, pruritus

SERIOUS REACTIONS
! Impurities in preparation may cause a rare allergic reaction.
! Peripheral vascular thrombosis, pulmonary edema, hypokalemia, and CHF may occur.

DENTAL CONSIDERATIONS
General:
- Deficiency in vitamin B_{12} and other B-complex vitamins may cause oral symptomatology.

cyclobenzaprine hydrochloride
sye-kloe-ben′-za-preen
(Flexeril, Flexitec[CAN], Novo-Cycloprine[CAN])
Do not confuse cyclobenzaprine with cycloserine or cyproheptadine, or Flexeril with Floxin.

CATEGORY AND SCHEDULE
Pregnancy Risk Category: B

MECHANISM OF ACTION
A centrally acting skeletal muscle relaxant that reduces tonic somatic muscle activity at the level of the brainstem. ***Therapeutic Effect:*** Relieves local skeletal muscle spasm.

PHARMACOKINETICS
Route	Onset	Peak	Duration
PO	1 hr	3–4 hr	12–24 hr

Well but slowly absorbed from the GI tract. Protein binding: 93%. Metabolized in the GI tract and the liver. Primarily excreted in urine. ***Half-life:*** 1–3 days.

AVAILABILITY
Tablets: 5 mg, 10 mg.

INDICATIONS AND DOSAGES
▸ **Acute, Painful Musculoskeletal Conditions**
PO
Adults. Initially, 5 mg 3 times a day. May increase to 10 mg 3 times a day.
Elderly. 5 mg 3 times a day.
▸ **Dosage in Hepatic Impairment**
Mild: 5 mg 3 times a day.
Moderate and severe: Not recommended.

C

OFF-LABEL USES
Treatment of fibromyalgia

CONTRAINDICATIONS
Acute recovery phase of MI, arrhythmias, CHF, heart block, conduction disturbances, hyperthyroidism, use within 14 days of MAOIs

INTERACTIONS
Drug
Alcohol, other CNS depression-producing medications (such as tricyclic antidepressants): May increase CNS depression.
MAOIs: May increase the risk of hypertensive crisis and severe seizures.
Herbal
None known.
Food
None known.
Drug interactions of concern to dentistry
- Increased CNS depression: alcohol, narcotics, barbiturates, sedatives, hypnotics
- Increased effects of anticholinergic drugs

Increased effects of direct-acting sympathomimetics (epinephrine, levonordefrin)

DIAGNOSTIC TEST EFFECTS
None known.

SIDE EFFECTS
Frequent
Somnolence (39%), dry mouth (27%), dizziness (11%)
Rare (3%–1%)
Fatigue, asthenia, blurred vision, headache, nervousness, confusion, nausea, constipation, dyspepsia, unpleasant taste

SERIOUS REACTIONS
! Overdose may result in visual hallucinations, hyperactive reflexes, muscle rigidity, vomiting, and hyperpyrexia.

DENTAL CONSIDERATIONS
General:
- Monitor vital signs at every appointment because of cardiovascular side effects.
- Assess salivary flow as a factor in caries, periodontal disease, and candidiasis.
- After supine positioning, have patient sit upright for at least 2 min to avoid orthostatic hypotension.
- Use vasoconstrictors with caution, in low doses, and with careful aspiration. Avoid use of gingival retraction cord with epinephrine.
- Place on frequent recall because of oral side effects.
- Consider drug in diagnosis of taste alterations.

Consultations:
- Medical consultation may be required to assess disease control.

Teach Patient/Family:
- *When chronic dry mouth occurs, advise patient:*
  - To avoid mouth rinses with high alcohol content because of drying effects
  - To use daily home fluoride products for anticaries effect
  - To use sugarless gum, frequent sips of water, or saliva substitutes

cyclopentolate hydrochloride

sye-kloe-pen′-toe-late
hye-droe-klor′-ide
(AK-Pentolate, Cyclogyl, Cylate, Diopentolate[CAN], Ocu-Pentolate, Pentolair)

CATEGORY AND SCHEDULE

Pregnancy Risk Category: C

MECHANISM OF ACTION

An antimuscarinic similar to atropine that competes with acetylcholine. Blocks the responses of the sphincter muscle of the iris and the accommodative muscle of the ciliary body to cholinergic stimulation. ***Therapeutic Effect:*** Results in mydriasis and cycloplegia.

PHARMACOKINETICS

Rapid systemic absorption following ophthalmic administration. Shorter duration of action than atropine. Complete recovery takes 6–24 hours.

AVAILABILITY

Ophthalmic Solution: 0.5% (Cyclogyl), 1% (AK-Pentolate, Cyclogyl, Cylate, Ocu-Pentolate, Pentolair), 2% (AK-Pentolate, Cyclogyl).

INDICATIONS AND DOSAGES

▸ Cycloplegia Induction, Mydriasis Induction

OPHTHALMIC

Adults, Elderly, Children. Instill 1–2 drops of 0.5%–2% solution in eye(s). May repeat with 0.5% or 1% solution in 5–10 minutes as needed.
Neonates, infants. Instill 1 drop of 0.5%–2% solution in eye(s) followed by 1 drop of 0.5% or 1% in 5 minutes as needed.

CONTRAINDICATIONS

Narrow-angle glaucoma, anatomical narrow angles, hypersensitivity to cyclopentolate or any component of the formulation.

INTERACTIONS

Drug

Belladonna, belladonna alkaloids: May increase anticholinergic effects.
Cisapride: May decrease cisapride efficacy.

Herbal

None known.

Food

None known.

Drug interactions of concern to dentistry

- None reported

DIAGNOSTIC TEST EFFECTS

None known.

SIDE EFFECTS

Occasional

Blurred vision, burning of eye, photophobia.

Rare

Conjunctivitis, increased intraocular pressure.

SERIOUS REACTIONS

! Systemic absorption, which includes signs and symptoms of confusion, psychosis, and ataxia; tachycardia and vasodilation occur rarely.

DENTAL CONSIDERATIONS

General:

- Not likely to be encountered in the dental office; used for diagnostic procedures.
- Question patient about eye health, including the presence of glaucoma.

C

cyclophosphamide

sye-kloe-foss′-fa-mide
(Cycloblastin[AUS], Cytoxan, Endoxan Asta[AUS], Endoxon Asta[AUS], Neosar, Procytox[CAN])
Do not confuse Cytoxan with cefoxitin, Ciloxan, cyclosporine, or Cytotec.

CATEGORY AND SCHEDULE

Pregnancy Risk Category: D

MECHANISM OF ACTION

An alkylating agent that inhibits DNA and RNA protein synthesis by cross-linking with DNA and RNA strands, preventing cell growth. Cell cycle-phase nonspecific.
Therapeutic Effect: Potent immunosuppressant.

PHARMACOKINETICS

Well absorbed from the GI tract. Protein binding: Low. Crosses the blood-brain barrier. Metabolized in the liver to active metabolites. Primarily excreted in urine. Removed by hemodialysis. ***Half-life:*** 3–12 hr.

AVAILABILITY

Tablets (Cytoxan): 25 mg, 50 mg.
Powder for Injection (Neosar): 100 mg, 200 mg.
Powder for Injection (Cytoxan, Neosar): 500 mg, 1 g, 2 g.

INDICATIONS AND DOSAGES

▸ Ovarian Adenocarcinoma, Breast Carcinoma, Hodgkin's Disease, Non-Hodgkin's Lymphoma, Multiple Myeloma, Leukemia (acute lymphoblastic, acute myelogenous, acute monocytic, chronic granulocytic, chronic lymphocytic), Mycosis Fungoides, Disseminated Neuroblastoma, Retinoblastoma

PO
Adults. 1–5 mg/kg/day.
Children. Initially, 2–8 mg/kg/day. Maintenance: 2–5 mg/kg twice a week.
IV
Adults. 40–50 mg/kg in divided doses over 2–5 days; or 10–15 mg/kg every 7–10 days or 3–5 mg/kg twice a week.
Children. 2–8 mg/kg/day for 6 days or total dose for 7 days once a week.

▸ Biopsy-Proven Minimal-Change Nephrotic Syndrome

PO
Adults, Children. 2.5–3 mg/kg/day for 60–90 days.

OFF-LABEL USES

Treatment of carcinoma of bladder, cervix, endometrium, lung, prostate, or testicles; germ cell ovarian tumors; osteosarcoma; rheumatoid arthritis; systemic lupus erythematosus

CONTRAINDICATIONS

None known.

INTERACTIONS

Drug

Allopurinol, bone marrow depressants: May increase myelosuppression.
Antigout medications: May decrease the effects of these drugs.
Cytarabine: May increase the risk of cardiomyopathy.
Immunosuppressants: May increase the risk of infection and development of neoplasms.
Live-virus vaccines: May potentiate virus replication, increase vaccine side effects, and decrease the patient's antibody response to the vaccine.

Herbal

None known.

Food

None known.

Drug interactions of concern to dentistry

- Increased blood dyscrasia: NSAIDs, dapsone, phenothiazines, corticosteroids
- Increased metabolism: phenobarbital

DIAGNOSTIC TEST EFFECTS

May increase serum uric acid levels.

IV INCOMPATIBILITIES

Amphotericin B complex (Abelcet, AmBisome, Amphotec)

IV COMPATIBILITIES

Granisetron (Kytril), heparin, hydromorphone (Dilaudid), lorazepam (Ativan), morphine, ondansetron (Zofran), propofol (Diprivan)

SIDE EFFECTS

Expected

Marked leukopenia 8–15 days after initial therapy

Frequent

Nausea, vomiting (beginning about 6 hr after administration and lasting about 4 hr); alopecia (33%)

Occasional

Diarrhea, darkening of skin and fingernails, stomatitis, headache, diaphoresis

Rare

Pain or redness at injection site

SERIOUS REACTIONS

! Cyclophosphamide's major toxic effect is myelosuppression resulting in blood dyscrasias, such as leukopenia, anemia, thrombocytopenia, and hypoprothrombinemia.

! Expect leukopenia to resolve in 17 to 28 days. Anemia generally occurs after large doses or prolonged therapy. Thrombocytopenia may occur 10–15 days after drug initiation.

! Hemorrhagic cystitis occurs commonly in long-term therapy, especially in pediatric patients.

! Pulmonary fibrosis and cardiotoxicity have been noted with high doses.

! Amenorrhea, azoospermia, and hyperkalemia may also occur.

DENTAL CONSIDERATIONS

General:

- Monitor vital signs at every appointment because of cardiovascular and respiratory side effects.
- Patients on chronic drug therapy may rarely have symptoms of blood dyscrasias, which can include infection, bleeding, and poor healing.
- Avoid prescribing aspirin-containing products.
- Prophylactic antibiotics may be indicated to prevent infection if surgery or deep scaling is planned because of leukopenic drug side effects.
- Patients receiving chemotherapy may require palliative treatment for stomatitis.

Consultations:

- In a patient with symptoms of blood dyscrasias, request a medical consultation for blood studies and postpone dental treatment until normal values are reestablished.
- Take precautions if dental surgery is anticipated and anesthesia is required.

Teach Patient/Family:

- Importance of good oral hygiene to prevent soft tissue inflammation
- Caution to prevent injury when using oral hygiene aids

C

cycloserine

sye-kloe-ser′-een
(Closina[AUS], Seromycin)

CATEGORY AND SCHEDULE

Pregnancy Risk Category: C

MECHANISM OF ACTION

An antitubercular that inhibits cell wall synthesis by competing with the amino acid, D-alanine, for incorporation into the bacterial cell wall. ***Therapeutic Effect:*** Causes disruption of bacterial cell wall. Bactericidal or bacteriostatic.

PHARMACOKINETICS

Readily absorbed from the gastrointestinal (GI) tract. No protein binding. Widely distributed (including cerebrospinal fluid [CSF]). Metabolized in liver. Primarily excreted in urine. Removed by hemodialysis. ***Half-life:*** 10 hrs.

AVAILABILITY

Capsules: 250 mg (Seromycin).

INDICATIONS AND DOSAGES

▸ **Tuberculosis**

Adults, Elderly. 250 mg q12h for 14 days, then 500 mg to 1g/day in 2 divided doses for 18–24 months. Maximum: 1 g as a single daily dose.
Children. 10–20 mg/kg/day in 2 divided doses. Maximum: 1000 mg/day for 18–24 months.
Dosage in renal impairment

Creatinine Clearance	Dosage Interval
10–50 ml/min	q24h
less than 10 ml/min	q36–48h

OFF-LABEL USES

Gaucher's disease, acute urinary tract infections

CONTRAINDICATIONS

Epilepsy, depression, severe anxiety, psychosis, severe renal insufficiency, excessive concurrent use of alcohol, history of hypersensitivity reactions with previous cycloserine therapy

INTERACTIONS

Drug

Alcohol: May increase central nervous system (CNS) effects.
Isoniazid, ethionamide: May increase cycloserine toxicity.
Phenytoin: May increase the risk of epileptic seizures.

Herbal

Vitamin B_{12}: May decrease vitamin B_{12}.
Folic acid: May decrease folic acid.

Food

None known.

Drug interactions of concern to dentistry

- Seizures: alcohol
- Drowsiness is a common side effect; although no drug interactions with sedatives are reported, increased drowsiness is possible

DIAGNOSTIC TEST EFFECTS

None known.

SIDE EFFECTS

Occasional

Drowsiness, headache, dizziness, vertigo, seizures, confusion, psychosis, paresis, tremor, vitamin B_{12} deficiency, folate deficiency, cardiac arrhythmias, increased liver enzymes

SERIOUS REACTIONS

! Neurotoxicity, as evidenced by confusion, agitation, CNS depression, psychosis, coma, and seizures, occur rarely.
! Neurotoxic effects of cycloserine may be treated and prevented with the administration of 200 to 300 mg of pyridoxine daily.

DENTAL CONSIDERATIONS

General:

- Patients on chronic drug therapy may rarely have symptoms of blood dyscrasias, which can include infection, bleeding, and poor healing.
- Examine for evidence of oral signs of disease.
- Determine why the patient is taking the drug (i.e., for preventive or therapeutic therapy).

Consultation:

- Medical consultation may be required to assess patient's ability to tolerate stress.
- In a patient with symptoms of blood dyscrasias, request a medical consultation for blood studies and postpone dental treatment until normal values are reestablished.
- *Determine that noninfectious status exists by ensuring that:*
  - Anti-TB drugs have been taken for more than 3 wk
  - Culture confirms antibiotic susceptibility to TB microorganism
  - Patient has had three consecutive negative sputum smears
  - Patient is not in the coughing stage

Teach Patient/Family:

- To avoid mouth rinses with high alcohol content
- Caution to prevent injury when using oral hygiene aids
- Importance of good oral hygiene to prevent soft tissue inflammation
- Importance of taking medication for full length of prescribed therapy to ensure effectiveness of treatment and prevent the emergence of resistant forms of microbe

cyclosporine

sye-kloe-spor′-in
(Cysporin[AUS], Gengraf, Neoral, Restasis, Sandimmune, Sandimmune Neoral[AUS])
Do not confuse cyclosporine with cycloserine, cyclophosphamide, or Cyklokapron.

CATEGORY AND SCHEDULE

Pregnancy Risk Category: C

MECHANISM OF ACTION

A cyclic polypeptide that inhibits both cellular and humoral immune responses by inhibiting interleukin-2, a proliferative factor needed for T-cell activity. ***Therapeutic Effect:*** Prevents organ rejection and relieves symptoms of psoriasis and arthritis.

PHARMACOKINETICS

Variably absorbed from the GI tract. Protein binding: 90%. Widely distributed. Metabolized in the liver. Eliminated primarily by biliary or fecal excretion. Not removed by hemodialysis. ***Half-life:*** Adults, 10–27 hr; children, 7–19 hr.

AVAILABILITY

Capsules (Softgel [Gengraf, Neoral, Sandimmune]): 25 mg, 100 mg.
Oral Solution (Sandimmune): 50-ml bottle with calibrated liquid measuring device.
Injection (Sandimmune): 50 mg/ml.
Ophthalmic Emulsion (Restasis): 0.05%.

INDICATIONS AND DOSAGES

▸ **Transplantation, Prevention of Organ Rejection**

PO

Adults, Elderly, Children. 10–18 mg/kg/dose given 4–12 hr prior to organ

transplantation. Maintenance: 5–15 mg/kg/day in divided doses then tapered to 3–10 mg/kg/day.
IV
Adults, Elderly, Children. Initially, 5–6 mg/kg/dose given 4–12 hr prior to organ transplantation. Maintenance: 2–10 mg/kg/day in divided doses.

▸ **Rheumatoid Arthritis**
PO
Adults, Elderly. Initially, 2.5 mg/kg a day in 2 divided doses. May increase by 0.5–0.75 mg/kg/day. Maximum: 4 mg/kg/day.

▸ **Psoriasis**
PO
Adults, Elderly. Initially, 2.5 mg/kg/day in 2 divided doses. May increase by 0.5 mg/kg/day. Maximum: 4 mg/kg/day.

▸ **Dry eye**
OPHTHALMIC
Adults, Elderly. Instill 1 drip in each affected eye q12h.

OFF-LABEL USES

Treatment of alopecia areata, aplastic anemia, atopic dermatitis, Behçet's disease, biliary cirrhosis, prevention of corneal transplant rejection

CONTRAINDICATIONS

History of hypersensitivity to cyclosporine or polyoxyethylated castor oil

INTERACTIONS

Drug

ACE inhibitors, potassium-sparing diuretics, potassium supplements: May cause hyperkalemia.
Cimetidine, danazol, diltiazem, erythromycin, ketoconazole: May increase cyclosporine concentration and risk of hepatotoxicity and nephrotoxicity.
Immunosuppressants: May increase risk of infection and lymphoproliferative disorders.
Live-virus vaccines: May increase vaccine side effects, potentiate virus replication, and decrease the patient's antibody response to the vaccine.
Lovastatin: May increase the risk of acute renal failure and rhabdomyolysis.

Herbal

St. John's wort: May alter cyclosporine absorption.

Food

Grapefruit, grapefruit juice: May increase the absorption and risk of toxicity of cyclosporine.

Drug interactions of concern to dentistry for systemic form:

- Hepatotoxicity/nephrotoxicity: erythromycin, azithromycin, clarithromycin
- Decreased action: barbiturates, carbamazepine
- Possibly reduced blood levels: clindamycin
- Increased infection and immunosuppression: corticosteroids
- Increased blood levels and risk of toxicity: fluconazole, ketoconazole, and itraconazole

DIAGNOSTIC TEST EFFECTS

May increase BUN and serum alkaline phosphatase, amylase, bilirubin, creatinine, potassium, uric acid, AST, and ALT levels. May decrease serum magnesium level. Therapeutic peak serum level is 50–300 ng/ml; toxic serum level is greater than 400 ng/ml.

IV INCOMPATIBILITIES

Amphotericin B complex (Abelcet, AmBisome, Amphotec), magnesium

IV COMPATIBILITIES

Propofol (Diprivan)

SIDE EFFECTS

Frequent

Mild to moderate hypertension (26%), hirsutism (21%), tremor (12%)

Occasional (4%–2%)
Acne, leg cramps, gingival hyperplasia (marked by red, bleeding, and tender gums), paresthesia, diarrhea, nausea, vomiting, headache
Rare (less than 1%)
Hypersensitivity reaction, abdominal discomfort, gynecomastia, sinusitis

SERIOUS REACTIONS

! Mild nephrotoxicity occurs in 25% of renal transplant patients, 38% of cardiac transplant patients, and 37% of liver transplant patients, generally 2 to 3 months after transplantation (more severe toxicity is generally occurs soon after transplantation). Hepatotoxicity occurs in 4% of renal transplant patients, 7% of cardiac transplant patients, and 4% of liver transplant patients, generally within the first month after transplantation. Both toxicities usually respond to dosage reduction.
! Severe hyperkalemia and hyperuricemia occur occasionally.

DENTAL CONSIDERATIONS

SYSTEMIC FORM

General:
• Monitor vital signs at every appointment because of cardiovascular side effects.
• Patients on chronic drug therapy may rarely have symptoms of blood dyscrasias, which can include infection, bleeding, and poor healing.
• Place on frequent recall to evaluate gingival condition and healing response.
• Monitor time since organ/tissue transplant.

Consultations:
• Antibiotic prophylaxis usually is recommended in patients with organ transplants and immunosuppression.
• In a patient with symptoms of blood dyscrasias, request a medical consultation for blood studies and postpone dental treatment until normal values are reestablished.
• Request baseline blood pressure in renal transplant patients for patient evaluation before dental treatment.

Teach Patient/Family:
• Importance of good oral hygiene to prevent soft tissue inflammation
• Caution to prevent injury when using oral hygiene aids

Drug interactions of concern to dentistry for ophthalmic-dose form:
• None reported

DENTAL CONSIDERATIONS

OPHTHALMIC-DOSE FORM

General:
• Determine why the patient is taking the drug.
• Protect the patient's eyes from accidental spatter during dental treatment.
• Avoid dental light in the patient's eyes; offer dark glasses for patient comfort.

Teach Patient/Family:
• *When chronic dry mouth occurs, advise patient:*
  • To avoid mouth rinses with high alcohol content because of drying effects
  • To use daily home fluoride products for anticaries effect
  • To use sugarless gum, frequent sips of water, or saliva substitutes

C

C

cyproheptadine
si-proe-hep′-ta-deen
(Periactin)

CATEGORY AND SCHEDULE
Pregnancy Risk Category: B

MECHANISM OF ACTION
An antihistamine that competes with histamine at histaminic receptor sites. Anticholinergic effects cause drying of nasal mucosa. ***Therapeutic Effect:*** Relieves allergic conditions (urticaria, pruritus).

PHARMACOKINETICS
Well absorbed from GI tract. Metabolized in liver. Primarily eliminated in feces. ***Half-life:*** 16 hrs.

AVAILABILITY
Syrup: 2 mg/5 ml (Periactin).
Tablets: 4 mg (Periactin).

INDICATIONS AND DOSAGES
▸ **Allergic Condition**
PO
Adults, Children older than 15 yrs. 4 mg 3 times/day. May increase dose but do not exceed 0.5 mg/kg/day.
Children 7–14 yrs. 4 mg 2–3 times/day, or 0.25 mg/kg daily in divided doses.
Children 2–6 yrs. 2 mg 2–3 times/day, or 0.25 mg/kg daily in divided doses.
Usual elderly dosage
PO
Initially, 4 mg 2 times/day.

CONTRAINDICATIONS
Acute asthmatic attack, patients receiving MAO inhibitors, history of hypersensitivity to antihistamines

INTERACTIONS
Drug
Alcohol, central nervous system (CNS) depressants: May increase CNS depression.
Fluoxetine, paroxetine: May decrease fluoxetine efficacy.
MAOIs: May increase anticholinergic and CNS depressant effects.
Protirelin: May decrease TSH response.
Herbal
None known.
Food
None known.
Drug interactions of concern to dentistry
- Increased CNS depression: alcohol, CNS depressants
- Increased effect of anticholinergic drugs

DIAGNOSTIC TEST EFFECTS
May suppress flare and wheal reaction to antigen skin testing unless drug is discontinued 4 days before testing. May increase SGPT (AST) levels.

SIDE EFFECTS
Frequent
Drowsiness, dizziness, muscular weakness, dry mouth/nose/throat/lips, urinary retention, thickening of bronchial secretions
Elderly
Frequent
Sedation, dizziness, hypotension
Occasional
Epigastric distress, flushing, visual disturbances, hearing disturbances, paresthesia, sweating, chills

SERIOUS REACTIONS
! Children may experience dominant paradoxical reaction (restlessness,

insomnia, euphoria, nervousness, tremors).

! Overdosage in children may result in hallucinations, convulsions, death.

! Hypersensitivity reaction (eczema, pruritus, rash, cardiac disturbances, angioedema, photosensitivity) may occur.

! Overdosage may vary from CNS depression (sedation, apnea, cardiovascular collapse, death) to severe paradoxical reaction (hallucinations, tremor, seizures).

DENTAL CONSIDERATIONS

General:

- Assess salivary flow as a factor in caries, periodontal disease, and candidiasis.
- Determine why the patient is taking the drug.

cysteamine bitartrate

sis-**tee**-a-meen bye-**tar**-trate
(Cystagon)

CATEGORY AND SCHEDULE

Pregnancy Risk Category: C

MECHANISM OF ACTION

An aminothiol that participates within lysosomes in a thiol-disulfide interchange reaction converting cystine into cysteine and cysteine-cysteamine mixed disulfide, both of which can exit cystinotic lysosomes. ***Therapeutic Effect:*** Lowers the cystine content in cells.

PHARMACOKINETICS

Poorly bound to plasma proteins. **Half-life:** Unknown.

AVAILABILITY

Capsules: 50 mg, 150 mg (Cystagon).

INDICATIONS AND DOSAGES

Cystinosis

PO

Adults. Initially, 1/4–1/6 of maintenance dose. Gradually, increase dose over 4–6 wk. *Maintenance.* 2 g/day in 4 divided doses.

Children older then 12 yr and over 110 lb. 2 g/day in 4 divided doses.

Children 6–12 yr. 1.30 g/m^2/day of the free base, given in 4 divided doses.

CONTRAINDICATIONS

Hypersensitivity to cysteamine or penicillamine

INTERACTIONS

Drug

None known.

Herbal

None known.

Food

None known.

Drug interactions of concern to dentistry

- Dental drug interactions have not been studied

DIAGNOSTIC TEST EFFECTS

None known.

SIDE EFFECTS

Frequent

Rash, loss of appetite, fever, vomiting, diarrhea, lethargy

Occasional

Dehydration, hypertension, nausea, abdominal pain, somnolence, nervousness, nightmares, urticaria

C

SERIOUS REACTIONS

! Leukopenia, abnormal liver function, and anemia occur rarely.
! Sudden deaths have been reported.

DENTAL CONSIDERATIONS

General:

• Patients taking this medication may have significant renal disease; thoroughly review medical and drug history.

Consultations:

• Specific consultation depends on type of renal disease.

Teach Patient/Family:

• Importance of good oral hygiene to prevent soft tissue inflammation
• To prevent trauma when using oral hygiene aids
• Importance of updating health and medication history if physician makes any changes in evaluation or drug regimens; include OTC, herbal, and nonherbal remedies in the update

cytarabine

sigh-tar′-ah-bean
(Ara-C, Cytosar[CAN], Cytosar-U)
Do not confuse cytarabine with Cytadren, Cytovene, or vidarabine.

CATEGORY AND SCHEDULE

Pregnancy Risk Category: D

MECHANISM OF ACTION

An antimetabolite that is converted intracellularly to a nucleotide. Cell cycle-specific for S phase of cell division. ***Therapeutic Effect:*** May inhibit DNA synthesis. Potent immunosuppressive activity.

PHARMACOKINETICS

Widely distributed; moderate amount crosses the blood-brain barrier. Protein binding: 15%. Primarily excreted in urine. ***Half-life:*** 1–3 hr.

AVAILABILITY

Injection Powder: 100 mg, 500 mg, 1 g, 2 g.
Injection Solution: 20 mg/ml, 100 mg/ml.

INDICATIONS AND DOSAGES

▸ To Induce Remission in Acute Lymphocytic Leukemia, Acute and Chronic Myelocytic Leukemia, Meningeal Leukemia, or Non-Hodgkin's Lymphoma in Children

IV
Adults, Elderly, Children.
200 mg/m^2/day for 5 days q2wk as monotherapy or 100–200 mg/m^2/day for 5- to 10-day course of therapy every q2–4wk in combination therapy.
INTRATHECAL
Adults, Elderly, Children.
5–7.5 mg/m^2 every 2–7 days.

▸ To Maintain Remission in Acute Lymphocytic Leukemia, Acute and Chronic Myelocytic Leukemia, Meningeal Leukemia, or Non-Hodgkin's Lymphoma in Children

IV
Adults, Elderly, Children.
70–200 mg/m^2/day for 2–5 days every month.
IM, SUBCUTANEOUS
Adults, Elderly, Children.
1–1.5 mg/m^2 as single dose q1–4wk.
INTRATHECAL
Adults, Elderly, Children.
5–7.5 mg/m^2 every 2–7 days.

OFF-LABEL USES

Treatment of Hodgkin's disease, myelodysplastic syndrome

CONTRAINDICATIONS

None known.

INTERACTIONS

Drug

Antigout medications: May decrease the effects of these drugs.
Bone marrow depressants: May increase myelosuppression.
Cyclophosphamide: May increase the risk of cardiomyopathy.
Live-virus vaccines: May potentiate virus replication, increase vaccine side effects, and decrease the patient's antibody response to the vaccine.

Herbal

None known.

Food

None known.

Drug interactions of concern to dentistry

- Increased risk of bleeding: drugs that interfere with coagulation or platelet function, such as NSAIDs and aspirin
- Increase risk of infection; glucocorticoids

DIAGNOSTIC TEST EFFECTS

May increase serum alkaline phosphatase, bilirubin, uric acid, and AST (SGOT) levels.

IV INCOMPATIBILITIES

Amphotericin B complex (Abelcet, AmBisome, Amphotec), ganciclovir (Cytovene), heparin, insulin (regular)

IV COMPATIBILITIES

Dexamethasone (Decadron), diphenhydramine (Benadryl), filgrastim (Neupogen), granisetron (Kytril), hydromorphone (Dilaudid), lorazepam (Ativan), morphine, ondansetron (Zofran), potassium chloride, propofol (Diprivan)

SIDE EFFECTS

Frequent

IV, Subcutaneous (33%–16%): Asthenia, fever, pain, altered taste and smell, nausea, vomiting (risk greater with IV push than with continuous IV infusion)
Intrathecal (28%–11%): Headache, asthenia, altered taste and smell, confusion, somnolence, nausea, vomiting

Occasional

IV, Subcutaneous (11%–7%): Abnormal gait, somnolence, constipation, back pain, urinary incontinence, peripheral edema, headache, confusion
Intrathecal (7%–3%): Peripheral edema, back pain, constipation, abnormal gait, urinary incontinence

SERIOUS REACTIONS

! Myelosuppression may result in blood dyscrasias, such as leukopenia, anemia, thrombocytopenia, megaloblastosis, and reticulocytopenia, after a single IV dose.
! Leukopenia, anemia, and thrombocytopenia should be expected with daily or continuous IV therapy.
! Cytarabine syndrome, (as evidenced by fever, myalgia, rash, conjunctivitis, malaise, and chest pain) and hyperuricemia may occur.
! High-dose cytarabine therapy may produce severe CNS, GI, and pulmonary toxicity.

DENTAL CONSIDERATIONS

General:

- Determine why patient is taking the drug.
- If additional analgesia is required for dental pain, consider alternative analgesics (NSAIDs) in patients taking narcotics for acute or chronic pain.
- Avoid prescribing aspirin-containing products.
- This drug may be used in the hospital or on an outpatient basis.

Confirm the patient's disease and treatment status.

- Patient on chronic drug therapy may rarely present with symptoms of blood dyscrasias, which can include infection, bleeding, and poor healing. If dyscrasia is present, caution patient to prevent oral tissue trauma when using oral hygiene aids.
- Short appointments and a stress reduction protocol may be required for anxious patients.
- Patients may have received other chemotherapy or radiation; confirm medical and drug history.
- Patients may be at risk of infection.
- Patients may be taking a prophylactic antiinfective.
- Patients are at risk of bleeding, so check for oral signs.
- Oral infections should be eliminated and/or treated aggressively.

Consultations:

- Medical consultation should include routine blood counts including platelet counts and bleeding time.
- Consult physician; prophylactic or therapeutic antiinfectives may be indicated if surgery or periodontal treatment is required.
- Medical consultation may be required to assess immunologic status during cancer chemotherapy and determine safety risk, if any, posed by the required dental treatment.
- Medical consultation may be required to assess disease control and patient's ability to tolerate stress.

Teach Patient/Family:

- Importance of good oral hygiene to prevent soft tissue inflammation
- To report oral lesions, soreness, or bleeding to dentist
- To prevent trauma when using oral hygiene aids
- Importance of updating health and medication history if physician makes any changes in evaluation or drug regimens; include OTC, herbal, and nonherbal remedies in the update

daclizumab

day-cly′-zu-mab
(Zenapax)

CATEGORY AND SCHEDULE

Pregnancy Risk Category: C

MECHANISM OF ACTION

A monoclonal antibody that binds to the interleukin-2 (IL-2) receptor complex, inhibiting the IL-2–mediated activation of T lymphocytes, a critical pathway in the cellular immune response involved in allograft rejection. ***Therapeutic Effect:*** Prevents organ rejection.

PHARMACOKINETICS

Half-life: Adults, 20 days.

AVAILABILITY

Injection: 25 mg/5 ml.

INDICATIONS AND DOSAGES

▸ Prevention of Acute Renal Transplant Rejection (in Combination with an Immunosuppressive)

IV

Adults, Children. 1 mg/kg over 15 min q14 days for 5 doses, beginning no more than 24 hr before transplantation. Maximum: 100 mg.

OFF-LABEL USES

Treatment of graft vs. host disease

CONTRAINDICATIONS

None known.

INTERACTIONS

Drug

None known.

Herbal

None known.

Food

None known.

Drug interactions of concern to dentistry

- None reported

DIAGNOSTIC TEST EFFECTS

None known.

IV INCOMPATIBILITIES

Don't mix daclizumab with any other drugs.

SIDE EFFECTS

Occasional (> 2%)

Constipation, nausea, diarrhea, vomiting, abdominal pain, edema, headache, dizziness, fever, pain, fatigue, insomnia, weakness, arthralgia, myalgia, diaphoresis

SERIOUS REACTIONS

! Hypersensitivity reaction, which occurs rarely, is characterized by dyspnea, tachycardia, dysphagia, peripheral edema, rash, and pruritus.

DENTAL CONSIDERATIONS

General:

- This is a hospital-type drug, but because some dosing is continued, patients may appear in the dental office while receiving this drug.
- Transplant patients may also be taking cyclosporine and glucocorticoids; review each transplant patient's medications.
- Short appointments and a stress reduction protocol may be required for anxious patients.

Consultations:

- Antibiotic prophylaxis usually is recommended in patients with organ transplants and immunosuppression.
- Medical consultation may be required to assess disease control and patient's ability to tolerate stress.

Teach Patient/Family:

- Importance of good oral hygiene to prevent soft tissue inflammation

• To prevent trauma when using oral hygiene aids
• Importance of updating health and drug history if physician makes any changes in evaluation or drug regimens

dalteparin sodium

doll′-teh-pare-in
(Fragmin)

CATEGORY AND SCHEDULE

Pregnancy Risk Category: B

MECHANISM OF ACTION

An antithrombin that inhibits factor Xa and thrombin in the presence of low-molecular-weight heparin. Only slightly influences platelet aggregation, PT, and aPTT. ***Therapeutic Effect:*** Produces anticoagulation.

PHARMACOKINETICS

Route	Onset	Peak	Duration
Subcutaneous	N/A	4 hr	N/A

Protein binding: less than 10%. ***Half-life:*** 3–5 hr.

AVAILABILITY

Syringe: 2,500 international units/0.2 ml, 5,000 international units/0.2 ml, 7,500 international units/0.3 ml, 10,000 international units/ml.
Vial: 10,000 international units/ml, 25,000 international units/ml.

INDICATIONS AND DOSAGES

▸ **Low- to Moderate-Risk Abdominal Surgery**
SUBCUTANEOUS
Adults, Elderly. 2,500 international units 1–2 hr before surgery, then daily for 5–10 days.

▸ **High-Risk Abdominal Surgery**
SUBCUTANEOUS
Adults, Elderly. 5,000 international units 1–2 hr before surgery, then daily for 5–10 days.

▸ **Total Hip Surgery**
SUBCUTANEOUS
Adults, Elderly. 2,500 international units 1–2 hr before surgery, then 2,500 units 6 hrs after surgery, then 5,000 units/day for 7–10 days.

▸ **Unstable Angina, Non-Q-Wave MI**
SUBCUTANEOUS
Adults, Elderly. 120 international units/kg q12h (maximum: 10,000 international units/dose) given with aspirin until clinically stable.

▸ **Prevention of DVT or PE in the Acutely Ill Patient**
SUBCUTANEOUS
Adults, Elderly. 5,000 international units once a day.

CONTRAINDICATIONS

Active major bleeding; concurrent heparin therapy; hypersensitivity to dalteparin, heparin, or pork products; thrombocytopenia associated with positive in vitro test for antiplatelet antibody

INTERACTIONS

Drug

Anticoagulants, platelet inhibitors: May increase risk of bleeding.

Herbal

None known.

Food

None known.

Drug interactions of concern to dentistry

• Avoid concurrent use of aspirin (except as noted), NSAIDs, dipyridamole, and sulfinpyrazone

DIAGNOSTIC TEST EFFECTS

Increases (reversible) LDH, serum alkaline phosphatase, AST(SGOT), and ALT(SGPT) levels.

SIDE EFFECTS

Occasional (7%–3%)
Hematoma at injection site
Rare (< 1%)
Hypersensitivity reaction (chills, fever, pruritus, urticaria, asthma, rhinitis, lacrimation, headache); mild, local skin irritation

SERIOUS REACTIONS

! Overdose may lead to bleeding complications ranging from local ecchymoses to major hemorrhage.
! Thrombocytopenia occurs rarely.

DENTAL CONSIDERATIONS

General:
- Product may be used in outpatient therapy. Delay elective dental treatment until patient completes anticoagulant therapy.
- Determine why patient is taking the drug.
- Consider local hemostasis measures to prevent excessive bleeding.
- Avoid prescribing aspirin-containing products.

Consultations:
- Medical consultation should include routine blood counts, including platelet counts and bleeding time.

Teach Patient/Family:
- Importance of good oral hygiene to prevent soft tissue inflammation
- To prevent trauma when using oral hygiene aids
- To report oral lesions, soreness, or bleeding to dentist

danazol

da′-na-zole
(Cyclomen[CAN], Danocrine)

CATEGORY AND SCHEDULE

Pregnancy Risk Category: X

MECHANISM OF ACTION

A testosterone derivative that suppresses the pituitary-ovarian axis by inhibiting the output of pituitary gonadotropins. Causes atrophy of both normal and ectopic endometrial tissue in endometriosis. Follicle-stimulating hormone (FSH) and luteinizing hormone (LH) are depressed in fibrocystic breast disease. Inhibits steroid synthesis and binding of steroids to their receptors in breast tissues. Increases serum levels of esterase inhibitor.
Therapeutic Effect: Produces anovulation and amenorrhea, reduces the production of estrogen, corrects biochemical deficiency as seen in hereditary angioedema.

PHARMACOKINETICS

Well absorbed from gastrointestinal (GI) tract. Metabolized in liver, primarily to 2-hydroxymethylethisterone. Excreted in urine.
Half-life: 4.5 hrs.

AVAILABILITY

Capsules: 50 mg, 100 mg, 200 mg (Danocrine).

INDICATIONS AND DOSAGES

▸ **Endometriosis**
PO
Adults. 200–800 mg/day in 2 divided doses for 3–9 mos.

▸ **Fibrocystic Breast Disease**
PO
Adults. 100–400 mg/day in 2 divided doses.

▸ Hereditary Angioedema
PO
Adults. Initially, 200 mg 2–3 times/day. Decrease dose by 50% or less at 1–3 mo intervals. If attack occurs, increase dose by up to 200 mg/day.

OFF-LABEL USES
Treatment of gynecomastia, menorrhagia, precocious puberty

CONTRAINDICATIONS
Cardiac impairment, hypercalcemia, pregnancy, prostatic or breast cancer in males, severe liver or renal disease

INTERACTIONS
Drug
Carbamazepine, cyclosporine, tacrolimus, and warfarin: May increase serum levels and increase risk of toxicity of these drugs.
HMG-CoA reductase inhibitors: May increase chance of developing myopathy or rhabdomyolysis.
Hormonal contraceptives: May decrease effectiveness of contraceptives.
Hypoglycemic agents: May increase the risk of hypoglycemia.
Herbal
None known.
Food
Food may delay time to peak. High fat meal increases plasma concentration.
Drug interactions of concern to dentistry
• Increased serum concentration of carbamazepine; consider avoiding concurrent administration

DIAGNOSTIC TEST EFFECTS
May increase blood Hgb and Hct, LDL concentrations, serum alkaline phosphatase, bilirubin, calcium, potassium, SGOT (AST) levels, and sodium levels. May decrease HDL concentrations. May alter levels of testosterone, androstenedione, dehydroepiandrosterone.

SIDE EFFECTS
Frequent
Females: Amenorrhea, breakthrough bleeding/spotting, decreased breast size, increased weight, irregular menstrual period.
Occasional
Males/females: Edema, rhabdomyolysis (muscle cramps, unusual fatigue), virilism (acne, oily skin), flushed skin, altered moods
Rare
Males/females: Hematuria, gingivitis, carpal tunnel syndrome, cataracts, severe headache, vomiting, rash, photosensitivity
Females: Enlarged clitoris, hoarseness, deepening voice, hair growth, monilial vaginitis
Males: Decreased testicle size.

SERIOUS REACTIONS
! Jaundice may occur in those receiving 400 mg/day or more. Liver dysfunction, eosinophilia, thrombocytopenia, pancreatitis occur rarely.

DENTAL CONSIDERATIONS
General:
• Patients on chronic drug therapy may rarely have symptoms of blood dyscrasias, which can include infection, bleeding, and poor healing.
Consultations:
• In a patient with symptoms of blood dyscrasias, request a medical consultation for blood studies and postpone dental treatment until normal values are reestablished.
Teach Patient/Family:
• Importance of good oral hygiene to prevent soft tissue inflammation

• To avoid mouth rinses with high alcohol content because of drying and irritating effects

danaparoid

da-nah-pah-roid **soe**-dee-um
(Organ k)

CATEGORY AND SCHEDULE

Pregnancy Risk Category: B

MECHANISM OF ACTION

An antithrombotic agent that inhibits thrombin formation through factor anti-Xa and anti-IIa effects. Does not significantly influence bleeding time, PT, aPTT, or platelet function. Possesses greater antithrombotic activity than anticoagulant activity.
Therapeutic Effect: Produces antithrombotic activity, anticoagulation.

PHARMACOKINETICS

Well absorbed following subcutaneous administration. Eliminated primarily in the urine.
Half-life: 24 hr (half-life prolonged with severe renal impairment).

AVAILABILITY

Injection: 750 anti-Xa units/0.6 ml.

INDICATIONS AND DOSAGES

Note: Give initial dose as soon as possible after surgery but not more than 24 hr after surgery.

▸ **Prevention of Deep Vein Thrombosis (DVT)**

SUBCUTANEOUS

Adults, Elderly. 750 anti-Xa units twice daily beginning 1–4 hr preoperatively and then not sooner than 2 hr after surgery. Continue treatment throughout postoperative care until risk of DVT has diminished (average duration 7–14 days).

UNLABELED USES

Heparin-induced thrombocytopenia

CONTRAINDICATIONS

Severe hemorrhagic diathesis (hemophilia, idiopathic thrombocytopenic purpura), active major bleeding state, including hemorrhagic stroke in the acute phase, type II phase thrombocytopenia associated with positive in vitro test for antiplatelet antibody in presence of danaparoid, hypersensitivity to pork products, danaparoid, or any component of the formulation

INTERACTIONS

Drug

Anticoagulants, platelet inhibitors: May increase bleeding (use with care).

Herbal

None known.

Food

None known.

Drug interactions of concern to dentistry

• Avoid concurrent use of platelet aggregation antagonist, such as aspirin, NSAIDs, dipyridamole

DIAGNOSTIC TEST EFFECTS

None known.

SIDE EFFECTS

Frequent (13%)

Injection site pain

Occasional (9%–4%)

Fever, pain, nausea, UTI, constipation

Rare (< 2%)

Rash, pruritus, infection

SERIOUS REACTIONS

Accidental overdosage may lead to bleeding complications ranging from minor ecchymosis to major hemorrhage. An unexplained fall in Hct or fall in BP should lead to consideration of a hemorrhagic event. The antidote protamine sulfate only partially neutralizes danaparoid activity and is incapable of reducing severe nonsurgical bleeding during treatment. If serious bleeding occurs, discontinue danaparoid; give blood or blood product transfusions.

DENTAL CONSIDERATIONS

General:

- Determine why patient is taking the drug.
- Consider local hemostasis measures to prevent excessive bleeding if dental treatment must be performed.
- Antibiotic prophylaxis before dental treatment may be required for joint prosthesis (see 2003 ADA guidelines).
- Delay elective dental treatment until patient completes danaparoid therapy.

Consultations:

- Medical consultation should include routine blood counts, including platelet counts and bleeding time.

Teach Patient/Family:

- Importance of good oral hygiene to prevent soft tissue inflammation
- Caution to prevent trauma when using oral hygiene aids
- To report oral lesions, soreness, or bleeding to dentist

dantrolene sodium

dan′-troe-leen

(Dantrium)

Do not confuse Dantrium with Daraprim.

CATEGORY AND SCHEDULE

Pregnancy Risk Category: C

MECHANISM OF ACTION

A skeletal muscle relaxant that reduces muscle contraction by interfering with release of calcium ion. Reduces calcium ion concentration. ***Therapeutic Effect:*** Dissociates excitation-contraction coupling. Interferes with catabolic process associated with malignant hyperthermic crisis.

PHARMACOKINETICS

Poorly absorbed from the GI tract. Protein binding: High. Metabolized in the liver. Primarily excreted in urine. ***Half-life:*** IV: 4–8 hr; PO: 8.7 hr.

AVAILABILITY

Capsules: 25 mg, 50 mg, 100 mg.
Powder for Injection: 20-mg vial.

INDICATIONS AND DOSAGES

▸ Spasticity

PO

Adults, Elderly. Initially, 25 mg/day. Increase to 25 mg 2–4 times a day, then by 25-mg increments up to 100 mg 2–4 times a day.

Children. Initially, 0.5 mg/kg twice a day. Increase to 0.5 mg/kg 3–4 times a day, then in increments of 0.5 mg/kg/day up to 3 mg/kg 2–4 times a day. Maximum: 400 mg/day.

▸ Prevention of Malignant Hyperthermic Crisis

PO

Adults, Elderly, Children. 4–8 mg/kg/day in 3–4 divided doses

1–2 days before surgery; give last dose 3–4 hr before surgery.
IV
Adults, Elderly, Children. 2.5 mg/kg about 1.25 hr before surgery.

▸ Management of Malignant Hyperthermic Crisis
IV
Adults, Elderly, Children. Initially a minimum of 1 mg/kg rapid IV; may repeat up to total cumulative dose of 10 mg/kg. May follow with 4–8 mg/kg/day PO in 4 divided doses up to 3 days after crisis.

OFF-LABEL USES
Relief of exercise-induced pain in patients with muscular dystrophy, treatment of flexor spasms and neuroleptic malignant syndrome

CONTRAINDICATIONS
Active hepatic disease

INTERACTIONS
Drug
Central nervous system (CNS) depressants: May increase CNS depression with short-term use.
Liver toxic medications: May increase the risk of liver toxicity with chronic use.
Herbal
None known.
Food
None known.
Drug interactions of concern to dentistry
- None reported

DIAGNOSTIC TEST EFFECTS
May alter liver function test results.

IV INCOMPATIBILITIES
None known.

SIDE EFFECTS
Frequent
Drowsiness, dizziness, weakness, general malaise, diarrhea (mild)
Occasional
Confusion, diarrhea (may be severe), headache, insomnia, constipation, urinary frequency
Rare
Paradoxical CNS excitement or restlessness, paresthesia, tinnitus, slurred speech, tremor, blurred vision, dry mouth, nocturia, impotence, rash, pruritus

SERIOUS REACTIONS
! There is a risk of liver toxicity, most notably in females, those 35 years of age and older, and those taking other medications concurrently.
! Overt hepatitis noted most frequently between 3rd and 12th month of therapy.
! Overdosage results in vomiting, muscular hypotonia, muscle twitching, respiratory depression, and seizures.

DENTAL CONSIDERATIONS
General:
- Monitor vital signs at every appointment because of cardiovascular and respiratory side effects.
- Patients on chronic drug therapy may rarely have symptoms of blood dyscrasias, which can include infection, bleeding, and poor healing.
- Requires proficiency in IV administration technique when used for emergency treatment of malignant hyperthermia.

Consultations:
- In a patient with symptoms of blood dyscrasias, request a medical consultation for blood studies and postpone dental treatment until normal values are reestablished.

Teach Patient/Family:

- Importance of good oral hygiene to prevent soft tissue inflammation
- To avoid mouth rinses with high alcohol content because of drying effects

dapiprazole hydrochloride

da′-pi-prah-zohl
hye-droh-klor′-ide
(Rev-Eyes)

CATEGORY AND SCHEDULE

Pregnancy Risk Category: B

MECHANISM OF ACTION

An alpha-adrenergic blocker that primarily affects alpha-1 adrenoceptors. Does not significantly affect intraocular pressure. ***Therapeutic Effect:*** Induces miosis via relaxation of the smooth dilator (radial) muscle of the iris, which causes papillary constriction.

PHARMACOKINETICS

Well absorbed. Mydriasis reversal begins in 1 hour and occurs in about 6 hours.

AVAILABILITY

Powder for reconstitution: 0.5% (Rev-Eyes).

INDICATIONS AND DOSAGES

▸ Drug-Induced Mydriasis

OPHTHALMIC

Adults, Elderly, Children. 2 drops applied topically to the conjunctiva of each eye. Repeat after 5 min. Do not use more than once per week.

CONTRAINDICATIONS

Acute iritis, hypersensitivity to dapiprazole or any component of the formulation

INTERACTIONS

Drug

None known.

Herbal

None known.

Food

None known.

Drug interactions of concern to dentistry

- None reported

DIAGNOSTIC TEST EFFECTS

None known.

SIDE EFFECTS

Occasional

Burning, eyelid edema, photophobia

SERIOUS REACTIONS

! None reported.

DENTAL CONSIDERATIONS

General:

- Used in ophthalmic examinations.
- Protect patient's eyes from accidental spatter during dental treatment.
- Avoid dental light in patient's eyes; offer dark glasses for patient comfort.

dapsone

dap′-sone
(Dapsone)

CATEGORY AND SCHEDULE

Pregnancy Risk Category: C

MECHANISM OF ACTION
An antibiotic that is a competitive antagonist of para-aminobenzoic acid (PABA); it prevents normal bacterial utilization of PABA for synthesis of folic acid. ***Therapeutic Effect:*** Inhibits bacterial growth.

AVAILABILITY
Tablets: 25 mg, 100 mg.

INDICATIONS AND DOSAGES
▸ **Leprosy**

PO

Adults, Elderly. 50–100 mg/day for 3–10 yr.

Children. 1–2 mg/kg/24 hr. Maximum: 100 mg/day.

▸ **Dermatitis Herpetiformis**

PO

Adults, Elderly. Initially, 50 mg/day. May increase up to 300 mg/day.

▸ **Pneumocystis Carinii Pneumonia (PCP)**

PO

Adults, Elderly. 100 mg/day in combination with trimethoprim for 21 days.

▸ **Prevention of PCP**

PO

Adults, Elderly. 100 mg/day.

Children older than 1 mo. 2 mg/kg/day. Maximum: 100 mg/day.

OFF-LABEL USES
Treatment of inflammatory bowel disorders, malaria

CONTRAINDICATIONS
None significant.

INTERACTIONS
Drug
Methotrexate: May increase hematologic reactions.

Probenecid: May decrease the excretion of dapsone.

Protease inhibitors (including ritonavir): May increase dapsone blood concentration.

Rifampin: May decrease rifampin blood concentration.

Trimethoprim: May increase the risk of toxic effects.

Herbal
St. John's wort: May decrease dapsone blood concentration.

Food
None significant.

Drug interactions of concern to dentistry
- None reported

DIAGNOSTIC TEST EFFECTS
None significant.

SIDE EFFECTS
Frequent (> 10%)
Hemolytic anemia, methemoglobinemia, rash

Occasional (10%–1%)
Hemolysis, photosensitivity reaction

SERIOUS REACTIONS
! Agranulocytosis and blood dyscrasias may occur.

DENTAL CONSIDERATIONS
General:
- Patients on chronic drug therapy may rarely have symptoms of blood dyscrasias, which can include infection, bleeding, and poor healing.
- Avoid dental light in patient's eyes; offer dark glasses for patient comfort.
- Advise patient if dental drugs prescribed have a potential for photosensitivity.

Consultations:
- In a patient with symptoms of blood dyscrasias, request a medical consultation for blood studies and postpone dental treatment until normal values are reestablished.

Teach Patient/Family:
• Importance of good oral hygiene to prevent soft tissue inflammation
• Caution to prevent injury when using oral hygiene aids

Daptomycin

dap′-toe-my-sin
(Cubicin)

CATEGORY AND SCHEDULE

Pregnancy Risk Category: B

MECHANISM OF ACTION

A lipopeptide antibacterial agent that binds to bacterial membranes and causes a rapid depolarization of the membrane potential. The loss of membrane potential leads to inhibition of protein, DNA, and RNA synthesis. ***Therapeutic Effect:*** Bactericidal.

PHARMACOKINETICS

Widely distributed. Protein binding: 90%. Primarily excreted unchanged in urine. Moderately removed by hemodialysis. ***Half-life:*** 7–8 hr (increased in impaired renal function).

AVAILABILITY

Powder for Injection: 250 mg/vial, 500 mg/vial.

INDICATIONS AND DOSAGES

▸ Complicated Skin and Skin-Structure Infections

IV

Adults, Elderly. 4 mg/kg every 24 hr for 7–14 days.

▸ Dosage in Renal Impairment

For patients with creatinine clearance of less than 30 ml/min, dosage is 4 mg/kg q48h for 7–14 days.

CONTRAINDICATIONS

None known.

INTERACTIONS

Drug

HMG-CoA reductase inhibitors: May cause myopathy.
Tobramycin: Increases the serum concentration of daptomycin.

Herbal

None known.

Food

None known.

Drug interactions of concern to dentistry

• None reported

DIAGNOSTIC TEST EFFECTS

May increase serum CPK levels. May alter liver function test results.

IV INCOMPATIBILITIES

Diluents containing dextrose. If the same IV line is used to administer different drugs, the line should be flushed with 0.9% NaCl.

SIDE EFFECTS

Frequent (6%–5%)

Constipation, nausea, peripheral injection site reactions, headache, diarrhea

Occasional (4%–3%)

Insomnia, rash, vomiting

Rare (< 3%)

Pruritus, dizziness, hypotension

SERIOUS REACTIONS

! Skeletal muscle myopathy, characterized by muscle pain and weakness, particularly of the distal extremities, occurs rarely.
! Antibiotic-associated colitis and other superinfections may result from altered bacterial balance.

DENTAL CONSIDERATIONS

General:

- Used in the hospital environment for serious infections.
- Determine why patient is taking the drug.
- Monitor vital signs, including temperature, blood pressure, and respiration characteristics and rate, at every appointment.

Consultations:

- Consult with patient's physician if an acute dental infection occurs and another antiinfective is required.

darbepoetin alfa

dar-beh-poe′-ee-tin
(Aranesp)
Do not confuse Aranesp with Aricept.

CATEGORY AND SCHEDULE

Pregnancy Risk Category: C

MECHANISM OF ACTION

A glycoprotein that stimulates formation of RBCs in bone marrow; increases serum half-life of epoetin. ***Therapeutic Effect:*** Induces erythropoiesis and release of reticulocytes from bone marrow.

PHARMACOKINETICS

Well absorbed after subcutaneous administration. ***Half-life:*** 48.5 hr.

AVAILABILITY

Injection: 25 mcg/ml, 40 mcg/ml, 60 mcg/ml, 100 mcg/ml, 150 mcg/ml, 200 mcg/ml, 300 mcg/ml.

INDICATIONS AND DOSAGES

▸ Anemia in Chronic Renal Failure

IV BOLUS, SUBCUTANEOUS
Adults, Elderly. Initially, 0.45 mcg/kg once weekly. Adjust dosage to achieve and maintain a target Hgb not to exceed 12 g/dl. Do not increase dosage more frequently than once monthly. Limit increases in Hgb by less than 1 g/dl over any 2-week period.

▸ Anemia Associated with Chemotherapy

IV, SUBCUTANEOUS
Adults, Elderly. 2.25 mcg/kg/dose once a week.

CONTRAINDICATIONS

History of sensitivity to mammalian cell-derived products or human albumin, uncontrolled hypertension

INTERACTIONS

Drug

None known.

Herbal

None known.

Food

None known.

Drug interactions of concern to dentistry

- No studies reported

DIAGNOSTIC TEST EFFECTS

May increase BUN, serum phosphorus, potassium, serum creatinine, serum uric acid, and sodium levels. May decrease bleeding time, serum iron concentration, and serum ferritin.

IV INCOMPATIBILITIES

Do not mix with other medications.

SIDE EFFECTS

Frequent

Myalgia, hypertension or hypotension, headache, diarrhea

Occasional
Fatigue, edema, vomiting, reaction at administration site, asthenia, dizziness

SERIOUS REACTIONS
! Vascular access thrombosis, CHF, sepsis, arrhythmias, and anaphylactic reaction occur rarely.

DENTAL CONSIDERATIONS
General:
- Monitor vital signs at every appointment because of cardiovascular side effects.
- Consider semisupine chair position for patient comfort if GI side effects occur.
- Monitor disease control and date of last dialysis.
- Prophylactic antibiotics may be indicated to prevent infection if surgery or deep scaling is planned.

Consultations:
- Medical consultation may be required to assess disease control and patient's ability to tolerate stress.

Teach Patient/Family:
- Importance of good oral hygiene to prevent soft tissue inflammation, infection
- Importance of updating health and drug history if physician makes any changes in evaluation or drug regimens

daunorubicin citrate liposome
dawn-oh-rue′-bih-sin
(DaunoXome)
Do not confuse with dactinomycin or doxorubicin.

CATEGORY AND SCHEDULE
Pregnancy Risk Category: D

MECHANISM OF ACTION
An anthracycline antibiotic that is cell cycle-phase nonspecific. Most active in S phase of cell division. Appears to bind to DNA.
Therapeutic Effect: Inhibits DNA, DNA-dependent RNA synthesis.

PHARMACOKINETICS
Widely distributed. Does not cross blood-brain barrier. Protein binding: High. Metabolized in liver to active metabolite. Excreted in urine, eliminated by biliary excretion.
Half-life: 18.5 hrs; metabolite: 26.7 hrs.

AVAILABILITY
Injection: 2 mg/ml (DaunoXome).

INDICATIONS AND DOSAGES
▸ Kaposi's Sarcoma
IV
Adults. 20–40 mg/m^2 over 1 hour. Repeat q2wk or 100 mg/m^2 q3wk.

OFF-LABEL USES
Treatment of chronic myelocytic leukemia, Ewing's sarcoma, neuroblastoma, non-Hodgkin's lymphoma, Wilms' tumor

CONTRAINDICATIONS
Arrhythmias, congestive heart failure (CHF), left ventricular ejection fraction less than 40%, preexisting bone marrow suppression

INTERACTIONS
Drug
Antigout medications: May decrease the effects of these drugs.
Bone marrow depressants: May enhance myelosuppression.
Live virus vaccines: May potentiate virus replication, increase vaccine side effects, and decrease the patient's antibody response to vaccine.

Herbal
None known.
Food
None known.
Drug interactions of concern to dentistry
- Dental drug interactions have not been studied

DIAGNOSTIC TEST EFFECTS
May increase serum alkaline phosphatase, serum bilirubin, serum uric acid, and serum glutamate oxaloacetate (SGOT) (aspartate aminotransferase [AST]) levels.

IV INCOMPATIBILITIES
Do not mix with any other solution, especially NaCl or bacteriostatic agents (e.g., benzyl alcohol).

SIDE EFFECTS
Frequent
Mild to moderate nausea, fatigue, fever
Occasional
Diarrhea, abdominal pain, esophagitis, stomatitis (redness or burning of oral mucous membranes, inflammation of gums or tongue), transverse pigmentation of fingernails and toenails
Rare
Transient fever, chills

SERIOUS REACTIONS
! Bone marrow depression manifested as hematologic toxicity (severe leukopenia, anemia, and thrombocytopenia) may occur.
! Decreases in platelet and white blood cell (WBC) counts occur in 10 to 14 days and return to normal levels by the third week of daunorubicin treatment.
! Cardiotoxicity noted as either acute with transient abnormal ECG findings or as chronic with cardiomyopathy manifested as congestive heart failure (CHF). The risk of cardiotoxicity increases when the cumulative dose exceeds 550 mg/m^2 in adults and 300 mg/m^2 in children older than 2 years or when the total dosage is greater than 10 mg/kg in children younger than 2 years.

DENTAL CONSIDERATIONS
General:
- Determine why patient is taking the drug.
- Assess salivary flow as a factor in caries, periodontal disease, and candidiasis.
- Administered in the hospital; AIDS patients will be taking many other medications; confirm medical and drug history.

Consultations:
- In a patient with symptoms of blood dyscrasias, request a medical consultation for blood studies and postpone treatment until normal values are reestablished.
- Medical consultation may be required to assess disease control and patient's ability to tolerate stress.

Teach Patient/Family:
- Importance of good oral hygiene to prevent soft tissue inflammation
- To prevent trauma when using oral hygiene aids
- To report oral lesions, soreness, or bleeding to dentist
- *When chronic dry mouth occurs advise patient:*
  - To avoid mouth rinses with high alcohol content due to drying effects
  - To use daily home fluoride products for anticaries effect
  - To use sugarless gum, frequent sips of water or saliva substitutes
- Importance of updating health and medication history if physician makes any changes in evaluation or drug regimens; include OTC, herbal, and nonherbal remedies in the update

delavirdine mesylate

deh-la′-ver-deen
(Rescriptor)

CATEGORY AND SCHEDULE

Pregnancy Risk Category: C
Do not confuse Rescriptor with Retrovin or Ritonavir.

MECHANISM OF ACTION

A nonnucleoside reverse transcriptase inhibitor that binds directly to HIV-1 reverse transcriptase and blocks RNA- and DNA-dependent DNA polymerase activities. ***Therapeutic Effect:*** Interrupts HIV replication, slowing the progression of HIV infection.

PHARMACOKINETICS

Rapidly absorbed after PO administration. Protein binding: 98%. Primarily distributed in plasma. Metabolized in the liver. Eliminated in feces and urine. ***Half-life:*** 2–11 hr.

AVAILABILITY

Tablets: 100 mg, 200 mg.

INDICATIONS AND DOSAGES

▸ **HIV Infection (in Combination with Other Antiretrovirals)**

PO

Adults. 400 mg 3 times a day.

CONTRAINDICATIONS

None known.

INTERACTIONS

Drug

Benzodiazepines, calcium channel blockers: May cause life-threatening adverse reactions.
Carbamazepine, phenobarbital, phenytoin: May decrease delavirdine blood concentration.
H_2 blockers: May decrease delavirdine absorption.
Rifampin: May decrease delavirdine blood concentrations.

Herbal

None known.

Food

None known.

Drug interactions of concern to dentistry

- Reduced absorption: antacids, cimetidine, other H_2-receptor antagonists
- Increased plasma levels of both delavirdine and clarithromycin
- Increased plasma levels of alprazolam, triazolam, midazolam
- Avoid coadministration with carbamazepine, phenobarbital, ketoconazole, fluoxetine

DIAGNOSTIC TEST EFFECTS

May increase AST (SGOT) and ALT (SGPT) levels. May decrease neutrophil count.

SIDE EFFECTS

Frequent (18%)
Rash, pruritus
Occasional (> 2%)
Headache, nausea, diarrhea, fatigue, anorexia

SERIOUS REACTIONS

! None known.

DENTAL CONSIDERATIONS

General:

- Examine for oral manifestation of opportunistic infection.
- Patients on chronic drug therapy may rarely have symptoms of blood dyscrasias, which can include infection, bleeding, and poor healing.
- Assess salivary flow as a factor in caries, periodontal disease, and candidiasis.

- After supine positioning, have patient sit upright for at least 2 min before standing to avoid orthostatic hypotension.
- Do not use ingestible sodium bicarbonate products, such as the Prophy-Jet air polishing system, within 2 hr of drug use.

Consultations:

- In a patient with symptoms of blood dyscrasias, request a medical consultation for blood studies and postpone treatment until normal values are reestablished.
- Medical consultation may be required to assess disease control and patient's ability to tolerate stress.

Teach Patient/Family:

- Importance of good oral hygiene to prevent soft tissue inflammation
- Caution to prevent trauma when using oral hygiene aids
- That secondary oral infection may occur; must see dentist immediately if infection occurs
- *When chronic dry mouth occurs, advise patient:*
  - To avoid mouth rinses with high alcohol content because of drying effects
  - To use daily home fluoride products for anticaries effect
  - To use sugarless gum, frequent sips of water, or saliva substitutes

demecarium bromide

de-mi-kare′-ee-um bro′-mide
(Humorsol Ocumeter)

CATEGORY AND SCHEDULE

Pregnancy Risk Category: X

MECHANISM OF ACTION

A cholinesterase inhibitor that increases the concentration of acetylcholine at cholinergic receptor sites and produces effects equivalent to excessive stimulation of cholinergic receptors. ***Therapeutic Effect:*** Reduces intraocular pressure due to facilitation of outflow of aqueous humor.

PHARMACOKINETICS

Decreases intraocular pressure within a few hours. The duration is variable among individuals.

AVAILABILITY

Ophthalmic solution: 0.125%, 0.25% (Humorsol).

INDICATIONS AND DOSAGES

▸ **Glaucoma**

OPHTHALMIC, TOPICAL

Adults, Elderly. 1–2 drops of the 0.125% or 0.25% solution in affected eye(s) twice daily to twice weekly.

▸ **Cyclostimulant**

OPHTHALMIC, TOPICAL

Adults, Elderly. 1 drop of 0.125% or 0.25% solution in each eye daily for 2 to 3 weeks, followed by 1 drop every 2 days for 4 weeks.

▸ **Diagnostic Aid (Accommodative Esotropia)**

OPHTHALMIC, TOPICAL

Adults, Elderly. 1 drop of 0.125% or 0.25% solution once a day for 2 weeks, then 1 drop every 2 days for 2–3 weeks.

CONTRAINDICATIONS

Pregnancy, active uveal inflammation and/or glaucoma associated with iridocyclitis, hypersensitivity to demecarium or any component of the formulation.

INTERACTIONS

Drug

Succinylcholine, other anticholinesterase agents: May cause additive effects.

Herbal

None known.

Food

None known.

Drug interactions of concern to dentistry

- Avoid use of succinylcholine in general anesthesia
- Possible inhibition of the metabolism of: ester-type local and topical anesthetics
- Avoid use of anticholinergics, such as systemic atropine or related drugs

DIAGNOSTIC TEST EFFECTS

None known.

SIDE EFFECTS

Occasional

Browache, nausea, vomiting, abdominal cramps, diarrhea, hypersalivation, urinary incontinence, lid muscle twitching, redness, myopia blurred vision, increase in intraocular pressure, iris cysts, breathing difficulties, increased sweating

SERIOUS REACTIONS

! Systemic absorption has been associated with demecarium resulting in anticholinesterase toxicity.

! Overdosage can produce cholinergic crisis characterized by cardiac arrhythmias, diarrhea, muscle weakness, profuse sweating, respiratory difficulties, urinary incontinence, and shock.

DENTAL CONSIDERATIONS

General:

- Determine why patient is taking the drug.
- Avoid drugs with anticholinergic activity, such as antihistamines, opioids, benzodiazepines, propantheline, atropine, and scopolamine.
- Avoid dental light in patient's eyes; offer dark glasses for patient comfort.
- Protect patient's eyes from accidental spatter during dental treatment.
- Question glaucoma patient about compliance with prescribed drug regimen.

Consultations:

- Medical consultation may be required to assess disease control.

Teach Patient/Family:

- Importance of updating health and medication history if physician makes any changes in evaluation or drug regimens; include OTC, herbal, and nonherbal remedies in the update

demeclocycline hydrochloride

dem-e-kloe-sye′-kleen
(Declomycin, Ledermycin[AUS])

CATEGORY AND SCHEDULE

Pregnancy Risk Category: D

MECHANISM OF ACTION

A tetracycline antibiotic that inhibits bacterial protein synthesis by binding to ribosomal receptor sites; also inhibits ADH-induced water reabsorption. ***Therapeutic Effect:*** Bacteriostatic; also produces water diuresis.

AVAILABILITY

Tablets: 150 mg, 300 mg.

INDICATIONS AND DOSAGES

▸ Mild to Moderate Infections, Including Acne, Pertussis, Chronic Bronchitis, and UTIs

PO

Adults, Elderly. 150 mg 4 times a day or 300 mg 2 times a day.
Children older than 8 yr.
8–12 mg/kg/day in 2–4 divided doses.

▸ Uncomplicated Gonorrhea

PO

Adults. Initially, 600 mg, then 300 mg q12h for 4 days for total of 3 g.

▸ Syndrome of Inappropriate ADH Secretion (SIADH)

PO

Adults, Elderly. Initially, 900–1200 mg/day in 3–4 divided doses, then decrease dose to 600–900 mg/day in divided doses.

CONTRAINDICATIONS

Children 8 years and younger, last half of pregnancy

INTERACTIONS

Drug

Antacids containing aluminum, calcium, or magnesium; laxatives containing magnesium; oral iron preparations: Impair the absorption of demeclocycline.
Cholestyramine, colestipol: May decrease demeclocycline absorption.
Oral contraceptives: May decrease the effects of oral contraceptives.

Herbal

None known.

Food

Dairy products: May decrease demeclocycline absorption.

Drug interactions of concern to dentistry

- Decreased effect of penicillins, cephalosporins, oral contraceptives
- Oral contraceptives: advise patient of a potential risk for decreased contraceptive action, to maintain compliance with oral contraceptive use while using antibiotics, and to consider the use of additional nonhormonal contraception
- Contraindicated with isotretinoin (Accutane)

DIAGNOSTIC TEST EFFECTS

May increase BUN and serum alkaline phosphatase, amylase, bilirubin, AST (SGOT), and ALT (SGPT) levels.

SIDE EFFECTS

Frequent

Anorexia, nausea, vomiting, diarrhea, dysphagia, possibly severe photosensitivity (with moderate to high demeclocycline dosage).

Occasional

Urticaria, rash; diabetes insipidus syndrome, marked by polydipsia, polyuria, and weakness (with long-term therapy).

SERIOUS REACTIONS

! Superinfection (especially fungal), anaphylaxis, and benign intracranial hypertension occur rarely.
! Bulging fontanelles occur rarely in infants.

DENTAL CONSIDERATIONS

General:

- Examine oral cavity for side effects if on long-term drug therapy.
- Determine why the patient is taking the drug.
- Do not prescribe during pregnancy or before age 8 yr because of tooth discoloration.
- Absorption is reduced by dairy products, metals, and antacids.

Consultations:

- Medical consultation may be required to assess disease control.

Teach Patient/Family:
- Importance of good oral hygiene to prevent soft tissue inflammation
- Caution to prevent injury when using oral hygiene aids
- *When used for dental infection, advise patient:*
  - To report sore throat, oral burning sensation, fever, and fatigue, any of which could indicate superinfection
  - To take at prescribed intervals and complete dosage regimen
  - To immediately notify the dentist if signs or symptoms of infection increase

desipramine hydrochloride

dess-ip′-ra-meen
(Apo-Desipramine[CAN], Norpramin, Novo-Desipramine[CAN], Pertofran[AUS])
Do not confuse desipramine with clomipramine, disopyramide, imipramine, or nortriptyline.

CATEGORY AND SCHEDULE
Pregnancy Risk Category: C

MECHANISM OF ACTION
A tricyclic antidepressant that blocks the reuptake of neurotransmitters, such as norepinephrine and serotonin, at presynaptic membranes, increasing their availability at postsynaptic receptor sites. Also has strong anticholinergic activity.
Therapeutic Effect: Relieves depression.

PHARMACOKINETICS
Rapidly, and well absorbed from the GI tract. Protein binding: 90%. Metabolized in the liver. Primarily excreted in urine. Minimally removed by hemodialysis. ***Half-life:*** 12–27 hr.

AVAILABILITY
Tablets: 10 mg, 25 mg, 50 mg, 75 mg, 100 mg, 150 mg.

INDICATIONS AND DOSAGES
▸ **Depression**
PO
Adults. 75 mg/day. May gradually increase to 150–200 mg/day. Maximum: 300 mg/day.
Elderly. Initially, 10–25 mg/day. May gradually increase to 75–100 mg/day. Maximum: 300 mg/day.
Children older than 12 yr. Initially, 25–50 mg/day. May gradually increase to 100 mg/day. Maximum: 150 mg/day.
Children 6–12 yr. 1–3 mg/kg/day. Maximum: 5 mg/kg/day.

OFF-LABEL USES
Treatment of attention deficit hyperactivity disorder, bulimia nervosa, cataplexy associated with narcolepsy, cocaine withdrawal, neurogenic pain, panic disorder

CONTRAINDICATIONS
Angle-closure glaucoma, use within 14 days of MAOIs

INTERACTIONS
Drug
Alcohol, other CNS depressants: May increase CNS and respiratory depression and the hypotensive effects of desipramine.
Antithyroid agents: May increase the risk of agranulocytosis.

Cimetidine: May increase desipramine blood concentration and risk of toxicity.
Clonidine, guanadrel: May decrease the effects of these drugs.
MAOIs: May increase the risk of neuroleptic malignant syndrome, hyperpyrexia, hypertensive crisis, and seizures.
Phenothiazines: May increase the anticholinergic and sedative effects of desipramine.
Phenytoin: May decrease the desipramine blood concentration.
Sympathomimetics: May increase the risk of cardiac effects.

Herbal

St. John's wort: May increase desipramine's pharmacologic effects and risk of toxicity.

Food

None known.

Drug interactions of concern to dentistry

- Increased anticholinergic effects: muscarinic blockers, antihistamines, phenothiazines
- Increased effects of direct-acting sympathomimetics: epinephrine, levonordefrin
- Potential risk for increased CNS depression: alcohol, barbiturates, benzodiazepines, and other CNS depressants
- Decreased antihypertensive effects: clonidine, guanadrel, guanethidine
- At higher tricyclic doses, serum levels of fluconazole and ketoconazole may be elevated
- Avoid concurrent use with St. John's wort (herb)

DIAGNOSTIC TEST EFFECTS

May alter blood glucose level and ECG readings. Therapeutic serum drug level is 115–300 ng/ml; toxic serum drug level is greater than 400 ng/ml.

SIDE EFFECTS

Frequent

Somnolence, fatigue, dry mouth, blurred vision, constipation, delayed micturition, orthostatic hypotension, diaphoresis, impaired concentration, increased appetite, urine retention

Occasional

GI disturbances (such as nausea, GI distress, metallic taste)

Rare

Paradoxical reactions (agitation, restlessness, nightmares, insomnia), extrapyramidal symptoms (particularly fine hand tremor)

SERIOUS REACTIONS

! Overdose may produce confusion, seizures, somnolence, arrhythmias, fever, hallucinations, dyspnea, vomiting, and unusual fatigue or weakness.
! Abrupt discontinuation after prolonged therapy may produce severe headache, malaise, nausea, vomiting, and vivid dreams.

DENTAL CONSIDERATIONS

General:

- Take vital signs at every appointment because of cardiovascular side effects.
- Assess salivary flow as a factor in caries, periodontal disease, and candidiasis.
- Patients on chronic drug therapy may rarely have symptoms of blood dyscrasias, which can include infection, bleeding, and poor healing.
- After supine positioning, have patient sit upright for at least 2 min to avoid orthostatic hypotension.
- Use vasoconstrictors with caution, in low doses, and with careful aspiration.

Avoid use of gingival retraction cord with epinephrine.
• Place on frequent recall because of oral side effects.

Consultations:
• In a patient with symptoms of blood dyscrasias, request a medical consultation for blood studies and postpone dental treatment until normal values are reestablished.
• Medical consultation may be required to assess disease control.
• Physician should be informed if significant xerostomic side effects occur (e.g., increased caries, sore tongue, problems eating or swallowing, difficulty wearing prosthesis) so that a medication change can be considered.

Teach Patient/Family:
• Importance of good oral hygiene to prevent soft tissue inflammation
• Caution to prevent injury when using oral hygiene aids
• *When chronic dry mouth occurs, advise patient:*
  • To avoid mouth rinses with high alcohol content because of drying effects
  • To use daily home fluoride products for anticaries effect
  • To use sugarless gum, frequent sips of water, or saliva substitutes

desirudin
deh-sear′-ew-din
(Iprivask)

CATEGORY AND SCHEDULE
Pregnancy Risk Category: C

MECHANISM OF ACTION
An anticoagulant that binds specifically and directly to thrombin, inhibiting free circulating and clot-bound thrombin. ***Therapeutic Effect:*** Prolongs the clotting time of human plasma.

PHARMACOKINETICS
Completely absorbed. Distributed in extracellular space. Metabolized and eliminated by the kidney. ***Half-life:*** 2–3 hr.

AVAILABILITY
Powder for Injection: 15-mg vial with diluent (diluent includes 0.6 ml mannitol [3%] in water for injection).

INDICATIONS AND DOSAGES
▸ **Prevention of Deep Vein Thrombosis in Patients Nndergoing Hip Replacement Surgery**
SUBCUTANEOUS
Adults, Elderly. Initially, 15 mg q12h given 5–15 min before surgery but following induction of regional block anesthesia, if used. May administer up to 12 days post surgery.
▸ **Moderate Renal Impairment (Creatinine Clearance 31–60 ml/min or Higher)**
SUBCUTANEOUS
Adults, Elderly. 5 mg q12h.
▸ **Severe Renal Impairment (Creatinine Clearance < 31 ml/min)**
SUBCUTANEOUS
Adults, Elderly. 1.7 mg q12h.

CONTRAINDICATIONS
Hypersensitivity to natural or recombinant hirudins (anticoagulation factors), active bleeding, irreversible coagulation disorders

INTERACTIONS
Drug
Anticoagulants, dextran 40, systemic glucocorticoids, thrombolytics: Increase the risk of

bleeding and should be discontinued before start of desirudin therapy.

Herbal

None known.

Food

None known.

Drug interactions of concern to dentistry

- Increased risk of bleeding: salicylates, NSAIDs, or any drug that affects coagulation

DIAGNOSTIC TEST EFFECTS

May increase aPTT. May decrease Hgb, and Hct concentrations.

SIDE EFFECTS

Frequent (6%)

Hematoma

Occasional (4%–2%)

Injection site mass, wound secretion, nausea, hypersensitivity reaction

SERIOUS REACTIONS

! Serious or major hemorrhage and anaphylactic reaction occur rarely.

DENTAL CONSIDERATIONS

General:

- Patients are at risk of bleeding, so check for oral signs.
- Product may be used in outpatient therapy. Delay elective dental treatment until patient completes anticoagulant therapy.
- Determine why patient is taking the drug.
- Avoid products that affect platelet function, such as aspirin and NSAIDs.
- Consider local hemostasis measures to prevent excessive bleeding.

Consultations:

- Medical consultation should include partial prothrombin time, prothrombin time, or INR.
- Medical consultation may be required to assess disease control and patient's ability to tolerate stress.

Teach Patient/Family:

- To use soft tooth brush to reduce risk of bleeding
- Importance of good oral hygiene to prevent soft tissue inflammation
- To report oral lesions, soreness, or bleeding to dentist
- To prevent trauma when using oral hygiene aids
- Importance of updating health and medication history if physician makes any changes in evaluation or drug regimens; include OTC, herbal, and nonherbal remedies in the update

desloratadine

des-loer-at′-ah-deen

(Aerius[CAN], Clarinex, Clarinex Redi-Tabs)

CATEGORY AND SCHEDULE

Pregnancy Risk Category: C

Do not confuse Clarinex with Claritin.

MECHANISM OF ACTION

A nonsedating antihistamine that exhibits selective peripheral histamine H_1 receptor blocking action. Competes with histamine at receptor sites. ***Therapeutic Effect:*** Prevents allergic responses mediated by histamine, such as rhinitis and urticaria.

PHARMACOKINETICS

Rapidly and almost completely absorbed from the GI tract. Distributed mainly in liver, lungs, GI tract, and bile. Metabolized in the liver to active metabolite and undergoes extensive first-pass metabolism. Eliminated in urine and feces. ***Half-life:*** 27 hr (increased in the elderly and in renal or hepatic impairment).

AVAILABILITY

Tablets: 5 mg.
Tablets (Orally Disintegrating [Reditabs]): 5 mg.
Syrup: 2.5 mg/5 ml.

INDICATIONS AND DOSAGES

▸ Allergic Rhinitis, Urticaria

PO
Adults, Elderly, Children older than 12 yr. 5 mg once a day.

▸ Dosage in Hepatic or Renal Impairment

Dosage is decreased to 5 mg every other day.

CONTRAINDICATIONS

None known.

INTERACTIONS

Drug

Erythromycin, ketoconazole: May increase desloratidine blood concentration.

Herbal

None known.

Food

None known.

Drug interactions of concern to dentistry

- Limited studies with concurrent doses of erythromycin; ketoconazole and azithromycin show slight elevations of plasma levels, but no clinically relevant changes in electrocardiographic parameters
- One report indicated a potential for increased anticholinergic effects with other anticholinergic drugs and increased somnolence with CNS depressants; however, data are lacking

DIAGNOSTIC TEST EFFECTS

May suppress wheal and flare reactions to antigen skin testing unless the drug is discontinued 4 days before testing.

SIDE EFFECTS

Frequent (12%)
Headache
Occasional (3%)
Dry mouth, somnolence
Rare (< 3%)
Fatigue, dizziness, diarrhea, nausea

SERIOUS REACTIONS

! None known.

DENTAL CONSIDERATIONS

General:

- Assess salivary flow as a factor in caries, periodontal disease, and candidiasis.

Teach Patient/Family:

- Importance of good oral hygiene to prevent soft tissue inflammation
- *When chronic dry mouth occurs, advise patient:*
  - To avoid mouth rinses with high alcohol content because of drying effects
  - To use sugarless gum, frequent sips of water, or saliva substitutes
  - To use daily home fluoride products for anticaries effect

desmopressin

des-moe-press′-in
(DDAVP, Minirin[AUS], Octostim[CAN], Stimate)

CATEGORY AND SCHEDULE

Pregnancy Risk Category: B

MECHANISM OF ACTION
A synthetic pituitary hormone that increases reabsorption of water by increasing permeability of collecting ducts of the kidneys. Also serves as a plasminogen activator. ***Therapeutic Effect:*** Increases plasma factor VIII (antihemophilic factor). Decreases urinary output.

PHARMACOKINETICS

Route	Onset	Peak	Duration
PO	1 hr	2–7 hr	6–8 hr
IV	15–30 min	1.5–3 hr	N/A
Intranasal	15 min–1 hr	1–5 hr	5–21 hr

Poorly absorbed after oral or nasal administration. Metabolism: Unknown. ***Half-life:*** Oral: 1.5–2.5 hr. Intranasal: 3.3–3.5 hr. IV: 0.4–4 hr.

AVAILABILITY
Tablets (DDAVP): 0.1 mg, 0.2 mg.
Injection (DDAVP): 4 mcg/ml.
Nasal Solution (DDAVP): 100 mcg/ml.
Nasal Spray (Stimate): 1.5 mg/ml (150 mcg/spray).
NAsal Spray (DDAVP): 100 mcg/ml (10 mcg/spray).

INDICATIONS AND DOSAGES
▸ Primary Nocturnal Enuresis
PO
Children 12 yr and older. 0.2–0.6 mg once before bedtime.
INTRANASAL
Children 6 yr and older. Initially, 20 mcg (0.2 ml) at bedtime; use one-half dose in each nostril. Adjust to maximum of 40 mcg/day.
▸ Central Cranial Diabetes Insipidus
PO
Adults, Elderly, Children 12 yr and older. Initially, 0.05 mg twice a day. Range: 0.1–1.2 mg/day in 2–3 divided doses.
Children younger than 12 yr. Initially, 0.05 mg; then twice a day. Range: 0.1–0.8 mg daily.
IV, SUBCUTANEOUS
Adults, Elderly, Children 12 yr and older. 2–4 mcg/day in 2 divided doses or 1/10 of maintenance intranasal dose.
INTRANASAL
Adults, Elderly, Children older than 12 yr. 5–40 mcg (0.05–0.4 ml) in 1–3 doses/day.
Children 3 mo–12 yr. Initially, 5 mcg (0.05 ml)/day. Range: 5–30 mcg (0.05–0.3 ml)/day.
▸ Hemophilia A, Von Willebrand's Disease (Type I)
IV INFUSION
Adults, Elderly, Children weighing more than 10 kg. 0.3 mcg/kg diluted in 50 ml 0.9% NaCl.
Children weighing 10 kg and less. 0.3 mcg/kg diluted in 10 ml 0.9% NaCl.
INTRANASAL
Adults, Elderly, Children 12 yr and older weighing more than 50 kg. 300 mcg; use 1 spray in each nostril.
Adults, Elderly, Children 12 yr and older weighing 50 kg or less. 150 mcg as a single spray.

CONTRAINDICATIONS
Hemophilia A with factor VIII levels less than 5%; hemophilia B; severe type I, type IIB, or platelet-type von Willebrand's disease

INTERACTIONS
Drug
Carbamazepine, chlorpropamide, clofibrate: May increase the effects of desmopressin.
Demeclocycline, lithium, norepinephrine: May decrease effects of desmopressin.
Herbal
None known.

Food
None known.

Drug interactions of concern to dentistry
- Decreased antidiuretic effects: demeclocycline
- Increased antidiuretic effects: carbamazepine

DIAGNOSTIC TEST EFFECTS
None known.

SIDE EFFECTS
Occasional
IV: Pain, redness, or swelling at injection site; headache; abdominal cramps; vulval pain; flushed skin; mild BP elevation; nausea with high dosages
Nasal: Rhinorrhea, nasal congestion, slight BP elevation

SERIOUS REACTIONS
! Water intoxication or hyponatremia, marked by headache, somnolence, confusion, decreased urination, rapid weight gain, seizures, and coma, may occur in overhydration. Children, elderly patients, and infants are especially at risk.

DENTAL CONSIDERATIONS
General:
- Monitor vital signs at every appointment because of cardiovascular side effects.
- Avoid prescribing aspirin-containing products if treatment is for bleeding disorder.
- Consider local hemostasis measures to prevent excessive bleeding.
- Determine why the patient is taking the drug.
- Consider semisupine chair position for patient comfort because of GI effects of disease.

Consultations:
- Medical consultation may be required to assess disease control; definite consultation for patients with chronic bleeding disorders.
- Medical consultation should include partial prothrombin time or PT.

Teach Patient/Family:
- To advise dentist if excessive bleeding occurs or continues after dental treatment

desonide
dess′-oh-nide
(Delonide, Desocrot[CAN], DesOwen, Scheinpharm Desonide[CAN], Tridesilon)

CATEGORY AND SCHEDULE
Pregnancy Risk Category: C

MECHANISM OF ACTION
A topical corticosteroid that has anti-inflammatory, antipruritic, and vasoconstrictive properties. The exact mechanism of the anti-inflammatory process is unclear.
Therapeutic Effect: Reduces or prevents tissue response to the inflammatory process.

PHARMACOKINETICS
Large variation in absorption determined by many factors. Metabolized in the liver. Primarily excreted by the kidneys and small amounts in the bile.

AVAILABILITY
Lotion: 0.05% (DesOwen).
Cream: 0.05% (DesOwen).
Ointment: 0.05% (DesOwen, Tridesilon).

INDICATIONS AND DOSAGES

▸ Dermatoses

TOPICAL

Adults, Elderly. Apply sparingly 2–3 times/day.

▸ Otitis Externa

AURAL

Adults, Elderly, Children. Instill 3 to 4 drops into the ear 3–4 times/day.

CONTRAINDICATIONS

Perforated eardrum, history of hypersensitivity to desonide or other corticosteroids

INTERACTIONS

Drug

Bupropion: May lower the seizure threshold.

Herbal

None known.

Food

None known.

DIAGNOSTIC TEST EFFECTS

None known.

SIDE EFFECTS

Occasional

Burning and stinging at site of application, dryness, skin peeling, contact dermatitis

SERIOUS REACTIONS

! The serious reactions of long-term therapy and the addition of occlusive dressings are reversible hypothalamic-pituitary-adrenal (HPA) axis suppression, manifestations of Cushing's syndrome, hyperglycemia and glucosuria.

DENTAL CONSIDERATIONS

General:

- Determine why the patient is taking the drug.
- Place on frequent recall to evaluate healing response if used on chronic basis.
- Apply lubricant to dry lips for patient comfort before dental procedures.

desoximetasone

des-ox-i-met′-a-sone

(Taro-Desoximetason[CAN], Topicort, Topicort-LP)

Do not confuse with dexamethasone.

CATEGORY AND SCHEDULE

Pregnancy Risk Category: C

MECHANISM OF ACTION

A high-potency, fluoronated topical corticosteroid that has anti-inflammatory, antipruritic, and vasoconstrictive properties. The exact mechanism of the anti-inflammatory process is unclear. ***Therapeutic Effect:*** Reduces tissue response to the inflammatory process.

PHARMACOKINETICS

Large variation in absorption among sites. Protein binding in varying degrees. Metabolized in liver. Primarily excreted in urine.

AVAILABILITY

Cream: 0.25% (Topicort), 0.05% (Topicort-LP).
Gel: 0.05% (Topicort).
Ointment: 0.25% (Topicort).

INDICATIONS AND DOSAGES

▸ Dermatoses

TOPICAL

Adults, Elderly. Apply sparingly 2 times/day.

Children. Apply sparingly 1–2 times/day.

OFF-LABEL USES
Eczema, psoriasis vulgaris

CONTRAINDICATIONS
History of hypersensitivity to desoximetasone or other corticosteroids

INTERACTIONS
Drug
None known.
Herbal
None known.
Food
None known.

DIAGNOSTIC TEST EFFECTS
None known.

SIDE EFFECTS
Frequent
Itching, redness, irritation, burning at site of application
Occasional
Dryness, folliculitis, hypertrichosis, acneiform eruptions, hypopigmentation, perioral dermatitis
Rare
Allergic contact dermatitis, adrenal suppression, atrophy, striae, miliaria, photosensitivity

SERIOUS REACTIONS
! Serious reactions of long-term therapy and addition of occlusive dressings are reversible hypothalamic-pituitary-adrenal (HPA) axis suppression, manifestations of Cushing's syndrome, hyperglycemia, and glucosuria.
! Abruptly withdrawing the drug after long-term therapy may require supplemental systemic corticosteroids.

DENTAL CONSIDERATIONS
General:
- Gel formulations are used in the treatment of oral lichen planus lesions when the diagnosis has been confirmed by immunofluorescent biopsy testing.
- Place on frequent recall to evaluate healing response.

Teach Patient/Family:
- When used for oral lesions, advise patient to return for oral evaluation if response of oral tissues has not occurred in 7–14 days
- Importance of good oral hygiene to prevent soft tissue inflammation
- That use on oral herpetic ulcerations is contraindicated
- To apply at bedtime or after meals for maximum effect
- To apply with cotton-tipped applicator, dabbing gently, not rubbing medication on lesion

dexamethasone
dex-a-meth′-a-sone
(Decadron, Desamethasone Intensol, Dexasone, Dexasone LA, Dexmethsone[AUS], Diodex[CAN], Hexadrol[CAN], Maxidex, Solurex, Solurex LA)
Do not confuse dexamethasone with desoximetasone or dextramethophan, or Maxidex with Maxzide.

CATEGORY AND SCHEDULE
Pregnancy Risk Category: C
(D if used in the first trimester)

MECHANISM OF ACTION
A long-acting glucocorticoid that inhibits accumulation of

inflammatory cells at inflammation sites, phagocytosis, lysosomal enzyme release and synthesis, and release of mediators of inflammation. ***Therapeutic Effect:*** Prevents and suppresses cell and tissue immune reactions and inflammatory process.

PHARMACOKINETICS

Rapidly, completely absorbed from the GI tract after oral administration. Widely distributed. Protein binding: High. Metabolized in the liver. Primarily excreted in urine. Minimally removed by hemodialysis. ***Half-life:*** 3–4.5 hr.

AVAILABILITY

Elixir: 0.5 mg/5 ml, 1 mg/ml.
Inhalant Ointment.
Inhalant Solution.
Inhalant Suspension.
Intranasal Ointment.
Intranasal Solution.
Intranasal Suspension.
Ophthalmic Ointment.
Ophthalmic Solution.
Oral Solution: 0.5 mg/5 ml, 0.5 mg/0.5 ml.
Tablets: 0.25 mg, 0.5 mg, 0.75 mg, 1 mg, 1.5 mg, 2 mg, 4 mg, 6 mg.
Topical Aerosol.
Topical Cream.
Injection: 4 mg/ml.

INDICATIONS AND DOSAGES

▸ Anti-inflammatory

PO, IV, IM

Adults, Elderly. 0.75–9 mg/day in divided doses q6–12h.
Children. 0.08–0.3 mg/kg/day in divided doses q6–12h.

▸ Cerebral Edema

IV

Adults, Elderly. Initially, 10 mg, then 4 mg (IV or IM) q6h.

PO, IV, IM

Children. Loading dose of 1–2 mg/kg, then 1–1.5 mg/kg/day in divided doses q4–6h.

▸ Nausea and Vomiting in Chemotherapy Patients

IV

Adults, Elderly. 8–20 mg once, then 4 mg (PO) q4–6h or 8 mg q8h.
Children. 10 mg/m²/dose (Maximum: 20 mg), then 5 mg/m²/dose q6h.

▸ Physiologic Replacement

PO, IV, IM

Children. 0.03–0.15 mg/kg/day in divided doses q6–12h.

▸ Usual Ophthalmic Dosage, Ocular Inflammatory Conditions

OINTMENT

Adults, Elderly, Children. Thin coating 3–4 times/day.

SUSPENSION

Adults, Elderly, Children. Initially, 2 drops q1h while awake and q2h at night for 1 day, then reduce to 3–4 times/day.

CONTRAINDICATIONS

Active untreated infections, fungal, tuberculosis, or viral diseases of the eye

INTERACTIONS

Drug

Amphotericin: May increase hypokalemia.
Digoxin: May increase digoxin toxicity caused by hypokalemia.
Diuretics, insulin, oral hypoglycemics, potassium supplements: May decrease the effects of these drugs.
Hepatic enzyme inducers: May decrease the effects of dexamethasone.
Live-virus vaccines: May decrease the patient's antibody response to vaccine, increase vaccine side effects, and potentiate virus replication.

Herbal
None known.
Food
None known.

DIAGNOSTIC TEST EFFECTS

May increase blood glucose and serum lipid, amylase, and sodium levels. May decrease serum calcium, potassium, and thyroxine levels.

IV INCOMPATIBILITIES

Ciprofloxacin (Cipro), daunorubicin (Cerubidine), idarubicin (Idamycin), midazolam (Versed)

IV COMPATIBILITIES

Aminophylline, cimetidine (Tagamet), cisplatin (Platinol), cyclophosphamide (Cytoxan), cytarabine (Cytosar), docetaxel (Taxotere), doxorubicin (Adriamycin), etoposide (VePesid), granisetron (Kytril), heparin, hydromorphone (Dilaudid), lorazepam (Ativan), morphine, ondansetron (Zofran), paclitaxel (Taxol), potassium chloride, propofol (Diprivan)

SIDE EFFECTS

Frequent
Inhalation: Cough, dry mouth, hoarseness, throat irritation
Intranasal: Burning, mucosal dryness
Ophthalmic: Blurred vision
Systemic: Insomnia, facial swelling or cushingoid appearance, moderate abdominal distention, indigestion, increased appetite, nervousness, facial flushing, diaphoresis
Occasional
Inhalation: Localized fungal infection, such as thrush
Intranasal: Crusting inside nose, nosebleed, sore throat, ulceration of nasal mucosa.
Ophthalmic: Decreased vision, watering of eyes, eye pain, burning, stinging, redness of eyes, nausea, vomiting
Systemic: Dizziness, decreased or blurred vision
Topical: Allergic contact dermatitis, purpura or blood-containing blisters, thinning of skin with easy bruising, telangiectasis or raised dark red spots on skin
Rare
Inhalation: Increased bronchospasm, esophageal candidiasis
Intranasal: Nasal and pharyngeal candidiasis, eye pain
Systemic: General allergic reaction (such as rash and hives); pain, redness, or swelling at injection site; psychological changes; false sense of well-being; hallucinations; depression

SERIOUS REACTIONS

! Long-term therapy may cause muscle wasting (especially in the arms and legs), osteoporosis, spontaneous fractures, amenorrhea, cataracts, glaucoma, peptic ulcer disease, and CHF.
! The ophthalmic form may cause glaucoma, ocular hypertension, and cataracts.
! Abrupt withdrawal following long-term therapy may cause severe joint pain, severe headache, anorexia, nausea, fever, rebound inflammation, fatigue, weakness, lethargy, dizziness, and orthostatic hypotension.

DENTAL CONSIDERATIONS

General:
- Monitor vital signs at every appointment because of cardiovascular side effects.
- Patients on chronic drug therapy may rarely have symptoms of blood dyscrasias, which can include infection, bleeding, and poor healing.
- Symptoms of oral infections may be masked.

• Patients who have been or are currently on chronic steroid therapy (>2 wk) may require supplemental steroids for dental treatment.
• Avoid prescribing aspirin-containing products.
• Place on frequent recall to evaluate healing response.
• Prophylactic antibiotics may be indicated to prevent infection if surgery or deep scaling is planned.

Consultations:

• In a patient with symptoms of blood dyscrasias, request a medical consultation for blood studies and postpone dental treatment until normal values are reestablished.
• Medical consultation may be required to assess disease control.
• Consultation may be required to confirm steroid dose and duration of use.

Teach Patient/Family:

• Importance of good oral hygiene to prevent soft tissue inflammation
• Caution to prevent injury when using oral hygiene aids
• To avoid mouth rinses with high alcohol content because of drug interaction

Dexamethasone sodium phosphate

dex-a-meth′-a-sone soe′-dee-um foss′-fate
(AK-Dex, Decadron Phosphate Ophthalmic, Dexamthasone Ophthalmic, Maxidex, Ocu-Dex, Diodex[CAN])
Do not confuse with desoximetasone, dextramethophan, or Maxzide.

CATEGORY AND SCHEDULE

Pregnancy Risk Category: C (D if used in the first trimester)

MECHANISM OF ACTION

A corticosteroid that inhibits accumulation of inflammatory cells at inflammation sites, phagocytosis, lysosomal enzyme release and synthesis and release of mediators of inflammation. ***Therapeutic Effect:*** Prevents and suppresses cell and tissue immune reactions, inflammatory process.

PHARMACOKINETICS

Absorbed into aqueous humor, cornea, iris, choroids, ciliary body, and retina. Systemic absorption may occur and is more likely at higher doses or in pediatric therapy.

AVAILABILITY

Ointment, Ophthalmic: 0.05% (AK-Dex, Decadron Phosphate, Ocu-Dex, Dexamethasone Ophthalmic).
Solution, Ophthalmic: 0.1% (Ocu-Dex, Dexamthasone Ophthalmic)
Suspension, Ophthalmic: 0.1% (Maxidex).

INDICATIONS AND DOSAGES

▸ Ocular Inflammatory Conditions

OPHTHALMIC, OINTMENT
Adults, Elderly. Apply thin strip 3–4 times/day.
OPHTHALMIC, SOLUTION AND SUSPENSION
Adults, Elderly. Instill 1 or 2 drops up to 6 times/day.

CONTRAINDICATIONS

Epithelial herpes simplex keratitis (dendritic keratitis), vaccinia, varicella or other viral diseases of the cornea and conjunctiva, mycobacterial infection of the eye, fungal diseases of ocular structures, hypersensitivity to any component of the medication.

INTERACTIONS

Drug
None known.
Herbal
None known.
Food
None known.
Drug interactions of concern to dentistry
- Decreased action: barbiturates
- Increased side effects: alcohol, salicylates, other NSAIDs
- Increased action: ketoconazole, macrolide antibiotics

DIAGNOSTIC TEST EFFECTS

None known.

SIDE EFFECTS

Frequent
Blurred vision, increase intraocular pressure
Occasional
Decreased vision, watering of eyes, eye pain, burning, stinging, redness of eyes, nausea, vomiting
Rare
Optic nerve damage, posterior subcapsular cataract formation, delayed wound healing

SERIOUS REACTIONS

! The serious reactions of the ophthalmic form of dexamethasone sodium phosphate are glaucoma, ocular hypertension, and cataracts.
! May promote development and spread of secondary infection (usually fungal).

DENTAL CONSIDERATIONS

General:
- Place on frequent recall to evaluate healing response.

Teach Patient/Family:
- When used for oral lesions, advise patient to return for oral evaluation if response of oral tissues has not occurred in 7–14 days
- Importance of good oral hygiene to prevent soft tissue inflammation
- To apply approximately 0.25 inch; measure and apply with cotton-tipped applicator by gently dabbing, not rubbing, medication on lesion
- To apply at bedtime or after meals for maximum effect

That use on oral herpetic ulcerations is contraindicated

dexchlorpheniramine

dex′-klor-fen-eer′-a-meen
(Polaramine, Polaramine Repetabs)

CATEGORY AND SCHEDULE

Pregnancy Risk Category: B

MECHANISM OF ACTION

A propylamine derivative that competes with histamine for H1-receptor sites on effector cells in the gastrointestinal (GI) tract, blood vessels, and respiratory tract. Dexchlorpheniramine is the dextro-isomer of chlorpheniramine and is approximately two times more active. ***Therapeutic Effect:*** Prevents allergic response, produces mild bronchodilation, blocks histamine-induced bronchitis.

PHARMACOKINETICS

Route	Onset	Peak	Duration
PO	0.5 hr	1–2 hr	3–6 hr

Well absorbed from the gastrointestinal (GI) tract. Protein binding: 70%. Widely distributed. Metabolized in liver to active metabolite, undergoes extensive first-pass metabolism. Excreted primarily in urine. Not removed by hemodialysis. ***Half-life:*** 20 hrs.

AVAILABILITY

Tablets: 2 mg (Polaramine [DSC]).
Extended-release Tablets: 4 mg, 6 mg (Polaramine Repetabs).
Syrup: 2 mg/5 ml (Polaramine).

INDICATIONS AND DOSAGES

▸ **Allergic Rhinitis, Common Cold**

PO

Adults, Elderly, Children 12 yrs or older. 2 mg q4–6h or 4–6 mg timed release at bedtime or q8–10h.
Children 6–11 yrs. 4 mg timed release at bedtime or 1 mg q4–6h.
Children 2–5 yrs. 0.5 mg q4–6h. Do not use timed release.

OFF-LABEL USES

Asthma, chemotherapy-induced stomatitis, dermographia, familial immunodeficiency disease, malaria, mastocytosi, Meniere's disease, nausea, neurocysticercosis, otitis media, psoriasis, radiocontrast media reactions, urticaria

CONTRAINDICATIONS

History of hypersensitivity to antihistamines, newborn or premature infants, nursing mothers, third trimester of pregnancy

INTERACTIONS

Drug

Alcohol, central nervous system (CNS) depressants: May increase CNS depression.
Methacholine: May interfere with interpretation of pulmonary function tests after a methacholine bronchial challenge.
Procarbazine: May increase CNS depression.

Herbal

None known.

Food

None known.

Drug interactions of concern to dentistry

- Increased CNS depression: barbiturates, narcotics, hypnotics, tricyclic antidepressants, alcohol
- Increased anticholinergic effect: anticholinergic drugs

DIAGNOSTIC TEST EFFECTS

May interfere with the interpretation of the pulmonary function tests after a methacholine bronchial challenge test.

SIDE EFFECTS

Frequent

Drowsiness, dizziness, headache, dry mouth, nose, or throat, urinary retention, thickening of bronchial secretions, sedation, hypotension

Occasional

Epigastric distress, flushing, blurred vision, tinnitus, paresthesia, sweating, chills

SERIOUS REACTIONS

! Children may experience dominant paradoxical reactions, including restlessness, insomnia, euphoria, nervousness, and tremors.
! Hypersensitivity reaction, such as eczema, pruritus, rash, cardiac disturbances, and photosensitivity, may occur.
! Overdosage may vary from CNS depression, including sedation, apnea, hypotension, cardiovascular collapse, or death to severe paradoxical reaction, such as hallucinations, tremor, and seizures.

DENTAL CONSIDERATIONS

General:

- Assess salivary flow as a factor in caries, periodontal disease, and candidiasis.

• Consider semisupine chair position for patient comfort because of respiratory effects of disease.

Teach Patient/Family:

• *When chronic dry mouth occurs, advise patient:*
  • To avoid mouth rinses with high alcohol content because of drying effects
  • To use sugarless gum, frequent sips of water, or saliva substitutes
  • To use daily home fluoride products for anticaries effect

dexmethylphenidate hydrochloride

dex-meth-ill-fen′-i-date
(Focalin)

CATEGORY AND SCHEDULE

Pregnancy Risk Category: C
Controlled Substance: Schedule II

MECHANISM OF ACTION

A CNS stimulant that blocks the reuptake of norepinephrine and dopamine into presynaptic neurons, increasing the release of these neurotransmitters into the synaptic cleft.
Therapeutic Effect: Decreases motor restlessness and fatigue; increases motor activity, mental alertness, and attention span; elevates mood.

PHARMACOKINETICS

Route	Onset	Peak	Duration
PO	N/A	N/A	4–5 hr

Readily absorbed from the GI tract. Plasma concentrations increase rapidly. Metabolized in the liver. Excreted unchanged in urine. ***Half-life:*** 2.2 hr.

AVAILABILITY

Tablets: 2.5 mg, 5 mg, 10 mg.

INDICATIONS AND DOSAGES

▸ Attention Deficit Hyperactivity Disorder (ADHD)

PO

Patients new to dexmethylphenidate or methylphenidate. 2.5 mg twice a day (5 mg/day). May adjust dosage in 2.5- to 5-mg increments. Maximum: 20 mg/day.

Patients currently taking methylphenidate. Half the methylphenidate dosage. Maximum: 20 mg/day.

CONTRAINDICATIONS

Diagnosis or family history of Tourette syndrome; glaucoma; history of marked agitation, anxiety, or tension; motor tics; use within 14 days of MAOIs

INTERACTIONS

Drug

Amitriptyline, phenobarbital, phenytoin, primidone: Dosage of these drugs may need to be decreased.
MAOIs: May increase the effects of dexmethylphenidate.
Other CNS stimulants: May have an additive effect.
Warfarin: May inhibit the metabolism of warfarin.

Herbal

None known.

Food

None known.

Drug interactions of concern to dentistry

• May inhibit metabolism of phenobarbital, tricyclic antidepressants, and SSRIs
• Increased effects of anticholinergics, CNS stimulants, tricyclic antidepressants, and sympathomimetics

DIAGNOSTIC TEST EFFECTS

None known.

SIDE EFFECTS

Frequent

Abdominal pain, nausea, anorexia, fever

Occasional

Tachycardia, arrhythmias, palpitations, insomnia, twitching

Rare

Blurred vision, rash, arthralgia

SERIOUS REACTIONS

! Withdrawal after prolonged therapy may unmask symptoms of the underlying disorder.

! Dexmethylphenidate may lower the seizure threshold in those with a history of seizures.

! Overdose produces excessive sympathomimetic effects, including vomiting, tremor, hyperreflexia, seizures, confusion, hallucinations, and diaphoresis.

! Prolonged administration to children may delay growth.

DENTAL CONSIDERATIONS

General:

- Monitor vital signs at every appointment because of cardiovascular side effects.
- Assess salivary flow as a factor in caries, periodontal disease, and candidiasis.
- Patients on chronic drug therapy may rarely have symptoms of blood dyscrasias, which can include infection, bleeding, and poor healing.
- Use vasoconstrictor with caution, in low doses, and with careful aspiration.
- Determine why the patient is taking the drug.

Consultations:

- In a patient with symptoms of blood dyscrasias, request a medical consultation for blood studies and postpone treatment until normal values are reestablished.
- Medical consultation may be required to assess disease control.

Teach Patient/Family:

- Importance of good oral hygiene to prevent soft tissue inflammation, infection
- To prevent injury when using oral hygiene aids
- Importance of updating health and drug history if physician makes any changes in evaluation or drug regimens
- *When chronic dry mouth occurs, advise patient:*
  - To avoid mouth rinses with high alcohol content because of drying effects
  - To use daily home fluoride products for anticaries effect
  - To use sugarless gum, frequent sips of water, or saliva substitutes

dextroamphetamine sulfate

dex-troe-am-fet′-a-meen

Schedule II

(Dexamphetamine[AUS], Dexedrine, Dexedrine Spansule, Dextrostat)

Do not confuse dextroamphetamine with dextromethorphan, or Dexedrine with Dextran or Excedrin.

CATEGORY AND SCHEDULE

Pregnancy Risk Category: C

Controlled Substance: Schedule II

MECHANISM OF ACTION

An amphetamine that enhances the action of dopamine and norepinephrine by blocking their reuptake from synapses; also inhibits

monoamine oxidase and facilitates the release of catecholamines.
Therapeutic Effect: Increases motor activity and mental alertness; decreases motor restlessness, drowsiness, and fatigue; suppresses appetite.

AVAILABILITY

Capsules (Sustained-Release [Dexedrine, Spansule]): 5 mg, 10 mg, 15 mg.
Tablets (Dexedrine): 5 mg.
Tablets (Dextrostat): 5 mg, 10 mg.

INDICATIONS AND DOSAGES

▸ Narcolepsy

PO

Adults, Children older than 12 yr. Initially, 10 mg/day. Increase by 10 mg/day at weekly intervals until therapeutic response is achieved.
Children 6–12 yr. Initially, 5 mg/day. Increase by 5 mg/day at weekly intervals until therapeutic response is achieved.
Maximum: 60 mg/day.

▸ Attention Deficit Hyperactivity Disorder (ADHD)

PO

Children 6 yr and older. Initially, 5 mg once or twice a day. Increase by 5 mg/day at weekly intervals until therapeutic response is achieved.
Children 3–5 yr. Initially, 2.5 mg/day. Increase by 2.5 mg/day at weekly intervals until therapeutic response is achieved. Maximum: 40 mg/day.

▸ Appetite Suppressant

PO

Adults. 5–30 mg daily in divided doses of 5–10 mg each, given 30–60 min before meals; or 1 extended-release capsule in the morning.

CONTRAINDICATIONS

Advanced arteriosclerosis, agitated states, glaucoma, history of drug abuse, hypersensitivity to sympathomimetic amines, hyperthyroidism, moderate to severe hypertension, symptomatic cardiovascular disease, use within 14 days of MAOIs

INTERACTIONS

Drug

Beta blockers: May increase the risk of bradycardia, heart block, and hypertension.
Digoxin: May increase the risk of arrhythmias.
MAOIs: May prolong and intensify the effects of dextroamphetamine.
Meperidine: May increase the risk of hypotension, respiratory depression, seizures, and vascular collapse.
Other CNS stimulants: May increase the effects of dextroamphetamine.
Thyroid hormones: May increase the effects of either drug.
Tricyclic antidepressants: May increase cardiovascular effects.

Herbal

None known.

Food

None known.

Drug interactions of concern to dentistry

- Increased risk of serious side effects: meperidine, propoxyphene, tricyclic antidepressants

DIAGNOSTIC TEST EFFECTS

May increase plasma corticosteroid concentrations.

SIDE EFFECTS

Frequent

Irregular pulse, increased motor activity, talkativeness, nervousness, mild euphoria, insomnia

Occasional

Headache, chills, dry mouth, GI distress, worsening depression in patients who are clinically depressed, tachycardia, palpitations, chest pain, dizziness, decreased appetite

SERIOUS REACTIONS

! Overdose may produce skin pallor or flushing, arrhythmias, and psychosis.
! Abrupt withdrawal after prolonged use of high doses may produce lethargy lasting for weeks.
! Prolonged administration to children with ADHD may inhibit growth.

DENTAL CONSIDERATIONS

General:

- Monitor vital signs at every appointment because of cardiovascular side effects.
- Assess salivary flow as a factor in caries, periodontal disease, and candidiasis.
- Psychologic and physical dependence may occur with chronic administration.

Consultations:

- Medical consultation may be required to assess disease control.

Teach Patient/Family:

- *When chronic dry mouth occurs, advise patient:*
  - To avoid mouth rinses with high alcohol content because of drying effects
  - To use daily home fluoride products for anticaries effect
  - To use sugarless gum, frequent sips of water, or saliva substitutes

dextromethorphan

dex-troe-meth-or′-fan
(Babee Cof Syrup, Benylin Adult, Benylin Pediatric, Creomulsion Cough, Creomulsion for Children, Creo-Terpin, Delsym, Dexalone, ElixSure Cough, Hold DM, PediaCare Infants' Long-Acting Cough, Robitussion[AUS], Robitussin CoughGels, Robitussin Honey Cough, Robitussin Maximum Strength Cough, Robitussin Pediatric Cough, Scot-Tussin DM Cough Chasers, Silphen DM, Simply Cough, Vicks 44 Cough Relief)

CATEGORY AND SCHEDULE

Pregnancy Risk Category: C
OTC

MECHANISM OF ACTION

A chemical relative of morphine without the narcotic properties that acts on the cough center in the medulla oblongata by elevating the threshold for coughing.
Therapeutic Effect:
Suppresses cough.

PHARMACOKINETICS

Rapidly absorbed from the gastrointestinal (GI) tract. Distributed into cerebrospinal fluid (CSF). Extensively and poorly metabolized in liver to dextrorphan (active metabolite). Excreted unchanged in urine. ***Half-life:*** 1.4–3.9 hrs (parent compound), 3.4–5.6 hrs. (dextrorphan).

AVAILABILITY

Gelcap: 15 mg (Robitussin CoughGels), 30 mg (Dexalone).
Liquid: 5 mg/5ml (Simply Cough), 10 mg/5 ml (Vicks Cough Relief), 10 mg/15 ml (Creo-Terpin).

Liquid drops: 7.5 mg/0.8 ml (PediaCare Infants' Long-Acting Cough).
Lozenges: 5 mg (Hold DM, Scot-Tussin DM Cough Chasers).
Suspension (extended-release): 30 mg/5 ml (Delsym).
Syrup: 7.5 mg/5 ml (Babee Cof Syrup, Benylin Pediatric, ElixSure, Robitussin Pediatric Cough), 10 mg/5 ml (Robitussin Honey Cough, Silphen DM), 15 mg/5 ml (Benylin Adult, Robitussin Maximum Strength Cough), 20 mg/15 ml (Creomulsion Cough, Creomulsion for Children)

INDICATIONS AND DOSAGES

▶ Cough

PO
Adults, Elderly, Children 12 years and older. 10–20 mg q4h. Maximum: 120 mg/day.
Children 6– 12 yrs. 5–10 mg q4h. Maximum: 60 mg/day.
Children 2–5 yrs. 2.5–5 mg q4h. Maximum: 30 mg/day.

OFF-LABEL USES

N-methyl-D-aspartate (NMDA) antagonist in cerebral injury

CONTRAINDICATIONS

Coadministration with monoamine oxidase inhibitors (MAOIs), hypersensitivity to dextromethorphan or its components

INTERACTIONS

Drug

MAOIs, phenelzine, SSRIs, sibutramine: May increase the risk of serotonin syndrome.
Haloperidol, quinidine: May increase adverse effects associated with dextromethorphan.

Herbal

None known.

Food

None known.

Drug interactions of concern to dentistry

- Inhibition of metabolism: terbinafine

DIAGNOSTIC TEST EFFECTS

None known.

SIDE EFFECTS

Rare

Abdominal discomfort, constipation, dizziness, drowsiness, GI upset, nausea

SERIOUS REACTIONS

! Overdosage may result in muscle spasticity, increase or decrease in blood pressure (B/P), blurred vision, blue fingernails and lips, nausea, vomiting, hallucinations, and respiratory depression.

DENTAL CONSIDERATIONS

General:

- Consider semisupine chair position for patients with respiratory disease.

diazepam

dye-az′-e-pam
Schedule IV
(Antenex[AUS], Apo-Diazepam[CAN], Diastat, Diazemuls[CAN], Dizac, Ducene[AUS], Valium, Valpam[AUS], Vivol[CAN])
Do not confuse diazepam with diazoxide or Ditropan, or Valium with Valcyte.

CATEGORY AND SCHEDULE

Pregnancy Risk Category: D
Controlled Substance: Schedule IV

MECHANISM OF ACTION
A benzodiazepine that depresses all levels of the CNS by enhancing the action of gamma-aminobutyric acid, a major inhibitory neurotransmitter in the brain. ***Therapeutic Effect:*** Produces anxiolytic effect, elevates the seizure threshold, produces skeletal muscle relaxation.

PHARMACOKINETICS

Route	Onset	Peak	Duration
PO	30 min	1–2 hr	2–3 hr
IV	1–5 min	15 min	15–60 min
IM	15 min	30–90 min	30–90 min

Well absorbed from the GI tract. Widely distributed. Protein binding: 98%. Metabolized in the liver to active metabolite. Excreted in urine. Minimally removed by hemodialysis. ***Half-life:*** 20–70 hr (increased in hepatic dysfunction and the elderly).

AVAILABILITY
Oral Concentrate (Diazepam Intensol): 5 mg/ml.
Oral Solution: 5 mg/5 ml.
Tablets (Valium): 2 mg, 5 mg, 10 mg.
Injection: 5 mg/ml.
Rectal Gel (Diastat): 5 mg/ml.

INDICATIONS AND DOSAGES
▸ Anxiety, Skeletal Muscle Relaxation
PO
Adults. 2–10 mg 2–4 times a day.
Elderly. 2.5 mg twice a day.
Children. 0.12–0.8 mg/kg/day in divided doses q6–8h.
IV, IM
Adults. 2–10 mg repeated in 3–4 hr.
Children. 0.04–0.3 mg/kg/dose q2–4h. Maximum: 0.5 mg/kg in an 8-hr period.
▸ Preanesthesia
IV
Adults, Elderly. 5–15 mg 5–10 min before procedure.
Children. 0.2–0.3 mg/kg. Maximum: 10 mg.
▸ Alcohol Withdrawal
PO
Adults, Elderly. 10 mg 3–4 times during first 24 hr, then reduced to 5–10 mg 3–4 times a day as needed.
IV, IM
Adults, Elderly. Initially, 10 mg, followed by 5–10 mg q3–4h.
▸ Status Epilepticus
IV
Adults, Elderly. 5–10 mg q10–15min up to 30 mg/8 hr.
Children 5 yr and older. 0.05–0.3 mg/kg/dose q15–30min. Maximum: 10 mg/dose.
Children 1 mo to younger than 5 yr. 0.05–0.3 mg/kg/dose q15–30min. Maximum: 5 mg/dose.
▸ Control of Increased Seizure Activity in Patients with Refractory Epilepsy Who Are on Stable Regimens of Anticonvulsants
RECTAL GEL
Adults, Children 12 yr and older. 0.2 mg/kg; may be repeated in 4–12 hr.
Children 6–11 yr. 0.3 mg/kg; may be repeated in 4–12 hr.
Children 2–5 yr. 0.5 mg/kg; may be repeated in 4–12 hr.

OFF-LABEL USES
Treatment of panic disorder, tension headache, tremors

CONTRAINDICATIONS
Angle-closure glaucoma, coma, pre-existing CNS depression, respiratory depression, severe, uncontrolled pain

INTERACTIONS
Drug
Alcohol, other CNS depressants: May increase CNS depression.
Herbal
Kava kava, valerian: May increase CNS depression.

D

Food
None known.

Drug interactions of concern to dentistry
- Increased CNS depression of diazepam: alcohol, all CNS depressants, kava (herb)
- Increased serum levels and prolonged effect of benzodiazepines: erythromycin, clarithromycin, ketoconazole, itraconazole, fluconazole, miconazole (systemic), cimetidine, rifamycin
- Contraindicated with saquinavir
- Possible increase in CNS side effects: kava (herb)

DIAGNOSTIC TEST EFFECTS
May elevate serum LDH, alkaline phosphatase, bilirubin, AST (SGOT), and ALT (SGPT) levels. May produce abnormal renal function test results. Therapeutic serum drug level is 0.5–2 mcg/ml; toxic serum drug level is greater than 3 mcg/ml.

IV INCOMPATIBILITIES
Amphotericin B complex (Abelcet, AmBisome, Amphotec), cefepime (Maxipime), diltiazem (Cardizem), fluconazole (Diflucan), foscarnet (Foscavir), heparin, hydrocortisone (Solu-Cortef), hydromorphone (Dilaudid), meropenem (Merrem IV), potassium chloride, propofol (Diprivan), vitamins

IV COMPATIBILITIES
Dobutamine (Dobutrex), fentanyl, morphine

SIDE EFFECTS
Frequent
Pain with IM injection, somnolence, fatigue, ataxia

Occasional
Slurred speech, orthostatic hypotension, headache, hypoactivity, constipation, nausea, blurred vision

Rare
Paradoxical CNS reactions, such as hyperactivity or nervousness in children and excitement or restlessness in the elderly or debilitated (generally noted during first 2 weeks of therapy, particularly in presence of uncontrolled pain)

SERIOUS REACTIONS
! IV administration may produce pain, swelling, thrombophlebitis, and carpal tunnel syndrome.
! Abrupt or too-rapid withdrawal may result in pronounced restlessness, irritability, insomnia, hand tremor, abdominal or muscle cramps, diaphoresis, vomiting, and seizures.
! Abrupt withdrawal in patients with epilepsy may produce an increase in the frequency or severity of seizures.
! Overdose results in somnolence, confusion, diminished reflexes, and coma.

DENTAL CONSIDERATIONS
General:
- Assess salivary flow as a factor in caries, periodontal disease, and candidiasis.
- After supine positioning, have patient sit upright for at least 2 min before standing to avoid orthostatic hypotension.
- Psychologic and physical dependence may occur with chronic administration.
- Geriatric patients are more susceptible to drug effects; use lower dose.
- Have someone drive patient to and from dental appointment when drug used for conscious sedation.
- Provide assistance when escorting patient to and from dental chair when dizziness occurs.
- Avoid use of this drug in a patient with a history of drug abuse or alcoholism.

Teach Patient/Family:

- Importance of good oral hygiene to prevent soft tissue inflammation
- *When chronic dry mouth occurs, advise patient:*
  - To avoid mouth rinses with high alcohol content because of drying effects
  - To use daily home fluoride products for anticaries effect
  - To use sugarless gum, frequent sips of water, or saliva substitutes

diclofenac

dye-kloe′-fen-ak

(Cataflam, Diclohexal[AUS], Diclotek[CAN], Fenac[AUS], Novo-Difenac[CAN], Solaraze, Voltaren, Voltaren Emulgel[AUS], Voltaren Ophthalmic, Voltaren Rapid[AUS], Voltaren XR)

Do not confuse diclofenac with Diflucan or Duphalac, or Voltaren with Verelan.

CATEGORY AND SCHEDULE

Pregnancy Risk Category: B (D if used in third trimester or near delivery; C for ophthalmic solution)

MECHANISM OF ACTION

An NSAID that inhibits prostaglandin synthesis, reducing the intensity of pain. Also constricts the iris sphincter. May inhibit angiogenesis (the formation of blood vessels) by inhibiting substance P or blocking the angiogenic effects of prostaglandin E. ***Therapeutic Effect:*** Produces analgesic and anti-inflammatory effects. Prevents miosis during cataract surgery. May reduce angiogenesis in inflamed tissue.

PHARMACOKINETICS

Route	Onset	Peak	Duration
PO	30 min	2–3 hr	Up to 8 hr

Completely absorbed from the GI tract; penetrates cornea after ophthalmic administration (may be systemically absorbed). Protein binding: greater than 99%. Widely distributed. Metabolized in the liver. Primarily excreted in urine. Minimally removed by hemodialysis. ***Half-life:*** 1.2–2 hr.

AVAILABILITY

Topical Gel (Solaraze): 3%.
Tablets (Cataflam): 50 mg.
Tablets (Enteric-Coated [Voltaren]): 25 mg, 50 mg, 75 mg.
Tablets (Extended-Release [Voltaren XR]): 100 mg.
Ophthalmic Solution (Voltaren Ophthalmic): 0.1%.

INDICATIONS AND DOSAGES

▸ **Osteoarthritis**

PO (Cataflam, Voltaren)
Adults, Elderly. 50 mg 2–3 times a day.
PO (Voltaren XR)
Adults, Elderly. 100 mg/day as a single dose.

▸ **Rheumatoid Arthritis**

PO (Cataflam, Voltaren)
Adults, Elderly. 50 mg 2–4 times a day. Maximum: 225 mg/day.
PO (Voltaren XR)
Adults, Elderly. 100 mg once a day. Maximum: 100 mg twice a day.

▸ **Ankylosing Spondylitis**

PO (Voltaren)
Adults, Elderly. 100–125 mg/day in 4–5 divided doses.

▸ **Analgesia, Primary Dysmenorrhea**

PO (Cataflam)
Adults, Elderly. 30 mg 3 times a day.

▸ **Usual Pediatric Dosage**
Children. 2–3 mg/kg/day in 2–4 divided doses.

▸ **Actinic Keratoses**
TOPICAL
Adults, Adolescents. Apply twice a day to lesion for 60–90 days.

▸ **Cataract Surgery**
OPHTHALMIC
Adults, Elderly. Apply 1 drop to eye 4 times a day commencing 24 hr after cataract surgery. Continue for 2 wk afterward.

▸ **Pain, Relief of Photophobia in Patients Undergoing Corneal Refractive Surgery**
OPHTHALMIC
Adults, Elderly. Apply 1 drop to affected eye 1 hr before surgery, within 15 min after surgery, then 4 times a day for 3 days.

OFF-LABEL USES

Treatment of vascular headaches (oral); to reduce the occurrence and severity of cystoid macular edema after cataract surgery (ophthalmic form)

CONTRAINDICATIONS

Hypersensitivity to aspirin, diclofenac, and other NSAIDs; porphyria

INTERACTIONS

Drug

Acetylcholine, carbachol: May decrease the effects of these drugs (with ophthalmic diclofenac).
Antihypertensives, diuretics: May decrease the effects of these drugs.
Aspirin, other salicylates: May increase the risk of GI side effects such as bleeding.
Bone marrow depressants: May increase the risk of hematologic reactions.
Epinephrine, other antiglaucoma medications: May decrease the antiglaucoma effect of these drugs.
Heparin, oral anticoagulants, thrombolytics: May increase the effects of these drugs.
Lithium: May increase the blood concentration and risk of toxicity of lithium.
Methotrexate: May increase the risk of methotrexate toxicity.
Probenecid: May increase diclofenac blood concentration.

Herbal

Ginkgo biloba: May increase the risk of bleeding.

Food

None known.

Drug interactions of concern to dentistry

- GI ulceration, bleeding: aspirin, alcohol, corticosteroids, potassium supplements
- Nephrotoxicity: acetaminophen (prolonged use)
- Possible risk of decreased renal function: cyclosporine
- *When prescribed for dental pain:*
  - Risk of increased effects: oral anticoagulants, oral antidiabetics, lithium, methotrexate
  - Decreased antihypertensive effects of diuretics, β-adrenergic blockers, and ACE inhibitors
  - First-time users of SSRIs also taking NSAIDs may have a higher risk of GI side effects; until more data are available, it may be advisable to avoid use of NSAIDs in these patients (*Br J Clin Pharmacol* 55: 591–595, 2003)

DIAGNOSTIC TEST EFFECTS

May increase BUN level; urine protein level; and serum LDH, potassium, alkaline phosphatase, creatinine, AST (SGOT), and ALT (SGPT) levels. May decrease serum uric acid level.

SIDE EFFECTS

Frequent (9%–4%)

PO: Headache, abdominal cramps, constipation, diarrhea, nausea, dyspepsia

Ophthalmic: Burning or stinging on instillation, ocular discomfort

Occasional (3%–1%)

PO: Flatulence, dizziness, epigastric pain

Ophthalmic: Ocular itching or tearing

Rare (< 1%)

PO: Rash, peripheral edema or fluid retention, visual disturbances, vomiting, drowsiness

SERIOUS REACTIONS

! Overdose may result in acute renal failure.

! Rare reactions with long-term use include peptic ulcer disease, GI bleeding, gastritis, a severe hepatic reaction (jaundice), nephrotoxicity (hematuria, dysuria, proteinuria), and a severe hypersensitivity reaction (bronchospasm or angioedema).

DENTAL CONSIDERATIONS

General:

- Patients on chronic drug therapy may rarely have symptoms of blood dyscrasias, which can include infection, bleeding, and poor healing.
- Assess salivary flow as a factor in caries, periodontal disease, and candidiasis.
- Avoid prescribing for dental use in last trimester of pregnancy.
- Avoid prescribing aspirin-containing products.
- Consider semisupine chair position for patients with rheumatic disease.
- Advise patient if dental drugs prescribed have a potential for photosensitivity.

Consultations:

- In a patient with symptoms of blood dyscrasias, request a medical consultation for blood studies and postpone dental treatment until normal values are reestablished.
- Medical consultation may be required to assess disease control.

Teach Patient/Family:

- Importance of good oral hygiene to prevent soft tissue inflammation
- Caution to prevent injury when using oral hygiene aids
- *When chronic dry mouth occurs, advise patient:*
  - To avoid mouth rinses with high alcohol content because of drying effects
  - To use daily home fluoride products for anticaries effect
  - To use sugarless gum, frequent sips of water, or saliva substitutes

DICLOFENAC SODIUM (VOLTAREN)

Drug interactions of concern to dentistry

- None reported

DENTAL CONSIDERATIONS

General:

- Determine why patient is taking the drug.
- Protect patient's eyes from accidental spatter during dental treatment.
- Avoid dental light in patient's eyes; offer dark glasses for patient comfort.

dicloxacillin sodium

dye-klox′-a-sill-in soe′-dee-um

(Dycil, Pathocil)

CATEGORY AND SCHEDULE

Pregnancy Risk Category: B

MECHANISM OF ACTION
A penicillin that acts as a bactericidal in susceptible microorganisms. *Therapeutic Effect:* Inhibits bacterial cell wall synthesis..

PHARMACOKINETICS
Well absorbed from gastrointestinal (GI) tract. Rate and extent reduced by food. Distributed throughout body including CSF. Protein binding: 96%. Partially metabolized in liver. Primarily excreted in feces and urine. Not removed by hemodialysis. ***Half-life:*** 0.7 hrs.

AVAILABILITY
Capsules: 250 mg, 500 mg (Dycil, Pathocil).

INDICATIONS AND DOSAGES
▸ **Respiratory Tract Infection, Staphylococcal and Streptococcal Infections**

PO

Adults, Elderly, Children weighing > 40 kg. 125–250 mg q6h.

Children weighing < 40 kg. 12.5-25 mg/kg/day q6h.

CONTRAINDICATIONS
Hypersensitivity to any penicillin

INTERACTIONS
Drug
Allopurinol: May increase incidence of rash.
Aminoglycosides: May decrease aminoglycoside efficacy.
Oral contraceptives: May decrease effects of oral contraceptives.
Probenecid: May increase amoxicillin blood concentration and risk for dicloxacillin toxicity.
Warfarin: May decrease effects of warfarin.

Herbal
None known.

Food
None known.

DIAGNOSTIC TEST EFFECTS
May cause positive Coombs' test.

SIDE EFFECTS
Frequent
Gastrointestinal (GI) disturbances (mild diarrhea, nausea, or vomiting), headache

Occasional
Generalized rash, urticaria

SERIOUS REACTIONS
! Altered bacterial balance may result in potentially fatal superinfections and antibiotic-associated colitis as evidenced by abdominal cramps, watery or severe diarrhea, and fever.

! Severe hypersensitivity reactions, including anaphylaxis and acute interstitial nephritis occur rarely.

DENTAL CONSIDERATIONS
General:
- Take precautions regarding allergy to medication.
- Determine why the patient is taking the drug.

Consultations:
- Concern for drug of choice if dental infection is also present.

Teach Patient/Family:
- Importance of good oral hygiene to prevent soft tissue inflammation
- Caution to prevent trauma when using oral hygiene aids
- *When used for dental infection, advise patient:*
  - Taking birth control pill to use additional method of contraception for duration of cycle
  - To report sore throat, oral burning sensation, fever, and fatigue, any of which could indicate superinfection
  - To take at prescribed intervals and complete dosage regimen
  - To immediately notify the dentist if signs or symptoms of infection increase

dicyclomine hydrochloride

dye-sye′-kloe-meen
(Bentyl, Bentylol[CAN], Formulex[CAN], Lomine[CAN],Merbentyl[AUS])
Do not confuse dicyclomine with doxycycline or dyclonime, or Bentyl with Aventyl or Benadryl.

CATEGORY AND SCHEDULE
Pregnancy Risk Category: B

MECHANISM OF ACTION
A GI antispasmodic and anticholinergic agent that directly acts as a relaxant on smooth muscle. ***Therapeutic Effect:*** Reduces tone and motility of GI tract.

PHARMACOKINETICS

Route	Onset	Peak	Duration
PO	1–2 hr	N/A	4 hr

Readily absorbed from the GI tract. Widely distributed. Metabolized in the liver. ***Half-life:*** 9–10 hr.

AVAILABILITY
Capsules: 10 mg.
Tablets: 20 mg.
Syrup: 10 mg/5 ml.
Injection: 10 mg/ml.

INDICATIONS AND DOSAGES
▸ Functional Disturbances of GI Motility
PO
Adults. 10–20 mg 3–4 times a day up to 40 mg 4 times/day.
Children older than 2 yr. 10 mg 3–4 times a day.
Children 6 mos–2 yr. 5 mg 3–4 times a day.
Elderly. 10–20 mg 4 times a day. May increase up to 160 mg/day.
IM
Adults. 20 mg q4–6h.

CONTRAINDICATIONS
Bladder neck obstruction due to prostatic hyperplasia, coronary vasospasm, intestinal atony, myasthenia gravis in patients not treated with neostigmine, narrow-angle glaucoma, obstructive disease of the GI tract, paralytic ileus, severe ulcerative colitis, tachycardia secondary to cardiac insufficiency or thyrotoxicosis, toxic megacolon, unstable cardiovascular status in acute hemorrhage

INTERACTIONS
Drug
Antacids, antidiarrheals: May decrease the absorption of dicyclomine.
Ketoconazole: May decrease the absorption of ketoconazole.
Other anticholinergics: May increase the effects of dicyclomine.
Potassium chloride: May increase the severity of GI lesions with the wax matrix formulation of potassium chloride.
Herbal
None known.
Food
None known.
Drug interactions of concern to dentistry
- Increased anticholinergic effect: atropine, scopolamine, other anticholinergics, meperidine
- Decreased effect of ketoconazole

DIAGNOSTIC TEST EFFECTS
None known.

SIDE EFFECTS
Frequent
Dry mouth (sometimes severe), constipation, diminished sweating ability

D

Occasional
Blurred vision; photophobia; urinary hesitancy; somnolence (with high dosage); agitation, excitement, confusion, or somnolence noted in elderly (even with low dosages); transient light-headedness (with IM route), irritation at injection site (with IM route)
Rare
Confusion, hypersensitivity reaction, increased IOP, nausea, vomiting, unusual fatigue

SERIOUS REACTIONS

! Overdose may produce temporary paralysis of ciliary muscle; pupillary dilation; tachycardia; palpitations; hot, dry, or flushed skin; absence of bowel sounds; hyperthermia; increased respiratory rate; ECG abnormalities; nausea; vomiting; rash over face or upper trunk; CNS stimulation; and psychosis (marked by agitation, restlessness, rambling speech, visual hallucinations, paranoid behavior, and delusions, followed by depression).

DENTAL CONSIDERATIONS

General:
- Assess salivary flow as a factor in caries, periodontal disease, and candidiasis.
- Avoid dental light in patient's eyes; offer dark glasses for patient comfort.

Consultation:
- Physician should be informed if significant xerostomic side effects occur (e.g., increased caries, sore tongue, problems eating or swallowing, difficulty wearing prosthesis) so that a medication change can be considered.

Teach Patient/Family:
- Importance of good oral hygiene to prevent soft tissue inflammation
- *When chronic dry mouth occurs, advise patient:*
  - To avoid mouth rinses with high alcohol content because of drying effects
  - To use daily home fluoride products for anticaries effect
  - To use sugarless gum, frequent sips of water, or saliva substitutes

didanosine

dye-dan′-o-seen
(Videx, Videx-EC)

CATEGORY AND SCHEDULE

Pregnancy Risk Category: B

MECHANISM OF ACTION

A purine nucleoside analogue that is intracellularly converted into a triphosphate, which interferes with RNA-directed DNA polymerase (reverse transcriptase). ***Therapeutic Effect:*** Inhibits replication of retroviruses, including HIV.

PHARMACOKINETICS

Variably absorbed from the GI tract. Protein binding: less than 5%. Rapidly metabolized intracellularly to active form. Primarily excreted in urine. Partially (20%) removed by hemodialysis. ***Half-life:*** 1.5 hr; metabolite: 8–24 hr.

AVAILABILITY

Capsules (Delayed-Release): 125 mg, 200 mg, 250 mg, 400 mg.
Pediatric Powder for Oral Solution: 10 mg/ml.

Powder for Oral Solution (Single-Dose Packet): 100 mg.
Tablets (Chewable): 25 mg, 50 mg, 100 mg, 150 mg, 200 mg.

INDICATIONS AND DOSAGES

▸ HIV Infection (in Combination with Other Antiretrovirals)

PO (Chewable Tablets)
Adults, children 13 yr and older weighing 60 kg or more. 200 mg q12h or 400 mg once a day.
Adults, Children 13 yr and older weighing 60 kg or less. 125 mg q12h or 250 mg once a day.
Children 3 mo to less than 13 yr. 180–300 mg/m²/day in divided doses q12h.
Children younger than 3 mo. 50 mg/m²/day in divided doses q12h.
PO (Delayed-Release Capsules)
Adults, Children 13 yr and older, weighing 60 kg or more. 400 mg once a day.
Adults, Children 13 yr and older, weighing 60 kg or less. 250 mg once a day.
PO (Oral Solution)
Adults, Children 13 yr and older weighing 60 kg or more. 250 mg q12h.
Adults, Children 13 yr and older weighing 60 kg or less. 167 mg q12h.
PO (Pediatric Powder for Oral Solution)
Children 3 mo to younger than 13 yr. 180–300 mg/m²/day in divided doses q12h.
Children younger than 3 mo. 50 mg/m²/day in divided doses q12h.

▸ Dosage in Renal Impairment

Patients weighing less than 60 kg:

CrCl	Tablets	Oral Solution	Delayed-Release Capsules
30–59 ml/min	75 mg twice a day	100 mg twice a day	125 mg once a day
10–29 ml/min	100 mg once a day	100 mg once a day	125 mg once a day
less than 10 ml/min	75 mg once a day	100 mg once a day	N/A CrCl = creatinine clearance

Patients weighing 60 kg or more:

CrCl	Tablets	Oral Solution	Delayed-Release Capsules
30–59 ml/min	100 mg twice a day	100 mg twice a day	200 mg once a day
10–29 ml/min	150 mg once a day	167 mg once a day	125 mg once a day
less than 10 ml/min	100 mg once a day	100 mg once a day	125 mg once a day CrCl = creatinine clearance

CONTRAINDICATIONS

Hypersensitivity to didanosine or any of its components

INTERACTIONS

Drug

Dapsone, flouroquinolones, itraconazole, ketoconazole, tetracyclines: May decrease absorption of these drugs.
Medications producing pancreatitis or peripheral neuropathy: May increase the risk of pancreatitis or peripheral neuropathy.
Stavudine: May increase the risk of fatal lactic acidosis in pregnancy.

Herbal

None known.

Food

All foods: Decreases absorption of didanosine.

Drug interactions of concern to dentistry

- Decreased absorption of the following drugs: ketoconazole, dapsone, itraconazole, tetracyclines, fluoroquinolone antibiotics
- Increased risk of pancreatitis: metronidazole, sulfonamides, sulindac, tetracyclines
- Increased risk of peripheral neuropathy: metronidazole, nitrous oxide

DIAGNOSTIC TEST EFFECTS

May increase serum alkaline phosphatase, amylase, bilirubin, lipase, triglyceride, AST (SGOT), ALT (SGPT), and uric acid levels. May decrease serum potassium levels.

SIDE EFFECTS

Frequent

Adults (> 10%)

Diarrhea, neuropathy, chills and fever

Children (> 25%)

Chills, fever, decreased appetite, pain, malaise, nausea, vomiting, diarrhea, abdominal pain, headache, nervousness, cough, rhinitis, dyspnea, asthenia, rash, pruritus

Occasional

Adults (9%–2%)

Rash, pruritus, headache, abdominal pain, nausea, vomiting, pneumonia, myopathy, decreased appetite, dry mouth, dyspnea

Children (25%–10%)

Failure to thrive, weight loss, stomatitis, oral thrush, ecchymosis, arthritis, myalgia, insomnia, epistaxis, pharyngitis

SERIOUS REACTIONS

! Pneumonia and opportunistic infections occur occasionally.

! Peripheral neuropathy, potentially fatal pancreatitis, retinal changes, and optic neuritis are the major toxic effects.

DENTAL CONSIDERATIONS

General:

- Monitor vital signs at every appointment because of cardiovascular side effects.
- Avoid dental light in patient's eyes; offer dark glasses for patient comfort.
- Patients on chronic drug therapy may rarely have symptoms of blood dyscrasias, which can include infection, bleeding, and poor healing.

Consultations:

- Medical consultation may be required to assess patient's ability to tolerate stress.
- In a patient with symptoms of blood dyscrasias, request a medical consultation for blood studies and postpone dental treatment until normal values are reestablished.

Teach Patient/Family:

- Importance of good oral hygiene to prevent soft tissue inflammation
- Caution to prevent injury when using oral hygiene aids
- *When chronic dry mouth occurs, advise patient:*
  - To avoid mouth rinses with high alcohol content because of drying effects
  - To use daily home fluoride products for anticaries effect
  - To use sugarless gum, frequent sips of water, or saliva substitutes

diethylpropion

die-ethyl-prop′-ion
Schedule IV
Tenuate, Teunate Dospan

CATEGORY AND SCHEDULE

Pregnancy Risk Category: B
Controlled Substance: Schedule IV

MECHANISM OF ACTION

A sympathomimetic amine that stimulates the release of norepinephrine and dopamine.
Therapeutic Effect: Decreases appetite.

PHARMACOKINETICS

Rapidly absorbed from the gastrointestinal (GI) tract. Widely distributed. Metabolized in liver to active metabolite and undergoes extensive first-pass metabolism. Excreted in urine. Unknown if removed by hemodialysis.
Half-life: 4–6 hrs.

AVAILABILITY

Tablets: 25 mg (Tenuate).
Tablets (extended-release): 75 mg (Tenuate Dospan).

INDICATIONS AND DOSAGES

▸ Obesity

PO

Adults. 25 mg 3 times/day before meals. (Extended-release) 75 mg at midmorning.

OFF-LABEL USES

Migraines

CONTRAINDICATIONS

Agitated states, use of MAOIs within 14 days, glaucoma, history of drug abuse, hyperthyroidism, advanced arteriosclerosis or severe cardiovascular disease, severe hypertension, and hypersensitivity to sympathomimetic amines

INTERACTIONS

Drug

Anorectic agents: May increase the risk of cardiac effects of diethylpropion.
Anesthetics: May increase the risk of arrhythmias.
Antidiabetic agents, insulin: May alter blood glucose concentrations.
Guanethidine: May decrease the effects of guanethidine.
MAOIs: May increase the risk of hypertensive crisis.
Phenothiazines: May decrease the effects of diethylpropion.
Tricyclic antidepressants: May increase the cardiac and CNS effects of diethylpropion.

Herbal

None known.

Food

None known.

Drug interactions of concern to dentistry

- Dysrhythmia: hydrocarbon inhalation anesthetics
- Decreased effects: barbiturates, tricyclic antidepressants, phenothiazines

DIAGNOSTIC TEST EFFECTS

Urine screen for amphetamines.

SIDE EFFECTS

Frequent

Elevated blood pressure, nervousness, insomnia

Occasional

Dizziness, drowsiness, tremor, headache, nausea, stomach pain, fever, rash

Rare

Agranulocytosis, leukopenia, blurred vision, psychosis, CVA, seizure

SERIOUS REACTIONS

! Overdose may produce agitation, tachycardia, palpitations, cardiac irregularities, chest pain, psychotic episode, seizures, and coma.
! Hypersensitivity reactions and blood dyscrasias occur rarely.

DENTAL CONSIDERATIONS

General:

- Monitor vital signs at every appointment because of cardiovascular and respiratory side effects.
- Examine for evidence of oral manifestations of blood dyscrasias (infection, bleeding, poor healing).
- Assess salivary flow as a factor in caries, periodontal disease, and candidiasis.
- Psychologic and physical dependence may occur with chronic administration.
- Consider semisupine chair position for patient comfort because of GI effects of disease.

Consultations:

- Medical consultation for blood studies (CBC); leukopenic or thrombocytopenic side effects may result in infection, delayed healing, and excessive bleeding. Postpone dental treatment until normal values are maintained.

Teach Patient/Family:

- Importance of good oral hygiene to prevent soft tissue inflammation
- Caution in use of oral hygiene aids to prevent injury
- *When chronic dry mouth occurs, advise patient:*
  - To avoid mouth rinses with high alcohol content because of drying effects
  - To use daily home fluoride products for anticaries effect
  - To use sugarless gum, frequent sips of water, or saliva substitutes

diflorasone

die-floor′-a-sone
(Florone[CAN], Maxiflor, Psorcon, Psorcon-e)

CATEGORY AND SCHEDULE

Pregnancy Risk Category: C

MECHANISM OF ACTION

A high-potency, fluorinated corticosteroid that decreases inflammation by suppression of migration of polymorphonuclear leukocytes and reversal of increased capillary permeability. The exact mechanism of the anti-inflammatory process is unclear. ***Therapeutic Effect:*** Decreases or prevents tissue response to the inflammatory process.

PHARMACOKINETICS

Poor absorption; occlusive dressings increase absorption. Metabolized in liver. Primarily excreted in urine.

AVAILABILITY

Cream: 0.05% (Maxiflor, Psorcon).
Ointment: 0.05% (Maxiflor, Psorcon).
Ointment, emollient: 0.05% (Psorcon-e).

INDICATIONS AND DOSAGES

▸ Dermatoses

TOPICAL

Adults, Elderly. (Cream) Apply sparingly 2–4 times/day. (Ointment) Apply sparingly 1–3 times/day.

OFF-LABEL USES

Psoriasis

CONTRAINDICATIONS

History of hypersensitivity to diflorasone or other corticosteroids

INTERACTIONS
Drug
None known.
Herbal
None known.
Food
None known.

DIAGNOSTIC TEST EFFECTS
None known.

SIDE EFFECTS
Rare
Itching, redness, dryness, irritation, burning at site of application, arthralgia, folliculitis, maceration, muscle atrophy, secondary infection

SERIOUS REACTIONS
! Overdosage symptoms include moon face, central obesity, hypertension, diabetes, hyperlipidemia, peptic ulcer, increased susceptibility to infection, electrolyte and fluid imbalance, psychosis, and hallucinations.
! The serious reactions of long-term therapy and the addition of occlusive dressings are reversible hypothalamic-pituitary-adrenal (HPA) axis suppression, manifestations of Cushing's syndrome, hyperglycemia, and glucosuria.

DENTAL CONSIDERATIONS
General:
- Determine why the patient is taking the drug.
- Apply lubricant to dry lips for patient comfort before dental procedures.
- Place on frequent recall to evaluate healing response if used on chronic basis.

diflunisal
dye-floo′-ni-sal
(Apo-Diflunisal[CAN], Dolobid, Novo-Diflunisal[CAN])
Do not confuse diflunisal with Dicarbosil or Dolobid with Slo-bid.

CATEGORY AND SCHEDULE
Pregnancy Risk Category: C (D if used in third trimester or near delivery)

MECHANISM OF ACTION
A nonsteroidal anti-inflammatory that inhibits prostaglandin synthesis, reducing inflammatory response and intensity of pain stimulus reaching sensory nerve endings. ***Therapeutic Effect:*** Produces analgesic and anti-inflammatory effect.

PHARMACOKINETICS
Route	Onset	Peak	Duration
PO	1 hr	2–3 hr	8–12 hr

Completely absorbed from the GI tract. Widely distributed. Protein binding: greater than 99%. Metabolized in liver. Primarily excreted in urine. Not removed by hemodialysis. ***Half-life:*** 8–12 hr.

AVAILABILITY
Tablets: 250 mg, 500 mg.

INDICATIONS AND DOSAGES
▸ **Mild to Moderate Pain**
PO
Adults, Elderly. Initially, 0.5–1 g, then 250–500 mg q8–12h. Maximum: 1.5 g/day.
▸ **Rheumatoid Arthritis,**

Osteoarthritis
PO
Adults, Elderly. 0.5–1 g/day in 2 divided doses. Maximum: 1.5 g/day.

OFF-LABEL USES
Treatment of psoriatic arthritis, vascular headache

CONTRAINDICATIONS
Active GI bleeding, factor VII or factor IX deficiencies, hypersensitivity to aspirin or NSAIDs

INTERACTIONS
Drug
Antihypertensives, diuretics: May decrease the effects of these drugs.
Aspirin, salicylates: May increase the risk of GI bleeding and side effects.
Bone marrow depressants: May increase the risk of hematologic reactions.
Heparin, oral anticoagulants, thrombolytics: May increase the effects of these drugs.
Lithium: May increase the blood concentration and risk of toxicity of lithium.
Methotrexate: May increase the risk of toxicity of methotrexate.
Probenecid: May increase diflunisal blood concentration.
Herbal
Ginkgo biloba: May increase the risk of bleeding.
Food
None known.
Drug interactions of concern to dentistry
- Increased risk of GI ulceration and bleeding: aspirin, steroids, alcohol, indomethacin, other NSAIDs
- Hepatotoxicity, nephrotoxicity: acetaminophen (prolonged use)
- Suspected increase in potential toxic effects: probenecid

DIAGNOSTIC TEST EFFECTS
May increase serum AST (SGOT) and ALT (SGPT) levels. May decrease serum uric acid levels.

SIDE EFFECTS
Side effects are less common with short-term treatment.
Occasional (9%–3%)
Nausea, dyspepsia (heartburn, indigestion, epigastric pain), diarrhea, headache, rash
Rare (3%–1%)
Vomiting, constipation, flatulence, dizziness, somnolence, insomnia, fatigue, tinnitus

SERIOUS REACTIONS
! Overdosage may produce drowsiness, vomiting, nausea, diarrhea, hyperventilation, tachycardia, diaphoresis, stupor, and coma.
! Peptic ulcer, GI bleeding, gastritis, and severe hepatic reaction, including cholestasis, jaundice occur rarely.
! Nephrotoxicity, including dysuria, hematuria, proteinuria, and nephrotic syndrome, and severe hypersensitivity reaction, marked by bronchospasm and angioedema, occur rarely.

DENTAL CONSIDERATIONS
General:
- Patients on chronic drug therapy may rarely have symptoms of blood dyscrasias, which can include infection, bleeding, and poor healing.
- Assess salivary flow as a factor in caries, periodontal disease, and candidiasis.
- Avoid prescribing for dental use in first and last trimester of pregnancy.

Consultations:

- Medical consultation may be required to assess disease control.
- In a patient with symptoms of blood dyscrasias, request a medical consultation for blood studies and postpone dental treatment until normal values are reestablished.

Teach Patient/Family:

- Importance of good oral hygiene to prevent soft tissue inflammation
- Caution to prevent injury when using oral hygiene aids
- *When chronic dry mouth occurs, advise patient:*
  - To avoid mouth rinses with high alcohol content because of drying effects
  - To use daily home fluoride products for anticaries effect
  - To use sugarless gum, frequent sips of water, or saliva substitutes

digoxin

di-jox′-in

(Digitek, Lanoxicaps, Lanoxin, Sigmaxin[AUS])

Do not confuse digoxin with Desoxyn or doxepin, or Lanoxin with Levsinex or Lonox.

CATEGORY AND SCHEDULE

Pregnancy Risk Category: C

MECHANISM OF ACTION

A cardiac glycoside that increases the influx of calcium from extracellular to intracellular cytoplasm. ***Therapeutic Effect:*** Potentiates the activity of the contractile cardiac muscle fibers and increases the force of myocardial contraction. Slows the heart rate by decreasing conduction through the SA and AV nodes.

PHARMACOKINETICS

Route	Onset	Peak	Duration
PO	0.5–2 hr	28 hr	3–4 days
IV	5–30 min	1–4 hr	3–4 days

Readily absorbed from the GI tract. Widely distributed. Protein binding: 30%. Partially metabolized in the liver. Primarily excreted in urine. Minimally removed by hemodialysis. ***Half-life:*** 36–48 hr (increased with impaired renal function and in the elderly).

AVAILABILITY

Capsules (Lanoxicaps): 50 mcg, 100 mcg, 200 mcg.
Elixir (Lanoxin): 50 mcg/ml.
Tablets (Digitek, Lanoxin): 125 mcg, 250 mcg.
Injection (Lanoxin): 100 mcg/ml, 250 mcg/ml.

INDICATIONS AND DOSAGES

▸ **Rapid Loading Dose for the Management and Treatment of CHF; Control of Ventricular Rate in Patients with Atrial Fibrillation; Treatment and Prevention of Recurrent Paroxysmal Atrial Tachycardia**

PO

Adults, Elderly. Initially, 0.5–0.75 mg, additional doses of 0.125–0.375 mg at 6- to 8-hr intervals. Range: 0.75–1.25 mg.
Children 10 yr and older. 10–15 mcg/kg.
Children 5–9 yr. 20–35 mcg/kg.
Children 2–4 yr. 30–40 mcg/kg.
Children 1–23 mo. 35–60 mcg/kg.
Neonate, full-term. 25–35 mcg/kg.
Neonate, premature. 20–30 mcg/kg.

D

IV
Adults, Elderly. 0.6–1 mg.
Children 10 yr and older. 8–12 mcg/kg.
Children 5–9 yr. 15–30 mcg/kg.
Children 2–4 yr. 25–35 mcg/kg.
Children 1–23 mo. 30–50 mcg/kg.
Neonates, full-term. 20–30 mcg/kg.
Neonates, premature. 15–25 mcg/kg.

▸ Maintenance Dosage for CHF; Control of Ventricular Rate in Patients with Atrial Fibrillation; Treatment and Prevention of Recurrent Paroxysmal Atrial Tachycardia
PO, IV
Adults, Elderly. 0.125–0.375 mg/day.
Children. 25%–35% loading dose (20%–30% for premature neonates).

▸ Dosage in Renal Impairment
Dosage adjustment is based on creatinine clearance. Total digitalizing dose: decrease by 50% in end-stage renal disease.

Creatinine Clearance	Dosage
10–50 ml/min	25%–75% usual
less than 10 ml/min	10%–25% usual

CONTRAINDICATIONS
Ventricular fibrillation, ventricular tachycardia unrelated to CHF

INTERACTIONS
Drug
Amiodarone: May increase digoxin blood concentration and risk of toxicity; may have an additive effect on the SA and AV nodes.
Amphotericin, glucocorticoids, potassium-depleting diuretics: May increase risk of toxicity due to hypokalemia.
Antiarrhythmics, parenteral calcium, sympathomimetics: May increase risk of arrhythmias.
Antidiarrheals, cholestyramine, colestipol, sucralfate: May decrease absorption of digoxin.
Diltiazem, fluoxetine, quinidine, verapamil: May increase digoxin blood concentration.
Parenteral magnesium: May cause cardiac conduction changes and heart block.
Herbal
Siberian ginseng: May increase serum digoxin levels.
St. John's wort: May reduce digoxin efficacy.
Food
All food: May decrease peak digoxin concentrations.
Drug interactions of concern to dentistry
- Hypokalemia: corticosteroids
- Increased digoxin blood levels: erythromycin, clarithromycin, tetracyclines, itraconazole, propantheline
- Cardiac dysrhythmias: adrenergic agonists, succinylcholine

DIAGNOSTIC TEST EFFECTS
None known.

IV INCOMPATIBILITIES
Amphotericin B complex (Abelcet, Amphotec, AmBisome), fluconazole (Diflucan), foscarnet (Foscavir), propofol (Diprivan)
IV COMPATIBILITIES
Cimetidine (Tagamet), diltiazem (Cardizem), furosemide (Lasix), heparin, insulin (regular), lidocaine, midazolam (Versed), milrinone (Primacor), morphine, potassium chloride, propofol (Diprivan)

SIDE EFFECTS
None known. However, there is a very narrow margin of safety between a therapeutic and toxic result. Long-term therapy may

produce mammary gland enlargement in women but is reversible when drug is withdrawn.

SERIOUS REACTIONS

! The most common early manifestations of digoxin toxicity are GI disturbances (anorexia, nausea, vomiting) and neurologic abnormalities (fatigue, headache, depression, weakness, drowsiness, confusion, nightmares).
! Facial pain, personality change, and ocular disturbances (photophobia, light flashes, halos around bright objects, yellow or green color perception) may be noted.

DENTAL CONSIDERATIONS

General:

• Monitor vital signs at every appointment because of cardiovascular side effects.
• After supine positioning, have patient sit upright for at least 2 min to avoid orthostatic hypotension.
• Avoid dental light in patient's eyes; offer dark glasses for patient comfort.
• An increased gag reflex may make dental procedures, such as taking radiographs or impressions, difficult.
• Use vasoconstrictors with caution, in low doses, and with careful aspiration. Avoid use of gingival retraction cord with epinephrine.

Consultations:

• Stress from dental procedures may compromise cardiovascular function; determine patient risk.
• Medical consultation may be required to assess disease control and patient's ability to tolerate stress.

dihydrotachysterol

dye-hye-droe-tak-iss′-ter-ole
(DHT, DHT Intensol, Hytakerol)

CATEGORY AND SCHEDULE

Pregnancy Risk Category: A
(D if used in doses above RDA)

MECHANISM OF ACTION

A fat-soluble vitamin that is essential for absorption, utilization of calcium phosphate, and normal calcification of bone.
Therapeutic Effect: Stimulates calcium and phosphate absorption from small intestine, promotes secretion of calcium from bone to blood, promotes renal tubule phosphate resorption, acts on bone cells to stimulate skeletal growth and on parathyroid gland to suppress hormone synthesis and secretion.

PHARMACOKINETICS

Well absorbed from small intestine. Metabolized in liver. Eliminated via biliary system; excreted in urine.
Half-life: Unknown.

AVAILABILITY

Oral Solution: 0. 2 mg/ml (DHT Intensol).
Capsule: 0. 125 mg (Hytakerol).
Tablets: 0. 125 mg, 0. 2 mg, 0. 4 mg (DHT).

INDICATIONS AND DOSAGES

▸ **Hypoparathyroidism**

PO

Adults, Elderly, Older Children. Initially, 0.8–2.4 mg/day for several days. Maintenance: 0.2–1 mg/day.
Infants, Young Children. Initially, 1–5 mg/day for 4 days, then 0.1–0.5 mg/day.

▸ Nutritional Rickets
PO
Adults, Elderly, Children. 0.5 mg as a single dose or 13–50 mcg/day until healing occurs.
▸ Renal Osteodystorphy
PO
Adults, Elderly. 0.25–0.6 mg/24 hrs adjusted as needed to achieve normal serum calcium levels and promote bone healing.

CONTRAINDICATIONS
Hypercalcemia, malabsorption syndrome, vitamin D toxicity, hypersensitivity to vitamin D products or analogs

INTERACTIONS
Drug
Aluminum-containing antacid (long-term use): May increase aluminum concentration and aluminum bone toxicity.
Calcium-containing preparations, thiazide diuretics: May increase the risk of hypercalcemia.
Magnesium-containing antacids: May increase magnesium concentration.
Herbal
None known.
Food
None known.
Drug interactions of concern to dentistry
- Decreased effect of dihydrotachysterol: prolonged use of corticosteroids, barbiturates

DIAGNOSTIC TEST EFFECTS
May increase serum cholesterol, calcium, magnesium, and phosphate levels. May decrease serum alkaline phosphatase.

SIDE EFFECTS
Occasional
Nausea, vomiting

SERIOUS REACTIONS
! Early signs of overdosage are manifested as weakness, headache, somnolence, nausea, vomiting, dry mouth, constipation, muscle and bone pain, and metallic taste sensation.
! Later signs of overdosage are evidenced by polyuria, polydipsia, anorexia, weight loss, nocturia, photophobia, rhinorrhea, pruritus, disorientation, hallucinations, hyperthermia, hypertension, and cardiac arrhythmias.

DENTAL CONSIDERATIONS
General:
- Consider semisupine chair position for patient comfort because of GI effects of drug.
- Assess salivary flow as a factor in caries, periodontal disease, and candidiasis.

Teach Patient/Family:
- *When chronic dry mouth occurs, advise patient:*
  - To avoid mouth rinses with high alcohol content because of drying effects
  - Of need for daily home fluoride to prevent caries
  - To use sugarless gum, frequent sips of water, or saliva substitutes

diltiazem hydrochloride

dil-tye′-a-zem
(Apo-Diltiaz[CAN], Auscard[AUS], Cardcal[AUS], Cardizem, Cardizem CD, Cardizem LA, Cardizem SR, Cartia, Coras[AUS], Dilacor XR, Diltahexal[AUS], Diltia XT, Diltiamax[AUS], Dilzem[AUS], Novo-Diltiazem[CAN], Taztia XT, Tiazac, Vasocardal CD[AUS])

Do not confuse Cardizem with Cardene or Cardene SR, or Tiazac with Ziac.

CATEGORY AND SCHEDULE

Pregnancy Risk Category: C

MECHANISM OF ACTION

An antianginal, antihypertensive, and antiarrhythmic agent that inhibits calcium movement across cardiac and vascular smooth-muscle cell membranes. This action causes the dilation of coronary arteries, peripheral arteries, and arterioles. ***Therapeutic Effect:*** Decreases heart rate and myocardial contractility, slows SA and AV conduction and decreases total peripheral vascular resistance by vasodilation.

PHARMACOKINETICS

Route	Onset	Peak	Duration
PO	0.5–1 hr	N/A	N/A
PO (extended-release)	2–3 hr	N/A	N/A
IV	3 min	N/A	N/A

Well absorbed from the GI tract. Protein binding: 70%–80%. Undergoes first-pass metabolism in the liver to active metabolite. Primarily excreted in urine. Not removed by hemodialysis. ***Half-life:*** 3–8 hr.

AVAILABILITY

Capsules (Sustained-Release [Cardizem SR]): 60 mg, 90 mg, 120 mg.
Capsules (Extended-Release [Cardizem CD]): 120 mg, 180 mg, 240 mg, 300 mg, 360 mg.
Capsules (Extended-Release [Cartia XT]): 120 mg, 180 mg, 240 mg, 300 mg.
Capsules (Extended-Release [Dilacor XR]): 120 mg, 180 mg, 240 mg.
Capsules (Extended-Release [Diltia XT]): 120 mg, 180 mg, 240 mg.
Capsules (Extended-Release [Taztia XT]): 120 mg, 180 mg, 240 mg, 300 mg, 360 mg.
Caspules (Extended-Release [Tiazac]): 120 mg, 180 mg, 240 mg, 300 mg, 360 mg, 420 mg.
Tablets (Cardizem): 30 mg, 60 mg, 90 mg, 120 mg.
Tablets (Extended-Release [Cardizem LA]): 120 mg, 180 mg, 240 mg, 300 mg, 360 mg, 420 mg.
Injection (Ready-to-Hang Infusion): 1 mg/ml.

INDICATIONS AND DOSAGES

▸ Angina Related to Coronary Artery Spasm (Prinzmetal's Variant), Chronic Stable Angina (Effort-Associated)

PO

Adults, Elderly. Initially, 30 mg 4 times a day. Increase up to 180–360 mg/day in 3–4 divided doses at 1- to 2-day intervals.

PO (Cardizem LA)

Adults, Elderly. Initially, 180 mg/day. May increase at intervals of 7–14 days up to 360 mg/day.

PO (Cardizem CD)

Adults, Elderly. Initially, 120–180 mg/day; titrate over 7–14 days. Range: Up to 480 mg/day.

▸ **Essential Hypertension**
PO (Cardizem CD, Cartia XT)
Adults, Elderly. Initially, 180–240 mg once a day. May increase at 2-week intervals. Maintenance 240–360 mg/day. Maximum: 480 mg once a day.
PO (Cardizem SR)
Adults, Elderly. Initially, 60–120 mg twice a day. May increase at 2 week intervals.
Maintenance: 240–360 mg/day.
PO (Cardizem LA)
Adults, Elderly. Initially, 180–240 mg once a day. May increase at 2 week intervals.
Maintenance: 120–540 mg/day.
PO (Dilacor XR)
Adults, Elderly. 180–240 mg once a day.
PO (Dilacor XT)
Adults, Elderly. Initially, 180–240 mg a day. May increase at 2 week intervals. Maximum: 540 mg once a day.
PO (Taztia XT)
Adults, Elderly. Initially, 120–240 mg once a day. May increase at 2 week intervals. Maximum: 540 mg once a day.

▸ **Temporary Control of Rapid Ventricular Rate in Atrial Fibrillation or Flutter, Rapid Conversion of Paroxysmal Supraventricular Tachycardia to Normal Sinus Rhythm.**
IV PUSH
Adults, Elderly. Initially, 0.25 mg/kg actual body weight over 2 min. May repeat in 15 min at dose of 0.35 mg/kg actual body weight. Subsequent doses individualized.
IV INFUSION
Adults, Elderly. After initial bolus injection, may begin infusion at 5–10 mg/hr; may increase by 5 mg/hr up to a maximum of 15 mg/hr. Infusion duration should not exceed 24 hr.

CONTRAINDICATIONS
Acute MI, pulmonary congestion, severe hypotension (< 90 mm Hg, systolic), sick sinus syndrome, second- or third-degree AV block (except in the presence of a pacemaker)

INTERACTIONS
Drug
Beta blockers: May have additive effect.
Carbamazepine, quinidine, theophylline: May increase diltiazem blood concentration and risk of toxicity.
Digoxin: May increase serum digoxin concentration.
Procainamide, quinidine: May increase risk of QT-interval prolongation.
Herbal
None known.
Food
None known.
Drug interactions of concern to dentistry
• Decreased effect: indomethacin, possibly other NSAIDs, phenobarbital
• Increased effect: parenteral and inhalational general anesthetics, other drugs with hypotensive actions
• Increased effects of carbamazepine, midazolam, triazolam, buspirone

DIAGNOSTIC TEST EFFECTS
PR interval may be increased.

IV INCOMPATIBILITIES
Acetazolamide (Diamox), acyclovir (Zovirax), aminophylline, ampicillin, ampicillin/sulbactam (Unasyn), cefoperazone (Cefobid), diazepam (Valium), furosemide (Lasix), heparin, insulin, nafcillin, phenytoin (Dilantin), rifampin (Rifadin), sodium bicarbonate

IV COMPATIBILITIES

Albumin, aztreonam (Azactam), bumetanide (Bumex), cefazolin (Ancef), cefotaxime (Claforan), ceftazidime (Fortaz), ceftriaxone (Rocephin), cefuroxime (Zinacef), cimetidine (Tagamet), ciprofloxacin (Cipro), clindamycin (Cleocin), digoxin (Lanoxin), dobutamine (Dobutrex), dopamine (Intropin), gentamicin (Garamycin), hydromorphone (Dilaudid), lidocaine, lorazepam (Ativan), metoclopramide (Reglan), metronidazole (Flagyl), midazolam (Versed), morphine, multivitamins, nitroglycerin, norepinephrine (Levophed), potassium chloride, potassium phosphate, tobramycin (Nebcin), vancomycin (Vancocin)

SIDE EFFECTS

Frequent (10%–5%)
Peripheral edema, dizziness, light-headedness, headache, bradycardia, asthenia (loss of strength, weakness)

Occasional (5%–2%)
Nausea, constipation, flushing, ECG changes

Rare (< 2%)
Rash, micturition disorder (polyuria, nocturia, dysuria, frequency of urination), abdominal discomfort, somnolence

SERIOUS REACTIONS

! Abrupt withdrawal may increase frequency or duration of angina.

! CHF and second- and third-degree AV block occur rarely.

! Overdose produces nausea, somnolence, confusion, slurred speech, and profound bradycardia.

DENTAL CONSIDERATIONS

General:

- Monitor cardiac status; take vital signs at each appointment because of cardiovascular side effects. Consider a stress reduction protocol to prevent stress-induced angina during the dental appointment.
- After supine positioning, have patient sit upright for at least 2 min to avoid orthostatic hypotension.
- Place on frequent recall to monitor gingival condition.
- Limit use of sodium-containing products, such as saline IV fluids, for patients with a dietary salt restriction.
- Assess salivary flow as a factor in caries, periodontal disease, and candidiasis.
- Consider drug in diagnosis of taste alterations.

Consultations:

- Medical consultation may be required to assess disease control.

Teach Patient/Family:

- Importance of good oral hygiene to prevent soft tissue inflammation and minimize gingival overgrowth
- Need for frequent oral prophylaxis if gingival overgrowth occurs
- *When chronic dry mouth occurs, advise patient:*
  - To avoid mouth rinses with high alcohol content because of drying effects
  - To use daily home fluoride products for anticaries effect
  - To use sugarless gum, frequent sips of water, or saliva substitutes

D

dimenhydrinate

dye-men-hye′-dri-nate
(Dramamine)

CATEGORY AND SCHEDULE

Pregnancy Risk Category: B

MECHANISM OF ACTION

An antihistamine and anticholinergic that competes for H_1 receptor sites on effector cells of the GI tract, blood vessels, and respiratory tract. The anticholinergic action diminishes vestibular stimulation and depresses labyrinthine function.
Therapeutic Effect: Prevents symptoms of motion sickness.

AVAILABILITY

Tablets (Chewable): 50 mg.
Tablets: 50 mg.

INDICATIONS AND DOSAGES

▸ Motion Sickness

PO
Adults, Elderly, Children older than 12 yr. 50–100 mg q4–6h.
Maximum: 400 mg/day.
Children 6–12 yr. 25–50 mg q6–8h.
Maximum: 150 mg/day.
Children 2–5 yr. 12.5–25 mg q6–8h.
Maximum: 75 mg/day.

CONTRAINDICATIONS

None significant.

INTERACTIONS

Drug

Alcohol, other CNS suppressants: May increase CNS depression.
Aminoglycosides: Masks signs and symptoms of ototoxicity associated with aminoglycosides.
Other anticholinergics: Increases anticholinergic effect.

Herbal

None known.

Food

None known.

Drug interactions of concern to dentistry

- Increased photosensitization: tetracycline
- Increased effects of alcohol, other CNS depressants, anticholinergics

DIAGNOSTIC TEST EFFECTS

None known.

SIDE EFFECTS

Frequent

Dry mouth

Occasional

Hypotension, palpitations, tachycardia, headache, somnolence, dizziness, paradoxical stimulation (especially in children), anorexia, constipation, dysuria, blurred vision, tinnitus, wheezing, chest tightness

Rare

Photosensitivity, rash, urticaria

SERIOUS REACTIONS

! None significant.

DENTAL CONSIDERATIONS

General:

- Assess salivary flow as a factor in caries, periodontal disease, and candidiasis.

Teach Patient/Family:

- *When chronic dry mouth occurs, advise patient:*
  - To avoid mouth rinses with high alcohol content because of drying effects
  - To use daily home fluoride products for anticaries effect
  - To use sugarless gum, frequent sips of water, or saliva substitutes

diphenhydramine

dye-fen-hye′-dra-meen
(Allerdryl[CAN], Banophen, Benadryl, Diphen, Diphenhist, Genahist, Nytol[CAN], Unisom Sleepgels[AUS])

Do not confuse diphenhydramine with dimenhydrinate, or Benadryl with benazepril, Bentyl, or Benylin, or Banophen with baclofen.

CATEGORY AND SCHEDULE

Pregnancy Risk Category: B
OTC (capsules, tablets, chewable tablets, syrup, elixir, cream, spray)

MECHANISM OF ACTION

An ethanolamine that competitively blocks the effects of histamine at peripheral H_1 receptor sites. ***Therapeutic Effect:*** Produces anticholinergic, antipruritic, antitussive, antiemetic, antidyskinetic, and sedative effects.

PHARMACOKINETICS

Route	Onset	Peak	Duration
PO	15–30 min	1–4 hr	4–6 hr
IV, IM	less than 15 min	1–4 hr	4–6 hr

Well absorbed after PO or parenteral administration. Protein binding: 98%–99%. Widely distributed. Metabolized in the liver. Primarily excreted in urine. ***Half-life:*** 1–4 hr.

AVAILABILITY

Capsules (Banophen, Diphen, Genahist): 25 mg.
Capsules (Nytol): 50 mg.
Syrup (Diphen, Diphenhist): 12.5 mg/5 ml.
Tablets (Banophen, Benadryl, Genahist, Nytol): 25 mg, 50 mg.
Injection (Benadryl): 50 mg/ml.
Cream (Benadryl): 1%, 2%.
Spray: 1%, 2%.

INDICATIONS AND DOSAGES

▸ Moderate to Severe Allergic Reaction, Dystonic Reaction

PO, IV, IM
Adults, Elderly. 25–50 mg q4h. Maximum: 400 mg/day.
Children. 5 mg/kg/day in divided doses q6–8h. Maximum: 300 mg/day.

▸ Motion Sickness, Minor Allergic Rhinitis

PO, IV, IM
Adults, Elderly, Children 12 yr and older. 25–50 mg q4–6h. Maximum: 300 mg/day.
Children 6–11 yr. 12.5–25 mg q4–6h. Maximum: 150 mg/day.
Children 2–5 yr. 6.25 mg q4–6h. Maximum: 37.5 mg/day.

▸ Antitussive

PO
Adults, Elderly, Children 12 yr and older. 25 mg q4h. Maximum: 150 mg/day.
Children 6–11 yr. 12.5 mg q4h. Maximum: 75 mg/day.
Children 2–5 yr. 6.25 mg q4h. Maximum: 37.5 mg/day.

▸ Nighttime Sleep Aid

PO
Adults, Elderly, Children 12 yr and older. 50 mg at bedtime.
Children 2–11 yr. 1 mg/kg/dose. Maximum: 50 mg.

▸ Pruritus

TOPICAL
Adults, Elderly, Children 12 yr and older. Apply 1% or 2% cream or spray 3–4 times a day.
Children 2–11 yr. Apply 1% cream or spray 3–4 times a day.

CONTRAINDICATIONS

Acute exacerbation of asthma, use within 14 days of MAOIs

INTERACTIONS

Drug

Alcohol, other CNS depressants: May increase CNS depressant effects.
Anticholinergics: May increase anticholinergic effects.
MAOIs: May increase the anticholinergic and CNS depressant effects of diphenhydramine.

Herbal

None known.

Food

None known.

Drug interactions of concern to dentistry

- Increased CNS depression: all CNS depressants, alcohol
- Increased anticholinergic effect: anticholinergics
- Increased plasma levels of labetalol

DIAGNOSTIC TEST EFFECTS

May suppress wheal and flare reactions to antigen skin testing unless the drug is discontinued 4 days before testing.

IV INCOMPATIBILITIES

Allopurinol (Aloprim), amphotericin B complex (Abelcet, AmBisome, Amphotec), cefepime (Maxipime), dexamethasone (Decadron), foscarnet (Foscavir)

IV COMPATIBILITIES

Atropine, cisplatin (Platinol), cyclophosphamide (Cytoxan), cytarabine (Ara-C), droperidol (Inapsine), fentanyl, glycopyrrolate (Robinul), heparin, hydrocortisone (Solu-Cortef), hydromorphone (Dilaudid), hydroxyzine (Vistaril), lidocaine, metoclopramide (Reglan), ondansetron (Zofran), promethazine (Phenergan), potassium chloride, propofol (Diprivan)

SIDE EFFECTS

Frequent

Somnolence, dizziness, muscle weakness, hypotension, urine retention, thickening of bronchial secretions, dry mouth, nose, throat, or lips; in elderly, sedation, dizziness, hypotension

Occasional

Epigastric distress, flushing, visual or hearing disturbances, paresthesia, diaphoresis, chills

SERIOUS REACTIONS

! Hypersensitivity reactions, such as eczema, pruritus, rash, cardiac disturbances, and photosensitivity, may occur.
! Overdose symptoms may vary from CNS depression, including sedation, apnea, hypotension, cardiovascular collapse, and death, to severe paradoxical reactions, such as hallucinations, tremor, and seizures.
! Children and neonates may experience paradoxical reactions, including restlessness, insomnia, euphoria, nervousness, and tremors.
! Overdosage in children may result in hallucinations, seizures, and death.

DENTAL CONSIDERATIONS

General:

- Patients on chronic drug therapy may rarely have symptoms of blood dyscrasias, which can include infection, bleeding, and poor healing.
- Assess salivary flow as a factor in caries, periodontal disease, and candidiasis.
- Consider semisupine chair position for patients with respiratory disease.

Consultations:

- In a patient with symptoms of blood dyscrasias, request a medical consultation for blood studies and postpone dental treatment until normal values are reestablished.

Teach Patient/Family:

- Importance of good oral hygiene to prevent soft tissue inflammation
- Caution to prevent injury when using oral hygiene aids
- *When chronic dry mouth occurs, advise patient:*
  - To avoid mouth rinses with high alcohol content because of drying effects
  - To use daily home fluoride products for anticaries effect
  - To use sugarless gum, frequent sips of water, or saliva substitutes

dipivefrin hydrochloride

dye-pi′-ve-frin hye-droe-klor′-ide
(Propine)

CATEGORY AND SCHEDULE

Pregnancy Risk Category: B

MECHANISM OF ACTION

A prodrug of epinephrine that penetrates into anterior chamber of the eye through its lipophilic character. ***Therapeutic Effect:*** Reduces intraocular pressure.

PHARMACOKINETICS

Onset of action occurs within 30 minutes and peak effect in 1 hour. Dipivefrin is more lipophilic than epinephrine. Distributed to cornea. Dipivefrin is converted to epinephrine inside the eye by enzyme hydrolysis.

AVAILABILITY

Ophthalmic solution: 1 mg/ml (Propine).

INDICATIONS AND DOSAGES

▸ **Glaucoma, Open-Angle**

OPHTHALMIC, TOPICAL

Adults, Elderly. Instill 1 drop of 0.1% solution in affected eye(s) q12h.

CONTRAINDICATIONS

Narrow-angle glaucoma, hypersensitivity to dipivefrin or any component of the formulation

INTERACTIONS

Drug

Pilocarpine: May increase myopia.

Herbal

None known.

Food

None known.

Drug interactions of concern to dentistry

- Avoid use of anticholinergics such as atropine, scopolamine, and propantheline; use benzodiazepines with caution

DIAGNOSTIC TEST EFFECTS

None known.

SIDE EFFECTS

Occasional

Blurred vision, burning or stinging of eye, mydriasis, headache

Rare

Follicular conjunctivitis

SERIOUS REACTIONS

! Signs of systemic absorption include hypertension, arrhythmias, and tachycardia.

! Follicular conjunctivitis has been reported.

DENTAL CONSIDERATIONS

General:

- Avoid dental light in patient's eyes; offer dark glasses for patient comfort.

dipyridamole

dye-peer-id′-a-mole
(Apo-Dipyridamole[CAN], Novodipiradol[CAN], Persantin[AUS], Persantin 100[AUS], Persantin SR[AUS], Persantine)
Do not confuse Aggrenox with Aggrastat, or dipyridamole with disopyramide, or Persantin with Periactin.

CATEGORY AND SCHEDULE

Pregnancy Risk Category: C

MECHANISM OF ACTION

A blood modifier and platelet aggregation inhibitor that inhibits the activity of adenosine deaminase and phosphodiesterase, enzymes causing accumulation of adenosine and cyclic adenosine monophosphate. ***Therapeutic Effect:*** Inhibits platelet aggregation; may cause coronary vasodilation.

PHARMACOKINETICS

Slowly, variably absorbed from the GI tract. Widely distributed. Protein binding: 91%–99%. Metabolized in the liver. Primarily eliminated via biliary excretion. ***Half-life:*** 10–15 hr.

AVAILABILITY

Tablets: 25 mg, 50 mg, 75 mg.
Injection: 5 mg/ml.

INDICATIONS AND DOSAGES

▸ Prevention of Thromboembolic Disorders

PO

Adults, Elderly. 75–400 mg/day in combination with other medications.
Children. 3–6 mg/kg/day in 3 divided doses.

▸ Diagnostic Aid

IV

Adults, Elderly (based on weight). 0.142 mg/kg/min infused over 4 min; although a maximum hasn't been determined, doses greater than 60 mg have been determined to be unnecessary for any patient.

OFF-LABEL USES

Prevention of myocardial reinfarction, treatment of transient ischemic attacks

CONTRAINDICATIONS

None known.

INTERACTIONS

Drug

Anticoagulants, aspirin, heparin, salicylates, thrombolytics: May increase the risk of bleeding with these drugs.

Herbal

None known.

Food

None known.

Drug interactions of concern to dentistry

- Additive antiplatelet effects: aspirin, other NSAIDs

DIAGNOSTIC TEST EFFECTS

None known.

IV INCOMPATIBILITIES

No information available via Y-site administration.

SIDE EFFECTS

Frequent (14%)

Dizziness

Occasional (6%–2%)

Abdominal distress, headache, rash

Rare (less than 2%)

Diarrhea, vomiting, flushing, pruritus

SERIOUS REACTIONS

! Overdose produces peripheral vasodilation, resulting in hypotension.

DENTAL CONSIDERATIONS

General:

- Monitor vital signs at every appointment because of cardiovascular side effects.
- After supine positioning, have patient sit upright for at least 2 min to avoid orthostatic hypotension.
- Avoid prescribing aspirin-containing products, even though ASA/dipyridamole combination drugs are used in some patients.
- Patients with prosthetic valves require antibiotic prophylaxis
- Evaluate for clotting ability during gingival instrumentation because inhibition of platelet aggregation may occur.
- Consider local hemostatic measures to prevent excessive bleeding during instrumentation.

Consultations:

- Medical consultation should include partial prothrombin time or PT.
- Medical consultation may be required to assess disease control.

Teach Patient/Family:

- Importance of good oral hygiene to prevent gingival inflammation

dirithromycin

die-rith-ro-my′-sin

(Dynabac)

Do not confuse Dynabac with Dynacin or DynaCirc.

CATEGORY AND SCHEDULE

Pregnancy Risk Category: C

MECHANISM OF ACTION

A macrolide that binds to ribosomal receptor sites of susceptible organisms, inhibiting bacterial protein synthesis. ***Therapeutic Effect:*** Bactericidal or bacteriostatic, depending on drug dosage.

PHARMACOKINETICS

Rapidly absorbed from the GI tract. Protein binding: 15%–30%.Widely distributed into tissues and within cells. Eliminated primarily unchanged by biliary excretion. Not removed by hemodialysis. ***Half-life:*** 30–44 hr.

AVAILABILITY

Tablets (Enteric-Coated): 250 mg.

INDICATIONS AND DOSAGES

▸ Pharyngitis, Tonsillitis

PO

Adults, Elderly, Children 12 yr and older: 500 mg once a day for 10 days.

▸ Acute or Chronic Bronchitis, Skin and Skin-Structure Infections

PO

Adults, Elderly, Children 12 yr and older: 500 mg once a day for 7 days.

▸ Community-Acquired Pneumonia

PO

Adults, Elderly, Children 12 yr and older: 500 mg once a day for 14 days.

CONTRAINDICATIONS

Hypersensitivity to dirithromycin or other macrolide antibiotics

INTERACTIONS

Drug

Aluminum- and magnesium-containing antacids: May decrease dirithromycin blood concentration.

H_2 antagonists: Increase dirithromycin absorption.

Herbal
None known.
Food
None known.
Drug interactions of concern to dentistry
- Other drug interactions: data are limited; antacids and histamine H_2 antagonists tend to enhance absorption; refer to erythromycin for potential interacting drugs

DIAGNOSTIC TEST EFFECTS
May increase serum CK and potassium levels, as well as blood eosinophil, neutrophil, and platelet counts.

SIDE EFFECTS
Frequent (10%–8%)
Abdominal pain, headache, nausea, diarrhea
Occasional (3%–2%)
Vomiting, dyspepsia, dizziness, nonspecific pain, asthenia
Rare (< 2%)
Increased cough, flatulence, rash, dyspnea, pruritus and urticaria, insomnia

SERIOUS REACTIONS
! Antibiotic-associated colitis and other superinfections may result from altered bacterial balance.

DENTAL CONSIDERATIONS
General:
- Do not use in patients at risk for bacteremias caused by inadequate serum levels.
- Potential value in dental infections is unknown.
- Determine why the patient is taking the drug.
- Examine for oral manifestations of opportunistic infections.

Consultations:
- Medical consultation may be required to assess disease control.

Teach Patient/Family:
- To be aware of the possibility of secondary oral infection and the need to see dentist immediately if infection occurs

disopyramide phosphate
dye-soe-peer′-a-mide
(Norpace, Norpace CR, Rythmodan[CAN])
Do not confuse disopyramide with desipramine, dipyridamole, or Rythmol.

CATEGORY AND SCHEDULE
Pregnancy Risk Category: C

MECHANISM OF ACTION
An antiarrhythmic that prolongs the refractory period of the cardiac cell by direct effect, decreasing myocardial excitability and conduction velocity. ***Therapeutic Effect:*** Depresses myocardial contractility. Has anticholinergic and negative inotropic effects.

AVAILABILITY
Capsules (Norpace): 100 mg, 150 mg.
Capsules (Extended-Release [Norpace CR]): 100 mg, 150 mg.

INDICATIONS AND DOSAGES
▸ **Suppression and Prevention of Ventricular Ectopy, Unifocal or Multifocal Premature Ventricular Contractions, Paired Ventricular Contractions (Couplets), and**

Episodes of Ventricular Tachycardia
PO
Adults, Elderly weighing 50 kg and more. 150 mg q6h (300 mg ql2h with extended-release).
Adults, Elderly weighing less than 50 kg. 100 mg q6h (200 mg q12h with extended-release).

▸ **Rapid Control of Arrhythmias**
PO
Adults, Elderly weighing 50 kg and more. Initially, 300 mg, then 150 mg q6h or 300 mg (controlled release) q12h.
Adults, Elderly weighing less than 50 kg. Initially, 200 mg, then 100 mg q6h or 200 mg (controlled release) q12h.

▸ **Severe Refractory Arrhythmias**
PO
Adults, Elderly. Up to 400 mg q6h.
Children 12–18 yr. 6–15 mg/kg/day in divided doses q6h.
Children 5–11 yr. 10–15 mg/kg/day in divided doses q6h.
Children 1–4 yr. 10–20 mg/kg/day in divided doses q6h.
Children younger than 1 yr. 10–30 mg/kg/day in divided doses q6h.

▸ **Dosage in Renal Impairment**
With or without loading dose of 150 mg:

Creatinine Clearance	Dosage
40 ml/min and higher	100 mg q6h (extended-release 200 mg q12h)
30–39 ml/min	100 mg q8h
15–29 ml/min	100 mg q12h
less than 15 ml/min	100 mg q24h

▸ **Dosage in Liver Impairment**
Adults, Elderly weighing 50 kg and more. 100 mg q6h (200 mg q12h with extended-release).

▸ **Dosage in Cardiomyopathy, Cardiac Decompensation**
Adults, Elderly weighing 50 kg and more. No loading dose; 100 mg q6–8h with gradual dosage adjustments.

OFF-LABEL USES
Prophylaxis and treatment of supraventricular tachycardia

CONTRAINDICATIONS
Cardiogenic shock, narrow-angle glaucoma (unless patient is undergoing cholinergic therapy), pre-existing second- or third-degree AV block, pre-existing urinary retention

INTERACTIONS
Drug
Other antiarrhythmics, including diltiazem, propranolol, verapamil: May prolong cardiac conduction, decrease cardiac output.
Pimozide: May increase cardiac arrhythmias.
Herbal
None known.
Food
None known.
Drug interactions of concern to dentistry
- Possible increased risk of prolonged QT interval: clarithromycin, erythromycin
- Increased side effects: anticholinergics, alcohol
- Decreased effects: barbiturates, corticosteroids

DIAGNOSTIC TEST EFFECTS
May decrease blood glucose levels. May cause ECG changes. May increase serum cholesterol and triglyceride levels. Therapeutic serum level is 2 to 8 mcg/ml, and the toxic serum level is greater than 8 mcg/ml.

SIDE EFFECTS

Frequent (> 9%)
Dry mouth (32%), urinary hesitancy, constipation
Occasional (9%–3%)
Blurred vision, dry eyes, nose, or throat, urinary retention, headache, dizziness, fatigue, nausea
Rare (< 1%)
Impotence, hypotension, edema, weight gain, shortness of breath, syncope, chest pain, nervousness, diarrhea, vomiting, decreased appetite, rash, itching

SERIOUS REACTIONS

! May produce or aggravate CHF.
! May produce severe hypotension, shortness of breath, chest pain, syncope (especially in patients with primary cardiomyopathy or CHF).
! Hepatotoxicity occurs rarely.

DENTAL CONSIDERATIONS

General:
- Monitor vital signs at every appointment because of cardiovascular side effects.
- After supine positioning, have patient sit upright for at least 2 min before standing to avoid orthostatic hypotension.
- Patients on chronic drug therapy may rarely have symptoms of blood dyscrasias, which can include infection, bleeding, and poor healing.
- Assess salivary flow as a factor in caries, periodontal disease, and candidiasis.

Consultations:
- In a patient with symptoms of blood dyscrasias, request a medical consultation for blood studies and postpone dental treatment until normal values are reestablished.
- Medical consultation may be required to assess disease control and patient's ability to tolerate stress.

Teach Patient/Family:
- Importance of good oral hygiene to prevent soft tissue inflammation
- *When chronic dry mouth occurs, advise patient:*
  - To avoid mouth rinses with high alcohol content because of drying effects
  - To use daily home fluoride products for anticaries effect
  - To use sugarless gum, frequent sips of water, or saliva substitutes

disulfiram

dye-**sul**-fi-ram
(Antabuse)

CATEGORY AND SCHEDULE

Pregnancy Risk Category: C

MECHANISM OF ACTION

A thiuram derivative and an irreversible aldehyde dehydrogenase inhibitor. When taken with alcohol, there is an increase in serum acetaldehyde levels. ***Therapeutic Effect:*** Produces an acute sensitivity to alcohol.

PHARMACOKINETICS

Slowly absorbed from GI tract. Metabolized in liver. Primarily excreted in urine. Up to 20% of dose remains in body for at least 1 wk. ***Half-life:*** Unknown.

AVAILABILITY

Tablets (Antabuse): 250 mg, 500 mg.

INDICATIONS AND DOSAGES

Adjunct in management of selected chronic alcoholic patients who want to remain in state of enforced sobriety

PO

Adults, elderly. Initially, administer maximum of 500 mg daily given as a single dose for 1–2 wk. Maintenance: 250 mg daily (normal range: 125–500 mg). Do not exceed maximum daily dose of 500 mg.

CONTRAINDICATIONS

Severe heart disease, psychosis, hypersensitivity to disulfiram or any component of the formulation

INTERACTIONS

Drug

Alcohol: Within 14 days, results in disulfiram-alcohol reaction.

- Isoniazid: May increase CNS effects.
- Metronidazole: May increase toxicity.
- Oral anticoagulant: May increase the effect.
- Phenytoin: May increase concentration, toxicity of phenytoin.

Herbal

None known.

Food

None known.

Drug interactions of concern to dentistry

- Increased CNS depression: long-acting benzodiazepines
- Increased disulfiram reaction: alcohol
- Risk of psychosis: metronidazole (do not use), tricyclic antidepressants

DIAGNOSTIC TEST EFFECTS

May increase cholesterol concentrations. May decrease vanillylmandelic acid concentrations.

SIDE EFFECTS

Frequent

Drowsiness

Occasional

Headache, restlessness, optic neuritis (impaired color perception, altered vision), peripheral neuropathy, metallic or garlic taste, rash

SERIOUS EFFECTS

Disulfiram-alcohol reactions to ingestion of alcohol in any form include flushing/throbbing in head and neck, throbbing headache, nausea, copious vomiting, diaphoresis, dyspnea, hyperventilation, tachycardia, hypotension, marked uneasiness, vertigo, blurred vision, confusion, and death.

DENTAL CONSIDERATIONS

General:

- Be aware of the needs of patients who are in recovery from substance abuse.
- Avoid other addictive drugs, including opioids and benzodiazepines.

Consultations:

- Medical consultation may be required to assess disease control.

Teach Patient/Family:

- To avoid mouth rinses with high alcohol content because of drying effects and drug–drug interaction

dobutamine hydrochloride

doe-byoo′-ta-meen

(Dobutrex)

Do not confuse dobutamine with dopamine.

CATEGORY AND SCHEDULE

Pregnancy Risk Category: B

MECHANISM OF ACTION

A direct-acting inotropic agent acting primarily on $beta_1$-adrenergic receptors. ***Therapeutic Effect:*** Decreases preload and afterload, and enhances myocardial contractility, stroke volume, and cardiac output.

Improves renal blood flow and urine output.

PHARMACOKINETICS

Route	Onset	Peak	Duration
IV	1–2 min	10 min	Length of infusion

Metabolized in the liver. Primarily excreted in urine. Not removed by hemodialysis. ***Half-life:*** 2 min.

AVAILABILITY

Infusion (ready-to-use): 1 mg/ml, 2 mg/ml, 4 mg/ml.
Injection: 12.5-mg/ml vial.

INDICATIONS AND DOSAGES

▸ Short-Term Management of Cardiac Decompensation

IV INFUSION
Adults, Elderly, Children.
2.5–15 mcg/kg/min. Rarely, drug can be infused at a rate of up to 40 mcg/kg/min to increase cardiac output.
Neonates. 2–15 mcg/kg/min.

CONTRAINDICATIONS

Hypovolemia patients, idiopathic hypertrophic subaortic stenosis, sulfite sensitivity

INTERACTIONS

Drug

Beta blockers: May antagonize the effects of dobutamine.
Digoxin: May increase the risk of arrhythmias and enhance the inotropic effect of both drugs.
MAOIs, oxytocics, tricyclic antidepressants: May increase the adverse effects of dobutamine, such as arrhythmias and hypertension.

Herbal

None known.

Food

None known.

DIAGNOSTIC TEST EFFECTS

Decreases serum potassium level

IV INCOMPATIBILITIES

Acyclovir (Zovirax), alteplase (Activase), amphotericin B complex (Abelcet, AmBisome, Amphotec), bumetanide (Bumex), cefepime (Maxipime), foscarnet (Foscavir), furosemide (Lasix), heparin, piperacillin/tazobactam (Zosyn)

IV COMPATIBILITIES

Amiodarone (Cordarone), calcium chloride, calcium gluconate, diltiazem (Cardizem), dopamine (Intropin), enalapril (Vasotec), famotidine (Pepcid), hydromorphone (Dilaudid), insulin (regular), lidocaine, lorazepam (Ativan), magnesium sulfate, midazolam (Versed), milrinone (Primacor), morphine, nitroglycerin, norepinephrine (Levophed), potassium chloride, propofol (Diprivan)

SIDE EFFECTS

Frequent (> 5%)
Increased heart rate, increased BP
Occasional (5%–3%)
Pain at injection site
Rare (3%–1%)
Nausea, headache, anginal pain, shortness of breath, fever

SERIOUS REACTIONS

! Overdose may produce a marked increase in heart rate (by 30 beats/minute or higher) marked increase in BP (by 50 mm Hg or higher), anginal pain, and premature ventricular contractions (PVCs).

DENTAL CONSIDERATIONS

General:

- Acute-use drug for use in hospitals, cardiac labs, or emergency rooms

docetaxel
dox-eh-tax′-el
(Taxotere)
Do not confuse docetaxel with Taxol.

CATEGORY AND SCHEDULE
Pregnancy Risk Category: D

MECHANISM OF ACTION
An antimitotic agent belonging to the taxoid family that disrupts the microtubular cell network, which is essential for cellular function. ***Therapeutic Effect:*** Inhibits cellular mitosis.

PHARMACOKINETICS
Distributed into peripheral compartments. Protein binding: 94%. Extensively metabolized. Excreted primarily in feces, with lesser amount in urine. ***Half-life:*** 11.1 hr.

AVAILABILITY
Injection: 20 mg/0.5 ml with diluent, 80 mg/2 ml with diluent.

INDICATIONS AND DOSAGES
▸ Breast Carcinoma
IV
Adults. 60–100 mg/m² given over 1 hr q3wk. If patient develops febrile neutropenia, a neutrophil count less than 500 cells/mm³ for longer than 1 wk, severe or cumulative cutaneous reactions, or severe peripheral neuropathy with initial dose of 100 mg/m², dosage should be decreased to 75 mg/m². If reaction continues, dosage should be further reduced to 55 mg/m² or therapy should be discontinued. Patients who don't experience the above symptoms at a dose of 60 mg/m² may tolerate an increased docetaxel dose.

▸ Non–Small Cell Lung Carcinoma
IV
Adults. 75 mg/m² q3wk. Adjust dosage if toxicity occurs.

D

OFF-LABEL USES
Treatment of small cell-bladder, head and neck, lung, ovarian, or prostate cancer

CONTRAINDICATIONS
History of severe hypersensitivity to docetaxel or other drugs formulated with polysorbate 80, neutrophil count less than 1,500 cells/mm³

INTERACTIONS
Drug
Bone marrow depressants: May increase myelosuppression.
Cyclosporine, erythromycin, ketoconazole: May significantly inhibit docetaxel metabolism.
Live-virus vaccines: May potentiate replication, increase vaccine side effects, and decrease the patient's antibody response to the vaccine.

Herbal
None known.

Food
None known.

Drug interactions of concern to dentistry
- Significant risk of increased effects: drugs that inhibit CYP3A4 isoenzymes (including ketoconazole, itraconazole, erythromycin)
- Caution in use of any drugs that induce CYP3A4 isoenzymes

DIAGNOSTIC TEST EFFECTS
May significantly increase BUN level and serum alkaline phosphatase, bilirubin, creatinine, AST (SGOT), and ALT (SGPT) levels. Reduces blood neutrophil, thrombocyte, and WBC counts.

D

IV INCOMPATIBILITIES

Amphotericin B (Fungizone), doxorubicin liposomal (DaunoXome), methylprednisolone (Solu-Medrol), nalbuphine (Nubain)

IV COMPATIBILITIES

Bumetanide (Bumex), calcium gluconate, dexamethasone (Decadron), diphenhydramine (Benadryl), dobutamine (Dobutrex), dopamine (Inotropin), furosemide (Lasix), granisetron (Kytril), heparin, hydromorphone (Dilaudid), lorazepam (Ativan), magnesium sulfate, mannitol, morphine, ondansetron (Zofran), potassium chloride

SIDE EFFECTS

Frequent

Alopecia (80%), asthenia (62%), hypersensitivity reaction such as dermatitis (59% decreases to 16% in those pretreated with oral corticosteroids), fluid retention (49%), stomatitis (43%), nausea and diarrhea (40%), fever (30%), nail changes (28%), vomiting (24%), myalgia (19%)

Occasional

Hypotension, edema, anorexia, headache, weight gain, infection (urinary tract, injection site, indwelling catheter tip), dizziness

Rare

Dry skin, sensory disorders (vision, speech, taste), arthralgia, weight loss, conjunctivitis, hematuria, proteinuria

SERIOUS REACTIONS

! In patients with normal liver function tests, neutropenia (neutrophil count < 2,000 cells/mm^3) and leukopenia (WBC count < 4,000 cells/mm^3) occur in 96% of patients; anemia (hemoglobin level < 11 g/dl) occurs in 90% of patients; thrombocytopenia (platelet count < 100,000 cells/mm^3) occur in 8% of patients; and infection occurs in 28% of patients.

! Neurosensory and neuromotor effects, such as distal paresthesias and weakness, occur in 54% and 13% of patients, respectively.

DENTAL CONSIDERATIONS

General:

- If additional analgesia is required for dental pain, consider alternative analgesics (NSAIDs) in patients taking narcotics for acute or chronic pain.
- Examine for oral manifestation of opportunistic infection.
- Avoid products that affect platelet function, such as aspirin and NSAIDs.
- This drug may be used in the hospital or on an outpatient basis. Confirm the patient's disease and treatment status.
- Chlorhexidine mouth rinse prior to and during chemotherapy may reduce severity of mucositis.
- Patient on chronic drug therapy may rarely present with symptoms of blood dyscrasias, which can include infection, bleeding and poor healing. If dyscrasia is present, caution patient to prevent oral tissue trauma when using oral hygiene aids.
- Palliative medication may be required for management of oral side effects.
- Short appointments and a stress reduction protocol may be required for anxious patients.
- Patients may be at risk of bleeding, check for oral signs.
- Oral infections should be eliminated and/or treated aggressively.

Consultations:

- Medical consultation should include routine blood counts including platelet counts and bleeding time.

• Consult physician; prophylactic or therapeutic antiinfectives may be indicated if surgery or periodontal treatment is required.
• Medical consultation may be required to assess immunologic status during cancer chemotherapy and determine safety risk, if any, posed by the required dental treatment.
• Medical consultation may be required to assess disease control and patient's ability to tolerate stress.

Teach Patient/Family:
• To be aware of oral side effects
• Importance of good oral hygiene to prevent soft tissue inflammation
• To report oral lesions, soreness, or bleeding to dentist
• To prevent trauma when using oral hygiene aids
• Importance of updating health and medication history if physician makes any changes in evaluation or drug regimens; include OTC, herbal, and nonherbal remedies in the update

docusate

dok′-yoo-sate
(Apo-Docusate[CAN], Colace, Colax-C[CAN], Coloxyl[AUS], Diocto, Docusoft-S, Novo-Ducosate[CAN], PMS-Docusate [CAN], Pro-Cal-Sof, Regulex[CAN], Selax[CAN], Soflax[CAN], Surfak)

CATEGORY AND SCHEDULE
Pregnancy Risk Category: C
OTC

MECHANISM OF ACTION
A bulk-producing laxative that decreases surface film tension by mixing liquid and bowel contents.
Therapeutic Effect: Increases infiltration of liquid to form a softer stool.

PHARMACOKINETICS
Minimal absorption from the GI tract. Acts in small and large intestines. Results usually occur 1–2 days after first dose, but may take 3–5 days.

AVAILABILITY
Capsules (Colace): 50 mg, 100 mg.
Capsules (Docusoft-S): 100 mg.
Capsules (Surfak): 240 mg.
Liquid (Colace): 50 mg/5 ml (sodium).
Syrup (Colace, Diocto): 60 mg/15 ml.

INDICATIONS AND DOSAGES
▸ Stool Softener
PO
Adults, Elderly, Children 12 yr and older. 50–500 mg/day in 1–4 divided doses.
Children 6–11 yr. 40–150 mg/day in 1–4 divided doses.
Children 3–5 yr. 20–60 mg/day in 1–4 divided doses.
Children younger than 3 yr. 10–40 mg in 1–4 divided doses.

CONTRAINDICATIONS
Acute abdominal pain, concomitant use of mineral oil, intestinal obstruction, nausea, vomiting

INTERACTIONS
Drug
Danthron, mineral oil: May increase the absorption of danthron or mineral oil.
Herbal
None known.
Food
None known.
Drug interactions of concern to dentistry
• None reported

DIAGNOSTIC TEST EFFECTS
None known.

SIDE EFFECTS

Occasional

Mild GI cramping, throat irritation (with liquid preparation)

Rare

Rash

SERIOUS REACTIONS

! None known.

DENTAL CONSIDERATIONS

General:

- Determine why patient is taking the drug.
- Caution: prescribing medications that may aggravate constipation.

dofetilide

doe-fet′-ill-ide

(Tikosyn)

CATEGORY AND SCHEDULE

Pregnancy Risk Category: C

MECHANISM OF ACTION

A selective potassium channel blocker that prolongs repolarization without affecting conduction velocity by blocking one or more time-dependent potassium currents. Dofetilide has no effect on sodium channels or adrenergic alpha or beta receptors. ***Therapeutic Effect:*** Terminates reentrant tachyarrhythmias, preventing reinduction.

AVAILABILITY

Capsules: 125 mcg, 250 mcg, 500 mcg.

INDICATIONS AND DOSAGES

▸ Maintain Normal Sinus Rhythm after Conversion from Atrial Fibrillation or Flutter

PO

Adults, Elderly. Individualized using a seven-step dosing algorithm dependent upon calculated creatinine clearance and QT interval measurements.

CONTRAINDICATIONS

Concurrent use of drugs that prolong the QT interval; concurrent use of amiodarone, megestrol, prochlorperazine, or verapamil; congenital or acquired prolonged QT syndrome; paroxysmal atrial fibrillation; severe renal impairment

INTERACTIONS

Drug

Amiloride, megestrol, metformin, prochlorperazine, triamterene: May increase plasma levels of dofetilide.

Bepridil, phenothiazines, tricyclic antidepressants: May prolong the QT interval.

Cimetidine, verapamil: Increases levels of dofetilide.

Ketoconazole, trimethoprim: Increases plasma concentration of dofetilide.

Herbal

None known.

Food

Grapefruit juice: Can increase dofetilide plasma levels.

Drug interactions of concern to dentistry

- Decreased renal excretion: ketoconazole (contraindicated use)
- Not recommended with concurrent use of phenothiazines, tricyclic antidepressants, SSRIs, macrolide antiinfectives (erythromycin, clarithromycin), azole antifungals, or other drugs that inhibit CYP3A4 isoenzymes
- Contraindicated with cimetidine, trimethoprim, ketoconazole, prochlorperazine, megestrol, or verapamil

DIAGNOSTIC TEST EFFECTS

None known.

SIDE EFFECTS

Occasional (< 5%)

Headache, chest pain, dizziness, dyspnea, nausea, insomnia, back and abdominal pain, diarrhea, rash

SERIOUS REACTIONS

! Angioedema, bradycardia, cerebral ischemia, facial paralysis, and serious ventricular arrhythmias or various forms of heart block may be noted.

DENTAL CONSIDERATIONS

General:

- Monitor vital signs at every appointment because of cardiovascular side effects.
- Delay or avoid dental treatment if patient shows signs of cardiac symptoms or respiratory distress.
- Ensure that the patient is compliant with drug therapy.

Consultations:

- Patient's physician should be informed about use of any dental drugs.
- Medical consultation may be required to assess disease control and patient's ability to tolerate stress.

Teach Patient/Family:

- Importance of updating health and drug history if physician makes any changes in evaluation or drug regimens

dolasetron

doe-lass′-eh-tron

(Anzemet)

Do not confuse Anzemet with Aldomet.

CATEGORY AND SCHEDULE

Pregnancy Risk Category: B

MECHANISM OF ACTION

A 5-HT_3 receptor antagonist that acts centrally in the chemoreceptor trigger zone and peripherally at the vagal nerve terminals. ***Therapeutic Effect:*** Prevents nausea and vomiting.

PHARMACOKINETICS

Readily absorbed from the GI tract after PO administration. Protein binding: 69%–77%. Metabolized in the liver. Primarily excreted in urine. Unknown if removed by hemodialysis. ***Half-life:*** 5–10 hr.

AVAILABILITY

Tablets: 50 mg, 100 mg.
Injection: 20 mg/ml in single use 0.625 ml amps, 0.625 ml fill in 2 ml Carpuject and 5 ml vials.

INDICATIONS AND DOSAGES

▸ Prevention of Chemotherapy-Induced Nausea and Vomiting

PO

Adults. 100 mg within 1 hr of chemotherapy.
Children 2–16 yr. 1.8 mg/kg within 1 hr of chemotherapy. Maximum: 100 mg.

IV

Adults, Children 1–16 yr. 1.8 mg/kg as a single dose 30 min before chemotherapy. Maximum: 100 mg.

▸ Treatment or Prevention of Postoperative Nausea or Vomiting

PO

Adults. 100 mg within 2 hr of surgery.
Children 2–16 yr. 1.2 mg/kg within 2 hr of surgery. Maximum: 100 mg.

IV

Adults. 12.5 mg 15 min before cessation of anesthesia or as soon as nausea occurs.

Children 2–16 yr. 0.35 mg/kg 15 min before cessation of anesthesia or as soon as nausea occurs. Maximum: 12.5 mg.

OFF-LABEL USES

Radiation therapy–induced nausea and vomiting

CONTRAINDICATIONS

None known.

INTERACTIONS

Drug

None known.

Herbal

None known.

Food

None known.

Drug interactions of concern to dentistry

- Does not influence anesthesia recovery time

DIAGNOSTIC TEST EFFECTS

May transiently increase AST (SGOT) and ALT (SGPT) levels.

IV INCOMPATIBILITIES

No information available for Y-site administration.

SIDE EFFECTS

Frequent (10%–5%)

Headache, diarrhea, fatigue

Occasional (5%–1%)

Fever, dizziness, tachycardia, dyspepsia

SERIOUS REACTIONS

! Overdose may produce a combination of CNS stimulant and depressant effects.

DENTAL CONSIDERATIONS

General:

- Monitor patients in recovery to avoid untoward events.
- Patients taking opioids for acute or chronic pain should be given alternative analgesics for dental pain.
- Chlorhexidine mouth rinse before and during chemotherapy may reduce severity of mucositis.
- Palliative medication may be required for management of oral side effects from chemotherapy.

Teach Patient/Family:

- To be aware of possible oral side effects from concurrent cancer chemotherapy
- To report to dentist excessive nausea and vomiting in patients recovering from anesthesia after dental treatment

donepezil hydrochloride

dah-nep′-eh-zil

(Aricept)

Do not confuse Aricept with Aciphex or Ascriptin.

CATEGORY AND SCHEDULE

Pregnancy Risk Category: C

MECHANISM OF ACTION

A cholinesterase inhibitor that inhibits the enzyme acetylcholinesterase, thus increasing the concentration of acetylcholine at cholinergic synapses and enhancing cholinergic function in the CNS. ***Therapeutic Effect:*** Slows the progression of Alzheimer's disease.

PHARMACOKINETICS

Well absorbed after PO administration. Protein binding: 96%. Extensively metabolized. Eliminated in urine and feces. ***Half-life:*** 70 hr.

AVAILABILITY

Tablets: 5 mg, 10 mg.
Tablets (Orally Disintegrating): 5 mg, 10 mg.

INDICATIONS AND DOSAGES

Alzheimer's Disease

PO

Adults, Elderly. 5–10 mg/day as a single dose. If initial dose is 5 mg, do not increase to 10 mg for 4–6 wk.

OFF-LABEL USES

Treatment of autism

CONTRAINDICATIONS

History of hypersensitivity to donepezil or piperidine derivatives

INTERACTIONS

Drug

Anticholinergics: May decrease the effect of anticholinergics.
Cholinergic agonists, neuromuscular blockers, succinylcholine: May increase the synergistic effects of these drugs.
Ketoconazole, quinidine: May inhibit the metabolism of donepezil.
NSAIDs: May increase gastric acid secretion of NSAIDs.
Paroxetine: May decrease the metabolism and increase the blood concentration of donepezil.

Herbal

None known.

Food

None known.

Drug interactions of concern to dentistry

- Enhanced succinylcholine muscle relaxation during anesthesia
- Risk of GI side effects: NSAIDs
- Action may be inhibited by anticholinergic drugs or enhanced by cholinergic agonists
- Increased blood levels: ketoconazole, paroxetine
- Use with caution drugs that inhibit CYP3A4 or CYP2D6 isoenzymes

DIAGNOSTIC TEST EFFECTS

May increase blood glucose and serum creatine kinase and LDH concentrations. May decrease the serum potassium level.

SIDE EFFECTS

Frequent (11%–8%)
Nausea, diarrhea, headache, insomnia, nonspecific pain, dizziness
Occasional (6%–3%)
Mild muscle cramps, fatigue, vomiting, anorexia, ecchymosis
Rare (3%–2%)
Depression, abnormal dreams, weight loss, arthritis, somnolence, syncope, frequent urination

SERIOUS REACTIONS

! Overdose may result in cholinergic crisis, characterized by severe nausea, increased salivation, diaphoresis, bradycardia, hypotension, flushed skin, abdominal pain, respiratory depression, seizures, and cardiorespiratory collapse. Increasing muscle weakness may result in death if respiratory muscles are involved. The antidote is 1–2 mg IV atropine sulfate with subsequent doses based on therapeutic response.

DENTAL CONSIDERATIONS

General:

- Determine why patient is taking the drug.
- Monitor vital signs at every appointment because of cardiovascular side effects.
- After supine positioning, have patient sit upright for at least 2 min before standing to avoid orthostatic hypotension.

- Use precaution if sedation or general anesthesia is required.
- Patients on chronic drug therapy may rarely have symptoms of blood dyscrasias, which can include infection, bleeding, and poor healing.
- Drug is used early in the disease; ensure that patient or caregiver understands informed consent.
- Place on frequent recall because early attention to dental health is important for Alzheimer's patients.
- Assess salivary flow as factor in caries, periodontal disease, and candidiasis.
- Consider semisupine chair position for patient comfort if GI side effects occur.

Consultations:
- Consultation with physician may be necessary if sedation or general anesthesia is required.
- Medical consultation may be required to assess disease control and patient's ability to tolerate stress.
- In a patient with symptoms of blood dyscrasias, request a medical consultation for blood studies and postpone treatment until normal values are reestablished.

Teach Patient/Family:
- Importance of good oral hygiene to prevent soft tissue inflammation
- To prevent trauma when using oral hygiene aids
- Use of electric toothbrush if patient has difficulty holding conventional devices
- *When chronic dry mouth occurs, advise patient:*
  - To avoid mouth rinses with high alcohol content because of drying effects
  - To use daily home fluoride products for anticaries effect
  - To use sugarless gum, frequent sips of water, or saliva substitutes

dopamine hydrochloride

doe′-pa-meen

(Dopamine Injection[AUS], Intropin)

Do not confuse dopamine with dobutamine or Dopram, or Inotropin with Isoptin.

CATEGORY AND SCHEDULE

Pregnancy Risk Category: C

MECHANISM OF ACTION

A sympathomimetic (adrenergic agonist) that stimulates adrenergic receptors. Effects are dose dependent. Low dosages (less than 5 mcg/kg/min) stimulate dopaminergic receptors, causing renal vasodilation. Low to moderate dosages (≤ 10 mcg/kg/min) have a positive inotropic effect by direct action and release of norepinephrine. High dosages (> 10 mcg/kg/min) stimulate alpha-receptors.

Therapeutic Effect: With low dosages, increases renal blood flow, urine flow, and sodium excretion. With low to moderate dosages, increases myocardial contractility, stroke volume, and cardiac output. With high dosages, increases peripheral resistance, renal vasoconstriction, and systolic and diastolic BP.

PHARMACOKINETICS

Route	Onset	Peak	Duration
IV	1–2 min	N/A	less than 10 min

Widely distributed. Does not cross blood-brain barrier. Metabolized in the liver, kidney, and plasma. Primarily excreted in urine. Not removed by hemodialysis. ***Half-life:*** 2 min.

AVAILABILITY

Injection: 40 mg/ml, 80 mg/ml, 160 mg/ml.
Injection (Premix with dextrose): 80 mg/100 ml, 160 mg/100 ml, 320 mg/100 ml.

INDICATIONS AND DOSAGES

▸ Treatment and Prevention of Acute Hypotension; Shock (Associated with Cardiac Decompensation, MI, Open Heart Surgery, Renal Failure, or Trauma), Treatment of Low Cardiac Output, Treatment of CHF

IV

Adults, Elderly. 1 mcg/kg/min up to 50 mcg/kg/min titrated to desired response.
Children. 1–20 mcg/kg/min. Maximum: 50 mcg/kg/min.
Neonates. 1–20 mcg/kg/min.

CONTRAINDICATIONS

Pheochromocytoma, sulfite sensitivity, uncorrected tachyarrhythmias, ventricular fibrillation

INTERACTIONS

Drug

Beta blockers: May decrease the effects of dopamine.
Digoxin: May increase the risk of arrhythmias.
Ergot alkaloids: May increase vasoconstriction.
MAOIs: May increase cardiac stimulation and vasopressor effects.
Tricyclic antidepressants: May increase cardiovascular effects.

Herbal

None known.

Food

None known.

DIAGNOSTIC TEST EFFECTS

None known.

IV INCOMPATIBILITIES

Acyclovir (Zovirax), amphotericin B complex (Abelcet, AmBisome, Amphotec), cefepime (Maxipime), furosemide (Lasix), insulin, sodium bicarbonate

IV COMPATIBILITIES

Amiodarone (Cordarone), calcium chloride, diltiazem (Cardizem), dobutamine (Dobutrex), enalapril (Vasotec), heparin, hydromorphone (Dilaudid), labetalol (Trandate), levofloxacin (Levaquin), lidocaine, lorazepam (Ativan), methylprednisolone (Solu-Medrol), midazolam (Versed), milrinone (Primacor), morphine, nicardipine (Cardene), nitroglycerin, norepinephrine (Levophed), piperacillin/tazobactam (Zosyn), potassium chloride, propofol (Diprivan)

SIDE EFFECTS

Frequent

Headache, ectopic beats, tachycardia, anginal pain, palpitations, vasoconstriction, hypotension, nausea, vomiting, dyspnea

Occasional

Piloerection or goose bumps, bradycardia, widening of QRS complex.

SERIOUS REACTIONS

! High doses may produce ventricular arrhythmias.
! Patients with occlusive vascular disease are at high risk for further compromise of circulation to the extremities, which may result in gangrene.
! Tissue necrosis with sloughing may occur with extravasation of IV solution.

D

D

DENTAL CONSIDERATIONS

General:
- Acute-use drug for use in hospitals, cardiac labs, or emergency rooms.
- Inquire about cardiovascular disease and medications used.

dornase alfa

door′-nace al′-fa
(Pulmozyme)

CATEGORY AND SCHEDULE

Pregnancy Risk Category: B

MECHANISM OF ACTION

An enzyme that selectively splits and hydrolyzes DNA in sputum.
Therapeutic Effect: Reduces sputum viscosity and elasticity.

AVAILABILITY

Inhalation: 2.5 mg ampules for nebulization.

INDICATIONS AND DOSAGES

▸ To Improve Management of Pulmonary Function in Patients with Cystic Fibrosis

NEBULIZATION

Adults, Children older than 5 yr. 2.5 mg (1 ampule) once daily by recommended nebulizer. May increase to 2.5 mg twice daily.

CONTRAINDICATIONS

Sensitivity to dornase alfa or epoetin alfa

INTERACTIONS

Drug
None known.
Herbal
None known.
Food
None known.
Drug interactions of concern to dentistry
- None documented

DIAGNOSTIC TEST EFFECTS

None known.

SIDE EFFECTS

Frequent (> 10%)
Pharyngitis, chest pain or discomfort, voice changes
Occasional (10%–3%)
Conjunctivitis, hoarseness, rash

SERIOUS REACTIONS

! None significant.

DENTAL CONSIDERATIONS

General:
- Consider semisupine chair position for patients with respiratory disease.
- Monitor vital signs at every appointment because of respiratory and cardiovascular side effects.
- Stress reduction protocol may be required.

Consultations:
- Medical consultation may be required to assess disease control.

Teach Patient/Family:
- Importance of good oral hygiene to prevent soft tissue inflammation

dorzolamide hydrochloride

door-zol′-a-mide
hye-droe-klor′-ide
(Trusopt)

CATEGORY AND SCHEDULE

Pregnancy Risk Category: C

MECHANISM OF ACTION
An ophthalmic agent that inhibits carbonic anhydrase. ***Therapeutic Effect:*** Reduces intraocular pressure (IOP).

PHARMACOKINETICS
Peak response occurs in 2 hours and the duration of action is 8 to 12 hours. Systemically absorbed to some degree. Protein binding: 33%. Distributed in red blood cells. Sites of metabolism have not been established. Metabolized to active metabolite, N-desethyldorzolamide. Excreted in urine. ***Half-life:*** unknown; 147 days (terminal red blood cell).

AVAILABILITY
Ophthalmic Solution: 2% (Trusopt).

INDICATIONS AND DOSAGES
▸ **Glaucoma, Ocular Hypertension**
OPHTHALMIC
Adults, Elderly. 1 drop in affected eye(s) 3 times/day.

CONTRAINDICATIONS
Hypersensitivity to dorzolamide or any other component of the formulation

INTERACTIONS
Drug
Topiramate: May increase risk of nephrolithiasis.
Herbal
None known.
Food
None known.
Drug interactions of concern to dentistry
- Avoid drugs that may exacerbate glaucoma (anticholinergic drugs)
- High-dose salicylates to avoid systemic toxicity

DIAGNOSTIC TEST EFFECTS
None known.

SIDE EFFECTS
Frequent
Ocular burning, bitter taste
Occasional
Superficial punctuate keratitis, ocular allergic reaction

SERIOUS REACTIONS
! Iridocyclitis, skin rash, and urolithiasis occur rarely.
! Electrolyte imbalance, development of an acidotic state, and possible CNS effects may occur.

DENTAL CONSIDERATIONS
General:
- Avoid dental light in patient's eyes; offer dark glasses for patient comfort.
- Protect patient's eyes from accidental spatter during dental treatment.
- Check patient's compliance with prescribed drug regimen for glaucoma.

Consultations:
- Medical consultation may be required to assess disease control.

doxazosin mesylate
dox-ay′-zoe-sin
(Apo-Doxazosin[CAN], Cardura)
Do not confuse doxazosin with doxapram, doxepin, or doxorubicin, or Cardura with Cardene, Cordarone, Coumadin, K-Dur, or Ridaura.

CATEGORY AND SCHEDULE
Pregnancy Risk Category: C

MECHANISM OF ACTION
An antihypertensive that selectively blocks alpha$_1$-adrenergic receptors, decreasing peripheral vascular

resistance. ***Therapeutic Effect:*** Causes peripheral vasodilation and lowers of BP. Also relaxes smooth muscle of bladder and prostate.

PHARMACOKINETICS

Route	Onset	Peak	Duration
PO	N/A	2–6 hr	24 hr

Well absorbed from the GI tract. Protein binding: 98%–99%. Metabolized in the liver. Primarily eliminated in feces. Not removed by hemodialysis. ***Half-life:*** 19–22 hr.

AVAILABILITY

Tablets: 1 mg, 2 mg, 4 mg, 8 mg.

INDICATIONS AND DOSAGES

▸ Mild to Moderate Hypertension

PO

Adults. Initially, 1 mg once a day. May increase to a maximum of 16 mg/day.

Elderly. Initially, 0.5 mg once a day.

▸ Benign Prostatic Hyperplasia, Alone or in Combination with Finasteride (Proscar)

PO

Adults, Elderly. Initially, 1 mg/day. May increase q1–2 wk. Maximum: 8 mg/day.

CONTRAINDICATIONS

Hypersensitivity to other quinazolines

INTERACTIONS

Drug

Estrogen, NSAIDs: May decrease the effect of doxazosin.

Hypotension-producing medications, such as antihypertensives and diuretics: May increase the effect of doxazosin.

Sildenafil, tadalafil, vardenafil: May potentiate hypotensive effects.

Herbal

None known.

Food

None known.

Drug interactions of concern to dentistry

- Increased hypotensive effects: all CNS depressants
- Reduced effects with indomethacin, NSAIDs, sympathomimetics

Caution in use of drugs that may cause urinary retention: anticholinergics, opioids

DIAGNOSTIC TEST EFFECTS

None known.

SIDE EFFECTS

Frequent (20%–10%)

Dizziness, asthenia, headache, edema

Occasional (9%–3%)

Nausea, pharyngitis, rhinitis, pain in extremities, somnolence

Rare (3%–1%)

Palpitations, diarrhea, constipation, dyspnea, myalgia, altered vision, dizziness, nervousness

SERIOUS REACTIONS

! First-dose syncope (hypotension with sudden loss of consciousness) may occur 30 to 90 minutes following initial dose of 2 mg or greater, a too-rapid increase in dosage, or addition of another antihypertensive agent to therapy. First-dose syncope may be preceded by tachycardia (pulse rate of 120–160 beats/minute).

DENTAL CONSIDERATIONS

General:

- Monitor vital signs at every appointment because of cardiovascular side effects.

• After supine positioning, have patient sit upright for at least 2 min before standing to avoid orthostatic hypotension
• Assess salivary flow as a factor in caries, periodontal disease, and candidiasis.

Consultations:
• Medical consultation may be required to assess disease control and patient's ability to tolerate stress.

Teach Patient/Family:
• *When chronic dry mouth occurs, advise patient:*
  • To avoid mouth rinses with high alcohol content because of drying effects
  • To use daily home fluoride products for anticaries effect
  • To use sugarless gum, frequent sips of water, or saliva substitutes

doxepin hydrochloride

dox'-eh-pin
dox'-eh-pin
(Apo-Doxepin[CAN], Deptran[AUS], Novo-Doxepin[CAN], Prudoxin, Sinequan, Zonalon)
Do not confuse doxepin with doxapram, doxazosin, or Doxidan, or Sinequan with saquinavir.

CATEGORY AND SCHEDULE
Pregnancy Risk Category: C (B for topical form)

MECHANISM OF ACTION
A tricyclic antidepressant, antianxiety agent, antineuralgic agent, antipruritic, and antiulcer agent that increases synaptic concentrations of norepinephrine and serotonin. ***Therapeutic Effect:*** Produces antidepressant and anxiolytic effects.

PHARMACOKINETICS
Rapidly and well absorbed from the GI tract. Protein binding: 80%–85%. Metabolized in the liver to active metabolite. Primarily excreted in urine. Not removed by hemodialysis. ***Half-life:*** 6–8 hr. Topical: Absorbed through the skin. Distributed to body tissues. Metabolized to active metabolite. Excreted in urine.

AVAILABILITY
Capsules (Sinequan): 10 mg, 25 mg, 50 mg, 75 mg, 100 mg, 150 mg.
Oral Concentrate (Sinequan): 10 mg/ml.
Cream (Prudoxin, Zonalon): 5%.

INDICATIONS AND DOSAGES
▸ Depression, Anxiety
PO
Adults. 30–150 mg/day at bedtime or in 2–3 divided doses. May increase to 300 mg/day.
Elderly. Initially, 10–25 mg at bedtime. May increase by 10–25 mg/day every 3–7 days. Maximum: 75 mg/day.
Adolescents. Initially, 25–50 mg/day as a single dose or in divided doses. May increase to 100 mg/day.
Children 12 yr and younger. 1–3 mg/kg/day.
▸ Pruritus Associated with Eczema
TOPICAL
Adults, Elderly. Apply thin film 4 times a day.

OFF-LABEL USES
Treatment of neurogenic pain, panic disorder; prevention of vascular headache, pruritus in idiopathic urticaria

CONTRAINDICATIONS

Angle-closure glaucoma, hypersensitivity to other tricyclic antidepressants, urine retention

D

INTERACTIONS

Drug

Alcohol, other CNS depressants: May increase CNS and respiratory depression and the hypotensive effects of doxepin.
Antithyroid agents: May increase the risk of agranulocytosis.
Cimetidine: May increase doxepin blood concentration and risk of toxicity.
Clonidine, guanadrel: May decrease the effects of these drugs.
MAOIs: May increase the risk of seizures, hyperpyrexia, and hypertensive crisis.
Phenothiazines: May increase the anticholinergic and sedative effects of doxepin.
Sympathomimetics: May increase cardiac effects.

Herbal

St. John's wort: May increase the risk of serotonin syndrome.

Food

None known.

Drug interactions of concern to dentistry for topical form:

- Potential for interactions depends on how much drug is absorbed and duration of use (>8 days)
- Increased anticholinergic effects: anticholinergics, antihistamines, phenothiazines, other tricyclic antidepressants
- Potential risk for increased CNS depression: all CNS depressants
- Increased effects of direct-acting sympathomimetics: epinephrine, levonordefrin
- Avoid concurrent use with St. John's wort (herb)

Drug interactions of concern to dentistry for systemic-dose form:

- Increased anticholinergic effects: anticholinergic blockers, antihistamines, phenothiazines
- Increased effects of direct-acting sympathomimetics (epinephrine, levonordefrin)
- Potential risk of increased CNS depression: alcohol, barbiturates, benzodiazepines, other CNS depressants
- Decreased antihypertensive effects: clonidine, guanadrel, guanethidine

DIAGNOSTIC TEST EFFECTS

May alter blood glucose levels and ECG readings. Therapeutic serum drug level is 110–250 ng/ml; toxic serum drug level is greater than 300 ng/ml.

SIDE EFFECTS

Frequent

Oral: Orthostatic hypotension, somnolence, dry mouth, headache, increased appetite, weight gain, nausea, unusual fatigue, unpleasant taste
Topical: Edema; increased pruritus and eczema; burning, tingling, or stinging at application site; altered taste; dizziness; drowsiness; dry skin; dry mouth; fatigue; headache; thirst

Occasional

Oral: Blurred vision, confusion, constipation, hallucinations, difficult urination, eye pain, irregular heartbeat, fine muscle tremors, nervousness, impaired sexual function, diarrhea, diaphoresis, heartburn, insomnia
Topical: Anxiety, skin irritation or cracking, nausea

Rare

Oral: Allergic reaction, alopecia, tinnitus, breast enlargement
Topical: Fever, photosensitivity

SERIOUS REACTIONS

! Abrupt or too-rapid withdrawal may result in headache, malaise, nausea, vomiting, and vivid dreams.

! Overdose may produce seizures, dizziness, and cardiovascular effects, such as severe orthostatic hypotension, tachycardia, palpitations, and arrhythmias.

DENTAL CONSIDERATIONS

TOPICAL FORM

General:

- Doxepin may be absorbed and produce typical systemic side effects of tricyclic drugs.
- Monitor vital signs at every appointment because of cardiovascular side effects.
- Use vasoconstrictors with caution, in low doses, and with careful aspiration.
- Place on frequent recall because of oral side effects.
- Apply lubricant to dry lips for patient comfort before dental procedures.
- Assess salivary flow as a factor in caries, periodontal disease, and candidiasis.

Consultations:

- Medical consultation may be required to assess disease control.

Teach Patient/Family:

- To avoid mouth rinses with high alcohol content because of interaction with alcohol (see precautions) and drying effects
- *When chronic dry mouth occurs, advise patient:*
  - Of need for daily home fluoride for anticaries effect
  - To use sugarless gum, frequent sips of water, or saliva substitutes

SYSTEMIC-DOSE FORM

General:

- Monitor vital signs at every appointment because of cardiovascular side effects.
- Assess salivary flow as a factor in caries, periodontal disease, and candidiasis.
- Patients on chronic drug therapy may rarely have symptoms of blood dyscrasias, which can include infection, bleeding, and poor healing.
- After supine positioning, have patient sit upright for at least 2 min before standing to avoid orthostatic hypotension.
- Use vasoconstrictors with caution, in low doses, and with careful aspiration. Avoid use of gingival retraction cord with epinephrine.
- Place on frequent recall because of oral side effects.

Consultations:

- In a patient with symptoms of blood dyscrasias, request a medical consultation for blood studies and postpone dental treatment until normal values are reestablished.
- Medical consultation may be required to assess disease control.
- Physician should be informed if significant xerostomic side effects occur (e.g., increased caries, sore tongue, problems eating or swallowing, difficulty wearing prosthesis) so that a medication change can be considered.

Teach Patient/Family:

- Importance of good oral hygiene to prevent soft tissue inflammation
- *When chronic dry mouth occurs, advise patient:*
  - To avoid mouth rinses with high alcohol content because of drying effects
  - To use daily home fluoride products for anticaries effect

- To use sugarless gum, frequent sips of water, or saliva substitutes

D

doxorubicin

dox-o-roo′-bi-sin
(Doxil)
Do not confuse with Daunorubicin, Idamycin, or Idarubicin.

CATEGORY AND SCHEDULE
Pregnancy Risk Category: D

MECHANISM OF ACTION
An anthracycline antibiotic that inhibits DNA and DNA-dependent RNA synthesis by binding with DNA strands. Liposomal encapsulation increases uptake by tumors, prolongs action, and may decrease toxicity. ***Therapeutic Effect:*** Prevents cellular division.

PHARMACOKINETICS
Widely distributed. Protein binding: Unknown. Metabolized in liver. Minimal excretion in urine. ***Half-life:*** 45–55 hrs.

AVAILABILITY
Lipid Complex: 2 mg/ml (Doxil).

INDICATIONS AND DOSAGES
▸ AIDS-Related Kaposi's Sarcoma
IV INFUSION
Adults. 20 mg/m^2 over 30 minutes q3wks.
▸ Ovarian Cancer
IV INFUSION
Adults. 50 mg/m^2 q4wks.
▸ Dosage in Liver Impairment

Serum Bilirubin Concentration	Dosage
1.2–3 mg/dl	50% usual dose
> 3 mg/dl	25% usual dose

OFF-LABEL USES
Multiple myeloma

CONTRAINDICATIONS
Nursing mothers, hypersensitivity to doxorubicin compounds or daunorubicin

INTERACTIONS
Drug
Antigout medications: May decrease the effects of these drugs.
Bone marrow depressants: May increase bone marrow depression.
Daunorubicin: May increase the risk of cardiotoxicity.
Live virus vaccines: May potentiate virus replication, increase vaccine side effects, and decrease the patient's antibody response to vaccine.
Herbal
None known.
Food
None known.
Drug interactions of concern to dentistry
- None reported

DIAGNOSTIC TEST EFFECTS
May reduce neutrophil and red blood cell (RBC) count.

IV INCOMPATIBILITIES
Do not mix with any other medications.

SIDE EFFECTS
Frequent
Nausea
Occasional
Anorexia, diarrhea, hyperpigmentation of nailbeds, phalangeal and dermal creases
Rare
Fever, chills, conjunctivitis, lacrimation

SERIOUS REACTIONS

! Bone marrow depression manifested as hematologic toxicity (principally leukopenia and, to lesser extent, anemia, thrombocytopenia) may occur.

! Cardiotoxicity noted as either acute, transient abnormal ECG findings or cardiomyopathy manifested as CHF may occur.

DENTAL CONSIDERATIONS

General:

- If additional analgesia is required for dental pain, consider alternative analgesics (NSAIDs) in patients taking narcotics for acute or chronic pain.
- Avoid prescribing aspirin-containing products.
- Examine for oral manifestation of opportunistic infection.
- This drug usually is administered in a hospital, a cancer treatment center, or possibly a home IV service. Dentists are involved in the management of oral mucositis associated with the chemotherapy.
- Chlorhexidine mouth rinse prior to and during chemotherapy may reduce severity of mucositis.
- Patient on chronic drug therapy may rarely present with symptoms of blood dyscrasias, which can include infection, bleeding and poor healing. If dyscrasia is present, caution patient to prevent oral tissue trauma when using oral hygiene aids.
- Palliative medication may be required for management of oral side effects.
- Consider local hemostasis measures to prevent excessive bleeding.
- Patient may be at risk of bleeding; check oral signs.

Consultations:

- Medical consultation should include routine blood counts including platelet counts and bleeding time.
- Consult physician; prophylactic or therapeutic antiinfectives may be indicated if surgery or periodontal treatment is required.
- Medical consultation may be required to assess immunologic status during cancer chemotherapy and determine safety risk, if any, posed by the required dental treatment.
- Medical consultation may be required to assess disease control and patient's ability to tolerate stress.
- In a patient with symptoms of blood dyscrasias, request a medical consultation for blood studies and postpone treatment until normal values are reestablished.

Teach Patient/Family:

- To be aware of oral side effects
- Importance of good oral hygiene to prevent soft tissue inflammation
- Alert the patient to the possibility of secondary oral infection and the need to see dentist immediately if signs of infection occur
- To prevent trauma when using oral hygiene aids
- Importance of updating health and medication history if physician makes any changes in evaluation or drug regimens; include OTC, herbal, and nonherbal remedies in the update

doxorubicin

dox-o-roo′-bi-sin

(Adriamycin, Caelyx, Doxil, Rubex)

Do not confuse doxorubicin with daunorubicin, or Adriamycin with idamycin or idarubicin.

CATEGORY AND SCHEDULE

Pregnancy Risk Category: D

MECHANISM OF ACTION

An anthracycline antibiotic that inhibits DNA and DNA-dependent RNA synthesis by binding with DNA strands. Liposomal encapsulation increases uptake by tumors, prolongs drug action, and may decrease toxicity.
Therapeutic Effect: Prevents cell division.

PHARMACOKINETICS

Widely distributed. Protein binding: 74%–76%. Does not cross the blood-brain barrier. Metabolized rapidly in the liver to active metabolite. Primarily eliminated by biliary system. Not removed by hemodialysis. ***Half-life:*** 16 hr; metabolite, 32 hr.

AVAILABILITY

Injection, Powder for Reconstitution (Adriamycin RDF): 10 mg, 20 mg, 50 mg, 150 mg.
Injection, Powder for Reconstitution (Rubex): 50 mg, 100 mg.
Injection Solution (Adriamycin PFS): 2 mg/ml.
Lipid Complex (Doxil): 2 mg/ml.

INDICATIONS AND DOSAGES

▸ To Produce Regression in Acute Lymphoblastic and Myeloblastic Leukemia; Breast, Bronchogenic, Gastric, Ovarian, Thyroid, and Transitional Cell Bladder Carcinomas; Hodgkin's Disease; Non-Hodgkin's Lymphomas; Neuroblastoma; Primary Liver Cancer; Soft Tissue and Bone Sarcomas; and Wilms' Tumor

IV

Adults. 60–75 mg/m² as a single dose every 21 days, 20 mg/m² once weekly, or 25–30 mg/m²/day on 2–3 successive days q4wk. Because of the risk of cardiotoxicity, don't exceed a cumulative dose of 550 mg/m² (400–450 mg/m² for those previously treated with related compounds or irradiation of cardiac region).
Children. 35–75 mg/m² as a single dose q3wk or 20–30 mg/m² weekly, or 60–90 mg/m² as continuous infusion over 96 hr q3–4wk.

▸ Kaposi's Sarcoma

IV (Doxil)

Adults. 20 mg/m² q3wk infused over 30 min.

▸ Ovarian Cancer

IV (Doxil)

Adults. 50 mg/m² q4wk.

▸ Dosage in Hepatic Impairment

Dosage is modified on the basis of serum bilirubin level.

Serum Bilirubin Concentration	% of Normal Dose
1.2–3 mg/dl	50%
greater than 3 mg/dl	25%

OFF-LABEL USES

Treatment of cervical, head or neck, endometrial, liver, pancreatic, prostatic, and testicular carcinomas; germ cell tumors; multiple myeloma

CONTRAINDICATIONS

Cardiomyopathy; pre-existing myelosuppression; previous or concomitant treatment with cyclophosphamide, idarubicin, mitoxantrone, or irradiation of the cardiac region; severe CHF

INTERACTIONS

Drug

Antigout medications: May decrease the effects of these drugs.
Bone marrow depressants: May increase myelosuppression.

Daunorubicin: May increase the risk of cardiotoxicity.
Live-virus vaccines: May potentiate virus replication, increase vaccine side effects, and decrease the patient's antibody response to the vaccine.

Herbal

None known.

Food

None known.

Drug interactions of concern to dentistry

- None reported

DIAGNOSTIC TEST EFFECTS

May cause ECG changes and increase serum uric acid level. Doxil may reduce neutrophil and RBC counts.

IV INCOMPATIBILITIES

Doxorubicin: Allopurinol (Aloprim), amphotericin B complex (Abelcet, AmBisome, Amphotec), cefepime (Maxipime), furosemide (Lasix), ganciclovir (Cytovene), heparin, piperacillin and tazobactam (Zosyn), propofol (Diprivan)
Doxil: Don't mix with any other medications.

IV COMPATIBILITIES

Dexamethasone (Decadron), diphenhydramine (Benadryl), etoposide (VePesid), granisetron (Kytril), hydromorphone (Dilaudid), lorazepam (Ativan), morphine, ondansetron (Zofran), paclitaxel (Taxol)

SIDE EFFECTS

Frequent

Complete alopecia (scalp, axillary, pubic hair), nausea, vomiting, stomatitis, esophagitis (especially if drug is given on several successive days), reddish urine
Doxil: Nausea

Occasional

Anorexia, diarrhea; hyperpigmentation of skin, nailbeds, and phalangeal and dermal creases

Rare

Fever, chills, conjunctivitis, lacrimation

SERIOUS REACTIONS

! Myelosuppression may cause hematologic toxicity (manifested principally as leukopenia and, to lesser extent, anemia and thrombocytopenia), usually within 10–15 days of starting therapy. Blood counts typically return to normal levels by the third week.
! Cardiotoxicity (either acute, manifested as transient ECG abnormalities, or chronic, manifested as CHF) may occur.

DENTAL CONSIDERATIONS

General:

- If additional analgesia is required for dental pain, consider alternative analgesics (NSAIDs) in patients taking narcotics for acute or chronic pain.
- Avoid prescribing aspirin-containing products.
- Examine for oral manifestation of opportunistic infection.
- This drug usually is administered in a hospital, a cancer treatment center, or possibly a home IV service, dentists are involved in the management of oral mucositis associated with the chemotherapy.
- Chlorhexidine mouth rinse prior to and during chemotherapy may reduce severity of mucositis.
- Patient on chronic drug therapy may rarely present with symptoms of blood dyscrasias, which can include infection, bleeding and poor healing. If dyscrasia is present, caution

patient to prevent oral tissue trauma when using oral hygiene aids.
• Palliative medication may be required for management of oral side effects.
• Consider local hemostasis measures to prevent excessive bleeding.
• Patient may be at risk of bleeding; check oral signs.

Consultations:
• Medical consultation should include routine blood counts including platelet counts and bleeding time.
• Consult physician; prophylactic or therapeutic antiinfectives may be indicated if surgery or periodontal treatment is required.
• Medical consultation may be required to assess immunologic status during cancer chemotherapy and determine safety risk, if any, posed by the required dental treatment.
• Medical consultation may be required to assess disease control and patient's ability to tolerate stress.
• In a patient with symptoms of blood dyscrasias, request a medical consultation for blood studies and postpone treatment until normal values are reestablished.

Teach Patient/Family:
• To be aware of oral side effects
• Importance of good oral hygiene to prevent soft tissue inflammation
• Alert the patient to the possibility of secondary oral infection and the need to see dentist immediately if signs of infection occur
• To prevent trauma when using oral hygiene aids
• Importance of updating health and medication history if physician makes any changes in evaluation or drug regimens; include OTC, herbal, and nonherbal remedies in the update

doxycycline

dox-i-sye′-kleen
(Adoxa, Apo-Doxy[CAN], Doryx, Doxsig[AUS], Doxy-100, Doxycin[CAN], Doxyhexal[AUS], Doxylin[AUS], Monodox, Vibramycin, Vibra-Tabs)
Do not confuse doxycycline with Dicyclomine or doxylamine, or Monodox with Monopril.

CATEGORY AND SCHEDULE

Pregnancy Risk Category: D

MECHANISM OF ACTION

A tetracycline antibiotic that inhibits bacterial protein synthesis by binding to ribosomes. ***Therapeutic Effect:*** Bacteriostatic.

AVAILABILITY

Capsules (Doryx): 75 mg, 100 mg.
Capsules (Monodox): 50 mg, 100 mg.
Capsules (Vibramycin): 100 mg.
Oral Suspension (Vibramycin): 25 mg/5 ml.
Syrup (Vibramycin): 50 mg/5 ml.
Tablets (Adoxa): 50 mg, 75 mg, 100 mg.
Tablets (Periostat): 20 mg.
Tablets (Vibra-Tabs): 100 mg.
Injection, Powder for Reconstitution (Doxy-100): 100 mg.

INDICATIONS AND DOSAGES

▸ **Respiratory, Skin, and Soft-Tissue Infections; UTIs; Pelvic Inflammatory Disease (PID); Brucellosis; Trachoma; Rocky Mountain Spotted Fever; Typhus; Q Fever; Rickettsia; Severe Acne (Adoxa); Smallpox; Psittacosis; Ornithosis; Granuloma Inguinale; Lymphogranuloma Venereum; Intestinal Amebiasis (Adjunctive**

Treatment); Prevention of Rheumatic Fever
PO
Adults, Elderly. Initially, 100 mg q12h, then 100 mg/day as single dose or 50 mg q12h for severe infections.
Children 8 yr and older and weighing more than 45 kg. 2–4 mg/kg/day divided q12–24h. Maximum: 200 mg/day.
IV
Adults, Elderly. Initially, 200 mg as 1–2 infusions; then 100–200 mg/day in 1–2 divided doses.
Children 8 yr and older. 2–4 mg/kg/day divided q12–24h. Maximum: 200 mg/day.

▸ **Acute Gonococcal Infections**
PO
Adults. Initially, 200 mg, then 100 mg at bedtime on first day; then 100 mg twice a day for 14 days.

▸ **Syphilis**
PO, IV
Adults. 200 mg/day in divided doses for 14–28 days.

▸ **Traveler's Diarrhea**
PO
Adults, Elderly. 100 mg/day during a period of risk (up to 14 days) and for 2 days after returning home.

▸ **Periodontitis**
PO
Adults. 20 mg twice a day as an adjunct to scaling and root planning; may be administered for up to 9 mos exceeding the recommended dosage may increase risk of side effects, including the development of resistant organisms.

OFF-LABEL USES

Treatment of atypical mycobacterial infections, rheumatoid arthritis, gonorrhea and malaria; prevention of Lyme disease; prevention or treatment of traveler's diarrhea.

CONTRAINDICATIONS

Children 8 years and younger, hypersensitivity to tetracyclines or sulfites, last half of pregnancy, severe hepatic dysfunction

INTERACTIONS

Drug

Antacids containing aluminum, calcium, or magnesium; laxatives containing magnesium: Decrease doxycycline absorption.
Barbiturates, carbamazepine, phenytoin: May decrease doxycycline blood concentrations.
Cholestyramine, colestipol: May decrease doxycycline absorption.
Oral contraceptives: May decrease the effects of oral contraceptives.
Oral iron preparations: Impair absorption of doxycycline.

Herbal

None known.

Food

None known.

Drug interactions of concern to dentistry

- No data reported for this dose form; see doxycycline hyclate monograph for drug interactions reported with tetracyclines

Drug interactions of concern to dentistry for systemic form:

- Decreased absorption: $NaHCO_3$,other antacids
- Increased rate of metabolism: barbiturates, carbamazepine, hydantoins
- Decreased effect of penicillins, cephalosporins
- May increase the effectiveness of anticoagulants, methotrexate, digoxin
- Oral contraceptives: advise patient of a potential risk for decreased contraceptive action, to maintain compliance with oral contraceptive use while using antibiotics, and to

consider the use of additional nonhormonal contraception
• Contraindicated with isotretinoin (Accutane)

DIAGNOSTIC TEST EFFECTS

May increase serum alkaline phosphatase, amylase, bilirubin, AST (SGOT), and ALT (SGPT) levels. May alter CBC.

IV INCOMPATIBILITIES

Allopurinol (Aloprim), heparin, piperacillin and tazobactam (Zosyn)

IV COMPATIBILITIES

Amiodarone (Cordarone), diltiazem (Cardizem), hydromorphone (Dilaudid), magnesium sulfate, morphine, propofol (Diprivan)

SIDE EFFECTS

Frequent

Anorexia, nausea, vomiting, diarrhea, dysphagia, possibly severe photosensitivity

Occasional

Rash, urticaria

SERIOUS REACTIONS

! Superinfection (especially fungal) and benign intracranial hypertension (headache, visual changes) may occur.

! Hepatotoxicity, fatty degeneration of the liver, and pancreatitis occur rarely.

DENTAL CONSIDERATIONS

DOXYCYCLINE HYCLATE (DENTAL-SYSTEMIC)

General:

• Examine for oral manifestation of opportunistic infection
• Should be administered at least 1 hr before or 2 hr after morning or evening meals

Teach Patient/Family:

• To avoid using ingestible sodium bicarbonate products, such as the Prophy-Jet air polishing system, within 2 hr of drug use

DOXYCYCLINE HYCLATE/ DOXYCYCLINE CALCIUM SYSTEMIC FORM

General:

• Determine why the patient is taking tetracycline.
• Broad-spectrum antibiotics may promote oral or vaginal *Candida* infection.

Consultations:

• Medical consultation may be required to assess disease control.

Teach Patient/Family:

• That tetracycline can be taken with milk, food; take with a full glass of water
• To take tetracycline doses 1 hr before or 2 hr after air polishing device (Prophy-Jet), if used
• *When used for dental infection, advise patient:*
  • To report sore throat, oral burning sensation, fever, and fatigue, any of which could indicate superinfection
  • To take at prescribed intervals and complete dosage regimen
  • To immediately notify the dentist if signs or symptoms of infection increase

dronabinol

droe-nab′-i-nol
Schedule II Schedule III
(Marinol)
Do not confuse dronabinol with droperidol.

CATEGORY AND SCHEDULE

Pregnancy Risk Category: C
Controlled Substance Schedule: III

MECHANISM OF ACTION

An antiemetic and appetite stimulant that may act by inhibiting vomiting control mechanisms in the medulla oblongata. ***Therapeutic Effect:*** Inhibits vomiting and stimulates appetite.

PHARMACOKINETICS

Well absorbed after PO administration. Protein binding: 97%. Undergoes first-pass metabolism. Is highly lipid soluble. Primarily excreted in feces. ***Half-life:*** 4 hr.

AVAILABILITY

Capsules (Gelatin [Marinol]): 2.5 mg, 5 mg, 10 mg.

INDICATIONS AND DOSAGES

▸ Prevention of Chemotherapy-Induced Nausea and Vomiting

PO

Adults, Children. Initially, 5 mg/m^2 1–3 hr before chemotherapy, then q2–4h after chemotherapy for total of 4–6 doses a day. May increase by 2.5 mg/m^2 up to 15 mg/m^2 per dose.

▸ Appetite Stimulant

PO

Adults. Initially, 2.5 mg twice a day (before lunch and dinner). Range: 2.5–20 mg/day.

OFF-LABEL USES

Postoperative nausea and vomiting

CONTRAINDICATIONS

Treatment of nausea and vomiting not caused by chemotherapy, hypersensitivity to sesame oil or tetrahydrocannabinol products

INTERACTIONS

Drug

Alcohol, other CNS suppressants: May increase CNS depression.

Herbal

None known.

Food

None known.

Drug interactions of concern to dentistry

- Increased CNS depression: alcohol, CNS depressants, tricyclic antidepressants
- Additive hypertension, tachycardia, possible cardiotoxicity: tricyclic antidepressants, amphetamines, other sympathomimetics
- Additive tachycardia, drowsiness: atropine, scopolamine, antihistamines, anticholinergic drugs

DIAGNOSTIC TEST EFFECTS

None known.

SIDE EFFECTS

Frequent (24%–3%)

Euphoria, dizziness, paranoid reaction, somnolence

Occasional (3%–1%)

Asthenia, ataxia, confusion, abnormal thinking, depersonalization

Rare (less than 1%)

Diarrhea, depression, nightmares, speech difficulties, headache, anxiety, tinnitus, flushed skin

SERIOUS REACTIONS

! Mild intoxication may produce increased sensory awareness (including taste, smell, and sound), altered time perception, reddened conjunctiva, dry mouth, and tachycardia.
! Moderate intoxication may produce memory impairment and urine retention.
! Severe intoxication may produce lethargy, decreased motor coordination, slurred speech, and orthostatic hypotension.

DENTAL CONSIDERATIONS

General:

- Monitor vital signs at every appointment because of cardiovascular side effects.
- After supine positioning, have patient sit upright for at least 2 min to avoid orthostatic hypotension.
- Patients taking opioids for acute or chronic pain should be given alternative analgesics for dental pain.
- Assess salivary flow as a factor in caries, periodontal disease, and candidiasis.
- Consider semisupine chair position for patient comfort if GI side effects occur.

Teach Patient/Family:

- *When chronic dry mouth occurs, advise patient:*
  - To avoid mouth rinses with high alcohol content because of drying effects
  - To use daily home fluoride products for anticaries effect
  - To use sugarless gum, frequent sips of water, or saliva substitutes

droperidol

droe-pear-′-ih-dall
(Inapsine)

CATEGORY AND SCHEDULE

Pregnancy Risk Category: C

MECHANISM OF ACTION

A general anesthetic and antiemetic agent that antagonizes dopamine neurotransmission at synapses by blocking postsynaptic dopamine receptor sites; partially blocks adrenergic receptor binding sites.
Therapeutic Effect: Produces tranquilization, antiemetic effect.

PHARMACOKINETICS

Onset of action occurs within 30 minutes. Well absorbed. Metabolized in liver. Excreted in urine and feces. ***Half-life:*** 2.3 hrs.

AVAILABILITY

Injection: 2.5 mg/ml (Inapsine).

INDICATIONS AND DOSAGES

▸ Preoperative

IM/IV
Adults, Elderly, Children 12 yrs and older. 2.5–10 mg 30–60 min before induction of general anesthesia.
Children 2–12 yrs.
0.088–0.165 mg/kg.
Adjunct for induction of general anesthesia
IV
Adults, Elderly, Children 12 yrs and older. 0.22–0.275 mg/kg.
Children 2–12 yrs.
0.088–0.165 mg/kg.
Adjunct for maintenance of general anesthesia
IV
Adults, Elderly. 1.25–2.5 mg.
Diagnostic procedures w/o general anesthesia

IM
Adults, Elderly. 2.5–10 mg 30–60 min before procedure. If needed, may give additional doses of 1.25–2.5 mg (usually by IV injection).

CONTRAINDICATIONS

Known or suspected QT prolongation, hypersensitivity to droperidol or any component of the formulation

INTERACTIONS

Drug

CNS depressants: May increase CNS depressant effect.
Class I, IA or III antiarrhythmics, cisapride, cyclobenzaprine, phenothiazines, pimozide, quinolone antibiotics, tricylic antidepressants: May increase risk of QT prolongation.
Hypotensive agents: May increase hypotension.

Herbal

None known.

Food

None known.

Drug interactions of concern to dentistry

- Increased frequency of nausea/vomiting: propofol
- Increased CNS depression: all CNS depressants
- Prolonged QT interval: intravenous narcotics
- Increased hypotension: anesthetics, systemic or local
- Risk of hypotension: epinephrine
- Orthostatic hypotension: antihypertensive medications

SIDE EFFECTS

Frequent

Mild to moderate hypotension

Occasional

Tachycardia, postop drowsiness, dizziness, chills, shivering

Rare

Postop nightmares, facial sweating, bronchospasm

SERIOUS REACTIONS

! Extrapyramidal symptoms may appear as akathisia (motor restlessness) and dystonias: torticollis (neck muscle spasm), opisthotonos (rigidity of back muscles), and oculogyric crisis (rolling back of eyes).
! Overdosage includes symptoms of hypotension, tachycardia, hallucinations, and extrapyramidal symptoms.
! Prolonged QT interval, seizures, and arrhythmias have been reported.

DENTAL CONSIDERATIONS

General:

- Used in a hospital, emergency room, or cancer treatment center for acute need.
- Caution in the use of drugs that prolong the QT interval.
- Use precaution if sedation or general anesthesia is required; risk of hypotensive episode.
- After supine positioning, have patient sit upright for at least 2 min before standing to avoid orthostatic hypotension.
- Monitor vital signs at every appointment due to cardiovascular side effects.

Consultations:

- Consultation with physician may be necessary if sedation or general anesthesia is required.
- Medical consultation may be required to assess disease control.

dutasteride

do-tah-stir′-eyed
(Avodart)

D

CATEGORY AND SCHEDULE

Pregnancy Risk Category: X

MECHANISM OF ACTION

An androgen hormone inhibitor that inhibits 5-alpha reductase, an intracellular enzyme that converts testosterone into dihydrotestosterone (DHT) in the prostate gland, reducing the serum DHT level.
Therapeutic Effect: Reduces size of the prostate gland.

PHARMACOKINETICS

Route	Onset	Peak	Duration
PO	24 hr	N/A	3–8 wk

Moderately absorbed after PO administration. Widely distributed. Protein binding: 99%. Metabolized in the liver. Primarily excreted in feces. ***Half-life:*** Up to 5 wk.

AVAILABILITY

Capsule: 0.5 mg.

INDICATIONS AND DOSAGES

▸ Benign Prostatic Hyperplasia (BPH)

PO

Adults, Elderly. 0.5 mg once a day.

OFF-LABEL USES

Treatment of hair loss

CONTRAINDICATIONS

Females, physical handling of tablets by those who are or may be pregnant

INTERACTIONS

Drug

None known.

Herbal

None known.

Food

None known.

Drug interactions of concern to dentistry

• No drug interaction studies have been conducted; however, caution should be observed when used in combination with potent and chronically used CYP3A4 inhibitors
• Opioids and anticholinergic drugs may enhance urinary retention; use alternative analgesics (NSAIDs)

DIAGNOSTIC TEST EFFECTS

Decreases the serum prostate-specific antigen (PSA) level

SIDE EFFECTS

Occasional

Gynecomastia, sexual dysfunction (decreased libido, impotence, and decreased volume of ejaculate)

SERIOUS REACTIONS

! Toxicity may be manifested as rash, diarrhea, and abdominal pain.

DENTAL CONSIDERATIONS

DOXYCYCLINE HYCLATE GEL

General:

• Determine why patient is taking the drug.

Consultations:

• Medical consultation may be required to assess disease control.

Teach Patient/Family:

• Importance of updating health and drug history if physician makes any changes in evaluation or drug regimens

dyphylline
dye′-fi-lin
(Dilor, Lufyllin)
Do not confuse with Dilacor.

CATEGORY AND SCHEDULE
Pregnancy Risk Category: C

MECHANISM OF ACTION
A xanthine derivative that acts as a bronchodilator by directly relaxing smooth muscle of the bronchial airway and pulmonary blood vessels similar to theophylline. ***Therapeutic Effect:*** Relieves bronchospasm, increases vital capacity, produces cardiac, and skeletal muscle stimulation.

PHARMACOKINETICS
Rapid absorption after PO administration. Excreted in urine. ***Half-life:*** 2 hrs.

AVAILABILITY
Elixir: 100 mg/15 ml (Lufyllin).
Injection: 250 mg/ml (Dilor).
Tablet: 200 mg, 400 mg (Dilor, Lufyllin).

INDICATIONS AND DOSAGES
▸ Chronic Bronchospasm, Asthma
PO
Adults, Elderly. 15 mg/kg 4 times/day.
IM
Adults, Elderly. 250–500 mg. Maximum: 15 mg/kg q6h.
Children. 4.4–6.6 mg/kg/day in divided doses.
Dosage in renal impairment

Creatinine Clearance	Dosage Percent
50–80 ml/min	Administer 75% of dose
10–50 ml/min	Administer 50% of dose
<10 ml/min	Administer 25% of dose

CONTRAINDICATIONS
Uncontrolled arrhythmias, hyperthyroidism, history of hypersensitivity to dyphylline, related xanthine derivatives, or any component of the formulation

INTERACTIONS
Drug
Beta-blockers: May decrease effects of dyphylline.
Cimetidine, ciprofloxacin, erythromycin, norfloxacin: May increase dyphylline blood concentrations and risk of toxicity.
Glucocorticoids: May produce hypernatremia.
Phenytoin, primidone, rifampin: May increase dyphylline metabolism.
Smoking: May decrease dyphylline blood concentrations.
Drug interactions of concern to dentistry
- Increased action: erythromycin, ciprofloxacin, tetracyclines
- Increased risk of cardiac dysrhythmia: halothane-inhalation anesthesia, CNS stimulants
- Decreased effect: barbiturates, carbamazepine, ketoconazole
- May decrease sedative effects of benzodiazepines

SIDE EFFECTS
Frequent
Tachycardia, nervousness, restlessness
Occasional
Heartburn, vomiting, headache, mild diuresis, insomnia, nausea

SERIOUS REACTIONS

! Ventricular arrhythmias, hypotension, circulatory failure, seizures, hyperglycemia, and syndrome of inappropriate antidiuretic hormone (SIADH) have been reported.

DENTAL CONSIDERATIONS

General:

- Monitor vital signs at every appointment because of cardiovascular and respiratory side effects.
- Consider semisupine chair position for patients with respiratory disease.

echothiophate iodide

ek-oh-thye′-oh-fate eye′-oh-dide
(Phospholine Iodide)

CATEGORY AND SCHEDULE

Pregnancy Risk Category: C

MECHANISM OF ACTION

A cholinesterase inhibitor that causes acetylcholine to accumulate at cholinergic receptor sites and produce effects like excessive stimulation of cholinergic receptors. ***Therapeutic Effect:*** Causes conjunctival hyperemia and constriction of the sphincter pupillae and ciliary muscles, which results in miosis and paralysis of accommodation.

PHARMACOKINETICS

None reported.

AVAILABILITY

Powder for reconstitution, ophthalmic: 6.25 mg [0.125%] (Phospholine Iodide).

INDICATIONS AND DOSAGES

▸ **Glaucoma**

OPHTHALMIC

Adults, Elderly. Instill1 drop twice daily into eyes with 1 dose prior to bedtime.

▸ **Accommodative Esotropia, Diagnosis**

OPHTHALMIC

Children. Instill 1 drop once daily into both eyes at bedtime for 2–3 weeks.

▸ **Accommodative Esotropia, Treatment**

OPHTHALMIC

Children. Instill 1 drop once daily.

CONTRAINDICATIONS

Active uveal inflammation, angle-closure glaucoma, hypersensitivity to echothiophate products

INTERACTIONS

Drug

Succinylcholine: May increase neuromuscular blockade.

Herbal

None known.

Food

None known.

Drug interactions of concern to dentistry

- Avoid use of succinylcholine in general anesthesia
- Possible inhibition of the metabolism of: ester-type local and topical anesthetics
- Avoid use of anticholinergics, such as systemic atropine or related drugs

DIAGNOSTIC TEST EFFECTS

None known.

SIDE EFFECTS

Occasional

Headache, browache, blurred vision, burning and stinging of eyes, decreased night vision, intraocular pressure changes, iritis, uveitis

SERIOUS REACTIONS

! Cardiac irregularities have been reported.

DENTAL CONSIDERATIONS

General:

- Determine why patient is taking the drug.
- Avoid drugs with anticholinergic activity, such as antihistamines, opioids, benzodiazepines, propantheline, atropine, and scopolamine.
- Avoid dental light in patient's eyes; offer dark glasses for patient comfort.

• Protect patient's eyes from accidental spatter during dental treatment.
• Question glaucoma patient about compliance with prescribed drug regimen.

Consultations:

• Medical consultation may be required to assess disease control.

Teach Patient/Family:

• Importance of updating health and medication history if physician makes any changes in evaluation or drug regimens; include OTC, herbal, and nonherbal remedies in the update

efalizumab

ef-ah-liz′-ewe-mab
(Raptiva)

CATEGORY AND SCHEDULE

Pregnancy Risk Category: C

MECHANISM OF ACTION

A monoclonal antibody that interferes with lymphocyte activation by binding to the lymphocyte antigen, inhibiting the adhesion of leukocytes to other cell types. ***Therapeutic Effect:*** Prevents the release of cytokines and the growth and migration of circulating total lymphocytes, predominant in psoriatic lesions.

PHARMACOKINETICS

Clearance is affected by body weight, not by gender or race, after subcutaneous injection. Serum concentration reaches steady state at 4 wk. Mean time to elimination: 25 days.

AVAILABILITY

Powder for Injection: 150 mg, designed to deliver 125 mg/1.25 ml.

INDICATIONS AND DOSAGES

▸ **Psoriasis**

SUBCUTANEOUS

Adults, Elderly. Initially, 0.7 mg/kg followed by weekly doses of 1 mg/kg. Maximum: 200 mg (single dose).

CONTRAINDICATIONS

Concurrent use of immunosuppressive agents

INTERACTIONS

Drug

Immunosuppressive agents: Increase the risk of infection.
Live-virus vaccines: Decrease the immune response.

Herbal

None known.

Food

None known.

Drug interactions of concern to dentistry

• None reported

DIAGNOSTIC TEST EFFECTS

May increase the lymphocyte count.

SIDE EFFECTS

Frequent (32%–10%)

Headache, chills, nausea, injection site pain

Occasional (8%–7%)

Myalgia, flulike symptoms, fever

Rare (4%)

Back pain, acne

SERIOUS REACTIONS

! Hypersensitivity reaction, malignancies, serious infections (abscess, cellulitis, postoperative wound infection, pneumonia), thrombocytopenia, and worsening of psoriasis occur rarely.

DENTAL CONSIDERATIONS

General:

• Understand the disease and the patient's need to use this drug.
• Rarely oral lesions and geographic tongue may occur in patients with psoriasis.

efavirenz

e-fahv′-er-ins
(Stocrin[AUS], Sustiva)
Do not confuse Sustiva with Survanta.

CATEGORY AND SCHEDULE

Pregnancy Risk Category: C

MECHANISM OF ACTION

A nonnucleoside reverse transcriptase inhibitor that inhibits the activity of HIV reverse transcriptase of HIV-1 and the transcription of HIV-1 RNa to DNA. ***Therapeutic Effect:*** Interrupts HIV replication, slowing the progression of HIV infection.

PHARMACOKINETICS

Rapidly absorbed after PO administration. Protein binding: 99%. Metabolized to major isoenzymes in the liver. Eliminated in urine and feces. ***Half-life:*** 40–55 hr.

AVAILABILITY

Capsules: 50 mg, 100 mg, 200 mg.
Tablets: 600 mg.

INDICATIONS AND DOSAGES

▸ HIV Infection (in Combination with Other Antiretrovirals)

PO

Adults, Elderly, Children 3 yr and older weighing 40 kg or more. 600 mg once a day at bedtime.
Children 3 yr and older weighing 32.5 kg to less than 40 kg. 400 mg once a day.
Children 3 yr and older weighing 25 kg to less than 32.5 kg. 350 mg once a day.
Children 3 yr and older weighing 20 kg to less than 25 kg. 300 mg once a day.
Children 3 yr and older weighing 15 kg to less than 20 kg. 250 mg once a day.
Children 3 yr and older weighing 10 kg to less than 15 kg. 200 mg once a day.

CONTRAINDICATIONS

Concurrent use with ergot derivatives, midazolam, or triazolam; efavirenz as monotherapy; hypersensitivity to efavirenz

INTERACTIONS

Drug

Alcohol, psychoactive drugs: May produce additive CNS effects.
Clarithromycin: Decreases clarithromycin plasma levels.
Ergot derivatives, midazolam, triazolam: May cause serious or life-threatening reactions, such as arrhythmias, prolonged sedation, or respiratory depression.
Indinavir, saquinavir: Decreases the plasma concentrations of these drugs.
Nelfinavir, ritonavir: Increases the plasma concentrations of these drugs.

Phenobarbital, rifabutin, rifampin: Lowers efavirenz plasma concentration.
Warfarin: Alters warfarin plasma concentration.

Herbal

None known.

Food

High-fat meals: May increase drug absorption.

Drug interactions of concern to dentistry

- Contraindicated drugs: midazolam, triazolam
- Decreased plasma levels of clarithromycin, carbamazepine, St. John's wort (herb)
- Potential for increased levels with ketoconazole, itraconazole (no studies)
- Increased risk of CNS side effects with CNS depressants

DIAGNOSTIC TEST EFFECTS

May produce false-positive urine test results for cannabinoid and increase total cholesterol, AST (SGOT), ALT (SGPT), and serum triglyceride levels.

SIDE EFFECTS

Frequent (52%)

Mild to severe: Dizziness, vivid dreams, insomnia, confusion, impaired concentration, amnesia, agitation, depersonalization, hallucinations, euphoria, somnolence (mild symptoms don't interfere with daily activities; severe symptoms interrupt daily activities)

Occasional

Mild to moderate: Maculopapular rash (27%); nausea, fatigue, headache, diarrhea, fever, cough (< 26%) (moderate symptoms may interfere with daily activities)

SERIOUS REACTIONS

! None known.

DENTAL CONSIDERATIONS

General:

- Examine for oral manifestation of opportunistic infection.
- Monitor vital signs at every appointment because of cardiovascular and respiratory side effects.
- Consider semisupine chair position for patient comfort because of GI side effects of drug.
- Assess salivary flow as a factor in caries, periodontal disease, and candidiasis.
- Short appointments and a stress reduction protocol may be required for anxious patients.

Consultations:

- Medical consultation may be required to assess disease control.

Teach Patient/Family:

- To prevent trauma when using oral hygiene aids
- Importance of good oral hygiene to prevent soft tissue inflammation
- To be alert for the possibility of secondary oral infection and to see dentist immediately if signs of infection occur
- *When chronic dry mouth occurs, advise patient:*
  - To avoid mouth rinses with high alcohol content because of drying effects
  - To use daily home fluoride products for anticaries effect
  - To use sugarless gum, frequent sips of water, or saliva substitutes

eletriptan

el-eh-trip′-tan
(Relpax)

CATEGORY AND SCHEDULE

Pregnancy Risk Category: C

MECHANISM OF ACTION

A serotonin receptor agonist that binds selectively to vascular receptors, producing a vasoconstrictive effect on cranial blood vessels. ***Therapeutic Effect:*** Relieves migraine headache.

PHARMACOKINETICS

Well absorbed after PO administration. Metabolized by the liver to inactive metabolite. Eliminated in urine. ***Half-life:*** 4.4 hr (increased in hepatic impairment and the elderly [older than 65 yr]).

AVAILABILITY

Tablets: 20 mg, 40 mg.

INDICATIONS AND DOSAGES

▸ **Acute Migraine Headache**

PO

Adults, Elderly. 20–40 mg. If headache improves but then returns, dose may be repeated after 2 hr. Maximum: 80 mg/day.

CONTRAINDICATIONS

Arrhythmias associated with conduction disorders, coronary artery disease, ischemic heart disease, severe hepatic impairment, uncontrolled hypertension

INTERACTIONS

Drug

Clarithromycin, itraconazole, ketoconazole, nefazodone, nelfinavir, ritonavir: May decrease eletriptan metabolism.

Ergotamine-containing medications: May produce a vasospastic reaction.

Sibutramine: May produce serotonin syndrome (marked by altered LOC, CNS irritability, motor weakness, myoclonus, and shivering).

Herbal

None known.

Food

None known.

Drug interactions of concern to dentistry

• Avoid use of strong CYP3A4 drugs concurrently or within 72 hr of use of eletriptan: ketoconazole, itraconazole, erythromycin, clarithromycin, others

DIAGNOSTIC TEST EFFECTS

None known.

SIDE EFFECTS

Occasional (6%–5%)

Dizziness, somnolence, asthenia, nausea

Rare (3%–2%)

Paresthesia, headache, dry mouth, warm or hot sensation, dyspepsia, dysphagia

SERIOUS REACTIONS

! Cardiac reactions (including ischemia, coronary artery vasospasm, and MI) and noncardiac vasospasm-related reactions (such as hemorrhage and CVA) occur rarely, particularly in patients with hypertension, diabetes, or a strong family history of coronary artery disease; obese patients; smokers; males older than 40 years; and postmenopausal women.

DENTAL CONSIDERATIONS

General:

• This is an acute-use drug; it is doubtful that patients will seek

dental treatment during acute migraine attacks.
• Be aware of the patient's disease, its severity, and its frequency, when known.
• Monitor vital signs at every appointment because of cardiovascular side effects.
• Assess salivary flow as a factor in caries, periodontal disease, and candidiasis.
• Consider semisupine chair position for patient comfort if GI side effects occur.

Consultations:
• If treating chronic orofacial pain, consult with patient's physician.

Teach Patient/Family:
• That oral symptoms will disappear when drug is discontinued

emedastine

e-med′-a-steen
(Emadine)

CATEGORY AND SCHEDULE

Pregnancy Risk Category: B

MECHANISM OF ACTION

An ophthalmic H_1-receptor antagonist that inhibits histamine-stimulated vascular permeability in the conjunctiva. ***Therapeutic Effect:*** Relieves ocular itching associated with allergic conjunctivitis.

PHARMACOKINETICS

Negligible absorption after ophthalmic administration. Metabolized into inactive metabolites. Excreted in urine. ***Half-life:*** 6.6 hrs

AVAILABILITY

Ophthalmic Solution: 0.05% (Emadine).

INDICATIONS AND DOSAGES

▸ Allergic Conjunctivitis

OPHTHALMIC
Adults, Elderly, Children 3 yrs and older. 1–2 drops in affected eye(s) twice daily.

CONTRAINDICATIONS

Hypersensitivity to emedastine or any other component of the formulation

INTERACTIONS

Drug
None known.
Herbal
None known.
Food
None known.
Drug interactions of concern to dentistry
• None reported

DIAGNOSTIC TEST EFFECTS

None known.

SIDE EFFECTS

Frequent (11%)
Headache
Occasional (<5%)
Abnormal dreams, asthenia (loss of strength, energy) bad taste, blurred vision, burning or stinging, dry eyes, foreign body sensation, tearing

SERIOUS REACTIONS

! Somnolence and malaise occurs rarely.

DENTAL CONSIDERATIONS

General:
• Protect patient's eyes from accidental spatter during dental treatment.

emtricitabine

em-trih-sit′-ah-bean
(Emtriva)

CATEGORY AND SCHEDULE

Pregnancy Risk Category: B

MECHANISM OF ACTION

An antiretroviral that inhibits HIV-1 reverse transcriptase by incorporating itself into viral DNA, resulting in chain termination. ***Therapeutic Effect:*** Interrupts HIV replication, slowing the progression of HIV infection.

PHARMACOKINETICS

Rapidly and extensively absorbed from the GI tract. Excreted primarily in urine (86%) and, to a lesser extent, in feces (14%); 30% removed by hemodialysis. Unknown if removed by peritoneal dialysis. ***Half-life:*** 10 hr.

AVAILABILITY

Capsules: 200 mg.

INDICATIONS AND DOSAGES

▸ HIV Infection (in Combination with Other Antiretrovirals)

PO

Adults, Elderly. 200 mg once a day.

▸ Dosage in Renal Impairment

Dosage and frequency are modified on the basis of creatinine clearance.

Creatinine Clearance	Dosage
30–49 ml/min	200 mg q48h
15–29 ml/min	200 mg q72h
less than 15 ml/min, hemodialysis patients	200 mg q96h

CONTRAINDICATIONS

None known.

INTERACTIONS

Drug

None known.

Herbal

None known.

Food

None known.

Drug interactions of concern to dentistry

- None reported

DIAGNOSTIC TEST EFFECTS

May elevate serum amylase, lipase, ALT (SGPT), AST (SGOT), and triglyceride levels. May alter blood glucose levels.

SIDE EFFECTS

Frequent (23%–13%)

Headache, rhinitis, rash, diarrhea, nausea

Occasional (14%–4%)

Cough, vomiting, abdominal pain, insomnia, depression, paresthesia, dizziness, peripheral neuropathy, dyspepsia, myalgia

Rare (3%–2%)

Arthralgia, abnormal dreams

SERIOUS REACTIONS

! Lactic acidosis and hepatomegaly with steatosis occur rarely and may be severe.

DENTAL CONSIDERATIONS

General:

- Examine for oral manifestation of opportunistic infection.
- Consider semisupine chair position for patient comfort if GI side effects occur.
- Patient history should include all medications and herbal or nonherbal remedies taken by the patient.

Consultations:

- Medical consultation may be required to assess disease control and patient's ability to tolerate stress.

Teach Patient/Family:

- Importance of good oral hygiene to prevent soft tissue inflammation, infection
- To prevent trauma when using oral hygiene aids
- Importance of updating health and drug history, reporting changes in health status, drug regimen changes, or disease/treatment status

enalapril maleate

en-al'-a-pril

(Alphapril[AUS], Amprace[AUS], Apo-Enalapril[CAN], Auspril[AUS], Renitec[AUS], Vasotec)

Do not confuse enalapril with Anafranil, Eldepryl, or ramipril.

CATEGORY AND SCHEDULE

Pregnancy Risk Category: D (C if used in first trimester)

MECHANISM OF ACTION

This angiotensin-converting enzyme (ACE) inhibitor suppresses the renin-angiotensin-aldosterone system and prevents conversion of angiotensin I to angiotensin II, a potent vasoconstrictor; may inhibit angiotensin II at local vascular, renal sites. Decreases plasma angiotensin II, increases plasma renin activity, decreases aldosterone secretion. ***Therapeutic Effect:*** In hypertension, reduces peripheral arterial resistance. In congestive heart failure (CHF), increases cardiac output; decreases peripheral vascular resistance, BP, pulmonary capillary wedge pressure, heart size.

PHARMACOKINETICS

Route	Onset	Peak	Duration
PO	1 hr	4–6 hr	24 hr
IV	15 min	1–4 hr	6 hr

Readily absorbed from the GI tract (not affected by food). Protein binding: 50%–60%. Converted to active metabolite. Primarily excreted in urine. Removed by hemodialysis. ***Half-life:*** 11 hr (half-life is increased in those with impaired renal function).

AVAILABILITY

Tablets: 2.5 mg, 5 mg, 10 mg, 20 mg.
Injection: 1.25 mg/ml.

INDICATIONS AND DOSAGES

▸ **Hypertension Alone or in Combination with Other Antihypertensives**

PO

Adults, Elderly. Initially, 2.5–5 mg/day. Range: 10–40 mg/day in 1–2 divided doses.

Children. 0.1 mg/kg/day in 1–2 divided doses. Maximum: 0.5 mg/kg/day.

Neonates. 0.1 mg/kg/day q24h.

IV

Adults, Elderly. 0.625–1.25 mg q6h up to 5 mg q6h.

Children, Neonates. 5–10 mcg/kg/dose q8–24h.

▸ **Adjunctive Therapy for CHF**

PO

Adults, Elderly. Initially, 2.5–5 mg/day. Range: 5–20 mg/day in 2 divided doses.

▸ **Dosage in Renal Impairment**

Dosage is modified on the basis of creatinine clearance.

Creatinine Clearance	% Usual Dose
10–50 ml/min	75–100
less than 10 ml/min	50

OFF-LABEL USES

Treatment of diabetic nephropathy or renal crisis in scleroderma

CONTRAINDICATIONS

History of angioedema from previous treatment with ACE inhibitors

INTERACTIONS

Drug

Alcohol, antihypertensives, diuretics: May increase the effects of enalapril.

Herbal

None known.

Food

None known.

Drug interactions of concern to dentistry

- Increased hypotension: alcohol, phenothiazines
- Decreased hypotensive effects: indomethacin, possibly other NSAIDs, sympathomimetics
- Suspected reduction in the antihypertensive and vasodilator effects by salicylates; monitor blood pressure if used concurrently

DIAGNOSTIC TEST EFFECTS

May increase BUN and serum alkaline phosphatase, serum bilirubin, serum creatinine, serum potassium, AST (SGOT), and ALT (SGPT) levels. May decrease serum sodium levels. May cause positive ANA titer.

IV INCOMPATIBILITIES

Amphotericin B (Fungizone), amphotericin B complex (Abelcet, AmBisome, Amphotec), cefepime (Maxipime), phenytoin (Dilantin)

IV COMPATIBILITIES

Calcium gluconate, dobutamine (Dobutrex), dopamine (Inotropin), fentanyl (Sublimaze), heparin, lidocaine, magnesium sulfate, morphine, nitroglycerin, potassium chloride, potassium phosphate, propofol (Diprivan)

SIDE EFFECTS

Frequent (7%–5%)

Headache, dizziness

Occasional (3%–2%)

Orthostatic hypotension, fatigue, diarrhea, cough, syncope

Rare (<2%)

Angina, abdominal pain, vomiting, nausea, rash, asthenia (loss of strength, energy), syncope

SERIOUS REACTIONS

! Excessive hypotension ("first-dose syncope") may occur in patients with CHF and in those who are severely salt or volume depleted.

! Angioedema (swelling of face, lips) and hyperkalemia occur rarely.

! Agranulocytosis and neutropenia may be noted in patients with collagen vascular diseases, including scleroderma and systemic lupus erythematosus, and impaired renal function.

! Nephrotic syndrome may be noted in those with history of renal disease.

DENTAL CONSIDERATIONS

General:

- Monitor vital signs at every appointment because of cardiovascular side effects.
- After supine positioning, have patient sit upright for at least 2 min before standing to avoid orthostatic hypotension.
- Patients on chronic drug therapy may rarely have symptoms of blood dyscrasias, which can include infection, bleeding, and poor healing.

E

• Assess salivary flow as a factor in caries, periodontal disease, and candidiasis.
• Limit use of sodium-containing products, such as saline IV fluids, for those patients with a dietary salt restriction.
• Use vasoconstrictors with caution, in low doses, and with careful aspiration.
• Stress from dental procedures may compromise cardiovascular function; determine patient risk.
• Short appointments and a stress reduction protocol may be required for anxious patients.

Consultations:
• Medical consultation may be required to assess patient's ability to tolerate stress.
• In a patient with symptoms of blood dyscrasias, request a medical consultation for blood studies and postpone dental treatment until normal values are reestablished.
• Take precautions if dental surgery is anticipated and sedation or general anesthesia is required; risk of hypotensive episode.

Teach Patient/Family:
• Importance of good oral hygiene to prevent soft tissue inflammation
• *When chronic dry mouth occurs, advise patient:*
  • To avoid mouth rinses with high alcohol content because of drying effects
  • To use daily home fluoride products for anticaries effect
  • To use sugarless gum, frequent sips of water, or saliva substitutes

enfuvirtide

en-few′-vir-tide
(Fuzeon)
Do not confuse Fuzeon with Furoxone.

CATEGORY AND SCHEDULE

Pregnancy Risk Category: B

MECHANISM OF ACTION

A fusion inhibitor that interferes with the entry of HIV-1 into CD4+ cells by inhibiting the fusion of viral and cellular membranes.
Therapeutic Effect: Impairs HIV replication, slowing the progression of HIV infection.

PHARMACOKINETICS

Comparable absorption when injected into subcutaneous tissue of abdomen, arm, or thigh. Protein binding: 92%. Undergoes catabolism to amino acids. ***Half-life:*** 3.8 hr.

AVAILABILITY

Powder for Injection: 108-mg (approximately 90 mg/ml when reconstituted) vials.

INDICATIONS AND DOSAGES

▸ HIV Infection (in Combination with Other Antiretrovirals)
SUBCUTANEOUS
Adults, Elderly. 90 mg (1 ml) twice a day.
Children 6–16 yr. 2 mg/kg twice a day. Maximum 90 mg twice a day.

Pediatric dosing guidelines

Weight: kg (lb)	Dose: mg (ml)
11–15.5 (24–34)	27 (0.3)
15.6–20 (35–44)	36 (0.4)
20.1–24.5 (45–54)	45 (0.5)
24.6–29 (55–64)	54 (0.6)
29.1–33.5 (65–74)	63 (0.7)
33.6–38 (75–84)	72 (0.8)
38.1–42.5 (85–94)	81 (0.9)
greater than 42.5 (>94)	90 (1)

CONTRAINDICATIONS

None known.

INTERACTIONS

Drug

None known.

Herbal

None known.

Food

None known.

Drug interactions of concern to dentistry

- None reported

DIAGNOSTIC TEST EFFECTS

May elevate blood glucose and serum amylase, CK, lipase, triglyceride, AST (SGOT), and ALT (SGPT) levels. May decrease blood hemoglobin levels and WBC count.

SIDE EFFECTS

Expected (98%)

Local injection site reactions (pain, discomfort, induration, erythema, nodules, cysts, pruritus, ecchymosis)

Frequent (26%–16%)

Diarrhea, nausea, fatigue

Occasional (11%–4%)

Insomnia, peripheral neuropathy, depression, cough, decreased appetite or weight loss, sinusitis, anxiety, asthenia, myalgia, cold sores

Rare (3%–2%)

Constipation, influenza, upper abdominal pain, anorexia, conjunctivitis

SERIOUS REACTIONS

! Enfuvirtide use may potentiate bacterial pneumonia.

! Hypersensitivity (rash, fever, chills, rigors, hypotension), thrombocytopenia, neutropenia, and renal insufficiency or failure may occur rarely.

DENTAL CONSIDERATIONS

General:

- Patients taking this drug will be taking other antiviral drugs that may interact with some dental drugs. Be sure to take a complete drug history.
- Patients on chronic drug therapy may rarely have symptoms of blood dyscrasias, which can include infection, bleeding, and poor healing.
- Examine for oral manifestation of opportunistic infection.

Consultations:

- Medical consultation may be required to assess disease control in the patient.
- In a patient with symptoms of blood dyscrasias, request a medical consultation for blood studies and postpone treatment until normal values are reestablished.

Teach Patient/Family:

- Importance of good oral hygiene to prevent soft tissue inflammation
- To prevent trauma when using oral hygiene aids
- Importance of updating health and drug history if physician makes any changes in evaluation or drug regimens

enoxaparin sodium

e-nox-ah-pair′-in
(Clexane[AUS], Klexane[CAN], Lovenox)
Do not confuse Lovenox with Lotronex.

CATEGORY AND SCHEDULE

Pregnancy Risk Category: B

MECHANISM OF ACTION

A low-molecular-weight heparin that potentiates the action of antithrombin III and inactivates coagulation factor Xa. ***Therapeutic Effect:*** Produces anticoagulation. Does not significantly influence bleeding time, PT, or aPTT.

PHARMACOKINETICS

Route	Onset	Peak	Duration
Subcutaneous	N/A	3–5 hr	12 hr

Well absorbed after subcutaneous administration. Eliminated primarily in urine. Not removed by hemodialysis. ***Half-life:*** 4.5 hr.

AVAILABILITY

Injection: 30 mg/0.3 ml, 40 mg/0.4 ml, 60 mg/0.6 ml, 80 mg/0.8 ml, 100 mg/ml, 120 mg/0.8 ml, 150 mg/ml in prefilled syringes.

INDICATIONS AND DOSAGES

▶ **Prevention of Deep Vein Thrombosis (DVT) after Hip and Knee Surgery**

SUBCUTANEOUS

Adults, Elderly. 30 mg twice a day, generally for 7–10 days.

▶ **Prevention of DVT After Abdominal Surgery**

SUBCUTANEOUS

Adults, Elderly. 40 mg a day for 7–10 days.

▶ **Prevention of Long-Term DVT in Nonsurgical Acute Illness**

SUBCUTANEOUS

Adults, Elderly. 40 mg once a day for 3 wk.

▶ **Prevention of Ischemic Complications of Unstable Angina and Non-Q-Wave MI (with Oral Aspirin Therapy)**

SUBCUTANEOUS

Adults, Elderly. 1 mg/kg q12h.

▶ **Acute DVT**

SUBCUTANEOUS

Adults, Elderly. 1 mg/kg q12h or 1.5 mg/kg once daily.

▶ **Usual Pediatric Dosage**

SUBCUTANEOUS

Children. 0.5 mg/kg q12h (prophylaxis); 1 mg/kg q12h (treatment).

▶ **Dosage in Renal Impairment**

Clearance of enoxaparin is decreased when creatinine clearance is less than 30 ml/min. Monitor patient and adjust dosage as necessary. When enoxaparin is used in abdomonal, hip, or knee surgery or acute illness, the dosage in renal impairment is 30 mg once a day. When enoxaparin is used to treat DVT, angina, or MI the dosage in renal impairment is 1 mg/kg once a day.

OFF-LABEL USES

Prevention of DVT following general surgical procedures

CONTRAINDICATIONS

Active major bleeding, concurrent heparin therapy, hypersensitivity to heparin or pork products, thrombocytopenia associated with positive in vitro test for antiplatelet antibodies

INTERACTIONS

Drug

Anticoagulants, platelet inhibitors: May increase bleeding.

Herbal
None known.
Food
None known.
Drug interactions of concern to dentistry
• Avoid concurrent use of aspirin, NSAIDs, dipyridamole, sulfinpyrazone
• Use with caution in patients taking olanzapine

DIAGNOSTIC TEST EFFECTS
Increases (reversible) LDH, serum alkaline phosphatase, AST(SGOT), and ALT(SGPT) levels.

SIDE EFFECTS
Occasional (4%–1%)
Injection site hematoma, nausea, peripheral edema

SERIOUS REACTIONS
! Overdose may lead to bleeding complications ranging from local ecchymoses to major hemorrhage. Antidote: Protamine sulfate (1% solution) equal to the dose of enoxaparin injected. One mg protamine sulfate neutralizes 1 mg enoxaparin. A second dose of 0.5 mg protamine sulfate per 1 mg enoxaparin may be given if aPTT tested 2–4 hr after first injection remains prolonged.

DENTAL CONSIDERATIONS
General:
• Determine why patient is taking the drug.
• Product may be used in outpatient therapy. Delay elective dental treatment until patient completes enoxaparin therapy.
• Consider local hemostasis measures to prevent excessive bleeding if dental treatment must be performed.
• Avoid products that affect platelet function, such as aspirin and NSAIDs.
• Antibiotic prophylaxis before dental treatment may be required for joint prosthesis (see 2003 ADA guidelines).
Consultations:
• Medical consultation should include routine blood counts, including platelet counts and bleeding time.
Teach Patient/Family:
• Importance of good oral hygiene to prevent soft tissue inflammation
• Caution to prevent trauma when using oral hygiene aids
• To report oral lesions, soreness, or bleeding to dentist

E

entacapone
en-tak′-a-pone
(Comtan)

CATEGORY AND SCHEDULE
Pregnancy Risk Category: C

MECHANISM OF ACTION
An antiparkinson agent that inhibits the enzyme, catechol-*O*-methyltransferase (COMT), potentiating dopamine activity and increasing the duration of action of levodopa.
Therapeutic Effect: Decreases signs and symptoms of Parkinson's disease.

PHARMACOKINETICS
Rapidly absorbed after PO administration. Protein binding: 98%. Metabolized in the liver. Primarily eliminated by biliary excretion. Not removed by hemodialysis. ***Half-life:*** 2.4 hr.

AVAILABILITY
Tablets: 200 mg.

E

INDICATIONS AND DOSAGES

▸ Adjunctive Treatment of Parkinson's Disease

PO

Adults, Elderly. 200 mg concomitantly with each dose of carbidopa and levodopa up to a maximum of 8 times a day (1,600 mg).

CONTRAINDICATIONS

Hypersensitivity, use within 14 days of MAOIs

INTERACTIONS

Drug

Ampicillin, cholestyramine, erythromycin, probenecid: May decrease the excretion of entacapone.

Bitolterol, dobutamine, dopamine, epinephrine, isoetharine, isoproterenol, epinephrine, methyldopa, norepinephrine: May increase the risk of arrhythmias and changes in BP.

Nonselective MAOIs (including phenelzine): May inhibit catecholamine metabolism.

Other CNS depressants: May increase CNS depression.

Herbal

None known.

Food

None known.

Drug interactions of concern to dentistry

- Increased heart rate, arrhythmias, hypertension: epinephrine, norepinephrine, levonordefrin, other sympathomimetics metabolized by catechol-*O*-methyltransferase (COMT)
- Possible decrease in urinary excretion: erythromycin

DIAGNOSTIC TEST EFFECTS

None known.

SIDE EFFECTS

Frequent (>10%)

Dyskinesia, nausea, dark yellow or orange urine and sweat, diarrhea

Occasional (9%–3%)

Abdominal pain, vomiting, constipation, dry mouth, fatigue, back pain

Rare (<2%)

Anxiety, somnolence, agitation, dyspepsia, flatulence, diaphoresis, asthenia, dyspnea

SERIOUS REACTIONS

! None known.

DENTAL CONSIDERATIONS

General:

- Monitor vital signs at every appointment because of cardiovascular side effects.
- Short appointments and a stress reduction protocol may be required for anxious patients.
- Consider semisupine chair position for patient comfort if GI side effects occur.
- Use vasoconstrictor with caution, in low doses, and with careful aspiration. Avoid using gingival retraction cord containing epinephrine.
- Assess for presence of extrapyramidal motor symptoms, such as tardive dyskinesia and akathisia. Extrapyramidal motor activity may complicate dental treatment.
- After supine positioning, have patient sit upright for at least 2 min to avoid orthostatic hypotension.
- Assess salivary flow as a factor in caries, periodontal disease, and candidiasis.

Consultations:

- Medical consultation may be required to assess disease control and patient's ability to tolerate stress.

Teach Patient/Family:

- Use of electric toothbrush if patient has difficulty holding conventional devices

- Importance of updating health and drug history if physician makes any changes in evaluation or drug regimens
- *When chronic dry mouth occurs, advise patient:*
  - To avoid mouth rinses with high alcohol content because of drying effects
  - To use daily home fluoride products for anticaries effect
  - To use sugarless gum, frequent sips of water, or saliva substitutes

ephedrine

eh-fed′-rin
(Pretz-D)
Do not confuse with epinephrine.

CATEGORY AND SCHEDULE

Pregnancy Risk Category: C

MECHANISM OF ACTION

A adrenergic agonist that stimulates alpha-adrenergic receptors causing vasoconstriction and pressor effects, $beta_1$-adrenergic receptors, resulting in cardiac stimulation, and $beta_2$-adrenergic receptors, resulting in bronchial dilation and vasodilation.
Therapeutic Effect: Increases blood pressure (B/P) and pulse rate.

PHARMACOKINETICS

Well absorbed after nasal and parenteral absorption. Metabolized in liver. Excreted in urine. ***Half-life:*** 3–6 hrs.

AVAILABILITY

Capsules: 25 mg.
Injection: 50 mg/ml.
Intranasal spray: 0.25% (Pretz-D).

INDICATIONS AND DOSAGES

▸ Asthma

PO

Adults. 25–50 mg q3–4h as needed.
Children. 3 mg/kg/day in 4 divided doses.

▸ Hypotension

IM

Adults. 25–50 mg as a single dose. Maximum 150 mg/day.
Children. 0.2–0.3 mg/kg/dose q4–6h.

IV

Adults. 5 mg/dose slow IVP as prevention. 10–25 mg/dose slow IVP repeated q5–10min as treatment. Maximum: 150 mg/day.
Children. 0.2–0.3 mg/kg/dose slow IVP q4–6h

SC

Adults. 25–50 q4–6h. Maximum 150 mg/day.
Children. 3 mg/kg/day q4–6h.

▸ Nasal Congestion

PO

Adults. 25–50 mg q6h as needed.
Children. 3 mg/kg/day in 4 divided doses.

NASAL

Adults, Children 12 years and older. 2–3 sprays into each nostril q4h
Children 6–12 yrs. 1–2 sprays into each nostril q4h

OFF-LABEL USES

Obesity, propofol-induced pain, radiocontrast media reactions

CONTRAINDICATIONS

Anesthesia with cyclopropane or halothane, diabetes (ephedrine injection), hypersensitivity to ephedrine or other sympathomimetic amines, hypertension or other cardiovascular disorders, pregnancy with maternal blood pressure above 130/80, thyrotoxicosis

INTERACTIONS

Drug

Caffeine: May increase cardiac stimulation.
Cardiac glycosides, sympathomimetics, theophylline, general anesthetics: May increase toxic cardiac stimulation.
Atropine, MAOIs, oxytocics, tricyclic antidepressants: May increase cardiovascular effects.

Herbal

Ephedra, bitter orange, yohimbe: May increase central nervous system (CNS) and cardiovascular stimulation and effects.

Food

None known.

Drug interactions of concern to dentistry

- Decreased pressor effect: haloperidol, phenothiazines, thioxanthenes
- Dysrhythmia: halogenated general anesthetics

DIAGNOSTIC TEST EFFECTS

May result in false-positive amphetamine EMIT assay. Lactic acid serum values may be increase.

IV INCOMPATIBILITIES

Phenobarbital (Luminal), secobarbital (Seconal)

IV COMPATIBILITIES

Chloramphenicol, fenoldopam (Corlopam), lidocaine, metaraminol (Aramine), nafcillin (Unipen), penicillin G, propofol (Diprivan), tetracycline

SIDE EFFECTS

Frequent

Hypertension, anxiety

Occasional

Nausea, vomiting, palpitations, tremor
Nasal: Burning, stinging, runny nose

Rare

Psychosis, decreased urination, necrosis at injection site from repeated injections

SERIOUS REACTIONS

! Excessive doses may cause hypertension, intracranial hemorrhage, anginal pain, and fatal arrhythmias.
! Prolonged or excessive use may result in metabolic acidosis due to increased serum lactic acid concentrations.
! Observe for disorientation, weakness, hyperventilation, headache, nausea, vomiting, and diarrhea.

DENTAL CONSIDERATIONS

General:

- Monitor vital signs at every appointment because of cardiovascular side effects.
- Assess salivary flow as a factor in caries, periodontal disease, and candidiasis.
- Consider semisupine chair position for patients with respiratory disease.
- Consider short appointments and a stress reduction protocol for anxious patients.

Consultations:

- Medical consultation may be required to assess disease control and patient's tolerance for stress.

Teach Patient/Family:

- *When chronic dry mouth occurs, advise patient:*
  - To avoid mouth rinses with high alcohol content because of drying effects
  - To use daily home fluoride products for anticaries effect
  - To use sugarless gum, frequent sips of water, or saliva substitutes

epinastine

eh-pin-ass′-teen
(Elestat)

CATEGORY AND SCHEDULE

Pregnancy Risk Category: C

MECHANISM OF ACTION

An ophthalmic H_1 receptor antagonist that inhibits the release of histamine from the mast cell. ***Therapeutic Effect:*** Prevents pruritus associated with allergic conjunctivitis.

PHARMACOKINETICS

Low systemic exposure. Protein binding: 64%. Less than 10% is metabolized. Excreted primarily in urine and, to a lesser extent, in feces. ***Half-life:*** 12 hr.

AVAILABILITY

Ophthalmic Solution: 0.05%.

INDICATIONS AND DOSAGES

▸ Allergic Conjunctivitis

OPHTHALMIC

Adults, Elderly, Children 3 yr and older. 1 drop in each eye twice a day. Continue treatment until period of exposure (pollen season, exposure to offending allergen) is over.

CONTRAINDICATIONS

None known.

INTERACTIONS

Drug

None known.

Herbal

None known.

Food

None known.

Drug interactions of concern to dentistry

- None reported

DIAGNOSTIC TEST EFFECTS

None known.

SIDE EFFECTS

Occasional

Ocular (10%–1%): Burning sensation in the eye, hyperemia, pruritus
Non-ocular (10%): Cold symptoms, upper respiratory tract infection

Rare (3%–1%)

Headache, rhinitis, sinusitis, increased cough, pharyngitis

SERIOUS REACTIONS

! None known.

DENTAL CONSIDERATIONS

General:

- Protect patient's eyes from accidental spatter during dental treatment.
- Avoid dental light in patient's eyes; offer dark glasses for patient comfort.

epinephrine

ep-i-nef′-rin
(Adrenalin, Adrenaline Injection[AUS], EpiPen, EpiPen Jr. 0.15 Adrenaline Autoinjector[AUS], Primatene)
Do not confuse epinephrine with ephedrine.

CATEGORY AND SCHEDULE

Pregnancy Risk Category: C

MECHANISM OF ACTION

A sympathomimetic, adrenergic agonist that stimulates alpha-adrenergic receptors causing vasoconstriction and pressor effects, $beta_1$-adrenergic receptors, resulting in cardiac stimulation, and $beta_2$-adrenergic receptors, resulting in bronchial dilation and vasodilation. With ophthalmic form, increases outflow of aqueous humor from anterior eye chamber. ***Therapeutic Effect:*** Relaxes smooth muscle of the bronchial tree, produces cardiac stimulation, and dilates skeletal muscle vasculature. The ophthalmic form dilates pupils and constricts conjunctival blood vessels.

E

PHARMACOKINETICS

Route	Onset	Peak	Duration
IM	5–10 min	20 min	1–4 hr
Subcutaneous	5–10 min	20 min	1–4 hr
Inhalation	3–5 min	20 min	1–3 hr
Ophthalmic	1 hr	4–8 hr	12–24 hr

Well absorbed after parenteral administration; minimally absorbed after inhalation. Metabolized in the liver, other tissues, and sympathetic nerve endings. Excreted in urine. The ophthalmic form may be systemically absorbed as a result of drainage into nasal pharyngeal passages. Mydriasis occurs within several min and persists several hr; vasoconstriction occurs within 5 min, and lasts less than 1 hr.

AVAILABILITY

Injection: 0.1 mg/ml, 1 mg/ml.
Injection (Epi-Pen): 0.3 mg/0.3 ml, 0.15 mg/0.3 ml.
*Inhalation (Aerosol [Primatene Mist]):*0.2 mg/inhalation.
Inhalation Solution: 1%, 2.25%.
Ophthalmic Solution (Epifrin): 0.5%, 1%, 2%.

INDICATIONS AND DOSAGES

▸ Asystole

IV

Adults, Elderly. 1 mg q3–5min up to 0.1 mg/kg q3–5min.
Children. 0.01 mg/kg (0.1 ml/kg of 1:10,000 solution). May repeat q3–5min. Subsequent doses of 0.1 mg/kg (0.1 ml/kg) of a 1:1000 solution q3–5min.

▸ Bradycardia

IV Infusion

Adults, Elderly. 1–10 mcg/min titrated to desired effect.

IV

Children. 0.01 mg/kg (0.1 mg/kg of 1:10,000 solution) q3–5min. Maximum: 1 mg/10 ml.

▸ Bronchodilation

IM, SUBCUTANEOUS

Adults, Elderly. 0.1–0.5 mg (1:1000) q10–15min to 4 hrs.

SUBCUTANEOUS

Children. 10 mcg/kg (0.01 ml/kg of 1:1,000) Maximum: 0.5 mg or suspension (1:200) 0.005 ml/kg/dose (0.025 mg/kg/dose) to a maximum of 0.15 ml (0.75 mg for single dose) q8–12h.

▸ Hypersensitivity Reaction

IM, SUBCUTANEOUS

Adults, Elderly. 0.3–0.5 mg q15–20min.

SUBCUTANEOUS

Children. 0.01 mg/kg q15min for 2 doses, then q4h. Maximum single dose: 0.5 mg.

INHALATION

Adults, Elderly, Children 4 yr and older. 1 inhalation, may repeat in at least 1 min. Give subsequent doses no sooner than 3 hr.

NEBULIZER

Adults, Elderly, Children 4 yr and older. 1–3 deep inhalations. Give subsequent doses no sooner than 3 hr.

▸ Glaucoma

OPHTHALMIC

Adults, Elderly. 1–2 drops 1–2 times a day.

OFF-LABEL USES

Systemic: Treatment of gingival or pulpal hemorrhage, priapism
Ophthalmic: Treatment of conjunctival congestion during surgery, secondary glaucoma

CONTRAINDICATIONS
Cardiac arrhythmias, cerebrovascular insufficiency, hypertension, hyperthyroidism, ischemic heart disease, narrow-angle glaucoma, shock

INTERACTIONS
Drug
Beta blockers: May decrease the effects of beta blockers.
Digoxin, sympathomimetics: May increase risk of arrhythmias.
Ergonovine, methergine, oxytocin: May increase vasoconstriction.
MAOIs, tricyclic antidepressants: May increase cardiovascular effects.
Herbal
None known.
Food
None known.
Drug interactions of concern to dentistry
- Hypotension, tachycardia: haloperidol, loxapine, phenothiazines, thioxanthenes
- Ventricular dysrhythmia: hydrocarbon-inhalation anesthetics, CNS stimulants, tricyclic antidepressants
- With larger doses of epinephrine risk of hypertension followed by bradycardia with β-adrenergic antagonists

DIAGNOSTIC TEST EFFECTS
May decrease serum potassium level.

IV INCOMPATIBILITIES
Ampicillin (Omnipen, Polycillin)
IV COMPATIBILITIES
Calcium chloride, calcium gluconate, diltiazem (Cardizem), dobutamine (Dobutrex), dopamine (Intropin), fentanyl (Sublimaze), heparin, hydromorphone (Dilaudid), lorazepam (Ativan), midazolam (Versed), milrinone (Primacor), morphine, nitroglycerin, norepinephrine (Levophed), potassium chloride, propofol (Diprivan)

SIDE EFFECTS
Frequent
Systemic: Tachycardia, palpitations, nervousness
Ophthalmic: Headache, eye irritation, watering of eyes
Occasional
Systemic: Dizziness, light-headedness, facial flushing, headache, diaphoresis, increased BP, nausea, trembling, insomnia, vomiting, fatigue
Ophthalmic: Blurred or decreased vision, eye pain
Rare
Systemic: Chest discomfort or pain, arrhythmias, bronchospasm, dry mouth or throat

SERIOUS REACTIONS
! Excessive doses may cause acute hypertension or arrhythmias.
! Prolonged or excessive use may result in metabolic acidosis due to increased serum lactic acid concentrations. Metabolic acidosis may cause disorientation, fatigue, hyperventilation, headache, nausea, vomiting, and diarrhea.

DENTAL CONSIDERATIONS
General:
- Monitor vital signs at every appointment because of cardiovascular side effects.
- Assess salivary flow as a factor in caries, periodontal disease, and candidiasis.
- Consider semisupine chair position for patients with respiratory disease.
- Acute asthmatic episodes may be precipitated in the dental office. Sympathomimetic inhalants should be available for emergency use; a stress reduction protocol may be required.

epinephryl borate

ep-i-nef′-rill bor′-ate
(Epifrin, Epinal, Eppy/N)

CATEGORY AND SCHEDULE

Pregnancy Risk Category: C

MECHANISM OF ACTION

A direct-acting sympathomimetic amine whose mechanism of action is unknown. ***Therapeutic Effect:*** Increases outflow of aqueous humor from anterior eye chamber.

PHARMACOKINETICS

May have systemic absorption from drainage into nasal pharyngeal passages. Mydriasis occurs within several minutes, persists several hours; vasoconstriction occurs within 5 min, lasts less than 1 hr.

AVAILABILITY

Ophthalmic solution: 0.5%, 1%, 2% (Epifrin).
Ophthalmic solution (borate): 0.5% (Epinal), 1% (Epinal, Eppy/N), 2% (Eppy/N).

INDICATIONS AND DOSAGES

▶ **Glaucoma**

OPHTHALMIC

Adults, Elderly. Instill 1 drop 1–2 times/day.

OFF-LABEL USES

Ophthalmic: Treatment of conjunctival congestion during surgery, secondary glaucoma

CONTRAINDICATIONS

Cardiac arrhythmias, cerebrovascular insufficiency, hypertension, hyperthyroidism, ischemic heart disease, narrow-angle glaucoma, shock, hypersensitivity to epinephryl borate or any component of the formulation

INTERACTIONS

Drug

Beta-blockers: May decrease the effects of beta blockers.
Digoxin, sympathomimetics: May increase risk of arrhythmias.
Ergonovine, methergine, oxytocin: May increase vasoconstriction.
MAOIs, tricyclic antidepressants: May increase cardiovascular effects.

Herbal

None known.

Food

None known.

Drug interactions of concern to dentistry

- Risk of arrhythmias: halogenated hydrocarbon anesthetics, tricyclic antidepressants, amphetamine-like drugs

DIAGNOSTIC TEST EFFECTS

None known.

SIDE EFFECTS

Frequent

Headache, stinging, burning or other eye irritation, watering of eyes

Occasional

Blurred or decreased vision, eye pain

SERIOUS REACTIONS

! Systemic absorption occurs rarely. These effects include fast, irregular, or pounding heartbeat, feeling faint, increased sweating, paleness, trembling, and increased blood pressure.

DENTAL CONSIDERATIONS

General:

- Determine why patient is taking the drug.
- Avoid drugs with anticholinergic activity, such as antihistamines,

opioids, benzodiazepines, propantheline, atropine, and scopolamine.

- Avoid dental light in patient's eyes; offer dark glasses for patient comfort.
- Protect patient's eyes from accidental spatter during dental treatment.
- Question glaucoma patient about compliance with prescribed drug regimen.

Consultations:

- Medical consultation may be required to assess disease control.

Teach Patient/Family:

- Importance of updating health and medication history if physician makes any changes in evaluation or drug regimens; include OTC, herbal, and nonherbal remedies in the update

epirubicin

eh-pea-rew-bih-sin
(Ellence, Pharmorubicin)

CATEGORY AND SCHEDULE

Pregnancy Risk Category: D

MECHANISM OF ACTION

An anthracycline antibiotic whose exact mechanism is unknown but may include formation of a complex with DNA and subsequent inhibition of DNA, RNA, and protein synthesis. Also inhibits DNA helicase activity, preventing enzymatic separation of double-stranded DNA and interfering with replication and transcription. ***Therapeutic Effect:*** Produces antiproliferative and cytotoxic activity.

PHARMACOKINETICS

Widely distributed into tissues. Protein binding: 77%. Metabolized in the liver and RBCs. Primarily eliminated through biliary excretion. Not removed by hemodialysis. ***Half-life:*** 33 hr.

AVAILABILITY

Injection: 2-mg/ml single-use vials.

INDICATIONS AND DOSAGES

▸ **Breast Cancer**

IV

Adults. Initially, 100–120 mg/m^2 in repeated cycles of 3–4 wk, in combination with fluorouracil (5-FU) and Cytoxan. Total dose may be given on day 1 of each cycle or in equally divided doses on days 1 and 8 of each cycle.

OFF-LABEL USES

Treatment of lung or ovarian carcinoma, non-Hodgkin's lymphoma, sarcomas

CONTRAINDICATIONS

Baseline neutrophil count less than 1,500/mm^3, hypersensitivity to epirubicin, previous treatment with anthracyclines up to maximum cumulative dose, recent MI, severe hepatic impairment, severe myocardial insufficiency

INTERACTIONS

Drug

Blood dyscrasia-causing medications: May increase the patient's risk of developing leukopenia or thrombocytopenia.
Bone marrow depressants: May cause additive bone marrow suppression.
Calcium channel blockers: May increase the patient's risk of developing heart failure.
Cimetidine: May increase epirubicin serum concentration and toxicity.

Hepatotoxic medications: May increase the risk of hepatotoxicity.
Live-virus vaccines: May potentiate virus replication, increase vaccine side effects, and decrease the patient's antibody response to the vaccine.

Herbal

None known.

Food

None known.

Drug interactions of concern to dentistry

- None reported

DIAGNOSTIC TEST EFFECTS

None known.

IV INCOMPATIBILITIES

Heparin, fluorouracil (5-FU). Don't mix epirubicin in same syringe with other medications.

SIDE EFFECTS

Frequent (83%–70%)

Nausea, vomiting alopecia, amenorrhea

Occasional (9%–%)

Stomatitis, diarrhea, hot flashes

Rare (2%–1%)

Rash, pruritus, fever, lethargy, conjunctivitis

SERIOUS REACTIONS

! The risk of cardiotoxicity (either acute, manifested as transient ECG abnormalities, or chronic, manifested as CHF) increases when the total cumulative dose exceeds 900 mg/m^2.

! Extravasation during administration may result in severe local tissue necrosis.

! Myelosuppression may cause hematologic toxicity, manifested principally as leukopenia and, to lesser extent, anemia and thrombocytopenia.

DENTAL CONSIDERATIONS

General:

- If additional analgesia is required for dental pain, consider alternative analgesics (NSAIDs) in patients taking narcotics for acute or chronic pain.
- Examine for oral manifestation of opportunistic infection.
- This drug may be used in the hospital or on an outpatient basis. Confirm the patient's disease and treatment status.
- Chlorhexidine mouth rinse prior to and during chemotherapy may reduce severity of mucositis.
- Patient on chronic drug therapy may rarely present with symptoms of blood dyscrasias, which can include infection, bleeding, and poor healing. If dyscrasia is present, caution patient to prevent oral tissue trauma when using oral hygiene aids.
- Palliative medication may be required for management of oral side effects.
- Patient may be at risk of bleeding; check oral signs.
- Patient may be at risk of infection.

Consultations:

- Medical consultation should include routine blood counts including platelet counts and bleeding time.
- In a patient with symptoms of blood dyscrasias, request a medical consultation for blood studies and postpone treatment until normal values are reestablished.
- Consult physician; prophylactic or therapeutic antiinfectives may be indicated if surgery or periodontal treatment is required.
- Medical consultation may be required to assess immunologic status during cancer chemotherapy and determine safety risk, if any, posed by the required dental treatment.

• Medical consultation may be required to assess disease control and patient's ability to tolerate stress.

Teach Patient/Family:

• To be aware of oral side effects
• Importance of good oral hygiene to prevent soft tissue inflammation
• To report oral lesions, soreness, or bleeding to dentist
• To prevent trauma when using oral hygiene aids
• Importance of updating health and medication history if physician makes any changes in evaluation or drug regimens; include OTC, herbal, and nonherbal remedies in the update

eplerenone

e-plear′-a-nown
(Inspra)

CATEGORY AND SCHEDULE

Pregnancy Risk Category: B

MECHANISM OF ACTION

An aldosterone receptor antagonist that binds to the mineralocorticoid receptors in the kidney, heart, blood vessels, and brain, blocking the binding of aldosterone. ***Therapeutic Effect:*** Reduces BP.

PHARMACOKINETICS

Absorption unaffected by food. Protein binding: 50%. No active metabolites. Excreted in the urine with a lesser amount eliminated in the feces. Not removed by hemodialysis. ***Half-life:*** 4–6 hr.

AVAILABILITY

Tablets: 25 mg, 50 mg.

INDICATIONS AND DOSAGES

▸ Hypertension

PO

Adults, Elderly. 50 mg once a day. If 50 mg once a day produces an inadequate BP response, may increase dosage to 50 mg twice a day. If patient is concurrently receiving erythromycin, saquinavir, verapamil, or fluconazole, reduce initial dose to 25 mg once a day.

▸ CHF Following MI

PO

Adults, Elderly. Initially, 25 mg once a day. If tolerated, titrate up to 50 mg once a day within 4 wk.

CONTRAINDICATIONS

Concurrent use of potassium supplements or potassium-sparing diuretics (such as amiloride, spironolactone, and triamterene), or strong inhibitors of the cytochrome P450 3A4 enzyme system (including ketoconazole and itraconazole), creatinine clearance less than 50 ml/min, serum creatinine level greater than 2 mg/dl in males or 1.8 mg/dl in females, serum potassium level greater than 5.5 mEq/L, type 2 diabetes mellitus with microalbuminuria

INTERACTIONS

Drug

ACE inhibitors, angiotensin II antagonists, erythromycin, fluconazole, saquinavir, verapamil: Increases risk of hyperkalemia.

Herbal

St. John's wort: Decreases eplerenone effectiveness.

Food

Grapefruit, grapefruit juice: Produces small increase in serum potassium level.

Drug interactions of concern to dentistry

- See contraindications; use with caution in patients taking strong inhibitors of CYP3A4 isoenzymes (erythromycin)
- Monitor blood pressure if NSAIDs are required

DIAGNOSTIC TEST EFFECTS

May increase serum potassium level. May decrease serum sodium level.

SIDE EFFECTS

Rare (3%–1%)

Dizziness, diarrhea, cough, fatigue, flu-like symptoms, abdominal pain

SERIOUS REACTIONS

! Hyperkalemia may occur, particularly in patients with type 2 diabetes mellitus and microalbuminuria.

DENTAL CONSIDERATIONS

General:

- Monitor vital signs at every appointment because of cardiovascular side effects.
- Short appointments and a stress reduction protocol may be required for anxious patients.
- Take precautions if dental surgery is anticipated and general anesthesia is required.

Consultations:

- Medical consultation may be required to assess disease control and patient's ability to tolerate stress.
- Consultation with physician may be necessary if sedation or general anesthesia is required.

Teach Patient/Family:

- Importance of updating health and drug history if physician makes any changes in evaluation or drug regimens

epoetin alfa

eh-poh′-ee-tin al′-fa

(Epogen, Eprex[CAN], Procrit)

Do not confuse Epogen with Neupogen.

CATEGORY AND SCHEDULE

Pregnancy Risk Category: C

MECHANISM OF ACTION

A glycoprotein that stimulates division and differentiation of erythroid progenitor cells in bone marrow. ***Therapeutic Effect:*** Induces erythropoiesis and releases reticulocytes from bone marrow.

PHARMACOKINETICS

Well absorbed after subcutaneous administration. Following administration, an increase in reticulocyte count occurs within 10 days, and increases in Hgb, Hct, and RBC count are seen within 2–6 wk. ***Half-life:*** 4–13 hr.

AVAILABILITY

Injection: 2,000 units/ml, 3,000 units/ml, 4,000 units/ml, 10,000 units/ml, 20,000 units/ml, 40,000 units/ml.

INDICATIONS AND DOSAGES

▸ **Treatment of Anemia in Chemotherapy Patients**

IV, SUBCUTANEOUS

Adults, Elderly, Children.
150 units/kg/dose 3 times a wk. Maximum: 1,200 units/kg/wk.

▸ **Reduction of Allogenic Blood Transfusions in Elective Surgery**

SUBCUTANEOUS

Adults, Elderly. 300 units/kg/day 10 days before day of and 4 days after surgery.

▸ Chronic Renal Failure

IV BOLUS, SUBCUTANEOUS

Adults, Elderly. Initially, 50–100 units/kg 3 times a wk. Target Hct range: 30%–36%. Adjust dosage no earlier than 1-mo intervals unless prescribed. Decrease dosage if Hct is increasing and approaching 36%. Plan to temporarily withhold doses if Hct continues to rise and to reinstate lower dosage when Hct begins to decrease. If Hct increases by more than 4 points in 2 wk, monitor Hct twice a wk for 2–6 wk. Increase dose if Hct does not increase 5–6 points after 8 wk (with adequate iron stores) and if Hct is below target range. Maintenance: *For patients on dialysis:* 75 units/kg 3 times a wk. Range: 12.5–525 units/kg. *For patients not on dialysis:* 75–150 units/kg/wk.

▸ HIV Infection in Patients Treated with AZT

IV, SUBCUTANEOUS

Adults. Initially, 100 units/kg 3 times a wk for 8 wk; may increase by 50–100 units/kg 3 times a wk. Evaluate response q4–8wk thereafter. Adjust dosage by 50–100 units/kg 3 times a wk. If dosages larger than 300 units/kg 3 times a wk are not eliciting response, it is unlikely patient will respond. Maintenance: Titrate to maintain desired Hct.

OFF-LABEL USES

Prevention of anemia in patients donating blood before elective surgery or autologous transfusion, treatment of anemia associated with neoplastic diseases.

CONTRAINDICATIONS

History of sensitivity to mammalian cell-derived products or human albumin, uncontrolled hypertension

INTERACTIONS

Drug

Heparin: An increase in RBC volume may enhance blood clotting. Heparin dosage may need to be increased.

Herbal

None known.

Food

None known.

Drug interactions of concern to dentistry

- None reported

DIAGNOSTIC TEST EFFECTS

May increase BUN, serum phosphorus, serum potassium, serum creatinine, serum uric acid, and sodium levels. May decrease bleeding time, iron concentration, and serum ferritin levels.

IV INCOMPATIBILITIES

Do not mix with other medications.

SIDE EFFECTS

PATIENTS RECEIVING CHEMOTHERAPY

Frequent (20%–17%)

Fever, diarrhea, nausea, vomiting, edema

Occasional (13%–11%)

Asthenia, shortness of breath, paresthesia

Rare (5%–3%)

Dizziness, trunk pain

PATIENTS WITH CHRONIC RENAL FAILURE

Frequent (24%–11%)

Hypertension, headache, nausea, arthralgia

Occasional (9%–7%)

Fatigue, edema, diarrhea, vomiting, chest pain, skin reactions at administration site, asthenia, dizziness

PATIENTS WITH HIV INFECTION TREATED WITH AZT

Frequent (38%–15%)
Fever, fatigue, headache, cough, diarrhea, rash, nausea
Occasional (14%–9%)
Shortness of breath, asthenia, skin reaction at injection site, dizziness

E

SERIOUS REACTIONS

! Hypertensive encephalopathy, thrombosis, cerebrovascular accident, MI, and seizures have occurred rarely.
! Hyperkalemia occurs occasionally in patients with chronic renal failure, usually in those who do not conform to medication regimen, dietary guidelines, and frequency of dialysis regimen.

DENTAL CONSIDERATIONS

General:

- Patient's disease, treatment history, and use of other drugs will affect patient evaluation and management.
- Determine why patient is taking the drug.
- Monitor vital signs at every appointment because of cardiovascular and respiratory side effects.
- Take precautions if dental surgery is anticipated and general anesthesia is required.
- Patient history should include all medications and herbal or nonherbal remedies taken by the patient.
- Consider semisupine chair position for patient comfort if GI side effects occur.
- Place on frequent recall because of oral side effects, depending on chemotherapy regimen or human immunodeficiency virus (HIV) immunologic status.

Consultations:

- Medical consultation should include hematocrit and routine blood counts, including platelet counts and bleeding time.
- Consultation with physician may be necessary if sedation or general anesthesia is required.
- Medical consultation may be required to assess disease control and patient's ability to tolerate stress.

Teach Patient/Family:

- Importance of good oral hygiene to prevent soft tissue inflammation, infection

epoprostenol sodium, prostacyclin

e-poe-pros′-ten-ol
(Flolan)

CATEGORY AND SCHEDULE

Pregnancy Risk Category: B

MECHANISM OF ACTION

An antihypertensive that directly dilates pulmonary and systemic arterial vascular beds and inhibits platelet aggregation. ***Therapeutic Effect:*** Reduces right and left ventricular afterload; increases cardiac output and stroke volume.

AVAILABILITY

Injection, Powder for Reconstitution: 0.5 mg, 1.5 mg.

INDICATIONS AND DOSAGES

▸ **Long-term Treatment of New York Heart Association Class III and IV Primary Pulmonary Hypertension**

IV Infusion

Adults, Elderly. Procedure to determine dose range: Initially, 2 ng/kg/min, increased in increments

of 2 ng/kg/min q15min until dose-limiting adverse effects occur.
Chronic infusion: Start at 4 ng/kg/min less than the maximum dose rate tolerated during acute dose ranging (or one half of the maximum rate if rate was <5 ng/kg/min).

OFF-LABEL USES

Cardiopulmonary bypass surgery; hemodialysis; pulmonary hypertension associated with acute respiratory distress syndrome, systemic lupus erythematosus, or congenital heart disease; neonatal pulmonary hypertension, refractory CHF; severe community-acquired pneumonia

CONTRAINDICATIONS

Long-term use in patients with CHF (severe ventricular systolic dysfunction)

INTERACTIONS

Drug

Acetate in dialysis fluids, other vasodilators: May increase hypotensive effect.
Anticoagulants, antiplatelets: May increase the risk of bleeding.
Vasoconstrictors: May decrease effects of epoprostenol.

Herbal

None known.

Food

None known.

Drug interactions of concern to dentistry

• Increased risk of bleeding: drugs which interfere with coagulation or platelet function; such as NSAIDs and aspirin

DIAGNOSTIC TEST EFFECTS

None known.

IV INCOMPATIBILITIES

Don't mix epoprostenol with other medications.

SIDE EFFECTS

Frequent

Acute phase: Flushing (58%), headache (49%), nausea (32%), vomiting (32%), hypotension (16%), anxiety (11%), chest pain (11%), dizziness (8%)
Chronic phase (>20%): Dyspnea, asthenia, dizziness, headache, chest pain, nausea, vomiting, palpitations, edema, jaw pain, tachycardia, flushing, myalgia, nonspecific muscle pain, paresthesia, diarrhea, anxiety, chills, fever, or flu-like symptoms

Occasional

Acute phase (5%–2%): Bradycardia, abdominal pain, muscle pain, dyspnea, back pain
Chronic phase (20%–10%): Rash, depression, hypotension, pallor, syncope, bradycardia, ascites

Rare

Acute phase: Paresthesia
Chronic phase (<2%): Diaphoresis, dyspepsia, tachycardia

SERIOUS REACTIONS

! Overdose may cause hyperglycemia or ketoacidosis manifested as increased urination, thirst, and fruitlike breath odor.
! Angina, MI, and thrombocytopenia occur rarely.
! Abrupt withdrawal, including a large reduction in dosage or interruption in drug delivery, may produce rebound pulmonary hypertension as evidenced by dyspnea, dizziness, and asthenia.

DENTAL CONSIDERATIONS

General:

• Continuous-use drug for patients with severe cardiovascular disease. Provide palliative emergency dental care as required.
• Determine why patient is taking the drug.

• Monitor vital signs at every appointment due to cardiovascular side effects.
• Avoid products that affect platelet function, such as aspirin and NSAIDs.
• Stress from dental procedures may compromise cardiovascular function, determine patient risk.
• Postpone elective dental treatment if patient shows signs of cardiac symptoms or respiratory distress.
• Use vasoconstrictor with caution, in low doses, and with careful aspiration. Avoid using gingival retraction cord containing epinephrine.

Consultations:
• Medical consultation may be required to assess disease control and patient's ability to tolerate stress.
• Medical consultation should include routine blood counts including platelet counts and bleeding time.

Teach Patient/Family:
• Importance of good oral hygiene to prevent soft tissue inflammation
• To prevent trauma when using oral hygiene aids
• Importance of updating health and medication history if physician makes any changes in evaluation or drug regimens; include OTC, herbal, and nonherbal remedies in the update

eprosartan
eh-pro-sar′-tan
(Teveten)

CATEGORY AND SCHEDULE
Pregnancy Risk Category: C (D if used in second or third trimester)

MECHANISM OF ACTION
An angiotensin II receptor antagonist that blocks the vasoconstrictor and aldosterone-secreting effects of angiotensin II, inhibiting the binding of angiotensin II to the AT_1 receptors. ***Therapeutic Effect:*** Causes vasodilation, decreases peripheral resistance, and decreases BP.

PHARMACOKINETICS
Rapidly absorbed after PO administration. Protein binding: 98%. Undergoes first-pass metabolism in the liver to active metabolites. Excreted in urine and biliary system. Minimally removed by hemodialysis. ***Half-life:*** 5–9 hr.

AVAILABILITY
Tablets: 400 mg, 600 mg.

INDICATIONS AND DOSAGES
▸ Hypertension
PO
Adults, Elderly. Initially, 600 mg/day. Range: 400–800 mg/day.

CONTRAINDICATIONS
Bilateral renal artery stenosis, hyperaldosteronism

INTERACTIONS
Drug
None known.
Herbal
None known.
Food
None known.
Drug interactions of concern to dentistry
• None reported

DIAGNOSTIC TEST EFFECTS
May increase BUN, serum alkaline phosphatase, serum bilirubin, serum creatinine, AST(SGOT), and ALT (SGPT) levels. May decrease blood Hgb and Hgb levels.

SIDE EFFECTS
Occasional (5%–2%)
Headache, cough, dizziness
Rare (<2%)
Muscle pain, fatigue, diarrhea, upper respiratory tract infection, dyspepsia

SERIOUS REACTIONS
! Overdosage may manifest as hypotension and tachycardia. Bradycardia occurs less often.

DENTAL CONSIDERATIONS
General:
- Monitor vital signs at every appointment because of cardiovascular side effects.
- Stress from dental procedures may compromise cardiovascular function; determine patient risk.
- Limit use of sodium-containing products, such as saline IV fluids, for those patients with a dietary salt restriction.
- Short appointments and a stress reduction protocol may be required for anxious patients.
- Use precaution if sedation or general anesthesia is required; risk of hypotensive episode.
- Assess salivary flow as a factor in caries, periodontal disease, and candidiasis.
- After supine positioning, have patient sit upright for at least 2 min before standing to avoid orthostatic hypotension.

Consultations:
- Medical consultation may be required to assess disease control and patient's ability to tolerate stress.

Teach Patient/Family:
- Importance of updating health and drug history if physician makes any changes in evaluation or drug regimens
- *When chronic dry mouth occurs, advise patient:*
  - To avoid mouth rinses with high alcohol content because of drying effects
  - To use daily home fluoride products for anticaries effect
  - To use sugarless gum, frequent sips of water, or saliva substitutes

eptifibatide
ep-tih-fib′-ah-tide
(Integrilin)

CATEGORY AND SCHEDULE
Pregnancy Risk Category: B

MECHANISM OF ACTION
A glycoprotein IIb/IIIa inhibitor that rapidly inhibits platelet aggregation by preventing binding of fibrinogen to receptor sites on platelets.
Therapeutic Effect: Prevents closure of treated coronary arteries. Also prevents acute cardiac ischemic complications.

AVAILABILITY
Injection solution: 0.75 mg/ml, 2 mg/ml.

INDICATIONS AND DOSAGES
▸ **Adjunct to Percutaneous Coronary Intervention**
IV BOLUS, IV INFUSION
Adults, Elderly. 180 mcg/kg before PCI initiation; then continuous drip of 2 mcg/kg/min and a second 180 mcg/kg bolus 10 min after the first. Maximum: 15 mg/h. Continue until hospital discharge or for up to 18–24 hours. Minimum 12 hours is recommended. Concurrent aspirin

and heparin therapy is recommended.

▸ **Acute Coronary Syndrome**

IV BOLUS, IV INFUSION

Adults, Elderly. 180 mcg/kg bolus then 2 mcg/kg/min until discharge or coronary artery bypass graft, up to 72 hr. Maximum: 15 mg/h. Concurrent aspirin and heparin therapy is recommended.

▸ **Dosage in Renal Impairment**

Creatinine clearance less than 50 ml/min. Use 180 mcg/kg bolus (maximum 22.6 mg) and 1 mcg/kg/min infusion (maximum: 7.5 mg/h).

CONTRAINDICATIONS

Active internal bleeding, AV malformation or aneurysm, history of cerebrovascular accident (CVA) within 2 years or CVA with residual neurologic defect, history of vasculitis, intracranial neoplasm, oral anticoagulant use within last 7 days unless PT is less than 1.22 times the control, recent (6 wk≤) GI or GU bleeding, recent (6 wk≤) surgery or trauma, prior IV dextran use before or during PTCA, severe uncontrolled hypertension, thrombocytopenia (< 100,000 cells/mcl)

INTERACTIONS

Drug

Anticoagulants, heparin: May increase the risk of hemorrhage.
Dextran, other platelet aggregation inhibitors (such as aspirin), thrombolytic agents: May increase the risk of bleeding.

Herbal

None known.

Food

None known.

Drug interactions of concern to dentistry

- Increased risk of bleeding: drugs that interfere with coagulation or platelet function, such as NSAIDs and aspirin

DIAGNOSTIC TEST EFFECTS

Increases aPTT, PT, and clotting time. Decreases platelet count.

IV INCOMPATIBILITIES

Administer in separate line; do not add other medications to infusion solution.

SIDE EFFECTS

Occasional (7%)

Hypotension

SERIOUS REACTIONS

! Minor to major bleeding complications may occur, most commonly at arterial access site for cardiac catheterization.

DENTAL CONSIDERATIONS

General:

- Monitor vital signs at every appointment due to cardiovascular side effects.
- Avoid products that affect platelet function, such as aspirin and NSAIDs.
- Consider local hemostasis measures to prevent excessive bleeding.
- For acute use in emergency rooms or hospitals.
- Provide palliative emergency dental care only during drug use.
- Patients may be at risk of bleeding, check for oral signs.
- Confirm patient's medical and drug history.

Consultations:

- Medical consultation may be required to assess disease control and patient's ability to tolerate stress.
- Medical consultation should include routine blood counts including platelet counts and bleeding time.

- Medical consultation should include partial prothrombin time, prothrombin time, or INR

Teach Patient/Family:

- Importance of good oral hygiene to prevent soft tissue inflammation
- To prevent trauma when using oral hygiene aids
- To report oral lesions, soreness, or bleeding to dentist
- Importance of updating health and medication history if physician makes any changes in evaluation or drug regimens; include OTC, herbal, and nonherbal remedies in the update
- To use soft tooth brush to reduce risk of bleeding

ergoloid mesylates

ur-go-loyd mess-ah-lates
(Gerimal, Hydergine, Hydergine[CAN])

CATEGORY AND SCHEDULE

Pregnancy Risk Category: C

MECHANISM OF ACTION

An ergot alkaloid that centrally acts and decreases vascular tone, slows heart rate. Peripheral action blocks alpha adrenergic receptors. ***Therapeutic Effect:*** Improved O_2 uptake and improves cerebral metabolism.

PHARMACOKINETICS

Rapidly, incompletely absorbed from GI tract. Metabolized in liver. Eliminated primarily in feces. ***Half-life:*** 2–5 hrs.

AVAILABILITY

Capsules: 1 mg (Hydergine).
Oral solution: 1 mg/ml (Hydergine).
Tablets: 1 mg (Germinal, Hydergine).
Tablets, sublingual: 1 mg (Germinal, Hydergine).

INDICATIONS AND DOSAGES

▸ Age-Related Decline in Mental Capacity

PO

Adults, Elderly. Initially, 1 mg 3 times/day. Range: 1.5–12 mg/day.

CONTRAINDICATIONS

Acute or chronic psychosis (regardless or etiology), hypersensitivity to ergoloid mesylates or any component of the formulation

INTERACTIONS

Drug

Potent CYP450 3A4 inhibitors: May increase risk of ergotism (nausea, vomiting, vasospastic ischemia).
Frovatriptan, naratriptan, rizatriptan, sumatriptan, zolmitriptan: May prolong vasospastic reactions.

Herbal

None known.

Food

Grapefruit juice: May increase risk of ergotism (nausea, vomiting, vasospastic ischemia).

INTERACTIONS

Drug

Potent CYP450 3A4 inhibitors: May increase risk of ergotism (nausea, vomiting, vasospastic ischemia).
Frovatriptan, naratriptan, rizatriptan, sumatriptan, zolmitriptan: May prolong vasospastic reactions.

Food

Grapefruit juice: May increase risk of ergotism (nausea, vomiting, vasospastic ischemia).

E

SIDE EFFECTS

Occasional

GI distress, transient nausea, sublingual irritation

SERIOUS REACTIONS

! Overdose may produce blurred vision, dizziness, syncope, headache, flushed face, nausea, vomiting, decreased appetite, stomach cramps, and stuffy nose.

DENTAL CONSIDERATIONS

General:

- Monitor vital signs at every appointment because of cardiovascular side effects.
- After supine positioning, have patient sit upright for at least 2 min before standing to avoid orthostatic hypotension.
- Consider semisupine chair position for patient comfort because of GI effects of drug.

Teach Patient/Family:

- Use of electric toothbrush if patient is unable to carry out oral hygiene procedures

ergotamine tartrate/ dihydroergotamine

er-got′-a-meen

(ergotamine tartrate) Cafergot[CAN], Ergodryl Mono[AUS], Ergomar, Ergostat, Gynergen(dihyrdoergotamine) D.H.E. 45, Dihydergot[AUS], Dihydroergotamine Sandoz[CAN], Migranal

CATEGORY AND SCHEDULE

Pregnancy Risk Category: X

MECHANISM OF ACTION

An ergotamine derivative and alpha-adrenergic blocker that directly stimulates vascular smooth muscle, resulting in peripheral and cerebral vasoconstriction. May also have antagonist effects on serotonin. ***Therapeutic Effect:*** Suppresses vascular headaches.

PHARMACOKINETICS

Slowly and incompletely absorbed from the GI tract; rapidly and extensively absorbed after rectal administration. Protein binding: greater than 90%. Undergoes extensive first-pass metabolism in the liver to active metabolite. Eliminated in feces by the biliary system. ***Half-life:*** 21 hr.

AVAILABILITY

Tablets (Sublingual [Ergomar]): 2 mg.
Injection (DHE 45): 1 mg/ml.
Nasal Spray (Migranal): 0.5 mg/spray.
Suppositories (ergotamine and caffeine): 2 mg, with 100 mg caffeine.

INDICATIONS AND DOSAGES

▸ Vascular Headaches

PO (Cafergot [fixed-combination of ergotamine and caffeine])

Adults, Elderly. 2 mg at onset of headache, then 1–2 mg q30min. Maximum: 6 mg/episode; 10 mg/wk.

PO, Sublingual

Children. 1 mg at onset of headache, then 1 mg q30min. Maximum: 3 mg/episode.

IV

Adults, Elderly. 1 mg at onset of headache; may repeat hourly. Maximum: 2 mg/day; 6 mg/wk.

SUBLINGUAL

Adults, Elderly. 1 tablet at onset of headache, then 1 tablet q30min.

Maximum: 3 tablets/24 hr; 5 tablets/wk.
IM, SUBCUTANEOUS (dihydroergotamine)
Adults, Elderly. 1 mg at onset of headache; may repeat hourly. Maximum: 3 mg/day; 6 mg/wk.
INTRANASAL
Adults, Elderly. 1 spray (0.5 mg) into each nostril; may repeat in 15 min. Maximum: 4 sprays/day; 8 sprays/wk.
RECTAL
Adults, Elderly. 1 suppository at onset of headache; may repeat dose in 1 hr. Maximum: 2 suppositories/episode; 5 suppositories/wk.

CONTRAINDICATIONS

Coronary artery disease, hypertension, impaired hepatic or renal function, malnutrition, peripheral vascular diseases (such as thromboangiitis obliterans, syphilitic arteritis, severe arteriosclerosis, thrombophlebitis, and Raynaud's disease), sepsis, severe pruritus

INTERACTIONS

Drug

Beta blockers, erythromycin: May increase the risk of vasospasm.
Ergot alkaloids, systemic vasoconstrictors: May increase pressor effect.
Nitroglycerin: May decrease the effects of nitroglycerin.

Herbal

None known.

Food

None known.

Drug interactions of concern to dentistry

- Increased vasoconstriction: vasoconstrictor in local anesthetics
- Suspected increased risk of ergotism: erythromycin, clarithromycin, troleandomycin
- Use anticholinergic with caution in the elderly

DIAGNOSTIC TEST EFFECTS

None known.

SIDE EFFECTS

Occasional (5%–2%)

Cough, dizziness

Rare (<2%)

Myalgia, fatigue, diarrhea, upper respiratory tract infection, dyspepsia

SERIOUS REACTIONS

! Prolonged administration or excessive dosage may produce ergotamine poisoning, manifested as nausea and vomiting; paresthesia, muscle pain or weakness; precordial pain; tachycardia or bradycardia; and hypertension or hypotension. Vasoconstriction of peripheral arteries and arterioles may result in localized edema and pruritus. Muscle pain will occur when walking and later, even at rest. Other rare effects include confusion, depression, drowsiness, seizures, and gangrene.

DENTAL CONSIDERATIONS

General:

- This is an acute-use drug; patients are unlikely to seek dental treatment while using this drug.
- Monitor vital signs at every appointment because of cardiovascular side effects.

Teach Patient/Family:

- Use of electric toothbrush if patient has difficulty holding conventional devices

E

erlotinib

er-low′-tih-nib
(Tarceva)

CATEGORY AND SCHEDULE

Pregnancy Risk Category: D

E

MECHANISM OF ACTION

A human epidermal growth factor that inhibits tyrosine kinases (TK) associated with transmembrane cell surface receptors found on both normal and cancer cells. One such receptor is epidermal growth factor receptor (EGFR). ***Therapeutic Effect:*** TK activity appears to be vitally important to cell proliferation and survival.

AVAILABILITY

Tablets: 25 mg, 100 mg, 150 mg.

INDICATIONS AND DOSAGES

▸ **Overactive Bladder**

PO

Adults, Elderly. Initially, 7.5 mg once a day. If response is not adequate after a minimum of 2 weeks, dosage may be increased to 15 mg once daily. Do not exceed 7.5 mg once a day in patients with moderate hepatic impairment.

CONTRAINDICATIONS

Pregnancy

INTERACTIONS

Drug

Aminoglutethimide, carbamazepine, nafcillin, nevirapine, phenobarbital, phenytoin: May decrease the levels and effects of erlotinib.
Azole antifungals, ciprofloxacin, clarithromycin, diclofenac, doxycycline, erythromycin, imatinib, isoniazid, nefazodone, nicardipine, propofol, protease inhibitors, quinidine, verapamil: May increase the levels and effects of erlotinib.
Ketoconazole: May increase serum erlotinib concentration.
Rifampin: May decrease serum erlotinib concentration.

Herbal

St. John's wort: May increase metabolism and decrease serum erlotinib concentration.

Food

All foods: Give erlotinib at least 1 hr before or 2 hrs after ingestion of food.

Drug interactions of concern to dentistry

- Increased blood levels and effects: potent inhibitors of CYP3A4 isoenzymes (ketoconazole, itraconazole, erythromycin, clarithromycin, diclofenac, doxycycline, protease inhibitors)
- Decreased effects: potent inducers of CYP3A4 isoenzymes (carbamazepine, phenobarbital, St. John's wort [herb])

DIAGNOSTIC TEST EFFECTS

May increase hepatic enzyme levels.

SIDE EFFECTS

Frequent (35%–21%)
Dry mouth, constipation
Occasional (8%–4%)
Dyspepsia, headache, nausea, abdominal pain
Rare (3%–2%)
Asthenia, diarrhea, dizziness, ocular dryness

SERIOUS REACTIONS

! Urinary tract infection occurs occasionally.

DENTAL CONSIDERATIONS

General:

- Note interactions with drugs commonly prescribed in dentistry.

- For longer dental appointments, offer patient frequent breaks.
- Consider semisupine chair position for patient comfort if GI side effects occur.
- Protect patient's eyes from accidental spatter during dental treatment.
- Avoid dental light in patient's eyes; offer dark glasses for patient comfort.
- Examine for oral manifestation of opportunistic infection.
- Assess salivary flow as a factor in caries, periodontal disease, and candidiasis.
- Place on frequent recall due to oral side effects.

Consultations:

- Physician should be informed if significant xerostomic side effects occur (increased caries, sore tongue, problems eating or swallowing, difficulty wearing prosthesis) so that a medication change can be considered.

Teach Patient/Family:

- *When chronic dry mouth occurs advise patient:*
  - To avoid mouth rinses with high alcohol content due to drying effects
  - To use daily home fluoride products for anticaries effect
  - To use sugarless gum, frequent sips of water or saliva substitutes
- Importance of good oral hygiene to prevent soft tissue inflammation
- Importance of updating health and medication history if physician makes any changes in evaluation or drug regimens; include OTC, herbal, and nonherbal remedies in the update

ertapenem

er-ta-pen′-em
(Invanz)

CATEGORY AND SCHEDULE

Pregnancy Risk Category: B

MECHANISM OF ACTION

A carbapenem that penetrates the bacterial cell wall of microorganisms and binds to penicillin-binding proteins, inhibiting cell wall synthesis. ***Therapeutic Effect:*** Produces bacterial cell death.

PHARMACOKINETICS

Almost completely absorbed after IM administration. Protein binding: 85%–95%. Widely distributed. Primarily excreted in urine with smaller amount eliminated in feces. Removed by hemodialysis. ***Half-life:*** 4 hr.

AVAILABILITY

Injection Powder for Reconstitution: 1-g.

INDICATIONS AND DOSAGES

▸ Intra-Abdominal Infection

IV, IM

Adults, Elderly. 1 g/day for 5–14 days.

▸ Skin and Skin Structure Infection

IV, IM

Adults, Elderly. 1 g/day for 7–14 days.

▸ Pneumonia, Urinary Tract Infection (UTI)

IV, IM

Adults, Elderly. 1 g/day for 10–14 days.

▸ Pelvic Infection

IV, IM

Adults, Elderly. 1 g/day for 3–10 days.

▸ Dosage in Renal Impairment

For adults and elderly patients with creatinine clearance less than 30 ml/min dosage is 500 mg once a day.

CONTRAINDICATIONS
History of hypersensitivity to beta-lactams (imipenem and cilastin, meropenem), hypersensitivity to amide-type local anesthetics (IM)

INTERACTIONS
Drug
Probenecid: Reduces renal excretion of ertapenem.
Herbal
None known.
Food
None known.
Drug interactions of concern to dentistry
- Increased or prolonged plasma levels: probenecid
- Dental drug interactions have not been studied

DIAGNOSTIC TEST EFFECTS
May increase serum alkaline phosphatase, AST (SGOT) and ALT (SGPT) levels. May decrease platelet count, blood Hct and Hgb levels, and serum potassium level.

IV INCOMPATIBILITIES
Do not mix or infuse ertapenem with any other medications. Do not use diluents or IV solutions containing dextrose.

IV COMPATIBILITIES
Sterile water for injection, 0.9% NaCl

SIDE EFFECTS
Frequent (10%–6%)
Diarrhea, nausea, headache
Occasional (5%–2%)
Altered mental status, insomnia, rash, abdominal pain, constipation, vomiting, edema, fever
Rare (<2%)
Dizziness, cough, oral candidiasis, anxiety, tachycardia, phlebitis at IV site

SERIOUS REACTIONS
! Antibiotic-associated colitis and other superinfections may occur.
! Anaphylactic reactions have been reported.
! Seizures may occur in those with CNS disorders (including patients with brain lesions or a history of seizures), bacterial meningitis, or severe renal impairment.

DENTAL CONSIDERATIONS
General:
- For selected infections in the hospital setting; provide palliative emergency dental treatment only.
- Examine for oral manifestation of opportunistic infection.
- Determine why patient is taking the drug.
- Caution regarding allergy to medication.
Consultations:
- CONIF
- Medical consultation may be required to assess disease control and patient's ability to tolerate stress.
Teach Patient/Family:
- Importance of good oral hygiene to prevent soft tissue inflammation
- To report sore throat, oral burning sensation, fever, or fatigue, any of which could indicate presence of a superinfection

erythromycin

er-ith-roe-mye′-sin
(A/T/S, Akne-Mycin, Apo-Erythro Base[CAN], EES, Emgel, Eryacne[AUS], Erybid[CAN], Eryc, Eryc LD[AUS], EryDerm, Erygel, EryPed, Ery-Tab, Erythra-Derm, Erythrocin, Erythromid[CAN], PCE)
Do not confuse erythromycin with azithromycin or Ethmozine, or Eryc with Emct.

CATEGORY AND SCHEDULE

Pregnancy Risk Category: B

MECHANISM OF ACTION

A macrolide that reversibly binds to bacterial ribosomes, inhibiting bacterial protein synthesis. ***Therapeutic Effect:*** Bacteriostatic.

PHARMACOKINETICS

Variably absorbed from the GI tract (depending on dosage form used). Protein binding: 70%–90%. Widely distributed. Metabolized in the liver. Primarily eliminated in feces by bile. Not removed by hemodialysis. ***Half-life:*** 1.4–2 hr (increased in impaired renal function).

AVAILABILITY

Topical Gel (A/T/S, Emgel, Erygel): 2%.
*Injection Powder for Reconstitution (Erythrocin):*500 mg, 1 g.
Ophthalmic Ointment: 5 mg/g.
Topical Ointment (Akne-Mycin): 2%.
Oral Suspension (EryPed, EES): 200 mg/5 ml, 400 mg/5 ml.
Topical Solution (Staticin): 1.5%.
Topical Solution (A/T/S, EryDerm, Erythra-Derm): 2%.
Tablet (Chewable [Ery-Ped]): 200 mg.
Tablets (Ery-Tab): 250 mg, 333 mg, 500 mg.
Tablets (EES): 400 mg.
Tablets (Erythrocin): 250 mg, 500 mg.
Tablets (PCE): 333 mg, 500 mg.

INDICATIONS AND DOSAGES

▸ **Mild to Moderate Infections of the Upper and Lower Respiratory Tract, Pharyngitis, Skin Infections**

PO

Adults, Elderly. 250 mg q6h, 500 mg q12h, or 333 mg q8h. Maximum: 4 g/day.
Children. 30–50 mg/kg/day in divided doses up to 60–100 mg/kg/day for severe infections.
Neonates. 20–40 mg/kg/day in divided doses q6–12h.

IV

Adults, Elderly, Children. 15–20 mg/kg/day in divided doses. Maximum: 4 g/day.

▸ **Preoperative Intestinal Antisepsis**

PO

Adults, Elderly. 1 g at 1 pm, 2 pm, and 11 pm on day before surgery (with neomycin).
Children. 20 mg/kg at 1pm, 2pm, and 11 pm on day before surgery (with neomycin).

▸ **Acne Vulgaris**

TOPICAL

Adults. Apply thin layer to affected area twice a day.

▸ **Gonococcal Ophthalmia Neonatorum**

OPHTHALMIC

Neonates. 0.5–2 cm no later than 1 hr after delivery.

OFF-LABEL USES

Systemic: Treatment of acne vulgaris, chancroid, *Campylobacter* enteritis, gastroparesis, Lyme disease
Topical: Treatment of minor bacterial skin infections

Ophthalmic: Treatment of blepharitis, conjunctivitis, keratitis, chlamydial trachoma

CONTRAINDICATIONS

Administration of fixed-combination product, Pediazole, to infants younger than 2 months; history of hepatitis due to macrolides; hypersensitivity to macrolides; pre-existing hepatic disease.

INTERACTIONS

Drug

Buspirone, cyclosporine, felodipine, lovastatin, simvastatin: May increase the blood concentration and toxicity of these drugs.
Carbamazepine: May inhibit the metabolism of carbamazepine.
Chloramphenicol, clindamycin: May decrease the effects of these drugs.
Hepatotoxic medications: May increase the risk of hepatotoxicity.
Theophylline: May increase the risk of theophylline toxicity.
Warfarin: May increase warfarin's effects.

Herbal

None known.

Food

None known.

Drug interactions of concern to dentistry

- Increased duration of alfentanil, cyclosporine
- Increased serum levels: indinavir, digoxin
- Decreased action of clindamycin, penicillins, lincomycin
- Increased serum levels of alfentanil, carbamazepine, theophylline (and other methylxanthines) and felodipine (possibly with other calcium blockers in the dihydropyridine class), ergot alkaloids, oral anticoagulants, buspirone, tacrolimus
- Risk of rhabdomyolysis: HMG-CoA reductase inhibitors
- Oral contraceptives: advise patient of a potential risk for decreased contraceptive action, to maintain compliance with oral contraceptive use while using antibiotics, and to consider the use of additional nonhormonal contraception
- May increase the effects of certain benzodiazepines: alprazolam, diazepam, midazolam, triazolam
- Risk of prolonged QT interval; use with caution in patients taking gatifloxacin, moxifloxacin, pimozide, disopyramide
- Possible serotonin syndrome with SSRIs
- Suspected increase in plasma levels of repaglinide

DIAGNOSTIC TEST EFFECTS

May increase serum alkaline phosphatase, bilirubin, AST (SGOT), and ALT (SGPT) levels.

IV INCOMPATIBILITIES

Fluconazole (Diflucan)

IV COMPATIBILITIES

Aminophylline, amiodarone (Cordarone), diltiazem (Cardizem), heparin, hydromorphone (Dilaudid), lidocaine, lorazepam (Ativan), magnesium sulfate, midazolam (Versed), morphine, multivitamins, potassium chloride

SIDE EFFECTS

Frequent

IV: Abdominal cramping or discomfort, phlebitis or thrombophlebitis
Topical: Dry skin (50%)

Occasional

Nausea, vomiting, diarrhea, rash, urticaria

Rare

Ophthalmic: Sensitivity reaction with increased irritation, burning, itching, and inflammation
Topical: Urticaria

SERIOUS REACTIONS

! Antibiotic-associated colitis and other superinfections may occur.
! High dosages in patients with renal impairment may lead to reversible hearing loss.
! Anaphylaxis and hepatotoxicity occur rarely.
! Ventricular arrhythmias and prolonged QT interval occur rarely with the IV drug form.

DENTAL CONSIDERATIONS

ERYTHROMYCIN (OPHTHALMIC)

General:

- Avoid dental light in patient's eyes; offer dark glasses for patient comfort.
- Protect patient's eyes from accidental spatter during dental treatment.

ERYTHROMYCIN (TOPICAL)

DENTAL CONSIDERATIONS

- None indicated

ERYTHROMYCIN BASE/ ERYTHROMYCIN ESTOLATE/ ERYTHROMYCIN ETHYLSUCCINATE/ ERYTHROMYCIN GLUCEPTATE/ ERYTHROMYCIN LACTOBIONATE/ ERYTHROMYCIN STEARATE

DENTAL CONSIDERATIONS

General:

- Alternative drug of choice for mild infection caused by a susceptible organism in patients who are allergic to penicillin.
- Determine why the patient is taking the drug.
- Estolate salt form is not indicated for adults because of risk of cholestatic jaundice.

Teach Patient/Family:

- To take oral drug with full glass of water; take with food if GI symptoms occur (estolate, ethylsuccinate, coated tabs only)
- *When used for dental infection, advise patient:*
  - To report sore throat, oral burning sensation, fever, and fatigue, any of which could indicate superinfection
  - To take at prescribed intervals and complete dosage regimen
  - To immediately notify the dentist if signs or symptoms of infection increase

escitalopram

es-sy-tal′-oh-pram
(Lexapro)

CATEGORY AND SCHEDULE

Pregnancy Risk Category: C

MECHANISM OF ACTION

A selective serotonin reuptake inhibitor that blocks the uptake of the neurotransmitter serotonin at neuronal presynaptic membranes, increasing its availability at post-synaptic receptor sites. ***Therapeutic Effect:*** Relieves depression.

PHARMACOKINETICS

Well absorbed after PO administration. Primarily metabolized in the liver. Primarily excreted in feces with a lesser amount eliminated in urine. ***Half-life:*** 35 hr.

AVAILABILITY

Oral Solution: 5 mg/5 ml.
Tablets: 5 mg, 10 mg, 20 mg.

INDICATIONS AND DOSAGES

▸ Depression, General Anxiety Disorder (GAD)

PO

Adults. Initially, 10 mg once a day in the morning or evening. May increase to 20 mg after a minimum of 1 wk.

Elderly, Patients with hepatic impairment. 10 mg/day.

CONTRAINDICATIONS

Breast-feeding, use within 14 days of MAOIs

INTERACTIONS

Drug

Alcohol, other CNS suppressants: May increase CNS depression.

Antifungals, cimetidine, macrolide antibiotics: May increase plasma level of escitalopram.

Carbamazepine: May decrease plasma level of escitalopram.

MAOIs: May cause serotonin syndrome, marked by autonomic hyperactivity, coma, diaphoresis, excitement, hyperthermia, and rigidity, and neuroleptic malignant syndrome.

Metoprolol: Increases plasma level of metoprolol.

Herbal

None known.

Food

None known.

Drug interactions of concern to dentistry

- Increased sedation: alcohol, other CNS depressants
- Drugs that inhibit CYP3A4 or other CYP isoenzymes may or may not affect plasma levels; should be used with observation and caution
- Modest inhibitor of CYP2D6
- First-time users of SSRIs also taking NSAIDs may have a higher risk of GI side effects; until more data are available, it may be advisable to avoid use of NSAIDs in these patients (*Br J Clin Pharmacol* 55:591–595, 2003)

DIAGNOSTIC TEST EFFECTS

May reduce serum sodium level.

SIDE EFFECTS

Frequent (21%–11%)

Nausea, dry mouth, somnolence, insomnia, diaphoresis

Occasional (8%–4%)

Tremor, diarrhea, abnormal ejaculation, dyspepsia, fatigue, anxiety, vomiting, anorexia

Rare (3%–2%)

Sinusitis, sexual dysfunction, menstrual disorder, abdominal pain, agitation, decreased libido

SERIOUS REACTIONS

! Overdose is manifested as dizziness, drowsiness, tachycardia, somnolence, confusion, and seizures.

DENTAL CONSIDERATIONS

General:

- Assess salivary flow as a factor in caries, periodontal disease, and candidiasis.
- Consider semisupine chair position for patient comfort if GI side effects occur.
- Question patient about tolerance of NSAIDs or aspirin related to GI disease.
- Evaluate respiration characteristics and rate.

Consultations:

- Medical consultation may be required to assess disease control and patient's ability to tolerate stress.
- Physician should be informed if significant xerostomia occurs

(e.g., increased caries, sore tongue, problems eating or swallowing, difficulty wearing prosthesis) so that a medication change can be considered.

Teach Patient/Family:

- Importance of good oral hygiene to prevent soft tissue inflammation, infection
- *When chronic dry mouth occurs, advise patient:*
  - To avoid mouth rinses with high alcohol content because of drying effects
  - To use daily home fluoride products for anticaries effect
  - To use sugarless gum, frequent sips of water, or saliva substitutes
  - Importance of compliance with recommended regimens for oral care

esomeprazole

es-om-eh-pray′-zole
(Nexium, Nexium IV)

CATEGORY AND SCHEDULE

Pregnancy Risk Category: B

MECHANISM OF ACTION

A proton pump inhibitor that is converted to active metabolites that irreversibly bind to and inhibit hydrogen-potassium adenosine triphosphates, an enzyme on the surface of gastric parietal cells. Inhibits hydrogen ion transport into gastric lumen. ***Therapeutic Effect:*** Increases gastric pH, reducing gastric acid production.

PHARMACOKINETICS

Well absorbed after oral administration. Protein binding: 97%. Extensively metabolized by the liver. Primarily excreted in urine. ***Half-life:*** 1–1.5 hrs.

AVAILABILITY

Capsules (Delayed-Release, Magnesium [Nexium]): 20 mg, 40 mg.
*Powder for Solution (Sodium [Nexium IV]):*20 mg, 40 mg.

INDICATIONS AND DOSAGES

▸ Erosive Esophagitis

PO

Adults, Elderly. 20–40 mg once daily for 4–8 wk.

IV

Adults, Elderly. 20 or 40 mg once daily by IV injection over at least 3 minutes or IV infusion over 10–30 minutes.

▸ To Maintain Healing of Erosive Esophagitis

PO

Adults, Elderly. 20 mg/day.

▸ Gastroesophageal Reflux Disease, to Reduce the Risk of NSAID-Induced Gastric Ulcer

PO

Adults, Elderly. 20 mg once a day for 4 wk.

▸ Duodenal Ulcer Caused by *Helicobacter Pylori*

PO

Adults, Elderly. 40 mg (esomeprazole) once a day, with amoxicillin 1,000 mg and clarithromycin 500 mg twice a day for 10 days.

CONTRAINDICATIONS

Hypersensitivity to benzimidazoles

IV INCOMPATIBILITIES

Don't mix esomeprazole with any other medications through the same IV line or tubing.

INTERACTIONS

Drug

Digoxin, iron, ketoconazole: May decrease the concentration of digoxin, iron, and ketoconazole.

Herbal

None known.

E

Food
None known.
Drug interactions of concern to dentistry
- May interfere with absorption of drugs where gastric pH is an important factor in bioavailability (e.g., iron products, ketoconazole, trovafloxacin, ampicillin)

DIAGNOSTIC TEST EFFECTS
None known.

SIDE EFFECTS
Frequent (7%)
Headache
Occasional (3%–2%)
Diarrhea, abdominal pain, nausea
Rare (<2%)
Dizziness, asthenia or loss of strength, vomiting, constipation, rash, cough

SERIOUS REACTIONS
! None known.

DENTAL CONSIDERATIONS
General:
- Assess salivary flow as a factor in caries, periodontal disease, and candidiasis.
- Question patient about tolerance of NSAIDs or aspirin related to GI disease.
- Consider semisupine chair position for patient comfort because of GI side effects of disease.
- Patients on chronic drug therapy may rarely have symptoms of blood dyscrasias, which can include infection, bleeding, and poor healing.
- Place on frequent recall because of oral side effects and oral effects of reflux disease

Consultations:
- In a patient with symptoms of blood dyscrasias, request a medical consult for blood studies and postpone treatment until normal values are reestablished.

Teach Patient/Family:
- To be aware of oral side effects and potential sequelae.
- To prevent trauma when using oral hygiene aids
- Importance of good oral hygiene to prevent soft tissue inflammation, infection
- *When chronic dry mouth occurs, advise patient:*
  - To avoid mouth rinses with high alcohol content because of drying effects
  - To use daily home fluoride products for anticaries effect
  - To use sugarless gum, frequent sips of water, or saliva substitutes

estazolam
es-tay-zoe-lam
Schedule IV
(ProSom)

CATEGORY AND SCHEDULE
Pregnancy Risk Category: X
Controlled Substance: Schedule IV

MECHANISM OF ACTION
A benzodiazepine that enhances action of gamma aminobutyric acid (GABA) neurotransmission in the central nervous system (CNS). ***Therapeutic Effect:*** Produces depressant effect at all levels of central nervous system (CNS).

PHARMACOKINETICS
Rapidly absorbed from gastrointestinal (GI) tract. Protein binding: 93%. Metabolized in liver.

Primarily excreted in urine, minimal in feces. ***Half-life:*** 10–24 hrs.

AVAILABILITY

Tablets: 1 mg, 2 mg (ProSom).

INDICATIONS AND DOSAGES

▸ Insomnia

PO

Adults (older than 18 yrs). 1–2 mg at bedtime.
Elderly, debilitated, liver disease, low serum albumin. 0.5–1 mg at bedtime.

CONTRAINDICATIONS

Pregnancy, hypersensitivity to other benzodiazepines

INTERACTIONS

Drug

Alcohol, CNS depressants: May increase central nervous system (CNS) and respiratory depression, and have hypotensive effects.

Herbal

Kava kava, valerian: May increase CNS depressant effect of alprazolam.

Food

None known.

Drug interactions of concern to dentistry

- Increased CNS depression: alcohol, all CNS depressants
- Increased serum levels and prolonged effect of benzodiazepines: ketoconazole, itraconazole, fluconazole, miconazole (systemic), indinavir
- Contraindicated with saquinavir
- Possible increase in CNS side effects: kava (herb)
- Decreased plasma levels: St. John's wort (herb)

SIDE EFFECTS

Frequent

Drowsiness, sedation, rebound insomnia (may occur for 1–2 nights after drug is discontinued), dizziness, confusion, euphoria

Occasional

Weakness, anorexia, diarrhea

Rare

Paradoxical CNS excitement, restlessness (particularly noted in elderly/debilitated)

SERIOUS REACTIONS

! Overdosage results in somnolence, confusion, diminished reflexes, and coma.

DENTAL CONSIDERATIONS

General:

- Psychologic and physical dependence may occur with chronic administration.
- Geriatric patients are more susceptible to drug effects; use lower dose.
- Avoid the use of this drug in a patient with a history of drug abuse or alcoholism.

Teach Patient/Family:

- To avoid mouth rinses with high alcohol content because of drying effects

E

estradiol

ess-tra-dye′-ole
(Aerodil[AUS], Alora, Climara, Delestrogen, Depo-Estradiol, Esclim, Estrace, Estraderm, Estraderm MX[AUS], Estradot[CAN], Estrasorb, Estrogel, Estring, Femring, Kliovance[AUS], Menostar, Oesclim[CAN], Primogyn Depot[AUS], Progynova[AUS], Sandrena Gel[AUS], Vagifem, Vivelle, Vivelle Dot, Zumenon[AUS])
Do not confuse Estraderm with Testoderm.

CATEGORY AND SCHEDULE

Pregnancy Risk Category: X

MECHANISM OF ACTION

An estrogen that increases synthesis of DNA, RNA, and proteins in target tissues; reduces release of gonadotropin-releasing hormone from the hypothalamus; and reduces follicle-stimulating hormone and luteinizing hormone (LH) release from the pituitary. ***Therapeutic Effect:*** Promotes normal growth, promotes development of female sex organs, and maintains GU function and vasomotor stability. Prevents accelerated bone loss by inhibiting bone resorption, restoring balance of bone resorption and formation. Inhibits LH and decreases serum testosterone concentration.

PHARMACOKINETICS

Well absorbed from the GI tract. Widely distributed. Protein binding: 50%–80%. Metabolized in the liver. Primarily excreted in urine. ***Half-life:*** Unknown.

AVAILABILITY

Tablets (Estrace): 0.5 mg, 1 mg, 2 mg.
Emulsion (Topical [Estrasorb]): 2.5 mg/g.
Injection (Cypionate [Depo-Estradiol]): 5 mg/ml.
Injection (Valerate [Delestrogen]): 10 mg/ml.
Topical Gel (EstroGel): 1.25 g.
Transdermal System (Alora): twice weekly: 0.025 mg, 0.05 mg, 0.075 mg, 0.1 mg.
Transdermal System (Climara): once weekly: 0.025 mg, 0.0375 mg, 0.05 mg, 0.06 mg, 0.075 mg, 0.1 mg.
Transdermal System (Esclim): twice weekly: 0.025 mg, 0.0375 mg, 0.05 mg, 0.075 mg, 0.1 mg.
Transdermal System (Estraderm): twice weekly: 0.05 mg, 0.1 mg.
Transdermal System (Menostar): once a week: 1 mg.
Transdermal System (Vivelle): twice weekly: 0.025 mg, 0.0375 mg, 0.05 mg, 0.075 mg, 0.1 mg.
Transdermal System (Vivelle Dot): twice weekly: 0.0375 mg, 0.05 mg, 0.075 mg, 0.1 mg.
Vaginal Cream (Estrace): 0.1 mg/g.
Vaginal Ring (Estring): 2 mg.
Vaginal Ring (Femring): 0.05 mg.
Vaginal Tablet (Vagifem): 25 mcg.

INDICATIONS AND DOSAGES

▸ **Prostate Cancer**
IM (estradiol valerate)
Adults, Elderly. 30 mg or more q1–2 wk.
PO
Adults, Elderly. 10 mg 3 times a day for at least 3 mo.
▸ **Breast Cancer**
PO
Adults, Elderly. 10 mg 3 times a day for at least 3 mo.
▸ **Osteoporosis Prophylaxis in Postmenopausal Females**
PO
Adults, Elderly. 0.5 mg/day cyclically (3 weeks on, 1 week off).

Transdermal (Climara)
Adults, Elderly. Initially, 0.025 mg weekly, adjust dose as needed.
Transdermal (Alora, Vivelle, Vivelle-Dot)
Adults, Elderly. Initially, 0.025 mg patch twice weekly, adjust dose as needed.
Transdermal (Estraderm)
Adults, Elderly. 0.05 mg twice weekly.
Transdermal (Menostar)
Adults, Elderly. 1 mg weekly.

▸ Female Hypoestrogenism
PO
Adults, Elderly. 1–2 mg/day, adjust dose as needed.
IM (cypionate)
Adults, Elderly. 1.5–2 mg monthly.
IM (estradiol valerate)
Adults, Elderly. 10–20 mg q4wk.

▸ Vasomotor Symptoms Associated With Menopause
PO
Adults, Elderly. 1–2 mg/day cyclically (3 weeks on, 1 week off), adjust dose as needed.
IM (estradiol cypionate)
Adults, Elderly. 1–5 mg q3–4wk.
IM (estradiol valerate)
Adults, Elderly. 10–20 mg q4wk.
Topical emulsion (Estrasorb)
Adults, Elderly. 3.84 g once a day in the morning.
Topical Gel (Estrogel)
Adults, Elderly. 1.25 g/day.
Transdermal (Climara)
Adults, Elderly. 0.025 mg weekly. Adjust dose as needed.
Transdermal (Alora, Esclim, Estrader, Vivelle-Dot)
Adults, Elderly. 0.05 mg twice a week.
Transdermal (Vivelle)
Adults, Elderly. 0.0375 mg twice a week.
Vaginal Ring (Femring)
Adults, Elderly. 0.05 mg. May increase to 0.1 mg if needed.

▸ Vaginal Atrophy
Vaginal Ring (Estring)
Adults, Elderly. 2 mg.

▸ Atrophic Vaginitis
Vaginal Tablet (Vagifem)
Adults, Elderly. Initially, 1 tablet/day for 2 weeks. Maintenance: 1 tablet twice a week.

OFF-LABEL USES
Treatment of Turner's syndrome

CONTRAINDICATIONS
Abnormal vaginal bleeding, active arterial thrombosis, blood dyscrasias, estrogen-dependent cancer, known or suspected breast cancer, pregnancy, thrombophlebitis or thromboembolic disorders, thyroid dysfunction

INTERACTIONS
Drug
Bromocriptine: May interfere with the effects of bromocriptine.
Cyclosporine: May increase blood cyclosporine concentration and the risk of hepatotoxicity and nephrotoxicity.
Hepatotoxic medications: May increase the risk of hepatotoxicity.

Herbal
Saw palmetto: Increases the effects of saw palmetto.
St. John's wort: May decrease plasma concentrations and effectiveness of estrogens.

Food
None known.

Drug interactions of concern to dentistry
- Increased action of corticosteroids

ESTRADIOL/TRANSDERMAL SYSTEM
Drug interactions of concern to dentistry
- Increased action of corticosteroids

E

DIAGNOSTIC TEST EFFECTS

May increase blood glucose, HDL, serum calcium, and triglyceride levels. May decrease serum cholesterol levels and LDH concentrations. May affect metapyrone testing and thyroid function tests.

SIDE EFFECTS

Frequent

Anorexia, nausea, swelling of breasts, peripheral edema marked by swollen ankles and feet

Transdermal: Skin irritation, redness

Occasional

Vomiting, especially with high doses; headache that may be severe; intolerance to contact lenses; hypertension; glucose intolerance; brown spots on exposed skin

Vaginal: Local irritation, vaginal discharge, changes in vaginal bleeding, including spotting, and breakthrough or prolonged bleeding

Rare

Chorea or involuntary movements, hirsutism or abnormal hairiness, loss of scalp hair, depression

SERIOUS REACTIONS

! Estrogen therapy may increase the risk of developing coronary heart disease, hypercalcemia, gallbladder disease, cerebrovascular disease, and breast cancer.

! Prolonged administration increases the risk of gallbladder disease, thromboembolic disease, and breast, cervical, vaginal, endometrial, and hepatic carcinoma.

! Cholestatic jaundice occurs rarely.

DENTAL CONSIDERATIONS

ESTRADIOL/ESTRADIOL CYPIONATE/ESTRADIOL VALERATE

General:

- Place on frequent recall to evaluate gingival condition.
- Monitor vital signs because of cardiovascular side effects.

Teach Patient/Family:

- Importance of good oral hygiene to prevent gingival inflammation

DENTAL CONSIDERATIONS

General:

- Place on frequent recall to evaluate gingival condition.
- Monitor vital signs because of cardiovascular side effects.

Teach Patient/Family:

- Importance of good oral hygiene to prevent gingival inflammation

estramustine phosphate sodium

es-trah-mew′-steen

(Emcyt)

Do not confuse Emcyt with Eryc.

CATEGORY AND SCHEDULE

Pregnancy Risk Category: C

MECHANISM OF ACTION

An alkylating agent, estrogen and nitrogen mustard that binds to microtubule-associated proteins, causing their disassembly.

Therapeutic Effect: Reduces serum testosterone concentration.

PHARMACOKINETICS

Well absorbed from the GI tract. Highly localized in prostatic tissue. Rapidly dephosphorylated during absorption into peripheral circulation. Metabolized in the liver. Primarily eliminated in feces by biliary system. ***Half-life:*** 20 hr.

AVAILABILITY

Capsules: 140 mg.

INDICATIONS AND DOSAGES

▸ Prostatic Carcinoma

PO

Adults, Elderly. 10–16 mg/kg/day or 140 mg 4 times/day.

CONTRAINDICATIONS

Active thrombophlebitis or thromboembolic disorders (unless the tumor is the cause of the thromboembolic disorder and the benefits outweigh the risk), hypersensitivity to estradiol or nitrogen mustard

INTERACTIONS

Drug

Calcium-containing antacids: May impair estramustine absorption.
Hepatotoxic medications: May increase the risk of hepatotoxicity.

Herbal

None known.

Food

Milk, dairy products, and other calcium-rich foods: May impair estramustine absorption.

Drug interactions of concern to dentistry

- Increased risk of hepatoxicity: hepatoxic drugs
- Impaired absorption: calcium-containing products

DIAGNOSTIC TEST EFFECTS

May increase blood glucose level and serum bilirubin, cortisol, LDH, phospholipid, prolactin, AST (SGOT), sodium, and triglyceride levels. May decrease urine pregnanediol level and serum antithrombin III, folate, and phosphate levels. May alter thyroid function test results.

SIDE EFFECTS

Frequent

Peripheral edema of lower extremities, breast tenderness or enlargement, diarrhea, flatulence, nausea

Occasional

Increase in BP, thirst, dry skin, ecchymosis, flushing, alopecia, night sweats

Rare

Headache, rash, fatigue, insomnia, vomiting

SERIOUS REACTIONS

! Estramustine use may exacerbate CHF and increase the risk of pulmonary emboli, thrombophlebitis, and cerebrovascular accident.

DENTAL CONSIDERATIONS

General:

- Patients with prostate disease may experience urinary retention; caution with use of anticholinergic drugs that could aggravate urinary retention.
- Patients may have received other chemotherapy or radiation; confirm medical and drug history.
- Determine why patient is taking the drug.
- Monitor vital signs at every appointment due to cardiovascular side effects.
- Consider semisupine chair position for patient comfort if GI side effects occur.
- Patient may need assistance in getting into and out of dental chair. Adjust chair position for patient comfort.
- Short appointments and a stress reduction protocol may be required for anxious patients.

Consultations:

- Consultation with physician may be needed if sedation or general anesthesia is required.

• Medical consultation may be required to assess disease control.

Teach Patient/Family:

• Importance of good oral hygiene to prevent soft tissue inflammation

• Importance of updating health and medication history if physician makes any changes in evaluation or drug regimens; include OTC, herbal, and nonherbal remedies in the update

E

estrogens, conjugated; medroxyprogesterone acetate

ess′-troe-jens, kon′-joo-gay-ted; me-drox′-ee-proe-jes′-ter-rone ass′-eh-tayte

(Premphase, Prempro, Prempro Low Dose)

CATEGORY AND SCHEDULE

Pregnancy Risk Category: X

MECHANISM OF ACTION

Conjugated estrogens are estrogens that increase synthesis of DNA, RNA, and various proteins in responsive tissues; reduces release of gonadotropin-releasing hormone, reducing follicle-stimulating hormone (FSH) and leuteinizing hormone (LH). Medroxyprogesterone acetate is a hormone that transforms endometrium from proliferative to secretory in an estrogen-primed endometrium; inhibits secretion of pituitary gonadotropins. ***Therapeutic Effect:*** Conjugated estrogens promote vasomotor stability, maintain genitourinary (GU) function, normal growth, development of female sex organs; prevents accelerated bone loss by inhibiting bone resorption, restoring balance of bone resorption and formation; inhibits LH, decreases serum concentration of testosterone. Medroxyprogesterone acetate prevents follicular maturation and ovulation; stimulates growth of mammary alveolar tissue; relaxes uterine smooth muscle; restores hormonal imbalance.

PHARMACOKINETICS

Conjugated estrogens are well absorbed from the gastrointestinal (GI) tract. Widely distributed. Protein binding: 50%–80%. Metabolized in liver. Primarily excreted in urine. ***Half-life:*** 4–10 hrs. Medroxyprogesterone's absorption varies depending on the patient but is generally low. Binds mainly to albumin or other plasma proteins. Metabolized in liver. Primarily excreted in urine. ***Half-life:*** 2–4 hrs.

AVAILABILITY

Tablets: 0.3 mg of conjugated estrogens and 1.5 mg of medroxyprogesterone acetate (Prempro Low Dose), 0.45 mg of conjugated estrogens and 1.5 mg of medroxyprogesterone acetate (Prempro), 0.625 mg of conjugated estrogens and 2.5 mg of medroxyprogesterone acetate (Prempro), 0.625 mg of conjugated estrogens and 5 mg of medroxyprogesterone acetate (Prempro), and 0.625 mg of conjugated estrogens and 5 mg of medroxyprogesterone acetate (Premphase).

INDICATIONS AND DOSAGES

▸ Menopausal Symptoms, Osteoporosis, Vulvar/Vaginal Atrophy

PO

(Prempro)Adults, Elderly. 1 tablet once daily.

▸ **Menopausal Symptoms, Osteoporosis, Vulvar/Vaginal Atrophy**
PO
(Premphase)Adults, Elderly. 1 maroon conjugated estrogen tablet on days 1 through 14 and 1 light blue conjugated estrogens/medroxyprogesterone tablet on days 15 through 28.

CONTRAINDICATIONS

Breast cancer with some exceptions, liver disease, thrombophlebitis, undiagnosed vaginal bleeding, estrogen-dependent neoplasia (known of suspected), pregnancy (known or suspected), hypersensitivity to conjugated estrogens, medroxyprogesterone acetate or any component of the formulation.

INTERACTIONS

Drug

Bromocriptine: May interfere with the effects of bromocriptine.
Cyclosporine: May increase the blood concentration and liver and nephrotoxicity of cyclosporine.
Liver toxic medications: May increase the risk of liver toxicity.
Phenobarbital, carbamazepine, and rifampin: May reduce plasma concentrations of estrogens.
Erythromycin, clarithromycin, ketoconazole, itraconazole, ritonavir: May increase plasma concentrations of estrogens.

Herbal

St. John's wort: May reduce plasma concentrations of estrogens.

Food

Grapefruit juice: May increase plasma concentration of estrogens.

Drug interactions of concern to dentistry

- Increased action of corticosteroids

ESTROGENS A, CONJUGATED SYNTHETIC

Drug interactions of concern to dentistry

- None reported

DIAGNOSTIC TEST EFFECTS

Conjugated estrogens may affect metapyrone testing, thyroid function tests. May decrease serum cholesterol levels, and LDH concentrations. May increase blood glucose levels, HDL concentrations, serum calcium, and triglyceride levels. Medroxyprogesterone may alter thyroid and liver function tests, prothrombin time, and metapyrone test.

SIDE EFFECTS

Frequent

Change in vaginal bleeding, such as spotting or breakthrough bleeding, breast pain or tenderness, gynecomastia

Occasional

Headache, increased blood pressure (B/P), intolerance to contact lenses, nausea, edema, weight change, breast tenderness, nervousness, insomnia, fatigue, dizziness

Rare

Loss of scalp hair, mental depression, dermatologic changes, headache, fever

SERIOUS REACTIONS

! Prolonged administration may increase risk of gallbladder, thromboembolic disease, or breast, cervical, vaginal, endometrial, and liver carcinoma.

DENTAL CONSIDERATIONS

General:

- Place on frequent recall to evaluate gingival condition.
- Monitor vital signs because of cardiovascular side effects.

Teach Patient/Family:

- Importance of good oral hygiene to prevent gingival

DENTAL CONSIDERATIONS

General:

- Consider semisupine chair position for patient comfort if GI side effects occur.

Teach Patient/Family:

- Importance of good oral hygiene to prevent soft tissue inflammation

E

estropipate

es-tro-pip′-ate
(Genoral[AUS], Ogen, Ortho-Est)

CATEGORY AND SCHEDULE

Pregnancy Risk Category: X

MECHANISM OF ACTION

An estrogen that increases synthesis of DNA, RNA, abd proteins in target tissues; reduces release of gonadotropin-releasing hormone from the hypothalamus; and reduces follicle-stimulating hormone (FSH) and luteinizing hormone (LH) from the pituitary. ***Therapeutic Effect:*** Promotes normal growth, promotes development of female sex organs, and maintains GU function and vasomotor stability. Prevents accelerated bone loss by inhibiting bone resorption, restoring balance of bone resorption and formation. Inhibits LH and decreases serum testosterone concentration.

AVAILABILITY

Tablets (Ogen, Ortho-Est): 0.625 mg (0.75 mg estropipate), 1.25 mg (1.5 mg estropipate), 2.5 mg (3 mg estropipate).
Vaginal Cream (Ogen): 1.5 mg/g.

INDICATIONS AND DOSAGES

▸ Vasomotor Symptoms, Atrophic Vaginitis, Kraurosis Vulvae

PO

Adults, Elderly. 0.625–5 mg/day cyclically.

▸ Atrophic Vaginitis, Kraurosis Vulvae

INTRAVAGINAL

Adults, Elderly. 2–4 g/day cyclically.

▸ Female Hypogonadism, Castration, Primary Ovarian Failure

PO

Adults, Elderly. 1.25–7.5 mg/day for 21 days; then off for 8–10 days. Repeat if bleeding does not occur by end of off cycle.

▸ Prevention of Osteoporosis

PO

Adults, Elderly. 0.625 mg/day (25 days of 31-day cycle/mo).

CONTRAINDICATIONS

Abnormal vaginal bleeding, active arterial thrombosis, blood dyscrasias, estrogen-dependent cancer, known or suspected breast cancer, pregnancy, thrombophlebitis or thromboembolic disorders, thyroid dysfunction

INTERACTIONS

Drug

Bromocriptine: May interfere with the effects of bromocriptine.
Cyclosporine: May increase blood cyclosporine concentration and the risk of hepatotoxicity and nephrotoxicity.
Hepatotoxic medications: May increase the risk of hepatotoxicity.

Herbal

Saw palmetto: Increases the effects of saw palmetto.

Food

None known.

Drug interactions of concern to dentistry

- Increased action of corticosteroids

DIAGNOSTIC TEST EFFECTS

May increase blood glucose, HDL, serum calcium, and triglyceride levels. May decrease serum cholesterol and LDH concentrations. May affect metapyrone testing and thyroid function tests.

SIDE EFFECTS

Frequent

Anorexia, nausea, swelling of breasts, peripheral edema marked by swollen ankles and feet

Occasional

Vomiting, especially with high doses; headache that may be severe; intolerance to contact lenses; hypertension; glucose intolerance; brown spots on exposed skin

Vaginal: Local irritation, vaginal discharge, changes in vaginal bleeding, including spotting, and breakthrough or prolonged bleeding

Rare

Chorea or involuntary movements, hirsutism or abnormal hairiness, loss of scalp hair, depression

SERIOUS REACTIONS

! Prolonged administration increases the risk of gallbladder disease, thromboembolic disease and breast, cervical, vaginal, endometrial, and hepatic carcinoma.

! Cholestatic jaundice occurs rarely.

DENTAL CONSIDERATIONS

General:

- Place on frequent recall to evaluate gingival condition.
- Monitor vital signs because of cardiovascular side effects.

Teach Patient/Family:

- Importance of good oral hygiene to prevent gingival inflammation

etanercept

e-tan′-er-cept

(Enbrel)

CATEGORY AND SCHEDULE

Pregnancy Risk Category: B

E

MECHANISM OF ACTION

A protein that binds to tumor necrosis factor (TNF), blocking its interaction with cell surface receptors. Elevated levels of TNF, which is involved in inflammatory and immune responses, are found in the synovial fluid of rheumatoid arthritis patients. ***Therapeutic Effect:*** Relieves symptoms of rheumatoid arthritis.

PHARMACOKINETICS

Well absorbed after subcutaneous administration.

Half-life: 115 hr.

AVAILABILITY

Powder for Injection: 25 mg.

Prefilled Syringe: 50 mg.

INDICATIONS AND DOSAGES

▸ Rheumatoid Arthritis, Psoriatic Arthritis, Ankylosing Spondylitis

SUBCUTANEOUS

Adults, Elderly. 25 mg twice weekly given 72–96 hr apart. Alternative weekly dosing: 0.8 mg/kg/dose once a week. Maximum: 50 mg/week. Maximum: 25 mg/dose.

▸ Juvenile Rheumatoid Arthritis

SUBCUTANEOUS

Children 4–17 yr. 0.4 mg/kg (Maximum: 25 mg dose) twice weekly given 72–96 hr apart. Alternative weekly dosing: 50 mg once weekly. Maximum: 25 mg/dose.

▸ **Plaque Psoriasis**
SUBCUTANEOUS
Adults, Elderly. 50 mg twice a week (give 3–4 days apart) for 3 mo. Maintenance: 50 mg once a week.

E

OFF-LABEL USES
Treatment of Crohn's disease

CONTRAINDICATIONS
Serious active infection or sepsis

INTERACTIONS
Drug
None known.
Herbal
None known.
Food
None known.
Drug interactions of concern to dentistry
- No studies have been conducted.

DIAGNOSTIC TEST EFFECTS
None known.

SIDE EFFECTS
Frequent (37%)
Injection site erythema, pruritus, pain, and swelling; abdominal pain, vomiting (more common in children than adults)
Occasional (16%–4%)
Headache, rhinitis, dizziness, pharyngitis, cough, asthenia, abdominal pain, dyspepsia
Rare (<3%)
Sinusitis, allergic reaction

SERIOUS REACTIONS
! Infections (such as pyelonephritis, cellulitis, osteomyelitis, wound infection, leg ulcer, septic arthritis, diarrhea, bronchitis, and pneumonia), occur in 38%–29% of patients.
! Rare adverse effects include heart failure, hypertension, hypotension, pancreatitis, GI hemorrhage, and dyspnea. The patient also may develop autoimmune antibodies.

DENTAL CONSIDERATIONS
General:
- Monitor vital signs at every appointment because of potential cardiovascular side effects
- Consider semisupine chair position for patient comfort because of GI side effects of drug
- If acute oral infection occurs, inform physician.
- Note elevated antinuclear antibody (ANA) levels if diagnosing Sögren's syndrome.

Consultations:
- Medical consultation if needed.

Teach Patient/Family:
- Importance of good oral hygiene to prevent soft tissue inflammation
- Use of electric toothbrush if patient has difficulty holding conventional devices

ethambutol
e-tham′-byoo-tole
(Etibi[CAN], Myambutol)
Do not confuse ethambutol or Myambutol with Nembutal.

CATEGORY AND SCHEDULE
Pregnancy Risk Category: B

MECHANISM OF ACTION
An isonicotinic acid derivative that interferes with RNA synthesis.
Therapeutic Effect: Suppresses the multiplication of mycobacteria.

PHARMACOKINETICS
Rapidly and well absorbed from the GI tract. Protein binding: 20%–30%. Widely distributed. Metabolized in the liver. Primarily excreted in urine. Removed by hemodialysis. ***Half-life:*** 3–4 hr (increased in impaired renal function).

AVAILABILITY
Tablets: 100 mg, 400 mg.

INDICATIONS AND DOSAGES
▸ Tuberculosis

PO

Adults, Elderly, Children.

15–25 mg/kg/day as a single dose or 50 mg/kg 2 times/wk. Maximum: 2.5 g/dose.

▸ Atypical Mycobacterial Infections

PO

Adults, Elderly, Children.

15 mg/kg/day. Maximum: 1 g/day.

▸ Dosage in Renal Impairment

Dosage interval is modified on the basis of creatinine clearance.

Creatinine Clearance	Dosage Interval
10–50 ml/min	q24–36h
less than 10 ml/min	q48h

OFF-LABEL USES
Treatment of atypical mycobacterial infections

CONTRAINDICATIONS
Optic neuritis

INTERACTIONS
Drug

Neurotoxic medications: May increase the risk of neurotoxicity.

Herbal

None known.

Food

None known.

Drug interactions of concern to dentistry

- None reported

DIAGNOSTIC TEST EFFECTS
May increase serum uric acid levels.

SIDE EFFECTS
Occasional

Acute gouty arthritis (chills, pain, swelling of joints with hot skin), confusion, abdominal pain, nausea, vomiting, anorexia, headache

Rare

Rash, fever, blurred vision, eye pain, red-green color blindness

SERIOUS REACTIONS
! Optic neuritis (more common with high-dosage or long-term ethambutol therapy), peripheral neuritis, thrombocytopenia, and an anaphylactoid reaction occur rarely.

DENTAL CONSIDERATIONS
General:

- Examine for evidence of oral signs of disease.
- Avoid dental light in patient's eyes; offer dark glasses for patient comfort.
- Determine why the patient is taking the drug.

Consultations:

- Medical consultation is required to assess patient's current status; avoid elective dental procedures in active infections.
- *Determine that noninfectious status exists by ensuring the following:*
  - Anti-TB drugs have been taken for longer than 3 wk.

- Culture confirms antibiotic susceptibility to TB microorganisms.
- Patient has had three consecutive negative sputum smears.
- Patient is not in the coughing stage.

Teach Patient/Family:

- Importance of taking medication for full length of prescribed therapy to ensure effectiveness of treatment and to prevent the emergence of resistant forms of microbes

ethionamide

e-thye-on′-am-ide
(Trecator)
Do not confuse with Tricor.

CATEGORY AND SCHEDULE

Pregnancy Risk Category: C

MECHANISM OF ACTION

An antitubercular agent that inhibits peptide synthesis.
Therapeutic Effect: Suppresses mycobacterial multiplication. Bactericidal.

PHARMACOKINETICS

Rapidly absorbed from the gastrointestinal (GI) tract. Widely distributed. Protein binding: 10%. Metabolized in liver. Primarily excreted in urine. Removed by hemodialysis. ***Half-life:*** 2–3 hrs (half-life is increased with impaired renal function).

AVAILABILITY

Tablets: 250 mg (Trecator).

INDICATIONS AND DOSAGES

▸ **Tuberculosis**
PO
Adults, Elderly. 500–1000 mg/day as a single to 3 divided doses.
Children. 15–20 mg/kg/day. Maximum 1 g/day.

▸ **Dosage in Renal Impairment**
Creatinine clearance less than 50 ml/min, reduce dose by 50%.

OFF-LABEL USES

Treatment of atypical mycobacterial infections

CONTRAINDICATIONS

Severe hepatic impairment, hypersensitivity to ethionamide

INTERACTIONS

Drug
Cycloserine, isoniazid: May increase the risk of toxicity.
Rifampin: May increase the risk of hepatotoxicity.
Herbal
None known.
Food
None known.
Drug interactions of concern to dentistry

- None reported

DIAGNOSTIC TEST EFFECTS

May increase ALT and AST.

SIDE EFFECTS

Occasional
Abdominal pain, nausea, vomiting, weakness, postural hypotension, psychiatric disturbances, drowsiness, dizziness, headache, confusion, anorexia, headache, metallic taste, anorexia, diarrhea, stomatitis, peripheral neuritis
Rare
Rash, fever, blurred vision, optic neuritis, seizures, hypothyroidism,

hypoglycemia, gynecomastia, thrombocytopenia, jaundice

SERIOUS REACTIONS

! Peripheral neuropathy, anorexia, and joint pain rarely occur.

DENTAL CONSIDERATIONS

General:

- Monitor vital signs at every appointment because of cardiovascular side effects.
- After supine positioning, have patient sit upright for at least 2 min before standing to avoid orthostatic hypotension.
- Consider semisupine chair position for patient comfort because of GI effects of disease.
- Evaluate for clotting ability during gingival instrumentation.
- Examine for evidence of oral manifestations of blood dyscrasias (infection, bleeding, poor healing).
- Palliative treatment may be required for oral side effects.
- Examine for evidence of oral signs of disease.

Consultations:

- Medical consultation for blood studies (CBC); leukopenic or thrombocytopenic side effects may result in infection, delayed healing, and excessive bleeding. Postpone elective dental treatment until normal values are maintained. Instruct patient to take with meals to decrease GI symptoms.
- Medical consultation may be required to assess disease control and determine infectious nature of disease.

Teach Patient/Family:

- Importance of good oral hygiene to prevent soft tissue inflammation
- Caution in use of oral hygiene aids to prevent injury

ethosuximide

eth-oh-sux′-i-mide
(Zarontin)
Do not confuse with Zaroxolyn or Neurontin.

CATEGORY AND SCHEDULE

Pregnancy Risk Category: C

MECHANISM OF ACTION

An anticonvulsant that increases the seizure threshold and suppresses paroxysmal spike-and-wave pattern in absence seizures; depresses nerve transmission in the motor cortex.
Therapeutic Effect: Produces anticonvulsant activity.

PHARMACOKINETICS

Well absorbed from the gastrointestinal (GI) tract. Metabolized in liver. Excreted in urine. Removed by hemodialysis. ***Half-life:*** 50–60 hrs (in adults); 30 hrs (in children).

AVAILABILITY

Capsule: 250 mg, 100 mg, 150 mg, 200 mg (Zarontin).
Syrup: 250 mg/5 ml (Zarontin).

INDICATIONS AND DOSAGES

▸ Absence Seizures

PO

Adults, Elderly, Children older than 6 yrs. Initially, 250 mg/day or 15 mg/kg/day in 2 divided doses. Maintenance: 15–40 mg/kg/day in 2 divided doses.
Children 3–6 yrs. Initially, 250 mg in 2 divided doses, increased by 250 mg as needed every 4–7 days. Maintenance: 20–40 mg/kg/day in 2 divided doses.
Use with caution in patients with renal impairment.

E

OFF-LABEL USES
Treatment of learning problems

CONTRAINDICATIONS
Hypersensitivity to succinimides

INTERACTIONS
Drug
Alcohol, central nervous system (CNS) depressants: May increase CNS depression.
Carbamazepine, phenobarbital, phenytoin, primidone, valproic acid: May decreases ethosuximide blood concentration.
Azole antifungals, ciprofloxacin, clarithromycin, isoniazid, quinidine, protease inhibitors, verapamil: May increase ethosuximide blood concentration.
Herbal
Evening primrose oil: May decrease effectiveness of ethosuximide.
Ginkgo: May decrease effectiveness of ethosuximide.
St. John's Wort: May decrease ethosuximide blood concentrations.
Food
None known.
Drug interactions of concern to dentistry
- Enhanced CNS depression: CNS depressants, alcohol

DIAGNOSTIC TEST EFFECTS
None known.

SIDE EFFECTS
Occasional
Dizziness, drowsiness, double vision, headache, ataxia, nausea, diarrhea, vomiting, somnolence, urticaria
Rare
Arganulocytosis, gum hypertrophy, leucopenia, myopia, swelling of the tongue, systemic lupus erythematosus, vaginal bleeding

SERIOUS REACTIONS
! Abrupt withdrawal may increase seizure frequency.
! Overdosage results in nausea, vomiting, and CNS depression including coma with respiratory depression.

DENTAL CONSIDERATIONS
General:
- Patients on chronic drug therapy may rarely have symptoms of blood dyscrasias, which can include infection, bleeding, and poor healing.
- Talk with patient to ascertain seizure frequency and how well seizures are controlled. A stress reduction protocol may be required.

Consultations:
- In a patient with symptoms of blood dyscrasias, request a medical consultation for blood studies and postpone dental treatment until normal values are reestablished.
- Medical consultation may be required to assess disease control and patient's ability to tolerate stress.

Teach Patient/Family:
- Importance of good oral hygiene to prevent gingival inflammation
- To avoid mouth rinses with high alcohol content because of drying effects

etidronate disodium

ee-tid′-roe-nate
(Didronel)
Do not confuse etidronate with etidocaine or etomidate.

CATEGORY AND SCHEDULE

Pregnancy Risk Category: C (parenteral), B (oral)

MECHANISM OF ACTION

A bisphosphonate that decreases mineral release and matrix in bone and inhibits osteocytic osteolysis. ***Therapeutic Effect:*** Decreases bone resorption.

AVAILABILITY

Tablets: 200 mg, 400 mg.
Injection: 300-mg ampule (50 mg/ml).

INDICATIONS AND DOSAGES

▸ Paget's Disease

PO

Adults, Elderly. Initially, 5–10 mg/kg/day not to exceed 6 mo, or 11–20 mg/kg/day not to exceed 3 mo. Repeat only after drug-free period of at least 90 days.

▸ Heterotopic Ossification Caused by Spinal Cord Injury

PO

Adult, Elderly. 20 mg/kg/day for 2 wk; then 10 mg/kg/day for 10 wks.

▸ Heterotopic Ossification Complicating Total Hip Replacement

PO

Adults, Elderly. 20 mg/kg/day for 1 mo before surgery; then 20 mg/kg/day for 3 mo after surgery.

▸ Hypercalcemia Associated with Malignancy

IV

Adults, Elderly. 7.5 mg/kg/day for 3 days. For retreatment, allow 7 days between treatment courses. Follow with oral therapy on day after last infusion. Begin with 20 mg/kg/day for 30 days; may extend up to 90 days.

CONTRAINDICATIONS

Clinically overt osteomalacia

INTERACTIONS

Drug

Antacids containing aluminum, calcium, magnesium mineral supplements: May decrease the absorption of etidronate.

Herbal

None known.

Food

Foods with calcium: May decrease the absorption of etidronate.

Drug interactions of concern to dentistry

• Possible increased risk of gastric ulceration: NSAIDs

DIAGNOSTIC TEST EFFECTS

None known.

IV INCOMPATIBILITIES

Do not mix with other medications.

SIDE EFFECTS

Frequent

Nausea; diarrhea; continuing or more frequent bone pain in patients with Paget's disease

Occasional

Bone fractures, especially of the femur

Parenteral: Metallic, altered taste

Rare

Hypersensitivity reaction

SERIOUS REACTIONS

! Nephrotoxicity, including hematuria, dysuria, and proteinuria, has occurred with parenteral route.

DENTAL CONSIDERATIONS

General:

- Be aware of oral manifestations of Paget's disease (macrognathia, alveolar pain).

Consultations:

- Medical consultation may be required to assess disease control.

etodolac

e-toe-doe′-lak

(Apo-Etodolac[CAN], Lodine, Lodine XL, Ultradol[CAN])

Do not confuse Lodine with codeine or iodine.

CATEGORY AND SCHEDULE

Pregnancy Risk Category: C (D if used in third trimester or near delivery)

MECHANISM OF ACTION

An NSAID that produces analgesic and anti-inflammatory effects by inhibiting prostaglandin synthesis. ***Therapeutic Effect:*** Reduces the inflammatory response and intensity of pain.

PHARMACOKINETICS

Route	Onset	Peak	Duration
PO (analgesic)	30 min	N/A	4–12 hr

Completely absorbed from the GI tract. Protein binding: greater than 99%. Widely distributed. Metabolized in the liver. Primarily excreted in urine. Not removed by hemodialysis. ***Half-life:*** 6–7 hr.

AVAILABILITY

Capsules (Lodine): 200 mg, 300 mg.
Tablets (Lodine): 400 mg, 500 mg.
Tablets (Extended-Release [Lodine XL]): 400 mg, 500 mg, 600 mg.

INDICATIONS AND DOSAGES

▸ Osteoarthritis, Rheumatoid Arthritis

PO (Immediate-Release)
Adults, Elderly. Initially, 300 mg 2–3 times a day or 400–500 mg twice a day. Maintenance: 600–1000 mg/day in 2–4 divided doses.
PO (Extended-Release)
Adults, Elderly. 400–1000 mg once daily. Maximum: 1200 mg/day.

▸ Juvenile Rheumatoid Arthritis

PO (Extended-Release)
Children 6–16 yr. 1000 mg in children weighing more than 60 kg, 800 mg once daily in children weighing 46–60 kg, 600 mg once daily in children weighing 31–45 kg, 400 mg once daily in children weighing 20–30 kg.

▸ Analgesia

PO
Adults, Elderly. 200–400 mg q6–8h as needed. Maximum: 1,200 mg/day.

OFF-LABEL USES

Treatment of acute gouty arthritis, vascular headache

CONTRAINDICATIONS

Active peptic ulcer disease, chronic inflammation of GI tract, GI bleeding or ulceration, history of hypersensitivity to aspirin or NSAIDs

INTERACTIONS

Drug

Antihypertensives, diuretics: May decrease the effects of these drugs.
Aspirin, other salicylates: May increase the risk of GI side effects such as bleeding.
Bone marrow depressants: May increase the risk of hematologic reactions.

Heparin, oral anticoagulants, thrombolytics: May increase the effects of these drugs.
Lithium: May increase the blood concentration and risk of toxicity of lithium.
Methotrexate: May increase the risk of methotrexate toxicity.
Probenecid: May increase etodolac blood concentration.

Herbal

Feverfew, ginkgo biloba: May increase the risk of bleeding.

Food

None known.

Drug interactions of concern to dentistry

- GI ulceration, bleeding: aspirin, alcohol, corticosteroids, biphosphonates
- Decreased action: salicylates
- Nephrotoxicity: acetaminophen (prolonged use)
- Possible risk of decreased renal function: cyclosporine
- First-time users of SSRIs also taking NSAIDs may have a higher risk of GI side effects; until more data are available, it may be advisable to avoid use of NSAIDs in these patients (*Br J Clin Pharmacol* 55:591–595, 2003)
- *When prescribed for dental pain:*
  - Risk of increased effects: oral anticoagulants, oral antidiabetics, lithium, methotrexate
  - Decreased effects of diuretics
  - Increased risk of methotrexate toxicity

DIAGNOSTIC TEST EFFECTS

May increase bleeding time, liver function test results, and serum creatinine level. May decrease serum uric acid level.

SIDE EFFECTS

Occasional (9%–4%)

Dizziness, headache, abdominal pain or cramps, bloated feeling, diarrhea, nausea, indigestion

Rare (3%–1%)

Constipation, rash, pruritus, visual disturbances, tinnitus

SERIOUS REACTIONS

! Overdose may result in acute renal failure.
! There is an increased risk of cardiovascular events (including MI and CVA) and serious and potentially life-threatening GI bleeding.
! Rare reactions with long-term use include peptic ulcer disease, GI bleeding, gastritis, severe hepatic reactions (jaundice), nephrotoxicity (hematuria, dysuria, proteinuria), and a severe hypersensitivity reaction (bronchospasm, angioedema).

DENTAL CONSIDERATIONS

General:

- Patients on chronic drug therapy may rarely have symptoms of blood dyscrasias, which can include infection, bleeding, and poor healing.
- Assess salivary flow as a factor in caries, periodontal disease, and candidiasis.
- Avoid prescribing for dental use in last trimester of pregnancy.
- Avoid prescribing aspirin-containing products.
- Consider semisupine chair position for patients with arthritic disease.

Consultations:

- In a patient with symptoms of blood dyscrasias, request a medical consultation for blood studies and postpone dental treatment until normal values are reestablished.
- Medical consultation may be required to assess disease control.

Teach Patient/Family:

- To avoid mouth rinses with high alcohol content because of drying effects

E

etoposide, VP-16

e-toe′-poe-side
(Etopophos, Toposar, VePesid)
Do not confuse VePesid with Pepcid or Versed.

CATEGORY AND SCHEDULE

Pregnancy Risk Category: D

MECHANISM OF ACTION

An epipodophyllotoxin that induces single- and double-stranded breaks in DNA. Cell cycle-dependent and phase-specific; most effective in the S and G_2 phases of cell division. ***Therapeutic Effect:*** Inhibits or alters DNA synthesis.

PHARMACOKINETICS

Variably absorbed from the GI tract. Rapidly distributed, low concentrations in CSF. Protein binding: 97%. Metabolized in the liver. Primarily excreted in urine. Not removed by hemodialysis. ***Half-life:*** 3–12 hr.

AVAILABILITY

Capsules (VePesid): 50 mg.
Injection (Toposar, VePesid): 20 mg/ml.
Injection (Water-soluble [Etopophos]): 100 mg/ml.

INDICATIONS AND DOSAGES

▸ Refractory Testicular Tumors
IV
Adults. 50–100 mg/m²/day on days 1 to 5, or 100 mg/m²/day on days 1, 3, 5 (as combination therapy).

▸ Acute Myelocytic Leukemia
IV
Children. 150 mg/m²/day for 2–3 days and 2–3 cycles.

▸ Brain Tumor
IV
Children. 150 mg/m²/day on days 2 and 3 of treatment course.

▸ Neuroblastoma
IV
Children. 100 mg/m²/day on days 1–5 of treatment course; repeated q4wk.

▸ Small-Cell Lung Carcinoma
PO
Adults. Twice the IV dose rounded to nearest 50 mg. Give once a day for doses 400 mg or less, in divided doses for dosages greater than 400 mg.
IV
Adults. 35 mg/m²/day for 4 consecutive days up to 50 mg/m²/day for 5 consecutive days (as combination therapy).

▸ Leukemia, Rhabdomyosarcoma
Children. 60–150 mg/m²/day for 2–5 days q3–6wks.

▸ Dosage in Renal Impairment
Creatinine clearance 10–50 ml/min. 75% of normal dose.
Creatinine clearance less than 10 ml/min. 50% of normal dose.

OFF-LABEL USES

Treatment of acute myelocytic leukemia, AIDS-associated Kaposi's sarcoma, bladder carcinoma, Ewing's sarcoma, Hodgkin's disease, non-Hodgkin's lymphoma

CONTRAINDICATIONS

Pregnancy

INTERACTIONS

Drug

Bone marrow depressants: May increase myelosuppression.
Live-virus vaccines: May potentiate virus replication, increase vaccine side effects, and decrease the patient's antibody response to the vaccine.

Herbal

None known.

Food

None known.

Drug interactions of concern to dentistry

- None reported

DIAGNOSTIC TEST EFFECTS

None known.

IV INCOMPATIBILITIES

VePesid: Cefepime (Maxipime), filgrastim (Neupogen), idarubicin (Idamycin).
Etopophos: Amphotericin B (Fungizone), cefepime (Maxipime), chlorpromazine (Thorazine), methylprednisolone (Solu-Medrol), prochlorperazine (Compazine)

IV COMPATIBILITIES

VePesid: Carboplatin (Paraplatin), cisplatin (Platinol), cytarabine (Cytosar), daunorubicin (Cerubidine), doxorubicin (Adriamycin), granisetron (Kytril), mitoxantrone (Novantrone), ondansetron (Zofran)
Etopophos: Carboplatin (Paraplatin), cisplatin (Platinol), cytarabine (Cytosar), dacarbazine (DTIC-Dome), daunorubicin (Cerubidine), dexamethasone (Decadron), diphenhydramine (Benadryl), doxorubicin (Adriamycin), granisetron (Kytril), magnesium sulfate, mannitol, mitoxantrone (Novantrone), ondansetron (Zofran), potassium chloride

SIDE EFFECTS

Frequent (66%–43%)
Mild to moderate nausea and vomiting, alopecia
Occasional (13%–6%)
Diarrhea, anorexia, stomatitis
Rare (≤ 2%)
Hypotension, peripheral neuropathy

SERIOUS REACTIONS

! Myelosuppression may result in hematologic toxicity, manifested as anemia, leukopenia (occurring 7–14 days after drug administration), thrombocytopenia (occurring 9–16 days after administration) and, to lesser extent, pancytopenia. Bone marrow recovery occurs by day 20.
! Hepatotoxicity occurs occasionally.

E

DENTAL CONSIDERATIONS

General:

- Determine why patient is taking the drug.
- If additional analgesia is required for dental pain, consider alternative analgesics (NSAIDs) in patients taking narcotics for acute or chronic pain.
- Examine for oral manifestation of opportunistic infection.
- Avoid products that affect platelet function, such as aspirin and NSAIDs.
- This drug may be used in the hospital or on an outpatient basis. Confirm the patient's disease and treatment status.
- Chlorhexidine mouth rinse prior to and during chemotherapy may reduce severity of mucositis.
- Patient on chronic drug therapy may rarely present with symptoms of blood dyscrasias, which can include infection, bleeding and poor healing. If dyscrasia is present, caution patient to prevent oral tissue trauma when using oral hygiene aids.
- Palliative medication may be required for management of oral side effects.
- Short appointments and a stress reduction protocol may be required for anxious patients.
- Consider semisupine chair position for patient comfort if GI side effects occur.
- Patients may be at risk of bleeding, check for oral signs.
- Oral infections should be eliminated and/or treated aggressively.

Consultations:

- Medical consultation should include routine blood counts including platelet counts and bleeding time.
- Consult physician; prophylactic or therapeutic antiinfectives may be indicated if surgery or periodontal treatment is required.
- Medical consultation may be required to assess immunologic status during cancer chemotherapy and determine safety risk, if any, posed by the required dental treatment.
- Medical consultation may be required to assess disease control and patient's ability to tolerate stress.

Teach Patient/Family:

- Importance of good oral hygiene to prevent soft tissue inflammation
- To report oral lesions, soreness, or bleeding to dentist
- To prevent trauma when using oral hygiene aids
- Importance of updating health and medication history if physician makes any changes in evaluation or drug regimens; include OTC, herbal, and nonherbal remedies in the update

exemestane

x-eh-mess′-tane
(Aromasin)

CATEGORY AND SCHEDULE

Pregnancy Risk Category: D

MECHANISM OF ACTION

Inactivates aromatase, the principal enzyme that converts androgens to estrogens in both premenopausal and postmenopausal women, thereby lowering the circulating estrogen level. ***Therapeutic Effect:*** Inhibits the growth of breast cancers that are stimulated by estrogens.

PHARMACOKINETICS

Rapidly absorbed after PO administration. Protein binding: 90%. Distributed extensively into tissues. Metabolized in the liver; eliminated in urine and feces. ***Half-life:*** 24 hr.

AVAILABILITY

Tablets: 25 mg.

INDICATIONS AND DOSAGES

▸ Breast Cancer

PO

Adults, Elderly. 25 mg once a day after a meal.

OFF-LABEL USES

Prevention of prostate cancer

CONTRAINDICATIONS

Hypersensitivity to exemestane

INTERACTIONS

Drug

None known.

Herbal

None known.

Food

None known.

Drug interactions of concern to dentistry

- Data not available; however, possible reduction in plasma levels by inducers of CYP3A4 isoenzymes
- Ketoconazole had no significant effect

DIAGNOSTIC TEST EFFECTS

May increase serum alkaline phosphatase, AST (SGOT), and ALT (SGPT) levels.

SIDE EFFECTS

Frequent (22%–10%)

Fatigue, nausea, depression, hot flashes, pain, insomnia, anxiety, dyspnea

Occasional (8%–5%)
Headache, dizziness, vomiting, peripheral edema, abdominal pain, anorexia, flulike symptoms, diaphoresis, constipation, hypertension
Rare (4%)
Diarrhea

SERIOUS REACTIONS

! None known.

DENTAL CONSIDERATIONS

General:
- Monitor vital signs at every appointment due to cardiovascular side effects.
- If additional analgesia is required for dental pain, consider alternative analgesics (NSAIDs) in patients taking narcotics for acute or chronic pain.
- DHRDG
- Product may be used in outpatient therapy.
- If used in prostate cancer, consider urinary retention concern and avoid anticholinergic drugs that may aggravate retention.

Consultations:
- Medical consultation may be required to assess disease control and patient's ability to tolerate stress.

Teach Patient/Family:
- Importance of good oral hygiene to prevent soft tissue inflammation
- To prevent trauma when using oral hygiene aids
- Importance of updating health and medication history if physician makes any changes in evaluation or drug regimens; include OTC, herbal, and nonherbal remedies in the update

ezetimibe; simvastatin

ez-et′-i-mib; sim-vah-stay′-tin
(Vytorin)

CATEGORY AND SCHEDULE

Pregnancy Risk Category: X

MECHANISM OF ACTION

Ezetimibe is an antihyperlipidemic that inhibits cholesterol absorption in the small intestine, leading to a decrease in the delivery of intestinal cholesterol to the liver. ***Therapeutic Effect:*** Reduces total cholesterol and low-density lipoprotein (LDL) cholesterol and triglyceride levels and increases high-density lipoprotein (HDL) cholesterol level.
Simvastatin is a 3-hydroxy-3-methylglutaryl coenzyme A (HMG-CoA) reductase inhibitor that interferes with cholesterol biosynthesis by inhibiting the conversion of the enzyme HMG-CoA to mevalonate. ***Therapeutic Effect:*** Decreases LDL cholesterol, very low density lipoprotein (VLDL) cholesterol, and plasma triglyceride levels; slightly increases HDL concentration.

PHARMACOKINETICS

Ezetimibe: Well absorbed following oral administration. Protein binding: greater than 90%. Metabolized in the small intestine and liver. Excreted by the kidneys and bile. ***Half-life:*** 22 hrs.
Simvastatin: Well absorbed from the gastrointestinal (GI) tract. Protein binding: 95%. Undergoes extensive first-pass metabolism. Hydrolyzed to active metabolite. Primarily eliminated in feces. Unknown if removed by hemodialysis.

AVAILABILITY

Tablets: 10 mg ezetimibe/10 mg simvastatin, 10 mg ezetimibe/20 mg simvastatin, 10 mg ezetimibe/40 mg simvastatin, 10 mg ezetimibe/80 mg simvastatin (Vytorin).

E

INDICATIONS AND DOSAGES

▸ Homozygous Familial Hypercholesterolemia

PO

Adults. 10 mg/40 mg daily or 10 mg/80 mg daily.

▸ Primary Hypercholesterolemia

PO

Adults. Initially, 10 mg/20 mg daily. Initiate with a lower dose if the patient requires less aggressive LDL reductions. Initiate with a higher dose if the patient requires larger reduction in LDL.

CONTRAINDICATIONS

Active liver disease or unexplained, persistent elevations of liver function test results, age younger than 18 years, pregnancy

INTERACTIONS

Drug

Aluminum- and magnesium-containing antacids, cyclosporine, fenofibrate, gemfibrozil: Increase ezetimibe plasma concentration.
Cholestyramine: Decreases drug effectiveness.Cyclosporine, erythromycin, gemfibrozil, immunosuppressants, niacin: Increase the risk of acute renal failure and rhabdomyolysis.
Erythromycin, itraconazole, ketoconazole: May increase simvastatin blood concentration and cause muscle inflammation, pain, or weakness.

Herbal

None known.

Food

None known.

Drug interactions of concern to dentistry

- None reported

DIAGNOSTIC TEST EFFECTS

Ezetimibe may increase serum alkaline phosphatase, serum bilirubin, serum glutamate oxaloacetate (SGOT) (aspartate aminotransferase [AST]), and serum glutamate pyruvate transaminase (SGPT) (alanine aminotransferase [ALT]) levels. Simvastatin may increase serum creatine kinase and serum transaminase concentrations.

SIDE EFFECTS

Occasional

Headache, abdominal pain or cramps, constipation, upper respiratory tract infection, back pain, diarrhea, arthralgia, sinusitis

Rare

Cough, pharyngitis, fatigue, flatulence, asthenia (loss of strength and energy), nausea or vomiting

SERIOUS REACTIONS

! There is a potential for lens opacities.
! Hypersensitivity reaction and hepatitis occur rarely.

DENTAL CONSIDERATIONS

General:

- Consider semisupine chair position for patient comfort if GI, respiratory, or musculoskeletal side effects occur.
- Monitor vital signs at every appointment because of possible cardiovascular disease.

Teach Patient/Family:

- Importance of updating health and drug history if physician makes any changes in evaluation, drug regimens

famciclovir

fam-si′-klo-veer

(Famvir)

Do not confuse Famvir with Femhrt.

CATEGORY AND SCHEDULE

Pregnancy Risk Category: B

MECHANISM OF ACTION

A synthetic nucleoside that inhibits viral DNA synthesis. ***Therapeutic Effect:*** Suppresses replication of herpes simplex virus and varicella-zoster virus.

PHARMACOKINETICS

Rapidly and extensively absorbed after PO administration. Protein binding: 20%–25%. Rapidly metabolized to penciclovir by enzymes in the GI wall, liver, and plasma. Eliminated unchanged in urine. Removed by hemodialysis. ***Half-life:*** 2 hr.

AVAILABILITY

Tablets: 125 mg, 250 mg, 500 mg.

INDICATIONS AND DOSAGES

▸ Herpes Zoster

PO

Adults. 500 mg q8h for 7 days.

▸ Recurrent Genital Herpes

PO

Adults. 125 mg twice a day for 5 days.

▸ Suppression of Recurrent Genital Herpes

PO

Adults. 250 mg twice a day for up to 1 yr.

▸ Recurrent Herpes Simplex

PO

Adults. 500 mg twice a day for 7 days.

▸ Dosage in Renal Impairment

Dosage and frequency are modified on the basis of creatinine clearance.

Creatinine Clearance	Herpes Zoster	Genital Herpes
40–59 ml/min	500 mg q12h	125 mg q12h
20–39 ml/min	500 mg q24h	125 mg q24h
less than 20 ml/min	250 mg q24h	125 mg q24h

▸ Dosage in Hemodialysis Patients

For adults with herpes zoster, give 250 mg after each dialysis treatment; for adults with genital herpes, give 125 mg after each dialysis treatment.

CONTRAINDICATIONS

None known

INTERACTIONS

Drug

None known.

Herbal

None known.

Food

None known.

Drug interactions of concern to dentistry

- None reported in otherwise uncompromised patients

DIAGNOSTIC TEST EFFECTS

None known.

SIDE EFFECTS

Frequent

Headache (23%), nausea (12%)

Occasional (10%–2%)

Dizziness, somnolence, numbness of feet, diarrhea, vomiting, constipation, decreased appetite, fatigue, fever, pharyngitis, sinusitis, pruritus

Rare (<2%)

Insomnia, abdominal pain, dyspepsia, flatulence, back pain, arthralgia

F

SERIOUS REACTIONS

! None known.

DENTAL CONSIDERATIONS

General:

- Determine why the patient is taking the drug.
- Consider semisupine chair position for patient comfort because of GI effects of drug.
- Be aware of general discomfort associated with shingles; acute symptoms may preclude patient's routine dental visit or mandate short appointments.

Consultations:

- Medical consultation may be required to assess disease control and patient's ability to tolerate stress.

F

famotidine

fam-o′-tah-deen
(Amfamox[AUS], Novo-Famotidine[CAN] Pepcid, Pepcid AC, Pepcidine[AUS], Ulcidine[CAN])

CATEGORY AND SCHEDULE

Pregnancy Risk Category: B
OTC (10 mg tablets)

MECHANISM OF ACTION

An antiulcer agent and gastric acid secretion inhibitor that inhibits histamine action at histamine 2 receptors of parietal cells.
Therapeutic Effect: Inhibits gastric acid secretion when fasting, at night, or when stimulated by food, caffeine, or insulin.

PHARMACOKINETICS

Route	Onset	Peak	Duration
PO	1 hr	1–4 hr	10–12 hr
IV	1 hr	0.5–3 hr	10–12 hr

Rapidly, incompletely absorbed from the GI tract. Protein binding: 15%–20%. Partially metabolized in the liver. Primarily excreted in urine. Not removed by hemodialysis.
Half-life: 2.5–3.5 hr (increased with impaired renal function).

AVAILABILITY

Oral Suspension (Pepcid): 40 mg/5 ml.
Tablets (Pepcid): 20 mg, 40 mg.
Tablets (Pepcid AC): 10 mg, 20 mg.
Tablets (Chewable [Pepcid AC]): 10 mg.
Capsules (Pepcid AC): 10 mg.
Injection (Pepcid): 10 mg/ml.

INDICATIONS AND DOSAGES

▸ **Acute Treatment of Duodenal and Gastric Ulcers**

PO

Adults, Elderly, Children 12 yr and older. 40 mg/day at bedtime.
Children 1–11 yr. 0.5 mg/kg/day at bedtime. Maximum: 40 mg/day.

▸ **Duodenal Ulcer Maintenance**

PO

Adults, Elderly. 20 mg/day at bedtime.

▸ **Gastroesophageal Feflux Disease**

PO

Adults, Elderly, Children 12 yr and older. 20 mg twice a day.
Children 1–11 yr. 1 mg/kg/day in 2 divided doses.
Children 3 mo to 11 mo. 0.5 mg/kg/dose twice a day.
Children younger than 3 mo. 0.5 mg/kg/dose once a day.

▸ Esophagitis
PO
Adults, Elderly, Children 12 yr and older. 2–40 mg twice a day.
▸ Hypersecretory Conditions
PO
Adults, Elderly, Children 12 yr and older. Initially, 20 mg q6h. May increase up to 160 mg q6h.
▸ Acid Indigestion, Heartburn (Over-the-Counter)
PO
Adults, Elderly, Children 12 yr and older. 10–20 mg 15–60 min before eating. Maximum: 2 doses per day.
▸ Usual Parenteral Dosage
IV
Adults, Elderly, Children 12 yr and older. 20 mg q12h.
▸ Dosage in Renal Impairment
Dosing frequency is modified on the basis of creatinine clearance.

Creatinine Clearance	Dosing Frequency
10–50 ml/min	q24h
less than 10 ml/min	q36–48h

OFF-LABEL USES
Autism, prevention of aspiration pneumonitis

CONTRAINDICATIONS
None known.

INTERACTIONS
Drug
Antacids: May decrease the absorption of famotidine.
Ketoconazole: May decrease the absorption of ketoconazole.
Herbal
None known.
Food
None known.

Drug interactions of concern to dentistry
• Decreased absorption of ketoconazole or itraconazole (take doses 2 hr apart)

DIAGNOSTIC TEST EFFECTS
Interferes with skin tests using allergen extracts. May increase liver enzyme levels.

IV INCOMPATIBILITIES
Amphotericin B complex (Abelcet, Amphotec, AmBisome), cefepime (Maxipime), furosemide (Lasix), piperacillin/tazobactam (Zosyn)

IV COMPATIBILITIES
Calcium gluconate, dobutamine (Dobutrex), dopamine (Intropin), heparin, hydromorphone (Dilaudid), insulin (regular), lidocaine, lorazepam (Ativan), magnesium sulfate, midazolam (Versed), morphine, nitroglycerin, norepinephrine (Levophed), potassium chloride, potassium phosphate, propofol (Diprivan)

SIDE EFFECTS
Occasional (5%)
Headache
Rare (≤2%)
Constipation, diarrhea, dizziness

SERIOUS REACTIONS
! None known.

DENTAL CONSIDERATIONS
General:
• Avoid prescribing aspirin-containing products in patients with active GI disease.
• Consider semisupine chair position for patient comfort because of GI effects of disease.
• Assess salivary flow as a factor in caries, periodontal disease, and candidiasis.

Teach Patient/Family:
- Importance of good oral hygiene to prevent gingival inflammation
- *When chronic dry mouth occurs, advise patient:*
  - To avoid mouth rinses with high alcohol content because of drying effects
  - To use daily home fluoride products for anticaries effect
  - To use sugarless gum, frequent sips of water, or saliva substitutes

F

felbamate
fel-ba-mate
(Felbatol)

CATEGORY AND SCHEDULE
Pregnancy Risk Category: C

MECHANISM OF ACTION
An anticonvulsant, structurally similar to meprobamate, that weakly blocks repetitive, sustained firing of neurons by enhancing the ability of γ-aminobutyric acid (GABA), and antagonizes the strychnine-insensitive glycine recognition site of the *N*-methyl-D-aspartate receptor-ionophore complex.
Therapeutic Effect: Decreases seizure activity.

PHARMACOKINETICS
Rapidly and almost completely absorbed after PO administration. Protein binding: 22%–25%, primarily to albumin. Partially excreted unchanged in the urine.
Half-life: 20–23 hr.

AVAILABILITY
Tablets (Felbatol): 400 mg, 600 mg.
Oral Suspension (Felbatol): *600 mg/5 ml.*

INDICATIONS AND DOSAGES
▸ **Monotherapy or Adjunctive Therapy in the Treatment of Partial Seizures, with and without Generalization**
PO
Adults, children older than 14 yr. Initially, 1200 mg/day in divided doses 3–4 times daily.
At week 2, increase the felbamate dosage to 2400 mg/day while reducing the dosage of other antiepileptic drugs (AEDs) up to an additional one-third of their original dosage. At week 3, increase the felbamate dosage up to 3600 mg/day and continue to reduce the dosage of other AEDs as clinically indicated.
▸ **Adjunctive Therapy in the Treatment of Partial Seizures, with and without Generalization**
PO
Adults, children older than 14 yr. Add 1200 mg/day in divided doses 3–4 times daily while reducing present AEDs by 20% in order-control plasma concentrations of concurrent phenytoin, valproic acid, and carbamazepine and its metabolites. Increase dosage by 1200 mg/day increments at weekly intervals to 3600 mg/day.

CONTRAINDICATIONS
History of any blood dyscrasia or hepatic dysfunction, hypersensitivity to felbamate, its ingredients, or known sensitivity to other carbamates

INTERACTIONS
Drug
Carbamazepine, Phenytoin: May decrease blood concentration of felbamate.
Herbal
None known.
Food
None known.

Drug interactions of concern to dentistry

- Decreased effects of carbamazepine
- Increased photosensitization: drugs causing photosensitivity (e.g., tetracyclines)

DIAGNOSTIC TEST EFFECTS

None known.

SIDE EFFECTS

Frequent

Somnolence, dizziness, headache, fatigue, nausea, anorexia, vomiting, constipation

Occasional

Chest pain, palpitations, tachycardia, depression and behavioral changes, anxiety, nervousness, ataxia, malaise, agitation, rash, acne, pruritus, diarrhea, weight gain, tremors, abnormal vision, diplopia, sinusitis, difficulty with coordination, taste perversion

Rare

Delusion, bradycardia, hallucinations, urinary retention, acute renal failure

SERIOUS REACTIONS

! Alert

! Aplastic anemia has been reported during felbamate therapy.

! Hepatic failure resulting in death has been reported.

DENTAL CONSIDERATIONS

General:

- Examine for evidence of oral manifestations of blood dyscrasia (infection, bleeding, poor healing).
- Short appointments and a stress reduction protocol may be required for anxious patients.
- Determine type of epilepsy, seizure frequency, and quality of seizure control. A stress reduction protocol may be required.
- Assess salivary flow as a factor in caries, periodontal disease, and candidiasis.
- Monitor vital signs at every appointment because of cardiovascular side effects.
- Advise patient if dental drugs prescribed have a potential for photosensitivity.

Consultations:

- Medical consultation may be required to assess disease control and patient's ability to tolerate stress.

Teach Patient/Family:

- Importance of good oral hygiene to prevent soft tissue inflammation
- Caution to prevent injury when using oral hygiene aids
- Use of electric toothbrush if patient has difficulty holding conventional devices
- *When chronic dry mouth occurs, advise patient:*
  - To avoid mouth rinses with high alcohol content because of drying effects
  - To use daily home fluoride products for anticaries effect
  - To use sugarless gum, frequent sips of water, or saliva substitutes

felodipine

fell-o′-da-peen

(AGON SR[AUS], Felodur ER[AUS], Plendil, Plendil ER[AUS], Renedil[CAN])

Do not confuse Plendil with Pletal, or Renedil with Prinivil.

CATEGORY AND SCHEDULE

Pregnancy Risk Category: C

MECHANISM OF ACTION

An antihypertensive and antianginal agent that inhibits calcium movement

across cardiac and vascular smooth-muscle cell membranes. Potent peripheral vasodilator (does not depress SA or AV nodes).
Therapeutic Effect: Increases myocardial contractility, heart rate, and cardiac output; decreases peripheral vascular resistance and BP.

PHARMACOKINETICS

Route	Onset	Peak	Duration
PO	2–5 hr	N/A	N/A

Rapidly, completely absorbed from the GI tract. Protein binding: greater than 99%. Undergoes first-pass metabolism in the liver. Primarily excreted in urine. Not removed by hemodialysis. ***Half-life:*** 11–16 hr.

AVAILABILITY

Tablets (Extended-Release): 2.5 mg, 5 mg, 10 mg.

INDICATIONS AND DOSAGES

▸ Hypertension

PO

Adults. Initially, 5 mg/day as single dose.

Elderly, Patients with impaired hepatic function. Initially, 2.5 mg/day. Adjust dosage at no less than 2-wk intervals. Maintenance: 2.5–10 mg/day.

OFF-LABEL USES

Treatment of CHF, chronic angina pectoris, Raynaud's phenomenon

CONTRAINDICATIONS

None known.

INTERACTIONS

Drug

Beta blockers: May have additive effect.

Digoxin: May increase digoxin blood concentration.

Erythromycin: May increase felodipine blood concentration and risk of toxicity.

Hypokalemia-producing agents (such as fursosemide and certain other diuretics): May increase risk of arrhythmias.

Procainamide, quinidine: May increase risk of QT-interval prolongation.

Herbal

DHEA: May increase felodipine blood concentration.

Food

Grapefruit, grapefruit juice: May increase the absorption and blood concentration of felodipine.

Drug interactions of concern to dentistry

- Decreased effect: indomethacin, possibly other NSAIDs, phenobarbital, carbamazepine
- Increased effect: parenteral and inhalational general anesthetics, other drugs with hypotensive actions
- Increased effects of nondepolarizing muscle relaxants, diazepam, midazolam
- Increased plasma levels: itraconazole, erythromycin, carbamazepine

DIAGNOSTIC TEST EFFECTS

None known.

SIDE EFFECTS

Frequent (22%–18%)

Headache, peripheral edema

Occasional (6%–4%)

Flushing, respiratory infection, dizziness, light-headedness, asthenia (loss of strength, weakness)

Rare (<3%)

Paresthesia, abdominal discomfort, nervousness, muscle cramping, cough, diarrhea, constipation

SERIOUS REACTIONS

! Overdose produces nausea, somnolence, confusion, slurred speech, hypotension, and bradycardia.

DENTAL CONSIDERATIONS

General:

- Monitor cardiac status; take vital signs at each appointment because of cardiovascular side effects. Consider a stress reduction protocol to prevent stress-induced angina during the dental appointment.
- After supine positioning, have patient sit upright for at least 2 min before standing to avoid orthostatic hypotension at dismissal.
- Place on frequent recall to monitor gingival condition.
- Limit use of sodium-containing products, such as saline IV fluids, for patients with a dietary salt restriction.
- Assess salivary flow as a factor in caries, periodontal disease, and candidiasis.
- Use vasoconstrictors with caution, in low doses, and with careful aspiration. Avoid use of gingival retraction cord with epinephrine.
- Use precaution if sedation or general anesthesia is required; risk of hypotensive episode.

Consultations:

- Medical consultation may be required to assess disease control.
- Consultation with physician may be necessary if sedation or general anesthesia is required.

Teach Patient/Family:

- Importance of good oral hygiene to prevent gingival inflammation and minimize hyperplasia
- Need for frequent oral prophylaxis if hyperplasia occurs
- *When chronic dry mouth occurs, advise patient:*
  - To avoid mouth rinses with high alcohol content because of drying effects
  - To use daily home fluoride products for anticaries effect
  - To use sugarless gum, frequent sips of water, or saliva substitutes

F

fenofibrate

fee-no-fye′-brate

(Apo-Fenofibrate[CAN], Lafibra, Tricor)

Do not confuse Tricor with Tracleer.

CATEGORY AND SCHEDULE

Pregnancy Risk Category: C

MECHANISM OF ACTION

An antihyperlipidemic that enhances synthesis of lipoprotein lipase and reduces triglyceride-rich lipoproteins and VLDLs. ***Therapeutic Effect:*** Increases VLDL catabolism and reduces total plasma triglyceride levels.

PHARMACOKINETICS

Well absorbed from the GI tract. Absorption increased when given with food. Protein binding: 99%. Rapidly metabolized in the liver to active metabolite. Excreted primarily in urine; lesser amount in feces. Not removed by hemodialysis. ***Half-life:*** 20 hr.

AVAILABILITY

Capsules (Lafibra): 67 mg, 134 mg, 200 mg.
*Tablets (Tricor):*48 mg, 154 mg.

INDICATIONS AND DOSAGES

▸ Reduction of Very High Serum Triglyceride Levels in Patients at Risk for Pancreatitis

PO

Adults, Elderly. Initially, 67 mg/day(capsule); may increase to 200 mg/day. Or initially, 48 mg/day(tablet); may increase to 145 mg/day.

▸ Hypercholesterolemia

PO

Adults, Elderly. 200 mg/day (capsule) with meals. Or 145 mg/day(tablet) with meals.

CONTRAINDICATIONS

Gallbladder disease, hypersensitivity to fenofibrate, severe renal or hepatic dysfunction (including primary biliary cirrhosis, unexplained persistent liver function abnormality)

INTERACTIONS

Drug

Anticoagulants: Potentiates effects of these drugs.
Bile acid sequestrants: May impede fenofibrate absorption.
Cyclosporine: Increases risk of nephrotoxicity.
HMG-CoA reductase inhibitors: Increases risk of severe myopathy, rhabdomyolysis, and acute renal failure.

Herbal

None known.

Food

All foods: Increase absorption of fenofibrate.

Drug interactions of concern to dentistry

- None reported

DIAGNOSTIC TEST EFFECTS

May increase BUN and serum CK, AST(SGOT), and ALT(SGPT), levels. May decrease blood Hgb and Hct levels, serum uric acid level, and WBC count.

SIDE EFFECTS

Frequent (8%–4%)

Pain, rash, headache, asthenia or fatigue, flu symptoms, dyspepsia, nausea or vomiting, rhinitis

Occasional (3%–2%)

Diarrhea, abdominal pain, constipation, flatulence, arthralgia, decreased libido, dizziness, pruritus

Rare (<2%)

Increased appetite, insomnia, polyuria, cough, blurred vision, eye floaters, earache

SERIOUS REACTIONS

! Fenofibrate may increase excretion of cholesterol into bile, leading to cholelithiasis.
! Pancreatitis, hepatitis, thrombocytopenia, and agranulocytosis occur rarely.

DENTAL CONSIDERATIONS

General:

- Monitor vital signs at every appointment because of cardiovascular and respiratory side effects.
- Consider semisupine chair position for patient comfort because of GI side effects of drug.
- Patients on chronic drug therapy may rarely have symptoms of blood dyscrasias, which can include infection, bleeding, and poor healing.
- Avoid dental light in patient's eyes; offer dark glasses for patient comfort.

Consultations:

- In a patient with symptoms of blood dyscrasias, request a medical consultation for blood studies and postpone treatment until normal values are reestablished.

Teach Patient/Family:
- Use of electric toothbrush if patient has difficulty holding conventional devices
- To prevent trauma when using oral hygiene aids

fenoprofen calcium
fen-oh-proe′-fen
(Nalfon)
Do not confuse Nalfon with Naldecon.

CATEGORY AND SCHEDULE
Pregnancy Risk Category: B (D if used in third trimester or near delivery)

MECHANISM OF ACTION
An NSAID that produces analgesic and anti-inflammatory effects by inhibiting prostaglandin synthesis. ***Therapeutic Effect:*** Reduces the inflammatory response and intensity of pain.

AVAILABILITY
Capsules: 200 mg, 300 mg.
Tablets: 600 mg.

INDICATIONS AND DOSAGES
▸ Mild to Moderate Pain
PO
Adults, Elderly. 200 mg q4–6h as needed.
▸ Rheumatoid Arthritis, Osteoarthritis
PO
Adults, Elderly. 300–600 mg 3–4 times a day.

OFF-LABEL USES
Treatment of ankylosing spondylitis, psoriatic arthritis, vascular headaches

CONTRAINDICATIONS
Active peptic ulcer disease, chronic inflammation of GI tract, GI bleeding or ulceration, history of hypersensitivity to aspirin or NSAIDs, significant renal impairment

INTERACTIONS
Drug
Antihypertensives, diuretics: May decrease the effects of these drugs.
Aspirin, other salicylates: May increase the risk of GI side effects such as bleeding.
Bone marrow depressants: May increase the risk of hematologic reactions.
Heparin, oral anticoagulants, thrombolytics: May increase the effects of these drugs.
Lithium: May increase the blood concentration and risk of toxicity of lithium.
Methotrexate: May increase the risk of methotrexate toxicity.
Probenecid: May increase fenoprofen blood concentration.
Herbal
None known.
Food
None known.
Drug interactions of concern to dentistry
- GI bleeding, ulceration: salicylates, alcohol, corticosteroids, other NSAIDs, biphosphonates
- May decrease effects of fenoprofen: phenobarbital
- Nephrotoxicity: acetaminophen (prolonged use)
- Possible risk of decreased renal function: cyclosporine
- Probable increased bleeding risk: warfarin
- Suspected increased risk for methotrexate toxicity
- First-time users of SSRIs also taking NSAIDs may have a higher risk of GI side effects; until more

data are available, it may be advisable to avoid use of NSAIDs in these patients (*Br J Clin Pharmacol* 55:591–595, 2003)

DIAGNOSTIC TEST EFFECTS

May increase bleeding time, BUN and blood glucose levels, and serum protein, alkaline phosphatase, LDH, creatinine, AST (SGOT), and ALT (SGPT) levels.

SIDE EFFECTS

Frequent (9%–3%)

Headache, somnolence, dyspepsia, nausea, vomiting, constipation

Occasional (2%–1%)

Dizziness, pruritus, nervousness, asthenia, diarrhea, abdominal cramps, flatulence, tinnitus, blurred vision, peripheral edema and fluid retention

SERIOUS REACTIONS

! Overdose may result in acute hypotension and tachycardia.

! Rare reactions with long-term use include peptic ulcer disease, GI bleeding, gastritis, severe hepatic reaction (jaundice), nephrotoxicity (hematuria, dysuria, proteinuria), and a severe hypersensitivity reaction (bronchospasm, angioedema).

DENTAL CONSIDERATIONS

General:

- Assess salivary flow as a factor in caries, periodontal disease, and candidiasis.
- Avoid prescribing for dental use in pregnancy.
- Possibility of cross-allergenicity when patient is allergic to aspirin.

Consultations:

- Medical consultation may be required to assess disease control.

Teach Patient/Family:

- Importance of good oral hygiene to prevent gingival inflammation
- Caution to prevent injury when using oral hygiene aids
- *When chronic dry mouth occurs, advise patient:*
  - To avoid mouth rinses with high alcohol content because of drying effects
  - To use daily home fluoride products for anticaries effect
  - To use sugarless gum, frequent sips of water, or saliva substitutes

ferrous fumarate/ ferrous gluconate/ ferrous sulfate

fer′-rous fume′-ah-rate/fer′-rous glue′-kuh-nate/fer′-rous sul′-fate

(ferrous fumarate)Feostat, Femiron, Ferro-Sequels, Nephro-Fer, Palafer[CAN](ferrous gluconate)Apo-Ferrous Gluconate[CAN], Fergon(ferrous sulfate) Apo-Ferrous Sulfate[CAN], Fer-In-Sol, Fer-Iron, Ferro-Gradumet[AUS], Slow-Fe

CATEGORY AND SCHEDULE

Pregnancy Risk Category: A

OTC

MECHANISM OF ACTION

An enzymatic mineral that is an essential component in the formation of Hgb, myoglobin, and enzymes. Promotes effective erythropoiesis and transport and utilization of oxygen (O_2). ***Therapeutic Effect:*** Prevents iron deficiency.

PHARMACOKINETICS

Absorbed in the duodenum and upper jejunum. Ten percent absorbed in patients with normal iron stores; increased to 20%–30% in those with inadequate iron stores. Primarily bound to serum transferrin. Excreted in urine, sweat, and sloughing of intestinal mucosa and by menses. ***Half-life:*** 6 hr.

AVAILABILITY

Ferrous fumarate
Tablets (Femiron): 63 mg (20 mg elemental iron).
Tablets (Nephro-Fer): 350 mg (115 mg elemental iron).
Tablets (Chewable [Feostat]): 100 mg (33 mg elemental iron).
Tablet (Time-Release [Ferro-Sequels]): 150 mg (50 mg elemental iron).
Ferrous gluconate
Tablets: 325 mg (36 mg elemental iron).
Tablets (Fergon): 240 mg (27 mg elemental iron).
Ferrous sulfate
Tablets: 325 mg (65 mg elemental iron).
Tablets (Timed-Release [Slow FE]): 160 mg (50 mg elemental iron).
Elixir: 220 mg/5 ml (44 mg elemental iron per 5 ml).
Oral Drops (Ferr-In-Sol, Fer-Iron): 75 mg/0.6 ml.

INDICATIONS AND DOSAGES

▸ Iron Deficiency Anemia

Dosage is expressed in terms of milligrams of elemental iron, degree of anemia, patient weight, and presence of any bleeding. Expect to use periodic hematologic determinations as guide to therapy.
PO (ferrous fumarate)
Adults, Elderly. 60–100 mg twice a day.
Children. 3–6 mg/kg/day in 2–3 divided doses.
PO (ferrous gluconate)
Adults, Elderly. 60 mg 2–4 times a day.
Children. 3–6 mg/kg/day in 2–3 divided doses.
PO (ferrous sulfate)
Adults, Elderly. 325 mg 2–4 times a day.
Children. 3–6 mg/kg/day in 2–3 divided doses.

▸ Prevention of Iron Deficiency

PO (ferrous fumarate)
Adults, Elderly. 60–100 mg/day.
Children. 1–2 mg/kg/day.
PO (ferrous gluconate)
Adults, Elderly. 60 mg/day.
Children. 1–2 mg/kg/day.
PO (ferrous sulfate)
Adults, Elderly. 325 mg/day.
Children. 1–2 mg/kg/day.

CONTRAINDICATIONS

Hemochromatosis, hemosiderosis, hemolytic anemias, peptic ulcer disease, regional enteritis, ulcerative colitis

INTERACTIONS

Drug

Antacids, calcium supplements, pancreatin, pancrelipase: May decrease the absorption of ferrous fumarate, ferrous gluconate, and ferrous sulfate.
Etidronate, quinolones, tetracyclines: May decrease the absorption of etidronate, quinolones, and tetracyclines.

Herbal

None known.

Food

Eggs, milk: Inhibit ferrous fumarate absorption.

Drug interactions of concern to dentistry

- Decreased absorption of tetracycline, zinc, ciprofloxacin

DIAGNOSTIC TEST EFFECTS

May increase serum bilirubin and iron levels. May decrease serum calcium level. May obscure occult blood in stools.

F

SIDE EFFECTS

Occasional
Mild, transient nausea
Rare
Heartburn, anorexia, constipation, diarrhea

SERIOUS REACTIONS

! Large doses may aggravate existing GI tract disease, such as peptic ulcer disease, regional enteritis, and ulcerative colitis.
! Severe iron poisoning occurs most often in children and is manifested as vomiting, severe abdominal pain, diarrhea, and dehydration, followed by hyperventilation, pallor or cyanosis, and cardiovascular collapse.

DENTAL CONSIDERATIONS

Teach Patient/Family:
- If patient is using hydrogen peroxide as a dentifrice to remove extrinsic stain, caution against frequent use to avoid peroxide-related soft tissue injury
- That liquid iron preparation taken through straw followed by rinsing mouth can reduce staining

fexofenadine hydrochloride

fex-oh-fen′-eh-deen
(Allegra, Telfast[AUS])

CATEGORY AND SCHEDULE

Pregnancy Risk Category: C

MECHANISM OF ACTION

A piperidine that competes with histamine for H_1-receptor sites on effector cells. ***Therapeutic Effect:*** Relieves allergic rhinitis symptoms.

PHARMACOKINETICS

Rapidly absorbed after PO administration. Protein binding: 60%–70%. Does not cross the blood-brain barrier. Minimally metabolized. Eliminated in feces and urine. Not removed by hemodialysis. ***Half-life:*** 14.4 hr (increased in renal impairment).

AVAILABILITY

Tablets: 30 mg, 60 mg, 180 mg.

INDICATIONS AND DOSAGES

▸ Allergic Rhinitis, Urticaria

PO
Adults, Elderly, Children 12 yr and older. 60 mg twice a day or 180 mg once a day.
Children 6–11 yr. 30 mg twice a day.

▸ Dosage in Renal Impairment

For adults, elderly, and children 12 years and older, dosage is reduced to 60 mg once a day. For children 6–11 years, dosage is reduced to 30 mg once a day.

CONTRAINDICATIONS

None known.

INTERACTIONS

Drug
Antacids: May decrease fexofenadine absorption if given within 15 minutes of a fexofenadine dose.
Herbal
None known.
Food
None known.
Drug interactions of concern to dentistry
- Elevated plasma levels with erythromycin, ketoconazole
- Decreased absorption: grapefruit juice
- Suspected decreased antihistaminic effects: rifampin

DIAGNOSTIC TEST EFFECTS

May suppress wheal and flare reactions to antigen skin testing unless drug is discontinued at least 4 days before testing.

SIDE EFFECTS

Rare (<2%)
Somnolence, headache, fatigue, nausea, vomiting, abdominal distress, dysmenorrhea

SERIOUS REACTIONS

! None known.

DENTAL CONSIDERATIONS

General:

- Consider semisupine chair position for patient comfort because of GI effects of drug.

filgrastim

fill-grass′-tim
(Neupogen)
Do not confuse Neupogen with Epogen or Nutramigen.

CATEGORY AND SCHEDULE

Pregnancy Risk Category: C

MECHANISM OF ACTION

A biologic modifier that stimulates production, maturation, and activation of neutrophils to increase their migration and cytotoxicity. ***Therapeutic Effect:*** Decreases incidence of infection.

PHARMACOKINETICS

Readily absorbed after subcutaneous administration. Not removed by hemodialysis. ***Half-life:*** 3.5 hr.

AVAILABILITY

Injection: 300 mcg/ml, 480 mcg/0.8 ml.

INDICATIONS AND DOSAGES

▸ **Myelosuppression**
IV OR SUBCUTANEOUS INFUSION, SUBCUTANEOUS INJECTION
Adults, Elderly. Initially, 5 mcg/kg/day. May increase by 5 mcg/ kg for each chemotherapy cycle on the basis of duration or severity of absolute neutrophil count nadir.

▸ **Bone Marrow Transplant**
IV OR SUBCUTANEOUS INFUSION
Adults, Elderly. 5–10 mcg/kg/day. Adjust dosage daily during period of neutrophil recovery on the basis of neutrophil response.

▸ **Mobilization Progenitor Cells**
IV OR SUBCUTANEOUS INFUSION
Adults. 10 mcg/kg/day beginning at least 4 days before first leukapheresis and continuing until last leukapheresis.

▸ **Chronic Neutropenia, Congenital Neutropenia**
SUBCUTANEOUS
Adults, Children. 6 mcg/kg/dose twice a day.

▸ **Idiopathic or Cyclic Neutropenia**
SUBCUTANEOUS
Adults, Children. 5 mcg/kg/dose once a day.

OFF-LABEL USES

Treatment of AIDS-related neutropenia; drug-induced neutropenia; myelodysplastic syndrome

CONTRAINDICATIONS

Hypersensitivity to *Escherichia coli*–derived proteins, 24 hours before or after cytotoxic chemotherapy, concurrent use of other drugs that may result in lowered platelet count

F

INTERACTIONS

Drug

None known.

Herbal

None known.

Food

None known.

Drug interactions of concern to dentistry

- Dental drug interactions have not been studied

DIAGNOSTIC TEST EFFECTS

May increase LDH concentrations, leukocyte alkaline phosphatase (LAP) scores, and serum alkaline phosphatase and uric acid levels.

IV INCOMPATIBILITIES

Amphotericin (Fungizone), cefepime (Maxipime), cefotaxime (Claforan), cefoxitin (Mefoxin), ceftizoxime (Cefizox), ceftriaxone (Rocephin), cefuroxime (Zinacef), clindamycin (Cleocin), dactinomycin (Cosmegen), etoposide (VePesid), fluorouracil, furosemide (Lasix), heparin, mannitol, methylprednisolone (Solu-Medrol), mitomycin (Mutamycin), prochlorperazine (Compazine)

IV COMPATIBILITIES

Bumetanide (Bumex), calcium gluconate, hydromorphone (Dilaudid), lorazepam (Ativan), morphine, potassium chloride

SIDE EFFECTS

Frequent

Nausea or vomiting (57%), mild to severe bone pain (22%) that occurs more frequently with high-dose IV form and less frequently with low-dose subcutaneous form; alopecia (18%), diarrhea (14%), fever (12%), fatigue (11%)

Occasional (9%–5%)

Anorexia, dyspnea, headache, cough, rash

Rare (<5%)

Psoriasis, hematuria or proteinuria, osteoporosis

SERIOUS REACTIONS

! Long-term administration occasionally produces chronic neutropenia and splenomegaly.

! Thrombocytopenia, MI, and arrhythmias occur rarely.

! Adult respiratory distress syndrome may occur in patients with sepsis.

DENTAL CONSIDERATIONS

General:

- Determine why patient is taking the drug.
- Examine for oral manifestation of opportunistic infection.
- Monitor vital signs at every appointment due to cardiovascular side effects.
- Patient may need assistance in getting into and out of dental chair. Adjust chair position for patient comfort.
- Patients are at risk for infection.
- Oral infections should be eliminated and/or treated aggressively.
- Patients may have been treated with radiation and/or chemotherapy; confirm medical and drug history.

Consultations:

- Medical consultation may be required to assess disease control and patient's ability to tolerate stress.
- In a patient with symptoms of blood dyscrasias, request a medical consultation for blood studies and postpone treatment until normal values are reestablished.
- Medical consultation should include routine blood counts including platelet counts and bleeding time.

Teach Patient/Family:

- Importance of good oral hygiene to prevent soft tissue inflammation

• To prevent trauma when using oral hygiene aids
• Importance of updating health and medication history if physician makes any changes in evaluation or drug regimens; include OTC, herbal, and nonherbal remedies in the update
• To maintain fastidious oral hygiene

finasteride

feen-as′-ter-ide
(Propecia, Proscar)
Do not confuse Proscar with Posicor, ProSom, Prozac, or Psorcon.

CATEGORY AND SCHEDULE

Pregnancy Risk Category: X

MECHANISM OF ACTION

An androgen hormone inhibitor that inhibits 5-alpha reductase, an intracellular enzyme that converts testosterone into dihydrotestosterone (DHT) in the prostate gland, resulting in a decreased serum DHT level. ***Therapeutic Effect:*** Reduces size of the prostate gland.

PHARMACOKINETICS

Route	Onset	Peak	Duration
PO	24 hr	1–2 days	5–7 days

Rapidly absorbed from the GI tract. Protein binding: 90%. Widely distributed. Metabolized in the liver. ***Half-life:*** 6–8 hr. Onset of clinical effect: 3–6 mo of continued therapy.

AVAILABILITY

Tablets (Propecia): 1 mg.
Tablets (Proscar): 5 mg.

INDICATIONS AND DOSAGES

▸ **Benign Prostatic Hyperplasia (BPH)**
PO
Adults, Elderly. 5 mg once a day (for a minimum of 6 mo).
▸ **Hair Loss**
PO
Adults. 1 mg/day.

OFF-LABEL USES

Adjuvant monotherapy after radical prostatectomy in treatment of prostate cancer

CONTRAINDICATIONS

Exposure to the patient's semen or handling of finasteride tablets by those who are or may be pregnant

INTERACTIONS

Drug
None known.
Herbal
None known.
Food
None known.
Drug interactions of concern to dentistry
• Opioids and anticholinergic drugs may enhance urinary retention; use alternative analgesics (NSAIDs)

DIAGNOSTIC TEST EFFECTS

Decreases the serum prostate-specific antigen (PSA) level, even in patients with prostate cancer

SIDE EFFECTS

Rare (4%–2%)
Gynecomastia, sexual dysfunction (impotence, decreased libido, decreased volume of ejaculate)

SERIOUS REACTIONS

! None known.

DENTAL CONSIDERATIONS

Consultations:

- Determine why patient is taking the drug (for prostatic hyperplasia or male pattern baldness).
- Medical consultation may be required to assess disease control.

flavocoxid

flay-vox′-ah-sid
(Limbrel)

CATEGORY AND SCHEDULE

Pregnancy Risk Category: Not classified.

MECHANISM OF ACTION

An oral nutritional supplement that inhibits prostaglandin synthesis and arachidonic acid metabolism, reducing the production of leukotrienes. Also acts through an antioxidant mechanism. ***Therapeutic Effect:*** Produces anti-inflammatory and analgesic effects and increases mobility.

PHARMACOKINETICS

Undergoes hydrolysis at the gut mucosal border. Food decreases absorption. Little hepatic metabolism.

AVAILABILITY

Capsules: 250 mg.

INDICATIONS AND DOSAGES

▶ **Osteoarthritis**

PO

Adults 18 yr and older, Elderly. One 250-mg capsule q12h.

CONTRAINDICATIONS

History of peptic ulcer

INTERACTIONS

Drug

None known.

Herbal

None known.

Food

All foods: Decrease the absorption of flavocoxid.

Drug interactions of concern to dentistry

- None reported

DIAGNOSTIC TEST EFFECTS

None known.

SIDE EFFECTS

Rare (2%)

Increase in varicose veins, psoriasis, mild hypertension

SERIOUS REACTIONS

! GI bleeding, perforation, and ulceration occur rarely in patients currently or previously treated with NSAIDs or COX-2 inhibitors.

DENTAL CONSIDERATIONS

General:

- Determine why patient is taking the drug.
- Patient may need assistance in getting into and out of dental chair. Adjust chair position for patient comfort.
- Patients presenting with a history of osteoarthritis will be taking other agents; confirm medical and drug/herbal and nonherbal history.

Consultations:

- Medical consultation may be required to assess disease control and patient's ability to tolerate stress

Teach Patient/Family:
- Use of electric toothbrush if patient has difficulty holding conventional devices
- Importance of good oral hygiene to prevent soft tissue inflammation
- To prevent trauma when using oral hygiene aids
- Importance of updating health and medication history if physician makes any changes in evaluation or drug regimens; include OTC, herbal, and nonherbal remedies in the update

flavoxate

fla-vox′-ate
(Urispas)
Do not confuse Urispas with Urised.

CATEGORY AND SCHEDULE
Pregnancy Risk Category: B

MECHANISM OF ACTION
An anticholinergic that relaxes detrusor and other smooth muscle by cholinergic blockade, counteracting muscle spasm in the urinary tract. ***Therapeutic Effect:*** Produces anticholinergic, local anesthetic, and analgesic effects, relieving urinary symptoms.

AVAILABILITY
Tablets: 100 mg.

INDICATIONS AND DOSAGES
▸ To Relieve Symptoms of Cystitis, Prostatitis, Urethritis, Urethrocystitis, or Urethrotrigonitis
PO
Adults, Elderly, Adolescents. 100–200 mg 3–4 times a day.

CONTRAINDICATIONS
Duodenal or pyloric obstruction, GI hemorrhage or obstruction, ileus, lower urinary tract obstruction

INTERACTIONS
Drug
None known.
Herbal
None known.
Food
None known.
Drug interactions of concern to dentistry
- Increased anticholinergic effect: anticholinergic drugs
- Drug may cause drowsiness or blurred vision: advise patients when other CNS depressants are used

DIAGNOSTIC TEST EFFECTS
None known.

SIDE EFFECTS
Frequent
Somnolence, dry mouth and throat
Occasional
Constipation, difficult urination, blurred vision, dizziness, headache, increased light sensitivity, nausea, vomiting, abdominal pain
Rare
Confusion (primarily in elderly), hypersensitivity, increased IOP, leukopenia

SERIOUS REACTIONS
! Overdose may produce anticholinergic effects, including unsteadiness, severe dizziness, somnolence, fever, facial flushing, dyspnea, nervousness, and irritability.

DENTAL CONSIDERATIONS
General:
- Assess salivary flow as a factor in caries, periodontal disease, and candidiasis.

Teach Patient/Family:
- Importance of good oral hygiene to prevent gingival inflammation
- To avoid mouth rinses with high alcohol content because of drying effects

F

flecainide

fle′-kah-nide
(Flecatab[AUS], Tambocor)

CATEGORY AND SCHEDULE

Pregnancy Risk Category: C

MECHANISM OF ACTION

An antiarrhythmic that slows atrial, AV, His-Purkinje, and intraventricular conduction. Decreases excitability, conduction velocity, and automaticity. ***Therapeutic Effect:*** Controls atrial, supraventricular, and ventricular arrhythmias.

AVAILABILITY

Tablets: 50 mg, 100 mg.

INDICATIONS AND DOSAGES

▸ **Life-Threatening Ventricular Arrhythmias, Sustained Ventricular Tachycardia**

PO

Adults, Elderly. Initially, 100 mg q12h, increased by 100 mg (50 mg twice a day) every 4 days until effective dose or maximum of 400 mg/day is attained.

▸ **Paroxysmal Supraventricular Tachycardias (PSVT), Paroxysmal Atrial Fibrillation (PAF)**

PO

Adults, Elderly. Initially, 50 mg q12h, increased by 100 mg (50 mg twice a day) every 4 days until effective dose or maximum of 300 mg/day is attained.

CONTRAINDICATIONS

Cardiogenic shock, pre-existing second- or third-degree AV block, right bundle-branch block (without presence of a pacemaker)

INTERACTIONS

Drug

Beta blockers: May increase negative inotropic effects.
Digoxin: May increase blood concentration of digoxin.
Other antiarrhythmics: May have additive effects.
Urinary acidifiers: May increase the excretion of flecainide.
Urinary alkalinizers: May decrease the excretion of flecainide.

Herbal

None known.

Food

None known.

Drug interactions of concern to dentistry

- No specific interactions are reported with dental drugs; however, any drug that could affect the cardiac action of flecainide (e.g., other local anesthetics, vasoconstrictors, anticholinergics) should be used in the lowest effective dose.

DIAGNOSTIC TEST EFFECTS

None significant.

SIDE EFFECTS

Frequent (19%–10%)

Dizziness, dyspnea, headache

Occasional (9%–4%)

Nausea, fatigue, palpitations, chest pain, asthenia (loss of strength, energy), tremor, constipation

SERIOUS REACTIONS

! Flecainide may worsen existing arrhythmias or produce new ones.
! CHF may occur or existing CHF may worsen.
! Overdose may increase QRS duration, prolong QT interval, cause

conduction disturbances, reduce myocardial contractility, and cause hypotension.

DENTAL CONSIDERATIONS

General:

- Monitor vital signs at every appointment because of cardiovascular and respiratory side effects.
- Assess salivary flow as a factor in caries, periodontal disease, and candidiasis.
- Stress from dental procedures may compromise cardiovascular function; determine patient risk.
- Use vasoconstrictors with caution, in low doses, and with careful aspiration. Avoid use of gingival retraction cord with epinephrine.

Consultations:

- Medical consultation may be required to assess disease control and patient's ability to tolerate stress.

Teach Patient/Family:

- Importance of good oral hygiene to prevent gingival inflammation
- To avoid mouth rinses with high alcohol content because of drying effects

fluconazole

floo-con′-a-zole
(Apo-Fluconazole[CAN], Diflucan)
Do not confuse Diflucan with diclofenac.

CATEGORY AND SCHEDULE

Pregnancy Risk Category: C

MECHANISM OF ACTION

A fungistatic antifungal that interferes with cytochrome P-450, an enzyme necessary for ergosterol formation. ***Therapeutic Effect:*** Directly damages fungal membrane, altering its function.

PHARMACOKINETICS

Well absorbed from GI tract. Widely distributed, including to CSF. Protein binding: 11%. Partially metabolized in liver. Excreted unchanged primarily in urine. Partially removed by hemodialysis. ***Half-life:*** 20–30 hr (increased in impaired renal function).

AVAILABILITY

Tablets: 50 mg, 100 mg, 150 mg, 200 mg.
Powder for Oral Suspension: 10 mg/ml, 40 mg/ml.
Injection: 2 mg/ml (in 100- or 200-ml containers).

INDICATIONS AND DOSAGES

▸ Oropharyngeal Candidiasis

PO, IV

Adults, Elderly. 200 mg once, then 100 mg/day for at least 14 days.
Children. 6 mg/kg/day once, then 3 mg/kg/day.

▸ Esophageal Candidiasis

PO, IV

Adults, Elderly. 200 mg once, then 100 mg/day (up to 400 mg/day) for 21 days and at least 14 days following resolution of symptoms.
Children. 6 mg/kg/day once, then 3 mg/kg/day (up to 12 mg/kg/day) for 21 days at at least 14 days following resolution of symptoms.

▸ Vaginal Candidiasis

PO

Adults. 150 mg once.

▸ Prevention of Candidiasis in Patients Undergoing Bone Marrow Transplantation

PO

Adults. 400 mg/day.

F

▸ **Systemic Candidiasis**
PO, IV
Adults, Elderly. 400 mg once, then 200 mg/day (up to 400 mg/day) for at least 28 days and at least 14 days following resolution of symptoms.
Children. 6–12 mg/kg/day.

▸ **Cryptococcal Meningitis**
PO, IV
Adults, Elderly. 400 mg once, then 200 mg/day (up to 800 mg/day) for 10–12 wk after CSF becomes negative (200 mg/day for suppression of relapse in patients with AIDS).
Children. 12 mg/kg/day once, then 6–12 mg/kg/day (6 mg/kg/day for suppression of relapse in patients with AIDS).

▸ **Onychomycosis**
PO
Adults. 150 mg/wk.

▸ **Dosage in Renal Impairment**
After a loading dose of 400 mg, the daily dosage is based on creatinine clearance:

Creatinine Clearance	% of Recommended Dose
greater than 50 ml/min	100
21–50 ml/min	50
11–20 ml/min	25
Dialysis	Dose after dialysis

OFF-LABEL USES
Treatment of coccidioidomycosis, cryptococcosis, fungal pneumonia, onychomycosis, ringworm of the hand, septicemia

CONTRAINDICATIONS
None known.

INTERACTIONS
Drug
Cyclosporine: High fluconazole doses increase cyclosporine blood concentration.
Oral antidiabetics: May increase blood concentration and effects of oral antidiabetics.
Phenytoin, warfarin: May decrease the metabolism of these drugs.
Rifampin: May increase fluconazole metabolism.

Herbal
None known.

Food
None known.

Drug interactions of concern to dentistry
- Caution: potent inhibitor of cytochrome P450 3A4 isoenzymes
- Increased plasma levels of oral hypoglycemics: theophylline, cyclosporine, tacrolimus, corticosteroids
- Inhibits metabolism of certain benzodiazepines: alprazolam, chlordiazepoxide, clonazepam, clorazepate, diazepam, estazolam, flurazepam, halazepam, midazolam, triazolam, quazepam, zolpidem
- Increased anticoagulant effect: may inhibit metabolism of warfarin
- Suspected risk of increased neurologic side effects: haloperidol, tricyclic antidepressants
- May increase levels and side effects of HMG-CoA reductase inhibitors

Suspected increase in antihypertensive effects of losartan; monitor blood pressure if used concurrently
- Decreased renal clearance: hydrochlorothiazide
- Suspected decrease in oral contraceptive effectiveness; may want to suggest additional contraception

DIAGNOSTIC TEST EFFECTS
May increase serum alkaline phosphatase, serum bilirubin, AST(SGOT), and ALT(SGPT) levels.

IV INCOMPATIBILITIES

Amphotericin B (Fungizone), amphotericin B complex (Abelcet, Ambisome, Amphotec), ampicillin (Polycillin), calcium gluconate, cefotaxime (Claforan), ceftazidime (Fortaz), ceftriaxone (Rocephin), cefuroxime (Zinacef), chloramphenicol (Chloromycetin), clindamycin (Cleocin), co-trimoxazole (Bactrim), diazepam (Valium), digoxin (Lanoxin), erythromycin (Erythrocin), furosemide (Lasix), haloperidol (Haldol), hydroxyzine (Vistaril), imipenem and cilastatin (Primaxin)

IV COMPATIBILITIES

Diltiazem (Cardizem), dobutamine (Dobutrex), dopamine (Intropin), heparin, lorazepam (Ativan), midazolam (Versed), propofol (Diprivan)

SIDE EFFECTS

Occasional (4%–1%)

Hypersensitivity reaction (including chills, fever, pruritus, and rash), dizziness, drowsiness, headache, constipation, diarrhea, nausea, vomiting, abdominal pain

SERIOUS REACTIONS

! Exfoliative skin disorders, serious hepatic effects, and blood dyscrasias (such as eosinophilia, thrombocytopenia, anemia, and leukopenia) have been reported rarely.

DENTAL CONSIDERATIONS

General:

- Culture may be required to confirm fungal organism.
- Patients on chronic drug therapy may rarely have symptoms of blood dyscrasias, which can include infection, bleeding, and poor healing.

Consultations:

- In a patient with symptoms of blood dyscrasias, request a medical consultation for blood studies and postpone treatment until normal values are reestablished.

Teach Patient/Family:

- That long-term therapy may be necessary to clear infection
- To prevent reinoculation of *Candida* infection by disposing of toothbrush or other contaminated oral hygiene devices used during period of infection

flucytosine

floo-sye′-toe-seen
(Ancobon)

CATEGORY AND SCHEDULE

Pregnancy Risk Category: C

MECHANISM OF ACTION

An antifungal that penetrates fungal cells and is converted to fluorouracil which competes with uracil interfering with fungal RNA and protein synthesis. ***Therapeutic Effect:*** Damages fungal membrane.

PHARMACOKINETICS

Well absorbed from gastrointestinal (GI) tract. Widely distributed, including cerebrospinal fluid (CSF). Protein binding: 2–4%. Metabolized in liver. Partially removed by hemodialysis. ***Half-life:*** 3–8 hrs (half-life is increased with impaired renal function).

AVAILABILITY

Capsule: 250 mg, 500 mg.

INDICATIONS AND DOSAGES

▸ **Fungal Infections, Candidiasis, Cryptococcosis**

PO

Adults, Elderly, Children. 50 to 150 mg/kg/day in 4 equally divided doses.

▸ **Dosage in Renal Function Impairment**

Based on creatinine clearance:

Creatinine Clearance	Dosage Interval
20–40 ml/min	q12h
10–20 ml/min	q24h
0–10 ml/min	q24–48h

CONTRAINDICATIONS

Hypersensitivity to flucytosine.

INTERACTIONS

Drug

Amphotericin B: May increase the effects of flucytosine.

Levomethadyl: May increase risk of cardiotoxicity.

Zidovudine: May increase the risk of hematologic toxicity.

Herbal

None known.

Food

None known.

Drug interactions of concern to dentistry

- None reported

DIAGNOSTIC TEST EFFECTS

May increase creatinine values if determined by the ektachem method.

SIDE EFFECTS

Occasional

Pruritus, rash, photosensitivity, dizziness, drowsiness, headache, diarrhea, nausea, vomiting, abdominal pain, increased liver enzymes, jaundice, in creased BUN and creatinine, weakness, hearing loss

SERIOUS REACTIONS

! Hepatic dysfunction and severe bone marrow suppression occur rarely.

DENTAL CONSIDERATIONS

General:

- Patients on chronic drug therapy may rarely have symptoms of blood dyscrasias, which can include infection, bleeding, and poor healing.
- Examine for evidence of oral *Candida* infection.

Consultations:

- Medical consultation may be required to assess disease control.
- In a patient with symptoms of blood dyscrasias, request a medical consultation for blood studies and postpone dental treatment until normal values are reestablished.

Teach Patient/Family:

- Importance of good oral hygiene to prevent gingival inflammation

fludarabine phosphate

flew-dare′-ah-bean

(Fludara)

Do not confuse Fludara with FUDR.

CATEGORY AND SCHEDULE

Pregnancy Risk Category: D

MECHANISM OF ACTION

An antimetabolite that inhibits DNA synthesis by interfering with DNA polymerase alpha, ribonucleotide reductase, and

DNA primase. ***Therapeutic Effect:*** Induces cell death.

PHARMACOKINETICS
Rapidly dephosphorylated in serum, then phosphorylated intracellularly to active triphosphate. Primarily excreted in urine. ***Half-life:*** 7–20 hr.

AVAILABILITY
Injection Powder for Reconstitution: 50 mg.

INDICATIONS AND DOSAGES
▸ Chronic Lymphocytic Leukemia
IV
Adults. 25 mg/m^2 daily for 5 consecutive days. Continue for up to 3 additional cycles. Begin each course of treatment every 28 days.
▸ Non-Hodgkin's Lymphoma
IV
Adults, Elderly. Initially, 20 mg/m^2, then 30 mg/m^2/day for 48 hr.
▸ Dosage in Renal Impairment

Creatinine Clearance	Dosage
30–70 ml/min	decrease dose by 20%
less than 30 ml/min	not recommended

CONTRAINDICATIONS
Concurrent use with pentostatin

INTERACTIONS
Drug
Antigout medications: May decrease the effects of these drugs.
Bone marrow depressants: May increase the risk of myelosuppression.
Live-virus vaccines: May potentiate virus replication, increase vaccine side effects, and decrease the patient's antibody response to the vaccine.
Herbal
None known.
Food
None known.
Drug interactions of concern to dentistry
- None reported

DIAGNOSTIC TEST EFFECTS
May increase serum alkaline phosphatase, uric acid, and AST (SGOT) levels.

IV INCOMPATIBILITIES
Acyclovir (Zovirax), amphotericin B (Fungizone), hydroxyzine (Vistaril), prochlorperazine (Compazine)

IV COMPATIBILITIES
Heparin, hydromorphone (Dilaudid), lorazepam (Ativan), magnesium sulfate, morphine, multivitamins, potassium chloride

SIDE EFFECTS
Frequent
Fever (60%), nausea and vomiting (36%), chills (11%)
Occasional (20%–10%)
Fatigue, generalized pain, rash, diarrhea, cough, asthenia, stomatitis, dyspnea, peripheral edema
Rare (7%–3%)
Anorexia, sinusitis, dysuria, myalgia, paresthesia, headaches, visual disturbances

SERIOUS REACTIONS
! Pneumonia occurs frequently.
! Severe hematologic toxicity (as evidenced by anemia, thrombocytopenia, and neutropenia) and GI bleeding may occur.
! Tumor lysis syndrome may start with flank pain and hematuria and may include hypercalcemia, hyperphosphatemia, hyperuricemia and renal failure.
! High-dosage therapy may produce acute leukemia, blindness, and coma.

F

DENTAL CONSIDERATIONS

General:

- Monitor vital signs at every appointment due to cardiovascular side effects.
- If additional analgesia is required for dental pain, consider alternative analgesics (NSAIDs) in patients taking narcotics for acute or chronic pain.
- Examine for oral manifestation of opportunistic infection.
- Avoid products that affect platelet function, such as aspirin and NSAIDs.
- This drug may be used in the hospital or on an outpatient basis. Confirm the patient's disease and treatment status.
- Chlorhexidine mouth rinse prior to and during chemotherapy may reduce severity of mucositis.
- Patient on chronic drug therapy may rarely present with symptoms of blood dyscrasias, which can include infection, bleeding and poor healing. If dyscrasia is present, caution patient to prevent oral tissue trauma when using oral hygiene aids.
- Palliative medication may be required for management of oral side effects.
- Patients may be at risk of infection.
- Patients may be at risk of bleeding, check for oral signs.

Oral infections should be eliminated and/or treated aggressively.

Consultations:

- Medical consultation should include routine blood counts including platelet counts and bleeding time.
- Consult physician; prophylactic or therapeutic antiinfectives may be indicated if surgery or periodontal treatment is required.
- Medical consultation may be required to assess immunologic status during cancer chemotherapy and determine safety risk, if any, posed by the required dental treatment.
- Medical consultation may be required to assess disease control and patient's ability to tolerate stress.

Teach Patient/Family:

- To be aware of oral side effects
- Importance of good oral hygiene to prevent soft tissue inflammation
- To report oral lesions, soreness, or bleeding to dentist
- To prevent trauma when using oral hygiene aids
- Importance of updating health and medication history if physician makes any changes in evaluation or drug regimens; include OTC, herbal, and nonherbal remedies in the update

fludrocortisone

floo-droe-kor′-ti-sone
(Florinef)

Do not confuse Florinef with Fioricet or Florinal.

CATEGORY AND SCHEDULE

Pregnancy Risk Category: C

MECHANISM OF ACTION

A mineralocorticoid that acts at distal tubules. ***Therapeutic Effect:*** Increases potassium and hydrogen ion excretion. Replaces sodium loss and raises blood pressure (with low dosages). Inhibits endogenous adrenal cortical secretion, thymic activity, and secretion of corticotropin by pituitary gland (with higher dosages).

PHARMACOKINETICS

Well absorbed from the GI tract. Protein binding: 42%. Widely distributed. Metabolized in the liver and kidney. Primarily excreted in urine. ***Half-life:*** 3.5 hr.

AVAILABILITY
Tablets: 0.1 mg.

INDICATIONS AND DOSAGES
▸ Addison's Disease
PO
Adults, Elderly. 0.05–0.1 mg/day. Range: 0.1 mg 3 times a wk to 0.2 mg/day. Administration with cortisone or hydrocortisone preferred.
▸ Salt-Losing Adrenogenital Syndrome
PO
Adults, Elderly. 0.1–0.2 mg/day.
▸ Usual Pediatric Dosage
Children. 0.05–0.1 mg/day.

OFF-LABEL USES
Treatment of acidosis in renal tubular disorders, idiopathic orthostatic hypotension

CONTRAINDICATIONS
CHF, systemic fungal infection

INTERACTIONS
Drug
Digoxin: May increase the risk of digoxin toxicity caused by hypokalemia.
Hepatic enzyme inducers (such as phenytoin): May increase the metabolism of fludrocortisone.
Hypokalemia-causing medications: May increase the effects of fludrocortisone.
Sodium-containing medications: May increase BP, incidence of edema, and serum sodium level.
Herbal
None known.
Food
None known.
Drug interactions of concern to dentistry
- Decreased action: barbiturates
- Increased side effects: sodium-containing food, sodium-containing polishing devices
- Decreased effects of salicylates

DIAGNOSTIC TEST EFFECTS
May increase serum sodium level. May decrease Hct and serum potassium level.

SIDE EFFECTS
Frequent
Increased appetite, exaggerated sense of well-being, abdominal distention, weight gain, insomnia, mood swings
High dosages, prolonged therapy, too rapid withdrawal: Increased susceptibility to infection with masked signs and symptoms, delayed wound healing, hypokalemia, hypocalcemia, GI distress, diarrhea or constipation, hypertension
Occasional
Headache, dizziness, menstrual difficulty or amenorrhea, gastric ulcer development
Rare
Hypersensitivity reaction

SERIOUS REACTIONS
! Long-term therapy may cause muscle wasting (especially in the arms and legs), osteoporosis, spontaneous fractures, amenorrhea, cataracts, glaucoma, peptic ulcer disease, and CHF.
! Abruptly withdrawing the drug after long-term therapy may cause anorexia, nausea, fever, headache, joint pain, rebound inflammation, fatigue, weakness, lethargy, dizziness, and orthostatic hypotension.

DENTAL CONSIDERATIONS
General:
- Patients with Addison's disease are more susceptible to stress and may require supplemental systemic glucocorticoids before dental treatment.

• Patients who have been or are currently on chronic steroid therapy (>2 wk) may require supplemental steroids for dental treatment.
• Monitor vital signs at every appointment because of nature of disease.
• Short appointments and a stress reduction protocol may be required for anxious patients.
• Patients with Addison's disease must be evaluated closely for presence of oral infection.
• Do not use ingestible sodium bicarbonate products, such as the Prophy-Jet air polishing system, or IV saline fluids for patients on a salt-restricted regimen.
• Use precautions if dental surgery is anticipated and conscious sedation or general anesthesia is required.
• Monitor patient for any signs of inadequate management of disease, such as potassium depletion, muscle weakness, paresthesia, fatigue, nausea, depression, polyuria, and edema.

Consultations:
• Medical consultation is required to assess disease control and patient's ability to tolerate stress.
• Consultation may be required to confirm steroid dose and duration of use.

Teach Patient/Family:
• That identification as a steroid user should be carried
• To report to the dental office any signs that might indicate an oral infection

flumazenil
flew-maz′-ah-nil
(Anexate[CAN], Romazicon)

CATEGORY AND SCHEDULE
Pregnancy Risk Category: C

MECHANISM OF ACTION
An antidote that antagonizes the effect of benzodiazepines on the gamma-aminobutyric acid receptor complex in the CNS. ***Therapeutic Effect:*** Reverses sedative effect of benzodiazepines.

PHARMACOKINETICS

Route	Onset	Peak	Duration
IV	1–2 min	6–10 min	less than 1 hr

Duration and degree of benzodiazepine reversal depend on dosage and plasma concentration. Protein binding: 50%. Metabolized by the liver; excreted in urine.

AVAILABILITY
Injection: 0.1 mg/ml.

INDICATIONS AND DOSAGES
▸ Reversal of Conscious Sedation or General Anesthesia
IV
Adults, Elderly. Initially, 0.2 mg (2 ml) over 15 sec; may repeat dose in 45 sec; then at 60-sec intervals. Maximum: 1 mg (10-ml) total dose.
Children, Neonates. Initially, 0.01 mg/kg; may repeat in 45 sec, then at 60-sec intervals. Maximum: 0.2 mg single dose; 0.05 mg/kg or 1 mg cumulative dose.
▸ Benzodiazepine Overdose
IV
Adults, Elderly. Initially, 0.2 mg (2 ml) over 30 sec; if desired LOC

is not achieved after 30 sec, 0.3 mg (3 ml) may be given over 30 sec. Further doses of 0.5 mg (5 ml) may be administered over 30 sec at 60-sec intervals. Maximum: 3 mg (30 ml) total dose.
Children, Neonates. Initially, 0.01 mg/kg; may repeat in 45 sec, then at 60-sec intervals. Maximum: 0.2 mg single dose; 1 mg cumulative dose.

CONTRAINDICATIONS

Anticholinergic signs (such as mydriasis, dry mucosa, and hypoperistalsis), arrhythmias, cardiovascular collapse, history of hypersensitivity to benzodiazepines, patients with signs of serious cyclic antidepressant overdose (such as motor abnormalities), patients who have been given a benzodiazepine for control of a potentially life-threatening condition (such as control of status epilepticus or increased intracranial pressure)

INTERACTIONS

Drug

Tricyclic antidepressants: May produces seizures and arrhythmias as flumazenil reverses the sedative effects of tricyclic antidepressants.

Herbal

None known.

Food

None known.

Drug interactions of concern to dentistry

• May not be effective: mixed drug overdosage

DIAGNOSTIC TEST EFFECTS

None known.

IV INCOMPATIBILITIES

No information available for Y-site administration.

IV COMPATIBILITIES

Aminophylline, cimetidine (Tagamet), dobutamine (Dobutrex), dopamine (Intropin), famotidine (Pepcid), heparin, lidocaine, procainamide (Pronestyl), ranitidine (Zantac)

SIDE EFFECTS

Frequent (11%–4%)
Agitation, anxiety, dry mouth, dyspnea, insomnia, palpitations, tremors, headache, blurred vision, dizziness, ataxia, nausea, vomiting, pain at injection site, diaphoresis
Occasional (3%–1%)
Fatigue, flushing, auditory disturbances, thrombophlebitis, rash
Rare (<1%)
Urticaria, pruritus, hallucinations

SERIOUS REACTIONS

! Toxic effects, such as seizures and arrhythmias, of other drugs taken in overdose, especially tricyclic antidepressants, may emerge with reversal of sedative effect of benzodiazepines.
! Flumazenil may provoke a panic attack in those with a history of panic disorder.

DENTAL CONSIDERATIONS

General:

• Monitor vital signs at every appointment because of cardiovascular side effects.
• Monitor for resedation; duration of antagonism is short compared with benzodiazepines.

Teach Patient/Family:

• To be alert for possible resedation when discharged from office

flunisolide

floo-niss′-oh-lide
(AeroBid, Nasalide, Nasarel, Rhinalar[CAN])
Do not confuse flunisolide with fluocinonide, or Nasalide with Nasalcrom.

F

CATEGORY AND SCHEDULE

Pregnancy Risk Category: C

MECHANISM OF ACTION

An adrenocorticosteroid that controls the rate of protein synthesis, depresses migration of polymorphonuclear leukocytes, reverses capillary permeability, and stabilizes lysosomal membranes. ***Therapeutic Effect:*** Prevents or controls inflammation.

AVAILABILITY

Aerosol (AeroBid): 250 mcg/activation.
Nasal Spray (Nasalide, Nasarel): 25 mcg/activation.

INDICATIONS AND DOSAGES

▸ Long-Term Control of Bronchial Asthma, Assists in Reducing or Discontinuing Oral Corticosteroid Therapy

INHALATION

Adults, Elderly. 2 inhalations twice a day, morning and evening. Maximum: 4 inhalations twice a day.

Children 6–15 yr. 2 inhalations twice a day.

▸ Relief of Symptoms of Perennial and Seasonal Rhinitis

INTRANASAL

Adults, Elderly. Initially, 2 sprays each nostril twice a day, may increase at 4–7 day intervals to 2 sprays 3 times a day. Maximum: 8 sprays in each nostril daily.

Children 6–14 yr. Initially, 1 spray 3 times a day or 2 sprays twice a day. Maximum: 4 sprays in each nostril daily. Maintenance: 1 spray into each nostril each day.

OFF-LABEL USES

To prevent recurrence of nasal polyps after surgery

CONTRAINDICATIONS

Hypersensitivity to any corticosteroid, persistently positive sputum cultures for *Candida albicans,* primary treatment of status asthmaticus, systemic fungal infections

INTERACTIONS

Drug

None known.

Herbal

None known.

Food

None known.

DIAGNOSTIC TEST EFFECTS

None known.

SIDE EFFECTS

Frequent

Inhalation (25%–10%): Unpleasant taste, nausea, vomiting, sore throat, diarrhea, upset stomach, cold symptoms, nasal congestion

Occasional

Inhalation (9%–3%): Dizziness, irritability, nervousness, tremors, abdominal pain, heartburn, oropharynx candidiasis, edema
Nasal: Mild nasopharyngeal irritation or dryness, rebound congestion, bronchial asthma, rhinorrhea, altered taste

SERIOUS REACTIONS

! An acute hypersensitivity reaction, marked by urticaria, angioedema, and severe bronchospasm, occurs rarely.

! A transfer from systemic to local steroid therapy may unmask previously suppressed bronchial asthma condition.

DENTAL CONSIDERATIONS

General:

- Examine oral cavity for evidence of drug side effects.
- Assess salivary flow as a factor in caries, periodontal disease, and candidiasis.
- Evaluate respiration characteristics and rate.
- Consider semisupine chair position for patients with respiratory disease.
- Determine dose and duration of steroid therapy for each patient to assess risk for stress tolerance and immunosuppression.
- Acute asthmatic episodes may be precipitated in the dental office. Sympathomimetic inhalants should be available for emergency use. A stress reduction protocol may be required.
- Consider the drug in the diagnosis of taste alterations.

Consultations:

- Medical consultation may be required to assess disease control.

Teach Patient/Family:

- Importance of good oral hygiene to prevent soft tissue inflammation
- Caution to prevent injury when using oral hygiene aids
- Importance of gargling, rinsing mouth with water, and expectorating after each aerosol dose
- *When chronic dry mouth occurs, advise patient:*
  - To use daily home fluoride products for anticaries effect
  - To avoid mouth rinses with high alcohol content because of drying effects
  - To use sugarless gum, frequent sips of water, or saliva substitutes

fluocinolone acetonide

floo-oh-sin′-oh-lone a-seat′-oh-nide
(Capex, Derma-Smooth/FS, Fluoderm[CAN], Synalar)

CATEGORY AND SCHEDULE

Pregnancy Risk Category: C

F

MECHANISM OF ACTION

A fluorinated topical corticosteroid that controls the rate of protein synthesis; depresses migration of polymorphonuclear leukocytes and fibroblasts; reduces capillary permeability; prevents or controls inflammation. ***Therapeutic Effect:*** Decreases tissue response to inflammatory process.

PHARMACOKINETICS

Use of occlusive dressings may increase percutaneous absorption. Protein binding: more than 90%. Excreted in urine. ***Half-life:*** Unknown.

AVAILABILITY

Cream: 0.01%, 0.025% (Synalar).
Oil: 0.01% (Derma-Smoothe/FS).
Ointment: 0.025% (Synalar).
Shampoo: 0.01% (Capex).
Solution: 0.01% (Synalar).

INDICATIONS AND DOSAGES

▸ **Atopic Dermatitis**

TOPICAL

Adults, Elderly. Apply 3 times/day.
Children 2 yrs and older. Apply 2 times/day.

▸ **Scalp Psoriasis**

TOPICAL

Adults, Elderly. Apply to damp or wet hair and leave on overnight or for at least 4 hrs. Remove by washing hair with shampoo.

▸ **Seborrheic Dermatitis, Scalp**
SHAMPOO
Adults, Elderly. Apply once daily allowi to remain on scalp for at least 5 min.

OFF-LABEL USES
Vitiligo

F

CONTRAINDICATIONS
Hypersensitivity to fluocinolone or other corticosteroids

INTERACTIONS
Drug
None known.
Herbal
None known.
Food
None known.
Drug interactions of concern to dentistry
• None reported

DIAGNOSTIC TEST EFFECTS
None known.

SIDE EFFECTS
Occasional
Burning, dryness, itching, stinging
Rare
Allergic contact dermatitis, purpura or blood-containing blisters, thinning of skin with easy bruising, telangiectasis or raised dark red spots on skin

SERIOUS REACTIONS
! When taken in excessive quantities, systemic hypercorticism and adrenal suppression may occur.

DENTAL CONSIDERATIONS
General:
• Determine why patient is taking the drug.
Teach Patient/Family:
• Use on oral herpetic ulcerations is contraindicated.

fluocinonide
floo-oh-sin′-oh-nide
(Lidex, Lidex-E)

CATEGORY AND SCHEDULE
Pregnancy Risk Category: C

MECHANISM OF ACTION
A topical corticosteroid that has anti-inflammatory, antipruritic, and vasoconstrictive properties. The exact mechanism of the anti-inflammatory process is unclear. ***Therapeutic Effect:*** Reduces or prevents tissue response to the inflammatory process.

PHARMACOKINETICS
Well absorbed systemically. Large variation in absorption among sites. Protein binding: varies. Metabolized in liver. Primarily excreted in urine.

AVAILABILITY
Cream (anhydrous emollient): 0.05% (Lidex).
Cream (aqueous emollient): 0.05% (Lidex-E).
Gel: 0.05% (Lidex).
Ointment: 0.05% (Lidex).
Solution: 0.05% (Lidex).

INDICATIONS AND DOSAGES
▸ **Dermatoses**
TOPICAL
Adults, Elderly. Apply sparingly 2–4 times/day.

CONTRAINDICATIONS
History of hypersensitivity to fluocinonide or other corticosteroids

INTERACTIONS
Drug
None known.
Herbal
None known.

Food
None known.

DIAGNOSTIC TEST EFFECTS
None known.

SIDE EFFECTS
Occasional
Itching, redness, irritation, burning at site of application, dryness, folliculitis, acneiform eruptions, hypopigmentation
Rare
Allergic contact dermatitis, maceration of the skin, secondary infection, skin atrophy

SERIOUS REACTIONS
! The serious reactions of long-term therapy and the addition of occlusive dressings are reversible hypothalamic-pituitary-adrenal (HPA) axis suppression, manifestations of Cushing's syndrome, hyperglycemia, and glucosuria.

DENTAL CONSIDERATIONS
General:
- Place on frequent recall to evaluate healing response.

Teach Patient/Family:
- When used for oral lesions, advise patient to return for oral evaluation if response of oral tissues has not occurred in 7–14 days
- That use on oral herpetic ulcerations is contraindicated
- Importance of good oral hygiene to prevent soft tissue inflammation
- To apply at bedtime or after meals for maximum effect
- To apply with cotton-tipped applicator by pressing, not rubbing, paste on lesion

fluorometholone
flure-oh-meth′-oh-lone
(Eflone, Flarex, Fluor-Op, FML Forte Liquifilm, FML Liquifilm, FML S.O.P.)

CATEGORY AND SCHEDULE
Pregnancy Risk Category: C

F

MECHANISM OF ACTION
An ophthalmic corticosteroid that decreases inflammation by suppression of migration of polymorphonuclear leukocytes and reversal of increased capillary permeability. ***Therapeutic Effect:*** Decrease ocular inflammation.

PHARMACOKINETICS
Absorbed into aqueous humor with slight systemic absorption.

AVAILABILITY
Ophthalmic Suspension, as base: 0.1% (Eflone, FML Liquifilm, Flarex, Fluor-Op), 0.25% (FML Forte Liquifilm).
Ophthalmic Ointment: 0.1% (FML S.O.P).

INDICATIONS AND DOSAGES
▸ Treatment of Steroid-Responsive Inflammatory Conditions of the Eye
OPHTHALMIC OINTMENT
Adults, Elderly. Apply thin strip to conjunctival sac every 4 hours in severe cases or 1–3 times per day in mild to moderate cases.
OPHTHALMIC SOLUTION
Adults, Elderly, Children 2 yrs and older. Instill 1–2 drops into conjunctival sac every hour during the day, every 2 hours at night until favorable response is obtained. Then use 1 drop every 4 hours. For mild to moderate inflammation, instill 1–2 drops into conjunctival sac 2–4 times/day.

F

CONTRAINDICATIONS
Viral diseases of the cornea and conjunctiva, mycobacterial or fungal infections of the eye, untreated eye infections which may be masked or enhanced by steroids, hypersensitivity to fluorometholone or any component of the formulation

INTERACTIONS
Drug
None known.
Herbal
None known.
Food
None known.
Drug interactions of concern to dentistry
None reported

DIAGNOSTIC TEST EFFECTS
None known.

SIDE EFFECTS
Occasional
Burning, tearing, itching, blurred vision
Rare
Cataract formation, corneal ulcers, glaucoma with optic nerve damage

SERIOUS REACTIONS
! Hypercorticoidism and taste perversion occurs rarely.
! Superinfections, particularly with fungi, may result from bacterial imbalance via any route of administration.

DENTAL CONSIDERATIONS
General:
- Determine why patient is taking the drug.
- Avoid dental light in patient's eyes; offer dark glasses for patient comfort.
- Protect patient's eyes from accidental spatter during dental treatment.

fluorouracil, 5FU
fluorouracil
flure-oh-yoor′-a-sill
(Adrucil, Carac, Efudex, Efudix[AUS], Fluoroplex)
Do not confuse Efudex with Efidac.

CATEGORY AND SCHEDULE
Pregnancy Risk Category: D

MECHANISM OF ACTION
An antimetabolite that blocks formation of thymidylic acid. Cell cycle-specific for S phase of cell division. ***Therapeutic Effect:*** Inhibits DNA and RNA synthesis. Topical form destroys rapidly proliferating cells.

PHARMACOKINETICS
Widely distributed. Crosses the blood-brain barrier. Rapidly metabolized in tissues to active metabolite, which is localized intracellularly. Primarily excreted by lungs as carbon dioxide. Removed by hemodialysis. ***Half-life:*** 20 hr.

AVAILABILITY
Injection (Adrucil): 50 mg/ml.
Topical Cream (Carac, Fluoroplex): 1%.
Topical Cream (Efudex): 5%.
Topical Solution (Efudex): 2%.
Topical Solution (Fluoroplex): 1%.

INDICATIONS AND DOSAGES
▸ **Carcinoma of Breast, Colon, Pancreas, Rectum,**

and Stomach; in Combination with Levamisole after Surgical Resection in Patients with Duke's Stage C Colon Cancer
IV
Adults, Elderly, Children. Initially, 12 mg/kg/day for 4–5 days.
Maximum: 800 mg/day.
Maintenance: 6 mg/kg every other day for 4 doses repeated in 4 wk; or 15 mg/kg as a single bolus dosel; or 5–15 mg/kg/wk as a single dose, not to exceed 1 g.

▸ **Multiple Actinic or Solar Keratoses**
TOPICAL (Carac)
Adults, Elderly. Apply once a day.
Topical (Efudex, Fluoroplex)
Adults, Elderly. Apply twice a day.

▸ **Basal Cell Carcinoma**
TOPICAL (Efudex)
Adult, Elderly. Apply twice a day.

OFF-LABEL USES
Parenteral: Treatment of bladder, cervical, endometrial, head and neck, liver, lung, ovarian, or prostate carcinomas; pericardial, peritoneal, or pleural effusions
Topical: Treatment of actinic cheilitis, radiodermatitis

CONTRAINDICATIONS
Major surgery within previous month, myelosuppression, poor nutritional status, potentially serious infections

INTERACTIONS
Drug
Bone marrow depressants: May increase the risk of myelosuppression.
Live-virus vaccines: May potentiate virus replication, increase vaccine side effects, and decrease the patient's antibody response to the vaccine.

Herbal
None known.

Food
None known.

Drug interactions of concern to dentistry
• None reported, but limit drugs that may also produce photosensitivity reaction

DIAGNOSTIC TEST EFFECTS
May decrease serum albumin level. May increase excretion of 5-hydroxyindoleacetic acid (5-HIAA) in urine. Topical form may cause eosinophilia, leukocytosis, thrombocytopenia, and toxic granulation.

IV INCOMPATIBILITIES
Amphotericin B complex (Abelcet, AmBisome, Amphotec), droperidol (Inapsine), filgrastim (Neupogen), ondansetron (Zofran), vinorelbine (Navelbine)

IV COMPATIBILITIES
Granisetron (Kytril), heparin, hydromorphone (Dilaudid), leucovorin, morphine, potassium chloride, propofol (Diprivan)

SIDE EFFECTS
Occasional
Parenteral: Anorexia, diarrhea, minimal alopecia, fever, dry skin, skin fissures, scaling, erythema
Topical: Pain, pruritus, hyperpigmentation, irritation, inflammation, and burning at application site; photosensitivity

Rare
Nausea, vomiting, anemia, esophagitis, proctitis, GI ulcer, confusion, headache, lacrimation, visual disturbances, angina, allergic reactions

SERIOUS REACTIONS

! The earliest sign of toxicity, which may occur 4–8 days after beginning therapy, is stomatitis (as evidenced by dry mouth, burning sensation, mucosal erythema, and ulceration at inner margin of lips).
! Hematologic toxicity may be manifested as leukopenia (generally within 9–14 days after drug administration, but possibly as late as the 25th day), thrombocytopenia (within 7–17 days after administration), pancytopenia, or agranulocytosis.
! The most common dermatologic toxicity is a pruritic rash on the extremities or, less frequently, the trunk.

DENTAL CONSIDERATIONS

General:

- Be aware of patient's disease and avoid treated areas to prevent further irritation.

fluoxetine hydrochloride

floo-ox′-e-teen
(Auscap[AUS], Fluohexal[AUS], Lovan[AUS], Novo-Fluoxetine [CAN], Prozac, Prozac Weekly, Sarafem, Zactin[AUS])
Do not confuse fluoxetine with fluvastatin, Prozac with Prilosec, Proscar, or ProSom; or Sarafem with Serophene.

CATEGORY AND SCHEDULE

Pregnancy Risk Category: C

MECHANISM OF ACTION

A psychotherapeutic agent that selectively inhibits serotonin uptake in the CNS, enhancing serotonergic function. ***Therapeutic Effect:*** Relieves depression; reduces obsessive-compulsive and bulimic behavior.

PHARMACOKINETICS

Well absorbed from the GI tract. Crosses the blood-brain barrier. Protein binding: 94%. Metabolized in the liver to active metabolite. Primarily excreted in urine. Not removed by hemodialysis. ***Half-life:*** 2–3 days; metabolite 7–9 days.

AVAILABILITY

Capsules (Prozac): 10 mg, 20 mg, 40 mg.
Capsules (Sarafem): 10 mg, 20 mg.
Capsules (Delayed-Release[Prozac Weekly]): 90 mg.
Oral Solution (Prozac): 20 mg/5 ml.
Tablets (Prozac): 10 mg, 20 mg.

INDICATIONS AND DOSAGES

▸ **Depression, obsessive-compulsive disorder**

PO

Adults. Initially, 20 mg each morning. If therapeutic improvement does not occur after 2 wk, gradually increase to maximum of 80 mg/day in 2 equally divided doses in morning and at noon. Prozac Weekly: 90 mg/wk, begin 7 days after last dose of 20 mg.
Elderly. Initially, 10 mg/day. May increase by 10–20 mg q2wk.
Children 7–17 yr. Initially, 5–10 mg/day. Titrate upward as needed. Usual dosage is 20 mg/day.

▸ **Panic disorder**

PO

Adults, Elderly. Initially, 10 mg/day. May increase to 20 mg/day after 1 week. Maximum: 60 mg/day.

▸ **Bulimia nervosa**

PO

Adults. 60 mg each morning.

▸ **Premenstrual dysphoric disorder**
PO
Adults. 20 mg/day.

OFF-LABEL USES
Treatment of hot flashes

CONTRAINDICATIONS
Use within 14 days of MAOIs

INTERACTIONS
Drug
Alcohol, other CNS depressants: May increase CNS depression.
Highly protein-bound medications (including oral anticoagulants): May increase adverse effects.
MAOIs: May produce serotonin syndrome and neuroleptic malignant syndrome.
Phenytoin: May increase phenytoin blood concentration and risk of toxicity.
Herbal
St. John's wort: May increase fluoxetine's pharmacologic effects and risk of toxicity.
Food
None known.
Drug interactions of concern to dentistry
• Increased CNS depression: alcohol, all CNS depressants, tricyclic antidepressants, benzodiazepines, St. John's wort (herb)
• Increased side effects: highly protein-bound drugs (aspirin)
• Caution: can inhibit cytochrome P4502D6 isoenzymes
• Increased serum levels of carbamazepine
• Possible "serotonin syndrome" with macrolide antibiotics
• First-time users of SSRIs also taking NSAIDs may have a higher risk of GI side effects; until more data are available, it may be advisable to avoid use of NSAIDs in these patients (*Br J Clin Pharmacol* 55:591–595, 2003)

DIAGNOSTIC TEST EFFECTS
None known.

SIDE EFFECTS
Frequent (more than 10%)
Headache, asthenia, insomnia, anxiety, nervousness, somnolence, nausea, diarrhea, decreased appetite
Occasional (9%–2%)
Dizziness, tremor, fatigue, vomiting, constipation, dry mouth, abdominal pain, nasal congestion, diaphoresis, rash
Rare (<2%)
Flushed skin, light-headedness, impaired concentration

SERIOUS REACTIONS
! Overdose may produce seizures, nausea, vomiting, agitation, and restlessness.

DENTAL CONSIDERATIONS
General:
• Monitor vital signs at every appointment because of cardiovascular side effects.
• Assess salivary flow as a factor in caries, periodontal disease, and candidiasis.
Consultations:
• Medical consultation may be required to assess disease control and patient's ability to tolerate stress.
• Physician should be informed if significant xerostomic side effects occur (e.g., increased caries, sore tongue, problems eating or swallowing, difficulty wearing prosthesis) so that a medication change can be considered.
Teach patient/family:
• To use electric toothbrush if patient has difficulty holding conventional devices

- *When chronic dry mouth occurs, advise patient:*
  - To avoid mouth rinses with high alcohol content because of drying effects
  - To use daily home fluoride products for anticaries effect
  - To use sugarless gum, frequent sips of water, or saliva substitutes

F

fluoxymesterone

floo-ex-ih-mes-the-rone
Schedule III
(Android-F, Halotestin, Halotestin[CAN])

CATEGORY AND SCHEDULE

Pregnancy Risk Category: X
Controlled substance: Schedule III

MECHANISM OF ACTION

An androgen that suppresses gonadotropin-releasing hormone, LH, and FSH. ***Therapeutic Effect:*** Stimulates spermatogenesis, development of male secondary sex characteristics, and sexual maturation at puberty. Stimulates production of red blood cells (RBCs).

PHARMACOKINETICS

Rapidly absorbed from the gastrointestinal (GI) tract. Protein binding: 98%. Metabolized in liver. Excreted in urine. ***Half-life:*** 9.2 hrs.

AVAILABILITY

Tablets: 2 mg, 5 mg, 10 mg (Halotestin).

INDICATIONS AND DOSAGES

▸ **Males (Hypogonadism)**
PO
Adults. 5–20 mg/day.
Males (delayed puberty)
PO
Adults. 2.5–20 mg/day for 4–6 mos.
Females (inoperable breast cancer)
PO
Adults. 10–40 mg/day in divided doses for 1–3 mos.
Females (prevent postpartum breast pain/engorgement)
PO
Adults. Initially, 2.5 mg shortly after delivery, then 5–10 mg/day in divided doses for 4–5 days.

CONTRAINDICATIONS

Serious cardiac, renal, or hepatic dysfunction, men with carcinomas of the breast or prostate, hypersensitivity to fluoxymesterone or any component of the formulation including tartrazine

INTERACTIONS

Drug

Oral anticoagulants: May increase the effect of these drugs.
Hepatotoxic medications: May increase the risk of hepatotoxicity.
Cyclosporine: May increase the risk of cyclosporine toxicity.

Herbal

Chaparral, comfrey, eucalyptus, germander, Jin Bu Huan, kava kava, pennyroyal, skullcap, valerian: May increase the risk of liver damage.

Food

None known.

Drug interactions of concern to dentistry

- Edema: corticosteroids

DIAGNOSTIC TEST EFFECTS

May decrease levels of thyroxine-binding globulin, total T4 serum levels, and resin uptake of T3 and T4. May increase alkaline phosphatase, SGOT (AST), bilirubin, calcium, potassium, sodium, Hgb, Hct, LDL. May decrease HDL.

SIDE EFFECTS

Frequent

Females: Amenorrhea, virilism (e.g., acne, decreased breast size, enlarged clitoris, male pattern baldness), deepening voice

Males: UTI, breast soreness, gynecomastia, priapism, virilism (e.g., acne, early pubic hair growth)

Occasional

Edema, nausea, vomiting, mild acne, diarrhea, stomach pain

Males: Impotence, testicular atrophy

SERIOUS REACTIONS

! Peliosis hepatitis (liver, spleen replaced with blood-filled cysts), hepatic neoplasms, and hepatocellular carcinoma have been associated with prolonged high dosage.

DENTAL CONSIDERATIONS

General:

• Monitor vital signs at every appointment because of cardiovascular side effects.

• Patients receiving chemotherapy may require palliative treatment for stomatitis.

Teach Patient/Family:

• Importance of good oral hygiene to prevent soft tissue inflammation

• To prevent trauma when using oral hygiene aids

fluphenazine decanoate

(Apo-Fluphenazie[CAN], Modecate[AUS], Prolixin); fluphenazine enanthate (Moditen[CAN], Prolixin); fluphenazine hydrochloride (Prolixin, Permitil)

CATEGORY AND SCHEDULE

Pregnancy Risk Category: C

MECHANISM OF ACTION

A phenothiazine that blocks dopamine at postsynaptic receptor sites. Possesses weak anticholinergic, sedative and entimetic effects and strong extrapyramidal activity.

Therapeutic Effect: Decreases psychotic behavior.

PHARMACOKINETICS

Erratic and variable absorption from the gastrointestinal (GI) tract. Widely distributed. Metabolized in liver. Primarily excreted in urine.

Half-life: 163–232 hrs.

AVAILABILITY

Elixir, as hydrochloride: 2.5 mg/5 ml (Prolixin).

Injection, as decanoate: 25 mg/ml (Prolixin).

Injection, as enanthate: 25 mg/ ml (Prolixin).

Injection solution, as hydrochloride: 2.5 mg/ml (Prolixin).

Oral solution, as hydrochloride: 5 mg/ml (Prolixin).

Tablets, as hydrochloride: 1 mg, 2.5 mg, 5 mg, 10 mg (Prolixin).

INDICATIONS AND DOSAGES

▸ **Psychotic Disorders**

PO

Adults. Initially, 0.5–10 mg/day fluphenazine HCl in divided

doses q6–8h. Increase gradually until therapeutic response is achieved (usually under 20 mg daily); decrease gradually to maintenance level (1–5 mg/day).
Elderly. Initially, 1–2.5 mg/day.
IM
Adults. Initially, 1.25 mg, followed by 2.5–10 mg/day in divided doses q6–8h.

▸ Chronic Schizophrenic Disorder

IM
Adults. Initially, 12.5–25 mg of fluphenazine decanoate q1–6 wks, or 25 mg fluphenazine enanthate q2wks.
Usual elderly dosage (nonpsychotic)
PO
Initially, 1–2.5 mg/day. May increase by 1–2.5 mg/day q4–7 days. Maximum: 20 mg/day.

OFF-LABEL USES

Treatment of neurogenic pain (adjunct to tricyclic antidepressants)

CONTRAINDICATIONS

Severe CNS depression, comatose states, severe cardiovascular disease, bone marrow depression, subcortical brain damage, hypersensitivity to fluphenazine or any component of the formulation including tartrazine

INTERACTIONS

Drug

Alcohol, CNS depressants: May increase respiratory depression and the hypotensive effects of fluphenazine.
Antithyroid agents: May increase the risk of agranulocytosis.
Extrapyramidal symptom (EPS)-producing medications: May increase EPS.
Hypotensives: May increase hypotension.
Levodopa: May decrease the effects of levodopa.
Lithium: May decrease the absorption of fluphenazine and produce adverse neurologic effects.
MAOIs, tricyclic antidepressants: May increase the anticholinergic and sedative effects of fluphenazine.

Herbal

Dong quai, kava kava, gotu kola, St. John's Wort, valerian: May increase risk of photosensitization or CNS depression.

Food

None known.

Drug interactions of concern to dentistry

- Increased sedation: other CNS depressants, alcohol, barbiturate anesthetics, opioid analgesics
- Hypotension, tachycardia: epinephrine
- Increased extrapyramidal effects: phenothiazines and related drugs (haloperidol, droperidol), metoclopramide
- Additive photosensitization: tetracyclines
- Increased anticholinergic effects: anticholinergics

DIAGNOSTIC TEST EFFECTS

May produce false-positive pregnancy test, PKU. ECG changes may occur, including Q and T wave disturbances.

SIDE EFFECTS

Frequent

Hypotension, dizziness, and fainting occur frequently after first injection, occasionally after subsequent injections, and rarely with oral dosage

Occasional

Drowsiness during early therapy, dry mouth, blurred vision, lethargy, constipation or diarrhea, nasal congestion, peripheral edema, urinary retention

Rare
Ocular changes, skin pigmentation (those on high doses for prolonged periods)

SERIOUS REACTIONS

! Extrapyramidal symptoms appear dose related (particularly high dosage), divided into 3 categories: akathisia (inability to sit still, tapping of feet, urge to move around); parkinsonian symptoms (mask-like face, tremors, shuffling gait, hypersalivation); and acute dystonias: torticollis (neck muscle spasm), opisthotonos (rigidity of back muscles), and oculogyric crisis (rolling back of eyes).
! Dystonic reaction may also produce profuse sweating, and pallor.
! Tardive dyskinesia (protrusion of tongue, puffing of cheeks, chewing/puckering of the mouth) occurs rarely (may be irreversible).
! Abrupt withdrawal after long-term therapy may precipitate nausea, vomiting, gastritis, dizziness, and tremors.
! Blood dyscrasias, particularly agranulocytosis, or mild leukopenia (sore mouth/gums/throat) may occur.
! May lower seizure threshold

DENTAL CONSIDERATIONS

General:
- Monitor vital signs at every appointment because of cardiovascular side effects.
- Patients on chronic drug therapy may rarely have symptoms of blood dyscrasias, which can include infection, bleeding, and poor healing.
- After supine positioning, have patient sit upright for at least 2 min before standing to avoid orthostatic hypotension.
- Assess salivary flow as a factor in caries, periodontal disease, and candidiasis.
- Avoid dental light in patient's eyes; offer dark glasses for patient comfort.
- Assess for presence of extrapyramidal motor symptoms, such as tardive dyskinesia and akathisia. Extrapyramidal motor activity may complicate dental treatment.
- Geriatric patients are more susceptible to drug effects; use a lower dose.
- Use vasoconstrictors with caution, in low doses, and with careful aspiration.

Consultations:
- In a patient with symptoms of blood dyscrasias, request a medical consultation for blood studies and postpone dental treatment until normal values are reestablished.
- Take precautions if dental surgery is anticipated and anesthesia is required.
- If signs of tardive dyskinesia or akathisia are present, refer to physician.
- Physician should be informed if significant xerostomic side effects occur (e.g., increased caries, sore tongue, problems eating or swallowing, difficulty wearing prosthesis) so that a medication change can be considered.

Teach Patient/Family:
- Importance of good oral hygiene to prevent soft tissue inflammation
- Caution to prevent injury when using oral hygiene aids
- To use electric toothbrush if patient has difficulty holding conventional devices
- *When chronic dry mouth occurs, advise patient:*
  - To avoid mouth rinses with high alcohol content because of drying effects

- To use daily home fluoride products for anticaries effect
- To use sugarless gum, frequent sips of water, or saliva substitutes

F

flurandrenolide

flure-an-dren′-oh-lide
(Cordran, Cordran SP)

CATEGORY AND SCHEDULE

Pregnancy Risk Category: C

MECHANISM OF ACTION

A fluorinated orticosteroid that decreases inflammation by suppression the migration of polymorphonuclear leukocytes and reversal of increased capillary permeability. ***Therapeutic Effect:*** Decreases tissue response to inflammatory process.

PHARMACOKINETICS

Repeated applications may lead to percutaneous absorption. Absorption is about 36% from scrotal area, 7% from the forehead, 4% from scalp, and 1% from forearm. Metabolized in liver. Excreted in urine. ***Half-life:*** Unknown.

AVAILABILITY

Cream: 0.025%, 0.05% (Cordran SP).
Lotion: 0.05% (Cordran).
Ointment: 0.025%, 0.05% (Cordran).
Tape, topical: 4 mcg/cm^2 (Cordran).

INDICATIONS AND DOSAGES

▸ **Anti-inflammatory, Immunosuppressant, Corticosteroid Replacement Therapy**

TOPICAL
Adults, Elderly. Apply 2–3 times/day.
Children. Apply 1–2 times/day.

CONTRAINDICATIONS

Hypersensitivity to flurandrenolide or any componenet of the formulation, viral, fungal, or tubercular skin lesions

INTERACTIONS

Drug
None known.
Herbal
None known.
Food
None known.

DIAGNOSTIC TEST EFFECTS

None known.

SIDE EFFECTS

Occasional
Itching, dry skin, folliculitis
Rare
Intracranial hemorrhage, acne, striae, miliaria, allergic contact dermatitis, telangiectasis or raised dark red spots on skin

SERIOUS REACTIONS

! When taken in excessive quantities, systemic hypercorticism and adrenal suppression may occur.

DENTAL CONSIDERATIONS

General:

- Determine why the patient is taking the drug.
- Apply lubricant to dry lips for patient comfort before dental procedures.
- Place on frequent recall to evaluate healing response when used on chronic basis.

flurazepam hydrochloride

flure-az′-e-pam
Schedule IV
(Apo-Flurazepam[CAN], Dalmane)
Do not confuse Dalmane with Dialume.

CATEGORY AND SCHEDULE

Pregnancy Risk Category: X
Controlled Substance: Schedule IV

MECHANISM OF ACTION

A benzodiazepine that enhances action of inhibitory neurotransmitter gamma-aminobutyric acid (GABA). ***Therapeutic Effect:*** Produces hypnotic effect due to CNS depression.

PHARMACOKINETICS

Route	Onset	Peak	Duration
PO	15–20 min	3–6 hr	7–8 hr

Well absorbed from the GI tract. Protein binding: 97%. Crosses the blood-brain barrier. Widely distributed. Metabolized in liver to active metabolite. Primarily excreted in urine. Not removed by hemodialysis. ***Half-life:*** 2.3 hr; metabolite: 40–114 hr.

AVAILABILITY

Capsules: 15 mg, 30 mg.

INDICATIONS AND DOSAGES

▸ **Insomnia**

PO

Adults. 15–30 mg at bedtime.
Elderly, debilitated, liver disease, low serum albumin, Children 15 yr and older. 15 mg at bedtime.

CONTRAINDICATIONS

Acute alcohol intoxication, acute angle-closure glaucoma, pregnancy or breast-feeding

INTERACTIONS

Drug

Alcohol, CNS depressants: May increase CNS depression.

Herbal

Kava kava, valerian: May increase CNS depression.

Food

None known.

Drug interactions of concern to dentistry

- Increased sedation: alcohol, CNS depressants
- Increased serum levels and prolonged effect of benzodiazepines: ketoconazole, itraconazole, fluconazole, miconazole (systemic), indinavir
- Contraindicated with saquinavir
- Possible increase in CNS side effects: kava (herb)

DIAGNOSTIC TEST EFFECTS

None known.

SIDE EFFECTS

Frequent

Drowsiness, dizziness, ataxia, sedation
Morning drowsiness may occur initially.

Occasional

GI disturbances, nervousness, blurred vision, dry mouth, headache, confusion, skin rash, irritability, slurred speech

Rare

Paradoxical CNS excitement or restlessness, particularly noted in elderly or debilitated

SERIOUS REACTIONS

! Abrupt or too-rapid withdrawal after long-term use may result

in pronounced restlessness and irritability, insomnia, hand tremors, abdominal or muscle cramps, vomiting, diaphoresis, and seizures.
! Overdose results in somnolence, confusion, diminished reflexes, and coma.

DENTAL CONSIDERATIONS

General:

- Assess salivary flow as a factor in caries, periodontal disease, and candidiasis.
- Psychologic and physical dependence may occur with chronic administration.
- Geriatric patients are more susceptible to drug effects; use lower dose.

Consultations:

- Medical consultation may be required to assess disease control.

Teach Patient/Family:

- To avoid mouth rinses with high alcohol content because of drying effects

flurbiprofen

flure-bi′-proe-fen
(Ansaid, Froben[CAN], Ocufen, Strepfen[AUS])
Do not confuse Ocufen with Ocuflox.

CATEGORY AND SCHEDULE

Pregnancy Risk Category: B (D if used in third trimester or near delivery; C for ophthalmic solution)

MECHANISM OF ACTION

A phenylalkanoic acid that produces analgesic and anti-inflammatory effect by inhibiting prostaglandin synthesis. Also relaxes the iris sphincter. ***Therapeutic Effect:*** Reduces the inflammatory response and intensity of pain. Prevents or decreases miosis during cataract surgery.

PHARMACOKINETICS

Well absorbed from the GI tract; ophthalmic solution penetrates cornea after administration, and may be systemically absorbed. Protein binding: 99%. Widely distributed. Metabolized in the liver. Primarily excreted in urine. ***Half-life:*** 3–4 hr.

AVAILABILITY

Tablets (Ansaid): 50 mg, 100 mg.
Ophthalmic Solution (Ocufen): 0.03%.

INDICATIONS AND DOSAGES

▸ Rheumatoid Arthritis, Osteoarthritis

PO

Adults, Elderly. 200–300 mg/day in 2–4 divided doses. Maximum: 100 mg/dose or 300 mg/day.

▸ Dysmenorrhea, Pain

PO

Adults. 50 mg 4 times a day

▸ Usual Ophthalmic Dosage

Adults, Elderly, Children. Apply 1 drop q30min starting 2 hr before surgery for total of 4 doses.

CONTRAINDICATIONS

Active peptic ulcer, chronic inflammation of GI tract, GI bleeding or ulceration, history of hypersensitivity to aspirin or NSAIDs

INTERACTIONS

Drug

Acetylcholine, carbachol: May decrease the effects of these drugs (with ophthalmic flurbiprofen).
Antihypertensives, diuretics: May decrease the effects of these drugs.

Aspirin, other salicylates: May increase the risk of GI side effects such as bleeding.
Bone marrow depressants: May increase the risk of hematologic reactions.
Epinephrine, other antiglaucoma medications: May decrease the antiglaucoma effect of these drugs.
Heparin, oral anticoagulants, thrombolytics: May increase the effects of these drugs.
Lithium: May increase the blood concentration and risk of toxicity of lithium.
Methotrexate: May increase the risk of methotrexate toxicity.
Probenecid: May increase the flurbiprofen blood concentration.

Herbal

Feverfew: May decrease the effects of feverfew.
Ginkgo biloba: May increase the risk of bleeding.

Food

None known.

Drug interactions of concern to dentistry

- GI ulceration, bleeding: aspirin, alcohol, corticosteroids
- Decreased action: salicylates
- Nephrotoxicity: acetaminophen (prolonged use)
- *When prescribed for dental pain:*
  - Risk of increased effects: oral anticoagulants, oral antidiabetics, lithium, methotrexate
  - Decreased effects of diuretics
  - First-time users of SSRIs also taking NSAIDs may have a higher risk of GI side effects; until more data are available, it may be advisable to avoid use of NSAIDs in these patients (*Br J Clin Pharmacol* 55:591–595, 2003)

DIAGNOSTIC TEST EFFECTS

May increase bleeding time and serum LDH, alkaline phosphatase, AST (SGOT), and ALT (SGPT) levels.

SIDE EFFECTS

Occasional

PO (9%–3%): Headache, abdominal pain, diarrhea, indigestion, nausea, fluid retention
Ophthalmic: Burning or stinging on instillation, keratitis, elevated intraocular pressure

Rare (less than 3%)

PO: Blurred vision, flushed skin, dizziness, somnolence, nervousness, insomnia, unusual fatigue, constipation, decreased appetite, vomiting, confusion

SERIOUS REACTIONS

! Overdose may result in acute renal failure.

! Rare reactions with long-term use include peptic ulcer disease, GI bleeding, gastritis, severe hepatic reaction (jaundice), nephrotoxicity (hematuria, dysuria, proteinuria), a severe hypersensitivity reaction (angioedema, bronchospasm) and cardiac arrhythmias.

DENTAL CONSIDERATIONS

General:

- Patients on chronic drug therapy may rarely have symptoms of blood dyscrasias, which can include infection, bleeding, and poor healing.
- Assess salivary flow as a factor in caries, periodontal disease, and candidiasis.
- Avoid prescribing for dental use in last trimester of pregnancy.
- Avoid prescribing aspirin-containing products.
- Consider semisupine chair position for patients with arthritic disease.

Consultations:

- Medical consultation may be required to assess disease control.
- In a patient with symptoms of blood dyscrasias, request a medical consultation for blood studies and postpone dental treatment until normal values are reestablished.

Teach Patient/Family:

- Importance of good oral hygiene to prevent soft tissue inflammation
- Caution to prevent injury when using oral hygiene aids
- *When chronic dry mouth occurs, advise patient:*
  - To avoid mouth rinses with high alcohol content because of drying effects
  - To use daily home fluoride products for anticaries effect
  - To use sugarless gum, frequent sips of water, or saliva substitutes

FLURBIPROFEN SODIUM

DENTAL CONSIDERATIONS

General:

- Avoid dental light in patient's eyes; offer dark glasses for patient comfort.

flutamide

flew′-tah-myd

(Euflex[CAN], Eulexin, Flugerel[AUS], Flutamin[AUS], Fugerel[AUS], Novo-Flutamide[CAN])

Do not confuse flutamide with Flumadine.

CATEGORY AND SCHEDULE

Pregnancy Risk Category: D

MECHANISM OF ACTION

An antiandrogen hormone that inhibits androgen uptake and prevents androgen from binding to androgen receptors in target tissue. Used in conjuction with leuprolide to inhibit the stimulant effects of flutamide on serum testosterone levels. ***Therapeutic Effect:*** Suppresses testicular androgen production and decreases growth of prostate carcinoma.

PHARMACOKINETICS

Completely absorbed from the GI tract. Protein binding: 94%–96%. Metabolized in the liver to active metabolite. Primarily excreted in urine. Not removed by hemodialysis. ***Half-life:*** 6 hr (increased in elderly).

AVAILABILITY

Capsules: 125 mg.

INDICATIONS AND DOSAGES

▸ Prostatic Carcinoma (in Combination with Leuprolide)

PO

Adults, Elderly. 250 mg q8h.

CONTRAINDICATIONS

Severe hepatic impairment

INTERACTIONS

Drug

None known.

Herbal

None known.

Food

None known.

DIAGNOSTIC TEST EFFECTS

May increase blood glucose level and serum estradiol, testosterone, bilirubin, creatinine, AST (SGOT), and ALT (SGPT) levels.

SIDE EFFECTS

Frequent

Hot flashes (50%); decreased libido, diarrhea (24%); generalized pain (23%); asthenia (17%); constipation (12%); nausea, nocturia (11%)

Occasional (8%–6%)

Dizziness, paresthesia, insomnia, impotence, peripheral edema, gynecomastia

Rare (5%–4%)

Rash, diaphoresis, hypertension, hematuria, vomiting, urinary incontinence, headache, flulike syndromes, photosensitivity

SERIOUS REACTIONS

! Hepatoxicity, including hepatic encephalopathy, and hemolytic anemia may be noted.

DENTAL CONSIDERATIONS

General:

- Talk with patient about any pain medication being taken.
- Avoid drugs (anticholinergics) that could exacerbate urinary retention (if present).

fluticasone propionate

flu-tic′-a-zone

(Beconase Allergy 24 Hour[AUS], Beconase Hayfever[AUS], Cutivate, Flixotide Disks[AUS], Flixotide Inhaler[AUS], Flonase, Flovent, Flovent Diskus, Flovent HFA)

CATEGORY AND SCHEDULE

Pregnancy Risk Category: C

MECHANISM OF ACTION

A corticosteroid that controls the rate of protein synthesis, depresses migration of polymorphonuclear leukocytes, reverses capillary permeability, and stabilizes lysosomal membranes. ***Therapeutic Effect:*** Prevents or controls inflammation.

PHARMACOKINETICS

Inhalation/intranasal: Protein binding: 91%. Undergoes extensive first-pass metabolism in liver. Excreted in urine. ***Half-life:*** 3–7.8 hrs. Topical: Amount absorbed depends on affected area and skin condition (absorption increased with fever, hydration, inflamed or denuded skin).

AVAILABILITY

Aerosol for Oral Inhalation (Flovent, Flovent HFA): 44 mcg/inhalation, 110 mcg/inhalation, 220 mcg/inhalation.

Powder for Oral Inhalation (Flovent Diskus): 50 mcg, 100 mcg, 250 mcg.

Intranasal Spray (Flonase): 50 mcg/inhalation.

Topical Cream (Cutivate): 0.05%.

Topical Ointment (Cutivate): 0.005%.

INDICATIONS AND DOSAGES

▸ **Allergic Rhinitis**

INTRANASAL

Adults, Elderly. Initially, 200 mcg (2 sprays in each nostril once daily or 1 spray in each nostril q12h). Maintenance: 1 spray in each nostril once daily.
Maximum: 200 mcg/day.

Children 4 yr and older. Initially, 100 mcg (1 spray in each nostril once daily). Maximum: 200 mcg/day.

▸ **Relief of Inflammation and Pruritus Associated with Steroid-Responsive Disorders, Such as Contact Dermatitis and Eczema**

TOPICAL

Adults, Elderly, Children 3 mo and older. Apply sparingly to affected area once or twice a day.

▸ Maintenance Treatment for Asthma for Those Previously Treated with Bronchodilators
INHALATION POWDER (Flovent Diskus)
Adults, Elderly, Children 12 yr and older. Initially, 100 mcg q12h. Maximum: 500 mcg/day.
Inhalation (Oral [Flovent])
Adults, Elderly, Children 12 yr and older. 88 mcg twice a day. Maximum: 440 mcg twice a day.

▸ Maintenance Treatment for Asthma for Those Previously Treated with Inhaled Steroids
INHALATION POWDER (Flovent Diskus)
Adults, Elderly, Children 12 yr and older. Initially, 100–250 mcg q12h. Maximum: 500 mcg q12h.
INHALATION (Oral [Flovent])
Adults, Elderly, Children 12 yr and older. 88–220 mcg twice a day. Maximum: 440 mcg twice a day.

▸ Maintenance Treatment for Asthma for Those Previously Treated with Oral Steroids
INHALATION POWDER (Flovent Diskus)
Adults, Elderly, Children 12 yr and older. 500–1,000 mcg twice a day.
INHALATION (Oral [Flovent])
Adults, Elderly, Children 12 yrs and older. 880 mcg twice a day.

CONTRAINDICATIONS

Primary treatment of status asthmaticus or other acute asthma episodes (inhalation); untreated localized infection of nasal mucosa

INTERACTIONS

Drug

Bupropion: May lower the seizure threshold.

Herbal

None known.

Food

None known.

Drug interactions of concern to dentistry

• No specific interactions reported, but use CYP3A4 inhibitors with caution

DIAGNOSTIC TEST EFFECTS

None known.

SIDE EFFECTS

Frequent

Inhalation: Throat irritation, hoarseness, dry mouth, cough, temporary wheezing, oropharyngeal candidiasis (particularly if mouth is not rinsed with water after each administration)
Intranasal: Mild nasopharyngeal irritation; nasal burning, stinging, or dryness; rebound congestion; rhinorrhea; loss of taste

Occasional

Inhalation: Oral candidiasis
Intranasal: Nasal and pharyngeal candidiasis, headache
Topical: Skin burning, pruritus

SERIOUS REACTIONS

! Deaths due to adrenal insufficiency have occurred in asthma patients during and after transfer from use of long-term systemic corticosteroids to less systemically available inhaled corticosteroids.

DENTAL CONSIDERATIONS

General:

• Examine oral cavity for evidence of opportunistic candidiasis in patients using the inhaler.
• Allergic rhinitis may be a factor in mouth breathing and drying of oral tissues.
• Be aware that aspirin or sulfite preservatives in vasoconstrictor-containing products can exacerbate asthma.

• Acute asthmatic episodes may be precipitated in the dental office. Rapid-acting sympathomimetic inhalants should be available for emergency use. A stress reduction protocol may be required.
• Consider semisupine chair position for patients with respiratory disease.

Consultations:
• Consultation may be required to confirm steroid dose and duration of use.

Teach Patient/Family:
• Importance of updating health and drug history if physician makes any changes in drug regimens
• Importance of gargling, rinsing mouth with water, and expectorating after each aerosol use

FLUTICASONE PROPIONATE

DENTAL CONSIDERATIONS

Teach Patient/Family:
• That use of topical preparations on fungal or herpetic lesions is contraindicated

fluvastatin

floo′-va-sta-tin
(Lescol, Lescol XL, Vastin[AUS])
Do not confuse fluvastatin with fluoxetine.

CATEGORY AND SCHEDULE

Pregnancy Risk Category: X

MECHANISM OF ACTION

An antihyperlipidemic that inhibits HMG-CoA reductase, the enzyme that catalyzes the early step in cholesterol synthesis. ***Therapeutic Effect:*** Decreases LDL cholesterol, VLDL, and plasma triglyceride levels. Slightly increases HDL cholesterol concentration.

PHARMACOKINETICS

Well absorbed from the GI tract and is unaffected by food. Does not cross the blood-brain barrier. Protein binding: greater than 98%. Primarily eliminated in feces. ***Half-life:*** 1.2 hr.

AVAILABILITY

Capsules (Lescol): 20 mg, 40 mg.
Tablets (Extended-Release [Lescol XL]): 80 mg.

INDICATIONS AND DOSAGES

▸ Hyperlipoproteinemia

PO
Adults, Elderly. Initially, 20 mg/day (capsule) in the evening. May increase up to 40 mg/day. Maintenance: 20–40 mg/day in a single dose or divided doses.
Patients requiring more than a 25% decrease in LDL cholesterol. 40 mg (capsule) 1–2 times a day. Or 80 mg tablet once a day.

CONTRAINDICATIONS

Active hepatic disease, unexplained increased serum transaminase levels

INTERACTIONS

Drug
Cyclosporine, erythromycin, gemfibrozil, immunosuppressants, niacin: Increases the risk of acute renal failure and rhabdomyolysis with these drugs.

Herbal
None known.

Food
None known.

Drug interactions of concern to dentistry
• Increased plasma levels: alcohol, fluconazole, itraconazole, ketoconazole, erythromycin

DIAGNOSTIC TEST EFFECTS
May increase serum CK and transaminase concentrations

SIDE EFFECTS
Frequent (8%–5%)
Headache, dyspepsia, back pain, myalgia, arthralgia, diarrhea, abdominal cramping, rhinitis
Occasional (4%–2%)
Nausea, vomiting, insomnia, constipation, flatulence, rash, pruritus, fatigue, cough, dizziness

SERIOUS REACTIONS
! Myositis (inflammation of voluntary muscle) with or without increased CK, and muscle weakness, occur rarely. These conditions may progress to frank rhabdomyolysis and renal impairment.

DENTAL CONSIDERATIONS
General:
• Consider semisupine chair position for patient comfort because of GI, musculoskeletal, and respiratory side effects.

fluvoxamine maleate
floo-vox′-a-meen
(Faverin[AUS], Luvox)

CATEGORY AND SCHEDULE
Pregnancy Risk Category: C

MECHANISM OF ACTION
An antidepressant and antiobsessive agent that selectively inhibits neuronal reuptake of serotonin. ***Therapeutic Effect:*** Relieves depression and symptoms of obsessive-compulsive disorder.

AVAILABILITY
Tablets: 25 mg, 50 mg, 100 mg.

INDICATIONS AND DOSAGES
▸ **Obsessive-Compulsive Disorder**
PO
Adults. 50 mg at bedtime; may increase by 50 mg every 4–7 days. Dosages greater than 100 mg/day given in 2 divided doses. Maximum: 300 mg/day.
Children 8–17 yr. 25 mg at bedtime; may increase by 25 mg every 4–7 days. Dosages greater than 50 mg/day given in 2 divided doses. Maximum: 200 mg/day.

OFF-LABEL USES
Treatment of depression, panic disorder, anxiety disorders in children

CONTRAINDICATIONS
Use within 14 days of MAOIs

INTERACTIONS
Drug
Benzodiazepines, carbamazepine, clozapine, theophylline: May increase the blood concentration and risk of toxicity of these drugs.
Lithium, tryptophan: May enhance fluvoxamine's serotonergic effects.
MAOIs: May produce serious reactions, including hyperthermia, rigidity, and myoclonus.
Tricyclic antidepressants: May increase the fluvoxamine blood concentration.
Warfarin: May increase the effects of warfarin.
Herbal
St. John's wort: May increase fluvoxamine's pharmacologic effects and risk of toxicity.
Food
None known.
Drug interactions of concern to dentistry
• Increased plasma levels of tricyclic antidepressants, carbamazepine, benzodiazepine; reduce doses of

alprazolam, diazepam, midazolam, triazolam by half
- Risk of serotonin syndrome: SSRIs
- First-time users of SSRIs also taking NSAIDs may have a higher risk of GI side effects; until more data are available, it may be advisable to avoid use of NSAIDs in these patients (*Br J Clin Pharmacol* 55:591–595, 2003)

DIAGNOSTIC TEST EFFECTS
None known.

SIDE EFFECTS
Frequent
Nausea (40%), headache, somnolence, insomnia (21%–22%)
Occasional (14%–8%)
Dizziness, diarrhea, dry mouth, asthenia, weakness, dyspepsia, constipation, abnormal ejaculation
Rare (6%–3%)
Anorexia, anxiety, tremor, vomiting, flatulence, urinary frequency, sexual dysfunction, altered taste

SERIOUS REACTIONS
! Overdose may produce seizures, nausea, vomiting, and extreme agitation and restlessness.

DENTAL CONSIDERATIONS
General:
- After supine positioning, have patient sit upright for at least 2 min to avoid orthostatic hypotension.
- Assess salivary flow as a factor in caries, periodontal disease, and candidiasis.
- Consider semisupine chair position for patient comfort because of GI effects of drug.

Consultations:
- Medical consultation may be required to assess patient's ability to tolerate stress.
- Physician should be informed if significant xerostomic side effects occur (e.g., increased caries, sore tongue, problems eating or swallowing, difficulty wearing prosthesis) so that a medication change can be considered.

Teach Patient/Family:
- *When chronic dry mouth occurs, advise patient:*
  - To avoid mouth rinses with high alcohol content because of drying effects
  - To use daily home fluoride products for anticaries effect
  - To use sugarless gum, frequent sips of water, or saliva substitutes

F

folic acid/sodium folate (vitamin B_9)
foe′-lik
(folic acid) Apo-Folic[CAN], Folvite, Megafol[AUS](sodium folate) Folvite-parenteral
Do not confuse Folvite with Florvite.

CATEGORY AND SCHEDULE
Pregnancy Risk Category: A (C if used in doses above the recommended daily allowance)
OTC (0.4-mg and 0.8-mg tablets only)

MECHANISM OF ACTION
A coenzyme that stimulates production of platelets, RBCs, and WBCs.
Therapeutic Effect: Essential for nucleoprotein synthesis and maintenance of normal erythropoiesis.

PHARMACOKINETICS
PO form almost completely absorbed from the GI tract (upper duodenum).

Protein binding: High. Metabolized in the liver and plasma to active form. Excreted in urine. Removed by hemodialysis.

AVAILABILITY

Tablets: 0.4 mg, 0.8 mg, 1 mg.
Injection: 5 mg/ml.

INDICATIONS AND DOSAGES

▸ Vitamin B_9 Deficiency

PO, IV, IM, SUBCUTANEOUS
Adults, Elderly, Children 12 yr and older. Initially, 1 mg/day. Maintenance: 0.5 mg/day.
Children 1–11 yr. Initially 1 mg/day. Maintenance: 0.1–0.4 mg/day.
Infants. 50 mcg/day.

▸ Dietary Supplement

PO, IV, IM, SUBCUTANEOUS
Adults, Elderly, Children 4 yr and older. 0.4 mg/day.
Children 1–younger than 4 yr. 0.3 mg/day.
Children younger than 1 yr. 0.1 mg/day.
Pregnant women. 0.8 mg/day.

OFF-LABEL USES

To decrease the risk of colon cancer

CONTRAINDICATIONS

Anemias (aplastic, normocytic, pernicious, refractory)

INTERACTIONS

Drug

Analgesics, carbamazepine, estrogens: May increase folic acid requirements.
Antacids, cholestyramine: May decrease the absorption of folic acid.
Hydantoin anticonvulsants: May decrease the effects of these drugs.
Methotrexate, triamterene, trimethoprim: May antagonize the effects of folic acid.

Herbal

None known.

Food

None known.

Drug interactions of concern to dentistry

- Increased metabolism of phenobarbital

DIAGNOSTIC TEST EFFECTS

May decrease vitamin B_{12} concentration.

SIDE EFFECTS

None known.

SERIOUS REACTIONS

! Allergic hypersensitivity occurs rarely with parenteral form. Oral folic acid is nontoxic.

DENTAL CONSIDERATIONS

General:

- Deficiency in folic acid; glossitis may be a symptom of folic acid deficiency.

fondaparinux sodium

fawn-da-pear′-ih-nux
(Arixtra)

CATEGORY AND SCHEDULE

Pregnancy Risk Category: B

MECHANISM OF ACTION

A factor Xa inhibitor and pentasaccharide that selectively binds to antithrombin, and increases its affinity for factor Xa, thereby inhibiting factor Xa and stopping the blood coagulation cascade. ***Therapeutic Effect:*** Indirectly prevents formation of thrombin and subsequently the fibrin clot.

PHARMACOKINETICS

Well absorbed after subcutaneous administration. Undergoes minimal, if any, metabolism. Highly bound to antithrombin III. Distributed mainly in blood and to a minor extent in extravascular fluid. Excreted unchanged in urine. Removed by hemodialysis. ***Half-life:*** 17–21 hr (prolonged in patients with impaired renal function).

AVAILABILITY

Injection: 2.5 mg/0.5 ml prefilled syringe.

INDICATIONS AND DOSAGES

▸ Prevention of Venous Thromboembolism

SUBCUTANEOUS

Adults. 2.5 mg once a day for 5–9 days after surgery. Initial dose should be given 6–8 hr after surgery. Dosage should be adjusted in the elderly and in those with renal impairment.

CONTRAINDICATIONS

Active major bleeding, bacterial endocarditis, severe renal impairment (with creatinine clearance <30 ml/min), thrombocytopenia associated with antiplatelet antibody formation in the presence of fondaparinux, body weight <50 kg

INTERACTIONS

Drug

Anticoagulants, platelet inhibitors: May increase bleeding.

Herbal

None known.

Food

None known.

Drug interactions of concern to dentistry

- Avoid concurrent use of aspirin and NSAIDs

DIAGNOSTIC TEST EFFECTS

Increases reversible serum creatinine, AST(SGOT), and ALT(SGPT) levels. May decrease Hgb, Hct, and platelet count.

SIDE EFFECTS

Occasional (14%)

Fever

Rare (4%–1%)

Injection site hematoma, nausea, peripheral edema

SERIOUS REACTIONS

! Accidental overdose may lead to bleeding complications ranging from local ecchymoses to major hemorrhage.

! Thrombocytopenia occurs rarely.

DENTAL CONSIDERATIONS

General:

- Determine why patient is taking the drug.
- Monitor vital signs at every appointment because of cardiovascular side effects.
- Consider local hemostasis measures to prevent excessive bleeding.
- Antibiotic prophylaxis before dental treatment may be required for joint prosthesis (see 2003 ADA guidelines).
- Delay elective dental treatment until patient completes anticoagulant therapy.

Consultations:

- Medical consultation should include routine blood counts, including platelet counts and bleeding time.

Teach Patient/Family:

- Importance of good oral hygiene to prevent soft tissue inflammation, infection
- To prevent injury when using oral hygiene aids
- To report oral lesions, soreness, or bleeding to dentist

F

formoterol fumarate

for-moe′-ter-ol
(Foradil Aerolizer, Foradile[AUS], Oxis[AUS])

CATEGORY AND SCHEDULE

Pregnancy Risk Category: C

F

MECHANISM OF ACTION

A long-acting bronchodilator that stimulates beta2-adrenergic receptors in the lungs, resulting in relaxation of bronchial smooth muscle. Also inhibits release of mediators from various cells in the lungs, including mast cells, with little effect on heart rate. ***Therapeutic Effect:*** Relieves bronchospasm, reduces airway resistance. Improves bronchodilation, nighttime asthma control, and peak flow rates.

PHARMACOKINETICS

Route	Onset	Peak	Duration
Inhalation	1–3 min	0.5–1 hr	12 hr

Absorbed from bronchi after inhalation. Metabolized in the liver. Primarily excreted in urine. Unknown if removed by hemodialysis. ***Half-life:*** 10 hr.

AVAILABILITY

Inhalation Powder in Capsules: 12 mcg.

INDICATIONS AND DOSAGES

▸ **Asthma, Chronic Obstructive Pulmonary Disease (COPD)**

INHALATION

Adults, Elderly, Children 5 yrs and older. 12 mcg capsule q12h.

▸ **Exercise-Induced Bronchospasm**

INHALATION

Adults, Elderly, Children 5 yr and older. 12 mcg capsule at least 15 min before exercise. Do not repeat for another 12 hours.

CONTRAINDICATIONS

None known.

INTERACTIONS

Drug

Beta blockers: May antagonize formoterol's bronchodilating effects.
Diuretics, steroids, xanthine derivatives: May increase the risk of hypokalemia.
Drugs that can prolong QT interval (including erythromycin, quinidine, and thioridazine), MAOIs, tricyclic antidepressants: May potentiate cardiovascular effects.

Herbal

None known.

Food

None known.

Drug interactions of concern to dentistry

- Avoid MAOIs, tricyclic antidepressants, and drugs that prolong the QT interval (phenothiazines, procainamide)
- Adrenergic agents/sympathomimetics may potentiate effects
- β-Adrenergic blockers may antagonize sympathomimetic effects

DIAGNOSTIC TEST EFFECTS

May decrease serum potassium level. May increase blood glucose level.

SIDE EFFECTS

Occasional

Tremor, muscle cramps, tachycardia, insomnia, headache, irritability, irritation of mouth or throat

SERIOUS REACTIONS

! Excessive sympathomimetic stimulation may produce palpitations, extrasystole, and chest pain.

DENTAL CONSIDERATIONS

General:

- Monitor vital signs at every appointment because of cardiovascular side effects.
- Assess salivary flow as a factor in caries, periodontal disease, and candidiasis.
- Consider semisupine chair position for patient comfort because of respiratory side effects of disease.
- Short midday appointments and a stress reduction protocol may be required for anxious patients.
- Have patient bring personal short-acting bronchodilator to appointment for use in emergency.
- Acute asthmatic episodes may be precipitated in the dental office. Rapid-acting sympathomimetic inhalants should be available for emergency use.
- Avoid prescribing aspirin-containing products.

Consultations:

- Medical consultation may be required to assess disease control and patient's ability to tolerate stress.

Teach Patient/Family:

- Importance of gargling, rinsing mouth with water, and expectorating after each aerosol dose
- *When chronic dry mouth occurs, advise patient:*
  - To avoid mouth rinses with high alcohol content because of drying effects
  - To use daily home fluoride products for anticaries effect
  - To use sugarless gum, frequent sips of water, or saliva substitutes

fosamprenavir

foss-am-pren′-ah-vur
(Lexiva)

CATEGORY AND SCHEDULE

Pregnancy Risk Category: C

F

MECHANISM OF ACTION

An antiretroviral that is rapidly converted to amprenavir, which inhibits HIV-1 protease by binding to the enzyme's active site, thus preventing the processing of viral precursors and resulting in the formation of immature, noninfectious viral particles.
Therapeutic Effect: Impairs HIV replication and proliferation.

PHARMACOKINETICS

Rapidly absorbed after PO administration. Protein binding: 90%. Metabolized in the liver. Excreted in urine and feces. ***Half-life:*** 7.7 hr.

AVAILABILITY

Tablets: 700 mg (equivalent to 600 mg amprenavir)

INDICATIONS AND DOSAGES

▸ **HIV Infection in Patients Who Have Not Had Previous Protease Inhibitor Therapy**

PO

Adults, Elderly. 1,400 mg twice daily without ritonavir; or 1,400 mg twice daily plus ritonavir 200 mg once daily; or 700 mg twice daily plus ritonavir 100 mg twice daily.

▸ **HIV Infection in Patients Who Have Had Previous Protease Inhibitor Therapy**

PO

Adults, Elderly. 700 mg twice daily plus ritonavir 100 mg twice daily.

▸ Concurrent Therapy with Efavirenz

PO

Adults, Elderly. In patients receiving fosamprenavir plus once-daily ritonavir in combination with efavirenz, an additional 100 mg/day ritonavir (300 mg total/day) should be given.

F

CONTRAINDICATIONS

Concurrent use of amprenavir, dihydroergotamine, ergonovine, ergotamine, methylergonovine, pimozide, midazolam, or triazolam. If fosamprenavir is given concurrently with ritonavir, flecainide and propafenone are also contraindicated.

INTERACTIONS

Drug

Amiodarone, bepridil, ergotamine, lidocaine, midazolam, oral contraceptives, quinidine, triazolam, tricyclic antidepressants: May interfere with the metabolism of the these drugs.

Antacids, didanosine: May decrease the absorption of fosamprenavir.

Carbamazepine, phenobarbital, phenytoin, rifampin: May decrease the fosamprenavir blood concentration.

Clozapine, HMG-CoA reductase inhibitors (statins), warfarin: May increase the blood concentrations of these drugs.

Herbal

St. John's wort: May decrease the fosamprenavir blood concentration.

Food

None known.

Drug interactions of concern to dentistry

- Contraindicated with midazolam, triazolam
- Increased plasma levels of: tricyclic antidepressants, lidocaine, alprazolam, chlorazepate, diazepam, flurazepam, ketoconazole, itraconazole, sildenafil, vardenafil
- Reduced absorption: antacids, carbamazepine, phenobarbital, St. John's wort (herb)

DIAGNOSTIC TEST EFFECTS

May increase serum lipase, triglyceride, AST (SGOT), and ALT (SGPT) levels.

SIDE EFFECTS

Frequent (39%–35%)

Nausea, rash, diarrhea

Occasional (19%–8%)

Headache, vomiting, fatigue, depression

Rare (7%–2%)

Pruritus, abdominal pain, perioral paresthesia

SERIOUS REACTIONS

! Severe and possibly life-threatening dermatologic reactions occur rarely.

DENTAL CONSIDERATIONS

General:

- Caution significant drug interactions with drugs used in dentistry.
- Question patient about other drugs or herbals they may be taking.
- Patient on chronic drug therapy may rarely present with symptoms of blood dyscrasias, which can include infection, bleeding and poor healing. If dyscrasia is present, caution patient to prevent oral tissue trauma when using oral hygiene aids.
- Consider semisupine chair position for patient comfort if GI side effects occur.

Consultations:

- In a patient with symptoms of blood dyscrasias, request a medical consultation for blood studies and postpone treatment until normal values are reestablished.

• Medical consultation may be required to assess disease control and patient's ability to tolerate stress.

Teach Patient/Family:

• Importance of good oral hygiene to prevent soft tissue inflammation
• To prevent trauma when using oral hygiene aids
• Importance of updating health and medication history if physician makes any changes in evaluation or drug regimens; include OTC, herbal, and nonherbal remedies in the update

foscarnet sodium

foss-car′-net
(Foscavir)

CATEGORY AND SCHEDULE

Pregnancy Risk Category: C

MECHANISM OF ACTION

An antiviral that selectively inhibits binding sites on virus-specific DNA polymerase and reverse transcriptase. ***Therapeutic Effect:*** Inhibits replication of herpes virus.

PHARMACOKINETICS

Sequestered into bone and cartilage. Protein binding: 14%–17%. Primarily excreted unchanged in urine. Removed by hemodialysis. ***Half-life:*** 3.3–6.8 hr (increased in impaired renal function).

AVAILABILITY

Injection: 24 mg/ml.

INDICATIONS AND DOSAGES

▸ Cytomegalovirus (CMV) Retinitis

IV

Adults, Elderly. Initially, 60 mg/kg q8h or 100 mg/kg q12h for 2–3 wk. Maintenance: 90–120 mg/kg/day as a single IV infusion.

▸ Herpes Infection

IV

Adults. 40 mg/kg q8–12h for 2–3 wk or until healed.

▸ Dosage in Renal Impairment

Dosages are individualized on the basis of creatinine clearance. Refer to the dosing guide provided by the manufacturer.

F

CONTRAINDICATIONS

None known.

INTERACTIONS

Drug

Nephrotoxic medications: May increase the risk of nephrotoxicity.
Pentamidine (IV): May cause reversible hypocalcemia, hypomagnesemia, and nephrotoxicity.
Zidovudine (AZT): May increase the risk of anemia.

Herbal

None known.

Food

None known.

Drug interactions of concern to dentistry

• Avoid nephrotoxic drugs (amphotericin B)
• Possible increased risk of seizures: fluoroquinolones

DIAGNOSTIC TEST EFFECTS

May increase serum alkaline phosphatase, bilirubin, creatinine, AST (SGOT), and ALT (SGPT) levels. May decrease serum magnesium and potassium levels. May alter serum calcium and phosphate concentrations.

IV INCOMPATIBILITIES

Acyclovir (Zovirax), amphotericin B (Fungizone), co-trimoxazole (Bactrim), diazepam (Valium), digoxin (Lanoxin), diphenhydramine (Benadryl), dobutamine (Dobutrex), droperidol (Inapsine), ganciclovir (Cytovene), haloperidol (Haldol), leucovorin, midazolam (Versed), pentamidine (Pentam IV), prochlorperazine (Compazine), vancomycin (Vancocin)

IV COMPATIBILITIES

Dopamine (Intropin), heparin, hydromorphone (Dilaudid), lorazepam (Ativan), morphine, potassium chloride

F

SIDE EFFECTS

Frequent

Fever (65%); nausea (47%); vomiting, diarrhea (30%)

Occasional (≥5%)

Anorexia, pain and inflammation at injection site, fever, rigors, malaise, headache, paresthesia, dizziness, rash, diaphoresis, abdominal pain

Rare (5%–1%)

Back or chest pain, edema, flushing, pruritus, constipation, dry mouth

SERIOUS REACTIONS

! Nephrotoxicity occurs to some extent in most patients.

! Seizures and serum mineral or electrolyte imbalances may be life-threatening.

DENTAL CONSIDERATIONS

General:

- Examine for oral manifestations of opportunistic infections.
- Examine for evidence of oral manifestations of blood dyscrasias (infection, bleeding, poor healing).
- Consider local hemostasis measures to prevent excessive bleeding.
- Assess salivary flow as a factor in caries, periodontal disease, and candidiasis.
- Monitor vital signs at every appointment because of cardiovascular and respiratory side effects.
- Place on frequent recall to evaluate healing response.

Consultations:

- Medical consultation for blood studies (CBC); leukopenic or thrombocytopenic side effects may result in infection, delayed healing, and excessive bleeding. Postpone elective dental treatment until normal values are maintained.
- Medical consultation may be required to assess disease control.

Teach Patient/Family:

- Caution in use of oral hygiene aids to prevent injury
- That secondary oral infection may occur; must see dentist immediately if infection occurs
- Importance of good oral hygiene to prevent soft tissue inflammation
- Use of electric toothbrush if patient has difficulty holding conventional devices because of extrapyramidal side effects
- *When chronic dry mouth occurs, advise patient:*
  - To avoid mouth rinses with high alcohol content because of drying effects
  - To use daily home fluoride products for anticaries effect
  - To use sugarless gum, frequent sips of water, or saliva substitutes

fosfomycin tromethamine

foss-fo-mye′-sin

(Monurol)

Do not confuse Monurol with Monopril.

CATEGORY AND SCHEDULE

Pregnancy Risk Category: B

MECHANISM OF ACTION

An antibiotic that prevents bacterial cell wall formation by inhibiting the synthesis of peptidoglycan. ***Therapeutic Effect:*** Bactericidal.

AVAILABILITY

Powder for Oral Solution: 3 g.

INDICATIONS AND DOSAGES

▸ Uncomplicated UTIs

PO

Females. 3 g mixed in 4 oz water as a single dose.

Males. 3 g/day for 2–3 days.

CONTRAINDICATIONS

None known.

INTERACTIONS

Drug

Metoclopramide: Lowers serum concentration and urinary excretion of fosfomycin.

Herbal

None known.

Food

None known.

Drug interactions of concern to dentistry

- Lowered serum concentrations: metoclopramide

DIAGNOSTIC TEST EFFECTS

May increase blood eosinophil count and serum alkaline phosphatase, bilirubin, AST (SGOT), and ALT (SGPT) levels. May alter platelet and WBC counts. May decrease blood Hct and Hgb levels.

SIDE EFFECTS

Occasional (9%–3%)

Diarrhea, nausea, headache, back pain

Rare (less than 2%)

Dysmenorrhea, pharyngitis, abdominal pain, rash

SERIOUS REACTIONS

! None known.

DENTAL CONSIDERATIONS

General:

- Determine why patient is taking the drug.
- Consider semisupine chair position for patient comfort if GI side effects occur.

Teach Patient/Family:

- *When chronic dry mouth occurs, advise patient:*
  - To avoid mouth rinses with high alcohol content because of drying effects
  - To use daily home fluoride products for anticaries effect
  - To use sugarless gum, frequent sips of water, or saliva substitutes

fosinopril

fo-sin′-o-pril

(Monopril)

Do not confuse Monopril with Monurol.

CATEGORY AND SCHEDULE

Pregnancy Risk Category: C (D if used in second or third trimester)

MECHANISM OF ACTION

An ACE inhibitor that suppresses the renin-angiotensin-aldosterone system and prevents conversion of angiotensin I to angiotensin II, a potent vasoconstrictor; may also inhibit angiotensin II at local vascular and renal sites. Decreases plasma angiotensin II, increases plasma renin activity, and decreases aldosterone secretion. ***Therapeutic Effect:*** Reduces peripheral arterial resistance, pulmonary capillary wedge pressure; improves cardiac output, and exercise tolerance.

PHARMACOKINETICS

Route	Onset	Peak	Duration
PO	1 hr	2–6 hr	24 hr

Slowly absorbed from the GI tract. Protein binding: 97%–98%. Metabolized in the liver and GI mucosa to active metabolite. Primarily excreted in urine. Minimal removal by hemodialysis. ***Half-life:*** 11.5 hr.

F

AVAILABILITY

Tablets: 10 mg, 20 mg, 40 mg.

INDICATIONS AND DOSAGES

▸ Hypertension (Monotherapy)

PO

Adults, Elderly. Initially, 10 mg/day. Maintenance: 20–40 mg/day. Maximum: 80 mg/day.

▸ Hypertension (With Diuretic)

PO

Adults, Elderly. Initially, 10 mg/day titrated to patient's needs.

▸ Heart Failure

PO

Adults, Elderly. Initially, 5–10 mg. Maintenance: 20–40 mg/day.

OFF-LABEL USES

Treatment of diabetic and non-diabetic nephropathy, post-myocardial infarction left ventricular dysfunction, renal crisis in scleroderma

CONTRAINDICATIONS

History of angioedema from previous treatment with ACE inhibitors

INTERACTIONS

Drug

Alcohol, antihypertensives, diuretics: May increase the effects of fosinopril.

Lithium: May increase lithium blood concentration and risk of lithium toxicity.

NSAIDs: May decrease the effects of fosinopril.

Potassium-sparing diuretics, potassium supplements: May cause hyperkalemia.

Herbal

None known.

Food

None known.

Drug interactions of concern to dentistry

- Increased hypotension: alcohol, phenothiazines
- Decreased hypotensive effects: indomethacin, possibly other NSAIDs, sympathomimetics
- Suspected reduction in the antihypertensive and vasodilator effects by salicylates; monitor blood pressure if used concurrently

DIAGNOSTIC TEST EFFECTS

May increase BUN, serum alkaline phosphatase, serum bilirubin, serum creatinine, serum potassium, AST (SGOT), and ALT (SGPT) levels. May decrease serum sodium levels. May cause positive antinuclear antibody titer.

SIDE EFFECTS

Frequent (12%–9%)

Dizziness, cough

Occasional (4%–2%)

Hypotension, nausea, vomiting, upper respiratory tract infection

SERIOUS REACTIONS

! Excessive hypotension ("first-dose syncope") may occur in patients with CHF and in those who are severely salt and volume depleted.

! Angioedema (swelling of face and lips) and hyperkalemia occur rarely.

! Agranulocytosis and neutropenia may be noted in those with collagen vascular disease, including scleroderma and systemic lupus erythematosus, and impaired renal function.

! Nephrotic syndrome may be noted in those with history of renal disease.

DENTAL CONSIDERATIONS

General:

- Monitor vital signs at every appointment because of cardiovascular and respiratory side effects.
- After supine positioning, have patient sit upright for at least 2 min before standing to avoid orthostatic hypotension.
- Patients on chronic drug therapy may rarely have symptoms of blood dyscrasias, which can include infection, bleeding, and poor healing.
- Assess salivary flow as a factor in caries, periodontal disease, and candidiasis.
- Limit use of sodium-containing products, such as saline IV fluids, for patients with a dietary salt restriction.
- Stress from dental procedures may compromise cardiovascular function; determine patient risk.
- Short appointments and a stress reduction protocol may be required for anxious patients.

Consultations:

- Medical consultation may be required to assess disease control and patient's ability to tolerate stress.
- In a patient with symptoms of blood dyscrasias, request a medical consultation for blood studies and postpone dental treatment until normal values are reestablished.
- Take precautions if dental surgery is anticipated and sedation or general anesthesia is required; risk of hypotensive episode.

Teach Patient/Family:

- Importance of good oral hygiene to prevent soft tissue inflammation
- Caution to prevent injury when using oral hygiene aids
- *When chronic dry mouth occurs, advise patient:*
- To avoid mouth rinses with high alcohol content because of drying effects
- To use daily home fluoride products for anticaries effect
- To use sugarless gum, frequent sips of water, or saliva substitutes

F

fosphenytoin

fos-phen′-ih-toyn

(Cerebyx)

Do not confuse Cerebyx with Celebrex or Celexa.

CATEGORY AND SCHEDULE

Pregnancy Risk Category: D

MECHANISM OF ACTION

A hydantoin anticonvulsant that stabilizes neuronal membranes by decreasing sodium and calcium ion influx into the neurons. Also decreases post-tetanic potentiation and repetitive discharge.

Therapeutic Effect: Decreases seizure activity.

PHARMACOKINETICS

Completely absorbed after IM administration. Protein binding: 95%–99%. Rapidly and completely hydrolyzed to phenytoin after IM or IV administration. Time of complete conversion to phenytoin: 4 hr after IM injection; 2 hr after IV infusion. ***Half-life:*** 8–15 min (for conversion to phenytoin).

AVAILABILITY

Injection: 75 mg/ml (equivalent to 50 mg/ml phenytoin)

F

INDICATIONS AND DOSAGES

▸ Status Epilepticus

IV

Adults. Loading dose: 15–20 mg phenytoin equivalent (PE)/kg infused at rate of 100–150 mg PE/min.

▸ Nonemergent Seizures

IV, IM

Adults. Loading dose: 10–20 mg PE/kg. Maintenance: 4–6 mg PE/kg/day.

▸ Short-Term Substitution for Oral Phenytoin

IV, IM

Adults. May substitute for oral phenytoin at same total daily dose.

CONTRAINDICATIONS

Adams-Stokes syndrome, hypersensitivity to fosphenytoin or phenytoin, second- or third-degree AV block, severe bradycardia, sinoatrial block

INTERACTIONS

Drug

Alcohol, other CNS depressants: May increase CNS depression.
Amiodarone, anticoagulants, cimetidine, disulfiram, fluoxetine, isoniazid, sulfonamides: May increase fosphenytoin blood concentration, effects, and risk of toxicity.
Antacids: May decrease fosphenytoin absorption.
Fluconazole, ketoconazole, miconazole: May increase fosphenytoin blood concentration.
Glucocorticoids: May decrease the effects of glucocorticoids.
Lidocaine, propranolol: May increase cardiac depressant effects.
Valproic acid: May increase the blood concentration and decrease the metabolism of fosphenytoin.
Xanthines: May increase the metabolism of xanthines.

Herbal

None known.

Food

None known.

Drug interactions of concern to dentistry

- Increased phenytoin levels: benzodiazepines (chlordiazepoxide, diazepam), halothane, salicylates
- Increased CNS depression: benzodiazepines, H_1-blocker antihistamines, opiate agonists
- Decreased phenytoin levels: carbamazepine, ciprofloxacin
- Decreased effectiveness of corticosteroids
- Suspected risk of hepatic toxicity: chronic use of acetaminophen and phosphenytoin

DIAGNOSTIC TEST EFFECTS

May increase blood glucose, serum GGT, and serum alkaline phosphatase levels.

IV INCOMPATIBILITIES

Midazolam (Versed)

IV COMPATIBILITIES

Lorazepam (Ativan), phenobarbital, potassium chloride

SIDE EFFECTS

Frequent

Dizziness, paresthesia, tinnitus, pruritus, headache, somnolence

Occasional

Morbilliform rash

SERIOUS REACTIONS

! An elevated fosphenytoin blood concentration may produce ataxia, nystagmus, diplopia, lethargy, slurred speech, nausea, vomiting, and hypotension. As the drug level increases, extreme lethargy may progress to coma.

DENTAL CONSIDERATIONS

General:

- This drug is intended for short-term use in an emergency department or hospital setting. Patient probably will return to oral phenytoin or other anticonvulsant after hospital care.
- Use precaution if sedation or general anesthesia is required; risk of hypotensive episode.

Consultations:

- Determine type of epilepsy, seizure frequency, and quality of seizure control. A stress reduction protocol may be required.
- Medical consultation may be required to assess disease control and patient's ability to tolerate stress.

Teach Patient/Family:

- Importance of updating health and drug history if physician makes any changes in evaluation or drug regimens

frovatriptan

fro-va-trip′-tan
(Frovan)

CATEGORY AND SCHEDULE

Pregnancy Risk Category: C

MECHANISM OF ACTION

A serotonin receptor agonist that binds selectively to vascular receptors, producing a vasoconstrictive effect on cranial blood vessels. ***Therapeutic Effect:*** Relieves migraine headache.

PHARMACOKINETICS

Well absorbed after PO administration. Metabolized by the liver to inactive metabolite. Eliminated in urine. ***Half-life:*** 26 hr (increased in hepatic impairment).

AVAILABILITY

Tablets: 2.5 mg.

INDICATIONS AND DOSAGES

▸ Acute Migraine Attack

PO

Adults, Elderly. Initially 2.5 mg. If headache improves but then returns, dose may be repeated after 2 hr. Maximum: 7.5 mg/day.

CONTRAINDICATIONS

Basilar or hemiplegic migraine, cerebrovascular or peripheral vascular disease, coronary artery disease, ischemic heart disease (including angina pectoris, history of MI, silent ischemia, and Prinzmetal's angina), severe hepatic impairment (Child-Pugh grade C), uncontrolled hypertension, use within 24 hours of ergotamine-containing preparations or another serotonin receptor agonist, use within 14 days of MAOIs

INTERACTIONS

Drug

Ergotamine-containing medications: May produce a vasospastic reaction.
Fluoxetine, fluvoxamine, paroxetine, sertraline: May produce a vasospastic reaction.
Oral contraceptives: Decrease frovatriptan clearance and volume of distribution.
Propranolol: May dramatically increase frovatriptan plasma concentration.

Herbal

None known.

Food

None known.

Drug interactions of concern to dentistry
- Potential serotonin crisis: SSRIs, ergot-containing drugs (avoid use within 24 hr of taking this drug)
- Decreased plasma levels: cimetidine

DIAGNOSTIC TEST EFFECTS
None known.

SIDE EFFECTS
Occasional (8%–4%)
Dizziness, paresthesia, fatigue, flushing
Rare (3%–2%)
Hot or cold sensation, dry mouth, dyspepsia

SERIOUS REACTIONS
! Cardiac reactions (including ischemia, coronary artery vasospasm, and MI), and noncardiac vasospasm-related reactions (such as hemorrhage and CVA), occur rarely, particularly in patients with hypertension, diabetes, or a strong family history of coronary artery disease; obese patients; smokers; males older than 40 years; and postmenopausal women.

DENTAL CONSIDERATIONS
General:
- This is an acute-use drug; it is doubtful that patients will seek dental treatment during acute migraine attacks.
- Be aware of patient's disease, its severity, and its frequency, when known.
- Advise patient if dental drugs prescribed have a potential for photosensitivity.

Consultations:
- If treating chronic orofacial pain, consult with physician of record.
- Medical consultation may be required to assess disease control and patient's ability to tolerate stress.

Teach Patient/Family:
- That dryness of the mouth may occur when taking this drug; avoid mouth rinses with high alcohol content because of additional drying effects
- Importance of updating health and drug history if physician makes any changes in evaluation or drug regimens

furosemide
fur-oh′-se-mide
(Apo-Furosemide[CAN], Frusehexal[AUS], Frusid[AUS], Lasix, Uremide[AUS], Urex-M[AUS])
Do not confuse Lasix with Lidex, Luvox, or Luxiq, or furosemide with Torsemide.

CATEGORY AND SCHEDULE
Pregnancy Risk Category: C (D if used in pregnancy-induced hypertension)

MECHANISM OF ACTION
A loop diuretic that enhances excretion of sodium, chloride, and potassium by direct action at the ascending limb of the loop of Henle. ***Therapeutic Effect:*** Produces diuresis and lower BP.

PHARMACOKINETICS

Route	Onset	Peak	Duration
PO	30–60 min	1–2 hr	6–8 hr
IV	5 min	20–60 min	2 hr
IM	30 min	N/A	N/A

Well absorbed from the GI tract. Protein binding: 91%–97%. Partially metabolized in the liver. Primarily excreted in urine (nonrenal clearance increases in severe renal impairment). Not removed by hemodialysis. ***Half-life:*** 30–90 min (increased in renal or hepatic impairment, and in neonates).

AVAILABILITY

Oral Solution: 10 mg/ml, 40 mg/5 ml.
Tablets: 20 mg, 40 mg, 80 mg.
Injection: 10 mg/ml.

INDICATIONS AND DOSAGES

▸ Edema, Hypertension

PO
Adults, Elderly. Initially, 20–80 mg/dose; may increase by 20-40 mg/dose q6–8h. May titrate up to 600 mg/day in severe edematous states.
Children. 1–6 mg/kg/day in divided doses q6–12h.
IV, IM
Adults, Elderly. 20–40 mg/dose; may increase by 20 mg/dose q1–2h.
Children. 1–2 mg/kg/dose q6–12h.
Neonates. 1–2 mg/kg/dose q12–24h.
IV INFUSION
Adults, Elderly. Bolus of 0.1 mg/kg, followed by infusion of 0.1 mg/kg/hr; may double q2h. Maximum: 0.4 mg/kg/hr.
Children. 0.05 mg/kg/hr; titrate to desired effect.

OFF-LABEL USES

Hypercalcemia

CONTRAINDICATIONS

Anuria, hepatic coma, severe electrolyte depletion

INTERACTIONS

Drug

Amphotericin B, nephrotoxic and ototoxic medications: May increase the risk of nephrotoxicity and ototoxicity.
Anticoagulants, heparin: May decrease the effects of these drugs.
Lithium: May increase the risk of lithium toxicity.
Other hypokalemia-causing medications: May increase the risk of hypokalemia.
Probenecid: May increase furosemide blood concentration.

Herbal

None known.

Food

None known.

Drug interactions of concern to dentistry

- Increased electrolyte imbalance: corticosteroids
- Masked ototoxicity: phenothiazines
- Decreased antihypertensive effect: NSAIDs, especially indomethacin

DIAGNOSTIC TEST EFFECTS

May increase blood glucose, BUN, and serum uric acid levels. May decrease serum calcium, chloride, magnesium, potassium, and sodium levels.

IV INCOMPATIBILITIES

Ciprofloxacin (Cipro), diltiazem (Cardizem), dobutamine (Dobutrex), dopamine (Intropin), doxorubicin (Adriamycin), droperidol (Inapsine), esmolol (Brevibloc), famotidine (Pepcid), filgrastim (Neupogen), fluconazole (Diflucan), gemcitabine (Gemzar), gentamicin (Garamycin), idarubicin (Idamycin), labetalol (Trandate), meperidine (Demerol), metoclopramide (Reglan), midazolam (Versed), milrinone (Primacor), nicardipine (Cardene), ondansetron (Zofran), quinidine, thiopental (Pentothal), vecuronium (Norcuron), vinblastine (Velban), vincristine (Oncovin), vinorelbine (Navelbine)

IV COMPATIBILITIES

Aminophylline, amiodarone (Cordarone), bumetanide (Bumex), calcium gluconate, cimetidine

(Tagamet), heparin, hydromorphone (Dilaudid), lidocaine, morphine, nitroglycerin, norepinephrine (Levophed), potassium chloride, propofol (Diprivan)

SIDE EFFECTS

Expected

Increased urinary frequency and urine volume

Frequent

Nausea, dyspepsia, abdominal cramps, diarrhea or constipation, electrolyte disturbances

Occasional

Dizziness, light-headedness, headache, blurred vision, paresthesia, photosensitivity, rash, fatigue, bladder spasm, restlessness, diaphoresis

Rare

Flank pain

SERIOUS REACTIONS

! Vigorous diuresis may lead to profound water loss and electrolyte depletion, resulting in hypokalemia, hyponatremia, and dehydration.

! Sudden volume depletion may result in increased risk of thrombosis, circulatory collapse, and sudden death.

! Acute hypotensive episodes may occur, sometimes several days after beginning therapy.

! Ototoxicity - manifested as deafness, vertigo, or tinnitus - may occur, especially in patients with severe renal impairment.

! Furosemide use can exacerbate diabetes mellitus, systemic lupus erythematosus, gout, and pancreatitis.

! Blood dyscrasias have been reported.

DENTAL CONSIDERATIONS

General:

- Monitor vital signs at every appointment because of cardiovascular side effects.
- Patients on chronic drug therapy may rarely have symptoms of blood dyscrasias, which can include infection, bleeding, and poor healing.
- Assess salivary flow as a factor in caries, periodontal disease, and candidiasis.
- After supine positioning, have patient sit upright for at least 2 min before standing to avoid orthostatic hypotension.
- Patients on high-potency diuretics should be monitored for serum K^+ levels.

Consultations:

- In a patient with symptoms of blood dyscrasias, request a medical consultation for blood studies and postpone dental treatment until normal values are reestablished.
- Medical consultation may be required to assess disease control.

Teach Patient/Family:

- Importance of good oral hygiene to prevent soft tissue inflammation
- Caution to prevent injury when using oral hygiene aids
- *When chronic dry mouth occurs, advise patient:*
  - To use daily home fluoride products for anticaries effect
  - To avoid mouth rinses with high alcohol content because of drying effects
  - To use sugarless gum, frequent sips of water, or saliva substitutes

gabapentin
ga′-ba-pen-tin
(Gantin[AUS], Neurontin, Pendine[AUS])
Do not confuse Neurontin with Noroxin.

CATEGORY AND SCHEDULE
Pregnancy Risk Category: C

MECHANISM OF ACTION
An anticonvulsant and antineuralgic agent whose exact mechanism unknown. May increase the synthesis or accumulation of gamma-aminobutyric acid by binding to as-yet-undefined receptor sites in brain tissue. ***Therapeutic Effect:*** Reduces seizure activity and neuropathic pain.

PHARMACOKINETICS
Well absorbed from the GI tract (not affected by food). Protein binding: less than 5%. Widely distributed. Crosses the blood-brain barrier. Primarily excreted unchanged in urine. Removed by hemodialysis. ***Half-life:*** 5–7 hr (increased in impaired renal function and the elderly).

AVAILABILITY
Capsules: 100 mg, 300 mg, 400 mg.
Oral Solution: 250 mg/5 ml.
Tablets: 600 mg, 800 mg.

INDICATIONS AND DOSAGES
▸ Adjunctive Therapy for Seizure Control
PO
Adults, Elderly, Children Older than 12 yr. Initially, 300 mg 3 times a day. May titrate dosage. Range: 900–1800 mg/day in 3 divided doses. Maximum: 3,600 mg/day.
Children 3–12 yr. Initially, 10–15 mg/kg/day in 3 divided doses. May titrate up to 25–35 mg/kg/day (for children 5–12 yr) and 40 mg/kg/day (for children 3–4 yr) Maximum: 50 mg/kg/day.

▸ Adjunctive Therapy for Neuropathic Pain
PO
Adults, Elderly. Initially, 100 mg 3 times a day; may increase by 300 mg/day at weekly intervals. Maximum: 3,600 mg/day in 3 divided doses.
Children. Initially, 5 mg/kg/dose at bedtime, followed by 5 mg/kg/dose for 2 doses on day 2, then 5 mg/kg/dose for 3 doses on day 3. Range: 8–35 mg/kg/day in 3 divided doses.

▸ Postherpetic Neuralgia
PO
Adults, Elderly. 300 mg on day 1, 300 mg twice a day on day 2, and 300 mg 3 times a day on day 3. Titrate up to 1,800 mg/day.

▸ Dosage in Renal Impairment
Dosage and frequency are modified on the basis of creatinine clearance:

Creatinine Clearance	Dosage
60 ml/min or higher	400 mg q8h
30–59 ml/min	300 mg q12h
16–29 ml/min	300 mg daily
less than 16 ml/min	300 mg every other day
Hemodialysis	200–300 mg after each 4-hr hemodialysis session

OFF-LABEL USES
Treatment of essential tremor, hot flashes, hyperhidrosis, migraines, psychiatric disorders

CONTRAINDICATIONS
None known.

INTERACTIONS

Drug

None known.

Herbal

None known.

Food

None known.

Drug interactions of concern to dentistry

- None reported at this time, but, because CNS side effects are common, the use of anxiolytic sedative drugs may potentially increase the CNS side effects.

DIAGNOSTIC TEST EFFECTS

May decrease serum WBC count.

SIDE EFFECTS

Frequent (19%–10%)

Fatigue, somnolence, dizziness, ataxia

Occasional (8%–3%)

Nystagmus, tremor, diplopia, rhinitis, weight gain

Rare (< 2%)

Nervousness, dysarthria, memory loss, dyspepsia, pharyngitis, myalgia

SERIOUS REACTIONS

! Abrupt withdrawal may increase seizure frequency.

! Overdosage may result in diplopia, slurred speech, drowsiness, lethargy, and diarrhea.

DENTAL CONSIDERATIONS

General:

- Early-morning appointments and a stress reduction protocol may be required for anxious patients.
- Place on frequent recall because of oral side effects.
- Monitor vital signs at every appointment because of cardiovascular side effects.
- Assess salivary flow as a factor in caries, periodontal disease, and candidiasis.
- Determine type of epilepsy and quality of seizure control.

Consultations:

- Medical consultation may be required to assess disease control and patient's ability to tolerate stress.

Teach Patient/Family:

- Importance of good oral hygiene to prevent soft tissue inflammation
- Caution in use of oral hygiene aids to prevent injury
- *When chronic dry mouth occurs, advise patient:*
  - To avoid mouth rinses with high alcohol content because of drying effects
  - To use daily home fluoride products for anticaries effect
  - To use sugarless gum, frequent sips of water, or saliva substitutes

galantamine

ga-lan′-ta-mene

(Reminyl)

Do not confuse Reminyl with Remeron, Remicade, or Robinul.

CATEGORY AND SCHEDULE

Pregnancy Risk Category: B

MECHANISM OF ACTION

A cholinesterase inhibitor that inhibits the enzyme acetylcholinesterase, thus increasing the concentration of acetylcholine at cholinergic synapses and enhancing cholinergic function in the CNS. ***Therapeutic Effect:*** Slows the progression of Alzheimer's disease.

PHARMACOKINETICS

Rapidly absorbed from the GI tract. Protein binding: 18%. Distributed to blood cells; binds to plasma proteins, mainly albumin. Metabolized in the liver. Excreted in urine. ***Half-life:*** 7 hr.

AVAILABILITY

Oral Solution: 4 mg/ml.
Tablets: 4 mg, 8 mg, 12 mg.

INDICATIONS AND DOSAGES

Alzheimer's Disease

PO

Adults, Elderly. Initially, 4 mg twice a day (8 mg/day). After a minimum of 4 wk (if well tolerated), may increase to 8 mg twice a day (16 mg/day). After another 4 wk, may increase to 12 mg twice daily (24 mg/day). Range: 16–24 mg/day in 2 divided doses.

Dosage in Renal Impairment

For moderate impairment, maximum dosage is 16 mg/day. Drug is not recommended for patients with severe impairment.

CONTRAINDICATIONS

Severe hepatic or renal impairment

INTERACTIONS

Drug

Bethanechol, succinylcholine: May interfere with the effects of these drugs.
Cimetidine, erythromycin, ketoconazole, paroxetine: May increase the galantamine blood concentration.

Herbal

None known.

Food

None known.

Drug interactions of concern to dentistry

- Increased plasma levels: ketoconazole
- Increased bioavailability: cimetidine, paroxetine
- Enhanced succinylcholine muscle relaxation during anesthesia
- Action may be inhibited by anticholinergic drugs or enhanced by cholinergic agonists

DIAGNOSTIC TEST EFFECTS

None known.

SIDE EFFECTS

Frequent (17%–5%)
Nausea, vomiting, diarrhea, anorexia, weight loss
Occasional (9%–4%)
Abdominal pain, insomnia, depression, headache, dizziness, fatigue, rhinitis
Rare (< 3%)
Tremors, constipation, confusion, cough, anxiety, urinary incontinence

SERIOUS REACTIONS

! Overdose may cause cholinergic crisis, characterized by increased salivation, lacrimation, severe nausea and vomiting, bradycardia, respiratory depression, hypotension, and increased muscle weakness. Treatment usually consists of supportive measures and an anticholinergic such as atropine.

DENTAL CONSIDERATIONS

General:

- Monitor vital signs at every appointment because of cardiovascular side effects.
- After supine positioning, have patient sit upright for at least 2 min to avoid orthostatic hypotension.
- Drug is used early in the disease; ensure that patient or caregiver understands informed consent.
- Place on frequent recall because early attention to dental health is important for Alzheimer's patients.
- Consider semisupine chair position for patient comfort if GI side effects occur.

Consultations:

- Consultation with physician may be necessary if sedation or general anesthesia is required.

G

• Medical consultation may be required to assess disease control and patient's ability to tolerate stress.

Teach Patient/Family:

• Importance of good oral hygiene to prevent soft tissue inflammation
• To assist patient or caregiver with oral home-care regimen as cognitive ability declines
• Use of electric toothbrush if patient has difficulty holding conventional devices
• Importance of updating health and drug history if physician makes any changes in evaluation or drug regimens

G

ganciclovir sodium

gan-sy′-clo-ver
(Cymevene[AUS], Cytovene, Vitrasert)
Do not confuse Cytovene with Cytosar.

CATEGORY AND SCHEDULE

Pregnancy Risk Category: C

MECHANISM OF ACTION

This synthetic nucleoside competes with viral DNA polymerase and is incorporated into growing viral DNa chains. ***Therapeutic Effect:*** Interferes with synthesis and replication of viral DNA.

PHARMACOKINETICS

Widely distributed. Protein binding: 1%–2%. Undergoes minimal metabolism. Excreted unchanged primarily in urine. Removed by hemodialysis. ***Half-life:*** 2.5–3.6 hr (increased in impaired renal function).

AVAILABILITY

Capsules (Cytovene): 250 mg, 500 mg.
Powder for Injection (Cytovene): 500 mg.
Implant (Vitrasert): 4.5 mg.

INDICATIONS AND DOSAGES

▸ Cytomegalovirus (CMV) Retinitis

IV

Adults, Children 3 mo and older. 10 mg/kg/day in divided doses q12h for 14–21 days, then 5 mg/kg/day as a single daily dose.

▸ Prevention of CMV Disease in Transplant Patients

IV

Adults, Children. 10 mg/kg/day in divided doses q12h for 7–14 days, then 5 mg/kg/day as a single daily dose.

▸ Other CMV Infections

IV

Adults. Initially, 10 mg/kg/day in divided doses q12h for 14–21 days, then 5 mg/kg/day as a single daily dose. Maintenance: 1,000 mg 3 times a day or 500 mg q3h (6 times a day).
Children. Initially, 10 mg/kg/day in divided doses q12h for 14–21 days, then 5 mg/kg/day as a single daily dose. Maintenance: 30 mg/kg/dose q8h.

INTRAVITREAL IMPLANT

Adults. 1 implant q6–9mo plus oral ganciclovir.
Children 9 yr and older. 1 implant q6–9mo plus oral ganciclovir (30 mg/dose q8h).

▸ Adult Dosage in Renal Impairment

Dosage and frequency are modified on the basis of CrCl.

CrCl	Induction Dosage	Maintenance Dosage	Oral
50–69 ml/min	2.5 mg/kg q12h	2.5 mg/kg q24h	1,500 mg/day
25–49 ml/min	2.5 mg/kg q24h	1.25 mg/kg q24h	1,000 mg/day

10–24 ml/min	1.25 mg/kg q24h	0.625 mg/kg q24h	500 mg/day
less than 10 ml/min	1.25 mg/kg 3 times/wk	0.625 mg/kg 3 times/wk	500 mg 3 times/wk

CrCl = creatinine clearance

OFF-LABEL USES

Treatment of other CMV infections, such as gastroenteritis, hepatitis, and pneumonitis

CONTRAINDICATIONS

Absolute neutrophil count less than $500/mm^3$, platelet count less than $25,000/mm^3$, hypersensitivity to acyclovir or ganciclovir, immunocompetent patients, patients with congenital or neonatal CMV disease.

INTERACTIONS

Drug

Bone marrow depressants: May increase bone marrow depression.
Imipenem and cilastatin: May increase the risk of seizures.
Zidovudine (AZT): May increase the risk of hepatotoxicity.

Herbal

None known.

Food

None known.

Drug interactions of concern to dentistry

- Increased risk of blood dyscrasias: dapsone, carbamazepine, phenothiazines
- Increased risk of seizures: imipenem/cilastatin (Primaxin)
- Low platelet counts may prevent the use of aspirin, NSAIDs

DIAGNOSTIC TEST EFFECTS

May increase serum alkaline phosphatase, bilirubin, AST (SGOT), and ALT (SGPT) levels.

IV INCOMPATIBILITIES

Aldesleukin (Proleukin), amifostine (Ethyol), aztreonam (Azactam), cefepime (Maxipime), cytarabine (ARA-C), doxorubicin (Adriamycin), fludarabine (Fludara), foscarnet (Foscavir), gemcitabine (Gemzar), ondansetron (Zofran), piperacillin and tazobactam (Zosyn), sargramostim (Leukine), vinorelbine (Navelbine)

IV COMPATIBILITIES

Amphotericin B, enalapril (Vasotec), filgrastim (Neupogen), fluconazole (Diflucan), propofol (Diprivan)

SIDE EFFECTS

Frequent

Diarrhea (41%), fever (40%), nausea (25%), abdominal pain (17%), vomiting (13%)

Occasional (11%–6%)

Diaphoresis, infection, paresthesia, flatulence, pruritus

Rare (4%–2%)

Headache, stomatitis, dyspepsia, phlebitis

SERIOUS REACTIONS

! Hematologic toxicity occurs commonly: leukopenia in 41%–29% of patients and anemia in 25%–19%.
! Intra-ocular insertion occasionally results in visual acuity loss, vitreous hemorrhage, and retinal detachment.
! GI hemorrhage occurs rarely.

DENTAL CONSIDERATIONS

General:

- Examine for oral manifestations of opportunistic infection.
- Examine for evidence of oral manifestations of blood dyscrasias (infection, bleeding, poor healing).
- Place on frequent recall to evaluate healing healing response.
- Consider local hemostasis measures to prevent excessive bleeding.
- Monitor vital signs at every appointment because of cardiovascular and respiratory side effects.

Consultations:
- Medical consultation for blood studies (CBC); leukopenic or thrombocytopenic side effects may result in infection, delayed healing, and excessive bleeding. Postpone elective dental treatment until normal values are maintained.
- Medical consultation may be required to assess disease control.

Teach Patient/Family:
- Caution in use of oral hygiene aids to prevent injury
- That secondary oral infection may occur; must see dentist immediately if infection occurs
- Importance of good oral hygiene to prevent soft tissue inflammation

gatifloxacin

gah-tee-floks′-a-sin
(Tequin, Zymar)

CATEGORY AND SCHEDULE
Pregnancy Risk Category: C

MECHANISM OF ACTION
A fluoroquinolone that inhibits two enzymes, topoisomerase II and IV, in susceptible microorganisms.
Therapeutic Effect: Interferes with bacterial DNA replication. Prevents or delays resistance emergence. Bactericidal.

PHARMACOKINETICS
Well absorbed from the GI tract after PO administration. Protein binding: 20%. Widely distributed. Metabolized in liver. Primarily excreted in urine. ***Half-life:*** 7–14 hr.

AVAILABILITY
Tablets (Tequin): 200 mg, 400 mg.
Injection (Tequin): 200-mg, 400-mg vials.
Ophthalmic Solution (Zymar): 0.3%.

INDICATIONS AND DOSAGES

▸ Chronic Bronchitis, Complicated Urinary Tract Infections, Pyelonephritis, Skin Infections
PO, IV
Adults, Elderly. 400 mg/day for 7–10 days (5 days for chronic bronchitis).

▸ Sinusitis
PO, IV
Adults, Elderly. 400 mg/day for 10 days.

▸ Pneumonia
PO, IV
Adults, Elderly. 400 mg/day for 7–14 days.

▸ Cystitis
PO, IV
Adults, Elderly. 400 mg as a single dose or 200 mg/day for 3 days.

▸ Urethral Gonorrhea in Men and Women, Endocervical and Rectal Gonorrhea in Women
PO, IV
Adults, Elderly. 400 mg as a single dose.

▸ Topical Treatment of Bacterial Conjunctivitis Due to Susceptible Strains of Bacteria
OPHTHALMIC
Adults, Elderly, Children 1 yr and older. 1 drop q2h while awake for 2 days, then 1 drop up to 4 times/day for days 3–7.

▸ Dosage in Renal Impairment

Creatinine Clearance	Dosage
40 ml/min	400 mg/day
less than 40 ml/min	Initially, 400 mg/day then 200 mg/day
Hemodialysis	Initially, 400 mg/day then 200 mg/day
Peritoneal dialysis	Initially, 400 mg/day then 200 mg/day

CONTRAINDICATIONS
Hypersensitivity to quinolones

INTERACTIONS
Drug
Antacids, digoxin, iron preparations: May decrease gatifloxacin plasma concentration and half-life.
Probenecid: May increase gatifloxacin plasma concentration and half-life.
Herbal
None known.
Food
None known.
Drug interactions of concern to dentistry
- Caution: use with erythromycin and tricyclic antidepressants (no data, risk of prolonged QT interval)
- Decreased absorption: divalent and trivalent cations, iron and zinc salts
- Increased risk of CNS stimulation and seizures: NSAIDs
- Increased risk of life-threatening arrhythmias: procainamide

Drug interactions of concern to dentistry
- None reported

DIAGNOSTIC TEST EFFECTS
None known.

IV INCOMPATIBILITIES
Amphotericin (Fungizone), potassium phosphate
IV COMPATIBILITIES
Aminophylline, calcium gluconate, hydromorphone (Dilaudid), lidocaine, lorazepam (Ativan), magnesium sulfate, methylprednisolone (Solu-Medrol), metoclopramide (Reglan), midazolam (Versed), morphine, nitroglycerin, potassium chloride, sodium phosphate

SIDE EFFECTS
Occasional (8%–3%)
Nausea, vaginitis, diarrhea, headache, dizziness
Ophthalmic: conjunctival irritation, increased tearing, corneal inflammation
Rare (3%–0.1%)
Abdominal pain, constipation, dyspepsia, stomatitis, edema, insomnia, abnormal dreams, diaphoresis, altered taste, rash
Ophthalmic: corneal swelling, dry eye, eye pain, eyelid swelling, headache, red eye, reduced visual acuity, altered taste

SERIOUS REACTIONS
! Pseudomembranous colitis as evidenced by severe abdominal pain and cramps, severe watery diarrhea, and fever, may occur.
! Superinfection manifested as genital or anal pruritus, ulceration or changes in oral mucosa, and moderate to severe diarrhea, may occur.

DENTAL CONSIDERATIONS
General:
- Determine why patient is taking the drug.
- Monitor vital signs at every appointment because of cardiovascular side effects.
- Examine for oral manifestation of opportunistic infection.
- Advise patient if dental drugs prescribed have a potential for photosensitivity.
- Ruptures of the shoulder, hand, and Achilles tendons requiring surgical repair or resulting in prolonged disability have been reported with use of fluoroquinolones. Question patient about history of side effects associated with fluoroquinolone use.

Consultations:
- Physician consultation is advised in the presence of an acute dental infection requiring another antibiotic.

Teach Patient/Family:
- *If used for dental infection:*
  - To minimize exposure to sunlight and wear sunscreen if sun exposure is planned

G

• To discontinue treatment and inform dentist immediately if patient experiences pain or inflammation of a tendon, and to rest and refrain from exercise

DENTAL CONSIDERATIONS

GATIFLOXACIN OPHTHALMIC

General:

• Protect patient's eyes from accidental spatter during dental treatment.
• Avoid dental light in patient's eyes; offer dark glasses for patient comfort.

gefitinib

geh-fih′-tih-nib
(Iressa)

CATEGORY AND SCHEDULE

Pregnancy Risk Category: D

MECHANISM OF ACTION

Blocks the signaling pathway that binds to the epidermal growth factor receptor (EGFR) on the surface of normal and cancer cells. EGFR activates the enzyme tyrosine kinase, which sends signals instructing the cells to grow. ***Therapeutic Effect:*** Inhibits the growth of cancer cells.

PHARMACOKINETICS

Slowly absorbed and extensively distributed throughout the body. Protein binding: 90%. Undergoes extensive metabolism in the liver. Excreted in the feces. ***Half-life:*** 48 hr.

AVAILABILITY

Tablets: 250 mg.

INDICATIONS AND DOSAGES

▸ Non–Small Cell Lung Cancer

PO

Adults, Elderly. 250 mg/day; may increase to 500 mg/day for patients receiving drugs that may decrease gefitinib blood concentrations, such as rifampin and phenytoin

CONTRAINDICATIONS

None known.

INTERACTIONS

Drug

Cimetidine, phenytoin, ranitidine, rifampin, sodium bicarbonate: May decrease gefitinib blood concentration and effectiveness.
Itraconazole, ketoconazole: Increases gefitinib blood concentration.
Metoprolol: Increases the effect of metoprolol.
Warfarin: Increases the risk of bleeding.

Herbal

None known.

Food

None known.

Drug interactions of concern to dentistry

• Decreased plasma levels: sodium bicarbonate
• Decreased metabolism: potent inhibitors of CYP3A4 isoenzymes (ketoconazole, itraconazole, erythromycin)

DIAGNOSTIC TEST EFFECTS

May increase serum alkaline phosphatase, bilirubin, AST (SGOT), and ALT (SGPT) levels.

SIDE EFFECTS

Frequent (48%–25%)

Diarrhea, rash, acne

Occasional (13%–8%)

Dry skin, nausea, vomiting, pruritus

Rare (7%–2%)

Anorexia, asthenia, weight loss, peripheral edema, eye pain

SERIOUS REACTIONS

! Pancreatitis and ocular hemorrhage occur rarely.
! Hypersensitivity reaction produces angioedema and urticaria.

DENTAL CONSIDERATIONS

General:

- If additional analgesia is required for dental pain, consider alternative analgesics (NSAIDs) in patients taking narcotics for acute or chronic pain.
- This drug may be used in the hospital or on an outpatient basis. Confirm the patient's disease and treatment status.
- Consider semisupine chair position for patients with respiratory disease.
- Examine for oral manifestation of opportunistic infection.
- Patients may have received other chemotherapy or radiation: confirm medical and drug history.
- Caution drug interactions with drugs used in dentistry.

Consultations:

- Medical consultation may be required to assess disease control and patient's ability to tolerate stress.
- Medical consultation may be required to assess immunologic status during cancer chemotherapy and determine safety risk, if any, posed by the required dental treatment.

Teach Patient/Family:

- Importance of good oral hygiene to prevent soft tissue inflammation
- To prevent trauma when using oral hygiene aids
- Importance of updating health and medication history if physician makes any changes in evaluation or drug regimens; include OTC, herbal, and nonherbal remedies in the update

gemcitabine hydrochloride

gem-cih′-tah-bean
(Gemzar)

CATEGORY AND SCHEDULE

Pregnancy Risk Category: D

G

MECHANISM OF ACTION

An antimetabolite that inhibits ribonucleotide reductase, the enzyme necessary for catalyzing DNA synthesis. ***Therapeutic Effect:*** Produces death in cells undergoing DNA synthesis.

PHARMACOKINETICS

Not extensively distributed after IV infusion (increased with length of infusion). Protein binding: less than 10%. Excreted primarily in urine as metabolite. ***Half-life:*** 42–94 min (influenced by gender of patient and duration of infusion).

AVAILABILITY

Powder for Reconstitution: 200 mg, 1-g vials.

INDICATIONS AND DOSAGES

▸ **Non–Small Cell Lung Cancer (in combination with cisplatin)**

IV

Adults, Elderly, Children.
1,000 mg/m^2 on days 1, 8, and 15, repeated every 28 days; or 1,250 mg/m^2 on days 1 and 8. Repeat every 21 days.

▸ **Pancreatic Cancer**

IV

Adults. 1,000 mg/m^2 once weekly for up to 7 wk or until toxicity necessitates decreasing dosage or withholding the dose, followed by 1 wk of rest. Subsequent cycles should consist of once-weekly dose for 3 consecutive wk out of every 4 wk.

For patients completing cycles at 1,000 mg/m², increase dose to 1,250 mg/m² as tolerated. Dose for next cycle may be increased to 1,500 mg/m².

Dosage Reduction Guidelines

Dosage adjustments should be on the basis of granulocyte count and platelet count, as follows:

Absolute Granulocyte Counts (cells/mm³)	Platelet Count (cells/mm³)	% of Full Dose
1,000 and	100,000	100
500–999 or	50,000–99,000	75
less than 500 or	less than 50,000	Hold

OFF-LABEL USES

Treatment of biliary tract carcinoma, gallbladder carcinoma, Hodgkins lymphoma, non-Hodgskin's lymphoma, ovarian carcinoma

CONTRAINDICATIONS

None known.

INTERACTIONS

Drug

Bone marrow depressants: May increase the risk of myelosuppression.

Live-virus vaccines: May potentiate virus replication, increase vaccine side effects, and decrease the patient's antibody response to the vaccine.

Herbal

None known.

Food

None known.

Drug interactions of concern to dentistry

- None reported

DIAGNOSTIC TEST EFFECTS

May increase BUN level and serum alkaline phosphatase, bilirubin, creatinine, AST (SGOT), and ALT (SGPT) levels.

IV INCOMPATIBILITIES

Acyclovir (Zovirax), amphotericin B (Fungizone), cefoperazone (Cefobid), furosemide (Lasix), ganciclovir (Cytovene), imipenem and cilastatin (Primaxin), irinotecan (Camptosar), methotrexate, methylprednisolone (Solu-Medrol), mitomycin (Mutamycin), piperacillin and tazobactam (Zosyn), prochlorperazine (Compazine)

IV COMPATIBILITIES

Bumetanide (Bumex), calcium gluconate, dexamethasone (Decadron), diphenhydramine (Benadryl), dobutamine (Dobutrex), dopamine (Intropin), granisetron (Kytril), heparin, hydrocortisone (Solu-Cortef), lorazepam (Ativan), ondansetron (Zofran), potassium

SIDE EFFECTS

Frequent

Nausea and vomiting (69%); generalized pain (48%); fever (41%); mild to moderate pruritic rash (30%); mild to moderate dyspnea, constipation (23%); peripheral edema (20%)

Occasional (19%–10%)

Diarrhea, petechiae, alopecia, stomatitis, infection, somnolence, paresthesia

Rare

Diaphoresis, rhinitis, insomnia, malaise

SERIOUS REACTIONS

! Severe myelosuppression, as evidenced by anemia, thrombocytopenia, and leukopenia, is a common reaction

DENTAL CONSIDERATIONS

General:

- Monitor vital signs at every appointment due to cardiovascular side effects.

• Consider semisupine chair position for patients with respiratory disease.
• If additional analgesia is required for dental pain, consider alternative analgesics (NSAIDs) in patients taking narcotics for acute or chronic pain.
• Examine for oral manifestation of opportunistic infection.
• Avoid products that affect platelet function, such as aspirin and NSAIDs.
• This drug may be used in the hospital or on an outpatient basis. Confirm the patient's disease and treatment status.
• Chlorhexidine mouth rinse prior to and during chemotherapy may reduce severity of mucositis.
• Patient on chronic drug therapy may rarely present with symptoms of blood dyscrasias, which can include infection, bleeding and poor healing. If dyscrasia is present, caution patient to prevent oral tissue trauma when using oral hygiene aids.
• Palliative medication may be required for management of oral side effects.
• Short appointments and a stress reduction protocol may be required for anxious patients.
• Patients may be at risk of bleeding, check for oral signs.
• Oral infections should be eliminated and/or treated aggressively.

Consultations:
• Medical consultation should include routine blood counts including platelet counts and bleeding time.
• Consult physician; prophylactic or therapeutic antiinfectives may be indicated if surgery or periodontal treatment is required.
• Medical consultation may be required to assess immunologic status during cancer chemotherapy and determine safety risk, if any, posed by the required dental treatment.
• Medical consultation may be required to assess disease control and patient's ability to tolerate stress.

Teach Patient/Family:
• To be aware of oral side effects
• Importance of good oral hygiene to prevent soft tissue inflammation
• To report oral lesions, soreness, or bleeding to dentist
• To prevent trauma when using oral hygiene aids
• Importance of updating health and medication history if physician makes any changes in evaluation or drug regimens; include OTC, herbal, and nonherbal remedies in the update

G

gemfibrozil

gem-fi′-broe-zil
(Apo-Gemfibrozil[CAN], Ausgem[AUS], Gemfibromax[AUS], Jezil[AUS], Lipazil[AUS], Lopid, Novo-Gemfibrozil[CAN])
Do not confuse Lopid with Lorabid or Levbid.

CATEGORY AND SCHEDULE

Pregnancy Risk Category: C

MECHANISM OF ACTION

A fibric acid derivative that inhibits lipolysis of fat in adipose tissue; decreases liver uptake of free fatty acids and reduces hepatic triglyceride production. Inhibits synthesis of VLDL carrier apolipoprotein B. ***Therapeutic Effect:*** Lowers serum cholesterol and triglycerides (decreases VLDL, LDL; increases HDL).

PHARMACOKINETICS

Well absorbed from the GI tract. Protein binding: 99%. Metabolized in liver. Primarily excreted in urine.

Not removed by hemodialysis.
Half-life: 1.5 hr.

AVAILABILITY
Tablets: 600 mg.
Capsules: 300 mg.

INDICATIONS AND DOSAGES
▸ Hyperlipidemia
PO
Adults, Elderly. 1200 mg/day in 2 divided doses 30 min before breakfast and dinner.

CONTRAINDICATIONS
Liver dysfunction (including primary biliary cirrhosis), pre-existing gallbladder disease, severe renal dysfunction

INTERACTIONS
Drug
Lovastatin: May cause rhabdomyolysis, leading to acute renal failure.
Pioglitazone, repaglinide, warfarin: May increase the effect of these drugs.
Herbal
None known.
Food
None known.
Drug interactions of concern to dentistry
• None reported

DIAGNOSTIC TEST EFFECTS
May increase serum alkaline phosphatase, serum bilirubin, serum creatinine kinase, serum LDH concentrations, and AST (SGOT) and ALT (SGPT) levels. May decrease blood Hgb and Hct levels, leukocyte counts, and serum potassium levels.

SIDE EFFECTS
Frequent (20%)
Dyspepsia
Occasional (10%–2%)
Abdominal pain, diarrhea, nausea, vomiting, fatigue
Rare (< 2%)
Constipation, acute appendicitis, vertigo, headache, rash, pruritus, altered taste

SERIOUS REACTIONS
! Cholelithiasis, cholecystitis, acute appendicitis, pancreatitis, and malignancy occur rarely.

DENTAL CONSIDERATIONS
General:
• Patients on chronic drug therapy may rarely have symptoms of blood dyscrasias, which can include infection, bleeding, and poor healing.
Consultations:
• In a patient with symptoms of blood dyscrasias, request a medical consultation for blood studies and postpone dental treatment until normal values are reestablished.

gemifloxacin mesylate
gem-ih-flocks′-ah-sin
(Factive)

CATEGORY AND SCHEDULE
Pregnancy Risk Category: C

MECHANISM OF ACTION
A fluoroquinolone that inhibits the enzyme DNA gyrase in susceptible microorganisms, interfering with bacterial cell replication and repair.
Therapeutic Effect: Bactericidal.

PHARMACOKINETICS
Rapidly and well absorbed from the GI tract. Protein binding: 70%. Widely distributed. Penetrates well into lung tissue and fluid.

Undergoes limited metabolism in the liver. Primarily excreted in feces; lesser amount eliminated in urine. Partially removed by hemodialysis. ***Half-life:*** 4–12 hr.

AVAILABILITY

Tablets: 320 mg.

INDICATIONS AND DOSAGES

▸ Acute Bacterial Exacerbation of Chronic Bronchitis

PO

Adults, Elderly. 320 mg once a day for 5 days.

▸ Community-Acquired Pneumonia

PO

Adults, Elderly. 320 mg once a day for 7 days.

▸ Dosage in Renal Impairment

Dosage and frequency are modified on the basis of creatinine clearance.

Creatinine Clearance	Dosage
greater than 40 ml/min	320 mg once a day
40 ml/min or less	160 mg once a day

CONTRAINDICATIONS

Concurrent use of amiodarone, quinidine, procainamide, or sotalol; history of prolonged QTc interval; hypersensitivity to fluoroquinolones; uncorrected electrolyte disorders (such as hypokalemia and hypomagnesemia)

INTERACTIONS

Drug

Aluminum and magnesium-containing antacids, bismuth subsalicylate, didanosine, iron preparations and other metals, sucralfate, zinc preparations: May decrease the absorption of gemifloxacin.

Antipsychotics, class 1A and class III antiarrhythmics, erythromycin, tricyclic antidepressants: May increase the risk of prolonged QTc interval and life-threatening arrhythmias.

Cyclosporine: Increases the risk of nephrotoxicity.

Probenecid: Increases gemifloxacin serum concentration.

Herbal

None known.

Food

None known.

Drug interactions of concern to dentistry

- Decreased absorption: divalent or trivalent antacids, iron or zinc salts
- Use with caution or avoid drugs that affect QT interval: erythromycin, antipsychotics, tricyclic antidepressants

DIAGNOSTIC TEST EFFECTS

May increase BUN and serum alkaline phosphatase, bilirubin, LDH, creatinine, AST (SGOT), and ALT (SGPT) levels.

SIDE EFFECTS

Occasional (4%–2%)

Diarrhea, rash, nausea

Rare (≤ 1%)

Headache, abdominal pain, dizziness

SERIOUS REACTIONS

! Antibiotic-associated colitis may result from altered bacterial balance. Hypersensitivity reactions, including photosensitivity (as evidenced by rash, pruritus, blisters, edema, and burning skin), have occurred in patients receiving fluoroquinolones.

DENTAL CONSIDERATIONS

General:

- Determine why patient is taking the drug.

G

- Avoid dental light in patient's eyes; offer dark glasses for patient comfort.
- Examine for oral manifestation of opportunistic infection.
- Advise patient if dental drugs prescribed have a potential for photosensitivity.
- As with other fluoroquinolones there is a risk of tendinitis and tendon rupture.
- Consider semisupine chair position for patient comfort if GI side effects occur.

Consultations:

- Consult with patient's physician if an acute dental infection occurs and another antiinfective is required.

Teach Patient/Family:

- *When chronic dry mouth occurs, advise patient:*
  - To avoid mouth rinses with high alcohol content because of drying effects
  - To use daily home fluoride products for anticaries effect
  - To use sugarless gum, frequent sips of water, or saliva substitutes

gentamicin sulfate

jen-ta-mye′-sin
(Alcomicin[CAN], Cidomycin[CAN], Garamycin, Genoptic, Gentak, Gentacidin)

CATEGORY AND SCHEDULE

Pregnancy Risk Category: C

MECHANISM OF ACTION

An aminoglycoside antibiotic that irreversibly binds to the protein of bacterial ribosomes. ***Therapeutic Effect:*** Interferes with protein synthesis of susceptible microorganisms. Bactericidal.

PHARMACOKINETICS

Rapid, complete absorption after IM administration. Protein binding: less than 30%. Widely distributed (doesn't cross the blood-brain barrier, low concentrations in CSF). Excreted unchanged in urine. Removed by hemodialysis. ***Half-life:*** 2–4 hr (increased in impaired renal function and neonates; decreased in cystic fibrosis and burn or febrile patients).

AVAILABILITY

Injection (Garamycin): 10 mg/ml, 40 mg/ml.
Ophthalmic Solution (Gentacidin, Genoptic, Gentak): 0.3%.
Ophthalmic Ointment (Gentak): 0.3%.
Cream (Garamycin): 0.1%.
Ointment: 0.1%.

INDICATIONS AND DOSAGES

▸ **Acute Pelvic, Bone, Intra-Abdominal, Joint, Respiratory Tract, Burn Wound, Postoperative, and Skin or Skin-Structure Infections; Complicated UTIs; Septicemia; Meningitis**

IV, IM
Adults, Elderly. Usual dosage, 3–6 mg/kg/day in divided doses q8h or 4–6.6 mg/kg once a day.
Children 5–12 yr. Usual dosage 2–2.5 mg/kg/dose q8h.
Children younger than 5 yr. Usual dosage, 2.5 mg/kg/dose q8h.
Neonates. Usual dosage 2.5–3.5 mg/kg/dose q8–12h.

▸ **Hemodialysis**

IV, IM
Adults, Elderly. 0.5–0.7 mg/kg/dose after dialysis.
Children. 1.25–1.75 mg/kg/dose after dialysis.
INTRATHECAL
Adults. 4–8 mg/day.
Children 3 mo–12 yr. 1–2 mg/day.
Neonates. 1 mg/day.

Superficial Eye Infections
OPHTHALMIC OINTMENT
Adults, Elderly. Usual dosage, apply thin strip to conjunctiva 2–3 times a day.
OPHTHALMIC SOLUTION
Adults, Elderly, Children. Usual dosage, 1–2 drops q2–4h up to 2 drops/hr.

Superficial Skin Infections
TOPICAL
Adults, Elderly. Usual dosage, apply 3–4 times/day.

Dosage in Renal Impairment
Creatinine clearance greater than 41–60 ml/min. dosage interval q12h.
Creatinine clearance 20–40 ml/min. dosage interval q24h.
Creatinine clearance less than 20 ml/min. monitor levels to determine dosage interval.

OFF-LABEL USES
Topical: Prophylaxis of minor bacterial skin infections, treatment of dermal ulcer

CONTRAINDICATIONS
Hypersensitivity to gentamicin, other aminoglycosides (cross-sensitivity), or their components. Sulfite sensitivity may result in anaphylaxis, especially in asthmatic patients.

INTERACTIONS
Drug
Nephrotoxic mediations, other aminoglycosides, ototoxic medications: May increase the risk of nephrotoxicity or ototoxicity.
Neuromuscular blockers: May increase neuromuscular blockade.
Herbal
None known.
Food
None known.
Drug interactions of concern to dentistry
- Increased risk of nephrotoxicity: cephalsporins, vancomycin, enflurane
- Increased neuromuscular blockade: neuromuscular-blocking drugs

DIAGNOSTIC TEST EFFECTS
May increase serum creatinine, serum bilirubin, BUN, serum LDH, AST(SGOT), and ALT(SGPT) levels. May decrease serum calcium, magnesium, potassium, and sodium concentrations. Therapeutic peak serum level is 6–10 mcg/ml and trough is 0.5–2 mcg/ml. Toxic peak serum level is greater than 10 mcg/ml, and trough is greater than 2 mcg/ml.

IV INCOMPATIBILITIES
Allopurinol (Aloprim), amphotericin B complex (Abelcet, AmBisome, Amphotec), furosemide (Lasix), heparin, hetastarch (Hespan), idarubicin (Idamycin), indomethacin (Indocin), propofol (Diprivan)

IV COMPATIBILITIES
Amiodarone (Cordarone), diltiazem (Cardizem), enalapril (Vasotec), filgrastim (Neupogen), hydromorphone (Dilaudid), insulin, lorazepam (Ativan), magnesium sulfate, midazolam (Versed), morphine, multivitamins

SIDE EFFECTS
Occasional
IM: Pain, induration
IV: Phlebitis, thrombophlebitis, hypersensitivity reactions (fever, pruritus, rash, urticaria)
Ophthalmic: Burning, tearing, itching, blurred vision
Topical: Redness, itching
Rare
Alopecia, hypertension, weakness

SERIOUS REACTIONS
! Nephrotoxicity (as evidenced by increased BUN and serum creatinine levels and decreased creatinine clearance) may be reversible if the drug is stopped at the first sign of symptoms.

G

! Irreversible ototoxicity (manifested as tinnitus, dizziness, ringing or roaring in the ears, and diminished hearing), and neurotoxicity (as evidenced by headache, dizziness, lethargy, tremor, and visual disturbances) occur occasionally. The risk of these effects increases with higher dosages or prolonged therapy and when the solution is applied directly to the mucosa.
! Superinfections, particularly with fungal infections, may result from bacterial imbalance no matter which administration route is used.
! Ophthalmic application may cause paresthesia of conjunctiva or mydriasis.

DENTAL CONSIDERATIONS

General:

- For selected infections in the hospital setting; provide emergency dental treatment only.
- Examine for oral manifestation of opportunistic infection.
- Determine why patient is taking the drug.
- Caution regarding allergy to medication.

Consultations:

- CONIF
- Medical consultation may be required to assess disease control and patient's ability to tolerate stress.

Teach Patient/Family:

- Importance of good oral hygiene to prevent soft tissue inflammation
- To prevent trauma when using oral hygiene aids
- To report oral lesions, soreness, or bleeding to dentist

gentamicin sulfate; prednisolone acetate

(Pred-G, Pred-G S.O.P.)

CATEGORY AND SCHEDULE

Pregnancy Risk Category: C

MECHANISM OF ACTION

Gentamicin is an aminoglycoside that irreversibly binds to the protein of bacterial ribosomes. Prednisolone is an adrenal corticosteroid that inhibits accumulation of inflammatory cells at inflammation sites, phagocytosis, lysosomal enzyme release and synthesis, and release of mediators of inflammation. ***Therapeutic Effect:*** Interferes in protein synthesis of susceptible microorganisms. Prevents or suppresses cell-mediated immune reactions; decreases or prevents tissue response to inflammatory process.

PHARMACOKINETICS

None reported.

AVAILABILITY

Ophthalmic Suspension: 0.3 % gentamicin sulfate and 0.6% prednisolone acetate (Pred-G S.O.P.).
Ophthalmic Ointment: 0.3% gentamicin sulfate and 1% prednisolone acetate (Pred-G).

INDICATIONS AND DOSAGES

▸ **Treatment of Steroid Responsive Inflammatory Conditions, Superficial Ocular Infections**

OPHTHALMIC OINTMENT

Adults, Elderly. Apply 1/2 inch ribbon in the conjunctival sac 1–3 times/day.

OPHTHALMIC SUSPENSION

Adults, Elderly. Instill 1 drop 2–4 times/day. During the initial

24–48 hours, the dosing frequency may be increased if necessary up to 1 drop every hour.

CONTRAINDICATIONS

Viral disease of the cornea and conjunctiva (including epithelia herpes simplex keratitis, vaccinia, varicella), mycobacterial or fungal infection of the eye, uncomplicated removal of a corneal foreign body, hypersensitivity to gentamicin, prednisolone, other aminoglycosides or corticosteroids, or any component of the formulation

INTERACTIONS

Drug

None known.

Herbal

None known.

Food

None known.

DIAGNOSTIC TEST EFFECTS

None known.

SIDE EFFECTS

Occasional

Burning, tearing, itching, blurred vision

Rare

Delayed wound healing, secondary infection, intraocular pressure increased, glaucoma

SERIOUS REACTIONS

! Optic nerve damage occurs rarely.

DENTAL CONSIDERATIONS

General:

- Avoid dental light in patient's eyes; offer dark glasses for patient comfort.
- Protect patient's eyes from accidental spatter during dental treatment.

glatiramer

gla-teer′-a-mer

(Copaxone)

Do not confuse Copaxone with Compazine.

CATEGORY AND SCHEDULE

Pregnancy Risk Category: B

G

MECHANISM OF ACTION

An immunosuppressive whose exact mechanism is unknown. May act by modifying immune processes thought to be responsible for the pathogenesis of multiple sclerosis (MS). ***Therapeutic Effect:*** Slows progression of MS.

PHARMACOKINETICS

Substantial fraction of glatiramer is hydrolyzed locally. Some fraction of injected material enters lymphatic circulation, reaching regional lymph nodes; some may enter systemic circulation intact.

AVAILABILITY

Injection: 20 mg/ml in prefilled syringes.

INDICATIONS AND DOSAGES

▸ MS

SUBCUTANEOUS

Adults, Elderly. 20 mg once a day.

CONTRAINDICATIONS

Hypersensitivity to glatiramer or mannitol

INTERACTIONS

Drug

None known.

Herbal

None known.

Food

None known.

Drug interactions of concern to dentistry
• Dental drug interactions have not been studied

DIAGNOSTIC TEST EFFECTS
None known.

SIDE EFFECTS
Expected (73%–40%)
Pain, erythema, inflammation, or pruritus at injection site; asthenia
Frequent (27%–18%)
Arthralgia, vasodilation, anxiety, hypertonia, nausea, transient chest pain, dyspnea, flulike symptoms, rash, pruritus
Occasional (17%–10%)
Palpitations, back pain, diaphoresis, rhinitis, diarrhea, urinary urgency
Rare (8%–6%)
Anorexia, fever, neck pain, peripheral edema, ear pain, facial edema, vertigo, vomiting

SERIOUS REACTIONS
! Infection is a common effect.
! Lymphadenopathy occurs occasionally.

DENTAL CONSIDERATIONS
General:
• Monitor vital signs at every appointment due to cardiovascular side effects.
• Protect patient's eyes from accidental spatter during dental treatment.
• Avoid dental light in patient's eyes; offer dark glasses for patient comfort.
• Short appointments may be required due to effects of disease on musculature.
• Short appointments and a stress reduction protocol may be required for anxious patients.
• Advise patient if dental drugs prescribed have a potential for photosensitivity.
• Inquire about history of disease, any physical limitations, and other drugs the patient may be taking.
• For longer dental appointments, offer patient frequent breaks.

Consultations:
• Consultation with physician may be necessary if sedation or general anesthesia is required.
• Medical consultation may be required to assess disease control and patient's ability to tolerate stress.

Teach Patient/Family:
• Importance of good oral hygiene to prevent soft tissue inflammation
• To prevent trauma when using oral hygiene aids
• Importance of updating health and medication history if physician makes any changes in evaluation or drug regimens; include OTC, herbal, and nonherbal remedies in the update

glimepiride
gly-mep′-er-ide
(Amaryl)
Do not confuse glimepiride with glipizide or glyburide.

CATEGORY AND SCHEDULE
Pregnancy Risk Category: C

MECHANISM OF ACTION
A second-generation sulfonylurea that promotes release of insulin from beta cells of the pancreas and increases insulin sensitivity at peripheral sites. ***Therapeutic Effect:*** Lowers blood glucose concentration.

PHARMACOKINETICS
Route	Onset	Peak	Duration
PO	N/A	2–3 hr	24 hr

Completely absorbed from the GI tract. Protein binding: greater than 99%. Metabolized in the liver. Excreted in urine and eliminated in feces.
Half-life: 5–9.2 hr.

AVAILABILITY

Tablets: 1 mg, 2 mg, 4 mg.

INDICATIONS AND DOSAGES

▸ Diabetes Mellitus

PO

Adults, Elderly. Initially, 1–2 mg once a day, with breakfast or first main meal. Maintenance: 1–4 mg once a day. After dose of 2 mg is reached, dosage should be increased in increments of up to 2 mg q1–2wk, on the basis of blood glucose response. Maximum: 8 mg/day.

▸ Dosage in Renal Impairment

PO

Adults. 1 mg once/day.

CONTRAINDICATIONS

Diabetic complications, such as ketosis, acidosis, and diabetic coma; severe hepatic or renal impairment; monotherapy for type 1 diabetes mellitus; stress situations, including severe infection, trauma, and surgery

INTERACTIONS

Drug

Beta blockers: May increase the hypoglycemic effect of glimepiride and mask signs of hypoglycemia.
Cimetidine, ciprofloxacin, fluconazole, MAOIs, quinidine, ranitidine, large doses of salicylates: May increase the effects of glimepiride.
Corticosteroids, lithium, thiazide diuretics: May decrease the effects of glimepiride.
Oral anticoagulants: May increase the effects of oral anticoagulants.

Herbal

None known.

Food

None known.

Drug interactions of concern to dentistry

- Risk of potentiation of hypoglycemic effects: NSAIDs, salicylates, sulfonamides, β-adrenergic blockers, ketoconazole

DIAGNOSTIC TEST EFFECTS

May increase BUN and LDH concentrations and serum alkaline phosphatase, creatinine, and AST(SGOT) levels.

SIDE EFFECTS

Frequent

Altered taste sensation, dizziness, somnolence, weight gain, constipation, diarrhea, heartburn, nausea, vomiting, stomach fullness, headache

Occasional

Increased sensitivity of skin to sunlight, peeling of skin, itching, rash

SERIOUS REACTIONS

! Overdose or insufficient food intake may produce hypoglycemia, especially with increased glucose demands.
! GI hemorrhage, cholestatic hepatic jaundice, leukopenia, thrombocytopenia, pancytopenia, agranulocytosis, and aplastic or hemolytic anemia occur rarely.

DENTAL CONSIDERATIONS

General:

- Short appointments and a stress reduction protocol may be required for anxious patients.

• Question patient about self-monitoring of drug's antidiabetic effect, including blood glucose values or finger-stick records.
• Ensure that patient is following prescribed diet and regularly takes medication.
• Patients on chronic drug therapy may rarely have symptoms of blood dyscrasias, which can include infection, bleeding, and poor healing.
• Diabetics may be more susceptible to infection and have delayed wound healing.
• Place on frequent recall to evaluate healing response.
• Advise patient if dental drugs prescribed have a potential for photosensitivity.

Consultations:
• Medical consultation may be required to assess disease control.
• In a patient with symptoms of blood dyscrasias, request a medical consultation for blood studies and postpone treatment until normal values are reestablished.
• Medical consultation may include data from patient's blood glucose monitoring, including glycosylated hemoglobin or HbA_{1c} testing.

Teach Patient/Family:
• Importance of good oral hygiene to prevent soft tissue inflammation
• Caution to prevent trauma when using oral hygiene aids
• Importance of updating health and drug history if physician makes any changes in evaluation or drug regimens

glipizide
glip′-i-zide
(Glucotrol, Glucotrol XL, Melizide[AUS], Minidiab[AUS])
Do not confuse glipizide with glimepiride or glyburide.

CATEGORY AND SCHEDULE
Pregnancy Risk Category: C

MECHANISM OF ACTION
A second-generation sulfonylurea that promotes the release of insulin from beta cells of the pancreas and increases insulin sensitivity at peripheral sites. ***Therapeutic Effect:*** Lowers blood glucose concentration.

PHARMACOKINETICS

Route	Onset	Peak	Duration
PO	15–30 min	2–3 hr	12–24 hr
Extended-release	2–3 hr	6–12 hr	24 hr

Well absorbed from the GI tract. Protein binding: 99%. Metabolized in the liver. Excreted in urine. ***Half-life:*** 2–4 hr.

AVAILABILITY
Tablets (Glucotrol): 5 mg, 10 mg.
Tablets (Extended-Release [Glucotrol XL]): 2.5 mg, 5 mg, 10 mg.

INDICATIONS AND DOSAGES
▸ Diabetes Mellitus
PO
Adults. Initially, 5 mg/day or 2.5 mg in the elderly or those with hepatic disease. Adjust dosage in 2.5- to 5-mg increments at intervals of several days. Maximum single dose: 15 mg. Maximum dose/day: 40 mg. Maintenance (extended-release tablet): 20 mg/day.

Elderly. Initially, 2.5–5 mg/day. May increase by 2.5–5 mg/day q1–2wk.

CONTRAINDICATIONS

Diabetic ketoacidosis with or without coma, type 1 diabetes mellitus

INTERACTIONS

Drug

Beta blockers: May increase the hypoglycemic effect of glipizide and mask signs of hypoglycemia.
Cimetidine, ciprofloxacin, fluconazole, MAOIs, quinidine, ranitidine, large doses of salicylates: May increase the effects of glipizide.
Corticosteroids, lithium, thiazide diuretics: May decrease the effects of glipizide.
Oral anticoagulants: May increase the effects of oral anticoagulants.

Herbal

None known.

Food

None known.

Drug interactions of concern to dentistry

- Increased hypoglycemic effects: salicylates, ketoconazole
- Decreased action of glipizide: corticosteroids
- Disulfiram-like reaction: alcohol

DIAGNOSTIC TEST EFFECTS

May increase BUN and LDH concentrations and serum alkaline phosphatase, creatinine, and AST(SGOT) levels.

SIDE EFFECTS

Frequent

Altered taste sensation, dizziness, somnolence, weight gain, constipation, diarrhea, heartburn, nausea, vomiting, stomach fullness, headache

Occasional

Increased sensitivity of skin to sunlight, peeling of skin, itching, rash

SERIOUS REACTIONS

! Overdose or insufficiet food intake may produce hypoglycemia, especially with increased glucose demands.
! GI hemorrhage, cholestatic hepatic jaundice, leukopenia, thrombocytopenia, pancytopenia, agranulocytosis, and aplastic or hemolytic anemia occurs rarely.

DENTAL CONSIDERATIONS

General:

- Monitor vital signs at every appointment because of cardiovascular side effects.
- Patients on chronic drug therapy may rarely have symptoms of blood dyscrasias, which can include infection, bleeding, and poor healing.
- Short appointments and a stress reduction protocol may be required for anxious patients.
- Place on frequent recall to evaluate healing response.
- Diabetics may be more susceptible to infection and have delayed wound healing.
- Question patient about self-monitoring of drug's antidiabetic effect, including blood glucose values or finger-stick records.
- Ensure that patient is following prescribed diet and regularly takes medication.
- Avoid prescribing aspirin-containing products.

Consultations:

- In a patient with symptoms of blood dyscrasias, request a medical consultation for blood studies and postpone dental treatment until normal values are reestablished.

- Medical consultation may be required to assess disease control.
- Medical consultation may include data from patient's blood glucose monitoring, including glycosylated hemoglobin or HbA_{1c} testing.

Teach Patient/Family:

- Importance of good oral hygiene to prevent soft tissue inflammation
- Caution to prevent injury when using oral hygiene aids
- To avoid mouth rinses with high alcohol content because of drying effects

G

glucagon hydrochloride

glue′-ka-gon

(GlucaGen, GlucaGen Diagnostic Kit, Glucagen[AUS], Glucagon, Glucagon Diagnostic Kit, Glucagon Emergency Kit)

Do not confuse glucagon with Glaucon.

CATEGORY AND SCHEDULE

Pregnancy Risk Category: B

MECHANISM OF ACTION

A glucose elevating agent that promotes hepatic glycogenolysis, gluconeogenesis. Stimulates production of cyclic adenosine monophosphate (cAMP), which results in increased plasma glucose concentration, smooth muscle relaxation, and an inotropic myocardial effect. ***Therapeutic Effect:*** Increases plasma glucose level.

AVAILABILITY

Powder for Injection: 1 mg.

INDICATIONS AND DOSAGES

▸ **Hypoglycemia**

IV, IM, SUBCUTANEOUS

Adults, Elderly, Children weighing more than 20 kg. 0.5–1 mg. May give 1 or 2 additional doses if response is delayed.

Children weighing 20 kg or less. 0.5 mg.

▸ **Diagnostic Aid**

IV, IM

Adults, Elderly. 0.25–2 mg 10 min prior to procedure.

OFF-LABEL USES

Treatment of esophageal obstruction due to foreign bodies, toxicity associated with beta blockers or calcium channel blockers

CONTRAINDICATIONS

Hypersensitivity to glucagon or beef or pork proteins, known pheochromocytoma

INTERACTIONS

Drug

Anticoagulants: May increase the effects of these drugs.

Herbal

None known.

Food

None known.

Drug interactions of concern to dentistry

- Patients taking β-adrenergic blockers: may be expected to have a transient but greater increase in blood pressure and pulse

DIAGNOSTIC TEST EFFECTS

May decrease serum potassium level.

IV INCOMPATIBILITIES

Don't mix glucagon with any other medications.

SIDE EFFECTS

Occasional

Nausea, vomiting

Rare

Allergic reaction, such as urticaria, respiratory distress, and hypotension

SERIOUS REACTIONS

! Overdose may produce persistent nausea and vomiting and hypokalemia, marked by severe weakness, decreased appetite, irregular heartbeat, and muscle cramps.

DENTAL CONSIDERATIONS

General:

- Glucagon may be used as an emergency drug for severe hypoglycemia. Patients should be closely monitored and referred immediately for evaluation.
- IV glucose may be required for patients nonresponsive to glucagon.
- Unconscious patients should awaken within 15 min or less.

glyburide

glye′-byoor-ide
(Daonil[CAN], DiaBeta, Euglucon[CAN], Glimel[AUS], Glynase, Micronase, Semi-Daonil[AUS], Semi-Euglucon[AUS])
Do not confuse glyburide with glimepiride or glipizide, or Micronase with Micro-K, Micronor.

CATEGORY AND SCHEDULE

Pregnancy Risk Category: C

MECHANISM OF ACTION

A second-generation sulfonylurea that promotes release of insulin from beta cells of the pancreas and increases insulin sensitivity at peripheral sites.
Therapeutic Effect: Lowers blood glucose concentration.

PHARMACOKINETICS

Route	Onset	Peak	Duration
PO	0.25–1 hr	1–2 hr	12–24 hr

Well absorbed from the GI tract. Protein binding: 99%. Metabolized in the liver to weakly active metabolite. Primarily excreted in urine. Not removed by hemodialysis. ***Half-life:*** 1.4–1.8 hr.

AVAILABILITY

Tablets (DiaBeta, Micronase): 1.25 mg, 2.5 mg, 5 mg.
Tablets (Glynase): 1.5 mg, 3 mg, 6 mg.

INDICATIONS AND DOSAGES

▸ Diabetes Mellitus

PO
Adults. Initially 2.5–5 mg. May increase by 2.5 mg/day at weekly intervals. Maintenance: 1.25–20 mg/day. Maximum: 20 mg/day.
Elderly. Initially, 1.25–2.5 mg/day. May increase by 1.25–2.5 mg/day at 1- to 3-wk intervals.
PO (micronized tablets [Glynase])
Adults, Elderly. Initially 0.75–3 mg/day. May increase by 1.5 mg/day at weekly intervals. Maintenance: 0.75–12 mg/day as a single dose or in divided doses.

▸ Dosage in Renal Impairment

Glyburide is not recommended in patients with creatinine clearance less than 50 ml/min.

CONTRAINDICATIONS

Diabetic ketoacidosis with or without coma, monotherapy for type 1 diabetes mellitus

INTERACTIONS

Drug

Beta blockers: May increase the hypoglycemic effect of glyburide and mask signs of hypoglycemia.

G

Cimetidine, ciprofloxacin, fluconazole, MAOIs, quinidine, ranitidine, large doses of salicylates: May increase the effects of glyburide.
Corticosteroids, lithium, thiazide diuretics: May decrease the effects of glyburide.
Oral anticoagulants: May increase the effects of oral anticoagulants.

Herbal
None known.

Food
None known.

Drug interactions of concern to dentistry
- Increased hypoglycemic effects: NSAIDs, salicylates, ketoconazole
- Decreased action of glyburide: corticosteroids
- Disulfiram-like reaction: alcohol

DIAGNOSTIC TEST EFFECTS
May increase BUN and LDH concentrations and serum alkaline phosphatase, creatinine, and AST(SGOT) levels.

SIDE EFFECTS
Frequent
Altered taste sensation, dizziness, somnolence, weight gain, constipation, diarrhea, heartburn, nausea, vomiting, stomach fullness, headache

Occasional
Increased sensitivity of skin to sunlight, peeling of skin, itching, rash

SERIOUS REACTIONS
! Overdose or insufficient food intake may produce hypoglycemia, especially in patients with increased glucose demands.
! Cholestatic jaundice, leukopenia, thrombocytopenia, pancytopenia, agranulocytosis, and aplastic or hemolytic anemia occur rarely.

DENTAL CONSIDERATIONS
General:
- Monitor vital signs at every appointment because of cardiovascular side effects.
- Patients on chronic drug therapy may rarely have symptoms of blood dyscrasias, which can include infection, bleeding, and poor healing.
- Place on frequent recall to evaluate healing response.
- Ensure that patient is following prescribed diet and regularly takes medication.
- Short appointments and stress reduction protocol may be required for anxious patients.
- Patients with diabetes may be more susceptible to infection and have delayed wound healing.
- Question patient about self-monitoring of drug's antidiabetic effect, including blood glucose values or finger-stick records.
- Avoid prescribing aspirin-containing products.

Consultations:
- In a patient with symptoms of blood dyscrasias, request a medical consultation for blood studies and postpone dental treatment until normal values are reestablished.
- Medical consultation may be required to assess disease control.
- Medical consultation may include data from patient's blood glucose monitoring, including glycosylated hemoglobin or HbA_{1c} testing.

Teach Patient/Family:
- Importance of good oral hygiene to prevent soft tissue inflammation
- Caution to prevent injury when using oral hygiene aids
- To avoid mouth rinses with high alcohol content because of drying effects

glycopyrrolate

glye-koe-pye′-roe-late
(Robinul, Robinul Forte, Robinul Injection[AUS])
Do not confuse Robinul with Reminyl.

CATEGORY AND SCHEDULE
Pregnancy Risk Category: B

MECHANISM OF ACTION
A quaternary anticholinergic that inhibits action of acetylcholine at postganglionic parasympathetic sites in smooth muscle, secretory glands, and CNS. ***Therapeutic Effect:*** Reduces salivation and excessive secretions of respiratory tract; reduces gastric secretions and acidity.

PHARMACOKINETICS
Poorly and irregularly absorbed from GI tract after oral administration. Metabolized in the liver. Primarily excreted in urine. ***Half-life:*** 1.7 hr.

AVAILABILITY
Injection (Robinul): 0.2 mg/ml.
Tablets: 1 mg (Robinul), 2 mg (Robinul Forte).

INDICATIONS AND DOSAGES
▸ Preoperative Inhibition of Salivation and Excessive Respiratory Tract Secretions
IM
Adults, Elderly. 4 mcg/kg 30–60 min before procedure.
Children 2 yr and older. 4 mcg/kg.
Children younger than 2 yr. 4–9 mcg/kg.
▸ To Block Effects of Anticholinesterase Agents
IV
Adults, Elderly. 0.2 mg for each 1 mg neostigmine or 5 mg pyridostigmine.
▸ Peptic Ulcer Disease, Adjunct
IV, IM
Adults, Elderly. 0.1 mg IV or IM 3–4 times/day.
PO
Adults, Elderly. 1–2 mg 2–3 times/day. Maximum: 8 mg/day.

CONTRAINDICATIONS
Acute hemorrhage, myasthenia gravis, narrow-angle glaucoma, obstructive uropathy, paralytic ileus, tachycardia, ulcerative colitis

INTERACTIONS
Drug
Antacids, antidiarrheals: May decrease the absorption of glycopyrrolate.
Ketoconazole: May decrease the absorption of ketoconazole.
Other anticholinergics: May increase the effects of glycopyrrolate.
Potassium chloride: May increase the severity of GI lesions with the wax matrix formulation of potassium chloride.
Herbal
None known.
Food
None known.
Drug interactions of concern to dentistry
- Increased anticholinergic effect: antihistamines, phenothiazines, meperidine, haloperidol, scopolamine, atropine
- Do not mix with diazepam, pentobarbital, in syringe or solution
- Constipation, urinary retention: opioid analgesics
- Reduced absorption of ketoconazole

DIAGNOSTIC TEST EFFECTS
May decrease serum uric acid levels.

G

IV INCOMPATIBILITIES

None known.

IV COMPATIBILITIES

Diphenhydramine (Benadryl), droperidol (Inapsine), hydromorphone (Dilaudid), hydroxyzine (Vistaril), lidocaine, midazolam (Versed), morphine, promethazine (Phenergan)

G

SIDE EFFECTS

Frequent

Dry mouth, decreased sweating, constipation

Occasional

Blurred vision, gastric bloating, urinary hesitancy, somnolence (with high dosage), headache, intolerance to light, loss of taste, nervousness, flushing, insomnia, impotence, mental confusion or excitement (particularly in the elderly and children), temporary light-headedness (with parenteral form), local irritation (with parenteral form)

Rare

Dizziness, faintness

SERIOUS REACTIONS

! Overdose may produce temporary paralysis of ciliary muscle; pupillary dilation; tachycardia; palpitations; hot, dry, or flushed skin; absence of bowel sounds; hyperthermia; increased respiratory rate; ECG abnormalities; nausea; vomiting; rash over face or upper trunk; CNS stimulation; and psychosis (marked by agitation, restlessness, rambling speech, visual hallucinations, paranoid behavior, and delusions, followed by depression).

DENTAL CONSIDERATIONS

General:

- Avoid dental light in patient's eyes; offer dark glasses for patient comfort.
- Assess salivary flow as a factor in caries, periodontal disease, and candidiasis.

Consultation:

- Physician should be informed if significant xerostomic side effects occur (e.g., increased caries, sore tongue, problems eating or swallowing, difficulty wearing prosthesis) so that a medication change can be considered.

Teach Patient/Family:

- *When chronic dry mouth occurs, advise patient:*
  - To avoid mouth rinses with high alcohol content because of drying effects
  - To use daily home fluoride products for anticaries effect
  - To use sugarless gum, frequent sips of water, or saliva substitutes

goserelin acetate

gos-er′-ah-lin

(Zoladex, Zoladex Implant[AUS], Zoladex LA)

CATEGORY AND SCHEDULE

Pregnancy Risk Category: D (advanced breast cancer), X (endometriosis, endometrial thinning)

MECHANISM OF ACTION

A gonadotropin-releasing hormone analogue and antineoplastic agent that stimulates the release of luteinizing hormone (LH) and follicle-stimulating hormone (FSH) from the anterior pituitary gland. In males, increases testosterone concentrations initially, then suppresses secretion of LH and FSH, resuting in decreased testosterone levels. ***Therapeutic Effect:*** In females, causes a reduction in ovarian size and function, reduction in uterine and mammary gland size, and regression of sex-hormone-responsive tumors. In males, produces pharmacologic castration and decreases the growth of abnormal prostate tissue.

AVAILABILITY

Implant: 3.6 mg, 10.8 mg.

INDICATIONS AND DOSAGES

▸ **Prostatic Carcinoma**

IMPLANT

Adults older than 18 yr, Elderly. 3.6 mg every 28 days or 10.8 mg q12wk subcutaneously into upper abdominal wall.

▸ **Breast Carcinoma, Endometriosis**

IMPLANT

Adults. 3.6 mg every 28 days subcutaneously into upper abdominal wall.

▸ **Endometrial Thinning**

IMPLANT

Adults. 3.6 mg subcutaneously into upper abdominal wall as a single dose or in 2 doses 4 wk apart.

CONTRAINDICATIONS

Pregnancy

INTERACTIONS

Drug

None known.

Herbal

None known.

Food

None known.

Drug interactions of concern to dentistry

- None reported

DIAGNOSTIC TEST EFFECTS

May increase serum prostatic acid phosphatase and testosterone levels.

SIDE EFFECTS

Frequent

Headache (60%), hot flashes (55%), depression (54%), diaphoresis (45%), sexual dysfunction (21%), decreased erection (18%), lower urinary tract symptoms (13%)

Occasional (10%–5%)

Pain, lethargy, dizziness, insomnia, anorexia, nausea, rash, upper respiratory tract infection, hirsutism, abdominal pain

Rare

Pruritus

SERIOUS REACTIONS

! Arrhythmias, CHF, and hypertension occur rarely.

! Ureteral obstruction and spinal cord compression have been observed. An immediate orchiectomy may be necessary if these conditions occur.

DENTAL CONSIDERATIONS

General:

- Monitor vital signs at every appointment due to cardiovascular side effects.
- Determine why patient is taking the drug.
- If additional analgesia is required for dental pain, consider alternative analgesics (NSAIDs) in patients taking narcotics for acute or chronic pain.
- Consider semisupine chair position for patient comfort if GI side effects occur.
- Assess salivary flow as a factor in caries, periodontal disease, and candidiasis.
- If used in prostate cancer, consider urinary retention concern and avoid anticholinergic drugs that may aggravate retention.
- Patients may be taking other medications; see complete drug/herbal history.

Consultations:

- Medical consultation may be required to assess immunologic status during cancer chemotherapy and determine safety risk, if any, posed by the required dental treatment.
- Medical consultation may be required to assess disease control and patient's ability to tolerate stress.

Teach Patient/Family:

G

- *When chronic dry mouth occurs advise patient:*
  - To avoid mouth rinses with high alcohol content due to drying effects
  - To use daily home fluoride products for anticaries effect
  - To use sugarless gum, frequent sips of water or saliva substitutes
- Importance of good oral hygiene to prevent soft tissue inflammation
- To report oral lesions, soreness, or bleeding to dentist
- To prevent trauma when using oral hygiene aids
- Importance of updating health and medication history if physician makes any changes in evaluation or drug regimens; include OTC, herbal, and nonherbal remedies in the update

granisetron

gra-ni′-se-tron
(Kytril)

CATEGORY AND SCHEDULE

Pregnancy Risk Category: B

MECHANISM OF ACTION

A 5-HT_3 receptor antagonist that acts centrally in the chemoreceptor trigger zone or peripherally at the vagal nerve terminals. ***Therapeutic Effect:*** Prevents nausea and vomiting.

PHARMACOKINETICS

Route	Onset	Peak	Duration
IV	1–3 min	N/A	24 hr

Rapidly and widely distributed to tissues. Protein binding: 65%. Metabolized in the liver to active metabolite. Eliminated in urine and feces. ***Half-life:*** 10–12 hr (increased in the elderly).

AVAILABILITY

Oral Solution: 1 mg/5 ml.
Tablets: 1 mg.
Injection: 0.1 mg/ml, 1 mg/ml.

INDICATIONS AND DOSAGES

▸ Prevention of Chemotherapy-Induced Nausea and Vomiting

PO

Adults, Elderly. 2 mg once a day up to 1 hr before chemotherapy or 1 mg twice a day.

IV

Adults, Elderly, Children 2 yr and older. 10 mcg/kg/dose (or 1 mg/dose) within 30 min of chemotherapy.

▸ Prevention of Radiation-Induced Nausea and Vomiting

PO

Adults, Elderly. 2 mg once a day given 1 hr before radiation therapy.

▸ Postoperative Nausea or Vomiting

PO

Adults, Elderly, Children 4 yr and older. 20–40 mcg/kg as a single postoperative dose.

IV

Adults, Elderly. 1 mg as a single postoperative dose.
Children older than 4 yr. 20–40 mcg/kg. Maximum: 1 mg.

OFF-LABEL USES

PO: Prophylaxis of nausea or vomiting associated with radiation therapy

CONTRAINDICATIONS
None known.

INTERACTIONS
Drug
Hepatic enzyme inducers: May decrease the effects of granisetron.
Herbal
None known.
Food
None known.
Drug interactions of concern to dentistry
• Possible decreased effects: strong inducers of CYP3A4 isoenzymes
• Possible increased effects: strong inhibitors of CYP3A4 isoenzymes

DIAGNOSTIC TEST EFFECTS
May increase AST (SGOT) and ALT (SGPT) levels.

IV INCOMPATIBILITIES
Amphotericin B (Fungizone)
IV COMPATIBILITIES
Allopurinol (Aloprim), bumetanide (Bumex), calcium gluconate, carboplatin (Paraplatin), cisplatin (Platinol), cyclophosphamide (Cytoxan), cytarabine (Ara-C), dacarbazine (DTIC-Dome), dexamethasone (Decadron), diphenhydramine (Benadryl), docetaxel (Taxotere), doxorubicin (Adriamycin), etoposide (VePesid), gemcitabine (Gemzar), magnesium, mitoxantrone (Novantrone), paclitaxel (Taxol), potassium

SIDE EFFECTS
Frequent (21%–14%)
Headache, constipation, asthenia
Occasional (8%–6%)
Diarrhea, abdominal pain
Rare (< 2%)
Altered taste, hypersensitivity reaction

SERIOUS REACTIONS
! None known.

DENTAL CONSIDERATIONS
General:
• When used in anesthesia, monitor patients to prevent untoward events.
Teach Patient/Family:
• To be aware of possible oral side effects from concurrent cancer chemotherapy.
• To report troublesome nausea and vomiting to dentist for patients recovering from anesthesia after dental treatment.
• To assure patient alteration in taste is temporary.

griseofulvin
griz-ee-oh-full′-vin
(Fulvicin P/G, Fulvicin U/F, Grifulvin V, Gris-PEG, Grisovin[AUS])

CATEGORY AND SCHEDULE
Pregnancy Risk Category: C

MECHANISM OF ACTION
An antifungal that inhibits fungal cell mitosis by disrupting mitotic spindle structure.. ***Therapeutic Effect:*** Fungistatic.

AVAILABILITY
Oral Suspension (Grifulvin V): 125 mg/5 ml.
Tablets (Microsize [Fulvicin-U/F]): 250 mg, 500 mg.
Tablets (Ultramicrosize [Fulvicin P/G]): 125 mg, 165 mg, 250 mg, 330 mg.
Tablets (Ultramicrosize [Gris-PEG]): 125 mg, 250 mg.

INDICATIONS AND DOSAGES
▸ Tinea Capitis, Tinea Corporis, Tinea Cruris, Tinea Pedis, Tinea Unguium
PO (Microsize Tablets, Oral Suspension)

Adults. Usual dosage, 500–1,000 mg as a single dose or in divided doses.
Children 2 yr and older. Usual dosage, 10–20 mg/kg/day.
PO (Ultramicrosize Tablets)
Adults. Usual dosage, 330–750 mg/day as a single dose or in divided doses.
Children 2 yr and older. 5–10 mg/kg/day.

CONTRAINDICATIONS
Hepatocellular failure, porphyria

INTERACTIONS
Drug
Oral contraceptives, warfarin: May decrease the effects of these drugs.
Herbal
None known.
Food
None known.
Drug interactions of concern to dentistry
- Possible decreased effects: phenobarbital

DIAGNOSTIC TEST EFFECTS
None known.

SIDE EFFECTS
Occasional
Hypersensitivity reaction (including pruritus, rash, and urticaria), headache, nausea, diarrhea, excessive thirst, flatulence, oral thrush, dizziness, insomnia
Rare
Paresthesia of hands or feet, proteinuria, photosensitivity reaction

SERIOUS REACTIONS
! Granulocytopenia occurs rarely.

DENTAL CONSIDERATIONS
General:
- Determine why patient is taking the drug.
- Assess salivary flow as a factor in caries, periodontal disease, and candidiasis.
- Examine for oral manifestation of opportunistic infection.
- Advise patient if dental drugs prescribed have a potential for photosensitivity.

Teach Patient/Family:
- *When chronic dry mouth occurs advise patient:*
  - To avoid mouth rinses with high alcohol content due to drying effects
  - To use daily home fluoride products for anticaries effect
  - To use sugarless gum, frequent sips of water or saliva substitutes
- To report oral lesions, soreness, or bleeding to dentist
- Importance of good oral hygiene to prevent soft tissue inflammation
- To report sore throat, oral burning sensation, fever, or fatigue, any of which could indicate presence of a superinfection
- Importance of updating health and medication history if physician makes any changes in evaluation or drug regimens; include OTC, herbal, and nonherbal remedies in the update
- To avoid concurrent use of alcohol

guaifenesin
gwye-fen′-e-sin
(Balminil[CAN], Benylin E[CAN], Guiatuss, Humibid LA, Mucinex, Organidin, Robitussin, Tussin)
Do not confuse guaifenesin with guanfacine.

CATEGORY AND SCHEDULE
Pregnancy Risk Category: C
OTC

MECHANISM OF ACTION

An expectorant that stimulates respiratory tract secretions by decreasing adhesiveness and viscosity of phlegm. ***Therapeutic Effect:*** Promotes removal of viscous mucus.

PHARMACOKINETICS

Well absorbed from the GI tract. Metabolized in the liver. Excreted in urine.

AVAILABILITY

Tablets (Organidin): 200 mg.
Tablets (Extended-Release [Humibid LA, Mucinex]): 600 mg.
Syrup (Guiatuss, Robitussin, Tussin): 100 mg/5 ml.

INDICATIONS AND DOSAGES

▸ Expectorant

PO
Adults, Elderly, Children older than 12 yr. 200–400 mg q4h.
Children 6–12 yr. 100–200 mg q4h. Maximum: 1.2 g/day.
Children 2–5 yr. 50–100 mg q4h.
Children younger than 2 yr. 12 mg/kg/day in 6 divided doses.
PO (Extended-Release)
Adults, Elderly, Children older than 12 yr. 600–1200 mg q12h. Maximum: 2.4 g/day.
Children 2–5 yr. 600 mg q12h. Maximum: 600 mg/day.

CONTRAINDICATIONS

None known.

INTERACTIONS

Drug
None known.
Herbal
None known.
Food
None known.

DIAGNOSTIC TEST EFFECTS

None known.

SIDE EFFECTS

Rare
Dizziness, headache, rash, diarrhea, nausea, vomiting, abdominal pain

SERIOUS REACTIONS

! Overdose may produce nausea and vomiting.

DENTAL CONSIDERATIONS

General:
• Consider semisupine chair position for patients with respiratory disease.
• Elective dental treatment may be precluded by significant coughing episodes.

guanabenz

gwan′-a-benz
(Wytensin)

CATEGORY AND SCHEDULE

Pregnancy Risk Category: C

MECHANISM OF ACTION

An alpha-adrenergic agonist that stimulates alpha2-adrenergic receptors. Inhibits sympathetic cardioaccelerator and vasoconstrictor center to heart, kidneys, peripheral vasculature. ***Therapeutic Effect:*** Decreases systolic, diastolic blood pressure (B/P). Chronic use decreases peripheral vascular resistance.

PHARMACOKINETICS

Well absorbed from gastrointestinal (GI) tract. Widely distributed. Protein binding: 90%. Metabolized in liver. Excreted in urine and feces. Not removed by hemodialysis. ***Half-life:*** 6 hrs.

AVAILABILITY

Tablets: 4 mg, 8 mg (Wytensin).

INDICATIONS AND DOSAGES

▸ Hypertension

PO

Adults. Initially, 4 mg 2 times/day. Increase by 4–8 mg at 1–2 wk intervals. Elderly. Initially, 4 mg/day. May increase q1–2 wks. Maintenance: 8–16 mg/day. Maximum: 32 mg/day.

CONTRAINDICATIONS

History of hypersensitivity to guanabenz or any component of the formulation

INTERACTIONS

Drug

Beta-blockers, hypotensive-producing medications: May increase antihypertensive effect.

Herbal

Licorice, yohimbine: May decrease guanabenz effectiveness.

Food

None known.

Drug interactions of concern to dentistry

- Increased CNS depression: alcohol, all CNS depressants
- Decreased hypotensive effects: NSAIDs, especially indomethacin, sympathomimetics

DIAGNOSTIC TEST EFFECTS

May decrease cholesterol, total triglyceride concentrations.

SIDE EFFECTS

Frequent

Drowsiness, dry mouth, dizziness

Occasional

Weakness, headache, nausea, decreased sexual ability

Rare

Ataxia, sleep disturbances, rash, itching, diarrhea, constipation, altered taste, muscle aches

SERIOUS REACTIONS

! Abrupt withdrawal may result in rebound hypertension manifested as nervousness, agitation, anxiety, insomnia, hand tingling, tremor, flushing, and sweating.

! Overdosage produces hypotension, somnolence, lethargy, irritability, bradycardia, and miosis (pupillary constriction).

DENTAL CONSIDERATIONS

General:

- Monitor vital signs at every appointment because of cardiovascular side effects.
- Limit use of sodium-containing products, such as saline IV fluids, for patients with a dietary salt restriction.
- Assess salivary flow as a factor in caries, periodontal disease, and candidiasis.
- Stress from dental procedures may compromise cardiovascular function; determine patient risk.
- Short appointments and a stress reduction protocol may be required for anxious patients.

Consultations:

- Medical consultation may be required to assess disease control and patient's ability to tolerate stress.

Teach Patient/Family:

- *When chronic dry mouth occurs, advise patient:*
  - To avoid mouth rinses with high alcohol content because of drying effects
  - To use daily home fluoride products for anticaries effect
  - To use sugarless gum, frequent sips of water, or saliva substitutes

guanadrel sulfate
gwahn′-a-drel
(Hylorel)

CATEGORY AND SCHEDULE
Pregnancy Risk Category: C

MECHANISM OF ACTION
An adrenergic blocking agent that depletes norepinephrine from adrenergic nerve endings. Prevents release of norepinephrine normally produced by nerve stimulation.
Therapeutic Effect: Reduces blood pressure (B/P).

PHARMACOKINETICS
Rapidly and well absorbed from gastrointestinal (GI) tract.
Widely distributed. Protein binding: 20%. Primarily excreted in urine.
Half-life: 10 hrs.

AVAILABILITY
Tablets: 10 mg, 25 mg (Hylorel).

INDICATIONS AND DOSAGES
▸ Hypertension
PO
Adults. Initially, 5 mg 2 times/day. Increase at 1–4 wk intervals. Maintenance: 20–75 mg/day in 2 divided doses. Maximum: 400 mg/day.
Elderly. Initially, 5 mg/day. May gradually increase at 1–4 wk intervals. Maintenance: 20–75 mg/day in 2 divided doses.

CONTRAINDICATIONS
Frank CHF, pheochromocytoma, hypersensitivity to guanadrel or any component of the formulation

INTERACTIONS
Drug
Tricyclic antidepressants, MAOIs, phenothiazines, sympathomimetics: May decrease antihypertensive effect.
Herbal
Licorice, yohimbine: May reduce guanadrel effectiveness.
Ma huang: May decrease hypotensive effect of guanadrel.
Food
None known.
Drug interactions of concern to dentistry
- Increased orthostatic hypotension: alcohol, opioid analgesics, barbiturates, phenothiazines, haloperidol
- Decreased hypotensive effect: ephedrine, sympathomimetics, NSAIDs, indomethacin, tricyclic antidepressants

DIAGNOSTIC TEST EFFECTS
None known.

SIDE EFFECTS
Frequent (42–64%)
Fatigue, headache, faintness, drowsiness, nocturia, urinary frequency, change in weight, aching limbs, shortness of breath (resting)
Occasional (21–29%)
Cough, change in vision, paresthesia, confusion, indigestion, constipation, anorexia, peripheral edema, leg cramps
Rare (10%)
Depression, altered sleep, nausea, vomiting, dry mouth, throat, impotence, backache.

SERIOUS REACTIONS
! Overdose may produce blurred vision, severe dizziness/faintness.

DENTAL CONSIDERATIONS
General:
- Monitor vital signs at every appointment because of cardiovascular side effects.
- After supine positioning, have patient sit upright for at least 2 min

before standing to avoid orthostatic hypotension.
- Limit use of sodium-containing products, such as saline IV fluids, for patients with a dietary salt restriction.
- Stress from dental procedures may compromise cardiovascular function; determine patient risk.
- Short appointments and a stress reduction protocol may be required for anxious patients.
- Assess salivary flow as a factor in caries, periodontal disease, and candidiasis.

Consultations:
- Medical consultation may be required to assess disease control and patient's ability to tolerate stress.

Teach Patient/Family:
- *When chronic dry mouth occurs, advise patient:*
  - To avoid mouth rinses with high alcohol content because of drying effects
  - To use daily home fluoride products for anticaries effect
  - To use sugarless gum, frequent sips of water, or saliva substitutes

guanethidine monosulfate

gwahn-eth′-i-deen
(Ismelin)

CATEGORY AND SCHEDULE
Pregnancy Risk Category: C

MECHANISM OF ACTION
An adrenergic blocker that inhibits the release of catecholamines produced by sympathetic nerve stimulation, thus suppressing peripheral sympathetic vasoconstriction. ***Therapeutic Effect:*** Decreases blood pressure.

PHARMACOKINETICS
Absorption is highly variable among patients. Protein binding: 26%. Metabolized in liver. Excreted in urine and feces. ***Half-life:*** 5–10 days.

AVAILABILITY
Tablets: 10 mg, 25 mg (Ismelin).

INDICATIONS AND DOSAGES
▸ **Hypertension**

PO

Adults. Initially, 10 mg/day. May increase in 10–25 mg increments at 5–7 day intervals. Maximum: 100 mg/day. Lower initial doses are recommended for the elderly.

OFF-LABEL USES
Treatment of anxiety, chronic angina pectoris, hypertrophic cardiomyopathy, myocardial infarction, pheochromocytoma, syndrome of mitral valve prolapse, thyrotoxicosis, and tremors

CONTRAINDICATIONS
MAOI therapy within 1 week, overt congestive heart failure, pheochromocytoma, hypersensitivity to guanethidine or any component of the formulation

INTERACTIONS
Drug

Amphetamines, chlorpromazine, deithylpropion, epinephrine, imipramine, methylphenidate, MAOIs, prochlorperazine, tricyclic antidepressants, zotepine: May decrease antihypertensive effectiveness.
Etilefrine: May increase etilefrine effects.
Norepinephrine, phenylephrine: May cause hypertension and/or arrhythmias.
Phenylpropanolamine, pseudoephedrine: May cause

a loss of blood pressure control and possible hypertensive urgency.

Herbal

Licorice, Ma huang, yohimbine: May decrease hypotensive effect of guanethidine.

Food

None known.

Drug interactions of concern to dentistry

- Increased orthostatic hypotension: alcohol, opioid analgesics, barbiturates, phenothiazines, haloperidol
- Decreased hypotensive effect: ephedrine, NSAIDs, indomethacin, sympathomimetics, tricyclic antidepressants

DIAGNOSTIC TEST EFFECTS

None known.

SIDE EFFECTS

Frequent

Bradycardia, dizziness, blurred vision, orthostatic hypotension, fluid retention

Occasional

Impotence, inhibition of ejaculation, nasal stuffiness

Rare

Apnea, hypertension, renal dysfunction

SERIOUS REACTIONS

! Arrhythmias, angina, and pulmonary edema have been reported.

! Overdosage may produce bradycardia, diarrhea, nausea, orthostatic hypotension, and shock.

DENTAL CONSIDERATIONS

General:

- Monitor vital signs at every appointment because of cardiovascular and respiratory side effects.
- Patients on chronic drug therapy may rarely have symptoms of blood dyscrasias, which can include infection, bleeding, and poor healing.
- Assess salivary flow as a factor in caries, periodontal disease, and candidiasis.
- After supine positioning, have patient sit upright for at least 2 min before standing to avoid orthostatic hypotension.
- Limit use of sodium-containing products, such as saline IV fluids, for patients with a dietary salt restriction.
- Stress from dental procedures may compromise cardiovascular function; determine patient risk.
- Short appointments and a stress reduction protocol may be required for anxious patients.
- Use vasoconstrictors with caution, in low doses, and with careful aspiration. Avoid using gingival retraction cord with epinephrine.
- Consider semisupine chair position for patients with respiratory distress.

Consultations:

- Medical consultation may be required to assess disease control and patient's ability to tolerate stress.
- In a patient with symptoms of blood dyscrasias, request a medical consultation for blood studies and postpone dental treatment until normal values are reestablished.

Teach Patient/Family:

- Importance of good oral hygiene to prevent soft tissue inflammation
- Caution to prevent injury when using oral hygiene aids
- *When chronic dry mouth occurs, advise patient:*
  - To avoid mouth rinses with high alcohol content because of drying effects
  - To use daily home fluoride products for anticaries effect
  - To use sugarless gum, frequent sips of water, or saliva substitutes

G

guanfacine

gwan′-fa-seen
(Tenex)

CATEGORY AND SCHEDULE

Pregnancy Risk Category: B

MECHANISM OF ACTION

An alpha-adrenergic agonist that stimulates alpha2-adrenergic receptors and inhibits sympathetic cardioaccelerator and vasoconstrictor center to heart, kidneys, peripheral vasculature. ***Therapeutic Effect:*** Decreases systolic, diastolic blood pressure (B/P). Chronic use decreases peripheral vascular resistance.

PHARMACOKINETICS

Well absorbed from gastrointestinal (GI) tract. Widely distributed. Protein binding: 71%. Metabolized in liver. Excreted in urine and feces. Not removed by hemodialysis. ***Half-life:*** 17 hrs.

AVAILABILITY

Tablets: 1 mg, 2 mg (Tenex).

INDICATIONS AND DOSAGES

▸ Hypertension

PO

Adults, Elderly. Initially, 1 mg/day. Increase by 1 mg/day at intervals of 3–4 wks up to 3 mg/day in single or divided doses.

OFF-LABEL USES

Attention deficit hyperactivity disorder (ADHD), tic disorders

CONTRAINDICATIONS

History of hypersensitivity to guanfacine or any component of the formulation

INTERACTIONS

Drug

Beta-blockers, hypotensive-producing medications: May increase antihypertensive effect.
Bupropion: May increase risk of seizure activity.

Herbal

Licorice, yohimbine: May decrease guanfacine effectiveness.
Ma Huang: May increase blood pressure.

Food

None known.

Drug interactions of concern to dentistry

- Possible increase in CNS depression: alcohol and all CNS depressants
- Possible reduced antihypertensive effect: indomethacin and perhaps other NSAIDs
- Possible increase in antihypertensive effects: other antihypertensive drugs

DIAGNOSTIC TEST EFFECTS

May increase growth hormone concentration. May decrease urinary catecholamine and VMA excretion.

SIDE EFFECTS

Frequent

Dry mouth, somnolence

Occasional

Fatigue, headache, asthenia (loss of strength, energy), dizziness

SERIOUS REACTIONS

! Overdosage may produce difficult breathing, dizziness, faintness, severe drowsiness, bradycardia.

DENTAL CONSIDERATIONS

General:

- Monitor vital signs at every appointment due to cardiovascular side effects.

• Limit use of sodium-containing products, such as saline IV fluids, for patients with a dietary salt restriction.
• Assess salivary flow as a factor in caries, periodontal disease, and candidiasis.
• Short appointments and a stress reduction protocol may be required for anxious patients.
• Stress from dental procedures may compromise cardiovascular function, determine patient risk.
• Use precaution if sedation or general anesthesia is required; risk of hypotensive episode.

Consultations:

• Medical consultation may be required to assess disease control and patient's ability to tolerate stress.

Teach Patient/Family:

• *When chronic dry mouth occurs advise patient:*
  • To avoid mouth rinses with high alcohol content due to drying effects
  • To use daily home fluoride products for anticaries effect
  • To use sugarless gum, frequent sips of water or saliva substitutes
• Importance of updating health and medication history if physician makes any changes in evaluation or drug regimens; include OTC, herbal, and nonherbal remedies in the update
• Caution patients about driving or performing other tasks requiring mental alertness

halcinonide

hal-sin′-o-nide
(Halog, Halog-E)

CATEGORY AND SCHEDULE

Pregnancy Risk Category: C

MECHANISM OF ACTION

A topical corticosteroid that has anti-inflammatory, antipruritic, and vasoconstrictive properties. The exact mechanism of the anti-inflammatory process is unclear. ***Therapeutic Effect:*** Reduces or prevents tissue response to the inflammatory process.

PHARMACOKINETICS

Well absorbed systemically. Large variation in absorption among sites. Protein binding: varies. Metabolized in liver. Primarily excreted in urine.

AVAILABILITY

Cream: 0.1% (Halog).
Cream (emollient base): 0.1% (Halog-E).
Ointment: 0.1% (Halog).
Solution: 0.1% (Halog).

INDICATIONS AND DOSAGES

▸ Dermatoses

TOPICAL

Adults, Elderly. Apply sparingly 1–3 times/day.

CONTRAINDICATIONS

History of hypersensitivity to halcinonide or other corticosteroids

INTERACTIONS

Drug

None known.

Herbal

None known.

Food

None known.

DIAGNOSTIC TEST EFFECTS

None known.

SIDE EFFECTS

Occasional

Itching, redness, irritation, burning at site of application, dryness, folliculitis, acneiform eruptions, hypopigmentation

Rare

Allergic contact dermatitis, maceration of the skin, secondary infection, skin atrophy

SERIOUS REACTIONS

! The serious reactions of long-term therapy and the addition of occlusive dressings are reversible hypothalamic-pituitary-adrenal (HPA) axis suppression, manifestations of Cushing's syndrome, hyperglycemia, and glucosuria.

DENTAL CONSIDERATIONS

General:

- Place on frequent recall to evaluate healing response when used on chronic basis.

Teach Patient/Family:

- Importance of good oral hygiene to prevent soft tissue inflammation
- When used for oral lesions, advise patient to return for oral evaluation if response of oral tissues has not occurred in 7–14 days
- To apply at bedtime or after meals for maximum effect
- To apply with cotton-tipped applicator by pressing, not rubbing, paste on lesion
- That use on oral herpetic ulcerations is contraindicated

halobetasol

hal-oh-be′-ta-sol
(Ultravate)

CATEGORY AND SCHEDULE

Pregnancy Risk Category: C

MECHANISM OF ACTION

A corticosteroid that inhibits accumulation of inflammatory cells at inflammation sites, phagocytosis, lysosomal enzyme release and synthesis or release of mediators of inflammation. ***Therapeutic Effect:*** Decreases or prevents tissue response to inflammatory process.

PHARMACOKINETICS

Variation in absorption among individuals and sites: scrotum 36%, forehead 7%, scalp 4%, forearm 1%.

AVAILABILITY

Cream: 0.05% (Ultravate).
Ointment: 0.05% (Ultravate).

INDICATIONS AND DOSAGES

▸ Dermatoses, Corticosteroid-Unresponsive

TOPICAL

Adults, Elderly, Children older than 12 yrs and older. Apply 1–2 times/day. Maximum: 50 g for 2 weeks.

CONTRAINDICATIONS

Hypersensitivity to halobetasol or other corticosteroids.

INTERACTIONS

Drug

None known.

Herbal

None known.

Food

None known.

DIAGNOSTIC TEST EFFECTS

None known.

SIDE EFFECTS

Frequent

Burning, stinging, pruritus

Rare

Cushing's syndrome, hyperglycemia, glucosuria, hypothalamic-pituitary-adrenal axis suppression

SERIOUS REACTIONS

! Overdosage can occur from topically applied halobetasol absorbed in sufficient amounts to produce systemic effects producing reversible adrenal suppression, manifestations of Cushing's syndrome, hyperglycemia, and glucosuria in some patients.

DENTAL CONSIDERATIONS

Teach Patient/Family:

• That use on oral herpetic ulcerations is contraindicated

H

haloperidol

ha-loe-per′-idole
(Apo-Haloperidol[CAN], Haldol, Haldol Decanoate, Novoperidol[CAN], Peridol[CAN], Serenace[AUS])
Do not confuse Haldol with Halcion, Halog, or Stadol.

CATEGORY AND SCHEDULE

Pregnancy Risk Category: C

MECHANISM OF ACTION

An antipsychotic, antiemetic, and antidyskinetic agent that competitively blocks postsynaptic dopamine receptors, interrupts nerve impulse movement, and increases turnover of dopamine in the brain.

Has strong extrapyramidal and antiemetic effects; weak anticholinergic and sedative effects. ***Therapeutic Effect:*** Produces tranquilizing effect.

PHARMACOKINETICS

Readily absorbed from the GI tract. Protein binding: 92%. Extensively metabolized in the liver. Primarily excreted in urine. Not removed by hemodialysis. ***Half-life:*** 12–37 hr PO; 10–19 hr IV; 17–25 hr IM.

AVAILABILITY

Oral Concentrate: 2 mg/ml.
Tablets: 0.5 mg, 1 mg, 2 mg, 5 mg, 10 mg, 20 mg.
Injection (Lactate): 5 mg/ml.
Injection (Decanoate): 50 mg/ml, 100 mg/ml.

INDICATIONS AND DOSAGES

▸ Treatment of Psychotic Disorders

PO

Adults, Children 12 yr and older. Initially, 0.5–5 mg 2–3 times/day. Dosage gradually adjusted as needed.

Elderly. 0.5–2 mg 2–3 times/day. Dosage gradually adjusted as needed.

Children 3–12 yr or weighing 15–40 kg. Initially, 0.05 mg/kg/day in 2–3 divided doses. May increase by 0.5 mg increments at 5–7 day intervals. Maximum: 0.15 mg/kg/day in divided doses.

IM

Adults, Elderly, Children 12 yr and older. Initially, 2–5. May repeat at 1 hour intervals as needed. Maximum: 100 mg/day.

IM (Decanoate)

Adults, Elderly, Children 12 yr and older. Initially, 10–15 times previous daily oral dose up to maximum initial dose of 100 mg. Maximum: 300 mg/month.

▸ Treatment of Non-Psychotic Disorders, Tourette's Syndrome

PO

Children 3–12 yr or weighing 15–40 kg. Initially, 0.05 mg/kg/day in 2–3 divided doses. May increase by 0.5 mg at 5–7 day intervals. Maximum: 0.075 mg/kg/day.

OFF-LABEL USES

Treatment of Huntington's chorea, infantile autism, nausea, or vomiting associated with cancer chemotherapy

CONTRAINDICATIONS

Angle-closure glaucoma, CNS depression, myelosuppression, Parkinson's disease, severe cardiac or hepatic disease

INTERACTIONS

Drug

Alcohol, other CNS depressants: May increase CNS depression.
Epinephrine: May block alpha-adrenergic effects.
Extrapyramidal symptom-producing medications: May increase extrapyramidal symptoms.
Lithium: May increase neurologic toxicity.

Herbal

None known.

Food

None known.

Drug interactions of concern to dentistry

- Increased sedation: other CNS depressants, alcohol, barbiturate anesthetics, opioid analgesics
- Hypotension, tachycardia: epinephrine
- Increased extrapyramidal effects: phenothiazines and related drugs (haloperidol, droperidol), metoclopramide
- Additive photosensitization: tetracyclines

- Increased anticholinergic effects: anticholinergics
- Suspected increase in neurologic side effects: fluconazole, itraconazole, ketoconazole

DIAGNOSTIC TEST EFFECTS

None known. Therapeutic serum level is 0.2–1 mcg/ml; toxic serum level is greater than 1 mcg/ml.

IV INCOMPATIBILITIES

Allopurinol (Aloprim), amphotericin B complex (Abelcet, AmBisome, Amphotec), cefepime (Maxipime), fluconazole (Diflucan), foscarnet (Foscavir), heparin, nitroprusside (Nipride), piperacillin and tazobactam (Zosyn)

IV COMPATIBILITIES

Dobutamine (Dobutrex), dopamine (Intropin), fentanyl (Sublimaze), hydromorphone (Dilaudid), lidocaine, lorazepam (Ativan), midazolam (Versed), morphine, nitroglycerin, norepinephrine (Levophed), propofol (Diprivan)

SIDE EFFECTS

Frequent

Blurred vision, constipation, orthostatic hypotension, dry mouth, swelling or soreness of female breasts, peripheral edema

Occasional

Allergic reaction, difficulty urinating, decreased thirst, dizziness, decreased sexual function, drowsiness, nausea, vomiting, photosensitivity, lethargy

SERIOUS REACTIONS

! Extrapyramidal symptoms appear to be dose related and typically occur in the first few days of therapy. Marked drowsiness and lethargy, excessive salivation, and fixed stare occur frequently. Less common reactions include severe akathisia (motor restlessness) and acute dystonias (such as torticollis, opisthotonos, and oculogyric crisis).

! Tardive dyskinesia (tongue protrusion, puffing of the cheeks, chewing or puckering of the mouth) may occur during long-term therapy or after discontinuing the drug and may be irreversible. Elderly female patients have a greater risk of developing this reaction.

DENTAL CONSIDERATIONS

General:

- Monitor vital signs at every appointment because of cardiovascular side effects.
- After supine positioning, have patient sit upright for at least 2 min before standing to avoid orthostatic hypotension.
- Assess salivary flow as a factor in caries, periodontal disease, and candidiasis.
- Avoid dental light in patient's eyes; offer dark glasses for patient comfort.
- Assess for presence of extrapyramidal motor symptoms, such as tardive dyskinesia and akathisia. Extrapyramidal motor activity may complicate dental treatment.
- Geriatric patients are more susceptible to drug effects; use lower dose.
- Use vasoconstrictors with caution, in low doses, and with careful aspiration. Avoid use of gingival retraction cord with epinephrine.

Consultations:

- Take precautions if dental surgery is anticipated and anesthesia is required.
- Refer to physician if signs of tardive dyskinesia or akathisia are present.

• Physician should be informed if significant xerostomic side effects occur (e.g., increased caries, sore tongue, problems eating or swallowing, difficulty wearing prosthesis) so that a medication change can be considered.

Teach Patient/Family:

• Importance of good oral hygiene to prevent soft tissue inflammation
• Caution to prevent injury when using oral hygiene aids
• To use electric toothbrush if patient has difficulty holding conventional devices
• *When chronic dry mouth occurs, advise patient:*
  • To avoid mouth rinses with high alcohol content because of drying effects
  • To use daily home fluoride products for anticaries effect
  • To use sugarless gum, frequent sips of water, or saliva substitutes

heparin sodium

hep′-a-rin
(Hepalean[CAN], Heparin injection B.P.[AUS], Heparin Leo, Uniparin[AUS])
Do not confuse heparin with Hespan.

CATEGORY AND SCHEDULE

Pregnancy Risk Category: C

MECHANISM OF ACTION

A blood modifier that interferes with blood coagulation by blocking conversion of prothrombin to thrombin and fibrinogen to fibrin. ***Therapeutic Effect:*** Prevents further extension of existing thrombi or new clot formation. Has no effect on existing clots.

PHARMACOKINETICS

Well absorbed following subcutaneous administration. Protein binding: Very high. Metabolized in the liver. Removed from the circulation via uptake by the reticuloendothelial system. Primarily excreted in urine. Not removed by hemodialysis. ***Half-life:*** 1–6 hr.

AVAILABILITY

Injection: 10 units/ml, 100 units/ml, 1,000 units/ml, 2,500 units/ml, 5,000 units/ml, 7,500 units/ml, 10,000 units/ml, 20,000 units/ml, 25,000 units/500 ml infusion.

INDICATIONS AND DOSAGES

▸ Line Flushing

IV

Adults, Elderly, Children. 100 units q6–8h.
Infants weighing less than 10 kg. 10 units q6–8h.

▸ Treatment of Venous Thrombosis, Pulmonary Embolism, Peripheral Arterial Embolism, Atrial Fibrillation with Embolism

INTERMITTENT IV

Adults, Elderly. Initially, 10,000 units, then 50–70 units/kg (5,000–10,000 units) q4–6h.
Children 1 yr and older. Initially, 50–100 units/kg, then 50–100 units q4h.

IV INFUSION

Adults, Elderly. Loading dose: 80 units/kg, then 18 units/kg/hr, with adjustments based on aPTT. Range: 10–30 units/kg/hr.
Children 1 yr and older. Loading dose: 75 units/kg, then 20 units/kg/hr with adjustments based on aPTT.
Children younger than 1 yr. Loading dose: 75 units/kg, then 28 units/kg/hr.

▸ Prevention of Venous Thrombosis, Pulmonary Embolism, Peripheral Arterial Embolism, Atrial Fibrillation with Embolism
SUBCUTANEOUS
Adult, Elderly. 5,000 units q8–12h.

CONTRAINDICATIONS

Intracranial hemorrhage, severe hypotension, severe thrombocytopenia, subacute bacterial endocarditis, uncontrolled bleeding

INTERACTIONS

Drug

Antithyroid medications, cefoperazone, cefotetan, valproic acid: May cause hypoprothrombinemia.
Other anticoagulants, platelet aggregation inhibitors, thrombolytics: May increase the risk of bleeding.
Probenecid: May increase the effects of heparin.

Herbal

Feverfew, ginkgo biloba: May have additive effect.

Food

None known.

Drug interactions of concern to dentistry

• Increased risk of bleeding: salicylates, NSAIDs, parenteral penicillins, glucocorticoids, certain cephalosporins (cefamandole, cefoperazone, cefotetan)

DIAGNOSTIC TEST EFFECTS

May increase free fatty acid, AST(SGOT), and ALT(SGPT) levels. May decrease serum cholesterol and triglyceride levels.

IV INCOMPATIBILITIES

Amiodarone (Cordarone), amphotericin B complex (Abelcet, AmBisome, Amphotec), ciprofloxacin (Cipro), dacarbazine (DTIC), diazepam (Valium), dobutamine (Dobutrex), doxorubicin (Adriamycin), droperidol (Inapsine), filgrastim (Neupogen), gentamicin (Garamycin), haloperidol (Haldol), idarubicin (Idamycin), labetalol (Trandate), nicardipine (Cardene), phenytoin (Dilantin), quinidine, tobramycin (Nebcin), vancomycin (Vancocin)

IV COMPATIBILITIES

Aminophylline, ampicillin/sulbactam (Unasyn), aztreonam (Azactam), calcium gluconate, cefazolin (Ancef), ceftazidime (Fortaz), ceftriaxone (Rocephin), digoxin (Lanoxin), diltiazem (Cardizem), dopamine (Intropin), enalapril (Vasotec), famotidine (Pepcid), fentanyl (Sublimaze), furosemide (Lasix), hydromorphone (Dilaudid), insulin, lidocaine, lorazepam (Ativan), magnesium sulfate, methylprednisolone (Solu-Medrol), midazolam (Versed), milrinone (Primacor), morphine, nitroglycerin, norepinephrine (Levophed), oxytocin (Pitocin), piperacillin/tazobactam (Zosyn), procainamide (Pronestyl), propofol (Diprivan)

SIDE EFFECTS

Occasional

Itching, burning (particularly on soles of feet) caused by vasospastic reaction

Rare

Pain, cyanosis of extremity 6–10 days after initial therapy lasting 4–6 hours; hypersensitivity reaction, including chills, fever, pruritus, urticaria, asthma, rhinitis, lacrimation, and headache

SERIOUS REACTIONS

! Bleeding complications ranging from local ecchymoses to major hemorrhage occur more frequently in high-dose therapy, intermittent IV infusion, and in women 60 years of age and older.

! Antidote: Protamine sulfate 1–1.5 mg, IV, for every 100 units heparin subcutaneous within 30 minutes of overdose, 0.5–0.75 mg for every 100 units heparin subcutaneous if within 30–60 minutes of overdose, 0.25–0.375 mg for every 100 units heparin subcutaneous if 2 hours have elapsed since overdose, 25–50 mg if heparin was given by IV infusion.

DENTAL CONSIDERATIONS

General:

- Heparin is used only in hospitalized patients or during dialysis. A medical consultation is necessary if oral and maxillofacial surgery or trauma treatment is required. May need to defer treatment.
- Avoid products that affect platelet function, such as aspirin and NSAIDs.
- Consider local hemostasis measures to prevent excessive bleeding.
- Take precautions if dental surgery or intubation for general anesthesia is anticipated.

Consultations:

- Medical consultation may be required to assess disease control and patient's ability to tolerate stress.
- Medical consultation should include activated clotting time (ACT), partial prothrombin, and PT.

Teach Patient/Family:

- Caution to prevent trauma when using oral hygiene aids
- Importance of good oral hygiene to prevent soft tissue inflammation
- To report oral lesions, soreness, or bleeding

homatropine hydrobromide

hoe-ma′-troe-peen
(Isopto Homatropine, Minims Homatropine[CAN])

CATEGORY AND SCHEDULE

Pregnancy Risk Category: C

MECHANISM OF ACTION

An ophthalmic agent that blocks response of iris sphincter muscle and the accommodative muscle of the ciliary body to cholinergic stimulation, resulting in dilation and loss of accommodation.
Therapeutic Effect: Produces cycloplegia and mydriasis for refraction.

PHARMACOKINETICS

Maximum mydriatic effect occurs within 10–30 min; maximum cycloplegic effect occurs within 30–90 minutes. Duration of mydriasis is 6 hrs - 4 days; duration of cycloplegia is 10–48 hrs.

AVAILABILITY

Ophthalmic Solution: 2%, 5% (Isopto Homatropine).

INDICATIONS AND DOSAGES

▸ Mydriasis and Cycloplegia for Refraction

OPHTHALMIC

Adults, Elderly. Instill 1–2 drops of 2% solution or 1 drop of 5% solution before the procedure. Repeat at 5- to 10-minute intervals as needed. Maximum: 3 doses for refraction.

Children. Instill 1 drop of 2% solution immediately before the procedure. Repeat at 10-minute intervals as needed.

▸ **Uveitis**
OPHTHALMIC
Adults, Elderly. Instill 1–2 drops of 2% or 5% 2–3 times/day up to every 3–4 hours as needed.
Children. Instill 1 drop of 2% solution 2–3 times/day.

CONTRAINDICATIONS
Narrow-angle glaucoma, acute hemorrhage, hypersensitivity to homatropine or any component of the formulation

INTERACTIONS
Drug
None known.
Herbal
None known.
Food
None known.
Drug interactions of concern to dentistry
• Avoid concurrent use with pilocarpine
• Increased anticholinergic effects with other anticholinergic drugs (when significant absorption from the eye occurs)

DIAGNOSTIC TEST EFFECTS
None known.

SIDE EFFECTS
Frequent
Blurred vision, photophobia
Occasional
Irritation, increased intraocular pressure, congestion
Rare
Eczematoid dermatitis, edema, exudates, follicular conjunctivitis, somnolence, vascular congestion

SERIOUS REACTIONS
! Overdosage may produce symptoms of blurred vision, urinary retention, and tachycardia. Anticholinergic toxicity is caused by strong binding of the drug to cholinergic receptors.

DENTAL CONSIDERATIONS
General:
• Avoid dental light in patient's eyes; offer dark glasses for patient comfort.
• Protect patient's eyes from accidental spatter during dental treatment.

H

hydralazine hydrochloride
hye-dral′-a-zeen
(Alphapress[AUS], Apresoline, Novohylazin[CAN])
Do not confuse hydralazine with hydroxyzine.

CATEGORY AND SCHEDULE
Pregnancy Risk Category: C

MECHANISM OF ACTION
An antihypertensive with direct vasodilating effects on arterioles.
Therapeutic Effect: Decreases BP and systemic resistance.

PHARMACOKINETICS

Route	Onset	Peak	Duration
PO	20–30 min	N/A	2–4 hr
IV	5–20 min	N/A	2–6 hr

Well absorbed from the GI tract. Widely distributed. Protein binding: 85%–90%. Metabolized in the liver to active metabolite. Primarily excreted in urine. Not removed by hemodialysis. ***Half-life:*** 3–7 hr (increased with impaired renal function).

AVAILABILITY

Tablets: 10 mg, 25 mg, 50 mg, 100 mg.
Injection: 20 mg/ml.

INDICATIONS AND DOSAGES

▸ Moderate to Severe Hypertension

PO
Adults. Initially, 10 mg 4 times a day. May increase by 10–25 mg/dose q2–5 days. Maximum: 300 mg/day.
Children. Initially, 0.75–1 mg/kg/day in 2–4 divided doses, not to exceed 25 mg/dose. May increase over 3–4 wk. Maximum: 7.5 mg/kg/day (5 mg/kg/day in infants).
IV, IM
Adults, Elderly. Initially, 10–20 mg/dose q4–6h. May increase to 40 mg/dose.
Children. Initially, 0.1–0.2 mg/kg/dose (maximum: 20 mg) q4–6h, as needed, up to 1.7–3.5 mg/kg/day in divided doses q4–6h.

▸ Dosage in Renal Impairment

Dosage interval is based on creatinine clearance.

Creatinine Clearance	Dosage Interval
10–50 ml/min	q8h
less than 10 ml/min	q8–24h

OFF-LABEL USES

Treatment of CHF, hypertension secondary to eclampsia and preeclampsia, primary pulmonary hypertension.

CONTRAINDICATIONS

Coronary artery disease, lupus erythematosus, rheumatic heart disease

INTERACTIONS

Drug

Diuretics, other antihypertensives: May increase hypotensive effect.

Herbal

None known.

Food

None known.

Drug interactions of concern to dentistry

• Reduced effects: NSAIDs, indomethacin, sympathomimetics

DIAGNOSTIC TEST EFFECTS

May produce positive direct Coombs' test.

IV INCOMPATIBILITIES

Aminophylline, ampicillin (Polycillin), furosemide (Lasix)

IV COMPATIBILITIES

Dobutamine (Dobutrex), heparin, hydrocortisone (Solu-Cortef), nitroglycerin, potassium

SIDE EFFECTS

Frequent

Headache, palpitations, tachycardia (generally disappears in 7–10 days)

Occasional

GI disturbance (nausea, vomiting, diarrhea), paraesthesia, fluid retention, peripheral edema, dizziness, flushed face, nasal congestion

SERIOUS REACTIONS

! High dosage may produce lupus erythematosus-like reaction, including fever, facial rash, muscle and joint aches, and splenomegaly.
! Severe orthostatic hypotension, skin flushing, severe headache, myocardial ischemia, and cardiac arrhythmias may develop.
! Profound shock may occur with severe overdosage.

DENTAL CONSIDERATIONS

General:

• Monitor vital signs at every appointment because of cardiovascular side effects.

• Patients on chronic drug therapy may rarely have symptoms of blood dyscrasias, which can include infection, bleeding, and poor healing.
• Limit use of sodium-containing products, such as saline IV fluids, for patients with a dietary salt restriction.
• After supine positioning, have patient sit upright for at least 2 min to avoid orthostatic hypotension.

Consultations:

• In a patient with symptoms of blood dyscrasias, request a medical consultation for blood studies and postpone dental treatment until normal values are reestablished.
• Medical consultation may be required to assess disease control and patient's ability to tolerate stress.

Teach Patient/Family:

• Importance of good oral hygiene to prevent soft tissue inflammation
• Caution to prevent injury when using oral hygiene aids

hydrochlorothiazide

hye-droe-klor-oh-thye′-a-zide
(Apo-Hydro[CAN], Aquazide H, Dichlotride[AUS], Dithiazide[AUS], Esidrix, HydroDIURIL, Microzide, Oretic)

CATEGORY AND SCHEDULE

Pregnancy Risk Category: B
(D if used in pregnancy-induced hypertension)

MECHANISM OF ACTION

A sulfonamide derivative that acts as a thiazide diuretic and antihypertensive. As a diuretic blocks reabsorption of water, sodium, and potassium at the cortical diluting segment of the distal tubule. As an antihypertensive reduces plasma, extracellular fluid volume, and peripheral vascular resistance by direct effect on blood vessels. ***Therapeutic Effect:*** Promotes diuresis; reduces BP.

PHARMACOKINETICS

Route	Onset	Peak	Duration
PO (diuretic)	2 hr	4–6 hr	6–12 hr

Variably absorbed from the GI tract. Primarily excreted unchanged in urine. Not removed by hemodialysis. ***Half-life:*** 5.6–14.8 hr.

AVAILABILITY

Capsules (Microzide): 12.5 mg.
Oral Solution: 50 mg/5 ml.
Tablets (Aquazide, Oretic): 25 mg, 50 mg, 100 mg.

INDICATIONS AND DOSAGES

▸ **Edema, Hypertension**

PO

Adults. 12.5–100 mg/day. Maximum: 200 mg/day.

▸ **Usual Pediatric Dosage**

PO

Children 6 mo–12 yr. 2 mg/kg/day in 2 divided doses. Maximum: 200 mg/day.
Children younger than 6 mo. 2–4 mg/kg/day in 2 divided doses. Maximum: 37.5 mg/day.

OFF-LABEL USES

Treatment of diabetes insipidus, prevention of calcium-containing renal calculi

CONTRAINDICATIONS

Anuria, history of hypersensitivity to sulfonamides or thiazide diuretics, renal decompensation

H

INTERACTIONS

Drug

Cholestyramine, colestipol: May decrease the absorption and effects of hydrochlorothiazide.
Digoxin: May increase the risk of digoxin toxicity associated with hydrochlorothiazide-induced hypokalemia.
Lithium: May increase the risk of lithium toxicity.

Herbal

None known.

Food

None known.

Drug interactions of concern to dentistry

- Decreased hypotensive response: NSAIDs, especially indomethacin

DIAGNOSTIC TEST EFFECTS

May increase blood glucose and serum cholesterol, LDL, bilirubin, calcium, creatinine, uric acid, and triglyceride levels. May decrease urinary calcium, and serum magnesium, potassium, and sodium levels.

SIDE EFFECTS

Expected

Increase in urinary frequency and urine volume

Frequent

Potassium depletion

Occasional

Orthostatic hypotension, headache, GI disturbances, photosensitivity

SERIOUS REACTIONS

! Vigorous diuresis may lead to profound water and electrolyte depletion, resulting in hypokalemia, hyponatremia, and dehydration.
! Acute hypotensive episodes may occur.
! Hyperglycemia may occur during prolonged therapy.
! Pancreatitis, blood dyscrasias, pulmonary edema, allergic pneumonitis, and dermatologic reactions occur rarely.
! Overdose can lead to lethargy and coma without changes in electrolytes or hydration.

DENTAL CONSIDERATIONS

General:

- Monitor vital signs at every appointment because of cardiovascular side effects.
- Patients on chronic drug therapy may rarely have symptoms of blood dyscrasias, which can include infection, bleeding, and poor healing.
- After supine positioning, have patient sit upright for at least 2 min before standing to avoid orthostatic hypotension.
- Assess salivary flow as a factor in caries, periodontal disease, and candidiasis.
- Limit use of sodium-containing products, such as saline IV fluids, for patients with a dietary salt restriction.
- Stress from dental procedures may compromise cardiovascular function; determine patient risk.
- Short appointments and a stress reduction protocol may be required for anxious patients.
- Patients taking diuretics should be monitored for serum K^+ levels.

Consultations:

- In a patient with symptoms of blood dyscrasias, request a medical consultation for blood studies and postpone dental treatment until normal values are reestablished.
- Medical consultation may be required to assess disease control and patient's ability to tolerate stress.
- Physician should be informed if significant xerostomic side effects

occur (e.g., increased caries, sore tongue, problems eating or swallowing, difficulty wearing prosthesis) so that a medication change can be considered.

Teach Patient/Family:

- Importance of good oral hygiene to prevent soft tissue inflammation
- Caution to prevent injury when using oral hygiene aids
- *When chronic dry mouth occurs, advise patient:*
  - To avoid mouth rinses with high alcohol content because of drying effects
  - To use daily home fluoride products for anticaries effect
  - To use sugarless gum, frequent sips of water, or saliva substitutes

hydrocodone bitartrate

high-drough-koe′-doan
(Hycodan[CAN],
Robidone[CAN])

CATEGORY AND SCHEDULE

Pregnancy Risk Category: C
(D if used for prolonged periods or at high dosages at term)
Controlled Substance: Schedule III

MECHANISM OF ACTION

A narcotic analgesic and antitussive that binds with opioid receptors in the CNS. ***Therapeutic Effect:*** Alters the perception of and emotional response to pain; suppresses cough reflex.

PHARMACOKINETICS

Route	Onset	Peak	Duration
PO (analgesic)	10–20 min	30–60 min	4–6 hr
PO (antitussive)	N/A	N/A	4–6 hr

Well absorbed from the GI tract. Metabolized in the liver. Primarily excreted in urine. ***Half-life:*** 3.8 hr (increased in elderly).

INDICATIONS AND DOSAGES

▸ Analgesia

PO

Adults, Children older than 12 yr. 5–10 mg q4–6h.

Elderly. 2.5–5 mg q4–6h.

▸ Cough

PO

Adults. 5–10 mg q4–6h as needed. Maximum: 15 mg/dose.

Children. 0.6 mg/kg/day in 3–4 divided doses at intervals of at least 4 hr. Maximum single dose: 5 mg (children 2–12 yr), 1.25 mg (children younger than 2 yr).

PO (Extended-release)

Adults. 10 mg q12h.

Children 6–12 yr. 5 mg q12h.

CONTRAINDICATIONS

None known.

INTERACTIONS

Drug

Alcohol, other CNS depressants: May increase CNS or respiratory depression and hypotension.

MAOIs: May produce a severe, sometimes fatal reaction; plan to administer one quarter of usual hydrocodone dose.

Herbal

None known.

Food

None known.

Drug interactions of concern to dentistry

- Increased CNS depression: alcohol, other opioids, phenothiazines, sedative/hypnotics, skeletal muscle relaxants, general anesthetics
- Contraindication: MAOIs
- Increased effects of anticholinergics

DIAGNOSTIC TEST EFFECTS
May increase serum amylase and lipase levels.

SIDE EFFECTS
Frequent
Sedation, hypotension, diaphoresis, facial flushing, dizziness, somnolence
Occasional
Urine retention, blurred vision, constipation, dry mouth, headache, nausea, vomiting, difficult or painful urination, euphoria, dysphoria

H

SERIOUS REACTIONS
! Overdose results in respiratory depression, skeletal muscle flaccidity, cold or clammy skin, cyanosis, and extreme somnolence progressing to seizures, stupor, and coma.
! The patient who uses hydrocodone repeatedly may develop a tolerance to the drug's analgesic effect, as well as physical dependence.
! The drug may have a prolonged duration of action and cumulative effect in patients with hepatic or renal impairment.

DENTAL CONSIDERATIONS
General:
• Monitor vital signs at every appointment because of cardiovascular and respiratory side effects.
• After supine positioning, have patient sit upright for at least 2 min to avoid orthostatic hypotension.
• Psychologic and physical dependence may occur with chronic administration.
• Determine why the patient is taking the drug.

Teach Patient/Family:
• To avoid mouth rinses with high alcohol content because of drying effects

hydrocodone
hye-droe-koe-done

SCHEDULE III
Hydrocodone and acetaminophen, (Anexsia, Bancap HC, Ceta-Plus, Co-Gesic, Hydrocet, Hydrogesic, Lorcet 10/650, Lorcet-HD Lorcet Plus, Lortab, Margesic H, Maxidone, Norco, Stagesic, Vicodin, Vicodin ES, Vicodin HP, Zydone); hydrocodone and aspirin (Damason-P); hydrocodone and chlorpheniramine (Tussionex), hydrocodone and guaifenesin (Codiclear DH, Hycosin, Hycotuss, Kwelcof, Pneumotussin, Vicoden Tuss, Vitussin); hydrocodone and homatropin (Hycodan and Hydromet, Hydropane, Tussigon); hydrocodone and ibuprofen, (Vicoprofen); hydrocodone and pseudoephedrine (Detussin, Histussin D, P-V Tussin); hydrocodone, chlorpheniramine, phenylephrine, acetaminophen, and caffeine (Hycomine Compound)

CATEGORY AND SCHEDULE
Pregnancy Risk Category: C, D if used for prolonged periods, high dosages at term
Controlled substance: Schedule III

MECHANISM OF ACTION
Hydrocodone blocks pain perception in the cerebral cortex by binding to specific opiate receptors (mu and kappa) neuronal membranes of synapses. This binding results in a decreased synaptic chemical transmission throughout the CNS thus inhibiting the flow of pain sensations into the higher centers and cause analgesia.

Therapeutic Effect: Alters perception of pain and produces analgesic effect.

PHARMACOKINETICS

Well absorbed. Metabolized in liver. Excreted in urine. ***Half-life:*** 3.3–3.4 hrs.

AVAILABILITY

Hydrocodone & acetaminophen
Capsules: hydrocodone bitartrate 5 mg and acetaminophen 500 mg (Bancap HC, Ceta-Plus, Hydrocet, Hydrogesic, Lorcet-HD, Margesic H, Stagesic).
Elixir: hydrocodone bitartrate 7.5 mg and acetaminophen 500 mg /15 ml (Lortab).
Tablets: hydrocodone bitartrate 2.5 mg and acetaminophen 500 mg (Lortab), hydrocodone bitartrate 5 mg and acetaminophen 325 mg (Norco), hydrocodone bitartrate 5 mg and acetaminophen 400 mg (Zydone), hydrocodone bitartrate 5 mg and acetaminophen 500 mg (Anexsia, Co-Gesic, Lortab 5/500, Vicodin), hydrocodone bitartrate 7.5 mg and acetaminophen 325 mg (Norco), hydrocodone bitartrate 5 mg and acetaminophen 400 mg (Zydone), hydrocodone bitartrate 7.5 mg and acetaminophen 500 mg (Lortab 7.5/500), hydrocodone bitartrate 7.5 mg and acetaminophen 650 mg (Anexsia, Lorcet Plus), hydrocodone bitartrate 7.5 mg and acetaminophen 750 mg (Vicodin ES), hydrocodone bitartrate 10 mg and acetaminophen 325 mg (Norco), hydrocodone bitartrate 5 mg and acetaminophen 400 mg (Zydone), hydrocodone bitartrate 10 mg and acetaminophen 500 mg (Lortab 10/500), hydrocodone bitartrate 10 mg and acetaminophen 650 mg (Lorcet 10/650), hydrocodone bitartrate 10 mg and acetaminophen 660 mg (Vicodin HP), hydrocodone bitartrate 10 mg and acetaminophen 750 mg (Maxicodone).
Hydrocodone & aspirin
Tablets: hydrocodone bitartrate 5 mg and aspirin 500 mg (Damason-P).
Hydrocodone & chlorpheniramine
Syrup, extended release: hydrocodone polistirex 10 mg and chlorpheniramine polistirex 8 mg/5 ml (Tussionex).
Hydrocodone & guaifenesin
Liquid: hydrocodone bitartrate 2.5 mg and guaifenesin 200 mg/5 ml (Pneumotussin), hydrocodone bitartrate 5 mg and guaifenesin 100 mg/5 ml (Codiclear DH, Hycosin, Hycotuss, Kwelcof, Vicodin Tuss, Vitussin).
Tablets: hydrocodone bitartrate 2.5 mg and guaifenesin 300 mg (Pneumotussin).
Hydrocodone & homatropine
Syrup: hydrocodone bitartrate 5 mg and homatropine methylbromide 1.5 mg/5 ml (Hycodan, Hydromet, Hydropane)
Tablets: hydrocodone bitartrate 5 mg and homatropine methylbromide 1.5 mg (Hycodan, Tussigon).
Hydrocodone & ibuprofen
Tablets: hydrocodone bitartrate 7.5 mg and aspirin 200 mg (Vicoprofen).
Hydrocodone & pseudoephedrine
Liquid: hydrocodone bitartrate 5 mg and pseudoephedrine 60 mg/5 ml (Detussin, Histussin D).
Tablets: hydrocodone bitartrate 5 mg and pseudoephedrine 60 mg (P-V Tussin).
Hydrocodone, chlorpheniramine, phenylephrine, acetaminophen, & caffeine
Tablets: hydrocodone bitartrate 5 mg, chlorpheniramine maleate 2 mg, phenylephrine hydrochloride 10 mg, acetaminophen 250 mg, and caffeine 30 mg (Hycomine Compound).

INDICATIONS AND DOSAGES

▸ Hydrocodone & Acetaminophen

Analgesia

PO

Adults, Children older than 13 yrs or more than 50 kg. 2.5–10 mg q4–6h. Maximum: 60 mg/day hydrocodone. Maximum dose of acetaminophen: 4 g/day.

Elderly. 2.5–5 mg hydrocodone q4–6h. Titrate dose to appropriate analgesic effect. Maximum: 4 g/day acetaminophen.

Children 2–13 yrs or less than 50 kg. 0.135 mg/kg/dose hydrocodone q4–6h. Maximum: 6 doses/day of hydrocodone or maximum recommended dose of acetaminophen.

▸ Hydrocodone & Aspirin

PO

Adults. 2.5–10 mg q4–6h. Maximum: 60 mg/day hydrocodone.

Elderly. 2.5–5 mg hydrocodone q4–6h. Titrate dose to appropriate analgesic effect.

Children 2–13 yrs or less than 50 kg. 0.135 mg/kg/dose hydrocodone q4–6h.

▸ Hydrocodone & Chlorpheniramine

Adults, Elderly, Children 12 yrs and older. 5 ml q12h. Maximum: 10 ml/24h.

Children 6–12 yrs. 2.5 ml q12h. Maximum: 5 ml/24h.

▸ Hydrocodone & Guaifenesin

Adults, Elderly, Children 12 yrs and older. 5 ml q4h. Maximum: 30 ml/24h.

Children 2–12 yrs. 2.5 ml q4h.

Children less than 2 yrs. 0.3 mg/kg/day (hydrocodone) in 4 divided doses.

▸ Hydrocodone & Homatropine

Adults, Elderly. 10 mg (hydrocodone) q4–6h. A single dose should not exceed 15 mg and not more frequently than q4h.

Children. 0.6 mg/kg/day (hydrocodone) in 3–4 divided doses. Do not administer more frequently than q4h.

▸ Hydrocodone & Ibuprofen

Adults. 7.5–15 mg (hydrocodone) q4–6h as needed for pain. Maximum: 5 tablets/day.

▸ Hydrocodone & Pseudoephedrine

Adults, Elderly. 5 ml 4 times/day.

▸ Hydrocodone, Chlorpheniramine, Phenylephrine, Acetaminophen, & Caffeine

Adults, Elderly. 1 tablet q4h up to 4 times/day.

CONTRAINDICATIONS

CNS depression, severe respiratory depression, hypersensitivity to hydrocodone, or any component of the formulation

INTERACTIONS

Drug

Alcohol, central nervous system (CNS) depressants: May increase CNS or respiratory depression, and hypotension.

CYP2D6 inhibitors (e.g., chlorpromazine): May decrease the effects of hydrocodone.

Hepatotoxic medications (e.g., phenytoin), liver enzyme inducers (e.g., cimetidine): May increase risk of hepatotoxicity associated with acetaminophen with prolonged high dose or single toxic dose.

MAOIs, tricyclic antidepressants: May increase effects of MAOIs and TCAs and hydrocodone.

Warfarin: May increase the risk of bleeding with regular use.

Herbal

None known.

Food

None known.

H

Drug interactions of concern to dentistry

- Increased CNS depression: alcohol, other opioids, phenothiazines, sedative/hypnotics, skeletal muscle relaxants, general anesthetics
- Contraindication: MAOIs
- Increased effects of anticholinergics

DIAGNOSTIC TEST EFFECTS

None known.

SIDE EFFECTS

Frequent

Dizziness, sedation, drowsiness, bradycardia

Occasional

Anxiety, dysphoria, euphoria, fear, lethargy, lightheadedness, malaise, mental clouding, mental impairment, mood changes, physiological dependence, sedation, somnolence, constipation, bradycardia, heartburn, nausea, vomiting

Rare

Hypersensitivity reaction, rash

SERIOUS REACTIONS

! Cardiac arrest, circulatory collapse, coma, hypotension, hypoglycemic coma, ureteral spasm, urinary retention, vesical sphincter spasm, agranulocytosis, bleeding time prolonged, hemolytic anemia, iron deficiency anemia, occult blood loss, thrombocytopenia, hepatic necrosis, hepatitis, skeletal muscle rigidity, renal toxicity, renal tubular necrosis have been reported.

! Hearing impairment or loss have been reported with chronic overdose.

! Acute airway obstruction, apnea, dyspnea, and respiratory depression occur rarely and are usually dose related.

DENTAL CONSIDERATIONS

General:

- Monitor vital signs at every appointment because of cardiovascular and respiratory side effects.
- After supine positioning, have patient sit upright for at least 2 min to avoid orthostatic hypotension.
- Psychologic and physical dependence may occur with chronic administration.
- Determine why the patient is taking the drug.

Teach Patient/Family:

- To avoid mouth rinses with high alcohol content because of drying effects

hydrocortisone

hye-dro-kor′-ti-sone

(A-HydroCort, Anusol-HC, Colifoam[AUS], Cortaid, Cortef cream[AUS], Cortic cream[AUS], Cortic DS[AUS], Cortifoam, Cortizone-5, Cortizone-10, Derm-Aid cream[AUS], Dermaid[AUS], Dermaid soft cream[AUS], Egocort cream[AUS], Emcort, Hycor[AUS], Hycor Eye Oinment[AUS], Hysone[AUS], Hytone, Locoid, Nupercainal Hydrocortisone Cream, Preparation H Hydrocortisone, Protocort, Siquent Hycor[AUS], Solu-Cortef, Squibb HC[AUS], WestCort)

CATEGORY AND SCHEDULE

Pregnancy Risk Category: C (D if used in first trimester)

OTC (Hydrocortisone 0.5% and 1% Cream, Gel, and Ointment)

MECHANISM OF ACTION

An adrenocortical steroid that inhibits accumulation of

inflammatory cells at inflammation sites, phagocytosis, lysosomal enzyme release and synthesis and release of mediators of inflammation. ***Therapeutic Effect:*** Prevents or suppresses cell-mediated immune reactions. Decreases or prevents tissue response to inflammatory process.

PHARMACOKINETICS

Route	Onset	Peak	Duration
IV	N/A	4–6 hr	8–12 hr

Well absorbed after IM administration. Widely distributed. Metabolized in the liver. ***Half-life:*** Plasma, 1.5–2 hr; biologic, 8–12 hr.

AVAILABILITY

Tablet (Cortef): 5 mg, 10 mg, 20 mg.
Cream (Rectal [Nupercainal Hydrocortisone Cream, Cortizone-10, Preparation H Hydrocortisone]): 1%.
Cream (Topical [Cortizone-5]): 0.5%.
Cream (Topical [Caldecort, Cortizone-10]): 1%.
Cream (Topical [Hytone]): 2.5%.
Ointment (Topical [Locoid]): 0.1%.
Ointment (Topical [Westcort]): 0.2%.
Ointment (Topical [Cortizone-5]): 0.5%.
Ointment (Topical [Anusol-HC, Cortaid, Cortizone-10]): 1%.
Ointment (Topical [Hytone]): 2.5%.
Suppositories (Anusol-HC): 25 mg.
Suppositories (Emcort, Protocort): 30 mg.
Injection (A-hydro-Cort, Solu-Cortef): 100 mg, 250 mg, 500 mg, 1 g.

INDICATIONS AND DOSAGES

▸ Acute Adrenal Insufficiency

IV

Adults, Elderly. 100 mg IV bolus; then 300 mg/day in divided doses q8h.

Children. 1–2 mg/kg IV bolus; then 150–250 mg/day in divided doses q6–8h.

Infants. 1–2 mg/kg/dose IV bolus; then 25–150 mg/day in divided doses q6–8h.

▸ Anti-Inflammation, Immunosuppression

IV, IM

Adults, Elderly. 15–240 mg q12h.

Children. 1–5 mg/kg/day in divided doses q12h.

▸ Physiologic Replacement

PO

Children. 0.5–0.75 mg/kg/day in divided doses q8h.

IM

Children. 0.25–0.35 mg/kg/day as a single dose.

▸ Status Asthmaticus

IV

Adults, Elderly. 100–500 mg q6h.

Children. 2 mg/kg/dose q6h.

▸ Shock

IV

Adults, Elderly, Children 12 yr and older. 100–500 mg q6h.

Children younger than 12 yr. 50 mg/kg. May repeat in 4 hr, then q24h as needed.

▸ Adjunctive Treatment of Ulcerative Colitis

RECTAL

Adults, Elderly. 100 mg at bedtime for 21 nights or until clinical and proctologic remission occurs (may require 2–3 mo of therapy).

RECTAL (Cortifoam)

Adults, Elderly. 1 applicator 1–2 times a day for 2–3 wk, then every second day until therapy ends.

TOPICAL

Adults, Elderly. Apply sparingly 2–4 times a day.

CONTRAINDICATIONS

Fungal, tuberculosis, or viral skin lesions; serious infections

INTERACTIONS

Drug

Amphotericin: May increase hypokalemia.
Digoxin: May increase the risk of digoxin toxicity caused by hypokalemia.
Diuretics, insulin, oral hypoglycemics, potassium supplements: May decrease the effects of these drugs.
Hepatic enzyme inducers: May decrease the effects of hydrocortisone.
Live-virus vaccines: May decrease the patient's antibody response to vaccine, increase vaccine side effects, and potentiate virus replication.

Herbal

None known.

Food

None known.

DIAGNOSTIC TEST EFFECTS

May increase blood glucose and serum lipid, amylase, and sodium levels. May decrease serum calcium, potassium, and thyroxine levels.

IV INCOMPATIBILITIES

Ciprofloxacin (Cipro), diazepam (Valium), idarubicin (Idamycin), midazolam (Versed), phenytoin (Dilantin)

IV COMPATIBILITIES

Aminophylline, amphotericin, calcium gluconate, cefepime (Maxipime), digoxin (Lanoxin), diltiazem (Cardizem), diphenhydramine (Benadryl), dopamine (Intropin), insulin, lidocaine, lorazepam (Ativan), magnesium sulfate, morphine, norepinephrine (Levophed), procainamide (Pronestyl), potassium chloride, propofol (Diprivan)

SIDE EFFECTS

Frequent

Insomnia, heartburn, nervousness, abdominal distention, diaphoresis, acne, mood swings, increased appetite, facial flushing, delayed wound healing, increased susceptibility to infection, diarrhea or constipation

Occasional

Headache, edema, change in skin color, frequent urination
Topical: Itching, redness, irritation

Rare

Tachycardia, allergic reaction (such as rash and hives), psychological changes, hallucinations, depression
Topical: Allergic contact dermatitis, purpura
Systemic: Absorption more likely with use of occlusive dressings or extensive application in young children

SERIOUS REACTIONS

! Long-term therapy may cause hypocalcemia, hypokalemia, muscle wasting (especially in arms and legs), osteoporosis, spontaneous fractures, amenorrhea, cataracts, glaucoma, peptic ulcer disease, and CHF.
! Abruptly withdrawing the drug after long-term therapy may cause anorexia, nausea, fever, headache, sudden severe joint pain, rebound inflammation, fatigue, weakness, lethargy, dizziness, and orthostatic hypotension.

DENTAL CONSIDERATIONS

TOPICAL FORM

General:

- Place on frequent recall to evaluate healing response if used on a chronic basis.

Teach Patient/Family:

- Importance of good oral hygiene to prevent soft tissue inflammation
- To apply at bedtime or after meals for maximum effect

- That use on oral herpetic ulcerations is contraindicated
- To apply with cotton-tipped applicator by pressing, not rubbing, paste on lesion
- When used for oral lesions, advise patient to return for oral evaluation if response of oral tissues has not occurred in 7–14 days

hydrocortisone acetate; oxytetracycline hydrochloride

hye-droe-kor′-ti-sone as′-a-tate; ox-i-tet-ra-sye′-kleen hye-droe-klor′-ide
(Terra-Cortril Ophthalmic Suspension)

CATEGORY AND SCHEDULE

Pregnancy Risk Category: C

MECHANISM OF ACTION

Hydrocortisone is an adrenal corticosteroid that inhibits accumulation of inflammatory cells at inflammation sites, phagocytosis, lysosomal enzyme release and synthesis or release of mediators of inflammation. Oxytetracycline is an antibiotic that binds with the 30S and 50S ribosome subunits of susceptible bacterial; cell wall synthesis is not affected.
Therapeutic Effect: Hydrocortisone: prevents or suppresses cell-mediated immune reactions. Decreases or prevents tissue response to inflammatory process.
Oxytetracycline: inhibits bacterial cell wall synthesis.

PHARMACOKINETICS

None reported.

AVAILABILITY

Ophthalmic Suspension: 10 mg/5 ml (Terra-Cortril Ophthalmic Suspension).

INDICATIONS AND DOSAGES

▸ **Superficial Eye Infections**

OPHTHALMIC

Adults, Elderly. Instill 1 or 2 drops to the affected eye 3 times daily.

CONTRAINDICATIONS

Mycobacterial infection of the eye, viral disease of the cornea and conjunctiva, ocular fungal diseases, mechanical lacerations and abrasions of the eye, hypersensitivity to hydrocortisone, oxytetracycline or any component of the formulation

INTERACTIONS

Drug

None known.

Herbal

None known.

Food

None known.

DIAGNOSTIC TEST EFFECTS

None known.

SIDE EFFECTS

Occasional

Eye irritation, blurred vision, photophobia

SERIOUS REACTIONS

! None reported.

DENTAL CONSIDERATIONS

General

- Place on frequent recall to evaluate healing response if used on a chronic basis.

Teach patient/family:

- Importance of good oral hygiene to prevent soft tissue inflammation

- To apply at bedtime or after meals for maximum effect
- That use on oral herpetic ulcerations is contraindicated
- To apply with cotton-tipped applicator by pressing, not rubbing, paste on lesion
- That when used for oral lesions, to return for oral evaluation if response of oral tissues has not occurred in 7-14 days.

hydroflumethiazide

high-drow-floo-meth-eye-′-ah-zide
(Diucardin, Saluron)

CATEGORY AND SCHEDULE

Pregnancy Risk Category: C, D if used in pregnancy-induced hypertension

MECHANISM OF ACTION

A diuretic that blocks reabsorption of water, the electrolytes sodium and potassium at cortical diluting segment of distal tubule. As an antihypertensive it reduces plasma and extracellular fluid volume and decreases peripheral vascular resistance (PVR) by direct effect on blood vessels. ***Therapeutic Effect:*** Promotes diuresis, reduces blood pressure (B/P).

PHARMACOKINETICS

Rapidly but incompletely absorbed from the gastrointestinal (GI) tract. Metabolized to metabolite that is extensively bound to red blood cells and has a longer half-life than parent compound. Primarily excreted in urine. Not removed by hemodialysis. ***Half-life:*** 2–17 hrs.

AVAILABILITY

Tablets: 50 mg (Diucardin, Saluron).

INDICATIONS AND DOSAGES

▸ Edema

PO

Adults, Elderly. Initially, 50 mg 2 times/day. Maintenance: 25–200 mg/day.

▸ Hypertension

Adults, Elderly. Children.
1 mg/kg/day.
Initially, 50 mg 2 times/day.
Maintenance: 50–100 mg/day.

OFF-LABEL USES

Treatment of diabetes insipidus

CONTRAINDICATIONS

Anuria, history of hypersensitivity to sulfonamides or thiazide diuretics, renal decompensation, pregnancy

INTERACTIONS

Drug

Ace inhibitors: May increase the risk of postural hypotension.
Beta blockers: May increase hyperglycemic effects in patients with Type 2 diabetes mellitus.
Cylosporine, other thiazides: May increase the risk of gout or renal toxicity.
Cholestyramine, colestipol: May decrease the absorption and effects of hydroflumethiazide.
Digoxin: May increase the risk of toxicity of digoxin caused by hypokalemia.
Lithium: May increase the risk of toxicity of lithium
Neuromuscular blocking agents: May prolong neuromuscular blockade.
NSAIDS: May decrease the effects of hydroflumethiazide.

Herbal

Calcitriol: May increase the risk of hypercalcemia

Ginkgo biloba: May increase blood pressure.

Gossypol: May increase the risk of hypokalemia.

Licorice: May increase the risk of hypokalemia and/or reduce effectiveness of hydroflumethiazide.

Ma Huang: May decrease hypotensive effect of hydroflumethiazide.

Yohimbine: May decrease the effects of hydroflumethiazide.

Food

None known.

Drug interactions of concern to dentistry

• Decreased hypotensive response: NSAIDs, especially indomethacin

DIAGNOSTIC TEST EFFECTS

May increase blood glucose levels, serum cholesterol, LDL, bilirubin, calcium, creatinine, uric acid, and triglyceride levels. May decrease urinary calcium, and serum magnesium, potassium, and sodium levels.

IV INCOMPATIBILITIES

None known.

IV COMPATIBILITIES

None known.

SIDE EFFECTS

Expected

Increase in urine frequency and volume

Frequent

Potassium depletion

Occasional

Postural hypotension, headache, gastrointestinal (GI) disturbances, photosensitivity reaction

SERIOUS REACTIONS

! Vigorous diuresis may lead to profound water loss and electrolyte depletion, resulting in hypokalemia, hyponatremia, and dehydration.

! Acute hypotensive episodes may occur.

! Hyperglycemia may be noted during prolonged therapy.

! GI upset, pancreatitis, dizziness, paresthesias, headache, blood dyscrasias, pulmonary edema, allergic pneumonitis, and dermatologic reactions occur rarely.

! Overdosage can lead to lethargy and coma without changes in electrolytes or hydration.

DENTAL CONSIDERATIONS

General:

• Monitor vital signs at every appointment due to cardiovascular side effects.

• Patient on chronic drug therapy may rarely present with symptoms of blood dyscrasias, which can include infection, bleeding, and poor healing. If dyscrasia is present, caution patient to prevent oral tissue trauma when using oral hygiene aids.

• After supine positioning, have patient sit upright for at least 2 min before standing to avoid orthostatic hypotension.

• Assess salivary flow as a factor in caries, periodontal disease, and candidiasis.

• Limit use of sodium-containing products, such as saline IV fluids, for patients with a dietary salt restriction.

• Stress from dental procedures may compromise cardiovascular function, determine patient risk.

• Patients taking diuretics should be monitored for serum K^+ levels.

Consultations:

• In a patient with symptoms of blood dyscrasias, request a medical consultation for blood studies and postpone treatment until normal values are reestablished.
• Medical consultation may be required to assess disease control and patient's ability to tolerate stress.
• Physician should be informed if significant xerostomic side effects occur (increased caries, sore tongue, problems eating or swallowing, difficulty wearing prosthesis) so that a medication change can be considered.

Teach Patient/Family:

• Importance of good oral hygiene to prevent soft tissue inflammation
• To prevent trauma when using oral hygiene aids
• *When chronic dry mouth occurs advise patient:*
  • To avoid mouth rinses with high alcohol content due to drying effects
  • To use daily home fluoride products for anticaries effect
  • To use sugarless gum, frequent sips of water or saliva substitutes
• Importance of updating health and medication history if physician makes any changes in evaluation or drug regimens; include OTC, herbal, and nonherbal remedies in the update

hydromorphone hydrochloride

hye-droe-mor′-fone

SCHEDULE II

(Dilaudid, Dilaudid HP, Hydromorph Contin[CAN], Palladone)
Do not confuse with morphine or Dilantin.

CATEGORY AND SCHEDULE

Pregnancy Risk Category: B (D if used for prolonged periods or at high dosages at term)
Controlled Substance: Schedule II

MECHANISM OF ACTION

An opioid agonist that binds to opioid receptors in the CNS, reducing the intensity of pain stimuli from sensory nerve endings.
Therapeutic Effect: Alters the perception of and emotional response to pain; suppresses cough reflex.

PHARMACOKINETICS

Route	Onset	Peak	Duration
PO	30 min	90–120 min	4 hr
IV	10–15 min	15–30 min	2–3 hr
IM	15 min	30–60 min	4–5 hr
Subcutaneous	15 min	30–90 min	4 hr
Rectal	15–30 min	N/A	N/A

Well absorbed from the GI tract after IM administration. Widely distributed. Metabolized in the liver. Excreted in urine. ***Half-life:*** 1–3 hr.

AVAILABILITY

Liquid (Dilaudid): 5 mg/5 ml.
Capsules (Extended-Release [Palladone]): 12 mg, 16 mg, 24 mg, 32 mg.

Tablets (Dilaudid): 2 mg, 3 mg, 4 mg, 8 mg.
Injection (Dilaudid): 1 mg/ml, 2 mg/ml, 4 mg/ml.
Injection (Dilaudid HP): 10 mg/ml.
Suppository (Dilaudid): 3 mg.

INDICATIONS AND DOSAGES

▸ Analgesia

PO
Adults, Elderly, Children weighing 50 kg and more. 2–4 mg q3–4h. Range: 2–8 mg/dose.
Children older than 6 mo and weighing less than 50 kg. 0.03–0.08 mg/kg/dose q3–4h.
PO (Extended-Release)
Adults, Elderly. 12–32 mg once a day.
IV
Adults, Elderly, Children weighing more than 50 kg. 0.2–0.6 mg q2–3h.
Children weighing 50 kg or less. 0.015 mg/kg/dose q3–6h as needed.
RECTAL
Adults, Elderly. 3 mg q4–8h.

▸ Patient-Controlled Analgesia (PCA)

IV
Adults, Elderly. 0.05–0.5 mg at 5–15 min lockout. Maximum (4-hr): 4–6 mg.
EPIDURAL
Adults, Elderly. Bolus dose of 1–1.5 mg at rate of 0.04–0.4 mg/hr. Demand dose of 0.15 mg at 30 min lockout.

▸ Cough

PO
Adults, Elderly, Children older than 12 yr. 1 mg q3–4h.
Children 6–12 yr. 0.5 mg q3–4h.

CONTRAINDICATIONS

None known.

H

INTERACTIONS

Drug

Alcohol, other CNS depressants: May increase CNS or respiratory depression and hypotension.
MAOIs: May produce a severe, sometimes fatal reaction; plan to administer one quarter of usual hydromorphone dose.

Herbal

None known.

Food

None known.

Drug interactions of concern to dentistry

- Effects may be increased with other CNS depressants: alcohol, narcotics, sedative/hypnotics, skeletal muscle relaxants
- Increased effects of anticholinergic drugs

DIAGNOSTIC TEST EFFECTS

May increase serum amylase and lipase concentrations.

IV INCOMPATIBILITIES

Amphotericin B complex (Abelcet, AmBisome, Amphotec), cefazolin (Ancef, Kefzol), diazepam (Valium), phenobarbital, phenytoin (Dilantin)

IV COMPATIBILITIES

Diltiazem (Cardizem), diphenhydramine (Benadryl), dobutamine (Dobutrex), dopamine (Intropin), fentanyl (Sublimaze), furosemide (Lasix), heparin, lorazepam (Ativan), magnesium sulfate, metoclopramide (Reglan), midazolam (Versed), milrinone (Primacor), morphine, propofol (Diprivan)

SIDE EFFECTS

Frequent

Somnolence, dizziness, hypotension (including orthostatic hypotension), decreased appetite

Occasional
Confusion, diaphoresis, facial flushing, urine retention, constipation, dry mouth, nausea, vomiting, headache, pain at injection site
Rare
Allergic reaction, depression

SERIOUS REACTIONS

! Overdose results in respiratory depression, skeletal muscle flaccidity, cold or clammy skin, cyanosis, and extreme somnolence progressing to seizures, stupor, and coma.
! The patient who uses hydromorphone repeatedly may develop a tolerance to the drug's analgesic effect, as well as physical dependence.
! This drug may have a prolonged duration of action and cumulative effect in patients with hepatic or renal impairment.

DENTAL CONSIDERATIONS

General:
- Monitor vital signs at every appointment because of cardiovascular and respiratory side effects.
- After supine positioning, have patient sit upright for at least 2 min to avoid orthostatic hypotension.
- Assess salivary flow as a factor in caries, periodontal disease, and candidiasis.
- Psychologic and physical dependence may occur with chronic administration.
- Determine why the patient is taking the drug.
- Avoid in patients with chronic obstructive pulmonary disease.

Teach Patient/Family:
- To avoid mouth rinses with high alcohol content because of drying effects

hydroxychloroquine sulfate

hye-drox-ee-klor′-oh-kwin
(Apo-Hydroxyquine[CAN], Plaquenil)
Do not confuse hydroxychloroquine with hydrocortisone or hydroxyzine.

CATEGORY AND SCHEDULE

Pregnancy Risk Category: C

H

MECHANISM OF ACTION

An antimalarial and antirheumatic that concentrates in parasite acid vesicles, increasing the pH of the vesicles and interfering with parasite protein synthesis. Antirheumatic action may involve suppressing formation of antigens responsible for hypersensitivity reactions.
Therapeutic Effect: Inhibits parasite growth.

AVAILABILITY

Tablets: 200 mg (155 mg base).

INDICATIONS AND DOSAGES

▸ **Treatment of Acute Attack of Malaria (dosage in mg base)**
PO

Dose	Times	Adults	Children
Initial	Day 1	620 mg	10 mg/kg
Second	6 hr later	310 mg	5 mg/kg
Third	Day 2	310 mg	5 mg/kg
Fourth	Day 3	310 mg	5 mg/kg

▸ **Suppression of Malaria**
PO
Adults. 310 mg base weekly on same day each week, beginning 2 wk before entering an endemic area and continuing for 4–6 wk after leaving the area.
Children. 5 mg base/kg/wk, beginning 2 wk before entering an

endemic area and continuing for 4–6 wk after leaving the area. If therapy is not begun before exposure, administer a loading dose of 10 mg base/kg in 2 equally divided doses 6 hr apart, followed by the ususal dosage regimen.

▸ **Rheumatoid Arthritis**

PO

Adults. Initially, 400–600 mg (310–465 mg base) daily for 5–10 days, gradually increased to optimum response level. Maintenance (usually within 4–12 wk): Dosage decreased by 50% and then continued at maintenance dose of 200–400 mg/day. Maximum effect may not be seen for several months.

▸ **Lupus Erythematosus**

PO

Adults. Initially, 400 mg once or twice a day for several weeks or months. Maintenance: 200–400 mg/day.

OFF-LABEL USES

Treatment of juvenile arthritis, sarcoid-associated hypercalcemia

CONTRAINDICATIONS

Long-term therapy for children, porphyria, psoriasis, retinal or visual field changes

INTERACTIONS

Drug

Penicillamine: May increase blood penicillamine concentration and the risk of hematologic, renal, or severe skin reactions.

Herbal

None known.

Food

None known.

Drug interactions of concern to dentistry

- None reported

DIAGNOSTIC TEST EFFECTS

None known.

SIDE EFFECTS

Frequent

Mild, transient headache; anorexia; nausea; vomiting

Occasional

Visual disturbances, nervousness, fatigue, pruritus (especially of palms, soles, and scalp), irritability, personality changes, diarrhea

Rare

Stomatitis, dermatitis, impaired hearing

SERIOUS REACTIONS

! Ocular toxicity, especially retinopathy, may occur and may progress even after drug is discontinued.

! Prolonged therapy may result in peripheral neuritis, neuromyopathy, hypotension, ECG changes, agranulocytosis, aplastic anemia, thrombocytopenia, seizures, and psychosis.

! Overdosage may result in headache, vomiting, visual disturbances, drowsiness, seizures, and hypokalemia followed by cardiovascular collapse and death.

DENTAL CONSIDERATIONS

General:

- Patients on chronic drug therapy may rarely have symptoms of blood dyscrasias, which can include infection, bleeding, and poor healing.
- Avoid dental light in patient's eyes; offer dark glasses for patient comfort.
- Determine why the patient is taking the drug.

Consultations:
- In a patient with symptoms of blood dyscrasias, request a medical consultation for blood studies and postpone dental treatment until normal values are reestablished.

Teach Patient/Family:
- Importance of good oral hygiene to prevent soft tissue inflammation
- To avoid mouth rinses with high alcohol content because of drying effects

hydroxyurea

high-drocks′-ee-your-e-ah
(Droxia, Hydrea, Mylocel)

CATEGORY AND SCHEDULE

Pregnancy Risk Category: D

MECHANISM OF ACTION

A synthetic urea analogue that inhibits DNA synthesis without interfering with RNA synthesis or protein. ***Therapeutic Effect:*** Interferes with the normal repair process of cancer cells damaged by irradiation.

AVAILABILITY

Capsules (Droxia): 200 mg, 300 mg, 400 mg.
Capsules (Hydrea): 500 mg.
Tablets (Mylocel): 1,000 mg.

INDICATIONS AND DOSAGES

▸ **Melanoma; Recurrent, Metastatic, or Inoperable Ovarian Carcinoma**
PO
Adults, Elderly. 80 mg/kg every 3 days or 20–30 mg/kg/day as a single dose.

▸ **Control of Primary Squamous Cell Carcinoma of the Head and Neck, Excluding Lips (in combination with radiation therapy)**
PO
Adults, Elderly. 80 mg/kg every 3 days, beginning at least 7 days before starting radiation therapy.

▸ **Resistant Chronic Myelocytic Leukemia**
PO
Adults, Elderly. 20–30 mg/kg once a day.
Children. 10–20 mg/kg once a day.

▸ **HIV Infection**
PO
Adults, Elderly. 500 mg twice a day with didanosine.

▸ **Sickle Cell Anemia**
PO
Adults, Elderly, Children. Initially, 15 mg/kg once a day. May increase by 5 mg/kg/day. Maximum: 35 mg/kg/day.

OFF-LABEL USES

Treatment of cervical carcinoma, polycythemia vera; long-term suppression of HIV infection.

CONTRAINDICATIONS

WBC count less than 2,500/mm^3 or platelet count less than 100,000/mm^3

INTERACTIONS

Drug

Antigout medications: May decrease the effects of these drugs.
Bone marrow depressants: May increase myelosuppression.
Live-virus vaccines: May potentiate virus replication, increase vaccine side effects, and decrease the patient's antibody response to the vaccine.

Herbal

None known.

Food

None known.

Drug interactions of concern to dentistry
- None reported

DIAGNOSTIC TEST EFFECTS
May increase BUN and serum creatinine and uric acid levels.

SIDE EFFECTS
Frequent
Nausea, vomiting, anorexia, constipation or diarrhea
Occasional
Mild, reversible rash; facial flushing; pruritus; fever; chills; malaise
Rare
Alopecia, headache, drowsiness, dizziness, disorientation

SERIOUS REACTIONS
! Myelosuppression may cause hematologic toxicity (manifested as leukopenia and, to a lesser extent, thrombocytopenia and anemia).

DENTAL CONSIDERATIONS
General:
- Patients receiving chemotherapy may be taking chronic opioids for pain. Consider NSAIDs for dental pain management.
- Patients receiving chemotherapy may require palliative therapy for stomatitis.
- Patients on chronic drug therapy may rarely have symptoms of blood dyscrasias, which can include infection, bleeding, and poor healing.

Consultations:
- Medical consultation may be required to assess disease control.
- In a patient with symptoms of blood dyscrasias, request a medical consultation for blood studies and postpone dental treatment until normal values are reestablished.

Teach Patient/Family:
- That secondary oral infection may occur; must see dentist immediately if infection occurs
- *When chronic dry mouth occurs, advise patient:*
  - To avoid mouth rinses with high alcohol content because of drying effects
  - To use sugarless gum, frequent sips of water, or saliva substitutes
  - To use daily home fluoride products for anticaries effect

hydroxyzine
hye-drox′-i-zeen
(Apo-Hydroxyzine[CAN], Atarax, Novohydroxyzin[CAN], Vistaril)
Do not confuse hydroxyzine with hydralazine or hydroxyurea.

CATEGORY AND SCHEDULE
Pregnancy Risk Category: C

MECHANISM OF ACTION
A piperazine derivative that competes with histamine for receptor sites in the GI tract, blood vessels, and respiratory tract. May exert CNS depressant activity in subcortical areas. Diminishes vestibular stimulation and depresses labyrinthine function. ***Therapeutic Effect:*** Produces anxiolytic, anticholinergic, antihistaminic, and analgesic effects; relaxes skeletal muscle; controls nausea and vomiting.

PHARMACOKINETICS

Route	Onset	Peak	Duration
PO	15–30 min	N/A	4–6 hr

Well absorbed from the GI tract and after parenteral administration. Metabolized in the liver. Primarily excreted in urine. Not removed by hemodialysis. ***Half-life:*** 20–25 hr (increased in the elderly).

AVAILABILITY

Capsules (Vistaril): 25 mg, 50 mg, 100 mg.
*Oral Suspension (Vistaril):*25 mg/5 ml.
Syrup (Atarax): 10 mg/5 ml.
*Tablets (Atarax):*10 mg, 25 mg, 50 mg, 100 mg.
*Injection (Vistaril):*25 mg/ml, 50 mg/ml.

INDICATIONS AND DOSAGES

▸ Anxiety

PO
Adults, Elderly. 25–100 mg 4 times a day. Maximum: 600 mg/day.

▸ Nausea and Vomiting

IM
Adults, Elderly. 25–100 mg/dose q4–6h.

▸ Pruritus

PO
Adults, Elderly. 25 mg 3–4 times a day.

▸ Preoperative Sedation

PO
Adults, Elderly. 50–100 mg.
IM
Adults, Elderly. 25–100 mg.

▸ Usual Pediatric Dosage

PO
Children. 2 mg/kg/day in divided doses q6–8h.
IM
Children. 0.5–1 mg/kg/dose q4–6h.

CONTRAINDICATIONS

None known.

INTERACTIONS

Drug

Alcohol, other CNS depressants: May increase CNS depressant effects.
MAOIs: May increase anticholinergic and CNS depressant effects.

Herbal

None known.

Food

None known.

Drug interactions of concern to dentistry

- Increased CNS depressant effect: alcohol, all CNS depressants
- Increased anticholinergic effects: other antihistamines, anticholinergics, opioid analgesics

DIAGNOSTIC TEST EFFECTS

May cause false-positive urine 17-hydroxycorticosteroid determinations.

SIDE EFFECTS

Side effects are generally mild and transient.

Frequent

Somnolence, dry mouth, marked discomfort with IM injection

Occasional

Dizziness, ataxia, asthenia, slurred speech, headache, agitation, increased anxiety

Rare

Paradoxical CNS reactions, such as hyperactivity or nervousness in children and excitement or restlessness in elderly or debilitated patients (generally noted during first 2 weeks of therapy, particularly in presence of uncontrolled pain)

SERIOUS REACTIONS

! A hypersensitivity reaction, including wheezing, dyspnea, and chest tightness, may occur.

H

DENTAL CONSIDERATIONS

General:

- Potentiates other CNS depressant drugs. When used in combination, the dose of other CNS depressants should be reduced by half.
- Assess salivary flow as a factor in caries, periodontal disease, and candidiasis.
- Geriatric patients are more susceptible to drug effects; use lower dose.
- Have someone drive patient to and from dental appointment if the drug is prescribed for dental therapy.

Teach Patient/Family:

- *When chronic dry mouth occurs, advise patient:*
  - To avoid mouth rinses with high alcohol content because of drying effects
  - To use sugarless gum, frequent sips of water, or saliva substitutes
  - To use daily home fluoride products for anticaries effect

H

hyoscyamine

hye-oh-sye′-a-meen

(Anaspaz, Buscopan[CAN], Cystospaz, Cystospaz-M, Hyosine, Levbid, Levsin, Levsinex, Levsin S/L, NuLev, Spacol, Spacol T/S, Symax SL, Symax SR)

Do not confuse Anaspaz with Anaprox.

CATEGORY AND SCHEDULE

Pregnancy Risk Category: C

MECHANISM OF ACTION

A GI antispasmodic and anticholinergic agent that inhibits the action of acetylcholine at post-ganglionic (muscarinic) receptor sites. ***Therapeutic Effect:*** Decreases secretions (bronchial, salivary, sweat gland) and gastric juices and reduces motility of GI and urinary tract.

AVAILABILITY

Tablets (Anaspaz, Cystospaz, Levsin, Spacol): 0.125 mg.
Tablets (Oral-Disintegrating [NuLev]): 0.125 mg.
Tablets (Sublingual [Levsin S/L, Symax SL]): 0.125 mg.
Tablets (Extended-Release [Levbid, Spacol T/S, Symax SR]): 0.375 mg.
Capsules (Extended-Release [Cystospaz-M, Levsinex]): 0.375 mg.
Liquid (Hyosine, Spacol): 0.125 mg/5 ml.
Oral Solution (Hyosine, Levsin): 0.125 mg/5 ml

INDICATIONS AND DOSAGES

▸ GI Tract Disorders

PO

Adults, Elderly, Children 12 yr and older. 0.125–0.25 mg q4h as needed. Extended-release: 0.375–0.75 mg q12h. Maximum: 1.5 mg/day.
Children 2–11 yr. 0.0625–0.125 mg q4h as needed. Extended-release: 0.375 mg q12h. Maximum: 0.75 mg/day.

IV, IM

Adults, Elderly, Children 12 yr and older. 0.25–0.5 mg q4h for 1–4 doses.

▸ Hypermotility of Lower Urinary Tract

PO, Sublingual

Adults, Elderly. 0.15–0.3 mg 4 times a day; or extended-release 0.375 mg q12h.

Infant Colic
PO
Infants. Individualized drops dosed q4h as needed.

CONTRAINDICATIONS
GI or GU obstruction, myasthenia gravis, narrow-angle glaucoma, paralytic ileus, severe ulcerative colitis

INTERACTIONS
Drug
Antacids, antidiarrheals: May decrease the absorption of hyoscyamine.
Ketoconazole: May decrease the absorption of this drug.
Other anticholinergics: May increase the effects of hyoscyamine.
Potassium chloride: May increase the severity of GI lesions with the matrix formulation of potassium chloride.
Herbal
None known.
Food
None known.
Drug interactions of concern to dentistry
- Increased anticholinergic effect: other anticholinergics, opioid analgesics
- Decreased effect of phenothiazines

DIAGNOSTIC TEST EFFECTS
None known.

SIDE EFFECTS
Frequent
Dry mouth (sometimes severe), decreased sweating, constipation
Occasional
Blurred vision; bloated feeling; urinary hesitancy; somnolence (with high dosage); headache; intolerance to light; loss of taste; nervousness; flushing; insomnia; impotence; mental confusion or excitement (particularly in the elderly and children); temporary lightheadedness (with parenteral form); local irritation (with parenteral form)
Rare
Dizziness, faintness

SERIOUS REACTIONS
! Overdose may produce temporary paralysis of ciliary muscle; pupillary dilation; tachycardia; palpitations; hot, dry, or flushed skin; absence of bowel sounds; hyperthermia; increased respiratory rate; ECG abnormalities; nausea; vomiting; rash over face or upper trunk; CNS stimulation; and psychosis (marked by agitation, restlessness, rambling speech, visual hallucinations, paranoid behavior, and delusions, followed by depression).

DENTAL CONSIDERATIONS
General:
- After supine positioning, have patient sit upright for at least 2 min to avoid orthostatic hypotension.
- Assess salivary flow as a factor in caries, periodontal disease, and candidiasis.
- Avoid dental light in patient's eyes; offer dark glasses for patient comfort.

Consultation:
- Physician should be informed if significant xerostomic side effects occur (e.g., increased caries, sore tongue, problems eating or swallowing, difficulty wearing prosthesis) so that a medication change can be considered.

Teach Patient/Family:
- Importance of good oral hygiene to prevent soft tissue inflammation

- *When chronic dry mouth occurs, advise patient:*
  - To avoid mouth rinses with high alcohol content because of drying effects
  - To use sugarless gum, frequent sips of water, or artificial saliva substitutes
  - To use daily home fluoride products for anticaries effect

ibandronate sodium

eye-band′-droh-nate
(Boniva)

CATEGORY AND SCHEDULE

Pregnancy Risk Category: C

MECHANISM OF ACTION

A bisphosphonate that binds to bone hydroxyapatite (part of the mineral matrix of bone) and inhibits osteoclast activity. ***Therapeutic Effect:*** Reduces rate of bone turnover and bone resorption, resulting in a net gain in bone mass.

PHARMACOKINETICS

Absorbed in the upper GI tract. Extent of absorption impaired by food or beverages (other than plain water). Rapidly binds to bone. Unabsorbed portion is eliminated in urine. Protein binding: 90%. ***Half-life:*** 10–60 hr.

AVAILABILITY

Tablets: 2.5 mg

INDICATIONS AND DOSAGES

▸ **Osteoporosis**

PO

Adults, Elderly. 2.5 mg daily.

CONTRAINDICATIONS

Hypersensitivity to other bisphosphonates, including alendronate, etidronate, pamidronate, risedronate, and tiludronate; inability to stand or sit upright for at least 60 minutes; severe renal impairment with creatinine clearance less than 30 ml/min; uncorrected hypocalcemia

INTERACTIONS

Drug

Antacids containing aluminum, calcium, magnesium; vitamin D: Decrease the absorption of ibandronate.

Herbal

None known.

Food

Beverages other than plain water, dietary supplements, food: Interfere with the absorption of ibandronate.

Drug interactions of concern to dentistry

- Decreased absorption: antacids containing aluminum, calcium, or magnesium salts, vitamin D
- Use with monitoring, risk of increased GI side effects: aspirin and NSAIDs

DIAGNOSTIC TEST EFFECTS

May decrease serum alkaline phosphatase level. May increase blood cholesterol level.

SIDE EFFECTS

Frequent (13%–6%)

Back pain; dyspepsia, including epigastric distress and heartburn; peripheral discomfort; diarrhea; headache; myalgia

Occasional (4%–3%)

Dizziness, arthralgia, asthenia

Rare (≤ 2%)

Vomiting, hypersensitivity reaction

SERIOUS REACTIONS

! Upper respiratory tract infection occurs occasionally.

! Overdose causes hypocalcemia, hypophosphatemia, and significant GI disturbances

DENTAL CONSIDERATIONS

General:

- Consider semisupine chair position for patient comfort if GI side effects occur.
- Patient may need assistance in getting into and out of dental chair.

Adjust chair position for patient comfort.

Consultations:

• Medical consultation may be required to assess disease control and patient's ability to tolerate stress.

Teach Patient/Family:

• Importance of updating health and medication history if physician makes any changes in evaluation or drug regimens; include OTC, herbal, and nonherbal remedies in the update

I

ibuprofen

eye-byoo′-pro-fen

(Act-3[AUS], Advil, Apo-Ibuprofen, Brufen[AUS], Codral Period Pain[AUS], Motrin, Novoprofen[CAN], Nurofen[AUS], Rafen[AUS])

CATEGORY AND SCHEDULE

Pregnancy Risk Category: B (D if used in third trimester or near delivery)

OTC (Tablets: 200 mg, Oral Suspension: 100 mg/5 ml)

MECHANISM OF ACTION

An NSAID that inhibits prostaglandin synthesis. Also produces vasodilation by acting centrally on the heat-regulating center of the hypothalamus. ***Therapeutic Effect:*** Produces analgesic and anti-inflammatory effects and decreases fever.

PHARMACOKINETICS

Route	Onset	Peak	Duration
PO (analgesic)	0.5 hr	N/A	4–6 hr
PO (antirheumatic)	2 days	1–2 wk	N/A

Rapidly absorbed from the GI tract. Protein binding: greater than 90%. Metabolized in the liver. Primarily excreted in urine. Not removed by hemodialysis. ***Half-life:*** 2–4 hr.

AVAILABILITY

Caplets (Advil, Menadol, Motrin): 200 mg.
Capsules (Advil, Advil Migraine): 200 mg.
*Gelcaps (Advil, Motrin IB):*200 mg.
Tablets (Advil, Motrin IB): 200 mg.
Tablets (Motin): 400 mg, 600 mg, 800 mg.
Tablets (Chewable [Children's Advil, Children's Motrin]) : 50 mg.
Tablets (Chewable [Junior Advil, Junior Strength Motrin]): 100 mg.
Oral Suspension (Children's Advil, Children's Motrin): 100 mg/5 ml.
Oral Drops (Infant Advil, Infant Motrin): 40 mg/ml.

INDICATIONS AND DOSAGES

▸ **Acute or Chronic Rheumatoid Arthritis, Osteoarthritis, Migraine Pain, Gouty Arthritis**

PO

Adults, Elderly. 400–800 mg 3–4 times a day. Maximum: 3.2 g/day.

▸ **Mild to Moderate Pain, Primary Dysmenorrhea**

PO

Adults, Elderly. 200–400 mg q4–6h as needed. Maximum: 1.6 g/day.

▸ **Fever, Minor Aches or Pain**

PO

Adults, Elderly. 200–400 mg q4–6h. Maximum: 1.6 g/day.

Children. 5–10 mg/kg/dose q6–8h. Maximum: 40 mg/kg/day. OTC: 7.5 mg/kg/dose q6–8h. Maximum: 30 mg/kg/day.

▸ **Juvenile Arthritis**

PO

Children. 30–70 mg/kg/day in 3–4 divided doses. Maximum:

400 mg/day in children weighing less than 20 kg, 600 mg/day in children weighing 20–30 kg, 800 mg/day in children weighing greater than 30–40 kg.

OFF-LABEL USES

Treatment of psoriatic arthritis, vascular headaches

CONTRAINDICATIONS

Active peptic ulcer, chronic inflammation of GI tract, GI bleeding disorders or ulceration, history of hypersensitivity to aspirin or NSAIDs

INTERACTIONS

Drug

Antihypertensives, diuretics: May decrease the effects of these drugs.
Aspirin, other salicylates: May increase the risk of GI side effects such as bleeding.
Bone marrow depressants: May increase the risk of hematologic reactions.
Heparin, oral anticoagulants, thrombolytics: May increase the effects of these drugs.
Lithium: May increase the blood concentration and risk of toxicity of lithium.
Methotrexate: May increase the risk of methotrexate toxicity.
Probenecid: May increase the ibuprofen blood concentration.

Herbal

Feverfew: May decrease the effects of feverfew.
Ginkgo biloba: May increase the risk of bleeding.

Food

None known.

Drug interactions of concern to dentistry

- GI ulceration, bleeding: aspirin, alcohol (three or more drinks per day), corticosteroids
- Decreased action: salicylates
- Nephrotoxicity: acetaminophen (prolonged use)
- Possible risk of decreased renal function: cyclosporine
- First-time users of SSRIs also taking NSAIDs may have a higher risk of GI side effects; until more data are available, it may be advisable to avoid use of NSAIDs in these patients (*Br J Clin Pharmacol* 55:591–595, 2003)
- *When prescribed for dental pain:*
  - Risk of increased effects: oral anticoagulants, oral antidiabetics, lithium, methotrexate
  - Decreased antihypertensive effects of diuretics, β-adrenergic blockers, and ACE inhibitors

DIAGNOSTIC TEST EFFECTS

May prolong bleeding time. May alter blood glucose level. May increase BUN level, and serum creatinine, potassium, AST (SGOT), and ALT (SGPT) levels. May decrease blood Hgb and Hct.

SIDE EFFECTS

Occasional (9%–3%)
Nausea with or without vomiting, dyspepsia, dizziness, rash
Rare (< 3%)
Diarrhea or constipation, flatulence, abdominal cramps or pain, pruritus

SERIOUS REACTIONS

! Acute overdose may result in metabolic acidosis.
! Rare reactions with long-term use include peptic ulcer disease, GI bleeding, gastritis, a severe hepatic reaction (cholestasis, jaundice), nephrotoxicity (dysuria, hematuria, proteinuria, nephrotic syndrome), and a severe hypersensitivity reaction (particularly in patients with systemic lupus erythematosus or other collagen diseases).

DENTAL CONSIDERATIONS

General:

- Patients on chronic drug therapy may rarely have symptoms of blood dyscrasias, which can include infection, bleeding, and poor healing.
- Assess salivary flow as a factor in caries, periodontal disease, and candidiasis.
- Avoid prescribing aspirin-containing products.
- Consider semisupine chair position for patients with arthritic disease.

Consultations:

- In a patient with symptoms of blood dyscrasias, request a medical consultation for blood studies and postpone dental treatment until normal values are reestablished.
- Medical consultation may be required to assess disease control.

Teach Patient/Family:

- To follow labeled directions for OTC products
- Importance of good oral hygiene to prevent soft tissue inflammation
- Caution to prevent injury when using oral hygiene aids
- *When chronic dry mouth occurs, advise patient:*
  - To avoid mouth rinses with high alcohol content because of drying effects
  - To use sugarless gum, frequent sips of water, or saliva substitutes
  - To use daily home fluoride products for anticaries effect

ibutilide fumarate

eye-byoo′-ti-lide
(Corvert)

CATEGORY AND SCHEDULE

Pregnancy Risk Category: C

MECHANISM OF ACTION

An antiarrhythmic that prolongs both atrial and ventricular action potential duration and increases the atrial and ventricular refractory period. Activates slow, inward current (mostly of sodium), produces mild slowing of sinus node rate and AV conduction, and causes dose-related prolongation of QT interval.
Therapeutic Effect: Converts arrhythmias to sinus rhythm.

PHARMACOKINETICS

After IV administration, highly distributed, rapidly cleared. Protein binding: 40%. Primarily excreted in urine as metabolite. ***Half-life:*** 2–12 hr (average: 6 hr).

AVAILABILITY

Injection: 0.1 mg/ml solution.

INDICATIONS AND DOSAGES

▸ Rapid Conversion of Atrial Fibrillation or Flutter of Recent Onset to Normal Sinus Rhythm

IV INFUSION

Adults, Elderly weighing 60 kg and more. One vial (1 mg) given over 10 min. If arrhythmia does not stop within 10 min after end of initial infusion, a second 1 mg/10-min infusion may be given.
Adults, Elderly weighing less than 60 kg. 0.01 mg/kg given over 10 min. If arrhythmia does not stop within 10 min after end of initial infusion, a second 0.01 mg/kg, 10-min infusion may be given.

CONTRAINDICATIONS

None known.

INTERACTIONS

Drug

Class IA antiarrhythmics (disopyramide, moricizine, procainamide, quinidine), Class III antiarrhythmics (amiodarone, bretylium, sotalol): Do not give

ibutilide with these drugs or give these drugs within 4 hours after infusing ibutilide.
H_1 receptor antagonists, phenothiazines, tricyclic and tetracyclic antidepressants: May prolong QT interval.

Herbal
None known.

Food
None known.

Drug interactions of concern to dentistry
• Potential for arrhythmia: drugs that prolong the QT interval, such as antidepressants

DIAGNOSTIC TEST EFFECTS
None known.

IV INCOMPATIBILITIES
No information is available for Y-site administration.

SIDE EFFECTS
Ibutilide is generally well tolerated.

Occasional
Ventricular extrasystoles (5.1%), ventricular tachycardia (4.9%), headache (3.6%), hypotension, orthostatic hypotension (2%)

Rare
Bundle-branch block, AV block, bradycardia, hypertension

SERIOUS REACTIONS
! Sustained polymorphic ventricular tachycardia, occasionally with QT prolongation (torsades de pointes) occurs rarely.
! Overdose results in CNS toxicity, including CNS depression, rapid gasping breathing, and seizures.
! Expect prolongation of repolarization may be exaggerated.
! Existing arrhythmias may worsen or new arrhythmias may develop.

DENTAL CONSIDERATIONS

General:
• Acute-use drug for use in hospitals, emergency rooms, or cardiac labs.
• Patients who have received this drug for arrhythmias may be at risk when it is combined with other drugs that prolong the QT interval.

Consultations:
• Medical consultation may be required to assess disease control and patient's ability to tolerate stress.

Teach Patient/Family:
• Importance of updating health and medication history if physician makes any changes in evaluation or drug regimens; include OTC, herbal, and nonherbal remedies in the update

idarubicin hydrochloride
eye-dah-roo′-bi-sin
(Idamycin PFS, Zavedos)
Do not confuse idarubicin with doxorubicin, or Idamycin with Adriamycin.

CATEGORY AND SCHEDULE
Pregnancy Risk Category: D

MECHANISM OF ACTION
An anthracycline antibiotic that inhibits nucleic acid synthesis by interacting with the enzyme topoisomerase II, which promotes DNA strand supercoiling.
Therapeutic Effect: Causes death of rapidly dividing cells.

PHARMACOKINETICS
Widely distributed. Protein binding: 97%. Rapidly metabolized in the liver to active metabolite. Primarily eliminated by biliary excretion. Not removed by hemodialysis. ***Half-life:*** 4–46 hr; metabolite: 8–92 hr.

AVAILABILITY

Injection: 1 mg/ml in 5 ml, 10 ml vials.

INDICATIONS AND DOSAGES

▸ Acute Myeloid Leukemia

IV

Adults. 8–12 mg/m^2/day for 3 days in combination with Ara-C.
Children (solid tumor). 5 mg/m^2 once a day for 3 days.
Children (leukemia). 10–12 mg/m^2 once a day for 3 days.

▸ Dosage in Hepatic or Renal Impairment

Dosage is modified on the basis of serum creatinine or bilirubin level.

Serum Level	Dose Reduction
Serum creatinine 2 mg/dl or more	25%
Serum bilirubin greater than 2.5 mg/dl	50%
Serum bilirubin greater than 5 mg/dl	Do not give

CONTRAINDICATIONS

Pre-existing arrhythmias, cardiomyopathy, myelosuppression, pregnancy, severe CHF

INTERACTIONS

Drug

Antigout medications: May decrease the effects of these drugs.
Bone marrow depressants: May increase myelosuppression.
Live-virus vaccines: May potentiate virus replication, increase vaccine side effects, and decrease the patient's antibody response to the vaccine.

Herbal

None known.

Food

None known.

Drug interactions of concern to dentistry

- Dental drug interactions have not been studied

DIAGNOSTIC TEST EFFECTS

May increase serum alkaline phosphatase, bilirubin, uric acid, AST (SGOT), and ALT (SGPT) levels. May cause ECG changes.

IV INCOMPATIBILITIES

Acyclovir (Zovirax), allopurinol (Aloprim), ampicillin and sulbactam (Unasyn), cefazolin (Ancef, Kefzol), cefepime (Maxipime), ceftazidime (Fortaz), clindamycin (Cleocin), dexamethasone (Decadron), furosemide (Lasix), hydrocortisone (Solu-Cortef), lorazepam (Ativan), meperidine (Demerol), methotrexate, piperacillin and tazobactam (Zosyn), sodium bicarbonate, teniposide (Vumon), vancomycin (Vancocin), vincristine (Oncovin)

IV COMPATIBILITIES

Diphenhydramine (Benadryl), granisetron (Kytril), magnesium, potassium

SIDE EFFECTS

Frequent

Nausea, vomiting (82%); complete alopecia (scalp, axillary, pubic hair) (77%); abdominal cramping, diarrhea (73%); mucositis (50%)

Occasional

Hyperpigmentation of nailbeds, phalangeal and dermal creases (46%); fever (36%); headache (20%)

Rare

Conjunctivitis, neuropathy

SERIOUS REACTIONS

! Myelosuppression may cause hematologic toxicity (manifested principally as leukopenia and, to lesser extent, anemia and thrombocytopenia), usually within 10 to 15 days of starting therapy. Blood counts typically return to normal levels by the third week.

! Cardiotoxicity (either acute, manifested as transient ECG abnormalities, or chronic, manifested as CHF) may occur.

DENTAL CONSIDERATIONS

General:

- If additional analgesia is required for dental pain, consider alternative analgesics (NSAIDs) in patients taking narcotics for acute or chronic pain.
- Examine for oral manifestation of opportunistic infection.
- This drug may be used in the hospital or on an outpatient basis. Confirm the patient's disease and treatment status.
- Chlorhexidine mouth rinse prior to and during chemotherapy may reduce severity of mucositis.
- Patient on chronic drug therapy may rarely present with symptoms of blood dyscrasias, which can include infection, bleeding, and poor healing. If dyscrasia is present, caution patient to prevent oral tissue trauma when using oral hygiene aids.
- Palliative medication may be required for management of oral side effects.

Consultations:

- Consult physician; prophylactic or therapeutic antiinfectives may be indicated if surgery or periodontal treatment is required.
- Medical consultation may be required to assess immunologic status during cancer chemotherapy and determine safety risk, if any, posed by the required dental treatment.
- Medical consultation may be required to assess disease control and patient's ability to tolerate stress.

Teach Patient/Family:

- To be aware of oral side effects
- Importance of good oral hygiene to prevent soft tissue inflammation
- To report oral lesions, soreness, or bleeding to dentist
- To prevent trauma when using oral hygiene aids
- Importance of updating health and medication history if physician makes any changes in evaluation or drug regimens; include OTC, herbal, and nonherbal remedies in the update

ifosfamide

eye-fos′-fah-mide

(Holoxan[AUS], Ifex)

CATEGORY AND SCHEDULE

Pregnancy Risk Category: D

MECHANISM OF ACTION

An alkylating agent that inhibits DNA and RNA protein synthesis by cross-linking with DNA and RNA strands, preventing cell growth. Cell cycle-phase nonspecific. ***Therapeutic Effect:*** Interferes with DNA and RNA function.

PHARMACOKINETICS

Metabolized in the liver to active metabolite. Crosses the blood-brain barrier (to a limited extent). Primarily excreted in urine. Removed by hemodialysis. ***Half-life:*** 15 hr.

AVAILABILITY

Powder for Injection: 1 g, 3 g.

INDICATIONS AND DOSAGES

▸ Germ Cell Testicular Carcinoma

IV

Adults. 700–2,000 mg/m^2/day for 5 consecutive days. Repeat every 3wk or after recovery from hematologic toxicity. Administer with mesna.

Children. 1,200–1,800 mg/m^2/day for 5 days every 21–28 days.

OFF-LABEL USES
Treatment of Ewing's sarcoma; non-Hodgkin's lymphoma; and lung, pancreatic, and soft-tissue carcinoma

CONTRAINDICATIONS
Pregnancy, severe myelosuppression

INTERACTIONS
Drug
Bone marrow depressants: May increase myelosuppression.
Live-virus vaccines: May potentiate virus replication, increase vaccine side effects, and decrease the patient's antibody response to the vaccine.
Herbal
None known.
Food
None known.
Drug interactions of concern to dentistry
• Dental drug interactions have not been studied

DIAGNOSTIC TEST EFFECTS
May increase BUN and serum bilirubin, creatinine, uric acid, AST (SGOT), and ALT (SGPT) levels.

IV INCOMPATIBILITIES
Cefepime (Maxipime), methotrexate
IV COMPATIBILITIES
Granisetron (Kytril), ondansetron (Zofran)

SIDE EFFECTS
Frequent
Alopecia (83%); nausea, vomiting (58%)
Occasional (15%–5%)
Confusion, somnolence, hallucinations, infection
Rare (< 5%)
Dizziness, seizures, disorientation, fever, malaise, stomatitis

SERIOUS REACTIONS
! Hemorrhagic cystitis with hematuria and dysuria occurs frequently if a protective agent (mesna) is not used.
! Myelosuppression, characterized by leukopenia and, to a lesser extent, thrombocytopenia, occurs frequently.
! Pulmonary toxicity, hepatotoxicity, nephrotoxicity, cardiotoxicity, and CNS toxicity (manifested as confusion, hallucinations, somnolence, and coma) may require discontinuation of therapy.

DENTAL CONSIDERATIONS
General:
• Determine why patient is taking the drug.
• If additional analgesia is required for dental pain, consider alternative analgesics (NSAIDs) in patients taking narcotics for acute or chronic pain.
• Examine for oral manifestation of opportunistic infection.
• Avoid products that affect platelet function, such as aspirin and NSAIDs.
• This drug may be used in the hospital or on an outpatient basis. Confirm the patient's disease and treatment status.
• Chlorhexidine mouth rinse prior to and during chemotherapy may reduce severity of mucositis.
• Patient on chronic drug therapy may rarely present with symptoms of blood dyscrasias, which can include infection, bleeding, and poor healing. If dyscrasia is present, caution patient to prevent oral tissue trauma when using oral hygiene aids.
• Palliative medication may be required for management of oral side effects.
• Short appointments and a stress reduction protocol may be required for anxious patients.
• Patients may be at risk of bleeding, check for oral signs.

- Oral infections should be eliminated and/or treated aggressively.

Consultations:

- Medical consultation should include routine blood counts including platelet counts and bleeding time.
- Consult physician; prophylactic or therapeutic antiinfectives may be indicated if surgery or periodontal treatment is required.
- Medical consultation may be required to assess immunologic status during cancer chemotherapy and determine safety risk, if any, posed by the required dental treatment.
- Medical consultation may be required to assess disease control and patient's ability to tolerate stress.

Teach Patient/Family:

- To be aware of oral side effects
- Importance of good oral hygiene to prevent soft tissue inflammation
- To report oral lesions, soreness, or bleeding to dentist
- To prevent trauma when using oral hygiene aids
- Importance of updating health and medication history if physician makes any changes in evaluation or drug regimens; include OTC, herbal, and nonherbal remedies in the update

imatinib mesylate

im′-a-tin-ib
(Gleevec, Glivec[AUS])

CATEGORY AND SCHEDULE

Pregnancy Risk Category: D

MECHANISM OF ACTION

Inhibits Bcr-Abl tyrosine kinase, an enzyme created by the Philadelphia chromosome abnormality found in patients with chronic myeloid leukemia (CML). ***Therapeutic Effect:*** Suppresses tumor growth during the three stages of CML; blast crisis, accelerated phase, and chronic phase.

PHARMACOKINETICS

Well absorbed after PO administration. Binds to plasma proteins, particularly albumin. Metabolized in the liver. Eliminated mainly in the feces as metabolites. ***Half-life:*** 18 hr.

AVAILABILITY

Tablets: 100 mg, 400 mg.

INDICATIONS AND DOSAGES

▸ CML

PO

Adults, Elderly. 400 mg/day for patients in chronic-phase CML; 600 mg/day for patients in accelerated phase or blast crisis. May increase dosage from 400 to 600 mg/day for patients in chronic phase or from 600 to 800 mg (given as 300–400 mg twice a day) for patients in accelerated phase or blast crisis in the absence of a severe drug reaction or severe neutropenia or thrombocytopenia in the following circumstances: progression of the disease, failure to achieve a satisfactory hematologic response after 3 months or more of treatment, or loss of a previously achieved hematologic response.

Children. 260 mg/m^2 a day as a single daily dose or in 2 divided doses.

CONTRAINDICATIONS

Known hypersensitivity to imatinib

INTERACTIONS

Drug

Carbamazepine, dexamethasone, phenobarbital, phenytoin, rifampicin: Decrease imatinib plasma concentration.

Clarithromycin, erythromycin, itraconazole, ketoconazole: Increase imatinib plasma concentration.
Cyclosporine, pimozide: May alter the therapeutic effects of these drugs.
Dihydropyridine calcium channel blockers, simvastatin, triazolo-benzodiazepines: May increase the blood concentration of these drugs.
Live-virus vaccines: May potentiate viral replication, increase vaccine side effects, and decrease the patient's antibody response to the vaccine.
Warfarin: Reduces the effect of warfarin.

Herbal

St. John's wort: Decreases imatinib concentration.

Food

None known.

Drug interactions of concern to dentistry

- Increased plasma levels with CYP3A4 isoenzyme inhibitors: ketoconazole; possibly macrolide antibiotics, itraconazole, benzodiazepines
- Use acetaminophen with caution or avoid if hepatotoxicity is present
- Possible decrease in plasma concentrations: dexamethasone, carbamazepine, St. John's wort (herb)

DIAGNOSTIC TEST EFFECTS

May increase serum bilirubin AST (SGOT), and ALT (SGPT) levels. May decrease platelet count, WBC count, and serum potassium level.

SIDE EFFECTS

Frequent (68%–24%)

Nausea, diarrhea, vomiting, headache, fluid retention (periorbital, lower extremities), rash, musculoskeletal pain, muscle cramps, arthralgia

Occasional (23%–10%)

Abdominal pain, cough, myalgia, fatigue, fever, anorexia, dyspepsia, constipation, night sweats, pruritus

Rare (< 10%)

Nasopharyngitis, petechiae, asthenia, epistaxis

SERIOUS REACTIONS

! Severe fluid retention (manifested as pleural effusion, pericardial effusion, pulmonary edema, and ascites) and hepatotoxicity occur rarely.
! Neutropenia and thrombocytopenia are expected responses to the drug.
! Respiratory toxicity, manifested as dyspnea and pneumonia, may occur.

DENTAL CONSIDERATIONS

General:

- Prophylactic or therapeutic antibiotics may be indicated to prevent or treat infection if surgery or periodontal debridement is required.
- Patients taking opioids for acute or chronic pain should be given alternative analgesics for dental pain.
- Short appointments and a stress reduction protocol may be required for anxious patients.
- Consider local hemostasis measures to control excessive bleeding.
- Patients on chronic drug therapy may rarely have symptoms of blood dyscrasias, which can include infection, bleeding, and poor healing.
- Consider semisupine chair position for patient comfort if GI side effects occur.

Consultations:

- In a patient with symptoms of blood dyscrasias, request a medical consultation for blood studies and postpone treatment until normal values are reestablished.

- Consultation with physician may be necessary if sedation or general anesthesia is required.
- Medical consultation should include routine blood counts, including platelet counts and bleeding time.

Teach Patient/Family:

- Importance of good oral hygiene to prevent soft tissue inflammation, infection
- To inform dentist of unusual bleeding episodes following dental treatment

imipramine

ih-mih′-prah-meen
(Apo-Imipramine[CAN], Melipramine[AUS], Tofranil, Tofranil-PM)

Do not confuse imipramine with desipramine.

CATEGORY AND SCHEDULE

Pregnancy Risk Category: D

MECHANISM OF ACTION

A tricyclic antidepressant, antibulimic, anticataplectic, antinarcoleptic, antineuralgic, antineuritic, and antipanic agent that blocks the reuptake of neurotransmitters, such as norepinephrine and serotonin, at presynaptic membranes, increasing their concentration at postsynaptic receptor sites. ***Therapeutic Effect:*** Relieves depression and controls nocturnal enuresis.

AVAILABILITY

Tablets: 10 mg, 25 mg, 50 mg.
Capsules: 75 mg, 100 mg, 125 mg, 150 mg.

INDICATIONS AND DOSAGES

▸ Depression

PO

Adults. Initially, 75–100 mg/day. May gradually increase to 300 mg/day for hospitalized patients, or 200 mg/day for outpatients; then reduce dosage to effective maintenance level, 50–150 mg/day.
Elderly. Initially, 10–25 mg/day at bedtime. May increase by 10–25 mg every 3–7 days. Range: 50–150 mg/day.
Children. 1.5 mg/kg/day. May increase by 1 mg/kg every 3–4 days. Maximum: 5 mg/kg/day.

▸ Enuresis

PO

Children older than 6 yr. Initially, 10–25 mg at bedtime. May increase by 25 mg/day. Maximum: 50 mg for children older than 12 yr.

OFF-LABEL USES

Treatment of attention-deficit hyperactivity disorder, cataplexy associated with narcolepsy, neurogenic pain, panic disorder

CONTRAINDICATIONS

Acute recovery period after MI, use within 14 days of MAOIs

INTERACTIONS

Drug

Alcohol, other CNS depressants: May increase the hypotensive effects and CNS and respiratory depression caused by imipramine.
Antithyroid agents: May increase the risk of agranulocytosis.
Cimetidine: May increase imipramine blood concentration and risk of toxicity.
Clonidine, guanadrel: May decrease the effects of these drugs.
MAOIs: May increase the risk of neuroleptic malignant syndrome,

hyperpyrexia, hypertensive crisis, and seizures.
Phenothiazines: May increase the anticholinergic and sedative effects of imipramine.
Phenytoin: May decrease the imipramine blood concentration.
Sympathomimetics: May increase the risk of cardiac effects.

Herbal

Ginkgo biloba: May decrease seizure threshold.
St. John's wort: May increase imipramine's pharmacologic effects and risk of toxicity.

Food

None known.

Drug interactions of concern to dentistry

- Increased anticholinergic effects: muscarinic blockers, antihistamines, phenothiazines
- Increased effects of direct-acting sympathomimetics (epinephrine, levonordefrin)
- Potential risk of increased CNS depression: alcohol, barbiturates, benzodiazepines, other CNS depressants
- Decreased antihypertensive effects: clonidine, guanadrel, guanethidine
- Avoid concurrent use with St. John's wort (herb)
- Suspected increased tricyclic antidepressant effects: fluconazole, ketoconazole
- Increased serum levels of carbamazepine
- Caution in using drugs metabolized by CYP2D6: increased effects

DIAGNOSTIC TEST EFFECTS

May alter blood glucose levels and ECG readings. Therapeutic serum drug level is 225–300 ng/ml; toxic serum drug level is greater than 500 ng/ml.

SIDE EFFECTS

Frequent

Somnolence, fatigue, dry mouth, blurred vision, constipation, delayed micturition, orthostatic hypotension, diaphoresis, impaired concentration, increased appetite, urine retention, photosensitivity.

Occasional

GI disturbances (nausea, metallic taste).

Rare

Paradoxical reactions, (agitation, restlessness, nightmares, insomnia), extrapyramidal symptoms (particularly fine hand tremor).

SERIOUS REACTIONS

! Overdose may produce seizures; cardiovascular effects, such as severe orthostatic hypotension, dizziness, tachycardia, palpitations, and arrhythmias; and altered temperature regulation, including hyperpyrexia or hypothermia.

! Abrupt discontinuation after prolonged therapy may produce headache, malaise, nausea, vomiting, and vivid dreams.

DENTAL CONSIDERATIONS

General:

- Monitor vital signs at every appointment because of cardiovascular side effects.
- Assess salivary flow as a factor in caries, periodontal disease, and candidiasis.
- Patients on chronic drug therapy may rarely have symptoms of blood dyscrasias, which can include infection, bleeding, and poor healing.
- After supine positioning, have patient sit upright for at least 2 min to avoid orthostatic hypotension.
- Use vasoconstrictors with caution, in low doses, and with careful aspiration. Avoid use of gingival retraction cord with epinephrine.

- Place on frequent recall because of oral side effects.

Consultations:

- In a patient with symptoms of blood dyscrasias, request a medical consultation for blood studies and postpone dental treatment until normal values are reestablished.
- Medical consultation may be required to assess disease control.
- Physician should be informed if significant xerostomic side effects occur (e.g., increased caries, sore tongue, problems eating or swallowing, difficulty wearing prosthesis) so that a medication change can be considered.

Teach Patient/Family:

- Importance of good oral hygiene to prevent soft tissue inflammation
- Caution to prevent injury when using oral hygiene aids
- *When chronic dry mouth occurs, advise patient:*
  - To avoid mouth rinses with high alcohol content because of drying effects
  - To use sugarless gum, frequent sips of water, or saliva substitutes
  - To use daily home fluoride products for anticaries effect

imiquimod

im-ick′-wih-mod
(Aldara)

CATEGORY AND SCHEDULE

Pregnancy Risk Category: C

MECHANISM OF ACTION

An immune response modifier whose mechanism of action is uknown. ***Therapeutic Effect:*** Reduces genital and perianal warts.

PHARMACOKINETICS

Minimal absorption after topical administration. Minimal excretion in urine and feces.

AVAILABILITY

Cream: 5% (Aldara).

INDICATIONS AND DOSAGES

▸ Warts/Condyloma Acuminata

TOPICAL

Adults, Elderly, Children 12 yrs and older. Apply 3 times/wk before normal sleeping hours; leave on skin 6–10 hrs. Remove following treatment period. Continue therapy for maximum of 16 weeks.

CONTRAINDICATIONS

History of hypersensitivity to imiquimod

INTERACTIONS

Drug

None known.

Herbal

None known.

Food

None known.

Drug interactions of concern to dentistry

None reported

DIAGNOSTIC TEST EFFECTS

None known.

SIDE EFFECTS

Frequent

Local skin reactions: erythema, itching, burning, erosion, excoriation/flaking, fungal infections (women)

Occasional

Pain, induration, ulceration, scabbing, soreness, headache, flulike symptoms

SERIOUS REACTIONS

! None reported.

DENTAL CONSIDERATIONS

General:

- Oral manifestations of the disease may occur in the oral mucosa.
- Patient may have history of other sexually transmitted diseases (STDs).

Consultations:

- Medical consultation may be required to assess disease control.

Teach Patient/Family:

- To report oral lesions to the dentist
- Importance of updating health and drug history if physician makes any changes in evaluation or drug regimens

indapamide

in-dap′-a-mide
(Dapa-tabs[AUS], Indahexal[AUS], Insig[AUS], Lozide[CAN], Lozol, Natrilix[AUS], Natrilix SR[AUS])
Do not confuse indapamide with iodamide or iopamidol.

CATEGORY AND SCHEDULE

Pregnancy Risk Category: B (D if used in pregnancy-induced hypertension)

MECHANISM OF ACTION

A thiazide-like diuretic that blocks reabsorption of water, sodium, and potassium at the cortical diluting segment of the distal tubule; also reduces plasma and extracellular fluid volume and peripheral vascular resistance by direct effect on blood vessels. ***Therapeutic Effect:*** Promotes diuresis and reduces BP.

AVAILABILITY

Tablets: 1.25 mg, 2.5 mg.

INDICATIONS AND DOSAGES

▸ Edema

PO

Adults. Initially, 2.5 mg/day, may increase to 5 mg/day after 1 wk.

▸ Hypertension

PO

Adults, Elderly. Initially, 1.25 mg, may increase to 2.5 mg/day after 4 wk or 5 mg/day after additional 4 wk.

CONTRAINDICATIONS

None known.

INTERACTIONS

Drug

Digoxin: May increase the risk of digoxin toxicity associated with indapamide-induced hypokalemia.
Lithium: May increase the risk of lithium toxicity.

Herbal

None known.

Food

None known.

Drug interactions of concern to dentistry

- Decreased hypotensive response: NSAIDs, especially indomethacin

DIAGNOSTIC TEST EFFECTS

May increase plasma renin activity. May decrease protein-bound iodine and serum calcium, potassium, and sodium levels.

SIDE EFFECTS

Frequent (≥ 5%)

Fatigue, numbness of extremities, tension, irritability, agitation, headache, dizziness, lightheadedness, insomnia, muscle cramps

Occasional (< 5%)

Tingling of extremities, urinary frequency, urticaria, rhinorrhea, flushing, weight loss, orthostatic hypotension, depression, blurred vision, nausea, vomiting, diarrhea or constipation, dry mouth, impotence, rash, pruritus

SERIOUS REACTIONS

! Vigorous diuresis may lead to profound water and electrolyte depletion, resulting in hypokalemia, hyponatremia, and dehydration.
! Acute hypotensive episodes may occur.
! Hyperglycemia may occur during prolonged therapy.
! Pancreatitis, blood dyscrasias, pulmonary edema, allergic pneumonitis, and dermatologic reactions occur rarely.
! Overdose can lead to lethargy and coma without changes in electrolytes or hydration.

DENTAL CONSIDERATIONS

General:

- Monitor vital signs at every appointment because of cardiovascular side effects.
- Patients on chronic drug therapy may rarely have symptoms of blood dyscrasias, which can include infection, bleeding, and poor healing.
- After supine positioning, have patient sit upright for at least 2 min before standing to avoid orthostatic hypotension.
- Assess salivary flow as a factor in caries, periodontal disease, and candidiasis.
- Limit use of sodium-containing products, such as saline IV fluids, for patients with a dietary salt restriction.
- Stress from dental procedures may compromise cardiovascular function; determine patient risk.
- Short appointments and a stress reduction protocol may be required for anxious patients.
- Patients on diuretic therapy should be monitored for serum K^+ levels.

Consultations:

- In a patient with symptoms of blood dyscrasias, request a medical consultation for blood studies and postpone dental treatment until normal values are reestablished.
- Medical consultation may be required to assess disease control and patient's ability to tolerate stress.

Teach Patient/Family:

- Importance of good oral hygiene to prevent soft tissue inflammation
- Caution to prevent injury when using oral hygiene aids
- *When chronic dry mouth occurs, advise patient:*
    - To avoid mouth rinses with high alcohol content because of drying effects
    - To use sugarless gum, frequent sips of water, or saliva substitutes
    - To use daily home fluoride products for anticaries effect

indinavir

in-din′-ah-veer
(Crixivan)
Do not confuse indinavir with Denavir.

CATEGORY AND SCHEDULE

Pregnancy Risk Category: C

MECHANISM OF ACTION

A protease inhibitor that suppresses HIV protease, an enzyme necessary for splitting viral polyprotein precursors into mature and infectious viral particles. ***Therapeutic Effect:*** Interrupts HIV replication, slowing the progression of HIV infection.

PHARMACOKINETICS

Rapidly absorbed after PO administration. Protein binding: 60%. Metabolized in the liver.

Primarily excreted in urine. Unknown if removed by hemodialysis. ***Half-life:*** 1.8 hr (increased in impaired hepatic function).

AVAILABILITY

Capsules: 100 mg, 200 mg, 333 mg, 400 mg.

INDICATIONS AND DOSAGES

▸ HIV Infection (in combination with other antiretrovirals)

PO

Adults. 800 mg (two 400-mg capsules) q8h.

▸ HIV Infection in Patients with Hepatic Insufficiency

PO

Adults. 600 mg q8h.

OFF-LABEL USES

Prophylaxis following occupational exposure to HIV

CONTRAINDICATIONS

Hypersensitivity to indinavir; nephrolithiasis

INTERACTIONS

Drug

Midazolam, triazolam: Increases the risk of arrhythmias and prolonged sedation.

Herbal

St. John's wort: May decrease indinavir blood concentration and effect.

Food

Grapefruit, grapefruit juice: May decrease indinavir blood concentration and effect.

High-fat, high-calorie, and high-protein meals: May decrease indinavir blood concentration.

Drug interactions of concern to dentistry

- Contraindicated with triazolam, midazolam
- Reduce dose when given with ketoconazole

DIAGNOSTIC TEST EFFECTS

May increase serum bilirubin (in 10% of patients), AST (SGOT), and ALT (SGPT) levels.

SIDE EFFECTS

Frequent

Nausea (12%), abdominal pain (9%), headache (6%), diarrhea (5%)

Occasional

Vomiting, asthenia, fatigue (4%); insomnia; accumulation of fat in waist, abdomen, or back of neck

Rare

Abnormal taste sensation, heartburn, symptomatic urinary tract disease, transient renal dysfunction

SERIOUS REACTIONS

! Nephrolithiasis (flank pain with or without hematuria) occurs in 4% of patients.

DENTAL CONSIDERATIONS

General:

- Consider semisupine chair position when GI side effects occur.
- Assess salivary flow as a factor in caries, periodontal disease, and candidiasis.
- Monitor vital signs at every appointment because of cardiovascular side effects.
- Examine for oral manifestation of opportunistic infection.
- Patients with gastroesophageal reflux may have oral symptoms, including burning mouth, secondary candidiasis, and signs of tooth erosion.

Consultations:

- Medical consultation may be required to assess disease control.

Teach Patient/Family:

- Importance of good oral hygiene to prevent soft tissue inflammation

- To report oral lesions, soreness, or bleeding to dentist
- Importance of updating health history/drug record if physician makes any changes in evaluation or drug regimens
- *When chronic dry mouth occurs, advise patient:*
  - To avoid mouth rinses with high alcohol content because of drying effects
  - To use daily home fluoride products for anticaries effect
  - To use sugarless gum, frequent sips of water, or saliva substitutes

indomethacin

in-doe-meth′-a-sin
(Apo-Indomethacin[CAN], Arthrexin[AUS], Indocid[CAN], Indocin, Indocin-IV, Indocin-SR, Novomethacin[CAN])
Do not confuse Indocin with Imodium or Vicodin.

CATEGORY AND SCHEDULE

Pregnancy Risk Category: B (D if used after 34 weeks' gestation, close to delivery, or for longer than 48 hours)

MECHANISM OF ACTION

An NSAID that produces analgesic and anti-inflammatory effects by inhibiting prostaglandin synthesis. Also increases the sensitivity of the premature ductus to the dilating effects of prostaglandins. ***Therapeutic Effect:*** Reduces the inflammatory response and intensity of pain. Closure of the patent ductus arteriosus.

AVAILABILITY

Capsules (Indocin): 25 mg, 50 mg.
Capsules (Sustained-Release [Indocin SR]): 75 mg.
Oral Suspension (Indocin): 25 mg/5 ml.
Powder for Injection (Indocin IV): 1 mg.
Suppositories: 50 mg.

INDICATIONS AND DOSAGES

▸ Moderate to Severe Rheumatoid Arthritis, Osteoarthritis, Ankylosing Spondylitis

PO

Adults, Elderly. Initially, 25 mg 2–3 times a day; increased by 25–50 mg/wk up to 150–200 mg/day. Or 75 mg/day (extended-release) up to 75 mg twice a day.
Children. 1–2 mg/kg/day. Maximum: 150–200 mg/day.

▸ Acute Gouty Arthritis

PO

Adults, Elderly. Initially, 100 mg, then 50 mg 3 times a day.

▸ Acute Shoulder Pain

PO

Adults, Elderly. 75–150 mg/day in 3–4 divided doses.

▸ Usual Rectal Dosage

Adults, Elderly. 50 mg 4 times a day.
Children. Initially, 1.5–2.5 mg/kg/day, increased up to 4 mg/kg/day. Maximum: 150–200 mg/day.

▸ Patent Ductus Arteriosus

IV

Neonates. Initially, 0.2 mg/kg. Subsquent doses are on the basis of age, as follows:
Neonates older than 7 days. 0.25 mg/kg for 2nd and 3rd doses.
Neonates 2–7 days. 0.2 mg/kg for 2nd and 3rd doses.
Neonates less than 48 hr. 0.1 mg/kg for 2nd and 3rd doses.

OFF-LABEL USES

Treatment of fever due to malignancy, pericarditis, psoriatic arthritis, rheumatic complications associated with Paget's disease of bone, vascular headache

CONTRAINDICATIONS

Active GI bleeding or ulcerations; hypersensitivity to aspirin, indomethacin, or other NSAIDs; renal impairment, thrombocytopenia

INTERACTIONS

Drug

Aminoglycosides: May increase the blood concentration of these drugs in neonates.
Antihypertensives, diuretics: May decrease the effects of these drugs.
Aspirin, other salicylates: May increase the risk of GI side effects such as bleeding.
Bone marrow depressants: May increase the risk of hematologic reactions.
Heparin, oral anticoagulants, thrombolytics: May increase the effects of these drugs.
Lithium: May increase the blood concentration and risk of toxicity of lithium.
Methotrexate: May increase the risk of methotrexate toxicity.
Probenecid: May increase the indomethacin blood concentration.
Triamterene: May potentiate acute renal failure. Don't give concurrently.

Herbal

Feverfew: May decrease the effects of feverfew.
Ginkgo biloba: May increase the risk of bleeding.

Food

None known.

Drug interactions of concern to dentistry

- Increased GI bleeding, ulceration: corticosteroids, alcohol, aspirin, other NSAIDs
- Renal toxicity: acetaminophen (high doses, prolonged use)
- Possible risk of decreased renal function: cyclosporine
- *When prescribed for dental pain:*
  - Risk of increased effects: oral anticoagulants, oral antidiabetics, lithium, methotrexate
  - Decreased antihypertensive effects of diuretics, β-adrenergic blockers, ACE inhibitors
  - Increased toxicity of zidovudine
  - First-time users of SSRIs also taking NSAIDs may have a higher risk of GI side effects; until more data are available, it may be advisable to avoid use of NSAIDs in these patients (*Br J Clin Pharmacol* 55:591–595, 2003)

DIAGNOSTIC TEST EFFECTS

May prolong bleeding time. May alter blood glucose level. May increase BUN level, and serum creatinine, potassium, AST (SGOT), and ALT (SGPT) levels. May decrease serum sodium level and platelet count.

IV INCOMPATIBILITIES

Amino acid injection, calcium gluconate, cimetidine (Tagamet), dobutamine (Dobutrex), dopamine (Intropin), gentamicin (Garamycin), tobramycin (Nebcin)

IV COMPATIBILITIES

Insulin, potassium

SIDE EFFECTS

Frequent (11%–3%)

Headache, nausea, vomiting, dyspepsia, dizziness

Occasional (less than 3%)

Depression, tinnitus, diaphoresis, somnolence, constipation, diarrhea, bleeding disturbances in patent ductus arteriosus

Rare

Hypertension, confusion, urticaria, pruritus, rash, blurred vision

SERIOUS REACTIONS

! Paralytic ileus and ulceration of the esophagus, stomach, duodenum, or small intestine may occur.
! Patients with impaired renal function may develop hyperkalemia and worsening of renal impairment.
! Indomethacin use may aggravate epilepsy, parkinsonism, and depression or other psychiatric disturbances.
! Nephrotoxicity, including dysuria, hematuria, proteinuria, and nephrotic syndrome, occurs rarely.
! Metabolic acidosis or alkalosis, apnea, and bradycardia occur rarely in patients with patent ductus arteriosus.

DENTAL CONSIDERATIONS

General:

- Avoid prescribing aspirin-containing products.
- Patients on chronic drug therapy may rarely have symptoms of blood dyscrasias, which can include infection, bleeding, and poor healing.
- Assess salivary flow as a factor in caries, periodontal disease, and candidiasis.
- Consider semisupine chair position for patients with arthritic disease.

Consultations:

- In a patient with symptoms of blood dyscrasias, request a medical consultation for blood studies and postpone dental treatment until normal values are reestablished.
- Medical consultation may be required to assess disease control.

Teach Patient/Family:

- Importance of good oral hygiene to prevent soft tissue inflammation
- Caution to prevent injury when using oral hygiene aids
- *When chronic dry mouth occurs, advise patient:*
  - To avoid mouth rinses with high alcohol content because of drying effects
  - To use sugarless gum, frequent sips of water, or saliva substitutes
  - To use daily home fluoride products for anticaries effect

infliximab

in-flicks′-ih-mab
(Remicade)
Do not confuse Remicade with Reminyl.

CATEGORY AND SCHEDULE

Pregnancy Risk Category: C

I

MECHANISM OF ACTION

A monoclonal antibody that binds to tumor necrosis factor (TNF), inhibiting functional activity of TNF. Reduces infiltration of inflammatory cells. ***Therapeutic Effect:*** Decreases inflamed areas of the intestine.

PHARMACOKINETICS

Route	Onset	Peak	Duration
IV (Crohn's disease)	1–2 wk	N/A	8–48 wk
IV (Rheumatoid arthritis [RA])	3–7 days	N/A	6–12 wk

Absorbed into the GI tissue; primarily distributed in the vascular compartment. ***Half-life:*** 9.5 days.

AVAILABILITY

Powder for Injection: 100 mg.

INDICATIONS AND DOSAGES

▸ **Moderate to Severe Crohn's Disease**

IV INFUSION

Adults, Elderly. 5 mg/kg as a single IV infusion.

▸ **Fistulizing Crohn's Disease**

IV INFUSION

Adults, Elderly. Initially, 5 mg/kg followed by additional 5-mg/kg doses at 2 and 6 wk after first infusion.

▸ **RA**

IV INFUSION

Adults, Elderly. 3 mg/kg; followed by additional doses at 2 and 6 wk after first infusion: Then q8wk.

OFF-LABEL USES

Sciatica

CONTRAINDICATIONS

Sensitivity to infliximab or murine proteins, sepsis, serious active infection

INTERACTIONS

Drug

Immunosuppressants: May reduce frequency of infusion reactions and antibodies to infliximab.

Live vaccines: May decrease immune response.

Herbal

None known.

Food

None known.

Drug interactions of concern to dentistry

- No drug interaction studies conducted

DIAGNOSTIC TEST EFFECTS

None known.

IV INCOMPATIBILITIES

Do not infuse infliximab in the same IV line with other agents.

SIDE EFFECTS

Frequent (22%–10%)

Headache, nausea, fatigue, fever

Occasional (9%–5%)

Fever or chills during infusion, pharyngitis, vomiting, pain, dizziness, bronchitis, rash, rhinitis, cough, pruritus, sinusitis, myalgia, back pain

Rare (4%–1%)

Hypotension or hypertension, paresthesia, anxiety, depression, insomnia, diarrhea, urinary tract infection

SERIOUS REACTIONS

! Hypersensitivity reaction, lupus-like syndrome, and severe hepatic reactions may occur.

DENTAL CONSIDERATIONS

General:

- Determine why patient is taking the drug.
- Question patient about other drugs being taken.
- Examine for oral manifestation of opportunistic infection.
- Report oral infections to patient's physician; treat infections aggressively.

Consultations:

- Medical consultation may be required to assess disease control and patient's ability to tolerate stress.

Teach Patient/Family:

- Importance of good oral hygiene to prevent soft tissue inflammation, infection
- To immediately report any signs or symptoms of oral infection

insulin glargine

in′-su-lin glare′-jeen

(Lantus)

CATEGORY AND SCHEDULE

Pregnancy Risk Category: C

MECHANISM OF ACTION

An exogenous insulin that facilitates passage of glucose, potassium, magnesium across cellular membranes of skeletal and cardiac muscle, adipose tissue; controls storage and metabolism of carbohydrates, protein, fats. Promotes conversion of glucose to glycogen in liver. ***Therapeutic Effect:*** Controls glucose levels in diabetic patients.

PHARMACOKINETICS

Drug Form	Onset (hrs)	Peak (hrs)	Duration (hrs)
Insulin glargine	N/A	N/A	24

Metabolized at the carboxyl terminus of the B chain in the subcutaneous depot to form two active metabolites. Unchanged drug and degradation products are present throughout circulation.

AVAILABILITY

Injection, solution: 100 unit/ml, 3 ml cartridge system [package of 5] (Lantus).

INDICATIONS AND DOSAGES

▸ Treatment of Insulin-Dependent Type 1 Diabetes Mellitus, Non-Insulin-Dependent Type 2 Diabetes Mellitus When Diet or Weight Control Therapy Has Failed to Maintain Satisfactory Blood Glucose Levels or in Event of Fever, Infection, Pregnancy, Severe Endocrine, Liver or Renal Dysfunction, Surgery, or Trauma, Regular Insulin Used in Emergency Treatment of Ketoacidosis, to Promote Passage of Glucose Across Cell Membrane in Hyperalimentation, to Facilitate Intracellular Shift of Potassium in Hyperkalemia

SUBCUTANEOUS

Adults, Elderly, Children. 10 units once daily, preferably at bedtime, adjusted according to patient response.

CONTRAINDICATIONS

Hypersensitivity or insulin resistance may require change of type or species source of insulin

INTERACTIONS

Drug

Alcohol: May increase the effects of insulin.

Beta-adrenergic blockers: May increase the risk of hyperglycemia or hypoglycemia, mask signs of hypoglycemia, and prolong the period of hypoglycemia.

Glucocorticoids, thiazide diuretics: May increase blood glucose.

Herbal

Chromium, garlic, gymnema: May increase risk of hypoglycemia.

Food

None known.

Drug interactions of concern to dentistry

- Increased hypoglycemia: salicylates, NSAIDs (large doses and chronic use), alcohol
- Hyperglycemia: corticosteroids, epinephrine

DIAGNOSTIC TEST EFFECTS

May decrease serum magnesium, phosphate, and potassium concentrations.

SIDE EFFECTS

Frequent

Hypoglycemia

Occasional

Local redness, swelling, itching, caused by improper injection technique or allergy to cleansing solution or insulin

Infrequent

Systemic allergic reaction, marked by rash, angioedema, and anaphylaxis, lipodystrophy or depression at injection site due to breakdown of adipose tissue, lipohypertrophy or accumulation of subcutaneous tissue at injection site due to lack of adequate site rotation

Rare

Insulin resistance

SERIOUS REACTIONS

! Severe hypoglycemia caused by hyperinsulinism may occur in overdose of insulin, decrease or delay of food intake, excessive exercise, or those with brittle diabetes.

! Diabetic ketoacidosis may result from stress, illness, omission of insulin dose, or long-term poor insulin control.

I

DENTAL CONSIDERATIONS

General:

- Monitor vital signs at every appointment because of cardiovascular effects of hypoglycemia.
- Place on frequent recall to evaluate healing response.
- Diabetics may be more susceptible to infection and have delayed wound healing.
- Assess salivary flow as a factor in caries, periodontal disease, and candidiasis.
- Prophylactic antibiotics may be indicated in uncontrolled diabetics to prevent infection if surgery or deep scaling is planned.
- Ensure that patient is following prescribed diet and regularly takes medication.
- Question patient about self-monitoring of drug's antidiabetic effect, including blood glucose values or finger-stick records.
- Keep a readily available source of sugar or fruit juice in case of insulin overdose.

Consultations:

- Medical consultation may be required to assess disease control and patient's ability to tolerate stress.
- Medical consultation may include data from patient's blood glucose monitoring, including glycosylated hemoglobin or HbA_{1c} testing.

Teach Patient/Family:

- Importance of good oral hygiene to prevent soft tissue inflammation
- Caution to prevent injury when using oral hygiene aids
- To avoid mouth rinses with high alcohol content because of drying effects

insulin glulisine

(Apidra)

CATEGORY AND SCHEDULE

Pregnancy Risk Category: C

MECHANISM OF ACTION

A recombinant, rapid-acting insulin analog that facilitates passage of glucose, potassium, magnesium across cellular membranes of skeletal and cardiac muscle, adipose tissue; controls storage and metabolism of carbohydrates, protein, fats. Promotes conversion of glucose to glycogen in liver. ***Therapeutic Effect:*** Controls glucose levels in diabetic patients.

PHARMACOKINETICS

Drug Form	Onset (min)	Peak (min)	Duration (hrs)
Insulin Glulisine	20 min	55 min	5 hrs

AVAILABILITY

Injection: 100 IU/ml (Apidra).

INDICATIONS AND DOSAGES

▸ **Diabetes Mellitus (Type 1 and Type 2)**

SUBCUTANEOUS, INFUSION PUMP

Adults, Elderly, Children.
Individualize per patient needs.

CONTRAINDICATIONS

Current hypoglycemic episode, hypersensitivity or insulin resistance may require change of type or species source of insulin

INTERACTIONS

Drug

Alcohol: May increase the effects of insulin glulisine.
Beta-adrenergic blockers: May increase the risk of hyperglycemia or hypoglycemia, mask signs of hypoglycemia, and prolong the period of hypoglycemia.
Glucocorticoids, thiazide diuretics: May increase blood glucose.

Herbal

None known.

Food

None known.

Drug interactions of concern to dentistry

- Increased hypoglycemia: salicylates, NSAIDs (large doses and chronic use), alcohol
- Hyperglycemia: corticosteroids, epinephrine

DIAGNOSTIC TEST EFFECTS

May decrease serum magnesium, phosphate, and potassium concentrations.

IV INCOMPATIBILITIES

None known.

SIDE EFFECTS

Occasional

Local redness, swelling, itching, caused by improper injection technique or allergy to cleansing solution or insulin

Infrequent

Somogyi effect, including rebound hyperglycemia with chronically excessive insulin doses. Systemic allergic reaction, marked by rash, angioedema, and anaphylaxis, lipodystrophy or depression at injection site due to breakdown of adipose tissue, lipohypertrophy or accumulation of subcutaneous tissue at injection site due to lack of adequate site rotation

Rare

Insulin resistance

SERIOUS REACTIONS

! Severe hypoglycemia caused by hyperinsulinism may occur in overdose of insulin, decrease or delay of food intake, excessive exercise, or those with brittle diabetes.
! Diabetic ketoacidosis may result from stress, illness, omission of insulin dose, or long-term poor insulin control.

DENTAL CONSIDERATIONS

General:

- Monitor vital signs at every appointment because of cardiovascular effects of hypoglycemia.
- Place on frequent recall to evaluate healing response.
- Diabetics may be more susceptible to infection and have delayed wound healing.
- Assess salivary flow as a factor in caries, periodontal disease, and candidiasis.
- Prophylactic antibiotics may be indicated in uncontrolled diabetics to prevent infection if surgery or deep scaling is planned.
- Ensure that patient is following prescribed diet and regularly takes medication.
- Question patient about self-monitoring of drug's antidiabetic effect, including blood glucose values or finger-stick records.
- Keep a readily available source of sugar or fruit juice in case of insulin overdose.

I

Consultations:
• Medical consultation may be required to assess disease control and patient's ability to tolerate stress.
• Medical consultation may include data from patient's blood glucose monitoring, including glycosylated hemoglobin or HbA_{1c} testing.

Teach Patient/Family:
• Importance of good oral hygiene to prevent soft tissue inflammation
• Caution to prevent injury when using oral hygiene aids
• To avoid mouth rinses with high alcohol content because of drying effects

I

insulin

in′-sull-in
Rapid acting: Insulin Lispro (Humalog), Insulin Aspart (Novolog, NovoMix 30[AUS], Novorapid[AUS]), Regular Insulin (Actrapid[AUS], Humulin R, Novolin R, Regular Iletin II) Intermediate acting: NPH (Humulin N, Novolin N, NPH Iletin II) Lente: (Humulin L, Lente Iletin II, Monotard[AUS], Novolin L) Long acting: Insulin Glargine (Lantus)

CATEGORY AND SCHEDULE

Pregnancy Risk Category: B
OTC

MECHANISM OF ACTION

An exogenous insulin that facilitates passage of glucose, potassium, and magnesium across the cellular membranes of skeletal and cardiac muscle and adipose tissue. Controls storage and metabolism of carbohydrates, protein, and fats. Promotes conversion of glucose to glycogen in the liver. ***Therapeutic Effect:*** Controls glucose levels in diabetic patients.

PHARMACOKINETICS

Drug Form	Onset (hr)	Peak (hr)	Duration (hr)
Lispro	0.25	0.5–1.5	4–5
Insulin aspart	1/6	1–3	3–5
Regular	0.5–1	2–4	5–7
NPH	1–2	6–14	24+
Lente	1–3	6–14	24+
Insulin glargine	N/A	N/A	24

AVAILABILITY

All insulins are available as 100 units/ml concentrations.
Rapid Acting: Humulin R, Novolin R, Novolog, Humalog, Regular Iletin II.
Intermediate Acting: Humulin L, Novolin L, Lente Iletin II, Humulin N, Novolin N, NPH Illetin II.
Long Acting: Lantus.

INDICATIONS AND DOSAGES

▸ **Treatment of Insulin-Dependent Type 1 Diabetes Mellitus and Non-Insulin-Dependent Type 2 Diabetes Mellitus When Diet or Weight Control Has Failed to Maintain Satisfactory Blood Glucose Levels or in Event of Fever, Infection, Pregnancy, Surgery, or Trauma, or Severe Endocrine, Hepatic or Renal Dysfunction; Emergency Treatment of Ketoacidosis (regular insulin); to Promote Passage of Glucose Across Cell Membrane in Hyperalimentation (regular insulin): to Facilitate Intracellular Shift of Potassium in Hyperkalemia (regular insulin)**

SUBCUTANEOUS
Adults, Elderly, Children.
0.5–1 unit/kg/day.
Adolescents (during growth spurt).
0.8–1.2 unit/kg/day.

CONTRAINDICATIONS

Hypersensitivity or insulin resistance may require change of type or species source of insulin

INTERACTIONS

Drug

Alcohol: May increase the effects of insulin.
Beta-adrenergic blockers: May increase the risk of hyperglycemia or hypoglycemia; may mask signs and prolong periods of hypoglycemia.
Glucocorticoids, thiazide diuretics: May increase blood glucose level.

Herbal

None known.

Food

None known.

Drug interactions of concern to dentistry

- Increased hypoglycemia: salicylates, NSAIDs (large doses and chronic use), alcohol
- Hyperglycemia: corticosteroids, epinephrine

DIAGNOSTIC TEST EFFECTS

May decrease serum magnesium, phosphate, and potassium concentrations.

IV INCOMPATIBILITIES

Diltiazem (Cardizem), dopamine (Intropin), nafcillin (Nafcil)

IV COMPATIBILITIES

Amiodarone (Cordarone), ampicillin/sulbactam (Unasyn), cefazolin (Ancef), cimetidine (Tagamet), digoxin (Lanoxin), dobutamine (Dobutrex), famotidine (Pepcid), gentamicin, heparin, magnesium sulfate, metoclopramide (Reglan), midazolam (Versed), milrinone (Primacor), morphine, nitroglycerin, potassium chloride, propofol (Diprivan), vancomycin (Vancocin)

SIDE EFFECTS

Occasional

Localized redness, swelling, and itching caused by improper injection technique or allergy to cleansing solution or insulin

Infrequent

Somogyi effect, including rebound hyperglycemia with chronically excessive insulin dosages: systemic allergic reaction, marked by rash, angioedema, and anaphylaxis; lipodystrophy or depression at injection site due to breakdown of adipose tissue; lipohypertrophy or accumulation of subcutaneous tissue at injection site due to inadequate site rotation

Rare

Insulin resistance

SERIOUS REACTIONS

! Severe hypoglycemia caused by hyperinsulinism may occur with insulin overdose, decrease or delay of food intake, or excessive exercise and in those with brittle diabetes.
! Diabetic ketoacidosis may result from stress, illness, omission of insulin dose, or long-term poor insulin control.

DENTAL CONSIDERATIONS

General:

- Monitor vital signs at every appointment because of cardiovascular effects of hypoglycemia.
- Place on frequent recall to evaluate healing response.
- Diabetics may be more susceptible to infection and have delayed wound healing.
- Assess salivary flow as a factor in caries, periodontal disease, and candidiasis.
- Prophylactic antibiotics may be indicated in uncontrolled diabetics to prevent infection if surgery or deep scaling is planned.

• Ensure that patient is following prescribed diet and regularly takes medication.
• Question patient about self-monitoring of drug's antidiabetic effect, including blood glucose values or finger-stick records.
• Keep a readily available source of sugar or fruit juice in case of insulin overdose.

Consultations:

• Medical consultation may be required to assess disease control and patient's ability to tolerate stress.
• Medical consultation may include data from patient's blood glucose monitoring, including glycosylated hemoglobin or HbA_{1c} testing.

Teach Patient/Family:

• Importance of good oral hygiene to prevent soft tissue inflammation
• Caution to prevent injury when using oral hygiene aids
• To avoid mouth rinses with high alcohol content because of drying effects

interferon alfa-2a

inn-ter-fear′-on
(Roferon-A)
Do not confuse interferon alfa-2a with interferon alfa-2b.

CATEGORY AND SCHEDULE

Pregnancy Risk Category: C

MECHANISM OF ACTION

A biological response modifier that inhibits viral replication in virus-infected cells, suppresses cell proliferation, increases phagocytic action of macrophage, and augments specific lymphocytic cell toxicity.
Therapeutic Effect: Prevents rapid growth of malignant cells; inhibits hepatitis virus.

PHARMACOKINETICS

Well absorbed after IM and subcutaneous administration. Undergoes proteolytic degradation during reabsorption in kidneys.
Half-life: 2 hr (IM); 3 hr (subcutaneous).

AVAILABILITY

Injection, vial: 6 million units/ml.
*Injection (Pre-filled Syringe):*3 million units/0.5 ml, 6 million units/0.5 ml, 9 million units/0.5 ml.
Injection (Single Dose Vial): 36 million units/ml.

INDICATIONS AND DOSAGES

▸ Hairy Cell Leukemia

IM, SUBCUTANEOUS
Adults. Initially, 3 million units/day for 16–24 wk. Maintenance: 3 million units 3 times a wk. Do not use 36-million-unit vial.

▸ Chronic Myelocytic Leukemia

IM, SUBCUTANEOUS
Adults. 9 million units/day.

▸ Melanoma

IM, SUBCUTANEOUS
Adults, Elderly. 12 million units/m^2 3 times a week for 3 mo.

▸ AIDS-Related Kaposi's Sarcoma

IM, SUBCUTANEOUS
Adults. Initially, 36 million units/day for 10–12 wk, may give 3 million units on day 1, 9 million units on day 2, 18 million units on day 3, then 36 million units/day for remaining of 10–12 wk. Maintenance: 36 million units/day 3 times a wk.

▸ Chronic Hepatitis C

IM, SUBCUTANEOUS
Adults, Elderly. 6 million units 3 times a week for 3 mo, then 3 million units 3 times a week for 9 mo.

OFF-LABEL USES
Treatment of active, chronic hepatitis; bladder or renal carcinoma; malignant melanoma; multiple myeloma; mycosis fungoides; non-Hodgkin's lymphoma

CONTRAINDICATIONS
Autoimmune hepatitis

INTERACTIONS
Drug
Bone marrow depressants: May have increase myelosuppression.
Herbal
None known.
Food
None known.
Drug interactions of concern to dentistry
• Risk of hepatotoxicity in severe liver disease: acetaminophen

DIAGNOSTIC TEST EFFECTS
May increase serum LDH, alkaline phosphatase, AST(SGOT), and ALT(SGPT) levels. May decrease Hct, blood Hgb level, and leukocyte and platelet counts.

SIDE EFFECTS
Frequent (> 20%)
Flu-like symptoms, nausea, vomiting, cough, dyspnea, hypotension, edema, chest pain, dizziness, diarrhea, weight loss, altered taste, abdominal discomfort, confusion, paresthesia, depression, visual and sleep disturbances, diaphoresis, lethargy
Occasional (20%–5%)
Alopecia (partial), rash, dry throat or skin, pruritus, flatulence, constipation, hypertension, palpitations, sinusitis
Rare (< 5%)
Hot flashes, hypermotility, Raynaud's syndrome, bronchospasm, earache, ecchymosis

SERIOUS REACTIONS
! Arrhythmias, CVA, transient ischemic attacks, CHF, pulmonary edema, and MI occur rarely.

DENTAL CONSIDERATIONS
General:
• Determine why the patient is taking the drug.
• Monitor vital signs at every appointment because of cardiovascular side effects.
• Patients on chronic drug therapy may rarely have symptoms of blood dyscrasias, which can include infection, bleeding, and poor healing.
• Palliative medication may be required for oral side effects.
• Assess salivary flow as a factor in caries, periodontal disease, and candidiasis.
• Consider semisupine chair position for patient comfort if GI side effects occur.
• Avoid elective dental procedures if severe neutropenia (>500 cells/mm^3) or thrombocytopenia (>50,000 cell/mm^3) is present.
• Antibiotic prophylaxis is indicated in severely neutropenic patients.
• Patient history should include all medications and herbal or nonherbal remedies taken by the patient.
• Severe side effects may require deferring elective dental procedures until drug therapy is completed.
• Evaluate efficacy of oral hygiene home care; preventive appointments may be necessary.
Consultations:
• Medical consultation may be required to assess disease control.
• In a patient with symptoms of blood dyscrasias, request a medical consultation for blood studies and postpone treatment until normal values are reestablished.

- Liver function tests may be required to determine chronic liver disease.

Teach Patient/Family:

- Importance of good oral hygiene to prevent soft tissue inflammation
- To report oral lesions, soreness, or bleeding to dentist
- Importance of updating medical/drug records if physician makes any changes in evaluation or drug regimens
- *When chronic dry mouth occurs, advise patient:*
  - To avoid mouth rinses with high alcohol content because of drying effects
  - To use sugarless gum, frequent sips of water, or saliva substitutes
  - To use daily home fluoride products for anticaries effect

I

interferon alfa-2a/2b

(Roferon-A)/(Intron-A)

CATEGORY AND SCHEDULE

Pregnancy Risk Category: C

MECHANISM OF ACTION

A biologic response modifier that inhibits viral replication in virus-infected cells. ***Therapeutic Effect:*** Suppresses cell proliferation; increases phagocytic action of macrophages; augments specific lymphocytic cell toxicity.

PHARMACOKINETICS

Interferon alfa-2a
Well absorbed after IM, subcutaneous administration. Undergoes proteolytic degradation during reabsorption in kidney. ***Half-life:*** IM: 2 hrs; Subcutaneous: 3 hrs.
Interferon alfa-2b
Well absorbed after IM, subcutaneous administration. Undergoes proteolytic degradation during reabsorption in kidney. ***Half-life:*** 2–3 hrs.

AVAILABILITY

Interferon alfa-2a
Injection: 3 million units, 6 million units, 9 million units, 36 million units (Roferon-A).
Interferon alfa-2b
Injection Powder for Reconstitution: 3 million units, 5 million units, 6 million units, 10 million units, 18 million units, 25 million units, 50 million units (Intron-A).
Injection, Prefilled Syringes: 3 million units, 5 million units, 6 million units, 10 million units, 18 million units, 25 million units, 50 million units (Intron-A).

INDICATIONS AND DOSAGES

▸ **Hairy Cell Leukemia**
Interferon alfa-2a
SUBCUTANEOUS/IM
Adults. Initially, 3 million units/day for 16– 24 wks. Maintenance: 3 million units 3 times/wk. Do not use 36-million-unit vial.
Interferon alfa-2b
SUBCUTANEOUS/IM
Adults. 2 million units/m2 3 times/wk. If severe adverse reactions occur, modify dose or temporarily discontinue.

▸ **Chronic Myelocytic Leukemia (CML)**
Interferon alfa-2a
SUBCUTANEOUS/IM
Adults. 9 million units daily.

▸ **Condylomata Acuminate**
Interferon alfa-2b
INTRALESIONAL
Adults. 1 million units/lesion 3 times/wk for 3 wks. Use only 10-million-units vial, reconstitute with no more than 1 ml diluent. Use tuberculin (TB) syringe with 25- or 26-gauge needle. Give in evening

with acetaminophen, which alleviates side effects.

▸ **Melanoma**

Interferon alfa-2a
SUBCUTANEOUS/IM
Adults, Elderly. 12 million units/m^2 3 times/wk for 3 mos.
Interferon alfa-2b
IV
Adults. Initially, 20 million units/m^2 5 times/wk for 4 wks. Maintenance: 10 million units IM/Subcutaneous for 48 wks.

▸ **AIDS-Related Kaposi's Sarcoma**

Interferon alfa-2a
SUBCUTANEOUS/IM
Adults. Initially, 36 million units/day for 10–12 wks, may give 3 million units on day 1; 9 million units on day 2; 18 million units on day 3; then begin 36 million units/day for remainder of 10–12 wks. Maintenance: 36 million units/day 3 times/wk.
Interferon alfa-2b
SUBCUTANEOUS/IM
Adults. 30 million units/m2 3 times/wk. Use only 50 million units vials. If severe adverse reactions occur, modify dose or temporarily discontinue.

▸ **Chronic Hepatitis B**

Interferon alfa-2b
SUBCUTANEOUS/IM
Adults. 30–35 million units/wk, 5 million units/day or 10 million units 3 times/wk.

▸ **Chronic Hepatitis C**

Interferon alfa-2a
SUBCUTANEOUS/IM
Adults. Initially, 6 million units once a day for 3 wks, then 3 million units 3 times/wk for 6 mos.
Interferon alfa-2b
SUBCUTANEOUS/IM
Adults. 3 million units 3 times/wk for up to 6 mos, for up to 18–24 mos for chronic hepatitis C.

OFF-LABEL USES

Interferon alfa-2a
Treatment of active, chronic hepatitis, bladder or renal carcinoma, malignant melanoma, multiple myeloma, mycosis fungoides, non-Hodgkin's lymphoma
Interferon alfa-2b
Treatment of bladder, cervical, renal carcinoma, chronic myelocytic leukemia, laryngeal papillomatosis, multiple myeloma, mycosis fungoides

CONTRAINDICATIONS

Hypersensitivity to any component of the formulations

INTERACTIONS

Drug

Bone marrow depressants: May have additive effect.

Herbal

None known.

Food

None known.

Drug interactions of concern to dentistry

- Risk of hepatotoxicity in severe liver disease: acetaminophen

DIAGNOSTIC TEST EFFECTS

May increase LDH concentration, serum alkaline phosphatase, SGOT (AST), and SGPT (ALT) levels. May decrease blood Hgb and Hct, and leukocyte and platelet counts.

IV INCOMPATIBILITIES

No information available. Do not mix with other medications via Y-site administration.

SIDE EFFECTS

Frequent

Interferon alfa-2a: Flulike symptoms, including fever, fatigue, headache, aches, pains, anorexia, and chills, nausea, vomiting,

I

coughing, dyspnea, hypotension, edema, chest pain, dizziness, diarrhea, weight loss, taste change, abdominal discomfort, confusion, paresthesia, depression, visual and sleep disturbances, diaphoresis, lethargy
Interferon alfa-2b: Flulike symptoms, including fever, fatigue, headache, aches, pains, anorexia, and chills, rash with hairy cell leukemia (Kaposi's sarcoma only)
Kaposi's sarcoma: All previously mentioned side effects plus depression, dyspepsia, dry mouth or thirst, alopecia, rigors

Occasional

Interferon alfa-2a: Partial alopecia, rash, dry throat or skin, pruritus, flatulence, constipation, hypertension, palpitations, sinusitis
Interferon alfa-2b: Dizziness, pruritus, dry skin, dermatitis, alteration in taste

Rare

Interferon alfa-2a: Hot flashes, hypermotility, Raynaud's syndrome, bronchospasm, earache, ecchymosis
Interferon alfa-2b: Confusion, leg cramps, back pain, gingivitis, flushing, tremor, nervousness, eye pain

SERIOUS REACTIONS

! Arrhythmias, stroke, transient ischemic attacks, congestive heart failure (CHF), pulmonary edema, and myocardial infarction (MI) occur rarely with interferon alfa-2a.
! Hypersensitivity reaction occurs rarely with interferon alfa-2b.
! Severe adverse reactions of flu-like symptoms appear dose related with interferon alfa-2b.

DENTAL CONSIDERATIONS

General:

- Determine why the patient is taking the drug.
- Monitor vital signs at every appointment because of cardiovascular side effects.
- After supine positioning, have patient sit upright for at least 2 min to avoid orthostatic hypotension.
- Palliative medication may be required for oral side effects.
- Assess salivary flow as a factor in caries, periodontal disease, and candidiasis.
- Patients on chronic drug therapy may rarely have symptoms of blood dyscrasias, which can include infection, bleeding, and poor healing.
- Consider semisupine chair position for patient comfort if GI side effects occur.
- Avoid elective dental procedures if severe neutropenia (<500 cells/mm^3) or thrombocytopenia (<50,000 cell/mm^3) is present.
- Antibiotic prophylaxis is indicated in severely neutropenic patients.
- Patient history should include all medications and herbal or nonherbal remedies taken by the patient.
- Severe side effects may require deferring elective dental procedures until drug therapy is completed.
- Evaluate efficacy of oral hygiene home care; preventive appointments may be necessary.

Consultations:

- Medical consultation may be required to assess disease control.
- In a patient with symptoms of blood dyscrasias, request a medical consultation for blood studies and postpone treatment until normal values are reestablished
- Liver function tests may be required to determine chronic liver disease.

Teach Patient/Family:

- Importance of good oral hygiene to prevent soft tissue inflammation

- To report oral lesions, soreness, or bleeding to dentist
- Importance of updating medical/drug records if physician makes any changes in evaluation or drug regimens
- *When chronic dry mouth occurs, advise patient:*
  - To avoid mouth rinses with high alcohol content because of drying effects
  - To use sugarless gum, frequent sips of water, or saliva substitutes
  - To use daily home fluoride products for anticaries effect

interferon alfa-2b

inn-ter-fear′-on
(Intron-A)
Do not confuse interferon alfa-2b with interferon alfa-2a.

CATEGORY AND SCHEDULE

Pregnancy Risk Category: C

MECHANISM OF ACTION

A biological response modifier that inhibits viral replication in virus-infected cells, suppresses cell proliferation, increases phagocytic action of macrophages, and augments specific cytotoxicity of lymphocytes for target cells. ***Therapeutic Effect:*** Prevents rapid growth of malignant cells; inhibits hepatitis virus.

PHARMACOKINETICS

Well absorbed after IM and subcutaneous administration. Undergoes proteolytic degradation during reabsorption in kidneys. ***Half-life:*** 2–3 hr.

AVAILABILITY

Injection (Multidose Vial): 6 million units/ml, 10 million units/ml.
Injection (Single Dose Vial): 3 million units/0.5 ml, 5 million units/0.5 ml, 10 million units/ml.
Injection (Prefilled Solution): 3 million units/0.2 ml, 5 million units/0.2 ml, 10 million units/0.2 ml.

INDICATIONS AND DOSAGES

▸ **Hairy Cell Leukemia**
IM, SUBCUTANEOUS
Adults. 2 million units/m^2 3 times a week. If severe adverse reactions occur, modify dose or temporarily discontinue drug.

▸ **Condyloma Acuminatum**
INTRALESIONAL
Adults. 1 million units/lesion 3 times a week for 3 wk.
Use only 10-million-unit vial, and reconstitute with no more than 1 ml diluent.

▸ **AIDS-Related Kaposi's Sarcoma**
IM, SUBCUTANEOUS
Adults. 30 million units/m^2 3 times a week. Use only 50-million-unit vials. If severe adverse reactions occur, modify dose or temporarily discontinue drug.

▸ **Chronic Hepatitis C**
IM, SUBCUTANEOUS
Adults. 3 million units 3 times a week for up to 6 mo. For patients who tolerate therapy and whose ALT(SGPT) level normalizes within 16 weeks, therapy may be extended for up to 18–24 mo.

▸ **Chronic Hepatitis B**
IM, SUBCUTANEOUS
Adults. 30–35 million units weekly, either as 5 million units/day or 10 million units 3 times a week.

▸ **Malignant Melanoma**
IV
Adults. Initially, 20 million units/m^2 5 times a week for 4 wk.
Maintenance: 10 million units IM or subcutaneously 3 times a week for 48 wk.

I

▸ **Follicular Lymphoma**
SUBCUTANEOUS
Adults. 5 million units 3 times a week for up to 18 mo.

OFF-LABEL USES
Treatment of bladder, cervical, or renal carcinoma; chronic myelocytic leukemia; laryngeal papillomatosis; multiple myeloma; mycosis fungoides

CONTRAINDICATIONS
None known.

INTERACTIONS
Drug
Bone marrow depressants: May increase myelosuppression.
Herbal
None known.
Food
None known.
Drug interactions of concern to dentistry
• Risk of hepatotoxicity in severe liver disease: acetaminophen

DIAGNOSTIC TEST EFFECTS
May increase PT, aPTT, and serum LDH, alkaline phosphatase, AST(SGOT), and ALT(SGPT) levels. May decrease blood Hgb level, Hct, and leukocyte and platelet counts.

IV INCOMPATIBILITIES
No information available. Do not mix with other medications for Y-site administration.

SIDE EFFECTS
Frequent
Flulike symptoms, rash (only in patients with hairy cell leukemia Kaposi's sarcoma)
Patients with Kaposi's sarcoma: All previously mentioned side effects plus depression, dyspepsia, dry mouth or thirst, alopecia, rigors
Occasional
Dizziness, pruritus, dry skin, dermatitis, altered taste
Rare
Confusion, leg cramps, back pain, gingivitis, flushing, tremor, nervousness, eye pain

SERIOUS REACTIONS
! Hypersensitivity reactions occur rarely.
! Severe flulike symptoms may occur at higher doses.

DENTAL CONSIDERATIONS
General:
• Determine why the patient is taking the drug.
• Monitor vital signs at every appointment because of cardiovascular side effects.
• Palliative medication may be required for oral side effects.
• Assess salivary flow as a factor in caries, periodontal disease, and candidiasis.
• Patients on chronic drug therapy may rarely have symptoms of blood dyscrasias, which can include infection, bleeding, and poor healing.
• Consider semisupine chair position for patient comfort if GI side effects occur.
• Avoid elective dental procedures if severe neutropenia (>500 cells/mm^3) or thrombocytopenia (>50,000 cell/mm^3) is present.
• Antibiotic prophylaxis is indicated in severely neutropenic patients.
• Patient history should include all medications and herbal or nonherbal remedies taken by the patient.
• Severe side effects may require deferring elective dental procedures until drug therapy is completed.

• Evaluate efficacy of oral hygiene home care; preventive appointments may be necessary.

Consultations:

• Medical consultation may be required to assess disease control.
• In a patient with symptoms of blood dyscrasias, request a medical consultation for blood studies and postpone treatment until normal values are reestablished.
• Liver function tests may be required to determine chronic liver disease.

Teach Patient/Family:

• Importance of good oral hygiene to prevent soft tissue inflammation
• To report oral lesions, soreness, or bleeding to dentist
• Importance of updating medical/drug records if physician makes any changes in evaluation or drug regimens
• *When chronic dry mouth occurs, advise patient:*
  • To avoid mouth rinses with high alcohol content because of drying effects
  • To use sugarless gum, frequent sips of water, or saliva substitutes
  • To use daily home fluoride products for anticaries effect

interferon alfa-n3

inn-ter-fear′-on
(Alferon N)

CATEGORY AND SCHEDULE

Pregnancy Risk Category: C

MECHANISM OF ACTION

A biological response modifier that inhibits viral replication in virus-infected cells, suppresses cell proliferation, increases phagocytic action of macrophages, and augments specific cytotoxicity of lymphocytes for target cells.
Therapeutic Effect: Inhibits viral growth in condylomata acuminatum.

AVAILABILITY

Injection: 5 million international units/ml.

INDICATIONS AND DOSAGES

▸ **Condyloma Acuminatum**

INTRALESIONAL

Adults, Children 18 yr and older. 0.05 ml (250,000 international units) per wart twice a week up to 8 wk. Maximum dose/treatment session: 0.5 ml (2.5 million international units). Do not repeat for 3 mo after initial 8 wk course unless warts enlarge or new warts appear.

I

OFF-LABEL USES

Treatment of active chronic hepatitis, bladder carcinoma, chronic myelocytic leukemia, laryngeal papillomatosis, malignant melanoma, multiple myeloma, mycosis fungoides, non-Hodgkin's lymphoma

CONTRAINDICATIONS

Previous history of anaphylactic reaction to egg protein, mouse immunoglobulin, or neomycin

INTERACTIONS

Drug

Bone marrow depressants: May increase myelosuppression.

Herbal

None known.

Food

None known.

Drug interactions of concern to dentistry

• None reported

DIAGNOSTIC TEST EFFECTS

May increase serum LDH, alkaline phosphatase, AST(SGOT), and

ALT(SGPT) levels. May decrease blood Hgb level, Hct, and leukocyte and platelet counts.

SIDE EFFECTS

Frequent
Flulike symptoms

Occasional
Dizziness, pruritus, dry skin, dermatitis, altered taste

Rare
Confusion, leg cramps, back pain, gingivitis, flushing, tremor, nervousness, eye pain

SERIOUS REACTIONS

! Hypersensitivity reaction occurs rarely.
! Severe flulike symptoms may occur at higher doses.

DENTAL CONSIDERATIONS

General:
- Determine why the patient is taking the drug.
- Following injection, advise patient to take acetaminophen (if there are no contraindications for its use) in PM to ease flulike symptoms.
- Advise patient if dental drugs prescribed have a potential for photosensitivity.
- Consider semisupine chair position for patient comfort if GI side effects occur.

Consultations:
- Medical consultation may be required to assess disease control.

Teach Patient/Family:
- Importance of updating medical/drug records if physician makes any changes in evaluation or drug regimens

interferon gamma-1b

inn-ter-fear′-on
(Actimmune, Imukin[AUS])

CATEGORY AND SCHEDULE

Pregnancy Risk Category: C

MECHANISM OF ACTION

A biological response modifier that induces activation of macrophages in blood monocytes to phagocytes, which is necessary in the body's cellular immune response to intracellular and extracellular pathogens. Enhances phagocytic function and antimicrobial activity of monocytes. ***Therapeutic Effect:*** Decreases signs and symptoms of serious infections in chronic granulomatous disease.

PHARMACOKINETICS

Slowly absorbed after subcutaneous administration.

AVAILABILITY

Injection: 100 mcg (2 million units).

INDICATIONS AND DOSAGES

▸ Chronic Granulomatous Disease; Severe, Malignant Osteopetrosis
SUBCUTANEOUS
Adults, Children older than 1 yr.
50 mcg/m^2 (1.5 million units/m^2) in patients with body surface area (BSA) greater than 0.5 m^2;
1.5 mcg/kg/dose in patients with BSA 0.5 m^2 or less.
Give 3 times a week.

CONTRAINDICATIONS

Hypersensitivity to *Escherichia coli*-derived products

INTERACTIONS

Drug
Bone marrow depressants: May increase myelosuppression.

Herbal
None known.
Food
None known.
Drug interactions of concern to dentistry
• None reported

DIAGNOSTIC TEST EFFECTS
None known.

SIDE EFFECTS
Frequent
Fever (52%); headache (33%); rash (17%); chills, fatigue, diarrhea (14%)
Occasional (13%–10%)
Vomiting, nausea
Rare (6%–3%)
Weight loss, myalgia, anorexia

SERIOUS REACTIONS
! Interferon gamma-1b may exacerbate pre-existing CNS disturbances, including decreased mental status, gait disturbance, and dizziness, as well as cardiac disorders.

DENTAL CONSIDERATIONS
General:
• Determine why the patient is taking the drug.
• Patients on chronic drug therapy may rarely have symptoms of blood dyscrasias, which can include infection, bleeding, and poor healing.
• Ask patient about side effects associated with drug use (abnormal hematologic values).
• Consider semisupine chair position for patient comfort if GI side effects occur.
• Place on frequent recall to evaluate healing response.
• Severe side effects may require deferring elective dental procedures until drug therapy is completed.
• Antibiotic prophylaxis is indicated in severely neutropenic patients.
• Avoid elective dental procedures if severe neutropenia (<500 cells/mm^3) or thrombocytopenia (<50,000 cell/mm^3) is present.
Consultations:
• In a patient with symptoms of blood dyscrasias, request a medical consultation for blood studies and postpone dental treatment until normal values are reestablished.
• Medical consultation may be required to assess disease control and patient's ability to tolerate stress.
Teach Patient/Family:
• Importance of good oral hygiene to prevent soft tissue inflammation
• Caution to prevent trauma when using oral hygiene aids
• Importance of updating medical history/drug records if physician makes any changes in evaluation or drug regimens

ipratropium bromide
eye-pra-troep′-ee-um
(Apo-Ipravent[CAN], Aproven[AUS], Atrovent, Atrovent Aerosol[AUS], Atrovent Nasal[AUS], Atrovent NPH, Novo-Ipramide[CAN], Nu-Ipratropium[CAN], PMS-Ipratropium[CAN])
Do not confuse Atrovent with Alupent.

CATEGORY AND SCHEDULE
Pregnancy Risk Category: B

MECHANISM OF ACTION
An anticholinergic that blocks the action of acetylcholine at parasympathetic sites in bronchial smooth muscle. ***Therapeutic Effect:*** Causes bronchodilation and inhibits nasal secretions.

PHARMACOKINETICS

Route	Onset	Peak	Duration
Inhalation	1–3 min	1–2 hr	4–6 hr

Minimal systemic absorption after inhalation. Metabolized in the liver (systemic absorption). Primarily eliminated in feces. ***Half-life:*** 1.5–4 hr.

AVAILABILITY

Oral Inhalation: 18 mcg/actuation.
Aerosol Solution for Inhalation: 0.02%.
Nasal Spray: 0.03%, 0.06%.

INDICATIONS AND DOSAGES

▸ Bronchospasm, Acute Treatment

INHALATION
Adults, Elderly, Children. 4–8 puffs as needed.
NEBULIZATION
Adults, Elderly, Children 12 yr and older. 500 mcg q30min for 3 doses, then q2–4h as needed.
Children younger than 12 yr. 250 mcg q20min for 3 doses, then q2–4h as needed.

▸ Bronchospasm, Maintenance Treatment

INHALATION
Adults, Elderly, Children 12 yr and older. 2–3 puffs q6h.
Children younger than 12 yr. 1–2 puffs q6h.
NEBULIZATION
Adults, Elderly, Children 12 yr and older. 500 mcg q6h.
Children younger than 12 yr. 250–500 mcg q6h.

▸ Rhinorrhea

INTRANASAL
Adults, Children older than 5 yr. 2 sprays of 0.06% solution 3–4 times a day.
Adults, Children older than 6 yr. 2 sprays of (0.03%) solution 2–3 times a day.

CONTRAINDICATIONS

History of hypersensitivity to atropine

INTERACTIONS

Drug
Cromolyn inhalation solution: Avoid mixing these drugs because they form a precipitate.
Herbal
None known.
Food
None known.
Drug interactions of concern to dentistry
- Increased effects of anticholinergic drugs

DIAGNOSTIC TEST EFFECTS

None known.

SIDE EFFECTS

Frequent
Inhalation (6%–3%): Cough, dry mouth, headache, nausea
Nasal: Dry nose and mouth, headache, nasal irritation
Occasional
Inhalation (2%): Dizziness, transient increased bronchospasm
Rare (< 1%)
Inhalation: Hypotension, insomnia, metallic or unpleasant taste, palpitations, urine retention
Nasal: Diarrhea or constipation, dry throat, abdominal pain, stuffy nose

SERIOUS REACTIONS

! Worsening of angle-closure glaucoma, acute eye pain, and hypotension occur rarely.

DENTAL CONSIDERATIONS

General:
- Monitor vital signs at every appointment because of cardiovascular and respiratory side effects.
- Assess salivary flow as a factor in caries, periodontal disease, and candidiasis.

- Acute asthmatic episodes may be precipitated in the dental office. Sympathomimetic inhalants should be available for emergency use.
- Consider semisupine chair position for patients with respiratory disease.
- Place on frequent recall because of oral side effects.

Consultations:

- Medical consultation may be required to assess disease control and patient's ability to tolerate stress.

Teach Patient/Family:

- For inhalation dosage forms, rinse mouth with water after each dose to prevent dryness
- *When chronic dry mouth occurs, advise patient:*
  - To avoid mouth rinses with high alcohol content because of drying effects
  - To use sugarless gum, frequent sips of water, or saliva substitutes
  - To use daily home fluoride products for anticaries effect

irbesartan

erb′-ba-sar-tan

(Avapro, Karvea[AUS])

CATEGORY AND SCHEDULE

Pregnancy Risk Category: C (D if used in second or third trimester)

MECHANISM OF ACTION

An angiotensin II receptor, type AT_1, antagonist that blocks the vasoconstrictor and aldosterone-secreting effects of angiotensin II, inhibiting the binding of angiotensin II to the AT_1 receptors. ***Therapeutic Effect:*** Causes vasodilation, decreases peripheral resistance, and decreases BP.

PHARMACOKINETICS

Rapidly and completely absorbed after PO administration. Protein binding: 90%. Undergoes hepatic metabolism to inactive metabolite. Recovered primarily in feces and, to a lesser extent, in urine. Not removed by hemodialysis. ***Half-life:*** 11–15 hr.

AVAILABILITY

Tablets: 75 mg, 150 mg, 300 mg.

INDICATIONS AND DOSAGES

▸ Hypertension Alone or in Combination with Other Antihypertensives

PO

Adults, Elderly, Children 13 yr and older. Initially, 75–150 mg/day. May increase to 300 mg/day.

Children 6–12 yr. Initially, 75 mg/day. May increase to 150 mg/day.

▸ Nephropathy

PO

Adults, Elderly. Target dose of 300 mg/day.

OFF-LABEL USES

Treatment of heart failure

CONTRAINDICATIONS

Bilateral renal artery stenosis, biliary cirrhosis or obstruction, primary hyperaldosteronism, severe hepatic insufficiency

INTERACTIONS

Drug

Hydrochlorothiazide: Further reduces BP.

Herbal

None known.

Food

None known.

Drug interactions of concern to dentistry

- None reported

DIAGNOSTIC TEST EFFECTS
May slightly increase BUN and serum creatinine levels. May decrease blood Hgb level.

SIDE EFFECTS
Occasional (9%–3%)
Upper respiratory tract infection, fatigue, diarrhea, cough
Rare (2%–1%)
Heartburn, dizziness, headache, nausea, rash

SERIOUS REACTIONS
! Overdosage may manifest as hypotension and tachycardia. Bradycardia occurs less often.

I

DENTAL CONSIDERATIONS
General:
- Monitor vital signs at every appointment because of cardiovascular side effects.
- Limit use of sodium-containing products, such as saline IV fluids, for those patients with a dietary salt restriction.
- Stress from dental procedures may compromise cardiovascular function; determine patient risk.
- Short appointments and a stress reduction protocol may be required for anxious patients.
- Use precaution if sedation or general anesthesia is required; risk of hypotensive episode.
- After supine positioning, have patient sit upright for at least 2 min before standing to avoid orthostatic hypotension.
- Consider semisupine chair position for patient comfort if GI side effects occur.

Consultations:
- Consultation with physician may be necessary if sedation or general anesthesia is required.
- Medical consultation may be required to assess disease control and patient's ability to tolerate stress; risk of hypotensive episode.

Teach Patient/Family:
- Importance of updating health and drug history if physician makes any changes in evaluation or drug regimens

isocarboxazid
eye-soe-kar-box′-a-zid
(Marplan)

CATEGORY AND SCHEDULE
Pregnancy Risk Category: C

MECHANISM OF ACTION
An antidepressant that inhibits the MAO enzyme system at central nervous system (CNS) storage sites. The reduced MAO activity causes an increased concentration in epinephrine, norepinephrine, serotonin, and dopamine at neuron receptor sites.
Therapeutic Effect: Produces antidepressant effect.

AVAILABILITY
Tablets: 10 mg (Marplan).

INDICATIONS AND DOSAGES
▸ Depression Refractory to Other Antidepressants or Electroconvulsive Therapy
PO
Adults, Elderly. Initially, 10 mg 3 times/day. May increase to 60 mg/day.

OFF-LABEL USES
Treatment of panic disorder, vascular or tension headaches

CONTRAINDICATIONS
Cardiovascular disease (CVD), cerebrovascular disease, liver impairment, pheochromocytoma, liver impairment

INTERACTIONS

Drug

Alcohol, CNS depressants: May increase CNS depressant effects.
Buspirone: May increase blood pressure (B/P).
Caffeine-containing medications: May increase cardiac arrhythmias and hypertension.
Carbamazepine, cyclobenzaprine, maprotiline, other MAOIs: May precipitate hypertensive crises.
Fluoxetine, trazodone, tricyclic antidepressants: May cause serotonin syndrome.
Insulin, oral hypoglycemics: May increase effects of insulin and oral hypoglycemics.
Meperidine, other opioid analgesics: May produce coma, convulsions, death, diaphoresis, immediate excitation, rigidity, severe hypertension or hypotension, severe respiratory distress, or vascular collapse.
Methylphenidate: May increase the CNS stimulant effects of methylphenidate.
Sympathomimetics: May increase the cardiac stimulant and vasopressor effects of isocarboxazid.
Tyramine: May cause severe, sudden hypertension.

Herbal

None known.

Food

None known.

Drug interactions of concern to dentistry

- Increased pressor effects: indirect-acting sympathomimetics (ephedrine)
- Hyperpyretic crisis, convulsions, hypertensive episode: meperidine, possibly other opioids, carbamazepine
- Increased anticholinergic effects: anticholinergics, antihistamines
- Increased effects of alcohol, barbiturates, benzodiazepines, CNS depressants, SSRIs, tricyclic antidepressants, cyclobenzaprine, bupropion, buspirone, dextromethorphan, antihypertensives

DIAGNOSTIC TEST EFFECTS

None known.

SIDE EFFECTS

Frequent (> 10%)

Postural hypotension, drowsiness, decreased sexual ability, weakness, trembling, visual disturbances

Occasional (10%–1%)

Tachycardia, peripheral edema, nervousness, chills, diarrhea, anorexia, constipation, xerostomia

Rare (< 1%)

Hepatitis, leukopenia, parkinsonian syndrome

SERIOUS REACTIONS

! Hypertensive crisis, marked by severe hypertension, occipital headache radiating frontally, neck stiffness or soreness, nausea, vomiting, sweating, fever or chilliness, clammy skin, dilated pupils, palpitations, tachycardia or bradycardia, and constricting chest pain.

DENTAL CONSIDERATIONS

General:

- Monitor vital signs at every appointment because of cardiovascular side effects.
- After supine positioning, have patient sit upright for at least 2 min to avoid orthostatic hypotension.
- Patients on chronic drug therapy may rarely have symptoms of blood dyscrasias, which can include infection, bleeding, and poor healing.
- Consider semisupine chair position for patient comfort if GI side effects occur.
- Assess salivary flow as a factor in caries, periodontal disease, and candidiasis.
- Hypertensive episodes are possible even though there are no specific

contraindications to vasoconstrictor use in local anesthetics.
- Short appointments and a stress reduction protocol may be required for anxious patients.

Consultations:
- Medical consultation may be required to assess disease control and patient's ability to tolerate stress.
- In a patient with symptoms of blood dyscrasias, request a medical consultation for blood studies and postpone treatment until normal values are reestablished.

Teach Patient/Family:
- When chronic dry mouth occurs, advise patient:
  - To avoid mouth rinses with high alcohol content because of drying effects
  - To use daily home fluoride products for anticaries effect
  - To use sugarless gum, frequent sips of water, or saliva substitutes

isoetharine hydrochloride

eye-soe-eth′-a-reen
(Beta-2, Bronkosol, Dey-Lute)
(Bronkometer)

CATEGORY AND SCHEDULE
Pregnancy Risk Category: C

MECHANISM OF ACTION
A sympathomimetic (adrenergic agonist) that stimulates beta2-adrenergic receptors in the lungs, resulting in relaxation of bronchial smooth muscle. ***Therapeutic Effect:*** Relieves bronchospasm, reduces airway resistance.

PHARMACOKINETICS
Rapidly, well absorbed from the gastrointestinal (GI) tract. Extensive metabolism in GI tract. Unknown extent metabolized in liver and lungs. Excreted in urine.
Half-life: 4 hrs.

AVAILABILITY
Metered spray: 0.61% (Brokometer).
Solution for Inhalation: 0.08% (Dey-Lute), 0.1% (Dey-Lute), 0.17% (Dey-Lute), 1% (Beta-2, Brokosol).

INDICATIONS AND DOSAGES
▸ Bronchospasm

HAND-BULB NEBULIZER

Adults, Elderly. 4 inhalations (range: 3–7 inhalations) undiluted. May be repeated up to 5 times/day.

▸ Metered Dose Inhalation

Adults, Elderly. 1–2 inhalations q4h. Wait 1 min before administering 2nd inhalation.

▸ IPPB, Oxygen Aerolization

Adults, Elderly. 0.5–1 ml of a 0.5% or 0.5 ml of a 1% solution diluted 1:3.

CONTRAINDICATIONS
History of hypersensitivity to sympathomimetics

INTERACTIONS
Drug

Beta-adrenergic blocking agents (beta-blockers): Antagonizes effects of isoetharine.
Digoxin: May increase risk of arrhythmias with digoxin.
MAOIs, tricyclic antidepressants: May potentiate cardiovascular effects.

Herbal

None known.

Food

None known.

Drug interactions of concern to dentistry
- Increased effects of both drugs: other sympathomimetics
- Increased dysrhythmia: halogenated hydrocarbon anesthetics

DIAGNOSTIC TEST EFFECTS

May decrease serum potassium levels.

SIDE EFFECTS

Occasional

Tremor, nausea, nervousness, palpitations, tachycardia, peripheral vasodilation, dryness of mouth, throat, dizziness, vomiting, headache, increased B/P, insomnia.

SERIOUS REACTIONS

! Excessive sympathomimetic stimulation may produce palpitations, extrasystoles, tachycardia, chest pain, slight increase in B/P followed by a substantial decrease, chills, sweating, and blanching of skin.

! Too frequent or excessive use may lead to loss of bronchodilating effectiveness and severe and paradoxical bronchoconstriction.

DENTAL CONSIDERATIONS

General:

- Assess salivary flow as a factor in caries, periodontal disease, and candidiasis.
- Consider semisupine chair position for patients with respiratory disease.
- Acute asthmatic episodes may be precipitated in the dental office. Sympathomimetic inhalants should be available for emergency use.

Consultations:

- Medical consultation may be required to assess disease control and patient's ability to tolerate stress.

Teach Patient/Family:

- For inhalation dosage forms, rinse mouth with water after each dose to prevent dryness
- *When chronic dry mouth occurs, advise patient:*
  - To avoid mouth rinses with high alcohol content because of drying effects
  - To use sugarless gum, frequent sips of water, or saliva substitutes
  - To use daily home fluoride products for anticaries effect

isoniazid

eye-soe-nye′-a-zid

(INH, Isotamine[CAN], Nydrazid, PMS Isoniazid[CAN])

CATEGORY AND SCHEDULE

Pregnancy Risk Category: C

MECHANISM OF ACTION

An isonicotinic acid derivative that inhibits mycolic acid synthesis and causes disruption of the bacterial cell wall and loss of acid-fast properties in susceptible mycobacteria. Active only during bacterial cell division. ***Therapeutic Effect:*** Bactericidal against actively growing intracelleluar and extracellular susceptible mycobacteria.

PHARMACOKINETICS

Readily absorbed from the GI tract. Protein binding: 10%–15%. Widely distributed (including to CSF). Metabolized in the liver. Primarily excreted in urine. Removed by hemodialysis. ***Half-life:*** 0.5–5 hr.

AVAILABILITY

Tablets: 100 mg, 300 mg.
Syrup: 50 mg/5 ml.
Injection: 100 mg/ml.

INDICATIONS AND DOSAGES

▸ Tuberculosis (in combination with one or more antituberculars)

PO, IM

Adults, Elderly. 5 mg/kg/day as a single dose. Maximum 300 mg/day.
Children. 10–15 mg/kg/day as a single dose. Maximum 300 mg/day.

Prevention of Tuberculosis
PO, IM
Adults, Elderly. 300 mg/day as a single dose.
Children. 10 mg/kg/day as a single dose. Maximum 300 mg/day.

CONTRAINDICATIONS
Acute hepatic disease, history of hypersensitivity reactions or hepatic injury with previous isoniazid therapy

INTERACTIONS
Drug
Alcohol: May increase isoniazid metabolism and the risk of hepatotoxicity.
Carbamazepine, phenytoin: May increase the toxicity of these drugs.
Disulfiram: May increase CNS effects.
Hepatotoxic medications: May increase the risk of hepatotoxicity.
Ketoconazole: May decrease ketoconazole blood concentration.
Herbal
None known.
Food
Tyramine-containing foods: May cause a hypertensive crisis.
Drug interactions of concern to dentistry
- Increased hepatotoxicity: alcohol, acetaminophen, carbamazepine
- Decreased effectiveness: glucocorticoids, especially prednisolone
- Increased plasma concentration: benzodiazepines, alfentanil
- Decreased effect of ketoconazole, miconazole

DIAGNOSTIC TEST EFFECTS
May increase serum bilirubin, AST (SGOT), and ALT (SGPT) levels.

SIDE EFFECTS
Frequent
Nausea, vomiting, diarrhea, abdominal pain
Rare
Pain at injection site, hypersensitivity reaction

SERIOUS REACTIONS
! Rare reactions include neurotoxicity (as evidenced by ataxia and paraesthesia), optic neuritis, and hepatotoxicity.

DENTAL CONSIDERATIONS
General:
- Patients on chronic drug therapy may rarely have symptoms of blood dyscrasias, which can include infection, bleeding, and poor healing.
- Medical consultation may be required to assess disease control.
- Examine for evidence of oral signs of disease.

Consultations:
- In a patient with symptoms of blood dyscrasias, request a medical consultation for blood studies and postpone dental treatment until normal values are reestablished.

Teach Patient/Family:
- Caution to prevent injury when using oral hygiene aids

isoproterenol
eye-soe-proe-ter′-e-nole
(Isuprel)

CATEGORY AND SCHEDULE
Pregnancy Risk Category: C

MECHANISM OF ACTION
A sympathomimetic (adrenergic agonist) that stimulates beta1-adrenergic receptors.
Therapeutic Effect: Increases myocardial contractility, stroke volume, cardiac output.

PHARMACOKINETICS
Readily absorbed. Metabolized in liver. Primarily excreted in urine. ***Half-life:*** 2.5–5 min.

AVAILABILITY
Injection: 0.02 mg/ml (Isuprel).

INDICATIONS AND DOSAGES
▸ Arrhythmias
IV BOLUS
Adults, Elderly. Initially, 0.02–0.06 mg (1–3 ml of diluted solution). Subsequent dose range: 0.01–0.2 mg (0.5–10 ml of diluted solution).
IV INFUSION
Adults, Elderly. Initially, 5 mcg/min (1.25 ml/min of diluted solution). Subsequent dose range: 2–20 mcg/min.
Children. 2.5 mcg/min or 0.1 mcg/kg per min.

▸ Complete Heart Block Following Closure of Ventricular Septal Defects
IV
Adults, Elderly. 0.04–0.06 mg (2–3 ml of diluted solution).
Infants. 0.01–0.03 (0.5–1.5 ml of diluted solution).

▸ Shock
IV INFUSION
Adults, Elderly. Rate of 0.5–5 mcg/min (0.25–2.5 ml of 1:500,000 dilution); rate of infusion on the basis of clinical response (heart rate, central venous pressure, systemic B/P, urine flow measurements).

CONTRAINDICATIONS
Tachycardia due to digitalis toxicity, preexisting arrhythmias, angina, precordial distress, hypersensitivity to isoproterenol or any component of the formulation

INTERACTIONS
Drug
Beta-blockers: May antagonize the effects of isoproterenol. **Digoxin:** May increase the risk of arrhythmias. Tricyclic antidepressants: May increase cardiovascular effects.

Herbal
Ma huang: May increase CNS stimulation.

Food
None known.

Drug interactions of concern to dentistry
- Hypotension, tachycardia: haloperidol, loxapine, phenothiazines, thioxanthenes
- Increased dysrhythmia: halogenated-hydrocarbon anesthetics

DIAGNOSTIC TEST EFFECTS
Decreases serum potassium levels

IV INCOMPATIBILITIES
None known.

SIDE EFFECTS
Frequent
Palpitations, tachycardia, restlessness, nervousness, tremor, insomnia, anxiety

Occasional
Increased sweating, headache, nausea, flushed skin, dizziness, coughing

SERIOUS REACTIONS
! Excessive sympathomimetic stimulation may cause palpitations, extrasystoles, tachycardia, chest pain, slight increase in B/P followed by a substantial decrease, chills, sweating, and blanching of skin.
! Ventricular arrhythmias may occur if heart rate is above 130 beats/min.
! Parotid gland swelling may occur with prolonged use.

DENTAL CONSIDERATIONS
General:
- This drug is used only in conjunction with general anesthesia procedures.

isosorbide

eye-soe-sor′-bide

isosorbide dinitrate (Apo-ISDN[CAN], Cedocard[CAN], Dilatrate, Isogen[AUS], Isordil, Sorbidin[AUS])isosorbide mononitrate(Duride[AUS], Imdur, Imtrate[AUS], ISMO, Monodur Durules[AUS], Monoket)

Do not confuse with Inderal, Isuprel, K-Dur, or Plendil.

CATEGORY AND SCHEDULE

Pregnancy Risk Category: C

I

MECHANISM OF ACTION

A nitrate that stimulates intracellular cyclic guanosine monophosphate (GMP.) ***Therapeutic Effect:*** Relaxes vascular smooth muscle of both arterial and venous vasculature. Decreases preload and afterload.

PHARMACOKINETICS

Route	Onset	Peak	Duration
Sublingual	2–10 min	N/A	1–2 hrs
Chewable	3 min	N/A	0.5–2 hrs
PO	45–60 min	N/A	4–6 hrs
Sustained-release	30 min	N/A	6–12 hrs

Mononitrate well absorbed after PO administration. Dinitrate poorly absorbed and metabolized in the liver to its activate metabolite isosorbide mononitrate. Excreted in urine and feces. ***Half-life:*** Dinitrate is 1–4 hrs and mononitrate is 4 hrs.

AVAILABILITY

Tablets: 5 mg (Isordil), 10 mg (Isordil, Monoket), 20 mg (Isordil, Ismo, Monoket), 30 mg (Isordil), 40 mg (Isordil).
Tablets (chewable): 5 mg, 10 mg.
Tablets (sublingual): 10 mg (Isordil).
Capsules (sustained-release): 40 mg (Dilatrate-SR).
Tablets (extended-release): 30 mg, 60 mg, 120 mg (Imdur).

INDICATIONS AND DOSAGES

▸ **Acute Angina, Prophylactic Management in Situations Likely to Provoke Attack**

SUBLINGUAL

Adults, Elderly. Initially, 2.5–5 mg. Repeat at 5–10 min intervals. No more than 3 doses in 15–30 min period.

▸ **Acute Prophylactic Management of Angina**

SUBLINGUAL

Adults, Elderly. 5–10 mg q2–3h.

▸ **Long-Term Prophylaxis of Angina**

PO

Adults, Elderly. Initially, 5–20 mg 3–4 times/day. Maintenance: 10–40 mg q6h. Consider 2–3 times/day, last dose no later than 7 pm to minimize intolerance.

PO (Mononitrate)

Adults, Elderly. 20 mg 2 times/day, 7 hrs apart. First dose upon awakening in morning.

PO (extended-release)

Adults, Elderly. Initially, 40 mg. Maintenance: 40–80 mg 2–3 times/day. Consider 1–2 times/day, last dose at 2 pm to minimize intolerance.

PO (Imdur)

Adults, Elderly. 60–120 mg/day as single dose.

▸ **Congestive Heart Failure**

PO (Chewable)

Adults, Elderly. 5–10 mg every 2–3 hours.

OFF-LABEL USES

Congestive heart failure (CHF), dysphagia, pain relief, relief of esophageal spasm with gastroesophageal (GE) reflux

CONTRAINDICATIONS

Closed-angle glaucoma, gastrointestinal (GI) hypermotility or malabsorption (extended-release tablets), head trauma, hypersensitivity to nitrates, increased intracranial pressure, postural hypotension, severe anemia (extended-release tablets)

INTERACTIONS

Drug

Alcohol, antihypertensives, vasodilators: May increase risk of orthostatic hypotension.

Herbal

None known.

Food

None known.

Drug interactions of concern to dentistry

- Increased effects: alcohol, other vasodilator-type drugs
- Severe hypotension: sildenafil, vardenafil, tadalafil

DIAGNOSTIC TEST EFFECTS

May increase urine catecholamines, urine VMA (vanillylmandelic acid).

SIDE EFFECTS

Frequent

Burning and tingling at oral point of dissolution (sublingual), headache (may be severe) occurs mostly in early therapy, diminishes rapidly in intensity, usually disappears during continued treatment; transient flushing of face and neck, dizziness (especially if patient is standing immobile or is in a warm environment), weakness, postural hypotension, nausea, vomiting, restlessness

Occasional

GI upset, blurred vision, dry mouth

SERIOUS REACTIONS

! Blurred vision or dry mouth may occur (drug should be discontinued).

! Severe postural hypotension manifested by fainting, pulselessness, cold or clammy skin, and diaphoresis may occur.

! Tolerance may occur with repeated, prolonged therapy (minor tolerance with intermittent use of sublingual tablets). Tolerance may not occur with extended-release form.

! High dose tends to produce severe headache.

DENTAL CONSIDERATIONS

General:

- Monitor vital signs at every appointment because of cardiovascular side effects.
- After supine positioning, have patient sit upright for at least 2 min before standing to avoid orthostatic hypotension.
- Stress from dental procedures may compromise cardiovascular function; determine patient risk.
- Assess salivary flow as a factor in caries, periodontal disease, and candidiasis.
- Short appointments and a stress reduction protocol may be required for anxious patients.
- Consider semisupine chair position for patients with respiratory distress.
- Use vasoconstrictors with caution, in low doses, and with careful aspiration. Avoid use of gingival retraction cord with epinephrine.
- Nitroglycerin should be available in case of an acute anginal episode.

Consultations:

- Medical consultation may be required to assess disease control and patient's ability to tolerate stress.

Teach Patient/Family:

- *When chronic dry mouth occurs, advise patient:*
  - To avoid mouth rinses with high alcohol content because of drying effects

• To use sugarless gum, frequent sips of water, or saliva substitutes
• To use daily home fluoride products for anticaries effect

isosorbide dinitrate/isosorbide mononitrate

(isosorbide dinitrate) Apo-ISDN[CAN], Cedocard[CAN], Dilatrate, Isogen[AUS], Isordil, Sorbidin[AUS](isosorbide mononitrate) Duride[AUS], Imdur, Imdur Durules[AUS], Imtrate[AUS], ISMO, Monodur Durules[AUS], Monoket

Do not confuse Isordil with Isuprel or Plendil, or Imdur with Inderal or K-Dur.

CATEGORY AND SCHEDULE

Pregnancy Risk Category: C

MECHANISM OF ACTION

A nitrate that stimulates intracellular cyclic guanosine monophosphate. ***Therapeutic Effect:*** Relaxes vascular smooth muscle of both arterial and venous vasculature. Decreases preload and afterload.

PHARMACOKINETICS

Route	Onset	Peak	Duration
Dinitrate Sublingual	2–5 min	N/A	1–2 hr
Oral (Chewable)	2–5 min	N/A	1–2 hr
Oral	15–40 min	N/A	4–6 hr
Oral (Sustained-Release)	30 min	N/A	12 hr
Mononitrate Oral (Extended-Release)	60 min	N/A	N/A

Dinitrate poorly absorbed and metabolized in the liver to its activate metabolite isosorbide mononitrate. Mononitrate well absorbed after PO administration. Excreted in urine and feces. ***Half-life:*** Dinitrate, 1–4 hr; mononitrate, 4 hr.

AVAILABILITY

Capsules (Sustained-Release [Dilatrate]): 40 mg.
Tablets (Isordil): 5 mg, 10 mg, 20 mg, 30 mg, 40 mg.
Tablets (Ismo, Monoket): 10 mg, 20 mg.
Tablets (Chewable): 5 mg, 10 mg.
Tablets (Extended-Release [Imdur]): 30 mg, 60 mg, 120 mg.
Tablets (Sublingual [Isordil]): 10 mg.

INDICATIONS AND DOSAGES

▸ Angina

PO (isosorbide dinitrate)
Adults, Elderly. 5–40 mg 4 times a day. Sustained-release: 40 mg q8–12h.
PO (isosorbide mononitrate)
Adults, Elderly. 5–10 mg twice a day given 7 hours apart. Sustained-release: Initially, 30–60 mg/day in morning as a single dose. May increase dose at 3 day intervals. Maximum: 240 mg/day.

OFF-LABEL USES

CHF, dysphagia, pain relief, relief of esophageal spasm with gastroesophageal reflux

CONTRAINDICATIONS

Closed-angle glaucoma, GI hypermotility or malabsorption (extended-release tablets), head trauma, hypersensitivity to nitrates, increased intracranial pressure, orthostatic hypotension, severe anemia (extended-release tablets)

INTERACTIONS

Drug

Alcohol, antihypertensives, vasodilators: May increase risk of orthostatic hypotension.

Herbal

None known.

Food

None known.

Drug interactions of concern to dentistry

- Increased effects: alcohol and other drugs that can lower blood pressure
- Severe hypotension: sildenafil, vardenafil, tadalafil

DIAGNOSTIC TEST EFFECTS

May increase urine catecholamine and urine vanillylmandelic acid levels.

SIDE EFFECTS

Frequent

Burning and tingling at oral point of dissolution (sublingual), headache (possibly severe) occurs mostly in early therapy, diminishes rapidly in intensity, and usually disappears during continued treatment, transient flushing of face and neck, dizziness (especially if patient is standing immobile or is in a warm environment), weakness, orthostatic hypotension, nausea, vomiting, restlessness

Occasional

GI upset, blurred vision, dry mouth

SERIOUS REACTIONS

! Blurred vision or dry mouth may occur (drug should be discontinued).

! Isosorbide administration may cause severe orthostatic hypotension manifested by fainting, pulselessness, cold or clammy skin, and diaphoresis.

! Tolerance may occur with repeated, prolonged therapy, but may not occur with the extended-release form. Minor tolerance may be seen with intermittent use of sublingual tablets.

! High dosage tends to produce severe headache.

DENTAL CONSIDERATIONS

General:

- Monitor vital signs at every appointment because of cardiovascular side effects.
- After supine positioning, have patient sit upright for at least 2 min before standing to avoid orthostatic hypotension.
- Assess salivary flow as a factor in caries, periodontal disease, and candidiasis.
- Stress from dental procedures may compromise cardiovascular function; determine patient risk.
- Use vasoconstrictors with caution, in low doses, and with careful aspiration. Avoid use of gingival retraction cord with epinephrine.
- Short appointments and a stress reduction protocol may be required for anxious patients.
- Nitroglycerin should be available in case of acute anginal episode.

Consultations:

- Medical consultation may be required to assess disease control and patient's ability to tolerate stress.

Teach Patient/Family:

- Importance of good oral hygiene to prevent soft tissue inflammation
- *When chronic dry mouth occurs, advise patient:*
  - To avoid mouth rinses with high alcohol content because of drying effects
  - To use sugarless gum, frequent sips of water, or saliva substitutes
  - To use daily home fluoride products for anticaries effect

isotretinoin

eye-soe-tret′-i-noyn
(Accutane, Amnesteem, Claravis, Isotrex[CAN], Sotret)
Do not confuse Accutane with Accupril or Accurbron.

CATEGORY AND SCHEDULE
Pregnancy Risk Category: X

MECHANISM OF ACTION
Reduces the size of sebaceous glands and inhibits their activity.
Therapeutic Effect: Decreases sebum production; produces antikeratinizing and anti-inflammatory effects.

I

PHARMACOKINETICS
Metabolized in the liver; major metabolite active. Eliminated in urine and feces.
Half-life: 21 hr; metabolite, 21–24 hr.

AVAILABILITY
Capsules: 10 mg, 20 mg, 40 mg.

INDICATIONS AND DOSAGES
▸ Recalcitrant Cystic Acne That Is Unresponsive to Conventional Acne Therapies
PO
Adults. Initially, 0.5–2 mg/kg/day divided into 2 doses for 15–20 wk. May repeat after at least 2 mo off therapy.

OFF-LABEL USES
Treatment of gram-negative folliculitis, severe keratinization disorders, severe rosacea

CONTRAINDICATIONS
Hypersensitivity to isotretinoin or parabens (component of capsules)

INTERACTIONS
Drug
Etretinate, tretinoin, vitamin A: May increase toxic effects.
Tetracycline: May increase the risk of pseudotumor cerebri.
Herbal
Dong quai, St John's wort: May cause photosensitization.
Food
None known.
Drug interactions of concern to dentistry
- Additive photosensitization: tetracycline
- Pseudotumor cerebri, intracranial hypertension: minocycline, doxycycline, tetracycline
- Increased tissue drying: alcohol
- Contraindicated with all tetracyclines (demeclocycline, doxycycline, minocycline, tetracycline)
- Avoid additional vitamin A supplements

DIAGNOSTIC TEST EFFECTS
May increase serum alkaline phosphatase, total cholesterol, LDH, triglyceride, ALT (SGPT), and AST (SGOT) levels; urine uric acid level; erythrocyte sedimentation rate; and fasting blood glucose level. May decrease HDL level.

SIDE EFFECTS
Frequent (90%–20%)
Cheilitis (inflammation of lips), dry skin and mucous membranes, skin fragility, pruritus, epistaxis, dry nose and mouth, conjunctivitis, hypertriglyceridemia, nausea, vomiting, abdominal pain
Occasional (16%–5%)
Musculoskeletal symptoms (including bone pain, arthralgia, generalized myalgia), photosensitivity
Rare
Decreased night vision, depression

SERIOUS REACTIONS

! Inflammatory bowel disease and pseudotumor cerebri (benign intracranial hypertension) have been associated with isotretinoin therapy.

DENTAL CONSIDERATIONS

General:

- Patients on chronic drug therapy may rarely have symptoms of blood dyscrasias, which can include infection, bleeding, and poor healing.
- Assess salivary flow as a factor in caries, periodontal disease, and candidiasis.
- Exaggerated healing response characterized by exuberant granulation tissue has been reported.
- Apply lubricant to dry lips for patient comfort before dental procedures.

Consultations:

- In a patient with symptoms of blood dyscrasias, request a medical consultation for blood studies and postpone dental treatment until normal values are reestablished.

Teach Patient/Family:

- Importance of good oral hygiene to prevent soft tissue inflammation
- *When chronic dry mouth occurs, advise patient:*
  - To avoid mouth rinses with high alcohol content because of drying effects
  - To use sugarless gum, frequent sips of water, or saliva substitutes
  - To use daily home fluoride products for anticaries effect

isoxsuprine hydrochloride

eye-**sox**-soo-preen
(Vasodilan)

CATEGORY AND SCHEDULE

Pregnancy Risk Category: C

MECHANISM OF ACTION

The mechanism of action of isoxsuprine hydrochloride is not fully understood. Increases muscle blood flow. May have a direct action on vascular smooth muscle. β-Adrenergic stimulation of the uterus. ***Therapeutic Effect:*** Relieves symptoms associated with cerebral vascular insufficiency. Inhibits preterm labor.

PHARMACOKINETICS

The pharmacokinetics of isoxsuprine hydrochloride is not fully understood. ***Half-life:*** Unknown.

AVAILABILITY

Tablets (Vasodilan): 10 mg, 20 mg

INDICATIONS AND DOSAGES

Raynaud's Syndrome

IV INFUSION

Adults, Elderly. 10–20 mg 3–4 times per day.

UNLABELED USES

Dysmenorrhea, premature labor, threatened abortion

CONTRAINDICATIONS

Arterial bleeding (recent), immediately postpartum

INTERACTIONS

Drug

None known.

Herbal

None known.

Food

None known.

Drug interactions of concern to dentistry

- Increased effects: alcohol and drugs that also lower blood pressure

DIAGNOSTIC TEST EFFECTS

None known.

SIDE EFFECTS

Rare

Hypotension, tachyarrhythmia, rash, abdominal discomfort, nausea, dizziness

SERIOUS REACTIONS

! Pulmonary edema occurs rarely.

DENTAL CONSIDERATIONS

General:

- Monitor vital signs at every appointment because of cardiovascular and respiratory side effects.
- After supine positioning, have patient sit upright for at least 2 min before standing to avoid orthostatic hypotension.
- Short appointments and a stress reduction protocol may be required for anxious patients.
- Drugs used for conscious sedation that lower blood pressure may potentiate the hypotensive effects.
- Use vasoconstrictors with caution, in low doses, and with careful aspiration. Avoid use of gingival retraction cord with epinephrine.

Consultations:

- Medical consultation may be required to assess disease control and patient's ability to tolerate stress.

isradipine

is-rad′-i-peen

(DynaCirc, DynaCirc CR)

Do not confuse DynaCirc with Dynabac or Dynacin.

CATEGORY AND SCHEDULE

Pregnancy Risk Category: C

MECHANISM OF ACTION

An antihypertensive that inhibits calcium movement across cardiac and vascular smooth-muscle cell membranes. Potent peripheral vasodilator that does not depress SA or AV nodes. ***Therapeutic Effect:*** Produces relaxation of coronary vascular smooth muscle and coronary vasodilation. Increases myocardial oxygen delivery to those with vasospastic angina.

PHARMACOKINETICS

Route	Onset	Peak	Duration
PO	2–3 hr	2–4 wk (with multiple doses) 8–16 hr (with single dose)	N/A
PO (Controlled-release)	2 hr	8–10 hr	N/A

Well absorbed from the GI tract. Protein binding: 95%. Metabolized in the liver (undergoes first-pass effect). Primarily excreted in urine. Not removed by hemodialysis. ***Half-life:*** 8 hr.

AVAILABILITY

Capsules (Dynacirc): 2.5 mg, 5 mg.
Capsules (Controlled-Release [Dynacirc-CR]): 5 mg, 10 mg.

INDICATIONS AND DOSAGES

▸ **Hypertension**

PO

Adults, Elderly. Initially 2.5 mg twice a day. May increase by 2.5 mg at 2- to 4-wk intervals. Range: 5–20 mg/day

OFF-LABEL USES

Treatment of chronic angina pectoris, Raynaud's phenomenon

CONTRAINDICATIONS
Cardiogenic shock, CHF, heart block, hypotension, sinus bradycardia, ventricular tachycardia

INTERACTIONS
Drug
Beta blockers: May have additive effect.
Herbal
None known.
Food
Grapefruit, grapefruit juice: May increase the absorption of isradipine.
Drug interactions of concern to dentistry
• Decreased effect: indomethacin, possibly other NSAIDs, phenobarbital
• Increased effect: parenteral and inhalational general anesthetics, other drugs with hypotensive actions, itraconazole
• Increased effects of carbamazepine

DIAGNOSTIC TEST EFFECTS
None known.

SIDE EFFECTS
Frequent (7%–4%)
Peripheral edema, palpitations (higher frequency in females)
Occasional (3%)
Facial flushing, cough
Rare (2%–1%)
Angina, tachycardia, rash, pruritus

SERIOUS REACTIONS
! Overdose produces nausea, drowsiness, confusion, and slurred speech.
! CHF occurs rarely.

DENTAL CONSIDERATIONS
General:
• Monitor cardiac status; take vital signs at each appointment because of cardiovascular side effects. Consider a stress reduction protocol to prevent stress-induced angina during the dental appointment.
• After supine positioning, have patient sit upright for at least 2 min before standing to avoid orthostatic hypotension.
• Place on frequent recall to monitor gingival condition.
• Limit use of sodium-containing products, such as saline IV fluids, for patients with a dietary salt restriction.
• Assess salivary flow as a factor in caries, periodontal disease, and candidiasis.
• Use vasoconstrictors with caution, in low doses, and with careful aspiration. Avoid use of gingival retraction cord with epinephrine.
• Patients on chronic drug therapy may rarely have symptoms of blood dyscrasias, which can include infection, bleeding, and poor healing.
Consultations:
• In a patient with symptoms of blood dyscrasias, request a medical consultation for blood studies and postpone dental treatment until normal values are reestablished.
• Medical consultation may be required to assess disease control and patient's ability to tolerate stress.
Teach Patient/Family:
• Importance of good oral hygiene to prevent soft tissue inflammation and minimize gingival overgrowth
• Need for frequent oral prophylaxis if overgrowth occurs
• *When chronic dry mouth occurs, advise patient:*
  • To avoid mouth rinses with high alcohol content because of drying effects
  • To use sugarless gum, frequent sips of water, or saliva substitutes
  • To use daily home fluoride products for anticaries effect

itraconazole

it-ra-con′-a-zol
(Sporanox)
Do not confuse Sporanox with Suprax.

CATEGORY AND SCHEDULE

Pregnancy Risk Category: C

MECHANISM OF ACTION

A fungistatic antifungal that inhibits the synthesis of ergosterol, a vital component of fungal cell formation
Therapeutic Effect: Damages the fungal cell membrane, altering its function.

I

PHARMACOKINETICS

Moderately absorbed from the GI tract. Absorption is increased if the drug is taken with food.
Protein binding: 99%. Widely distributed, primarily in the fatty tissue, liver, and kidneys. Metabolized in the liver to active metabolite. Primarily excreted in urine. Not removed by hemodialysis. ***Half-life:*** 21 hr; metabolite, 12 hr.

AVAILABILITY

Capsules: 100 mg.
Oral Solution: 10 mg/ml.
Injection: 10 mg/ml (25-ml ampule).

INDICATIONS AND DOSAGES

▸ **Blastomycosis, Histoplasmosis**
PO
Adults, Elderly. Initially, 200 mg once a day. Maximum: 400 mg/day in 2 divided doses.
IV
Adults, Elderly. 200 mg twice a day for 4 doses, then 200 mg once a day.

▸ **Aspergillosis**
PO
Adults, Elderly. 600 mg/day in 3 divided doses for 3–4 days, then 200–400 mg/day in 2 divided doses.
IV
Adults, Elderly. 200 mg twice a day for 4 doses, then 200 mg once a day.

▸ **Esophageal Candidiasis**
PO
Adults, Elderly. Swish 10 ml in mouth for several seconds, then swallow. Maximum: 200 mg/day.

▸ **Oropharyngeal Candidiasis**
PO
Adults, Elderly. Vigorously swish 10 ml in mouth for several seconds (20 ml total daily dose) once a day.

OFF-LABEL USES

Suppression of histoplasmosis; treatment of disseminated sporotrichosis, fungal pneumonia and septicemia, or ringworm of the hand

CONTRAINDICATIONS

Hypersensitivity to itraconazole, fluconazole, ketoconazole, or miconazole

INTERACTIONS

Drug

Antacids, didanosine, H_2 antagonists: May decrease itraconazole absorption.
Buspirone, cyclosporine, digoxin, lovastatin, simvastatin: May increase blood concentration of these drugs.
Oral anticoagulants: May increase the effect of oral anticoagulants.
Phenytoin, rifampin: May decrease itraconazole blood concentration.

Herbal

None known.

Food

Grapefruit, grapefruit juice: May alter itraconazole absorption.

Drug interactions of concern to dentistry

- Increased risk of rhabdomyolysis: lovastatin, simvastatin
- Increased risk of hypoglycemia: oral antidiabetics
- Increased metabolism: phenobarbital, carbamazepine
- May increase plasma levels of cyclosporine
- Contraindicated with triazolam, midazolam
- Inhibits metabolism of certain benzodiazepines: alprazolam, chlordiazepoxide, clonazepam, clorazepate, diazepam, estazolam, flurazepam, halazepam, midazolam, quazepam, triazolam, buspirone, allopurinol (Zyloprim), felodipine
- Decreased effects: didanosine
- Increased plasma levels: saquinavir, nisoldipine, haloperidol, carbamazepine, erythromycin, clarithromycin
- Avoid itraconazole use with HMG-Co A reductase inhibitors or lower their dose
- May inhibit warfarin metabolism
- Suspected increase in plasma levels: cola beverages
- Decrease in plasma levels: grapefruit juice
- Decreased effects: didanosine (take 2 hr before didanosine tabs)
- May increase levels and side effects of HMG-Co A reductase inhibitors
- Increased plasma levels of alfentanil, buspirone, carbamazepine, corticosteroids, zolpidem
- Suspected decrease in oral contractive effectiveness; suggest alternative method of contraception

DIAGNOSTIC TEST EFFECTS

May increase serum LDH serum alkaline phosphatase, serum bilirubin, AST(SGOT), and ALT(SGPT) levels. May decrease serum potassium level.

IV INCOMPATIBILITIES

Alert Dilution compatibility of itraconazole with any solution other than 0.9% NaCI is unknown. Don't mix with D_5W or lactated Ringer's solution. Not for IV bolus administration. Don't administer any medication in same bag or through same IV line as itraconazole.

SIDE EFFECTS

Frequent (11%–9%)

Nausea, rash

Occasional (5%–3%)

Vomiting, headache, diarrhea, hypertension, peripheral edema, fatigue, fever

Rare (≤ 2%)

Abdominal pain, dizziness, anorexia, pruritus

SERIOUS REACTIONS

! Hepatitis (as evidenced by anorexia, abdominal pain, unusual fatigue or weakness, jaundice skin or sclera, and dark urine) occurs rarely.

DENTAL CONSIDERATIONS

General:

- Monitor vital signs at every appointment because of cardiovascular side effects.
- Determine why the patient is taking the drug.
- Consider semisupine chair position for patient comfort because of GI effects of drug.

Consultations:

- Medical consultation may be required to assess patient's ability to tolerate stress.

kanamycin sulfate

kan-a-mye′-sin
(Kantrex)

CATEGORY AND SCHEDULE

Pregnancy Risk Category: Unavailable for irrigating solution.

MECHANISM OF ACTION

An aminoglycoside antibiotic that irreversibly binds to protein on bacterial ribosomes. ***Therapeutic Effect:*** Interferes with protein synthesis of susceptible microorganisms.

AVAILABILITY

Injection: 1 g/3 ml.

INDICATIONS AND DOSAGES

▸ Wound and Surgical Site Irrigation

Adults, Elderly. 0.25% solution to irrigate pleural space, ventricular or abscess cavities, wounds, or surgical sites.

CONTRAINDICATIONS

Hypersensitivity to kanamycin, other aminoglycosides (cross-sensitivity), or their components.

INTERACTIONS

Drug

None significant.

Herbal

None significant.

Food

None significant.

Drug interactions of concern to dentistry

- Increased risk of nephrotoxicity, ototoxicity and neuromuscular blockade: concurrent use with other aminoglycosides
- Risk of inactivation: β-lactam antiinfectives

DIAGNOSTIC TEST EFFECTS

None known.

SIDE EFFECTS

Occasional

Hypersensitivity reactions (fever, pruritus, rash, urticaria)

Rare

Headache

SERIOUS REACTIONS

! None known.

DENTAL CONSIDERATIONS

General:

- For selected infections in the hospital setting, provide palliative emergency dental treatment only.
- Examine for oral manifestation of opportunistic infection.
- Determine why patient is taking the drug.
- Caution regarding allergy to medication.

Consultations:

- CONIF
- Medical consultation may be required to assess disease control.

Teach Patient/Family:

- Importance of good oral hygiene to prevent soft tissue inflammation
- To report oral lesions, soreness, or bleeding to dentist
- To prevent trauma when using oral hygiene aids

ketamine

key′-tah-meen
(Ketalar)

CATEGORY AND SCHEDULE

Pregnancy Risk Category: B

MECHANISM OF ACTION

A rapidly acting general anesthetic that selectively blocks afferent impulses and interacts with CNS transmitter systems. ***Therapeutic Effect:*** Produces an anesthetic state characterized by profound analgesia and normal pharyngeal-laryngeal reflexes.

PHARMACOKINETICS

Route	Onset	Peak	Duration
IM (anesthetic)	3–4 min	N/A	12–25 min
IM (analgesic)	30 min	N/A	15–30 min
IV (anesthetic)	30 sec	N/A	5–10 min
IV (analgesic)	10–15 min	N/A	N/A

Rapidly distributed. Metabolized in the liver. Primarily excreted in urine. ***Half-life:*** Distribution: 10–15 min, elimination: 2–3 hr.

AVAILABILITY

Injection: 10 mg/ml, 50 mg/ml, 100 mg/ml.

INDICATIONS AND DOSAGES

▸ Sole Anesthetic for Short Diagnostic and Surgical Procedures That Don't Require Skeletal Muscle Relaxation, Induction of Anesthesia Before Administering Other General Anesthetics, Supplement to Low-Potency Agents

IV

Adults, Elderly. 1–4.5 mg/kg.
Children. 0.5–2 mg/kg.

IM

Adults, Elderly. 3–8 mg/kg.
Children. 3–7 mg/kg.

CONTRAINDICATIONS

Aneurysms, angina, CHF, elevated ICP, hypertension, psychotic disorders, thyrotoxicosis

INTERACTIONS

Drug

Antihypertensives, CNS depressants: May increase the risk of hypotension and respiratory depression.

Herbal

None known.

Food

None known.

Drug interactions of concern to dentistry

• Increased risk of hypotension and respiratory depression: all CNS depressants

DIAGNOSTIC TEST EFFECTS

May increase IOP.

IV INCOMPATIBILITIES

No information available for Y-site administration.

IV COMPATIBILITIES

Bupivacaine (Marcaine), clonidine (Duraclon), fentanyl (Sublimaze), lidocaine, morphine, propofol (Diprivan)

SIDE EFFECTS

Frequent

Increased BP and pulse rate; emergence reaction (marked by dreamlike state, delirium, hallucinations, and vivid imagery and occasionally accompanied by confusion, excitement, and irrational behavior; lasts from few hours to 24 hours after ketamine administration)

Occasional

Pain at injection site

Rare

Rash

SERIOUS REACTIONS

! Continuous or repeated intermittent infusion may result in extreme somnolence and circulatory or respiratory depression.

! Too-rapid IV administration of ketamine may produce severe hypotension, respiratory depression, and irregular muscle movements.

K

• Prolonged respiratory depression: nondepolarizing muscle relaxants

DENTAL CONSIDERATIONS

• Warning: Ketamine should be administered by persons trained in the administration of general anesthesia. Patients must be continually monitored, and facilities for maintenance of a patent airway, ventilatory support, oxygen supplementation, and circulatory resuscitation must be immediately available. Strict aseptic technique must be followed in handling ketamine.
• Increased BP and pulse rate; emergence reactions including hallucinations, delirium, dreamlike states, vivid imagery often accompanied by confusion, excitement, and irrational behavior.
• Responsible person must drive the patient home after recovery.
• Use safety measures: side rails, night light, and call bell within reach.

Consultations:

• Consultation with physician may be necessary if sedation or general anesthesia is required.

Teach Patient/Family:

• Warning to avoid performing tasks that require mental alertness or motor skills for 24 hours after anesthesia has been discontinued

ketoconazole

kee-toe-koe′-na-zole
(Apo-Ketocomazole[CAN], Nizoral, Nizoral AD, Sebizole[AUS])
Do not confuse Nizoral with Nasarel.

CATEGORY AND SCHEDULE

Pregnancy Risk Category: C
OTC (1% shampoo only)

MECHANISM OF ACTION

A fungistatic antifungal that inhibits the synthesis of ergosterol, a vital component of fungal cell formation. ***Therapeutic Effect:*** Damages the fungal cell membrane, altering its function.

AVAILABILITY

Tablets (Nizoral): 200 mg.
Cream (Nizoral): 2%.
Shampoo (Nizoral AD): 1%.

INDICATIONS AND DOSAGES

▸ **Histoplasmosis, Blastomycosis, Systemic Candidiasis, Chronic Mucocutaneous Candidiasis, Coccidioidomycosis, Paracoccidioidomycosis, Chromomycosis, Seborrheic Dermatitis, Tinea Corporis, Tinea Capitis, Tinea Manus, Tinea Cruris, Tinea Pedis, Tinea Unguium (Onychomycosis), Oral Thrush, Candiduria**

PO
Adults, Elderly. 200–400 mg/day.
Children. 3.3–6.6 mg/kg/day. Maximum: 800 mg/day in 2 divided doses.
TOPICAL
Adults, Elderly. Apply to affected area 1–2 times a day for 2–4 wk.
SHAMPOO
Adults, Elderly. Use twice weekly for 4 wk, allowing at least 3 days between shampooing. Use intermittently to maintain control.

OFF-LABEL USES

Systemic: Treatment of fungal pneumonia, prostate cancer, septicemia

CONTRAINDICATIONS

None known.

INTERACTIONS

Drug

Alcohol, hepatotoxic medications: May increase hepatotoxicity of ketoconazole.

Antacids, anticholinergics, H_2 antagonists, omeprazole: May decrease ketoconazole absorption.
Cyclosporine, lovastatin, simvastatin: May increase blood concentration and risk of toxicity of these drugs.
Isoniazid, rifampin: May decrease blood concentration of ketoconazole.

Herbal
Echinacea: May have additive hepatotoxic effects.

Food
None known.

Drug interactions of concern to dentistry
- Hepatotoxicity: alcohol, high-dose long-term use, acetaminophen, carbamazepine, sulfonamides
- Decreased absorption: antacids (take 2 hr after ketoconazole), proton pump inhibitors
- Leukocyte disorders: tacrolimus
- Contraindicated with triazolam, lovastatin, dofetilide
- Inhibits the metabolism of certain benzodiazepines: alprazolam, chlordiazepoxide, clonazepam, clorazepate, diazepam, estazolam, flurazepam, halazepam, midazolam, quazepam, triazolam, zolpidem
- May inhibit metabolism of warfarin
- Decreased effects: didanosine (take 2 hr before didanosine tabs)
- May increase plasma levels and side effects of HMG-CoA reductase inhibitors, cyclosporine
- Increased serum levels of indinavir, saquinavir, ritonavir, nisoldipine, haloperidol, carbamazepine, tricyclic antidepressants, buspirone, zolpidem, corticosteroids
- Suspected decrease in oral contraceptive effectiveness; may need to suggest additional contraception

DIAGNOSTIC TEST EFFECTS
May increase serum alkaline phosphatase, serum bilirubin, AST(SGOT), and ALT(SGPT) levels. May decrease serum corticosteroid and testosterone concentrations.

SIDE EFFECTS
Occasional (10%–3%)
Nausea, vomiting
Rare (< 2%)
Abdominal pain, diarrhea, headache, dizziness, photophobia, pruritus
Topical: itching, burning, irritation

SERIOUS REACTIONS
! Hematologic toxicity (as evidenced by thrombocytopenia, hemolytic anemia, and leukopenia) occurs occasionally.
! Hepatotoxicity may occur within 1 week to several months after starting therapy.
! Anaphylaxis occurs rarely.

K

DENTAL CONSIDERATIONS
General:
- To prevent reinoculation of *Candida* infection, dispose of toothbrush or other contaminated oral hygiene devices used during period of infection.
- Determine if medication controls disease.
- Place on frequent recall to evaluate healing response.
- Assess salivary flow as a factor in caries, periodontal disease, and candidiasis.

Teach Patient/Family:
- To avoid mouth rinses with high alcohol content because of drying effects

ketoprofen

kee-toe-proe′-fen
(Apo-Keto[CAN], Novo-Keto-EC, Orudis[AUS], Orudis KT[CAN], Orudis SR[AUS], Oruvail, Oruvail SR[AUS], Rhodis[CAN])

CATEGORY AND SCHEDULE

Pregnancy Risk Category: B (D if used in third trimester or near delivery)
OTC (tablets)

MECHANISM OF ACTION

An NSAID that produces analgesic and anti-inflammatory effects by inhibiting prostaglandin synthesis. ***Therapeutic Effect:*** Reduces the inflammatory response and intensity of pain.

K

AVAILABILITY

Capsules: 50 mg, 75 mg.
Capsules (Extended-Release [Oruvail]): 100 mg, 150 mg, 200 mg.
Tablets (Orudis KT): 12.5 mg (OTC).

INDICATIONS AND DOSAGES

▸ Acute or Chronic Rheumatoid Arthritis and Osteoarthritis

PO

Adults. Initially, 75 mg 3 times a day or 50 mg 4 times a day.
Elderly. Initially, 25–50 mg 3–4 times a day. Maintenance: 150–300 mg/day in 3–4 divided doses.

PO (Extended-Release)

Adults, Elderly. 100–200 mg once a day.

▸ Mild to Moderate Pain, Dysmenorrhea

PO

Adults, Elderly. 25–50 mg q6–8h. Maximum: 300 mg/day.

▸ Over-the-Counter (OTC) Dosage

PO

Adults, Elderly. 12.5 mg q4–6h. Maximum: 6 tabs/day.

▸ Dosage in Renal Impairment

Mild. 150 mg/day maximum.
Severe. 100 mg/day maximum.

OFF-LABEL USES

Treatment of acute gouty arthritis, psoriatic arthritis, ankylosing spondylitis, vascular headache

CONTRAINDICATIONS

Active peptic ulcer disease, chronic inflammation of the GI tract, GI bleeding or ulceration, history of hypersensitivity to aspirin or NSAIDs

INTERACTIONS

Drug

Antihypertensives, diuretics: May decrease the effects of these drugs.
Aspirin, other salicylates: May increase the risk of GI side effects such as bleeding.
Bone marrow depressants: May increase the risk of hematologic reactions.
Heparin, oral anticoagulants, thrombolytics: May increase the effects of these drugs.
Lithium: May increase the blood concentration and risk of toxicity of lithium.
Methotrexate: May increase the risk of methotrexate toxicity.
Probenecid: May increase the ketoprofen blood concentration.

Herbal

Feverfew: May decrease the effects of feverfew.
Ginkgo biloba: May increase the risk of bleeding.

Food

None known.

Drug interactions of concern to dentistry

- GI ulceration, bleeding: aspirin, other NSAIDs, alcohol, corticosteroids
- Nephrotoxicity: acetaminophen (prolonged use)

- Possible risk of decreased renal function: cyclosporine
- Increased photosensitizing effect: tetracycline
- First-time users of SSRIs also taking NSAIDs may have a higher risk of GI side effects; until more data are available, it may be advisable to avoid use of NSAIDs in these patients (*Br J Clin Pharmacol* 55:591-595, 2003)
- *When prescribed for dental pain:*
  - Risk of increased effects: oral anticoagulants, oral antidiabetics, lithium, methotrexate
  - Decreased effects of diuretics

DIAGNOSTIC TEST EFFECTS

May prolong bleeding time. May increase serum alkaline phosphatase and levels and liver function test results. May decrease Hct, blood Hgb, and serum sodium levels.

SIDE EFFECTS

Frequent (11%)
Dyspepsia
Occasional (> 3%)
Nausea, diarrhea or constipation, flatulence, abdominal cramps, headache
Rare (< 2%)
Anorexia, vomiting, visual disturbances, fluid retention

SERIOUS REACTIONS

! Rare reactions with long-term use include peptic ulcer disease, GI bleeding, gastritis, and severe hepatic reactions (cholestasis, jaundice), nephrotoxicity (dysuria, hematuria, proteinuria, nephrotic syndrome), and severe hypersensitivity reaction (bronchospasm, angioedema).

DENTAL CONSIDERATIONS

General:

- Patients on chronic drug therapy may rarely have symptoms of blood dyscrasias, which can include infection, bleeding, and poor healing.
- Assess salivary flow as a factor in caries, periodontal disease, and candidiasis.
- Avoid prescribing for dental use in first and last trimesters of pregnancy.
- Avoid prescribing aspirin-containing products or giving to patient taking aspirin.
- Consider semisupine chair position for patients with arthritic disease.

Consultations:

- In a patient with symptoms of blood dyscrasias, request a medical consultation for blood studies and postpone dental treatment until normal values are reestablished.
- Medical consultation may be required to assess disease control.

Teach Patient/Family:

- Importance of good oral hygiene to prevent soft tissue inflammation
- Caution to prevent injury when using oral hygiene aids
- *When chronic dry mouth occurs, advise patient:*
  - To avoid mouth rinses with high alcohol content because of drying effects
  - To use sugarless gum, frequent sips of water, or saliva substitutes
  - To use daily home fluoride products for anticaries effect

ketorolac tromethamine

kee-toe′-role-ak
(Acular, Acular LS, Acular PF, Toradol)
Do not confuse Acular with Acthar or Ocular.

CATEGORY AND SCHEDULE

Pregnancy Risk Category: C
(D if used in third trimester)

MECHANISM OF ACTION

An NSAID that inhibits prostaglandin synthesis and reduces prostaglandin levels in the aqueous humor. ***Therapeutic Effect:*** Relieves pain stimulus and reduces intraocular inflammation.

PHARMACOKINETICS

Route	Onset	Peak	Duration
PO	30–60 min	1.5–4 hr	4–6 hr
IV/IM	30 min	1–2 hr	4–6 hr

Readily absorbed from the GI tract, after IM administration. Protein binding: 99%. Largely metabolized in the liver. Primarily excreted in urine. Not removed by hemodialysis. ***Half-life:*** 3.8–6.3 hr (increased with impaired renal function and in the elderly).

K

AVAILABILITY

Tablets (Toradol): 10 mg.
Injection (Toradol): 15 mg/ml, 30 mg/ml.
Ophthalmic Solution (Acular): 0.5%.
Ophthalmic Solution (Acular LS): 0.4%.
Ophthalmic Solution (Acular PF): 0.5%.

INDICATIONS AND DOSAGES

▸ Short-Term Relief of Mild to Moderate Pain (multiple doses)

PO

Adults, Elderly. 10 mg q4–6h. Maximum: 40 mg/24 hr.

IV, IM

Adults younger than 65 yr. 30 mg q6h. Maximum: 120 mg/24 hr.
Adults 65 yr and older, those with renal impairment, those weighing less than 50 kg. 15 mg q6h. Maximum: 60 mg/24 hr.
Children 2–16 yr. 0.5 mg/kg q6h.

▸ Short-Term Relief of Mild to Moderate Pain (single dose)

IV

Adults younger than 65 yr, Children 17 yr and older weighing more than 50 kg. 30 mg.
Adults 65 yr and older, with renal impairment, weighing less than 50 kg. 15 mg.
Children 2–16 yr. 0.5 mg/kg. Maximum: 15 mg.

IM

Adults younger than 65 yr, Children 17 yr and older, weighing more than 50 kg. 60 mg.
Adults 65 yrs and older, with renal impairment, weighing less than 50 kg. 30 mg.
Children 2–16 yr. 1 mg/kg. Maximum: 15 kg.

▸ Allergic Conjunctivitis

OPHTHALMIC

Adults, Elderly, Children 3 yr and older. 1 drop 4 times a day.

▸ Cataract Extraction

OPHTHALMIC

Adults, Elderly. 1 drop 4 times a day. Begin 24 hr after surgery and continue for 2 wk.

▸ Refractive Surgery

OPHTHALMIC

Adults, Elderly. 1 drop 4 times a day for 3 days.

OFF-LABEL USES

Prevention or treatment of ocular inflammation(ophthalmic form)

CONTRAINDICATIONS

Active peptic ulcer disease, chronic inflammation of GI tract, GI bleeding or ulceration, history of hypersensitivity to aspirin or NSAIDs

INTERACTIONS

Drug

Antihypertensives, diuretics: May decrease the effects of these drugs.
Aspirin, other salicylates: May increase the risk of GI side effects such as bleeding.

Bone marrow depressants: May increase the risk of hematologic reactions.
Heparin, oral anticoagulants, thrombolytics: May increase the effects of these drugs.
Lithium: May increase the blood concentration and risk of toxicity of lithium.
Methotrexate: May increase the risk of methotrexate toxicity.
Probenecid: May increase ketorolac blood concentration.

Herbal

Feverfew: May decrease the effects of feverfew.
Ginkgo biloba: May increase the risk of bleeding.

Food

None known.

Drug interactions of concern to dentistry

- GI ulceration, bleeding: aspirin, alcohol, corticosteroids
- Contraindicated with probenecid
- Possible risk of decreased renal function: cyclosporine
- First-time users of SSRIs also taking NSAIDs may have a higher risk of GI side effects; until more data are available, it may be advisable to avoid use of NSAIDs in these patients (*Br J Clin Pharmacol* 55:591–595, 2003)
- *When prescribed for dental pain:*
  - Risk of increased effects: oral anticoagulants, oral antidiabetics, lithium, methotrexate
  - Decreased antihypertensive effects of diuretics, β-blockers, ACE inhibitors

Drug interactions of concern to dentistry

- None reported

DIAGNOSTIC TEST EFFECTS

May prolong bleeding time.
May increase liver function test results.

IV INCOMPATIBILITIES

Promethazine (Phenergan)

IV COMPATIBILITIES

Fentanyl (Sublimaze), hydromorphone (Dilaudid), morphine, nalbuphine (Nubain)

SIDE EFFECTS

Frequent (17%–12%)

Headache, nausea, abdominal cramps or pain, dyspepsia, oral lichenoid reaction

Occasional (9%–3%)

Diarrhea
Ophthalmic: Transient stinging and burning

Rare (3%–1%)

Constipation, vomiting, flatulence, stomatitis, dizziness
Ophthalmic: Ocular irritation, allergic reactions, superficial ocular infection, keratitis

SERIOUS REACTIONS

! Rare reactions with long-term use include peptic ulcer disease, GI bleeding, gastritis, severe hepatic reactions (cholestasis, jaundice), nephrotoxicity (glomerular nephritis, interstitial nephritis, nephrotic syndrome), and an acute hypersensitivity reaction (including fever, chills, and joint pain).

DENTAL CONSIDERATIONS

General:

- Assess salivary flow as a factor in caries, periodontal disease, and candidiasis.
- Avoid prescribing for dental use in pregnancy.
- Avoid prescribing aspirin or other NSAIDs.
- Avoid long-term use for chronic pain syndromes; combined use of IV/IM and oral doses must not exceed 5 days.

Consultations:

• Medical consultation may be required to assess disease control.

Teach Patient/Family:

• To avoid mouth rinses with high alcohol content because of drying effects

DENTAL CONSIDERATIONS

KETOROLAC TROMETHAMINE (OCULAR)

General:

• Determine why patient is taking the drug.
• Protect patient's eyes from accidental spatter during dental treatment.
• Avoid dental light in patient's eyes; offer dark glasses for patient comfort.

K

ketotifen fumarate

kee-toe-tye′-fen fyoo′-mah-rate (Apo-Ketotifen[CAN], Novo-Ketotifen[CAN], Zaditen[CAN], Zaditor)

CATEGORY AND SCHEDULE

Pregnancy Risk Category: C

MECHANISM OF ACTION

Selective histamine H1-antagonist and mast cell stabilizer, suppresses release of mediators from cells involved in hypersensitivity reactions, and decreases chemotoxis and activation of eosinophils. ***Therapeutic Effect:*** Reduces symptoms of allergic conjunctivitis.

PHARMACOKINETICS

None reported.

AVAILABILITY

Ophthalmic Solution: 0.025% (Zaditor).

INDICATIONS AND DOSAGES

▸ **Allergic Conjunctivitis**

OPHTHALMIC

Adults, Elderly, Children 3 yrs or older: 1 drop into affected eye q8–12h.

CONTRAINDICATIONS

Hypersensitivity to ketotifen or any component of the formulation (the preservative is benzalkonium chloride)

INTERACTIONS

Drug

None known.

Herbal

None known.

Food

None known.

Drug interactions of concern to dentistry

• None reported

DIAGNOSTIC TEST EFFECTS

None known.

SIDE EFFECTS

Frequent (25%–10%)

Conjunctival infection, headache, rhinitis

Occasional (5%–1%)

Allergic reaction, burning, stinging, eyelid disorder, flulike syndrome, keratitis, mydriasis, ocular discharge/pain, pharyngitis, photophobia, rash

SERIOUS REACTIONS

! No serious signs and symptoms have been seen after ingestion up to 20 mg.

DENTAL CONSIDERATIONS

General:

• Protect patient's eyes from accidental spatter during dental treatment.
• Avoid dental light in patient's eyes; offer dark glasses for patient comfort.

labetalol hydrochloride

la-bet′-a-lole
(Normodyne, Presolol[AUS], Trandate)
Do not confuse Trandate with tramadol or Trental.

CATEGORY AND SCHEDULE

Pregnancy Risk Category: C (D if used in second or third trimester)

MECHANISM OF ACTION

An antihypertensive that blocks $alpha_1$-, $beta_1$-, and $beta_2$-(large doses) adrenergic receptor sites. Large doses increase airway resistance. ***Therapeutic Effect:*** Slows sinus heart rate; decreases peripheral vascular resistance, cardiac output, and BP.

PHARMACOKINETICS

Route	Onset	Peak	Duration
PO	0.5–2 hr	2–4 hr	8–12 hr
IV	2–5 min	5–15 min	2–4 hr

Completely absorbed from the GI tract. Protein binding: 50%. Undergoes first-pass metabolism. Metabolized in the liver. Primarily excreted in urine. Not removed by hemodialysis. ***Half-life:*** PO, 6–8 hr; IV, 5.5 hr.

AVAILABILITY

Tablets (Normodyne, Trandate): 100 mg, 200 mg, 300 mg.
Injection (Trandate): 5 mg/ml.

INDICATIONS AND DOSAGES

▸ Hypertension

PO

Adults. Initially, 100 mg twice a day adjusted in increments of 100 mg twice a day q2–3 days. Maintenance: 200–400 mg twice a day. Maximum: 2.4 g/day.
Elderly. Initially, 100 mg 1–2 times a day. May increase as needed.

▸ Severe Hypertension, Hypertensive Emergency

IV

Adults. Initially, 20 mg. Additional doses of 20–80 mg may be given at 10–min intervals, up to total dose of 300 mg.

IV INFUSION

Adults. Initially, 2 mg/min up to total dose of 300 mg.

PO (after IV therapy)

Adults. Initially, 200 mg; then, 200–400 mg in 6–12 hr. Increase dose at 1-day intervals to desired level.

OFF-LABEL USES

Control of hypotension during surgery, treatment of chronic angina pectoris

L

CONTRAINDICATIONS

Bronchial asthma, cardiogenic shock, second- or third-degree heart block, severe bradycardia, uncontrolled CHF

INTERACTIONS

Drug

Diuretics, other antihypertensives: May increase hypotensive effect.
Insulin, oral hypoglycemics: May mask symptoms of hypoglycemia and prolong hypoglycemic effect of these drugs.
MAOIs: May produce hypertension.
Sympathomimetics, xanthines: May mutually inhibit effects.

Herbal

None known.

Food

None known.

Drug interactions of concern to dentistry

- Decreased metabolism: lidocaine
- Decreased effect: sympathomimetics

• Decreased hypotensive effects: indomethacin and other NSAIDs
• Increased hypotension, myocardial depression: hydrocarbon-inhalation anesthetics
• Increased plasma levels: diphenhydramine

DIAGNOSTIC TEST EFFECTS

May increase serum antinuclear antibody titer and BUN, serum LDH, lipoprotein, alkaline phosphatase, bilirubin, creatinine, potassium, triglyceride, uric acid, AST (SGOT), and ALT (SGPT) levels.

IV INCOMPATIBILITIES

Amphotericin B complex (Abelcet, AmBisome, Amphotec), ceftriaxone (Rocephin), furosemide (Lasix), heparin, nafcillin (Nafcil), thiopental

IV COMPATIBILITIES

Aminophylline, amiodarone (Cordarone), calcium gluconate, diltiazem (Cardizem), dobutamine (Dobutrex), dopamine (Intropin), enalapril (Vasotec), fentanyl (Sublimaze), hydromorphone (Dilaudid), lidocaine, lorazepam (Ativan), magnesium sulfate, midazolam (Versed), milrinone (Primacor), morphine, nitroglycerin, norepinephrine (Levophed), potassium chloride, potassium phosphate, propofol (Diprivan)

SIDE EFFECTS

Frequent
Drowsiness, difficulty sleeping, unusual fatigue or weakness, diminished sexual ability, transient scalp tingling
Occasional
Dizziness, dyspnea, peripheral edema, depression, anxiety, constipation, diarrhea, nasal congestion, nausea, vomiting, abdominal discomfort
Rare
Altered taste, dry eyes, increased urination, paresthesia

SERIOUS REACTIONS

! Labetolol administration may precipitate or aggravate CHF beacause of decreased myocardial stimulation.
! Abrupt withdrawal may precipitate ischemic heart disease, producing sweating, palpitations, headache, and tremor.
! May mask signs and symptoms of acute hypoglycemia (tachycardia, BP changes) in patients with diabetes.

DENTAL CONSIDERATIONS

General:
• Monitor vital signs at every appointment because of cardiovascular (CV) side effects.
• Patients on chronic drug therapy may rarely have symptoms of blood dyscrasias, which can include infection, bleeding, and poor healing.
• Assess salivary flow as a factor in caries, periodontal disease, and candidiasis.
• After supine positioning, have patient sit upright for at least 2 min before standing to avoid orthostatic hypotension.
• Limit use of sodium-containing products, such as saline IV fluids, for patients with a dietary salt restriction.
• Stress from dental procedures may compromise CV function; determine patient risk.
• Short appointments and a stress reduction protocol may be required for anxious patients.

Consultations:
• Medical consultation may be required to assess disease control and patient's ability to tolerate stress.

• In a patient with symptoms of blood dyscrasias, request a medical consultation for blood studies and postpone dental treatment until normal values are reestablished.

Teach Patient/Family:

• *When chronic dry mouth occurs, advise patient:*

- To avoid mouth rinses with high alcohol content because of drying effects
- To use sugarless gum, frequent sips of water, or saliva substitutes
- To use daily home fluoride products for anticaries effect

lamivudine

la-miv′-yoo-deen
(Epivir, Epivir-HBV, Heptovir[CAN], Zeffix[AUS])
Do not confuse lamivudine with lamotrigine.

CATEGORY AND SCHEDULE

Pregnancy Risk Category: C

MECHANISM OF ACTION

An antiviral that inhibits HIV reverse transcriptase by viral DNA chain termination. Also inhibits RNA- and DNA-dependent DNA polymerase, an enzyme necessary for HIV replication. ***Therapeutic Effect:*** Interrupts HIV replication, slowing the progression of HIV infection.

PHARMACOKINETICS

Rapidly and completely absorbed from the GI tract. Protein binding: less than 36%. Widely distributed (crosses the blood-brain barrier). Primarily excreted unchanged in urine. Not removed by hemodialysis or peritoneal dialysis. ***Half-life:*** 11–15 hr (intracellular), 2–11 hr (serum, adults), 1.7–2 hr (serum, children). (increased in impaired renal function).

AVAILABILITY

Oral Solution (Epivir): 10 mg/ml.
Oral Solution (Epivir-HBV): 5 mg/ml.
Tablets (Epivir): 150 mg, 300 mg.
Tablets (Epivir-HBV): 100 mg.

INDICATIONS AND DOSAGES

▸ HIV Infection (in combination with other antiretrovirals)

PO

Adults, Children 12–16 yr, weighing 50 kg (100 lb) or more. 150 mg twice a day or 300 mg once a day.

Adults weighing less than 50 kg. 2 mg/kg twice a day.

Children 3 mo–11 yr. 4 mg/kg twice a day (up to 150 mg/dose).

▸ Chronic Hepatitis B

PO

Adults, Children 17 yr and older. 100 mg/day.

Children younger than 17 yr. 3 mg/kg/day. Maximum: 100 mg/day.

▸ Dosage in Renal Impairment

Dosage and frequency are modified on the basis of creatinine clearance.

Creatinine Clearance (ml/min)	Dosage
50 ml/min or higher	150 mg twice a day
30–49 ml/min	150 mg once a day
15–29 ml/min	150 mg first dose, then 100 mg once a day
5–14 ml/min	150 mg first dose, then 50 mg once a day
less than 5 ml/min	50 mg first dose, then 25 mg once a day

L

OFF-LABEL USES

Prophylaxis in health care workers at risk of acquiring HIV after occupational exposure.

CONTRAINDICATIONS

None known.

INTERACTIONS

Drug

Co-trimoxazole: Increases lamivudine blood concentration.

Herbal

St. John's wort: May decrease lamivudine blood concentration and effect.

Food

None known.

Drug interactions of concern to dentistry

- None reported

L

DIAGNOSTIC TEST EFFECTS

May increase blood Hgb values, neutrophil count, and serum amylase, AST (SGOT), and ALT (SGPT) levels.

SIDE EFFECTS

Frequent

Headache (35%), nausea (33%), malaise and fatigue (27%), nasal disturbances (20%), diarrhea, cough (18%), musculoskeletal pain, neuropathy (12%), insomnia (11%), anorexia, dizziness, fever or chills (10%)

Occasional

Depression (9%); myalgia (8%); abdominal cramps (6%); dyspepsia, arthralgia (5%)

SERIOUS REACTIONS

! Pancreatitis occurs in 13% of pediatric patients.

! Anemia, neutropenia, and thrombocytopenia occur rarely.

DENTAL CONSIDERATIONS

General:

- Patients on chronic drug therapy may rarely have symptoms of blood dyscrasias, which can include infection, bleeding, and poor healing.
- Examine for oral manifestation of opportunistic infections.

Consultations:

- In a patient with symptoms of blood dyscrasias, request a medical consultation for blood studies and postpone dental treatment until normal values are reestablished.
- Medical consultation may be required to assess disease control and patient's ability to tolerate stress.

Teach Patient/Family:

- Importance of good oral hygiene to prevent soft tissue inflammation
- Caution to prevent trauma when using oral hygiene aids
- That secondary oral infection may occur; must see dentist immediately if infection occurs

lamotrigine

la-moe-trih′-jeen

(Apo-Lamotrigine[CAN], Lamictal, Lamictal CD)

Do not confuse lamotrigine with lamivudine.

CATEGORY AND SCHEDULE

Pregnancy Risk Category: C

MECHANISM OF ACTION

An anticonvulsant whose exact mechanism is unknown. May block voltage-sensitive sodium channels, thus stabilizing neuronal membranes and regulating presynaptic transmitter release of excitatory amino acids. ***Therapeutic Effect:*** Reduces seizure activity.

PHARMACOKINETICS

Rapidly absorbed from the GI tract. Protein binding: 55%. Metabolized primarily by glucuronic acid conjugation. Excreted in the urine. ***Half-life:*** 13–30 hr.

AVAILABILITY

Tablets: 25 mg, 100 mg, 150 mg, 200 mg.
Tablets (Chewable): 2 mg, 5 mg, 25 mg.

INDICATIONS AND DOSAGES

▸ Seizure Control in Patients Receiving Enzyme-Inducing Antiepileptic Drug (EIAEDs), but not Valproic Acid

PO

Adults, Elderly, Children older than 12 yr. Recommended as add-on therapy: 50 mg once a day for 2 wk, followed by 100 mg/day in 2 divided doses for 2 wk. Maintenance: Dosage may be increased by 100 mg/day every week, up to 300–500 mg/day in 2 divided doses.
Children 2–12 yr. 0.6 mg/kg/day in 2 divided doses for 2 wk, then 1.2 mg/kg/day in 2 divided doses for wk 3 and 4. Maintenance: 5–15 mg/kg/day. Maximum: 400 mg/day.

▸ Seizure Control in Patients Receiving Combination Therapy of EIAEDs and Valproic Acid

PO

Adults, Elderly, Children older than 12 yr. 25 mg every other day for 2 wk, followed by 25 mg once a day for 2 wk. Maintenance: Dosage may be increased by 25–50 mg/day q1–2wk, up to 150 mg/day in 2 divided doses.
Children 2–12 yr. 0.15 mg/kg/day in 2 divided doses for 2 wk, then 0.3 mg/kg/day in 2 divided doses for wk 3 and 4. Maintenance: 1–5 mg/kg/day in 2 divided doses. Maximum: 200 mg/day.

▸ Conversion to Monotherapy for Patients Receiving EIAED

PO

Adults, Elderly, Children 16 yr and older. 500 mg/day in 2 divided doses. Titrate to desired dose while maintaining EIAED at fixed level, then withdraw EIAED by 20% each wk over a 4-wk period.

▸ Conversion to Monotherapy for Patients Receiving Valproic Acid

PO

Adults, Elderly, Children 16 yr and older. Titrate lamotrigine to 200 mg/day, maintaining valproic acid dose. Maintain lamotrigine dose and decrease valproic acid to 500 mg/day, no greater than 500 mg/day/wk, then maintain 500 mg/day for 1 wk. Increase lamotrigine to 300 mg/day and decrease valproic acid to 250 mg/day. Maintain for 1 wk, then discontinue valproic acid and increase lamotrigine by 100 mg/day each wk until maintenance dose of 500 mg/day reached.

▸ Bipolar Disorder in Patients Receiving EIAED

PO

Adults, Elderly. 50 mg/day for 2 wk, then 100 mg/day for 2 wk, then 200 mg/day for 1 wk, then 300 mg/day for 1 wk, then up to usual maintenance dose 400 mg/day in divided doses.

▸ Bipolar Disorder in Patients Receiving Valproic Acid

PO

Adults, Elderly. 25 mg/day every other day for 2 wk, then 25 mg/day for 2 wk, then 50 mg/day for 1 wk, then 100 mg/day. Usual maintenance dose with valproic acid: 100 mg/day.

▸ Discontinuation Therapy

Adults, Children older than 12 yr. A dosage reduction of approximately 50% per week over at least 2 wk is recommended.

CONTRAINDICATIONS
None known.

INTERACTIONS
Drug
Carbamazepine, phenobarbital, phenytoin, primidone, valproic acid: Decrease lamotrigine blood concentration.
Carbamazepine, valproic acid: May increase serum levels of these drugs.
Herbal
None known.
Food
None known.
Drug interactions of concern to dentistry
- Increased excretion: chronic, high-dose acetaminophen (900 mg tid), but significance is unclear; carbamazepine
- Increased blood levels of carbamazepine

L

DIAGNOSTIC TEST EFFECTS
None known.

SIDE EFFECTS
Frequent
Dizziness (38%), diplopia (28%), headache (29%), ataxia (22%), nausea (19%), blurred vision (16%), somnolence, rhinitis (14%), drymouth, halitosis
Occasional (10%–5%)
Rash, pharyngitis, vomiting, cough, flulike symptoms, diarrhea, dysmenorrhea, fever, insomnia, dyspepsia
Rare
Constipation, tremor, anxiety, pruritus, vaginitis, hypersensitivity reaction

SERIOUS REACTIONS
! Abrupt withdrawal may increase seizure frequency.
! Serious rashes, including Stevens-Johnson syndrome, requiring hospitalization and discontinuation of treatment have been reported.

DENTAL CONSIDERATIONS
General:
- Early-morning appointments and a stress reduction protocol may be required for anxious patients.
- Determine type of epilepsy, seizure frequency, and quality of seizure control. A stress reduction protocol may be required.
- Evaluate respiration characteristics and rate.
- Assess salivary flow as factor in caries, periodontal disease, and candidiasis.
- Patients on chronic drug therapy may rarely have symptoms of blood dyscrasias, which can include infection, bleeding, and poor healing.
- Place on frequent recall because of oral side effects.

Consultations:
- Medical consultation may be required to assess disease control and the patient's ability to tolerate stress.
- In a patient with symptoms of blood dyscrasias, request a medical consultation for blood studies and postpone dental treatment until normal values are reestablished.

Teach Patient/Family:
- Importance of good oral hygiene to prevent soft tissue inflammation
- Use of electric toothbrush if patient has difficulty holding conventional devices
- *When chronic dry mouth occurs, advise patient:*
  - To avoid mouth rinses with high alcohol content because of drying effects
  - To use daily home fluoride products for anticaries effect
  - To use sugarless gum, frequent sips of water, or saliva substitutes

lansoprazole

lan-soe-pray′-zole
(Prevacid, Prevacid IV, Prevacid Solu-Tab, Zoton[AUS])
Do not confuse Prevacid with Pepcid, Pravachol, or Prevpac.

CATEGORY AND SCHEDULE

Pregnancy Risk Category: B

MECHANISM OF ACTION

A proton pump inhibitor that selectively inhibits the parietal cell membrane enzyme system (hydrogen-potassium adenosine triphosphatase) or proton pump. ***Therapeutic Effect:*** Suppresses gastric acid secretion.

PHARMACOKINETICS

Route	Onset	Peak	Duration
PO (15 mg)	2–3 hr	N/A	24 hr
PO (30 mg)	1–2 hr	N/A	longer than 24 hr

Rapid and complete absorption (food may decrease absorption) once drug has left stomach. Protein binding: 97%. Distributed primarily to gastric parietal cells and converted to two active metabolites. Extensively metabolized in the liver. Eliminated in bile and urine. Not removed by hemodialysis. ***Half-life:*** 1.5 hr (increased in the elderly and in those with hepatic impairment).

AVAILABILITY

Capsules (Delayed-Release [Prevacid]): 15 mg, 30 mg.
Granules for Oral Suspension (Prevacid): 15 mg/pack; 30 mg/pack.
Injection Powder for Reconstitution (Prevacid IV): 30 mg.
Oral-disintegrating Tablets (Prevacid Solu-Tab): 15 mg, 30 mg.

INDICATIONS AND DOSAGES

▸ Duodenal Ulcer
PO
Adults, Elderly. 15 mg/day, before eating, preferably in the morning, for up to 4 wks.

▸ Erosive Esophagitis
PO
Adults, Elderly. 30 mg/day, before eating, for up to 8 wks. If healing does not occur within 8 wk (in 5%–10% of cases), may give for additional 8 wk. Maintenance: 15 mg/day.
IV
Adults, Elderly. 30 mg once a day for up to 7 days. Switch to oral lansoprazole therapy as soon as patient can tolerate oral route.

▸ Gastric Ulcer
PO
Adults. 30 mg/day for up to 8 wk.

▸ NSAID Gastric Ulcer
PO
Adults, Elderly. (Healing): 30 mg/day for up to 8 wk. (Prevention): 15 mg/day for up to 12 wk.

▸ Healed Duodenal Ulcer, Gastroesophageal Reflux Disease
PO
Adults. 15 mg/day.

▸ Usual Pediatric Dosage
Children 3 mo–14 yr, weighing more than 20 kg. 30 mg once daily.
Children 3 mo–14 yr, weighing 10–20 kg. 15 mg once daily.
Children 3 mo–14 yr, weighing less than 10 kg. 7.5 mg once daily.

▸ Helicobacter Pylori Infection
PO
Adults. 30 mg twice a day for 10 days (with amoxicillin and clarithromycin).

▸ Pathologic Hypersecretory Conditions (including Zollinger-Ellison syndrome)
PO
Adults, Elderly. 60 mg/day. Individualize dosage according to

L

patient needs and for as long as clinically indicated. Administer up to 120 mg/day in divided doses.

CONTRAINDICATIONS
None known.

INTERACTIONS
Drug
Ampicillin, digoxin, iron salts, ketoconazole: May interfere with the absorption of ampicillin, digoxin, iron salts, and ketoconazole.
Sucralfate: May delay the absorption of lansoprazole.
Herbal
None known.
Food
None known.
Drug interactions of concern to dentistry
- Drug interactions not established but potentially can interfere with absorption of amoxicillin, ketoconazole

DIAGNOSTIC TEST EFFECTS
May increase LDH, serum alkaline phosphatase, bilirubin, cholesterol, creatinine, AST(SGOT), ALT(SGPT), triglyceride, and uric acid levels. May produce abnormal albumin/globulin ratio, electrolyte balance, and platelet, RBC, and WBC counts. May increase Hgb and Hct.

SIDE EFFECTS
Occasional (3%–2%)
Diarrhea, abdominal pain, rash, pruritus, altered appetite
Rare (1%)
Nausea, headache

SERIOUS REACTIONS
! Bilirubinemia, eosinophilia, and hyperlipemia occur rarely.

DENTAL CONSIDERATIONS
General:
- Consider semisupine chair position for patient comfort because of GI effects of disease.
- Question the patient about tolerance of NSAIDs or aspirin related to GI problem.
- Patients with gastroesophageal reflux may have oral symptoms, including burning mouth, secondary candidiasis, and oral signs of dental erosion.
- Assess salivary flow as factor in caries, periodontal disease, and candidiasis.

Teach Patient/Family:
- *When chronic dry mouth occurs, advise patient:*
  - To avoid mouth rinses with high alcohol content because of drying effects
  - To use daily home fluoride products for anticaries effect
  - To use sugarless gum, frequent sips of water, or saliva substitutes

lanthanum carbonate
lan-thah′-num
(Fosrenol)

CATEGORY AND SCHEDULE
Pregnancy Risk Category: C

MECHANISM OF ACTION
A phosphate regulator that dissociates in the acidic environment of the upper GI tract to lanthanum ions, which bind to dietary phosphate released from food during digestion, forming highly insoluble lanthanum phosphate complexes.
Therapeutic Effect: Reduces phosphate absorption.

PHARMACOKINETICS
Phosphate complexes are eliminated in urine.

AVAILABILITY
Tablets (Chewable): 250 mg, 500 mg.

INDICATIONS AND DOSAGES
▸ Reduce Serum Phosphate in End-Stage Renal Disease
PO
Adults, Elderly. 750 mg–1,500 mg in divided doses, taken with or immediately after a meal. Dosage may be titrated in 750-mg increments q2–3wk on the basis of serum phosphate levels.

CONTRAINDICATIONS
None known.

INTERACTIONS
Drug
Antacids: Interact with lanthanum; separate administration by 2 hours.
Herbal
None known.
Food
All foods: Enhance lanthanum's effect and reduce phosphate absorption.
Drug interactions of concern to dentistry
None reported

DIAGNOSTIC TEST EFFECTS
None known.

SIDE EFFECTS
Frequent
Nausea (11%), vomiting (9%), dialysis graft occlusion (8%), abdominal pain (5%)

SERIOUS REACTIONS
! None known.

DENTAL CONSIDERATIONS
General:
- Question patient about renal dialysis history and use of other medications.
- Dental drugs known to interact with antacid products should not be taken within 2 hr of lanthanum carbonate.
- Question patient about coexisting cardiovascular disease, related medications, and any bleeding problems.
- Avoid nephrotoxic drugs; dose adjustment may be required for renal-excreted drugs.
- Oral infections should be eliminated and/or treated aggressively.
- Patient may have AV shunt in place.
- Monitor and record vital signs.
- Consider semisupine chair position for patient comfort if GI side effects occur.
- Question patient about tolerance of NSAIDS or aspirin related to GI disease.
- After supine positioning, have patient sit upright for at least 2 min before standing to avoid orthostatic hypotension.
- Antiinfective prophylaxis may be indicated for patient on dialysis; complete physician consultation.

Consultations:
- Consultation with physician may be necessary if sedation or general anesthesia is required.
- Medical consultation may be required to assess disease control and patient's ability to tolerate stress.

Teach Patient/Family:
- Importance of good oral hygiene to prevent soft tissue inflammation
- To prevent trauma when using oral hygiene aids
- Importance of updating health and medication history if physician

makes any changes in evaluation/drug regimens; include OTC, herbal, and nonherbal in the update

latanoprost

la-ta′-noe-prost

(Xalatan)

Do not confuse with Xanax.

CATEGORY AND SCHEDULE

Pregnancy Risk Category: C

MECHANISM OF ACTION

An ophthalmic agent that is a prostanoid selective FP receptor agonist. ***Therapeutic Effect:*** Reduces intraocular pressure (IOP) by reducing aqueous humor production.

L

PHARMACOKINETICS

Absorbed through the cornea where the isopropyl ester prodrug is hydrolyzed to acid form to become biologically active. Highly lipophilic. The acid of latanoprost can be measured in the aqueous humor during the first 4 hours and in the plasma only during the first hour after local administration. Cornea, latanoprost, is hydrolyzed to the biologically active acid. Metabolized in liver if it reaches systemic circulation. Metabolized to 1,2-dinor metabolite and 1,2,3,4-tetranor metabolite. Primarily eliminated by the kidneys. ***Half-life:*** 17 min.

AVAILABILITY

Ophthalmic Solution: 0.005% (Xalatan).

INDICATIONS AND DOSAGES

▸ **Glaucoma, Ocular Hypertension**

OPHTHALMIC

Adults, Elderly. 1 drop (1.5 mcg) in affected eye(s) once daily, in the evening.

CONTRAINDICATIONS

Hypersensitivity to latanoprost or benzalkonium chloride, or any other component of the formulation

INTERACTIONS

Drug

Pilocarpine: May decrease latanoprost efficacy.

Thimerosal: May cause precipitation in the eye.

Herbal

None known.

Food

None known.

Drug interactions of concern to dentistry

- None reported at this time; avoid use of anticholinergic drugs, atropine-like drugs, propantheline, and diazepam (benzodiazepines) in patient with glaucoma

DIAGNOSTIC TEST EFFECTS

None known.

SIDE EFFECTS

Frequent

Blurred vision

Occasional

Eyelash changes, eyelid skin darkening, iris pigmentation

Rare

Macular edema

SERIOUS REACTIONS

! Pigmentation is expected to increase as long as latanoprost is administered but after discontinuation, pigmentation of the iris is likely to be permanent while pigmentation of the periorbital tissue and eyelash changes has been reported as reversible.

! Inflammation (iritis/uveitis) and macular edema, including cystoid macular edema have been reported.

DENTAL CONSIDERATIONS

General:

• Check compliance of patient with prescribed drug regimen for glaucoma.
• Avoid dental light in patient's eyes; offer dark glasses for patient comfort.
• Protect patient's eyes from accidental spatter during dental treatment.

Consultations:

• Medical consultation may be required to assess disease control.

leflunomide

le-flu′-na-mide
(Arava)

CATEGORY AND SCHEDULE

Pregnancy Risk Category: X

MECHANISM OF ACTION

An immunomodulatory agent that inhibits dihydroorotate dehydrogenase, the enzyme involved in autoimmune process that leads to rheumatoid arthritis. ***Therapeutic Effect:*** Reduces signs and symptoms of rheumatoid arthritis and slows structural damage.

PHARMACOKINETICS

Well absorbed after PO administration. Protein binding: greater than 99%. Metabolized to active metabolite in the GI wall and liver. Excreted through both renal and biliary systems. Not removed by hemodialysis. ***Half-life:*** 16 days.

AVAILABILITY

Tablets: 10 mg, 20 mg.

INDICATIONS AND DOSAGES

▸Rheumatoid Arthritis

PO

Adults, Elderly. Initially, 100 mg/day for 3 days, then 10–20 mg/day.

CONTRAINDICATIONS

Pregnancy or plans to become pregnant

INTERACTIONS

Drug

Rifampin: Increases the blood concentration of leflunomide.
Warfarin: May increase the effects of warfarin.

Herbal

None known.

Food

None known.

Drug interactions of concern to dentistry

• None reported

DIAGNOSTIC TEST EFFECTS

May increase hepatic enzyme levels, especially AST (SGOT), and ALT (SGPT).

SIDE EFFECTS

Frequent (20%–10%)

Diarrhea, respiratory tract infection, alopecia, rash, nausea

SERIOUS REACTIONS

! Transient thrombocytopenia and leukopenia occur rarely.

DENTAL CONSIDERATIONS

General:

• Monitor vital signs at every appointment because of CV side effects.
• Consider semisupine chair position for patient comfort if GI side effects occur.
• Examine for oral manifestation of opportunistic infection.
• If acute oral infection occurs, inform physician.
• Assess salivary flow as a factor in caries, periodontal disease, and candidiasis.

Consultations:
- Consult if needed.

Teach Patient/Family:
- Importance of good oral hygiene to prevent soft tissue inflammation
- Use of electric toothbrush if patient has difficulty holding conventional devices
- *When chronic dry mouth occurs, advise patient:*
  - To avoid mouth rinses with high alcohol content because of drying effects
  - To use daily home fluoride products for anticaries effect
  - To use sugarless gum, frequent sips of water, or saliva substitutes

lepirudin

leh-peer′-u-din
(Refludan)

CATEGORY AND SCHEDULE

Pregnancy Risk Category: B

MECHANISM OF ACTION

An anticoagulant that inhibits thrombogenic action of thrombin (independent of antithrombin II and not inhibited by platelet factor 4). One molecule of lepirudin binds to one molecule of thrombin. ***Therapeutic Effect:*** Produces dose-dependent increases aPTT.

PHARMACOKINETICS

Distributed primarily in extracellular fluid. Primarily eliminated by the kidneys. ***Half-life:*** 1.3 hr (increased in impaired renal function).

AVAILABILITY

Powder for Injection: 50 mg.

INDICATIONS AND DOSAGES

▸ **Heparin-Induced Thrombocytopenia and Associated Thromboembolic Disease to Prevent Further Thromboembolic Complications**

IV, IV INFUSION

Adults, Elderly. 0.2–0.4 mg/kg, IV slowly over 15–20 sec, followed by IV infusion of 0.1–0.15 mg/kg/hr for 2–10 days or longer.

▸ **Dosage in Renal Impairment**

Initial dose is decreased to 0.2 mg/kg, with infusion rate adjusted on the basis of creatinine clearance.

Creatinine Clearance (ml/min)	% of standard infusion rate	Infusion rate (mg/kg/hr)
45–60	50	0.075
30–44	30	0.045
15–29	15	0.0225

CONTRAINDICATIONS

None known.

INTERACTIONS

Drug

Platelet aggregation inhibitors, thrombolytics, warfarin: May increase the risk of bleeding complications.

Herbal

Ginkgo biloba: May increase the risk of bleeding.

Food

None known.

Drug interactions of concern to dentistry

- Increased risk of bleeding: drugs that interfere with coagulation and platelet function, such as NSAIDs, aspirin, ginkgo biloba (herb)

DIAGNOSTIC TEST EFFECTS
Increases APTT and thrombin time.

IV INCOMPATIBILITIES
Do not mix with other medications.

SIDE EFFECTS
Frequent (14%–5%)
Bleeding from gums, puncture sites, or wounds, hematuria, fever, GI and rectal bleeding
Occasional (3%–1%)
Epistaxis; allergic reaction, such as rash and pruritus; vaginal bleeding

SERIOUS REACTIONS
! Overdose is characterized by excessively high aPTT.
! Intracranial bleeding occurs rarely.
! Abnormal hepatic function occurs in 6% of patients.

DENTAL CONSIDERATIONS
General:
- Patients are at risk of bleeding; check for oral signs.
- Provide palliative dental care for dental emergencies only.
- Determine why patient is taking the drug.
- Avoid products that affect platelet function, such as aspirin and NSAIDs.
- Consider local hemostasis measures to prevent excessive bleeding.

Consultations:
- Medical consultation should include partial prothrombin time, prothrombin time, or INR.
- Medical consultation may be required to assess disease control and patient's ability to tolerate stress.

Teach Patient/Family:
- Use soft tooth brush to reduce risk of bleeding
- Importance of good oral hygiene to prevent soft tissue inflammation
- To report oral lesions, soreness, or bleeding to dentist
- To prevent trauma when using oral hygiene aids
- Importance of updating health and medication history if physician makes any changes in evaluation or drug regimens; include OTC, herbal, and nonherbal in the update

letrozole
leh′-troe-zoll
(Femara)
Do not confuse Femara with FemHRT.

CATEGORY AND SCHEDULE
Pregnancy Risk Category: D

L

MECHANISM OF ACTION
Decreases the level of circulating estrogen by inhibiting aromatase, an enzyme that catalyzes the final step in estrogen production. ***Therapeutic Effect:*** Inhibits the growth of breast cancers that are stimulated by estrogens.

PHARMACOKINETICS
Rapidly and completely absorbed. Metabolized in the liver. Primarily eliminated by the kidneys. Unknown if removed by hemodialysis. ***Half-life:*** Approximately 2 days.

AVAILABILITY
Tablets: 2.5 mg.

INDICATIONS AND DOSAGES
▸ **Breast Cancer**
PO
Adults, Elderly. 2.5 mg/day. Continue until tumor progression is evident.

CONTRAINDICATIONS
None known.

INTERACTIONS

Drug
None known.

Herbal
None known.

Food
None known.

Drug interactions of concern to dentistry
- None reported

DIAGNOSTIC TEST EFFECTS
May increase serum calcium, cholesterol, GGT, AST (SGOT), and ALT (SGPT) levels.

SIDE EFFECTS

Frequent (21%–9%)
Musculoskeletal pain (back, arm, leg), nausea, headache

Occasional (8%–5%)
Constipation, arthralgia, fatigue, vomiting, hot flashes, diarrhea, abdominal pain, cough, rash, anorexia, hypertension, peripheral edema

Rare (4%–1%)
Asthenia, somnolence, dyspepsia, weight gain, pruritus

SERIOUS REACTIONS
! None known.

DENTAL CONSIDERATIONS

General:
- Patients taking opioids for acute or chronic pain should be given alternative analgesics for dental pain.
- Patients on chronic drug therapy may rarely have symptoms of blood dyscrasias, which can include infection, bleeding, and poor healing.
- Palliative medication may be required for management of oral side effects.
- Examine for oral manifestation of opportunistic infection.
- Consider semisupine chair position for patient comfort if GI side effects occur.
- Monitor vital signs at every appointment because of CV and respiratory side effects.

Consultations:
- In a patient with symptoms of blood dyscrasias, request a medical consultation for blood studies and postpone treatment until normal values are reestablished.

Teach Patient/Family:
- Importance of good oral hygiene to prevent soft tissue inflammation
- To be aware of the possibility of secondary oral infection and the need to see dentist immediately if signs of infection occur

leucovorin calcium (folinic acid, citrovorum factor)
loo-koe-vor′-in
(Calcium Leucovorin[AUS], Wellcovorin)
Do not confuse Wellcovorin with Wellbutrin or Wellferon.

CATEGORY AND SCHEDULE
Pregnancy Risk Category: C

MECHANISM OF ACTION
An antidote to folic acid antagonists that may limit methotrexate action on normal cells by competing with methotrexate for the same transport processes into the cells. ***Therapeutic Effect:*** Reverses toxic effects of folic acid antagonists. Reverses folic acid deficiency.

PHARMACOKINETICS
Readily absorbed from the GI tract. Widely distributed. Primarily concentrated in the liver.

Metabolized in the liver and intestinal mucosa to active metabolite. Primarily excreted in urine. ***Half-life:*** 15 min; metabolite, 30–35 min.

AVAILABILITY

Tablets: 5 mg, 10 mg, 15 mg, 25 mg.
Injection: 10 mg/ml.
Powder for Injection: 50 mg, 100 mg, 200 mg, 350 mg.

INDICATIONS AND DOSAGES

▸ Conventional Rescue Dosage in High-Dose Methotrexate Therapy

PO, IV, IM

Adults, Elderly, Children. 10 mg/m^2 IM or IV one time, then PO q6h until serum methotrexate level is less than 10^{-8} M. If 24-hr serum creatinine level increases by 50% or greater over baseline or methotrexate level exceeds 5×10^{-6} M or 48-hr level exceeds 9×10^{-7} M, increase to 100 mg/m^2 IV q3h until methotrexate level is less than 10^{-8} M.

▸ Folic Acid Antagonist Overdose

PO

Adults, Elderly, Children.
2–15 mg/day for 3 days or 5 mg every 3 days.

▸ Megaloblastic Anemia

IM

Adults, Elderly, Children.
3–6 mg/day.

▸ Megaloblastic Anemia Secondary to Folate Deficiency

IM

Adults, Elderly, Children. 1 mg/day.

▸ Prevention of Hematologic Toxicity (for toxoplasmosis), with Sulfadiazine

PO, IV

Adults, Elderly, Children.
5–10 mg/day, repeat every 3 days.

▸ Prevention of Hematologic Toxicity with Pyrimethamine, PCP

PO, IV

Adults, Children. 25 mg once weekly.

OFF-LABEL USES

Treatment of Ewing's sarcoma, gestational trophoblastic neoplasms, or non-Hodgkin's lymphoma; treatment adjunct for head and neck carcinoma

CONTRAINDICATIONS

Pernicious anemia, other megaloblastic anemias secondary to vitamin B_{12} deficiency

INTERACTIONS

Drug

Anticonvulsants: May decrease the effects of anticonvulsants.
Chemotherapeutic agents: May increase the effects and toxicity of these drugs when taken in combination.

Herbal

None known.

Food

None known.

Drug interactions of concern to dentistry

- None reported

DIAGNOSTIC TEST EFFECTS

None known.

IV INCOMPATIBILITIES

Amphotericin B complex (Abelcet, AmBisome, Amphotec), droperidol (Inapsine), foscarnet (Foscavir)

IV COMPATIBILITIES

Cisplatin (Platinol AQ), cyclophosphamide (Cytoxan), doxorubicin (Adriamycin), etoposide (VePesid), filgrastim (Neupogen), 5-fluorouracil, gemcitabine (Gemzar), granisetron (Kytril), heparin, methotrexate, metoclopramide (Reglan), mitomycin (Mutamycin), piperacillin and tazobactam (Zosyn), vinblastine (Velban), vincristine (Oncovin)

SIDE EFFECTS

Frequent

When combined with chemotherapeutic agents: Diarrhea, stomatitis, nausea, vomiting, lethargy or malaise or fatigue, alopecia, anorexia

Occasional

Urticaria, dermatitis

SERIOUS REACTIONS

! Excessive dosage may negate chemotherapeutic effects of folic acid antagonists.

! Anaphylaxis occurs rarely.

! Diarrhea may cause rapid clinical deterioration.

DENTAL CONSIDERATIONS

General:

- Signs of folate deficiency may appear in oral tissues.
- Determine why the patient is taking the drug.
- Patients with severe anemia or cancer or those receiving cancer chemotherapy may have oral complaints. Palliative therapy may be required.

Consultations:

- Medical consultation may be required to assess disease control.

Teach Patient/Family:

- Importance of good oral hygiene to prevent soft tissue inflammation
- Caution to prevent trauma when using oral hygiene aids
- To report oral lesions, soreness, or bleeding to dentist
- That secondary oral infection may occur; must see dentist immediately if infection occurs
- Importance of updating medical/drug records if physician makes any changes in evaluation or drug regimens

leuprolide acetate

loo′-proe-lide

(Eligard, Lucrin[AUS], Lucrin Depot Inj[AUS], Lupron, Lupron Depot, Lupron Depot Ped, Viadur)

Do not confuse leuprolide or Lupron with Lopurin or Nuprin.

CATEGORY AND SCHEDULE

Pregnancy Risk Category: X

MECHANISM OF ACTION

A gonadotropin-releasing hormone analogue and antineoplastic agent that stimulates the release of luteinizing hormone (LH) and follicle-stimulating hormone (FSH) from the anterior pituitary gland.

Therapeutic Effect: Produces pharmacologic castration and decreases the growth of abnormal prostate tissue in males; causes endometrial tissue to become inactive and atrophic in females; and decreases the rate of pubertal development in children with central precocious puberty.

PHARMACOKINETICS

Rapidly and well absorbed after subcutaneous administration. Absorbed slowly after IM administration. Protein binding: 43%–49%. ***Half-life:*** 3–4 hr.

AVAILABILITY

*Implant (Viadur):*65 mg.

Injection Depot Formulation (Eligard): 7.5 mg, 22.5 mg, 30 mg, 45 mg.

Injection Depot Formulation (Leupron Depot): 3.75 mg, 7.5 mg, 11.25 mg, 22.5 mg, 30 mg.

Injection Depot Formulation (Lupron Depot-Ped): 7.5 mg, 11.25 mg, 15 mg.

Injection solution (Lupron): 5 mg/ml.

INDICATIONS AND DOSAGES

▸ Advanced Prostatic Carcinoma

IM (Lupron Depot)
Adults, Elderly. 7.5 mg every month or 22.5 mg q3mo or 30 mg q4mo.
SUBCUTANEOUS (Eligard)
Adults, Elderly. 7.5 mg every month or 22.5 mg q3mo or 30 mg q4mo.
SUBCUTANEOUS (Lupron)
Adults, Elderly. 1 mg/day.
SUBCUTANEOUS (Viadur)
Adults, Elderly. 65 mg implanted q12mo.

▸ Endometriosis

IM (Lupron Depot)
Adults, Elderly. 3.75 mg/mo for up to 6 months or 11.25 mg q3mo for up to 2 doses.

▸ Uterine Leiomyomata

IM (with iron [Lupron Depot])
Adults, Elderly. 3.75 mg/mo for up to 3 months or 11.25 mg as a single injection.

▸ Precocious Puberty

IM (Lupron Depot)
Children. 0.3 mg/kg/dose every 28 days. Minimum: 7.5 mg. If down regulation is not achieved, titrate upward in 3.75-mg increments q4wk.
SUBCUTANEOUS (Lupron)
Children. 20–45 mcg/kg/day. Titrate upward by 10 mcg/kg/day if down regululation is not achieved.

CONTRAINDICATIONS

Pernicious anemia, pregnancy

INTERACTIONS

Drug
None known.
Herbal
None known.
Food
None known.

Drug interactions of concern to dentistry
• None reported

DIAGNOSTIC TEST EFFECTS

May increase serum prostatic acid phosphatase (PAP) levels. Initially increases, then decreases, serum testosterone concentration.

SIDE EFFECTS

Frequent
Hot flashes (ranging from mild flushing to diaphoresis)
Females: Amenorrhea, spotting
Occasional
Arrhythmias; palpitations; blurred vision; dizziness; edema; headache; burning or itching, or swelling at injection site; nausea; insomnia; weight gain
Females: Deepening voice, hirsutism, decreased libido, increased breast tenderness, vaginitis, altered mood
Males: Constipation, decreased testicle size, gynecomastia, impotence, decreased appetite, angina
Rare
Males: Thrombophlebitis

SERIOUS REACTIONS

! Signs and symptoms of metastatic prostatic carcinoma (such as bone pain, dysuria or hematuria, and weakness or paresthesia of the lower extremities) occasionally worsen 1 to 2 weeks after the initial dose but then subside with continued therapy.
! Pulmonary embolism and MI occur rarely.

DENTAL CONSIDERATIONS

General:
• If additional analgesia is required for dental pain, consider alternative analgesics (NSAIDs) in patients taking narcotics for acute or chronic pain.

L

• Monitor and record vital signs.
• This drug may be used in the hospital or on an outpatient basis. Confirm the patient's disease and treatment status.
• Consider semisupine chair position for patient comfort if GI side effects occur.
• Question patient about tolerance of NSAIDS or aspirin related to GI disease.
• Patient on chronic drug therapy may rarely present with symptoms of blood dyscrasias, which can include infection, bleeding, and poor healing. If dyscrasia is present, caution patient to prevent oral tissue trauma when using oral hygiene aids.
• Examine for oral manifestation of opportunistic infection.

L

Consultations:
• Medical consultation may be required to assess immunologic status during cancer chemotherapy and determine safety risk, if any, posed by the required dental treatment.
• Consider consulting with physician before prescribing drugs that may cause constipation (narcotics).
• Medical consultation may be required to assess disease control and patient's ability to tolerate stress.
• In a patient with symptoms of blood dyscrasias, request a medical consultation for blood studies and postpone treatment until normal values are reestablished.

Teach Patient/Family:
• *When chronic dry mouth occurs advise patient:*
  • To avoid mouth rinses with high alcohol content due to drying effects
  • To use daily home fluoride products for anticaries effect
  • To use sugarless gum, frequent sips of water or saliva substitutes
• Assess salivary flow as a factor in caries, periodontal disease and candidiasis
• To prevent trauma when using oral hygiene aids
• To report oral lesions, soreness, or bleeding to dentist
• Importance of updating health and medication history if physician makes any changes in evaluation or drug regimens; include OTC, herbal, and nonherbal in the update

levalbuterol

lee-val-bwet′-err-all
(Xopenex)
Do not confuse Xopenex with Xanax.

CATEGORY AND SCHEDULE

Pregnancy Risk Category: C

MECHANISM OF ACTION

A sympathomimetic that stimulates beta$_2$-adrenergic receptors in the lungs resulting in relaxation of bronchial smooth muscle.
Therapeutic Effect: Relieves bronchospasm and reduces airway resistance.

PHARMACOKINETICS

Route	Onset	Peak	Duration
Inhalation	10–17 min	1.5 hr	5–6 hr

Metabolized in the liver to inactive metabolite. ***Half-life:*** 3.3–4 hr.

AVAILABILITY

Solution for Nebulization: 0.31 in 3-ml vials, 0.63 mg in 3-ml vials, 1.25 mg in 3-ml vials.

INDICATIONS AND DOSAGES

Treatment and Prevention of Bronchospasm

NEBULIZATION

Adults, Elderly, Children 12 yr and older. Initially, 0.63 mg 3 times a day 6–8 hr apart. May increase to 1.25 mg 3 times a day with dose monitoring.

Children 3–11 yr. Initially 0.31 mg 3 times a day. Maximum: 0.63 mg 3 times a day

CONTRAINDICATIONS

History of hypersensitivity to sympathomimetics

INTERACTIONS

Drug

Beta blockers: Antagonize the effects of levalbuterol.

Digoxin: May increase the risk of arrhythmias.

MAOIs, tricyclic antidepressants: May potentiate cardiovascular effects.

Herbal

None known.

Food

None known.

Drug interactions of concern to dentistry

- Significant reduction of effects: β-adrenergic blockers
- Potentiation of CV effects: MAOIs, tricyclic antidepressants, methylxanthines
- No specific dental drug interactions reported

DIAGNOSTIC TEST EFFECTS

May increase serum potassium level.

SIDE EFFECTS

Frequent

Tremor, nervousness, headache, throat dryness and irritation

Occasional

Cough, bronchial irritation

Rare

Somnolence , diarrhea, dry mouth, flushing, diaphoresis, anorexia

SERIOUS REACTIONS

! Excessive sympathomimetic stimulation may produce palpitations, extrasystoles, tachycardia, chest pain, a slight increase in BP followed by a substantial decrease, chills, diaphoresis, and blanching of skin.

! Too-frequent or excessive use may lead to decreased bronchodilating effectiveness and severe, paradoxical bronchoconstriction.

DENTAL CONSIDERATIONS

General:

- Monitor vital signs at every appointment because of CV side effects.
- Assess salivary flow as a factor in caries, periodontal disease, and candidiasis.
- Consider semisupine chair position for patients with respiratory disease.
- Short midday appointments and a stress reduction protocol may be required for anxious patients.
- Be aware that aspirin or sulfite preservatives in vasoconstrictor-containing products can exacerbate asthma.
- Acute asthmatic episodes may be precipitated in the dental office. Rapid-acting sympathomimetic inhalants should be available for emergency use. A stress reduction protocol may be required.

Consultations:

- Medical consultation may be required to assess disease control and patient's ability to tolerate stress.

Teach Patient/Family:

- For inhalation dosage forms, rinse mouth with water after each dose to prevent dryness

• *When chronic dry mouth occurs, advise patient:*
  • To avoid mouth rinses with high alcohol content because of drying effects
  • To use daily home fluoride products for anticaries effect
  • To use sugarless gum, frequent sips of water, or saliva substitutes

levetiracetam

leva-tir-ass′-eh-tam
(Keppra)
Do not confuse Keppra with Kaletra.

CATEGORY AND SCHEDULE

Pregnancy Risk Category: C

L

MECHANISM OF ACTION

An anticonvulsant that inhibits burst firing without affecting normal neuronal excitability. ***Therapeutic Effect:*** Prevents seizure activity.

AVAILABILITY

Liquid: 100 mg/ml.
Tablets: 250 mg, 500 mg, 750 mg.

INDICATIONS AND DOSAGES

▸ Partial-Onset Seizures

PO

Adults, Elderly. Initially, 500 mg q12h. May increase by 1,000 mg/day q2wk. Maximum: 3,000 mg/day.
Children 4–16 yr. 10–20 mg/kg/day in 2 divided doses. May increase at weekly intervals by 10–20 mg/kg. Maximum: 60 mg/kg.

▸ Dosage in Renal Impairment

Dosage is modified on the basis of creatinine clearance.

Creatinine Clearance (ml/min)	Dosage
Higher than 80 ml/min	500–1500 mg q12h
50–80 ml/min	500–1000 mg q12h
30–50 ml/min	250–750 mg q12h
less than 30 ml/min	250–500 mg q12h
End stage renal disease using dialysis	500–1000 mg q12h, after dialysis, a 250- to 500-mg supplemental dose is recommended.

CONTRAINDICATIONS

Hypersensitivity reaction

INTERACTIONS

Drug
None known.
Herbal
None known.
Food
None significant.
Drug interactions of concern to dentistry
• None reported

DIAGNOSTIC TEST EFFECTS

May increase blood Hgb level, Hct, and RBC and WBC counts.

SIDE EFFECTS

Frequent (15%–10%)
Somnolence, asthenia, headache, infection
Occasional (9%–3%)
Dizziness, pharyngitis, pain, depression, nervousness, vertigo, rhinitis, anorexia
Rare (< 3%)
Amnesia, anxiety, emotional lability, cough, sinusitis, anorexia, diplopia

SERIOUS REACTIONS

! None known.

DENTAL CONSIDERATIONS

General:

• Short appointments and a stress reduction protocol may be required for anxious patients.
• Ask patient about type of epilepsy, seizure frequency, and quality of seizure control.

Consultation:

• Medical consultation may be required to assess disease control and patient's ability to tolerate stress.
• In patients with symptoms of blood dyscrasias, request a medical consultation for blood studies and postpone treatment until normal values are reestablished.

Teach Patient/Family:

• Importance of updating health and drug history if physician makes changes in evaluation or drug regimens

levobetaxolol hydrochloride

le-vo-bay-tax′-oh-lol
(Betaxon)
Do not confuse with levobunolol.

CATEGORY AND SCHEDULE

Pregnancy Risk Category: C

MECHANISM OF ACTION

An antiglaucoma agent that blocks beta1-adrenergic receptors. Reduces aqueous humor production.
Therapeutic Effect: Reduces intraocular pressure (IOP).

PHARMACOKINETICS

Route	Onset	Peak	Duration
Eye drops	30 min	2 hrs	12 hrs

May be systemically absorbed.

AVAILABILITY

Ophthalmic Solution: 0.5% (Betaxon).

INDICATIONS AND DOSAGES

▸ **Glaucoma, Ocular Hypertension**
OPHTHALMIC
Adults, Elderly. Instill 1 drop 2 times/day.

CONTRAINDICATIONS

Sinus bradycardia, second- or third-degree atrioventricular (AV) block, cardiogenic shock, overt heart failure, hypersensitivity to betaxolol, levobetaxolol, or any component of levobetaxolol formulations

INTERACTIONS

Drug

Fenoldopam: May exaggerate hypotensive response.

Herbal

Dong quai: May decrease blood pressure.
Licorice, Ma Huang, St. John's wort, yohimbine: May decrease effectiveness of levobetaxolol.

Food

None known.

Drug interactions of concern to dentistry

• None reported

DIAGNOSTIC TEST EFFECTS

None known.

SIDE EFFECTS

Frequent

Ocular discomfort

Occasional

Blurred vision

Rare

Anxiety, dizziness, vertigo, headache

SERIOUS REACTIONS

! Diabetes, hypothyroidism, bradycardia, tachycardia, hypertension, hypotension, heart block, alopecia, dermatitis, psoriasis, arthritis, tendonitis, dyspnea

L

and other respiratory symptoms (e.g. bronchitis, pneumonia, rhinitis, sinusitits, pharyngitis) occur rarely.
! Ophthalmic overdosage may produce bradycardia, hypotension, bronchospasm, and acute cardiac failure.

DENTAL CONSIDERATIONS

General:

- Determine why patient is taking the drug.
- Avoid drugs with anticholinergic activity, such as antihistamines, opioids, benzodiazepines, propantheline, atropine, and scopolamine.
- Avoid dental light in patient's eyes; offer dark glasses for patient comfort.
- Protect patient's eyes from accidental spatter during dental treatment.
- Question glaucoma patient about compliance with prescribed drug regimen.

Consultations:

- Medical consultation may be required to assess disease control.

Teach Patient/Family:

- Importance of updating health and medication history if physician makes any changes in evaluation or drug regimens; include OTC, herbal, and nonherbal in the update

levobunolol hydrochloride

lee-vo-byoo′-no-lol
(AK-Beta, Betagan, Novo-Levobunolol[CAN], Ohtho-Bunolol[CAN], PMS-Levobunolol[CAN])
Do not confuse with levobetaxolol.

CATEGORY AND SCHEDULE

Pregnancy Risk Category: C

MECHANISM OF ACTION

A nonselective beta-blocker that blocks beta1- and beta2-adrenergenic receptors. ***Therapeutic Effect:*** Reduces intraocular pressure. Decreases production of aqueous humor.

PHARMACOKINETICS

Well absorbed after administration. Metabolized in liver. Primarily excreted in urine. ***Half-life:*** 6.1 hrs.

AVAILABILITY

Ophthalmic Solution: 0.25%, 0.5% (AK-Beta, Betagan).

INDICATIONS AND DOSAGES

▸ Glaucoma, Ocular Hypertension

OPHTHALMIC

Adults, Elderly. Instill 1–2 drops in affected eye(s) once daily.

OFF-LABEL USES

Bronchial asthma, chronic obstructive pulmonary disease (COPD), cardiogenic shock, overt cardiac failure, second or third degree AV block, severe sinus bradycardia, hypersensitivity to levobunolol or any component of the formulation

CONTRAINDICATIONS

Cardiogenic shock, overt cardiac failure, second- or third-degree heart block, sinus bradycardia, hypersensitivity to levobunolol or any component of the formulation

INTERACTIONS

Drug

Amiodarone: May increase risk of hypotension, bradycardia, and cardiac arrest.

Diuretics, fentanyl, other hypotensives: May increase hypotensive effect.
NSAIDs: May decrease antihypertensive effect.
Sympathomimetics, xanthines: May mutually inhibit hypotensive effects and may mask symptoms of hypoglycemia.

Herbal

Dong quai: May increase hypotensive effect.
Licorice, Ma huang, St. John's wort, yohimbine: May decrease effectiveness of levobunolol.

Food

None known.

Drug interactions of concern to dentistry

- Patient with glaucoma: avoid use of anticholinergic drugs, atropine-like drugs, propantheline, and diazepam (benzodiazepines)

DIAGNOSTIC TEST EFFECTS

None known.

SIDE EFFECTS

Frequent

Burning/stinging, eye irritation, visual disturbances

Occasional

Increased light sensitivity, watering of eye

Rare

Dry eye, conjunctivitis, eye pain, diarrhea, dyspepsia

SERIOUS REACTIONS

! Abrupt withdrawal may result in sweating, headache, and fatigue.

! Ophthalmic overdosage may produce bradycardia, hypotension, bronchospasm, and acute cardiac failure.

DENTAL CONSIDERATIONS

General:

- Check compliance of patient with prescribed drug regimen for glaucoma.
- Avoid dental light in patient's eyes; offer dark glasses for patient comfort.

Consultations:

- Consultation with physician may be necessary if sedation or anesthesia is required.

levocabastine

levo-cab′-a-steen
(Livostin)

CATEGORY AND SCHEDULE

Pregnancy Risk Category: C

MECHANISM OF ACTION

An antiallergic agent that selectively antagonizes H1 receptor.
Therapeutic Effect: Blocks histamine-associated symptoms of seasonal allergic conjunctivitis.

PHARMACOKINETICS

Duration of action is about 2 hours. Minimal systemic absorbtion.

AVAILABILITY

Ophthalmic Suspension: 0.05% (Livostin).

INDICATIONS AND DOSAGES

▸ **Allergic Conjunctivitis**

OPHTHALMIC

Adults, Elderly, Children 12 yrs or older. 1 drop 4 times/day, for up to 2 wks.

CONTRAINDICATIONS

Wearing of soft contact lenses (product contains benzalkonium chloride), hypersensitivity to levocabastine or any component of the formulation

INTERACTIONS

Drug

None known.

Herbal

None known.

Food

None known.

Drug interactions of concern to dentistry

- None reported

DIAGNOSTIC TEST EFFECTS

None known.

SIDE EFFECTS

Frequent

Transient stinging, burning, discomfort, headache

Occasional

Dry mouth, fatigue, eye dryness, lacrimation/discharge, eyelid edema

Rare

Rash, erythema, nausea, dyspnea

SERIOUS REACTIONS

! None reported.

DENTAL CONSIDERATIONS

General:

- Question patient about history of allergy to avoid using other potential allergens.
- Avoid dental light in patient's eyes; offer dark glasses for patient comfort.
- Evaluate respiration characteristics and rate.
- Using for <2 wk should not present a problem with dry mouth.

Teach Patient/Family:

- *When chronic dry mouth occurs, advise patient:*
  - To avoid mouth rinses with high alcohol content because of drying effects
  - To use daily home fluoride products for anticaries effect
  - To use sugarless gum, frequent sips of water, or saliva substitutes

levodopa

lev-oh-dope-ah

(Dopar, Larodopa)

CATEGORY AND SCHEDULE

Pregnancy Risk Category: C

MECHANISM OF ACTION

A dopamine prodrug that is converted to dopamine in basal ganglia. Increases dopamine concentrations in the brain, inhibiting hyperactive cholinergic activity. ***Therapeutic Effect:*** Decreases signs and symptoms of Parkinson's disease.

PHARMACOKINETICS

About 30% absorbed. May be reduced with high-protein meal. Protein binding: minimal. Crosses blood-brain barrier. Converted to dopamine. Eliminated primarily in urine and to a lesser amount in feces and expired air. Not removed by hemodialysis. ***Half-life:*** 0.75–1.5 hrs.

AVAILABILITY

Capsules: 100 mg, 250 mg, 500 mg (Dopar).

Tablets: 100 mg, 250 mg, 500 mg (Larodopa).

INDICATIONS AND DOSAGES

▸ **Parkinsonism**

PO

Adults, Elderly. Initially, 0.5–1 g 2–4 times/day. May increase in increments not exceeding 0.75 g every 3–7 days, up to a maximum of 8 g/day.

CONTRAINDICATIONS

Nonselective MAOI therapy, hypersensitivity to levodopa or any component of its formulation.

INTERACTIONS

Drug

Alcohol: May increase the risk of CNS depression.
Anticonvulsants, benzodiazepines, bromperidol, droperidol, haloperidol, phenothiazines: May decrease the effects of levodopa.
Bupropion: May increase risk of nausea, vomiting, excitation, restlessness, and postural tremor.
Cisapride: May increase risk of levodopa adverse effects.
Ferric ammonium citrate: May decrease the effects of levodopa.
Indinavir: May increase dyskinesias.
Iron: May decrease the effects of levodopa.
Isoniazide: May increase symptomatic deterioration of Parkinson's disease.
MAOIs: May increase risk of hypertensive crises
Metoclopramide: May increase bioavailability and increase incidence of extrapyramidal symptoms.
Phenytoin: May decrease the effects of levodopa.
Selegiline: May increase dyskinesias, nausea, orthostatic hypotension, confusion, hallucinations.

Herbal

Kava kava: May decrease the effects of levodopa.
Pyridoxine: May decrease the effects of levodopa.

Food

High protein meals: May decrease peak levodopa concentrations.

Drug interactions of concern to dentistry

- Decreased absorption: anticholinergics
- Decreased therapeutic effect: benzodiazepines, pyridoxine (vitamin B_6), tricyclic antidepressants

DIAGNOSTIC TEST EFFECTS

May increase BUN, LDH concentrations, serum alkaline phosphatase and bilirubin, SGOT (AST), and SGPT (ALT) levels. May falsely increase acetaminophen levels. May result in false positive urine glucose measurements.

SIDE EFFECTS

Frequent

Uncontrolled body movements of the face, tongue, arms and upper body, nausea and vomiting, anorexia

Occasional

Depression, anxiety, confusion, nervousness, difficulty urinating, irregular heartbeats, hiccoughs, dizziness, lightheadedness, decreased appetite, blurred vision, constipation, dry mouth, flushed skin, headache, insomnia, diarrhea, unusual tiredness, darkening of urine, discolored sweat

Rare

Hypertension, ulcer, hemolytic anemia, marked by tiredness or weakness.

SERIOUS REACTIONS

! High incidence of involuntary dystonic, and dyskinetic movements may be noted in patients on long-term therapy.
! Mental changes, such as paranoid ideation, psychotic episodes and depression, may be noted.
! Numerous mild to severe central nervous system (CNS) psychiatric disturbances may include reduced attention span, anxiety, nightmares, daytime somnolence, euphoria, fatigue, paranoia, and hallucinations.

DENTAL CONSIDERATIONS

General:

- Patients on chronic drug therapy may rarely have symptoms of blood dyscrasias, which can include infection, bleeding, and poor healing.
- Assess salivary flow as a factor in caries, periodontal disease, and candidiasis.
- After supine positioning, have patient sit upright for at least 2 min before standing to avoid orthostatic hypotension.
- Avoid dental light in patient's eyes; offer dark glasses for patient comfort.

Consultations:

- In a patient with symptoms of blood dyscrasias, request a medical consultation for blood studies and postpone dental treatment until normal values are reestablished.
- Take precautions if dental surgery is anticipated and anesthesia is required.
- Medical consultation may be required to assess disease control.

Teach Patient/Family:

- To use electric toothbrush if patient has difficulty holding conventional devices
- *When chronic dry mouth occurs, advise patient:*
  - To avoid mouth rinses with high alcohol content because of drying effects
  - To use sugarless gum, frequent sips of water, or saliva substitutes
  - To use daily home fluoride products for anticaries effect.

levofloxacin

levo-flox′-a-sin
(Iquix, Levaquin, Quixin)

CATEGORY AND SCHEDULE

Pregnancy Risk Category: C

MECHANISM OF ACTION

A fluoroquinolone that inhibits the enzyme DNA enzyme gyrase in susceptible microorganisms, interfering with bacterial cell replication and repair. ***Therapeutic Effect:*** Bactericidal.

PHARMACOKINETICS

Well absorbed after both PO and IV administration. Protein binding: 24%–8%. Penetrates rapidly and extensively into leukocytes, epithelial cells, and macrophages. Lung concentrations are 2–5 times higher than those of plasma. Eliminated unchanged in the urine. Partially removed by hemodialysis. ***Half-life:*** 8 hr.

AVAILABILITY

Oral Solution: 25 mg/ml.
Tablets (Levaquin): 250 mg, 500 mg, 750 mg.
Injection (Levaquin): 500-mg/20-ml vials.
Premixed Solution (Levaquin): 250 mg/50 ml, 500 mg/100 ml, 750 mg/150 ml.
Ophthalmic Solution (Quixin): 1.5%
Ophthalmic Solution (Iquix): 0.5%.

INDICATIONS AND DOSAGES

▸ **Bronchitis**
PO, IV
Adults, Elderly. 500 mg q24h for 7 days.

▸ **Community-Acquired Pneumonia**
PO
Adults, Elderly. 750 mg/day for 5 days.

▸ **Pneumonia**
PO, IV
Adults, Elderly. 500 mg q24h for 7–14 days.

▸ **Acute Maxillary Sinusitis**
PO, IV
Adults, Elderly. 500 mg q24h for 10–14 days.

▸ Skin and Skin-Structure Infections
PO, IV
Adults, Elderly. 500 mg q24h for 7–10 days.

▸ UTIs, Acute Pyelonephritis
PO, IV
Adults, Elderly. 250 mg q24h for 10 days.

▸ Bacterial Conjunctivitis
OPHTHALMIC
Adults, Elderly, Children 1 yr and older. 1–2 drops q2h for 2 days (up to 8 times a day), then 1–2 drops q4h for 5 days.

▸ Corneal Ulcer
OPHTHALMIC
Adults, Elderly, Children older than 5 yr. Days 1–3: Instill 1–2 drops q30min to 2 hours while awake and 4–6 hours after retiring. Days 4 through completion: 1–2 drops q1–4h while awake.

▸ Dosage in Renal Impairment
For bronchitis, pneumonia, sinusitis, and skin and skin-structure infections, dosage and frequency are modified on the basis of creatinine clearance.

Creatinine Clearance	Dosage
50–80 ml/min	No change
20–49 ml/min	500 mg initially, then 250 mg q24h
10–19 ml/min	500 mg initially, then 250 mg q48h

Dialysis 500 mg initially, then 250 mg q48h
For UTIs and pyelonephritis, dosage and frequency are modified on the basis of creatinine clearance.

Creatinine Clearance	Dosage
20 ml/min	No change
10–19 ml/min	250 mg initially, then 250 mg q48h

CONTRAINDICATIONS
Hypersensitivity to levofloaxcin, other fluoroquinolones, or nalidixic acid

INTERACTIONS
Drug
Antacids, iron preparations, sucralfate, zinc: Decrease levofloxacin absorption.
NSAIDs: May increase the risk of CNS stimulation or seizures.
Herbal
None known.
Food
None known.
Drug interactions of concern to dentistry
- Interference with absorption: solutions with multivalent cations (e.g., Mg^{2+})
- Increased seizure risk: NSAIDs
- May increase effects of warfarin (monitor bleeding)

DIAGNOSTIC TEST EFFECTS
May alter blood glucose levels.

IV INCOMPATIBILITIES
Furosemide (Lasix), heparin, insulin, nitroglycerin, propofol (Diprivan)

IV COMPATIBILITIES
Aminophylline, dobutamine (Dobutrex), dopamine (Intron), fentanyl (Sublimaze), lidocaine, lorazepam (Ativan), morphine

SIDE EFFECTS
Occasional (3%–1%)
Diarrhea, nausea, abdominal pain, dizziness, drowsiness, headache, light-headedness
Ophthalmic: Local burning or discomfort, margin crusting, crystals or scales, foreign body sensation, ocular itching, altered taste
Rare (< 1%)
Flatulence; altered taste; pain; inflammation or swelling in calves,

hands, or shoulder; chest pain; difficulty breathing; palpitations; edema; tendon pain
Ophthalmic: Corneal staining, keratitis, allergic reaction, eyelid swelling, tearing, reduced visual acuity

SERIOUS REACTIONS

! Antibiotic-associated colitis and other superinfections may occur from altered bacterial balance. Hypersensitivity reactions, including photosensitivity (as evidenced by rash, pruritus, blisters, edema, and burning skin), have occurred in patients receiving fluoroquinolones.

DENTAL CONSIDERATIONS

General:
- Determine why patient is taking the drug.
- If dental drugs prescribed, advise patient of potential for photosensitivity.

Consultations:
- Consult with patient's physician if an acute dental infection occurs and another antiinfective is required.

Teach Patient/Family:
- To minimize exposure to sunlight and wear sunscreen if sun exposure is planned
- To discontinue treatment and inform dentist immediately if patient experiences pain or inflammation of a tendon, and to rest and refrain from exercise

levothyroxine

lee-voe-thye-rox′-een
(Droxine[AUS], Eltroxin[CAN], Eutroxsig[AUS], Levothroid, Levoxyl, Novothyrox[CAN], Oroxine[AUS], Synthroid, Unithroid)
Do not confuse levothyroxine with liothyronine.

CATEGORY AND SCHEDULE

Pregnancy Risk Category: A

MECHANISM OF ACTION

A synthetic isomer of thyroxine involved in normal metabolism, growth, and development, especially of the CNS in infants. Possesses catabolic and anabolic effects.
Therapeutic Effect: Increases basal metabolic rate, enhances gluconeogenesis and stimulates protein synthesis.

PHARMACOKINETICS

Variable, incomplete absorption from the GI tract. Protein binding: greater than 99%. Widely distributed. Deiodinated in peripheral tissues, minimal metabolism in the liver. Eliminated by biliary excretion. ***Half-life:*** 6–7 days.

AVAILABILITY

Tablets (Levo-T, Levothroid, Levoxyl, Synthroid, Unithroid): 0.025 mg, 0.05 mg, 0.075 mg, 0.088 mg, 0.1 mg, 0.112 mg, 0.125 mg, 0.137 mg, 0.15 mg, 0.175 mg, 0.2 mg, 0.3 mg.
Injection (Synthroid): 200 mcg, 500 mcg.

INDICATIONS AND DOSAGES

▸ **Hypothyroidism**

PO

Adults, Elderly. Initially, 12.5–50 mcg. May increase by

25–50 mcg/day q2–4wk.
Maintenance: 100–200 mcg/day.
Children 13 yr and older.
150 mcg/day.
Children 6–12 yr. 100–125 mcg/day.
Children 1–5 yr. 75–100 mcg/day.
Children 7–11 mo. 50–75 mcg/day.
Children older than 3–6 mo.
25–50 mcg/day.
Children 3 mo and younger.
10–15 mcg/day.

▸ Thyroid Suppression Therapy
PO
Adults, Elderly. 2–6 mcg/kg/day for 7–10 days.

▸ Thyroid Stimulating Hormone Suppression in Thyroid Cancer, Nodules, Euthyroid Goiters
PO
Adults, Elderly. 2–6 mcg/kg/day for 7–10 days.
IV
Adults, Elderly, Children. Initial dosage approximately half the previously established oral dosage.

CONTRAINDICATIONS

Hypersensitivity to tablet components, such as tartrazine; allergy to aspirin; lactose intolerance; MI and thyrotoxicosis uncomplicated by hypothyroidism; treatment of obesity

INTERACTIONS

Drug

Cholestyramine, colestipol: May decrease the absorption of levothyroxine.
Oral anticoagulants: May alter the effects of oral anticoagulants
Sympathomimetics: May increase the risk of coronary insufficiency and the effects of levothyroxine.

Herbal

None known.

Food

None known.

Drug interactions of concern to dentistry

Increased effects of sympathomimetics when thyroid doses are not carefully monitored or in patients with coronary artery disease

DIAGNOSTIC TEST EFFECTS

None known.

IV INCOMPATIBILITIES

Do not use or mix with other IV solutions.

SIDE EFFECTS

Occasional

Reversible hair loss at the start of therapy (in children)

Rare

Dry skin, GI intolerance, rash, hives, pseudotumor cerebri or severe headache in children

SERIOUS REACTIONS

! Excessive dosage produces signs and symptoms of hyperthyroidism, including weight loss, palpitations, increased appetite, tremors, nervousness, tachycardia, hypertension, headache, insomnia, and menstrual irregularities.
! Cardiac arrhythmias occur rarely.

DENTAL CONSIDERATIONS

General:

- Uncontrolled hypothyroid patients may be more responsive to CNS depressants.
- Increased nervousness, excitability, sweating, or tachycardia may indicate a patient with uncontrolled hyperthyroidism or a dose of medication that is too high. Uncontrolled patients should be referred for medical treatment.
- Monitor vital signs at every appointment because of CV side effects.

Consultations:

- Medical consultation may be required to assess disease control.

lidocaine hydrocloride

lye′-doe-kane
(Lidoderm, Lignocaine Gel[AUS], Xylocaine, Xylocaine Aerosol [AUS], Xylocaine Ointment[AUS], Xylocaine Viscous Topical Solution[AUS], Xylocard[CAN], Zilactin-L[CAN])

CATEGORY AND SCHEDULE

Pregnancy Risk Category: B

MECHANISM OF ACTION

An amide anesthetic that inhibits conduction of nerve impulses. ***Therapeutic Effect:*** Causes temporary loss of feeling and sensation. Also an antiarrhythmic that decreases depolarization, automaticity, excitability of the ventricle during diastole by direct action. ***Therapeutic Effect:*** Inhibits ventricular arrhythmias.

PHARMACOKINETICS

Route	Onset	Peak	Duration
IV	30–90 sec	N/A	10–20 min
Local anesthetic	2.5 min	N/A	30–60 min

Completely absorbed after IM administration. Protein binding: 60% to 80%. Widely distributed. Metabolized in the liver. Primarily excreted in urine. Minimally removed by hemodialysis. ***Half-life:*** 1–2 hr.

AVAILABILITY

IM Injection: 300 mg/3 ml.
Direct IV Injection: 10 mg/ml, 20 mg/ml.
IV Admixture Injection: 40 mg/ml, 100 mg/ml, 200 mg/ml.
IV Infusion: 2 mg/ml, 4 mg/ml, 8 mg/ml.
Injection (anesthesia): 0.5%, 1%, 1.5%, 2%, 4%.
Liquid: 2.5%, 5%.
Ointment: 2.5%, 5%.
Cream: 0.5%.
Gel: 0.5%, 2.5%.
Topical Spray: 0.5%.
Topical Solution: 2%, 4%.
Topical Jelly: 2%.
Dermal Patch: 5%.

INDICATIONS AND DOSAGES

▸ Rapid Control of Acute Ventricular Arrhythmias after an MI, Cardiac Catheterization, Cardiac Surgery, or Digitalis-Induced Ventricular Arrhythmias

IM

Adults, Elderly. 300 mg (or 4.3 mg/kg). May repeat in 60–90 min.

IV

Adults, Elderly. Initially, 50–100 mg (1 mg/kg) IV bolus at rate of 25–50 mg/min. May repeat in 5 min. Give no more than 200–300 mg in 1 hr. Maintenance: 20–50 mcg/kg/min (1–4 mg/min) as IV infusion.
Children, Infants. Initially, 0.5–1 mg/kg IV bolus; may repeat but total dose not to exceed 3–5 mg/kg. Maintenance: 10–50 mcg/kg/min as IV infusion.

▸ Dental or Surgical Procedures, Childbirth

INFILTRATION OR NERVE BLOCK

Adults. Local anesthetic dosage varies with procedure, degree of anesthesia, vascularity, duration. Maximum dose: 4.5 mg/kg. Do not repeat within 2 hrs.

▸ Local Skin Disorders (minor burns, insect bites, prickly heat, skin manifestations of chickenpox, abrasions), and Mucous Membrane Disorders (local anesthesia of oral, nasal, and laryngeal mucous membranes; local anesthesia of respiratory, urinary tract; relief of

discomfort of pruritus ani, hemorrhoids, pruritus vulvae)
TOPICAL
Adults, Elderly. Apply to affected areas as needed.

▸ **Treatment of Shingles-Related Skin Pain**
TOPICAL (Dermal patch)
Adults, Elderly. Apply to intact skin over most painful area (up to 3 applications once for up to 12 hrs in a 24-hr period).

CONTRAINDICATIONS

Adams-Stokes syndrome, hypersensitivity to amide-type local anesthetics, septicemia (spinal anesthesia), supraventricular arrhythmias, Wolff-Parkinson-White syndrome

INTERACTIONS

Drug

Anticonvulsants: May increase cardiac depressant effects.
Beta-adrenergic blockers: May increase risk of toxicity.
Other antiarrhythmics: May increase cardiac effects.

Herbal

None known.

Food

None known.

Drug interactions of concern to dentistry in patch form:

- None reported

DIAGNOSTIC TEST EFFECTS

IM lidocaine may increase creatine kinase level (used to diagnose acute MI). Therapeutic blood level is 1.5 to 6 mcg/ml; toxic blood level is greater than 6 mcg/ml.

IV INCOMPATIBILITIES

Amphotericin B complex (Abelcet, AmBisome, Amphotec), thiopental

IV COMPATIBILITIES

Aminophylline, amiodarone (Cordarone), calcium gluconate, digoxin (Lanoxin), diltiazem (Cardizem), dobutamine (Dobutrex), dopamine (Intropin), enalapril (Vasotec), furosemide (Lasix), heparin, insulin, nitroglycerin, potassium chloride

SIDE EFFECTS

CNS effects are generally dose related and of short duration.

Occasional

IM: Pain at injection site
Topical: Burning, stinging, tenderness at application site

Rare

Generally with high dose: Drowsiness; dizziness; disorientation; light-headedness; tremors; apprehension; euphoria; sensation of heat, cold, or numbness; blurred or double vision; ringing or roaring in ears (tinnitus); nausea

SERIOUS REACTIONS

! Although serious adverse reactions to lidocaine are uncommon, high dosage by any route may produce cardiovascular depression, bradycardia, hypotension, arrhythmias, heart block, cardiovascular collapse, and cardiac arrest.
! Potential for malignant hyperthermia.
! CNS toxicity may occur, especially with regional anesthesia use, progressing rapidly from mild side effects to tremors, somnolence, seizures, vomiting, and respiratory depression.
! Methemoglobinemia (evidenced by cyanosis) has occurred following topical application of lidocaine for teething discomfort and laryngeal anesthetic spray.

DENTAL CONSIDERATIONS

PATCH FORM

General:

- Use no more than one patch per area, remove after 15 min to avoid toxicity.

L

Teach Patient/Family:
- To prevent injury while numbness is present and to refrain from gum chewing and eating after dental treatment
- To report unresolved oral lesions to dentist

lincomycin HCl
lincomycin

lin-koe-**my**-sin
(Bactramycin, Lincocin, Lincomycin)

CATEGORY AND SCHEDULE
Pregnancy Risk Category: B

L

MECHANISM OF ACTION
A lincosamide antibiotic that specifically binds on the 50S subunit and affects the process of peptide chain initiation. ***Therapeutic Effect:*** Inhibits protein synthesis of the bacterial cell wall.

PHARMACOKINETICS
Rapidly absorbed from the GI tract. Protein binding: Unknown. Metabolized in liver. Primarily excreted in urine. Not removed by hemodialysis. ***Half-life:*** 5.4 hr (prolonged with renal or hepatic impairment).

AVAILABILITY
Injectable Solution (Bactramycin, Lincocin): 300 mg/ml.

INDICATIONS AND DOSAGES
▸ **Serious Infection Due to Susceptible Strains of Streptococci, Pneumococci, and Staphylococci**
PO
Adults. 500 mg 3 times per day (500 mg approximately q8h).
Children Older than 1 mo.
30 mg/kg/day (15 mg/lb/day) divided into 3 or 4 equal doses.

▸ **More Severe Infection Due to Susceptible Strains of Streptococci, Pneumococci, and staphylococci**
PO
Adults. 500 mg or more 4 times per day (500 mg or more approximately q6h).
Children Older Than 1 mo.
60 mg/kg/day (30 mg/lb/day) divided into 3 or 4 equal doses.

▸ **Serious Infection Due to Susceptible Strains of Streptococci, Pneumococci, and Staphylococci**
IM
Adults. 600 mg (2 ml) q24h.
Children Older Than 1 mo.
One injection of 10 mg/kg (5 mg/lb) q24h.

▸ **More Severe Infection Due to Susceptible Strains of Streptococci, Pneumococci, and Staphylococci**
IM
Adults. 600 mg (2 ml) q12h or more often.
Children Older Than 1 mo.
One injection of 10 mg/kg (5 mg/lb) q12h or more often.

▸ **Serious Infection Due to Susceptible Strains of Streptococci, Pneumococci, and Staphylococci**
IV
Adults. 600 mg (2 ml) to 1 g q8–12h
Children Older Than 1 mo.
One injection of 10 mg/kg (5 mg/lb) q12h or more often. Depending on the severity of the infection, 10–20 mg/kg/day (5–10 mg/lb/day) can be infused in divided doses as described for adults.

▸ **More Severe Infection Due to Susceptible Strains of Streptococci, Pneumococci, and Staphylococci**
IV
Adults. 600 mg (2 ml) to 1 g q8–12h. Maximum: 8 g/day. Intravenous doses are given on the

basis of 1 g lincomycin diluted in not less than 100 ml of appropriate solution and infused over a period of not less than 1 hr.

Subconjunctival Injection

Adults. Inject 0.25 ml (75 mg).

Dosage in Renal Impairment

An appropriate dose is 25%–30% of that recommended for patients with normally functioning kidneys.

CONTRAINDICATIONS

History of hypersensitivity to clindamycin or lincomycin

INTERACTIONS

Drug

Erythromycin: May antagonize the effects of lincomycin.

Kaolin-pectin mixtures: Inhibits the absorption of orally administered lincomycin.

Neuromuscular blockers: May increase the effects of these drugs.

Herbal

None known.

Food

None known.

Drug interactions of concern to dentistry

- Decreased action of erythromycin
- Oral contraceptives: advise patient of a potential risk for decreased contraceptive action, to maintain compliance with oral contraceptive use while using antibiotics, and to consider the use of additional nonhormonal contraception

DIAGNOSTIC TEST EFFECTS

None known.

IV INCOMPATIBILITIES

Novobiocin, kanamycin

IV COMPATIBILITIES

Vitamin B complex, vitamin B complex with ascorbic acid, penicillin G sodium (satisfactory for 4 hr), cephalothin, tetracycline HCl, cephaloridine, colistimethate (satisfactory for 4 hr), ampicillin, methicillin, chloramphenicol, polymyxin B sulfate

SIDE EFFECTS

Frequent

Abdominal pain, nausea, vomiting, diarrhea

Occasional

Phlebitis, thrombophlebitis with IV administration, pain, induration at IM injection site, allergic reaction, urticaria, pruritus, tinnitus, vertigo

Rare

Dermatitis

SERIOUS REACTIONS

Alert

! Antibiotic-associated colitis, as evidenced by severe abdominal pain and tenderness, fever, and watery and severe diarrhea, may occur during and several weeks after lincomycin therapy.

! Cardiopulmonary arrest and hypotension have been reported.

DENTAL CONSIDERATIONS

General:

- Determine why the patient is taking the drug.

Consultations:

- Medical consultation may be required to assess disease control.

Teach Patient/Family:

- Importance of good oral hygiene to prevent soft tissue inflammation
- Caution to prevent injury when using oral hygiene aids
- To notify dentist if diarrhea occurs
- *When used for dental infection, advise patient:*
  - To report sore throat, oral burning sensation, fever, fatigue, any of which could indicate superinfection
  - To take at prescribed intervals and complete dosage regimen
  - To immediately notify the dentist if signs or symptoms of infection increase

L

linezolid

li-nee′-zoh-lid
(Zyvox, Zyvoxam)
Do not confuse Zyvox with Zoverax.

CATEGORY AND SCHEDULE

Pregnancy Risk Category: C

MECHANISM OF ACTION

An oxalodinone anti-infective that binds to a site on bacterial 23S ribosomal RNA, preventing the formation of a complex that is essential for bacterial translation. ***Therapeutic Effect:*** Bacteriostatic against enterococci and staphylococci; bactericidal against streptococci.

L

PHARMACOKINETICS

Rapidly and extensively absorbed after PO administration. Protein binding: 31%. Metabolized in the liver by oxidation. Excreted in urine. ***Half-life:*** 4–5.4 hr.

AVAILABILITY

Powder for Oral Suspension: 100 mg/5 ml.
Tablets: 400 mg, 600 mg.
Injection: 2 mg/ml in 100-ml, 200-ml, 300-ml bags.

INDICATIONS AND DOSAGES

▸ Vancomycin-Resistant Infections
PO, IV
Adults, Elderly, Children older than 11 yr. 600 mg q12h for 14–28 days.

▸ Pneumonia, Complicated Skin and Skin Structure Infections
PO, IV
Adults, Elderly, Children older than 11 yr. 600 mg q12h for 10–14 days.

▸ Uncomplicated Skin and Skin Structure Infections
PO
Adults, Elderly. 400 mg q12h for 10–14 days.
Children older than 11 yr. 600 mg q12h for 10–14 days.
Children 5–11 yr. 10 mg/kg/dose q12h for 10–14 days.

▸ Usual Neonate Dosage
PO, IV
Neonates. 10 mg/kg/dose q8–12h.

CONTRAINDICATIONS

None known.

INTERACTIONS

Drug

Adrenergic agents (sympathomimetics): Increase the effects of linezolid.
MAOIs: Decrease the effects of MAOIs.

Herbal

None known.

Food

Tyramine-containing foods and beverages: Excessive amounts may cause significant hypertension.

Drug interactions of concern to dentistry

- Potential to increase pressor effects of indirect-action sympathomimetic drugs and vasopressors, such as dopaminergic drugs, phenylephrine, phenylpropanolamine, and pseudoephedrine
- Interactions with vasoconstrictors in local anesthetics has not been studied

DIAGNOSTIC TEST EFFECTS

May decrease blood Hgb, platelet count, WBC count, and ALT (SGPT) levels.

IV INCOMPATIBILITIES

Amphotericin B complex (Abelcet, AmBisome, Amphotec), chlorpromazine (Thorazine), co-trimoxazole (Bactrim), diazepam (Valium), erythromycin (Erythrocin), pentamidine (Pentam IV), phenytoin (Dilantin)

SIDE EFFECTS

Occasional (5%–2%)

Diarrhea, nausea, headache

Rare (< 2%)

Altered taste, vaginal candidiasis, fungal infection, dizziness, tongue discoloration

SERIOUS REACTIONS

! Thrombocytopenia and myelosuppression occur rarely.

! Antibiotic-associated colitis and other superinfections may result from altered bacterial balance.

DENTAL CONSIDERATIONS

General:

- Determine why patient is taking the drug.
- Use vasoconstrictor with caution, in low doses, and with careful aspiration. Avoid using gingival retraction cord containing epinephrine.
- Patients on chronic drug therapy may rarely have symptoms of blood dyscrasias, which can include infection, bleeding, and poor healing.
- Examine for oral manifestation of opportunistic infection.
- Consider semisupine chair position for patient comfort if GI side effects occur.

Consultations:

- In a patient with symptoms of blood dyscrasias, request a medical consultation for blood studies and postpone treatment until normal values are reestablished.
- Medical consultation may be required to assess disease control and patient's ability to tolerate stress.
- Physician consultation is advised in the presence of an acute dental infection requiring another antibiotic.

Teach Patient/Family:

- That secondary oral infection may occur; need to see dentist immediately if infection occurs
- To report sore throat, oral burning sensation, fever, fatigue, any of which could indicate presence of a superinfection

liothyronine (T3)

lye-oh-thye′-roe-neen

(Cytomel, Tertroxin[AUS], Triostat)

Do not confuse liothyronine with levothyroxine.

CATEGORY AND SCHEDULE

Pregnancy Risk Category: A

L

MECHANISM OF ACTION

A synthetic form of triiodothyronine (T_3), a thyroid hormone involved in normal metabolism, growth, and development, especially of the CNS in infants. Possesses catabolic and anabolic effects. ***Therapeutic Effect:*** Increases basal metabolic rate, enhances gluconeogenesis, and stimulates protein synthesis.

AVAILABILITY

Tablets (Cytomel): 5 mcg, 25 mcg, 50 mcg.

Injection (Triostat): 10 mcg/ml.

INDICATIONS AND DOSAGES

▸ **Hypothyroidism**

PO

Adults, Elderly. Initially, 25 mcg/day. May increase in increments of 12.5–25 mcg/day q1–2wk. Maximum 100 mcg/day.

Children. Initially, 5 mcg/day. May increase by 5 mcg/day q3–4wk.

Maintenance: 100 mcg/day (children older than 3 yr); 50 mcg/day (children 1–3 yr); 20 mcg/day (infants).

▸ **Myxedema**

PO

Adults, Elderly. Initially, 5 mcg/day. Increase by 5–10 mcg q1–2wk (after 25 mcg/day has been reached, may increase in 12.5-mcg increments). Maintenance: 50–100 mcg/day.

▸ **Nontoxic Goiter**

PO

Adults, Elderly. Initially, 5 mcg/day. Increase by 5–10 mcg/day q1–2wk. When 25 mcg/day has been reached, may increase by 12.5–25 mcg/day q1–2wk. Maintenance: 75 mcg/day.

Children. 5 mcg/day. May increase by 5 mcg q1–2wk. Maintenance: 15–20 mcg/day.

▸ **Congenital Hypothyroidism**

PO

Children. Initially, 5 mcg/day. Increase by 5 mcg/day q3–4 days. Maintenance: Full adult dosage (children older than 3 yr); 50 mcg/day (children 1–3 yr); 20 mcg/day (infants).

▸ **T_3 suppression Test**

PO

Adults, Elderly. 75–100 mcg/day for 7 days; then repeat I^{131} thyroid uptake test.

▸ **Myxedema Coma, Precoma**

IV

Adults, Elderly. Initially, 25–50 mcg (10–20 mcg in patients with cardiovascular disease). Total dose at least 65 mcg/day.

CONTRAINDICATIONS

MI and thyrotoxicosis uncomplicated by hypothyroidism; obesity

INTERACTIONS

Drug

Cholestyramine, colestipol: May decrease the absorption of liothyronine.

Oral anticoagulants: May alter the effects of these drugs.

Sympathomimetics: May increase the risk of coronary insufficiency and the effects of liothyronine.

Herbal

None known.

Food

None known.

Drug interactions of concern to dentistry

- Hypertension, tachycardia: ketamine
- Increased effects of sympathomimetics when thyroid doses are not carefully monitored or in patients with coronary artery disease

DIAGNOSTIC TEST EFFECTS

None known.

SIDE EFFECTS

Occasional

Reversible hair loss at start of therapy (in children)

Rare

Dry skin, GI intolerance, rash, hives, pseudotumor cerebri or severe headache in children

SERIOUS REACTIONS

! Excessive dosage produces signs and symptoms of hyperthyroidism, including weight loss, palpitations, increased appetite, tremors, nervousness, tachycardia, hypertension, headache, insomnia, and menstrual irregularities.

! Cardiac arrhythmias occur rarely.

DENTAL CONSIDERATIONS

General:

- Patients with uncontrolled hypothyroidism may be more responsive to CNS depressants.

• Increased nervousness, excitability, sweating, or tachycardia may indicate a patient with uncontrolled hyperthyroidism or a dose of medication that is too high. Uncontrolled patients should be referred for medical treatment.

Consultations:

• Medical consultation may be required to assess disease control.

liotrix

lye-oh-trix
(Thyrolar, Thyrolar-1, Thyrolar-1/2, Thyrolar-1/4, Thyrolar-2, Thyrolar-3)

CATEGORY AND SCHEDULE

Pregnancy Risk Category: A

MECHANISM OF ACTION

A synthetic form of levothyroxine (T_4) and triiodothyronine (T_3) involved in normal metabolism, growth, and development, especially the CNS of infants. Possesses catabolic and anabolic effects.
Therapeutic Effect: Increases basal metabolic rate, enhances gluconeogenesis, stimulates protein synthesis.

PHARMACOKINETICS

T_4 is partially absorbed from the GI tract. T_3 is almost completely absorbed. Widely distributed. Deiodinated in peripheral tissues, minimal metabolism in the liver.
Half-life: Unknown.

AVAILABILITY

Tablets (Thyrolar-1/4): 15 mg.
Tablets (Thyrolar-1/2): 30 mg.
Tablets (Thyrolar): 60 mg.
Tablets (Thyrolar, Thyrolar-2): 120 mg.
Tablets (Thyrolar-3): 180 mg.

INDICATIONS AND DOSAGES

▸ Hypothyroidism

PO

Adults, Elderly. Initially, 50 mcg (0.05 mg) levothyroxine and 12.5 mcg (0.0125 mg) liothyronine per day, with increments of a like amount at monthly intervals until the desired result is obtained. Maintenance: 50–100 mcg (0.05–0.1 mg) levothyroxine and 12.5–25 mcg (0.0125–0.025 mg) liothyronine per day.

▸ Congenital Hypothyroidism

PO

Children Older than 12 yr. Over 150 mcg of levothyroxine per day.
Children 6–12 yr. 100–150 mcg of levothyroxine per day.
Children 1–5 yr. 75–100 mcg of levothyroxine per day.
Children 6–12 mo. 50–75 mcg of levothyroxine per day.
Children 0–6 mo. 25–50 mcg of levothyroxine per day.

▸ Myxedema

PO

Adults, Elderly. Initially, 12.5 mcg (0.0125 mg) levothyroxine and 3.1 mcg (0.0031 mg) liothyronine per day, with increments of a like amount q2–3wk until the desired result is obtained. Maintenance: 50–100 mcg (0.05–0.1 mg) levothyroxine and 12.5–25 mcg (0.0125–0.025 mg) liothyronine per day.

▸ Thyroid Cancer

PO

Adults, Elderly. Larger amounts of thyroid hormone than those used for replacement therapy are required.

▸ Thyroid Suppression Therapy

PO

Adults, Elderly. Usual dosage of levothyroxine 2.6 mcg/kg/day for 7–10 days.

CONTRAINDICATIONS

Uncorrected adrenal cortical insufficiency, untreated thyrotoxicosis, or hypersensitivity to any of active constituents

INTERACTIONS

Drug

Cholestyramine, colestipol: May decrease absorption of liotrix.
Oral anticoagulants: May alter the effects of these drugs.
Sympathomimetics: May increase the effects and coronary insufficiency of liotrix.

Herbal

None known.

Food

None known.

Drug interactions of concern to dentistry

- Hypertension, tachycardia: ketamine
- Increased effects of sympathomimetics when thyroid doses are not carefully monitored or in patients with coronary artery disease

DIAGNOSTIC TEST EFFECTS

None known.

SIDE EFFECTS

Occasional

Reversible hair loss at the start of therapy (in children)

Rare

Dry skin, GI intolerance, rash, hives, pseudotumor cerebri or severe headache in children

SERIOUS REACTIONS

! Excessive dosage produces signs and symptoms of hyperthyroidism, including weight loss, palpitations, increased appetite, tremors, nervousness, tachycardia, hypertension, headache, insomnia, menstrual irregularities.
! Cardiac arrhythmias occur rarely.

DENTAL CONSIDERATIONS

General:

- Patients with uncontrolled hypothyroidism may be more responsive to CNS depressants.
- Increased nervousness, excitability, sweating, or tachycardia may indicate a patient with uncontrolled hyperthyroidism or a dose of medication that is too high. Uncontrolled patients should be referred for medical treatment.

Consultations:

- Medical consultation may be required to assess disease control.

Teach Patient/Family:

- Importance of good oral hygiene to prevent soft tissue inflammation
- To avoid mouth rinses with high alcohol content because of drying effects

lisinopril

ly-sin′-oh-pril
(Apo-Lisinopril[CAN], Fibsol[AUS], Lisodur[AUS], Prinivil, Zestril)

Do not confuse lisinopril with fosinopril; Prinivil with Desyrel, Plendil, Proventil, or Restoril; Fibsol with Lioresal; or Zestril with Zostrix. Do not confuse lisinopril's combination form Zestoretic with Prilosec.

CATEGORY AND SCHEDULE

Pregnancy Risk Category: C (D if used in second or third trimester)

MECHANISM OF ACTION

This angiotensin-converting enzyme (ACE) inhibitor suppresses the renin-angiotensin-aldosterone system and prevents conversion of angiotensin I to angiotensin II, a potent vasoconstrictor; may also inhibit angiotensin II at local vascular and renal sites. Decreases plasma angiotensin II, increases plasma renin activity, and decreases aldosterone secretion. ***Therapeutic Effect:*** Reduces peripheral arterial resistance, BP, afterload, pulmonary capillary wedge pressure (preload), and pulmonary vascular resistance. In those with heart failure, also decreases heart size, increases cardiac output, and exercise tolerance time.

PHARMACOKINETICS

Route	Onset	Peak	Duration
PO	1 hr	6 hr	24 hr

Incompletely absorbed from the GI tract. Protein binding: 25%. Primarily excreted unchanged in urine. Removed by hemodialysis. ***Half-life:*** 12 hr (half-life is prolonged in those with impaired renal function).

AVAILABILITY

Tablets (Prinivil, Zestril): 2.5 mg, 5 mg, 10 mg, 20 mg, 30 mg, 40 mg.

INDICATIONS AND DOSAGES

▸ **Hypertension (used alone)**

PO

Adults. Initially, 10 mg/day. May increase by 5–10 mcg/day at 1–2 wk intervals. Maximum: 40 mg/day.
Elderly. Initially, 2.5–5 mg/day. May increase by 2.5–5 mg/day at 1–to 2–wk intervals. Maximum: 40 mg/day.

▸ **Hypertension (used in combination with other antihypertensives)**

PO

Adults. Initially, 2.5–5 mg/day titrated to patient's needs.

▸ **Adjunctive Therapy for Management of Heart Failure**

PO

Adults, Elderly. Initially, 2.5–5 mg/day. May increase by no more than 10 mg/day at intervals of at least 2 wk. Maintenance: 5–40 mg/day.

▸ **Improve Survival in Patients after a Myocardial Infarction (MI)**

PO

Adults, Elderly. Initially, 5 mg, then 5 mg after 24 hr, 10 mg after 48 hr, then 10 mg/day for 6 wk. For patients with low systolic BP, give 2.5 mg/day for 3 days, then 2.5–5 mg/day.

▸ **Dosage in Renal Impairment**

Titrate to patient's needs after giving the following initial dose:

Creatinine Clearance	% Normal Dose
10–50 ml/min	50–75
less than 10 ml/min	25–50

OFF-LABEL USES

Treatment of hypertension or renal crises with scleroderma

CONTRAINDICATIONS

History of angioedema from previous treatment with ACE inhibitors

INTERACTIONS

Drug

Alcohol, diuretics, hypotensive agents: May increase the effects of lisinopril.
Lithium: May increase lithium blood concentration and risk of toxicity.
NSAIDs: May decrease the effects of lisinopril.

Potassium-sparing diuretics, potassium supplements: May cause hyperkalemia.

Herbal

None known.

Food

None known.

Drug interactions of concern to dentistry

- Increased hypotension: alcohol, phenothiazines
- Decreased hypotensive effects: indomethacin and possibly other NSAIDs, sympathomimetics
- Suspected reduction in the antihypertensive and vasodilator effects by salicylates; monitor blood pressure if used concurrently

DIAGNOSTIC TEST EFFECTS

May increase BUN, serum alkaline phosphatase, serum bilirubin, serum creatinine, serum potassium, AST, and ALT levels. May decrease serum sodium levels. May cause positive ANA titer.

SIDE EFFECTS

Frequent (12%–5%)

Headache, dizziness, postural hypotension

Occasional (4%–2%)

Chest discomfort, fatigue, rash, abdominal pain, nausea, diarrhea, upper respiratory infection

Rare (≤ 1%)

Palpitations, tachycardia, peripheral edema, insomnia, paresthesia, confusion, constipation, dry mouth, muscle cramps

SERIOUS REACTIONS

! Excessive hypotension ("first-dose syncope") may occur in patients with CHF and severe salt and volume depletion.

! Angioedema (swelling of face and lips) and hyperkalemia occurs rarely.

! Agranulocytosis and neutropenia may be noted in patients with collagen vascular disease, including scleroderma and systemic lupus erythematosus, and impaired renal function.

! Nephrotic syndrome may be noted in patients with history of renal disease.

DENTAL CONSIDERATIONS

General:

- Monitor vital signs at every appointment because of CV and respiratory side effects.
- After supine positioning, have patient sit upright for at least 2 min before standing to avoid orthostatic hypotension.
- Patients on chronic drug therapy may rarely have symptoms of blood dyscrasias, which can include infection, bleeding, and poor healing.
- Assess salivary flow as a factor in caries, periodontal disease, and candidiasis.
- Limit use of sodium-containing products, such as saline IV fluids, for patients with a dietary salt restriction.
- Use vasoconstrictors with caution, in low doses, and with careful aspiration.
- Short appointments and a stress reduction protocol may be required for anxious patients.

Consultations:

- Medical consultation may be required to assess disease control and patient's ability to tolerate stress.
- In a patient with symptoms of blood dyscrasias, request a medical consultation for blood studies and postpone dental treatment until normal values are reestablished.
- Take precautions if dental surgery is anticipated and sedation or general

anesthesia is required; risk of hypotensive episode.

Teach Patient/Family:

- Importance of good oral hygiene to prevent soft tissue inflammation
- Caution to prevent injury when using oral hygiene aids
- *When chronic dry mouth occurs, advise patient:*
  - To avoid mouth rinses with high alcohol content because of drying effects
  - To use sugarless gum, frequent sips of water, or saliva substitutes
  - To use daily home fluoride products for anticaries effect

lithium carbonate/lithium citrate

lith′-ee-um

(lithium carbonate) Duralith[CAN], Eskalith, Lithicarb[AUS], Lithobid, Quilonum SR[AUS] (lithium citrate) Cibalith-S

Do not confuse Lithobid with Levbid, Lithostat, or Lithotabs.

CATEGORY AND SCHEDULE

Pregnancy Risk Category: D

MECHANISM OF ACTION

A psychotherapeutic agent that affects the storage, release, and reuptake of neurotransmitters. Antimanic effect may result from increased norepinephrine reuptake and serotonin receptor sensitivity. ***Therapeutic Effect:*** Produces antimanic and antidepressant effects.

PHARMACOKINETICS

Rapidly and completely absorbed from the GI tract. Primarily excreted unchanged in urine. Removed by hemodialysis. ***Half-life:*** 18–24 hr (increased in elderly).

AVAILABILITY

Capsules: 150 mg, 300 mg, 600 mg.
Syrup: 300 mg/ml.
Tablets: 300 mg.
Tablets (Controlled-Release): 450 mg.
Tablets (Slow-Release): 300 mg.

INDICATIONS AND DOSAGES

Alert: During acute phase, a therapeutic serum lithium concentration of 1–1.4 mEq/L is required. For long-term control, the desired level is 0.5–1.3 mEq/L. Monitor serum drug concentration and clinical response.

▸ Prevention or Treatment of Acute Mania, Manic Phase of Bipolar Disorder (manic-depressive illness)

PO

Adults. 300 mg 3–4 times a day or 450–900 mg slow-release form twice a day. Maximum: 2.4 g/day.

Elderly. 300 mg twice a day. May increase by 300 mg/day q1wk. Maintenance: 900–1,200 mg/day.

Children 12 yr and older. 600–1,800 mg/day in 3–4 divided doses (2 doses/day for slow-release).

Children younger than 12 yr. 15–60 mg/kg/day in 3–4 divided doses.

OFF-LABEL USES

Prevention of vascular headache; treatment of depression, neutropenia

CONTRAINDICATIONS

Debilitated patients, severe cardiovascular disease, severe dehydration, severe renal disease, severe sodium depletion

INTERACTIONS

Drug

Antithyroid medications, iodinated glycerol, potassium iodide: May increase the effects of these drugs.

L

Diuretics, NSAIDs: May increase lithium serum concentration and risk of toxicity.
Haloperidol: May increase extrapyramidal symptoms and the risk of neurologic toxicity.
Molindone: May increase the risk of neurotoxicity.
Phenothiazines: May decrease the absorption of phenothiazines, increase the intracellular concentration and renal excretion of lithium, and increase delirium and extrapyramidal symptoms. Antiemetic effect of some phenothiazines may mask early signs of lithium toxicity.

Herbal

None known.

Food

None known.

Drug interactions of concern to dentistry

- Increased toxicity: aspirin, indomethacin, other NSAIDs, haloperidol, metronidazole, carbamazepine
- Increased effects of neuromuscular blocking agents

DIAGNOSTIC TEST EFFECTS

May increase blood glucose, immunoreactive parathyroid hormone, and serum calcium levels. Therapeutic serum level is 0.6–1.2 mEq/L; toxic serum level is greater than 1.5 mEq/L.

SIDE EFFECTS

Occasional

Fine hand tremor, polydipsia, polyuria, mild nausea, dry mouth

Rare

Weight gain, bradycardia or tachycardia, acne, rash, muscle twitching, cold and cyanotic extremities, pseudotumor cerebri (eye pain, headache, tinnitus, vision disturbances)

SERIOUS REACTIONS

! A lithium serum concentration of 1.5–2.0 mEq/L may produce vomiting, diarrhea, drowsiness, confusion, incoordination, coarse hand tremor, muscle twitching, and T-wave depression on ECG.

! A lithium serum concentration of 2.0–2.5 mEq/L may result in ataxia, giddiness, tinnitus, blurred vision, clonic movements, and severe hypotension.

! Acute toxicity may be characterized by seizures, oliguria, circulatory failure, coma, and death.

DENTAL CONSIDERATIONS

General:

- Assess salivary flow as a factor in caries, periodontal disease, and candidiasis.
- After supine positioning, have patient sit upright for at least 2 min before standing to avoid orthostatic hypotension.

Consultations:

- Medical consultation may be required to assess disease control.

Teach Patient/Family:

- Importance of good oral hygiene to prevent soft tissue inflammation
- Caution to prevent injury when using oral hygiene aids
- *When chronic dry mouth occurs, advise patient:*
  - To avoid mouth rinses with high alcohol content because of drying effects
  - To use sugarless gum, frequent sips of water, or saliva substitutes
  - To use daily home fluoride products for anticaries effect

lodoxamide

loe-dox′-a-mide
(Alomide)

CATEGORY AND SCHEDULE

Pregnancy Risk Category: B

MECHANISM OF ACTION

A mast cell stabilizer that prevents increase in cutaneous vascular permeability, antigen-stimulated histamine release and may prevent calcium influx into mast cells.
Therapeutic Effect: Inhibits sensitivity reaction.

PHARMACOKINETICS

Non-detectable absorption.
Half-life: 8.5 hrs.

AVAILABILITY

Ophthalmic Solution: 0.1% (Alomide).

INDICATIONS AND DOSAGES

▸ Treatment of Vernal Keratoconjunctivitis, Conjunctivitis, and Keratitis

OPHTHALMIC
Adults, Elderly, Children 2 yrs or older. 1–2 drops 4 times/day, for up to 3 mos.

CONTRAINDICATIONS

Wearing soft contact lenses (product contains benzalkonium chloride), hypersensitivity to lodoxamide tromethamine or any component of the formulation

INTERACTIONS

Drug
None known.
Herbal
None known.
Food
None known.
Drug interactions of concern to dentistry
- None reported

DIAGNOSTIC TEST EFFECTS

None known.

SIDE EFFECTS

Frequent
Transient stinging, burning, instillation discomfort
Occasional
Ocular itching, blurred vision, dry eye, tearing/discharge/foreign body sensation, headache, dry mouth
Rare
Scales on lid/lash, ocular swelling, sticky sensation, dizziness, somnolence, nausea, sneezing, dry nose, rash

SERIOUS REACTIONS

! None reported.

DENTAL CONSIDERATIONS

General:
- Question patient about history of allergy to avoid use of other potential allergens.
- Protect patient's eyes from accidental spatter during dental treatment.
- Avoid dental light in patient's eyes; offer dark glasses for patient comfort.
- Use for <2 wk should not present a problem with dry mouth.

Teach Patient/Family:
- *When chronic dry mouth occurs advise patient:*
  - To avoid mouth rinses with high alcohol content due to drying effects

L

- To use daily home fluoride products for anticaries effect
- To use sugarless gum, frequent sips of water or saliva substitutes

lomefloxacin hydrochloride

low-meh-flocks′-ah-sin
(Maxaquin)

CATEGORY AND SCHEDULE

Pregnancy Risk Category: C

MECHANISM OF ACTION

A quinolone that inhibits the enzyme DNA gyrase in susceptible microorganisms, interfering with bacterial cell replication and repair. ***Therapeutic Effect:*** Bactericidal.

PHARMACOKINETICS

Well absorbed from the GI tract. Protein binding: 10%. Widely distributed. Metabolized in the liver. Primarily excreted in urine. Not removed by hemodialysis. ***Half-life:*** 4–6 hr (increased with impaired renal function and in the elderly).

AVAILABILITY

Tablets: 400 mg.

INDICATIONS AND DOSAGES

▸ Complicated UTIs

PO

Adults, Elderly. 400 mg/day for 10–14 days.

▸ Uncomplicated UTIs

PO

Adults (females). 400 mg/day for 3 days.

▸ Lower Respiratory Tract Infections

PO

Adults, Elderly. 400 mg/day for 10 days.

▸ Surgical Prophylaxis

PO

Adults, Elderly. 400 mg 2–6 hr before surgery.

▸ Dosage in Renal Impairment

Dosage and frequency are modified on the basis of creatinine clearance.

Creatinine Clearance	Dosage
41 ml/min and higher	No change
10–40 ml/min	400 mg initially, then 200 mg/day for10–14 days

CONTRAINDICATIONS

Hypersensitivity to quinolones

INTERACTIONS

Drug

Antacids, iron preparations, sucralfate: May decrease lomefloxacin absorption.
Caffeine, oral anticoagulants: May increase the effects of these drugs.
Theophylline: Decreases clearance and may increase blood concentration and risk of toxicity of theophylline.

Herbal

None known.

Food

None known.

Drug interactions of concern to dentistry

- Decreased effects: antacids
- Increased levels of cyclosporine, caffeine

DIAGNOSTIC TEST EFFECTS

May increase BUN and serum alkaline phosphatase, bilirubin, creatinine, LDH, AST, and ALT levels.

SIDE EFFECTS

Occasional (3%–2%)
Nausea, headache, photosensitivity, dizziness
Rare (1%)
Diarrhea

SERIOUS REACTIONS

! Antibiotic-associated colitis and other superinfections may result from altered bacterial balance.
! Hypersensitivity reactions, including photosensitivity (as evidenced by rash, pruritus, blisters, edema, and burning skin), have occurred in patients receiving fluoroquinolones.
! Arthropathy may occur if the drug is given to children younger than 18 years.

DENTAL CONSIDERATIONS

General:
- Because of drug interactions, do not use ingestible sodium bicarbonate products, such as the Prophy-Jet air polishing system, until 2 hr after drug use.
- Use caution in prescribing caffeine-containing analgesics.
- Determine why the patient is taking the drug.
- Avoid dental light in patient's eyes; offer dark glasses for patient comfort.
- Ruptures of the shoulder, hand, and Achilles tendons that required surgical repair or resulted in prolonged disability have been reported with this drug.

Consultations:
- Consult with patient's physician if an acute dental infection occurs and another antiinfective is required.

Teach Patient/Family:
- Caution to prevent injury when using oral hygiene aids
- To avoid mouth rinses with high alcohol content because of drying effects
- To minimize exposure to sunlight and wear sunscreen if sun exposure is planned
- To discontinue treatment and inform dentist immediately if patient experiences pain or inflammation of a tendon, and to rest and refrain from exercise

lomustine

low-meuw′-steen
(CeeNU)

CATEGORY AND SCHEDULE

Pregnancy Risk Category: D

L

MECHANISM OF ACTION

An alkylating agent and nitrosourea that inhibits DNA and RNA protein synthesis by cross-linking with DNA and RNA strands, preventing cell division. Cell cycle-phase nonspecific.
Therapeutic Effect: Interferes with DNA and RNA function.

AVAILABILITY

Capsules: 10 mg, 40 mg, 100 mg.

INDICATIONS AND DOSAGES

▸ Disseminated Hodgkin's Disease, Primary and Metastatic Brain Tumors
PO
Adults, Elderly. 100–130 mg/m^2 as single dose. Repeat dose at intervals of at least 6 wk but not until circulating blood elements have returned to acceptable levels. Adjust dose on the basis of hematologic response to previous dose.
Children. 75–150 mg/m^2 as a single dose every 6wk.

OFF-LABEL USES
Breast, GI, lung, or renal carcinoma; malignant melanoma; multiple myeloma

CONTRAINDICATIONS
Pregnancy

INTERACTIONS
Drug
Bone marrow depressants: May increase myelosuppression.
Live-virus vaccines: May potentiate virus replication, increase vaccine side effects, and decrease the patient's antibody response to the vaccine.
Herbal
None known.
Food
None known.
Drug interactions of concern to dentistry
- This drug depresses bone marrow function, which may increase risk of bleeding; avoid drugs that can increase bleeding, such as aspirin, NSAIDs

L

DIAGNOSTIC TEST EFFECTS
May increase liver function test results.

SIDE EFFECTS
Frequent
Nausea, vomiting (occuring 45 min–6 hr after dose and lasting 12–24 hr); anorexia (often follows for 2–3 days).
Occasional
Neurotoxicity (confusion, slurred speech), stomatitis, darkening of skin, diarrhea, rash, pruritus, alopecia

SERIOUS REACTIONS
! Myelosuppression may result in hematologic toxicity, manifested principally as leukopenia, mild anemia, and thrombocytopenia. Leukopenia occurs about 6 weeks after a dose, thrombocytopenia about 4 weeks after a dose; both persist for 1–2 weeks.
! Refractory anemia and thrombocytopenia occur commonly if lomustine therapy continues for more than 1 year.
! Hepatotoxicity occurs infrequently.
! Large cumulative doses of lomustine may result in renal damage.

DENTAL CONSIDERATIONS
General:
- Patients on chronic drug therapy may rarely have symptoms of blood dyscrasias, which can include infection, bleeding, and poor healing.
- Consider semisupine chair position for patient comfort if GI side effects occur.
- Palliative medication may be required for oral side effects.
- Consider local hemostasis measures to prevent excessive bleeding.
- Prophylactic antibiotics may be indicated to prevent infection if surgery or deep scaling is planned.
- Patients taking opioids for acute or chronic pain should be given alternative analgesics for dental pain.
- Avoid prescribing aspirin-containing products.

Consultations:
- In a patient with symptoms of blood dyscrasias, request a medical consultation for blood studies and postpone dental treatment until normal values are reestablished.
- Patients on cancer chemotherapy should have an adequate WBC count before completing dental procedures that may produce a wound. Consult to determine blood count before appointment.

Teach Patient/Family:
- Importance of good oral hygiene to prevent soft tissue inflammation
- Caution to prevent trauma when using oral hygiene aids
- That secondary oral infection may occur; must see dentist immediately if infection occurs
- To report oral lesions, soreness, or bleeding to dentist
- To avoid mouth rinses with high alcohol content because of drying and irritating effects
- Importance of updating medical/drug records if physician makes any changes in evaluation or drug regimens

loperamide hydrochloride

loe-per′-a-mide
(Apo-Loperamide[CAN], Gastro-Stop[AUS], Imodium, Imodium A-D, Loperacap[CAN], Novo-Loperamide[CAN])
Do not confuse Imodium with Indocin or Ionamin.

CATEGORY AND SCHEDULE

Pregnancy Risk Category: B
OTC liquid, tablets

MECHANISM OF ACTION

An antidiarrheal that directly affects the intestinal wall muscles.
Therapeutic Effect: Slows intestinal motility and prolongs transit time of intestinal contents by reducing fecal volume, diminishing loss of fluid and electrolytes, and increasing viscosity and bulk of stool.

PHARMACOKINETICS

Poorly absorbed from the GI tract. Protein binding: 97%. Metabolized in the liver. Eliminated in feces and excreted in urine. Not removed by hemodialysis. ***Half-life:*** 9.1–14.4 hr.

AVAILABILITY

Capsules: 2 mg.
Liquid: 1 mg/5 ml.
Tablets: 2 mg.

INDICATIONS AND DOSAGES

▸ **Acute Diarrhea**

PO (capsules)
Adults, Elderly. Initially, 4 mg; then 2 mg after each unformed stool. Maximum: 16 mg/day.
Children 9–12 yr, weighing more than 30 kg. Initially, 2 mg 3 times a day for 24 hr.
Children 6–8 yr, weighing 20–30 kg. Initially, 2 mg twice a day for 24 hr.
Children 2–5 yrs, weighing 13–20 kg. Initially, 1 mg 3 times/day for 24 hrs. Maintenance: 1 mg/10 kg only after loose stool.

▸ **Chronic Diarrhea**

PO
Adults, Elderly. Initially, 4 mg; then 2 mg after each unformed stool until diarrhea is controlled.
Children. 0.08–0.24 mg/kg/day in 2–3 divided doses. Maximum: 2 mg/dose.

▸ **Traveler's Diarrhea**

PO
Adults, Elderly. Initially, 4 mg; then 2 mg after each loose bowel movement (LBM). Maximum: 8 mg/day for 2 days.
Children 9–11 yr. Initially, 2 mg; then 1 mg after each LBM. Maximum: 6 mg/day for 2 days.
Children 6–8 yr. Initially, 1 mg; then 1 mg after each LBM. Maximum: 4 mg/day for 2 days.

CONTRAINDICATIONS

Acute ulcerative colitis (may produce toxic megacolon), diarrhea associated with pseudomembranous enterocolitis due to broad-spectrum antibiotics or to organisms that invade intestinal mucosa (such as *Escherichia coli*, shigella, and salmonella), patients who must avoid constipation

INTERACTIONS

Drug

Opioid (narcotic) analgesics: May increase the risk of constipation.

Herbal

None known.

Food

None known.

Drug interactions of concern to dentistry

- Increased action: opioid analgesics

DIAGNOSTIC TEST EFFECTS

None known.

SIDE EFFECTS

Rare

Somnolence, abdominal discomfort, allergic reaction (such as rash and itching)

Common dry mouth

SERIOUS REACTIONS

! Toxicity results in constipation, GI irritation, including nausea and vomiting, and CNS depression. Activated charcoal is used to treat loperamide toxicity.

DENTAL CONSIDERATIONS

General:

- Assess salivary flow as a factor in caries, periodontal disease, and candidiasis.
- Evaluate respiration characteristics and rate.
- Consider semisupine chair position for patient comfort because of GI effects of drug.
- This drug product is normally used only for a few doses for acute problems; however, some patients may have to take it for longer time periods as dictated by contributing disease.

Teach Patient/Family:

- *When chronic dry mouth occurs, advise patient:*
  - To avoid mouth rinses with high alcohol content because of drying effects
  - To use sugarless gum, frequent sips of water, or saliva substitutes
  - To use daily home fluoride products for anticaries effect

loracarbef

lor-a-kar′-bef

(Lorabid)

Do not confuse loracarbef or Lorabid with Lortab.

CATEGORY AND SCHEDULE

Pregnancy Risk Category: B

MECHANISM OF ACTION

A second-generation cephalosporin that binds to bacterial cell membranes and inhibits cell wall synthesis.

Therapeutic Effect: Bactericidal.

AVAILABILITY

Capsules: 200 mg, 400 mg.

Powder for Oral Suspension: 100 mg/5 ml, 200 mg/5 ml.

INDICATIONS AND DOSAGES

▶ **Bronchitis**

PO

Adults, Elderly, Children 12 yr and older. 200–400 mg q12h for 7 days.

▶ **Pharyngitis**

PO

Adults, Elderly, Children 12 yr and older. 200 mg q12h for 10 days.
Children 6 mo–11 yr. 7.5 mg/kg q12h for 10 days.

▶ **Pneumonia**

PO

Adults, Elderly, Children 12 yr and older. 400 mg q12h for 14 days.

▶ **Sinusitis**

PO

Adults, Elderly, Children 12 yr and older. 400 mg q12h for 10 days.
Children 6 mo–11 yr. 15 mg/kg q12h for 10 days.

▶ **Skin and Soft-Tissue Infections**

PO

Adults, Elderly, Children 12 yr and older. 200 mg q12h for 7 days.
Children 6 mo–11 yr. 7.5 mg/kg q12h for 7 days.

▶ **UTIs**

PO

Adults, Elderly, Children 6 mo–12 yr. 200–400 mg q12h for 7–14 days.

▶ **Otitis Media**

PO

Children 6 mo–12 yr. 15 mg/kg q12h for 10 days.

CONTRAINDICATIONS

History of anaphylactic reaction to penicillins or hypersensitivity to cephalosporins

INTERACTIONS

Drug

Probenecid: Increases serum concentration and half-life of loracarbef.

Herbal

None known.

Food

None known.

Drug interactions of concern to dentistry

- Decreased effects: tetracyclines, erythromycins, lincomycins
- *When used for dental infection:* may reduce effect of oral contraceptives

DIAGNOSTIC TEST EFFECTS

May increase BUN level and serum alkaline phosphatase, creatinine, AST (SGOT), and ALT (SGPT) levels. May decrease blood leukocyte and platelet counts.

SIDE EFFECTS

Frequent

Abdominal pain, anorexia, nausea, vomiting, diarrhea

Occasional

Rash, pruritus

Rare

Dizziness, headache, vaginitis

SERIOUS REACTIONS

! Antibiotic-associated colitis and other superinfections may result from altered bacterial balance.

! Hypersensitivity reactions (ranging from rash, urticaria, and fever to anaphylaxis) occur in less than 5% of patients—most commonly in patients with a history of drug allergies, especially to penicillins.

DENTAL CONSIDERATIONS

General:

- Take precautions regarding allergy to medication.
- Determine why the patient is taking the drug.
- Examine for evidence of oral manifestations of blood dyscrasias (infection, bleeding, poor healing).

Consultations:
- Medical consultation may be required to assess disease control.
- Medical consultation for blood studies (CBC); leukopenic or thrombocytopenic side effects may result in infection, delayed healing, and excessive bleeding. Postpone elective dental treatment until normal values are maintained.

Teach Patient/Family:
- Importance of good oral hygiene to prevent soft tissue inflammation

loratadine

loer-at′-ah-deen
(Alavert, Claratyne[AUS], Claritin, Claritin RediTab, Dimetapp, Tavist ND)

L

CATEGORY AND SCHEDULE

Pregnancy Risk Category: B

MECHANISM OF ACTION

A long-acting antihistamine that competes with histamine for H_1 receptor sites on effector cells.
Therapeutic Effect: Prevents allergic responses mediated by histamine, such as rhinitis, urticaria, and pruritus.

PHARMACOKINETICS

Route	Onset	Peak	Duration
PO	1–3 hr	8–12 hr	longer than 24 hr

Rapidly and almost completely absorbed from the GI tract. Protein binding: 97%; metabolite, 73%–77%. Distributed mainly to the liver, lungs, GI tract, and bile. Metabolized in the liver to active metabolite; undergoes extensive first-pass metabolism. Eliminated in urine and feces. Not removed by hemodialysis. ***Half-life:*** 8.4 hr; metabolite, 28 hr (increased in elderly and hepatic impairment).

AVAILABILITY

Syrup (Claritin): 10 mg/10 ml.
Tablets (Alavert, Claritin, Tavist ND): 10 mg.
Tablets (Rapid-Disintegrating [Alavert, Claritin RediTab]): 10 mg.

INDICATIONS AND DOSAGES

▸ Allergic Rhinitis, Urticaria

PO
Adults, Elderly, Children 6 yr and older. 10 mg once a day.
Children 2–5 yr. 5 mg once a day.

▸ Dosage in Hepatic Impairment

For adults, elderly, and children 6 years and older dosage is reduced to 10 mg every other day.

OFF-LABEL USES

Adjunct treatment of bronchial asthma

CONTRAINDICATIONS

Hypersensitivity to loratadine or its ingredients

INTERACTIONS

Drug

Clarithromycin, erythromycin, fluconazole, ketoconazole: May increase the loratadine blood concentration.

Herbal

None known.

Food

All foods: Delay the absorption of loratadine.

Drug interactions of concern to dentistry

- Increased CNS depression: all CNS depressants, alcohol

• Increased anticholinergic effect: anticholinergics, antihistamines, antiparkinsonian drugs
• Increased plasma concentration: ketoconazole

DIAGNOSTIC TEST EFFECTS

May suppress wheal and flare reactions to antigen skin testing unless the drug is discontinued 4 days before testing.

SIDE EFFECTS

Frequent (12%–8%)
Headache, fatigue, somnolence
Occasional (3%)
Dry mouth, nose, or throat
Rare
Photosensitivity

SERIOUS REACTIONS

! None known.

DENTAL CONSIDERATIONS

General:

• Assess salivary flow as a factor in caries, periodontal disease, and candidiasis.
• Consider semisupine chair position for patients with respiratory disease.
• Conscious sedation drugs may produce synergistic, sedative action.

Teach Patient/Family:

• Importance of good oral hygiene to prevent soft tissue inflammation
• *When chronic dry mouth occurs, advise patient:*
  • To avoid mouth rinses with high alcohol content because of drying effects
  • To use sugarless gum, frequent sips of water, or saliva substitutes
  • To use daily home fluoride products for anticaries effect

lorazepam

lor-a′-ze-pam
Schedule IV
(Apo-Lorazepam[CAN], Ativan, Lorazepam Intensol, Novolorazepam[CAN])
Do not confuse lorazepam with Alprazolam.

CATEGORY AND SCHEDULE

Pregnancy Risk Category: D
Controlled Substance Schedule: IV

MECHANISM OF ACTION

A benzodiazepine that enhances the action of the inhibitory neurotransmitter gamma-aminobutyric acid in the CNS, affecting memory, as well as motor, sensory, and cognitive function. ***Therapeutic Effect:*** Produces anxiolytic, anticonvulsant, sedative, muscle relaxant, and antiemetic effects.

PHARMACOKINETICS

Route	Onset	Peak	Duration
PO	60 min	N/A	8–12 hr
IV	15–30 min	N/A	8–12 hr
IM	30–60 min	N/A	8–12 hr

Well absorbed after PO and IM administration. Protein binding: 85%. Widely distributed. Metabolized in the liver. Primarily excreted in urine. Not removed by hemodialysis. ***Half-life:*** 10–20 hr.

AVAILABILITY

Tablets (Ativan): 0.5 mg, 1 mg, 2 mg.
Injection (Ativan): 2 mg/ml, 4 mg/ml.
Oral solution (Lorazepam Intensol): 2 mg/ml.

INDICATIONS AND DOSAGES

▶ Anxiety

PO

Adults. 1–10 mg/day in 2–3 divided doses. Average: 2–6 mg/day.
Elderly. Initially, 0.5–1 mg/day. May increase gradually. Range: 0.5–4 mg.

IV

Adults, Elderly. 0.02–0.06 mg/kg q2–6h.

IV INFUSION

Adults, Elderly. 0.01–0.1 mg/kg/h.

PO, IV

Children. 0.05 mg/kg/dose q4–8h. Range: 0.02–0.1 mg/kg. Maximum: 2 mg/dose.

▶ Insomnia Due to Anxiety

PO

Adults. 2–4 mg at bedtime.
Elderly. 0.5–1 mg at bedtime.

▶ Preoperative Sedation

IV

Adults, Elderly. 0.044 mg/kg 15–20 min before surgery. Maximum total dose: 2 mg.

IM

Adults, Elderly. 0.05 mg/kg 2 hr before procedure. Maximum total dose: 4 mg.

▶ Status Epilepticus

IV

Adults, Elderly. 4 mg over 2–5 min. May repeat in 10–15 min. Maximum: 8 mg in 12-hr period.
Children. 0.1 mg/kg over 2–5 min. May give second dose of 0.05 mg/kg in 15–20 min. Maximum: 4 mg.
Neonates. 0.05 mg/kg. May repeat in 10–15 min.

OFF-LABEL USES

Treatment of alcohol withdrawal, panic disorders, skeletal muscle spasms, chemotherapy-induced nausea or vomiting, tension headache, tremors; adjunctive treatment before endoscopic procedures (diminishes patient recall)

CONTRAINDICATIONS

Angle-closure glaucoma; pre-existing CNS depression; severe hypotension; severe uncontrolled pain

INTERACTIONS

Drug

Alcohol, other CNS depressants: May increase CNS depression.

Herbal

Kava kava, valerian: May increase CNS depression.

Food

None known.

Drug interactions of concern to dentistry

- Increased effects: alcohol, all CNS depressants, probenecid
- Increased sedation, hallucination: scopolamine
- Possible increase in CNS side effects of kava (herb)

DIAGNOSTIC TEST EFFECTS

None known. Therapeutic serum drug level is 50–240 ng/ml; toxic serum drug level is unknown.

IV INCOMPATIBILITIES

Aldesleukin (Proleukin), aztreonam (Azactam), idarubicin (Idamycin), ondansetron (Zofran), sufentanil (Sufenta)

IV COMPATIBILITIES

Bumetanide (Bumex), cefepime (Maxipime), diltiazem (Cardizem), dobutamine (Dobutrex), dopamine (Intropin), heparin, labetalol (Normodyne, Trandate), milrinone (Primacor), norepinephrine (Levophed), piperacillin and tazobactam (Zosyn), potassium, propofol (Diprivan)

SIDE EFFECTS

Frequent
Somnolence (initially in the morning), ataxia, confusion
Occasional
Blurred vision, slurred speech, hypotension, headache
Rare
Paradoxical CNS restlessness or excitement in elderly or debilitated

SERIOUS REACTIONS

! Abrupt or too-rapid withdrawal may result in pronounced restlessness, irritability, insomnia, hand tremor, abdominal or muscle cramps, diaphoresis, vomiting, and seizures.
! Overdose results in somnolence, confusion, diminished reflexes, and coma.

DENTAL CONSIDERATIONS

General:
• After supine positioning, have patient sit upright for at least 2 min before standing to avoid orthostatic hypotension.
• Elderly persons are more prone to orthostatic hypotension and have increased sensitivity to anticholinergic and sedative effects; use lower dose.
• When administered with opioid analgesic, reduce dose of opioid by one third.
• Psychologic and physical dependence may occur with chronic administration.
• Have someone drive patient to and from dental office when drug used for conscious sedation.
Consultations:
• Medical consultation may be required to assess disease control.
Teach Patient/Family:
• Importance of good oral hygiene to prevent soft tissue inflammation
• To avoid mouth rinses with high alcohol content because of drying effects

losartan

lo-sar′-tan
(Cozaar)
Do not confuse Cozaar with Zocor.

CATEGORY AND SCHEDULE

Pregnancy Risk Category: C (D if used in second or third trimesters)

MECHANISM OF ACTION

An angiotensin II receptor, type AT_1, antagonist that blocks vasoconstrictor and aldosterone-secreting effects of angiotensin II, inhibiting the binding of angiotensin II to the AT_1 receptors.
Therapeutic Effect: Causes vasodilation, decreases peripheral resistance, and decreases BP.

PHARMACOKINETICS

Route	Onset	Peak	Duration
PO	N/A	6 hr	24 hr

Well absorbed after PO administration. Protein binding: 98%. Undergoes first-pass metabolism in the liver to active metabolites. Excreted in urine and via the biliary system. Not removed by hemodialysis. ***Half-life:*** 2 hr, metabolite: 6–9 hr.

AVAILABILITY

Tablets: 25 mg, 50 mg, 100 mg.

L

INDICATIONS AND DOSAGES

▸ Hypertension

PO

Adults, Elderly. Initially, 50 mg once a day. Maximum: May be given once or twice a day, with total daily doses ranging from 25–100 mg.

▸ Nephropathy

PO

Adults, Elderly. Initially, 50 mg/day. May increase to 100 mg/day based on BP response.

▸ Stroke Reduction

PO

Adults, Elderly. 50 mg/day. Maximum: 100 mg/day.

▸ Hypertension in Patients with Impaired Hepatic Function

PO

Adults, Elderly. Initially, 25 mg/day.

CONTRAINDICATIONS

None known.

INTERACTIONS

Drug

Cimetidine: May increase the effects of losartan.
Ketoconazole, troleandomycin: May inhibit the effects of these drugs.
Lithium: May increase lithium blood concentration and risk of lithium toxicity.
Phenobarbital, rifampin: May decrease the effects of losartan.

Herbal

None known.

Food

Grapefruit, grapefruit juice: May alter the absorption of losartan.

Drug interactions of concern to dentistry

- Potential for increased hypotensive effects with other hypotensive drugs and sedatives
- Suspected increase in antihypertensive effects: fluconazole, ketoconazole; monitor blood pressure if used concurrently

DIAGNOSTIC TEST EFFECTS

May increase BUN, serum alkaline phosphatase, serum bilirubin, serum creatinine, AST(SGOT), and ALT(SGPT) levels. May decrease blood Hgb and Hct levels.

SIDE EFFECTS

Frequent (8%)
Upper respiratory tract infection
Occasional (4%–2%)
Dizziness, diarrhea, cough
Rare (≤ 1%)
Insomnia, dyspepsia, heartburn, back and leg pain, muscle cramps, myalgia, nasal congestion, sinusitis

SERIOUS REACTIONS

! Overdosage may manifest as hypotension and tachycardia. Bradycardia occurs less often.

DENTAL CONSIDERATIONS

General:

- Monitor vital signs at every appointment because of CV effects.
- Limit use of sodium-containing products, such as saline IV fluids, for patients with a dietary salt restriction.
- Stress from dental procedures may compromise CV function; determine patient risk.
- Assess salivary flow as a factor in caries, periodontal disease, and candidiasis.
- Short appointments and a stress reduction protocol may be required for anxious patients.
- Consider semisupine chair position for patient comfort because of respiratory side effects of drug.
- Use precaution if sedation or general anesthesia is required; risk of hypotensive episode.

Consultations:

- Medical consultation may be required to assess disease control and patient's ability to tolerate stress.

Teach Patient/Family:

- Importance of updating health and drug history if physician makes any changes in evaluation or drug regimens
- *When chronic dry mouth occurs, advise patient:*
  - To avoid mouth rinses with high alcohol content because of drying effects
  - Of need for daily home fluoride use to prevent caries
  - To use sugarless gum, frequent sips of water, or saliva substitutes

loteprednol

loh-teh-pred′-nol
(Alrex, Lotemax)

CATEGORY AND SCHEDULE

Pregnancy Risk Category: C

MECHANISM OF ACTION

A glucocorticoid that inhibits accumulation of inflammatory cells at inflammation sites, phagocytosis, lysosomal enzyme release and synthesis and/or release of mediators of inflammation. ***Therapeutic Effect:*** Prevents and suppresses cell and tissue immune reactions, inflammatory process.

PHARMACOKINETICS

Metabolized by enzymes in the eye, minimizing systemic adverse effects.

AVAILABILITY

Ophthalmic Suspension: 0.2% (Alrex), 0.5% (Lotemax).

INDICATIONS AND DOSAGES

▸ **Treatment of Seasonal Allergic Conjunctivitis, Giant Papillary Conjunctivitis, Ureitis**

OPHTHALMIC

Adults, Elderly. Instill 1 drop 4 times/day for 4–6 weeks.

CONTRAINDICATIONS

Acute epithelial herpes simplex keratitis, fungal diseases of ocular structures, vaccinia, varicella, ocular tuberculosis, hypersensitivity, after removal of corneal foreign body, mycobacterial eye infection, acute, purulent, untreated eye infection

INTERACTIONS

Drug

None known.

Herbal

None known.

Food

None known.

Drug interactions of concern to dentistry

- None reported

DIAGNOSTIC TEST EFFECTS

None known.

SIDE EFFECTS

Frequent

Blurred vision

Occasional

Decreased vision, watering of eyes, eye pain, nausea, vomiting, burning, stinging, redness of eyes

SERIOUS REACTIONS

! Glaucoma with optic nerve damage, cataract formation, and secondary ocular infection occur rarely.

DENTAL CONSIDERATIONS

General:

- Avoid dental light in patient's eyes; offer dark glasses for patient comfort.
- Determine why patient is taking the drug.

loteprednol etabonate; tobramycin

loe-te-pred′-nol; toe-bra-mye′-sin
(Zylet)

CATEGORY AND SCHEDULE

Pregnancy Risk Category: C

MECHANISM OF ACTION

A combination ophthalmic product of an aminoglycoside and a glucocorticoid. Loteprednol is a glucocorticoid that inhibits accumulation of inflammatory cells at inflammation sites, phagocytosis, lysosomal enzyme release and synthesis, and/or release of mediators of inflammation. Tobramycin is an antibiotic that irreversibly binds to protein on bacterial ribosomes. ***Therapeutic Effect:*** Prevents and suppresses cell and tissue immune reactions and inflammatory process. Interferes with protein synthesis of susceptible microorganisms.

L

PHARMACOKINETICS

Limited systemic absorption.

AVAILABILITY

Ophthalmic Solution: 0.5% loteprednol etabonate and 0.3% tobramycin (Zylet).

INDICATIONS AND DOSAGES

▸ **Steroid-Responsive Inflammatory Ocular Conditions for Which a Corticosteroid Is Indicated and Where Superficial Bacterial Ocular Infection or a Risk of Bacterial Ocular Infection Exists**

OPHTHALMIC

Adults, Elderly. Apply 1 or 2 drops into the affected eye(s) q4–6h. During the initial 24 to 48 hours, the dosing may be increased to every 1 to 2 hours. Gradually decrease by improvement in clinical signs.

CONTRAINDICATIONS

Viral diseases of the cornea and conjunctiva including epithelial herpes simplex keratitis (dendritic keratitis), vaccinia, varicella, and mycobacterial infection of the eye and fungal diseases of ocular structures, hypersensitivity to any of loteprednol, tobramycin or any component of the formulation and to other corticosteroids

INTERACTIONS

Drug

None known.

Herbal

None known.

Food

None known.

Drug interactions of concern to dentistry

- None reported

DIAGNOSTIC TEST EFFECTS

None known.

SIDE EFFECTS

Frequent

Blurred vision

Occasional

Tearing, burning, itching, redness, swelling of eyelid, decreased vision, eye pain

Rare

Nausea, vomiting

SERIOUS REACTIONS

! Glaucoma with optic nerve damage, cataract formation, and secondary ocular infection occurs rarely.

! Secondary infection, especially fungal infections of the cornea, may occur after use of this medication. These infections are more frequent with long-term applications.

DENTAL CONSIDERATIONS

General:

- Avoid dental light in patient's eyes; offer dark glasses for patient comfort.
- Determine why patient is taking the drug.

lovastatin

lo′-va-sta-tin
(Altoprev, Lotrel, Mevacor)
Do not confuse lovastatin with Leustatin or Livostin, or Mevacor with Mivacron.

CATEGORY AND SCHEDULE

Pregnancy Risk Category: X

MECHANISM OF ACTION

An antihyperlipidemic that inhibits HMG-CoA reductase, the enzyme that catalyzes the early step in cholesterol synthesis. ***Therapeutic Effect:*** Decreases LDL cholesterol, VLDL cholesterol, plasma triglycerides; increases HDL cholesterol.

PHARMACOKINETICS

Route	Onset	Peak	Duration
PO	3 days	4–6 wk	N/A

Incompletely absorbed from the GI tract (increased on empty stomach). Protein binding: 95%. Hydrolyzed in the liver to active metabolite. Primarily eliminated in feces. Not removed by hemodialysis. ***Half-life:*** 1.1–1.7 hr.

AVAILABILITY

Tablets (Mevacor): 10 mg, 20 mg, 40 mg.
Tablets (Extended-Release [Altoprev]): 20 mg, 40 mg, 60 mg.

INDICATIONS AND DOSAGES

▸ Hyperlipoproteinemia, Primary Prevention of Coronary Artery Disease

PO

Adults, Elderly. Initially, 20–40 mg/day with evening meal. Increase at 4-wk intervals up to maximum of 80 mg/day. Maintenance: 20–80 mg/day in single or divided doses.

PO (Extended-Release)

Adults, Elderly. Initially, 20 mg/day. May increase at 4-wk intervals up to 60 mg/day.
Children 10–17 yr. 10–40 mg/day with evening meal.

▸ Heterozygous Familial Hypercholesterolemia

PO

Children 10–17 yr. Initially, 10 mg/day. May increase to 20 mg/day after 8 wk and 40 mg/day after 16 wk if needed.

CONTRAINDICATIONS

Active liver disease, pregnancy, unexplained elevated liver function tests

INTERACTIONS

Drug

Cyclosporine, erythromycin, gemfibrozil, immunosuppressants, niacin: Increases the risk of acute renal failure and rhabdomyolysis.
Erythromycin, itraconazole, ketoconazole: May increase lovastatin blood concentration causing severe muscle inflammation, myalgia, and weakness.

Herbal
None known.
Food
Grapefruit juice: Large amounts of grapefruit juice may increase risk of side effects, such as myalgia and weakness.
Drug interactions of concern to dentistry
- Increased myalgia, rhabdomyolysis: erythromycin, cyclosporine
- Contraindicated with itraconazole, ketoconazole, erythromycin

DIAGNOSTIC TEST EFFECTS
May increase serum creatine kinase and serum transaminase concentrations.

SIDE EFFECTS
Generally well tolerated. Side effects usually mild and transient.
Frequent (9%–5%)
Headache, flatulence, diarrhea, abdominal pain or cramps, rash and pruritus
Occasional (4%–3%)
Nausea, vomiting, constipation, dyspepsia
Rare (2%–1%)
Dizziness, heartburn, myalgia, blurred vision, eye irritation

SERIOUS REACTIONS
! There is a potential for cataract development.

DENTAL CONSIDERATIONS
General:
- Consider semisupine chair position for patient comfort because of GI side effects.

Teach Patient/Family:
- To avoid mouth rinses with high alcohol content because of drying effects

loxapine
lox′-a-peen
(Apo-Loxapine[CAN], Loxapac[CAN], Loxitane)

CATEGORY AND SCHEDULE
Pregnancy Risk Category: C

MECHANISM OF ACTION
A dibenzodiazepine derivative that interferes with the binding of dopamine at postysnaptic receptor sites in brain. Strong anticholinergic effects. ***Therapeutic Effect:*** Suppresses locomotor activity, produces tranquilization.

PHARMACOKINETICS
Onset of action occurs within 1 hours. Metabolized to active metabolites 8-hydroxyloxapine, 7-hydroxyloxapine, and 8-hydroxyamoxapine. Excreted in urine. ***Half-life:*** 4 hrs.

AVAILABILITY
Capsules: 5 mg, 10 mg, 25 mg, 50 mg (Loxitane).

INDICATIONS AND DOSAGES
▸ **Psychotic Disorders**
PO
Adults. 10 mg 2 times/day. Increase dosage rapidly during first week to 50 mg, if needed. Usual therapeutic, maintenance range: 60–100 mg daily in 2–4 divided doses. Maximum: 250 mg/day.

CONTRAINDICATIONS
Severe central nervous system (CNS) depression, comatose states, hypersensivitiy to loxapine or any component of the formulation

INTERACTIONS

Drug

Alcohol, CNS depressants: May increase CNS depressant effects.
Antacids, antidiarrheals: May decrease absorption of loxapine.
Extrapyramidal symptom (EPS)-producing medications: May increase risk of EPS.

Herbal

None known.

Food

None known.

Drug interactions of concern to dentistry

- Increased effects of both drugs: anticholinergics
- Increased CNS depression: alcohol, all CNS depressants
- Decreased effects of sympathomimetics, carbamazepine

DIAGNOSTIC TEST EFFECTS

None known.

SIDE EFFECTS

Frequent

Blurred vision, confusion, drowsiness, dry mouth, dizziness, lightheadedness

Occasional

Allergic reaction (rash, itching), decreased urination, constipation, decreased sexual ability, enlarged breasts, headache, photosensitivity, nausea, vomiting, insomnia, weight gain

SERIOUS REACTIONS

! Extrapyramidal symptoms frequently noted are akathisia (motor restlessness, anxiety). Less frequently noted are akinesia (rigidity, tremor, salivation, mask-like facial expression, reduced voluntary movements). Infrequently noted dystonias: torticollis (neck muscle spasm), opisthotonos (rigidity of back muscles), and oculogyric crisis (rolling back of eyes). Tardive dyskinesia (protrusion of tongue, puffing of cheeks, chewing/puckering of mouth) occurs rarely but may be irreversible. Risk is greater in female elderly patients.

DENTAL CONSIDERATIONS

General:

- Patients on chronic drug therapy may rarely have symptoms of blood dyscrasias, which can include infection, bleeding, and poor healing.
- Assess salivary flow as a factor in caries, periodontal disease, and candidiasis.
- Assess for presence of extrapyramidal motor symptoms, such as tardive dyskinesia and akathisia. Extrapyramidal motor activity may complicate dental treatment.
- After supine positioning, have patient sit upright for at least 2 min before standing to avoid orthostatic hypotension.

Consultations:

- In a patient with symptoms of blood dyscrasias, request a medical consultation for blood studies and postpone dental treatment until normal values are reestablished.
- If signs of tardive dyskinesia or akathisia are present, refer to physician.
- Physician should be informed if significant xerostomic side effects occur (e.g., increased caries, sore tongue, problems eating or swallowing, difficulty wearing prosthesis) so that a medication change can be considered.

Teach Patient/Family:

- Importance of good oral hygiene to prevent soft tissue inflammation
- Caution to prevent injury when using oral hygiene aids

- To use electric toothbrush if patient has difficulty holding conventional devices
- *When chronic dry mouth occurs, advise patient:*
  - To avoid mouth rinses with high alcohol content because of drying effects
  - To use sugarless gum, frequent sips of water, or saliva substitutes
  - To use daily home fluoride products for anticaries effect

mafenide
ma′-fe-nide
(Sulfamylon)

CATEGORY AND SCHEDULE
Pregnancy Risk Category: C

MECHANISM OF ACTION
A topical anti-infective that decreases number of bacteria avascular tissue of second- and third-degree burns. ***Therapeutic Effect:*** Bacteriostatic. Promotes spontaneous healing of deep partial-thickness burns.

PHARMACOKINETICS
Absorbed through devascularzied areas into systemic circulation following topical administration. Excreted in the form of its metabolite rho-carboxybenzenesulfonamide

AVAILABILITY
Cream: 85 mg base/g (Sulfamylon).

INDICATIONS AND DOSAGES
▸ Burns
TOPICAL
Adults, Elderly, Children. Apply 1–2 times/day.

CONTRAINDICATIONS
Hypersensitivity to mafenide or sulfite or any other component of the formulation

INTERACTIONS
Drug
None known.
Herbal
None known.
Food
None known.
Drug interactions of concern to dentistry
- None reported

DIAGNOSTIC TEST EFFECTS
None known.

SIDE EFFECTS
Difficult to distinguish side effects and effects of severe burn
Frequent
Pain, burning upon application
Occasional
Allergic reaction (usually 10–14 days after initiation): itching, rash, facial edema, swelling; unexplained syndrome of marked hyperventilation with respiratory alkalosis
Rare
Delay in eschar separation, excoriation of new skin

SERIOUS REACTIONS
! Hemolytic anemia, porphyria, bone marrow depression, superinfections (especially with fungi), metabolic acidosis occurs rarely.

DENTAL CONSIDERATIONS
General:
- Dental management depends on extent and severity of burns and patients ability to cooperate; above all use aseptic techniques.
- Provide palliative dental care for dental emergencies only.
- Monitor and record vital signs.

Consultations:
- Medical consultation may be required to assess disease control and patient's ability to tolerate stress.
- Consult patient's physician if an acute dental infection occurs and another antiinfective is required.

Teach Patient/Family:
- Importance of good oral hygiene to prevent soft tissue inflammation
- To prevent trauma when using oral hygiene aids

magaldrate

(Iosopan Plus, Lowsium Plus, Riopan Plus)

CATEGORY AND SCHEDULE

Pregnancy Risk Category: C

MECHANISM OF ACTION

An antacid that causes less hydrogen ion available for diffusion through the gastrointestinal (GI) mucosa.
Therapeutic Effect: Reduces and neutralizes gastric acid.

AVAILABILITY

Suspension: magaldrate 540 mg and simethicone 20 mg/5ml, magaldrate 540 mg and simethicone 40 mg/5ml, magaldrate 1080 mg and simethicone 40 mg/5 ml.
Tablets (chewable): magaldrate 540 mg and simethicone 20 mg, magaldrate 1080 mg and simethicone 20 mg.

M

INDICATIONS AND DOSAGES

▸Hyperacidity and Gas

PO

Adults, Elderly. 540 to 1080 mg between meals and at bedtime.

CONTRAINDICATIONS

Hypersensitivity to magaldrate, colostomy or ileostomy, appendicitis, ulcerative colitis, diverticulits

INTERACTIONS

Drug

Fluoroquinolones: May decrease the effects of fluoroquinolones.
Ketoconazole, methenamine: May decrease the effects of ketoconazole or methenamine.
Mecamylamine: May increase the effects of mecamylamine
Sodium polystyrene sulfonate resin: May decrease the effects of antacids.
Tetracyclines: May decrease the effects of both tetracyclines and antacids.

Herbal

None known.

Food

None known.

Drug interactions of concern to dentistry

• Decreased absorption of anticholinergics, corticosteroids, sodium fluoride, tetracycline, ketoconazole, chlordiazepoxide, ciprofloxacin, metronidazole

SIDE EFFECTS

Rare

Constipation, diarrhea, fluid retention, dizziness or lightheadedness, continuing discomfort, irregular heartbeat, loss of appetite, mood or mental changes, muscle weakness, unusual tiredness or weakness, weight loss, chalky taste

SERIOUS REACTIONS

! None known.

DENTAL CONSIDERATIONS

General:

• If prescribing oral form of a drug for which risk of decreased absorption is reported, advise taking doses at least 2 hr after or before antacid use.
• Avoid drugs that could exacerbate upper GI distress (aspirin and NSAIDs).
• Consider semisupine chair position for patient comfort because of GI effects of disease.

maprotiline

mah-pro-′-tih-leen
(Ludiomil)

CATEGORY AND SCHEDULE

Pregnancy Risk Category: B

MECHANISM OF ACTION

A tetracyclic compound that blocks reuptake norepinephrine by CNS presynaptic neuronal membranes, increasing availability at postsynaptic neuronal receptor sites, and enhances synaptic activity. ***Therapeutic Effect:*** Produces antidepressant effect, with prominent sedative effects and low anticholinergic activity.

PHARMACOKINETICS

Slowly and completely absorbed after PO administration. Protein binding: 88%. Metabolized in liver by hydroxylation and oxidative modification. Excreted in urine. Unknown if removed by hemodialysis. ***Half-life:*** 27–58 hrs.

AVAILABILITY

Tablets: 25 mg, 50 mg, 75 mg (Ludiomil).

INDICATIONS AND DOSAGES

▸ Mild to Moderate Depression

PO

Adults. 75 mg/day to start, in 1–4 divided doses.

Elderly. 50–75 mg/day. In 2 wks, increase dosage gradually in 25 mg increments until therapeutic response is achieved. Reduce to lowest effective maintenance level.

▸ Severe Depression

PO

Adults. 100–150 mg/day in 1–4 divided doses. May increase gradually to maximum 225 mg/day.

▸ Usual Elderly Dosage

PO

Initially, 25 mg at bedtime. May increase by 25 mg q3–7 days. Maintenance: 50–75 mg/day.

CONTRAINDICATIONS

Acute recovery period following myocardial infarction (MI), Within 14 days of MAOI ingestion, known or suspected seizure disorder, hypersensitivity to maprotiline or any component of the formulation

INTERACTIONS

Drug

Acute recovery period following myocardial infarction (MI), within 14 days of MAOI ingestion, known or suspected seizure disorder, hypersensitivity to maprotiline or any component of the formulation

MAOIs: May increase risk of hypertensive crisis and severe convulsions.

Sympathomimetics: May increase cardiovascular effects (arrhythmias, tachycardias, severe hypertension).

Herbal

None known.

Food

None known.

Drug interactions of concern to dentistry

- Increased effects of direct-acting sympathomimetics (epinephrine)
- Potential risk of increased CNS depression: alcohol, and all CNS depressants
- Decreased antihypertensive effect: clonidine, guanadrel, guanethidine

DIAGNOSTIC TEST EFFECTS

None known.

IV INCOMPATIBILITIES

None known.

IV COMPATIBILITIES

None known.

SIDE EFFECTS

Frequent

Drowsiness, fatigue, dry mouth, blurred vision, constipation, delayed micturition, postural hypotension, excessive sweating, disturbed concentration, increased appetite, urinary retention

M

Occasional
GI disturbances (nausea, GI distress, metallic taste sensation), photosensitivity
Rare
Paradoxical reaction (agitation, restlessness, nightmares, insomnia), extrapyramidal symptoms (particularly fine hand tremor)

SERIOUS REACTIONS

! Higher incidence of seizures than with tricyclic antidepressants, especially in those with no previous history of seizures.
! High dosage may produce cardiovascular effects, such as severe postural hypotension, dizziness, tachycardia, palpitations, and arrhythmias.
! May also result in altered temperature regulation (hyperpyrexia or hypothermia).
! Abrupt withdrawal from prolonged therapy may produce headache, malaise, nausea, vomiting, and vivid dreams.

M

DENTAL CONSIDERATIONS

General:
- Monitor vital signs at every appointment because of CV side effects.
- Patients on chronic drug therapy may rarely have symptoms of blood dyscrasias, which can include infection, bleeding, and poor healing.
- Assess salivary flow as a factor in caries, periodontal disease, and candidiasis.
- After supine positioning, have patient sit upright for at least 2 min before standing to avoid orthostatic hypotension.
- Use of epinephrine in gingival retraction cord is contraindicated. Use vasoconstrictors with caution, in low doses, and with careful aspiration.

Consultations:
- In a patient with symptoms of blood dyscrasias, request a medical consultation for blood studies and postpone dental treatment until normal values are reestablished.
- Take precautions if dental surgery is anticipated and anesthesia is required.
- Medical consultation may be required to assess disease control.
- Physician should be informed if significant xerostomic side effects occur (e.g., increased caries, sore tongue, problems eating or swallowing, difficulty wearing prosthesis) so that a medication change can be considered.

Teach Patient/Family:
- Importance of good oral hygiene to prevent soft tissue inflammation
- Caution to prevent injury when using oral hygiene aids
- *When chronic dry mouth occurs, advise patient:*
  - To avoid mouth rinses with high alcohol content because of drying effects
  - To use sugarless gum, frequent sips of water, or saliva substitutes
  - To use daily home fluoride products for anticaries effect

mebendazole

meh-ben′-dah-zole
(Vermox)

CATEGORY AND SCHEDULE

Pregnancy Risk Category: C

MECHANISM OF ACTION

A synthetic benzimidazole derivative that degrades parasite cytoplasmic microtubules and irreversibly blocks glucose uptake in helminthes and larvae. Vermicidal. ***Therapeutic Effect:*** depletes glycogen, decreases ATP, causes helminth death.

PHARMACOKINETICS

Poorly absorbed from GI tract (absorption increases with food). Metabolized in liver. Primarily eliminated in feces. ***Half-life:*** 2.5–9 hrs (half life increased with impaired renal function.

AVAILABILITY

Tablets, chewable: 100 mg (Vermox).

INDICATIONS AND DOSAGES

▸ Trichuriasis, Ascariasis, Hookworm

PO

Adults, Elderly, Children older than 2 yrs. 1 tablet in morning and at bedtime for 3 days.

▸ Enterobiasis

PO

Adults, Elderly, Children older than 2 yrs. 1 tablet one time.

OFF-LABEL USES

Ancylostoma duodenale or Necator americanus

CONTRAINDICATIONS

Hypersensitivity to mebendazole or any component of the formulation

INTERACTIONS

Drug

Carbamazepine: May decrease concentrations of mebendazole.

Herbal

None known.

Food

None known.

Drug interactions of concern to dentistry

• Decreased plasma levels: carbamazepine

DIAGNOSTIC TEST EFFECTS

May increase SGOT (AST), SGPT (ALT), alkaline phosphatase, BUN. May decrease Hgb.

IV INCOMPATIBILITIES

None known.

IV COMPATIBILITIES

None known.

SIDE EFFECTS

Occasional

Nausea, vomiting, headache, dizziness, transient abdominal pain, diarrhea with massive infection and expulsion of helminths

Rare

Fever

SERIOUS REACTIONS

! High dosage may produce reversible myelosuppression (granulocytopenia, leukopenia, neutropenia).

DENTAL CONSIDERATIONS

General:

• Determine why patient is taking the drug.

• Patient on chronic drug therapy may rarely present with symptoms of blood dyscrasias, which can include infection, bleeding, and poor healing. If dyscrasia is present, caution patient to prevent oral tissue trauma when using oral hygiene aids.

• Question patient about other drugs he/she is taking.

Consultations:

• In a patient with symptoms of blood dyscrasias, request a medical consultation for blood studies and postpone treatment until normal values are reestablished.

meclizine

mek′-li-zeen
(Antivert, Bonamine[CAN], Bonine)
Do not confuse Antivert with Axert.

CATEGORY AND SCHEDULE

Pregnancy Risk Category: B

MECHANISM OF ACTION

An anticholinergic that reduces labyrinthine excitability and diminishes vestibular stimulation of the labyrinth, affecting the chemoreceptor trigger zone. ***Therapeutic Effect:*** Reduces nausea, vomiting, and vertigo.

PHARMACOKINETICS

Route	Onset	Peak	Duration
PO	30–60 min	N/A	12–24 hr

Well absorbed from the GI tract. Widely distributed. Metabolized in the liver. Primarily excreted in urine. ***Half-life:*** 6 hr.

AVAILABILITY

Tablets (Antivert): 12.5 mg, 25 mg, 50 mg.
*Tablets (Chewable [Bonine]):*25 mg.

INDICATIONS AND DOSAGES

▸ **Motion Sickness**

PO

Adults, Elderly, Children 12 yr and older. 12.5–25 mg 1 hr before travel. May repeat q12–24h. May require a dose of 50 mg.

▸ **Vertigo**

PO

Adults, Elderly, Children 12 yr and older. 25–100 mg/day in divided doses, as needed.

CONTRAINDICATIONS

None known.

INTERACTIONS

Drug

Alcohol, CNS depression-producing medications: May increase CNS depressant effect.

Herbal

None known.

Food

None known.

Drug interactions of concern to dentistry

- Increased effect of alcohol, other CNS depressants, anticholinergics

DIAGNOSTIC TEST EFFECTS

May produce false-negative results in antigen skin testing unless meclizine is discontinued 4 days before testing.

SIDE EFFECTS

Frequent

Drowsiness

Occasional

Blurred vision; dry mouth, nose, or throat

SERIOUS REACTIONS

! A hypersensitivity reaction, marked by eczema, pruritus, rash, cardiac disturbances, and photosensitivity, may occur.

! Overdose may produce CNS depression (manifested as sedation, apnea, cardiovascular collapse, or death) or severe paradoxical reactions (such as hallucinations, tremor, and seizures).

! Children may experience paradoxical reactions, including restlessness, insomnia, euphoria, nervousness, and tremors.

! Overdose in children may result in hallucinations, seizures, and death.

M

DENTAL CONSIDERATIONS

General:

• Assess salivary flow as a factor in caries, periodontal disease, and candidiasis.

Teach Patient/Family:

• *When chronic dry mouth occurs, advise patient:*
  • To avoid mouth rinses with high alcohol content because of drying effects
  • To use daily home fluoride products for anticaries effect
  • To use sugarless gum, frequent sips of water, or saliva substitutes

meclofenamate

me′-kloe-fen-′-a-mate soe-dee-um
(Meclomen[CAN])
Do not confuse with meclizine.

CATEGORY AND SCHEDULE

Pregnancy Risk Category: B, D if used in third trimester or near delivery

MECHANISM OF ACTION

A nonsteroidal anti-inflammatory drug that inhibits prostaglandin synthesis by decreasing activity of the enzyme, cyclooxygenase, which results in decreased formation of prostaglandin precursors. ***Therapeutic Effect:*** Reduces inflammatory response and intensity of pain stimulus reaching sensory nerve endings.

PHARMACOKINETICS

PO route, onset 15 minutes, peak 0.5–1.5 hours, duration 2–4 hours. Completely absorbed from the gastrointestinal (GI) tract. Widely distributed. Protein binding: greater than 99%. Metabolized in liver. Primarily excreted in urine and feces as metabolites. Not removed by hemodialysis. ***Half-life:*** 2–3.3 hrs.

AVAILABILITY

Capsules: 50 mg, 100 mg.

INDICATIONS AND DOSAGES

▸ **Mild to Moderate Pain**

PO

Adults, Elderly. 50 mg q4–6h as needed.

▸ **Excessive Menstrual Blood Loss and Primary Dysmenorrhea**

PO

Adults, Elderly. 100 mg 3 times/day for 6 days, starting at the onset of menstrual flow.

▸ **Rheumatoid Arthritis, Osteoarthritis**

PO

Adults, Elderly. 200–400 mg 3–4 times/day.

CONTRAINDICATIONS

Active peptic ulcer disease, chronic inflammation of GI tract, GI bleeding disorders, GI ulceration, history of hypersensitivity to aspirin or NSAIDs

INTERACTIONS

Drug

Antihypertensives, diuretics: May decrease the effects of antihypertensives and diuretics.
Aspirin, salicylates: May increase the risk of GI bleeding and side effects.
Bone marrow depressants: May increase the risk of hematologic reactions.
Heparin, oral anticoagulants, thrombolytics: May increase the effects of heparin, oral anticoagulants, and thrombolytics.

Lithium: May increase the blood concentration and risk of toxicity of lithium.
Methotrexate: May increase the risk of toxicity with methotrexate.
Probenecid: May increase meclofenamate blood concentration.

Herbal

Feverfew: May increase the risk of bleeding.
Ginkgo biloba: May increase the risk of bleeding.

Food

None known.

Drug interactions of concern to dentistry

- GI ulceration, bleeding: aspirin, alcohol, corticosteroids, biphosphonates
- Nephrotoxicity: acetaminophen (prolonged use)
- Possible risk of decreased renal function: cyclosporine
- First-time users of SSRIs also taking NSAIDs may have a higher risk of GI side effects; until more data are available, it may be advisable to avoid use of NSAIDs in these patients (*Br J Clin Pharmacol* 55:591–595, 2003)
- *When prescribed for dental pain:*
  - Risk of increased effects: oral anticoagulants, oral antidiabetics, lithium, methotrexate
  - Decreased effects of diuretics, β-adrenergic blockers

DIAGNOSTIC TEST EFFECTS

May increase chloride and sodium test results. May increase BUN, serum LDH concentration, serum alkaline phosphatase, serum creatinine, potassium, and transaminase levels, and urine protein levels. May decrease serum uric acid levels.

SIDE EFFECTS

Frequent (33%–10%)

Diarrhea, nausea, abdominal cramping/pain, dyspepsia (heartburn, indigestion, epigastric pain), oral lichenoid reaction

Occasional (9%–1%)

Flatulence, rash, dizziness

Rare (<1%)

Constipation, anorexia, stomatitis, headache, ringing in the ears, rash

SERIOUS REACTIONS

! Overdosage may result in headache, seizure, vomiting, and cerebral edema.
! Peptic ulcer disease, GI bleeding, gastritis, severe hepatic reactions, such as jaundice, nephrotoxicity, marked by hematuria, dysuria, proteinuria, and severe hypersensitivity reaction, including bronchospasm, and facial edema occur rarely.

DENTAL CONSIDERATIONS

General:

- Patients on chronic drug therapy may rarely have symptoms of blood dyscrasias, which can include infection, bleeding, and poor healing.
- Assess salivary flow as a factor in caries, periodontal disease, and candidiasis.
- Avoid prescribing for dental use in last trimester of pregnancy.
- Avoid prescribing aspirin-containing products.
- Consider semisupine chair position for patients with rheumatic disease.

Consultations:

- In a patient with symptoms of blood dyscrasias, request a medical consultation for blood studies and postpone dental treatment until normal values are reestablished.
- Medical consultation may be required to assess disease control.

Teach Patient/Family:

- Importance of good oral hygiene to prevent soft tissue inflammation
- Caution to prevent injury when using oral hygiene aids

- *When chronic dry mouth occurs, advise patient:*
  - To avoid mouth rinses with high alcohol content because of drying effects
  - To use sugarless gum, frequent sips of water, or saliva substitutes
  - To use daily home fluoride products for anticaries effect

medroxyprogesterone acetate

me-drox′-ee-proe-jess′-te-rone
(Depo-Provera, Depo-Provera Contraceptive, Novo-Medrone[CAN], Provera, Ralovera[AUS])
Do not confuse medroxyprogesterone with hydroxyprogesterone, methylprednisolone, or methyltestosterone.

CATEGORY AND SCHEDULE

Pregnancy Risk Category: X

MECHANISM OF ACTION

A hormone that transforms endometrium from proliferative to secretory in an estrogen-primed endometrium. Inhibits secretion of pituitary gonadotropins. ***Therapeutic Effect:*** Prevents follicular maturation and ovulation. Stimulates growth of mammary alveolar tissue and relaxes uterine smooth muscle. Corrects hormonal imbalance.

PHARMACOKINETICS

Slowly absorbed after IM administration. Protein binding: 90%. Metabolized in the liver. Primarily excreted in urine. ***Half-life:*** 30 days.

AVAILABILITY

Tablets (Provera): 2.5 mg, 5 mg, 10 mg.
Injection (Depo-Provera Contraceptive): 150 mg/ml.
Injection (Depo-Provera): 400 mg/ml.

INDICATIONS AND DOSAGES

▸ Endometrial Hyperplasia
PO
Adults. 2.5–10 mg/day for 14 days.

▸ Secondary Amenorrhea
PO
Adults. 5–10 mg/day for 5–10 days, beginning at any time during menstrual cycle or 2.5 mg/day.

▸ Abnormal Uterine Bleeding
PO
Adults. 5–10 mg/day for 5–10 days, beginning on calculated day 16 or day 21 of menstrual cycle.

▸ Endometrial, Renal Carcinoma
IM
Adults, Elderly. Initially, 400–1,000 mg; repeat at 1-wk intervals. If improvement occurs and disease is stabilized, begin maintenance with as little as 400 mg/mo.

▸ Prevention of Pregnancy
IM
Adults. 150 mg q3mo.

OFF-LABEL USES

Hormone replacement therapy in estrogen-treated menopausal women, treatment of endometriosis

CONTRAINDICATIONS

Carcinoma of breast; estrogen-dependent neoplasm; history of or active thrombotic disorders, such as cerebral apoplexy, thrombophlebitis, or thromboembolic disorders; hypersensitivity to progestins; known or suspected pregnancy; missed abortion; severe hepatic dysfunction; undiagnosed abnormal genital bleeding; use as pregnancy test

INTERACTIONS

Drug

Bromocriptine: May interfere with the effects of bromocriptine.

Herbal

None known.

Food

None known.

DIAGNOSTIC TEST EFFECTS

May alter results for serum thyroid and liver function tests, prothrombin time, and metapyrone test

SIDE EFFECTS

Frequent

Transient menstrual abnormalities (including spotting, change in menstrual flow or cervical secretions, and amenorrhea) at initiation of therapy

Occasional

Edema, weight change, breast tenderness, nervousness, insomnia, fatigue, dizziness

Rare

Alopecia, depression, dermatologic changes, headache, fever, nausea

SERIOUS REACTIONS

! Thrombophlebitis, pulmonary or cerebral embolism, and retinal thrombosis occur rarely.

DENTAL CONSIDERATIONS

General:

- Place on frequent recall to evaluate inflammatory and healing response.

Teach Patient/Family:

- Importance of good oral hygiene to prevent soft tissue inflammation

medrysone

me′-dri-sone

(HMS Liquifilm)

CATEGORY AND SCHEDULE

Pregnancy Risk Category: C

MECHANISM OF ACTION

A topical synthetic corticosteroid that inhibits accumulation of inflammatory cells at inflammation sites. ***Therapeutic Effect:*** Inhibits inflammatory process.

PHARMACOKINETICS

Absorbed through aqueous humor. Metabolized in liver if absorbed. Excreted in urine and feces.

AVAILABILITY

Ophthalmic suspension: 1% (HMS Liquifilm).

INDICATIONS AND DOSAGES

▸ **Ophthalmic Disorders**

OPHTHALMIC

Adults, Elderly, Children 3 yrs and older. Instill 1 drop up to every 4 hours.

CONTRAINDICATIONS

Active superficial herpes simplex, conjunctival or corneal viral disease, fungal diseases of the eye, ocular tuberculosis, hypersensitivity to medrysone or any component of the formulation

INTERACTIONS

Drug

None known.

Herbal

None known.

Food

None known.

Drug interactions of concern to dentistry

- None reported

DIAGNOSTIC TEST EFFECTS

None known.

SIDE EFFECTS

Frequent

Blurred vision

Occasional

Decreased vision, watering of eyes, eye pain, burning, stinging, redness of eyes, nausea, vomiting

SERIOUS REACTIONS

! Systemic absorption may occur with topical application.
! Cataracts, corneal thinning, corneal ulcers, delayed wound healing, optic nerve damage, and glaucoma have been reported.

DENTAL CONSIDERATIONS

General:

- Determine why patient is taking the drug.
- Protect patient's eyes from accidental spatter during dental treatment.
- Avoid dental light in patient's eyes; offer dark glasses for patient comfort.

mefenamic acid

me-fe-nam′-ik
(Apo-Mefenamic[CAN], Nu-Mefenamic[CAN], PMS-Mefenamic Acid[CAN], Ponstan[CAN], Ponstel)

CATEGORY AND SCHEDULE

Pregnancy Risk Category: C, D if used in third trimester or near delivery

MECHANISM OF ACTION

A nonsteroidal anti-inflammatory that produces analgesic and anti-inflammatory effect by inhibiting prostaglandin synthesis. ***Therapeutic Effect:*** Reduces inflammatory response and intensity of pain stimulus reaching sensory nerve endings.

PHARMACOKINETICS

Rapidly absorbed from the gastrointestinal (GI) tract. Protein binding: high. Metabolized in liver. Partially excreted in urine and partially in the feces. Not removed by hemodialysis. ***Half-life:*** 3.5 hrs.

AVAILABILITY

Capsules: 250 mg (Ponstel).

INDICATIONS AND DOSAGES

▸ **Mild to Moderate Pain, Lower Back Pain, Dysmenorrhea**

PO

Adults, Elderly, Children 14 yrs and older. Initially, 500 mg to start, then 250 mg q4h as needed. Maximum: 1 week of therapy.

OFF-LABEL USES

Cataract prevention, menorrhagia, osteoarthritis, premenstrual syndrome, rheumatoid arthritis

M

CONTRAINDICATIONS

History of hypersensitivity to aspirin or NSAIDs, pregnancy

INTERACTIONS

Drug

Antihypertensives, diuretics: May decrease the effects of antihypertensives and diuretics.
Aspirin, salicylates: May increase the risk of GI bleeding and side effects.
Bone marrow depressants: May increase the risk of hematologic reactions.
Heparin, oral anticoagulants, thrombolytics: May increase the effects of heparin, oral anticoagulants, and thrombolytics.
Lithium: May increase the blood concentration and risk of toxicity of lithium.
Methotrexate: May increase the risk of toxicity of methotrexate.

Probenecid: May increase mefenamic acid blood concentration.

Drug interactions of concern to dentistry

- GI bleeding, ulceration: aspirin, alcohol, corticosteroids
- Nephrotoxicity: acetaminophen (prolonged use and high doses)
- Possible risk of decreased renal function: cyclosporine
- First-time users of SSRIs also taking NSAIDs may have a higher risk of GI side effects; until more data are available, it may be advisable to avoid use of NSAIDs in these patients (*Br J Clin Pharmacol* 55:591–595, 2003)
- *When prescribed for dental pain:*
  - Risk of increased effects of oral anticoagulants, oral antidiabetics, lithium, methotrexate
  - Decreased effects of diuretics

M

DIAGNOSTIC TEST EFFECTS

May increase chloride and sodium levels. May prolong bleeding time. May increase liver function tests.

SIDE EFFECTS

Occasional (10%–1%)

Dyspepsia, including heartburn, indigestion, flatulence, abdominal cramping, constipation, nausea, diarrhea, epigastric pain, vomiting, headache, nervousness, dizziness, bleeding, elevated liver function tests, tinnitus, oral lichenoid reaction

Rare (<1%)

Fluid retention, arrhythmias, tachycardia, confusion, drowsiness, rash, dry eyes, blurred vision, hot flashes

SERIOUS REACTIONS

! Peptic ulcer, GI bleeding, gastritis, and severe hepatic reaction, such as cholestasis and jaundice, occur rarely.

! Nephrotoxicity, including dysuria, hematuria, proteinuria, and nephrotic syndrome and severe hypersensitivity reaction, marked by bronchospasm, and angioedema occur rarely.

DENTAL CONSIDERATIONS

General:

- Avoid prescribing for dental use in last trimester of pregnancy.
- Avoid prescribing aspirin-containing products.

Consultations:

- Medical consultation may be required to assess disease control.

mefloquine

me′-flow-quine

(Lariam)

Do not confuse with Librium.

CATEGORY AND SCHEDULE

Pregnancy Risk Category: C

MECHANISM OF ACTION

A quinolone-methanol compound structurally similar to quinine that destroys the asexual blood forms of malarial pathogens, *Plasmodium falciparum, P. vivax, P. malariae, P. ovale*. ***Therapeutic Effect:*** Inhibits parasite growth.

PHARMACOKINETICS

Well absorbed from the gastrointestinal (GI) tract. Protein binding: 98%. Widely distributed, including cerebrospinal fluid (CSF). Metabolized in liver. Primarily excreted in urine. ***Half-life:*** 21–22 days.

AVAILABILITY

Tablets: 250 mg.

INDICATIONS AND DOSAGES

▸ Suppression of Malaria

PO

Adults. 250 mg base weekly starting 1 week before travel, continuing weekly during travel and for 4 weeks after leaving endemic area.
Children more than 45 kg. 250 mg weekly starting 1 week before travel, continuing weekly during travel and for 4 weeks after leaving endemic area.
Children 45–31kg. 187.5 mg (3/4 tablet) weekly starting 1 week before travel, continuing weekly during travel and for 4 weeks after leaving endemic area.
Children 30–20 kg. 125 mg (1/2 tablet) weekly starting 1 week before travel, continuing weekly during travel and for 4 weeks after leaving endemic area.
Children 19–15 kg. 62.5 mg (1/4 tablet) weekly starting 1 week before travel, continuing weekly during travel and for 4 weeks after leaving endemic area.

▸ Treatment of Malaria

PO

Adults. 1250 mg as a single dose.
Children. 15–25 mg/kg in a single dose. Maximum: 1250 mg.

CONTRAINDICATIONS

Cardiac abnormalities, severe psychiatric disorders, epilepsy, history of hypersensitivity to mefloquine

INTERACTIONS

Drug

Cytochrome P450 effect: Inhibits CYP 3A4.
Beta-blockers: May increase bradycardia with beta-blockers.
Chloroquine, quinine, quinidine: May increase the risk of toxicity with these drugs.
Valproic acid: May decrease the effect of valproic acid.

Herbal

None known.

Food

None known.

Drug interactions of concern to dentistry

- None reported

DIAGNOSTIC TEST EFFECTS

None known.

SIDE EFFECTS

Occasional

Mild transient headache, difficulty concentrating, insomnia, lightheadedness, vertigo, diarrhea, nausea, vomiting, visual disturbances, tinnitus

Rare

Aggressive behavior, anxiety, bradycardia, depression, hallucinations, hypotension, panic attacks, paranoia, psychosis, syncope, tremor

SERIOUS REACTIONS

! Prolonged therapy may result in peripheral neuritis, neuromyopathy, hypotension, electrocardiogram (ECG) changes, agranulocytosis, aplastic anemia, thrombocytopenia, seizures, and psychosis.
! Overdosage may result in headache, vomiting, visual disturbance, drowsiness, and seizures.

DENTAL CONSIDERATIONS

General:

- Consider semisupine chair position for patient comfort if GI side effects occur.
- Question patient about tolerance of NSAIDS or aspirin related to GI disease.
- Determine why patient is taking the drug.
- Be aware of patient's disease, its severity and frequency when known.
- TGB.
- Monitor and record vital signs.

Consultations:
- Medical consultation may be required to assess disease control and patient's ability to tolerate stress.

Teach Patient/Family:
- To prevent trauma when using oral hygiene aids
- Warn to avoid performing tasks that require mental alertness

megestrol acetate

me-jess'-trole
(Apo-Megestrol[CAN], Megace, Megostat[AUS])

CATEGORY AND SCHEDULE

Pregnancy Risk Category: X (for suspension), D (for tablets)

MECHANISM OF ACTION

A hormone and antineoplastic agent that suppresses the release of luteinizing hormone from the anterior pituitary gland by inhibiting pituitary function. ***Therapeutic Effect:*** Shrinks tumors. Also increases appetite by an unknown mechanism.

PHARMACOKINETICS

Well absorbed from the GI tract. Metabolized in the liver; excreted in urine.

AVAILABILITY

Tablets: 20 mg, 40 mg.
Suspension: 40 mg/ml.

INDICATIONS AND DOSAGES

▸ Palliative Treatment of Advanced Breast Cancer
PO
Adults, Elderly. 160 mg/day in 4 equally divided doses.

▸ Palliative Treatment of Advanced Endometrial Carcinoma
PO
Adults, Elderly. 40–320 mg/day in divided doses. Maximum: 800 mg/day in 1–4 divided doses.

▸ Anorexia, Cachexia, Weight Loss
PO
Adults, Elderly. 800 mg (20 ml)/day.

OFF-LABEL USES

Appetite stimulant, treatment of hormone-dependent or advanced prostate carcinoma

CONTRAINDICATIONS

None known.

INTERACTIONS

Drug
None known.
Herbal
None known.
Food
None known.

DIAGNOSTIC TEST EFFECTS

May increase blood glucose level.

SIDE EFFECTS

Frequent
Weight gain secondary to increased appetite
Occasional
Nausea, breakthrough bleeding, backache, headache, breast tenderness, carpal tunnel syndrome
Rare
Feeling of coldness

SERIOUS REACTIONS

! Thrombophlebitis and pulmonary embolism occur rarely.

DENTAL CONSIDERATIONS

General:
- Place on frequent recall to evaluate inflammatory and healing response.

• Patients receiving chemotherapy may require palliative treatment for stomatitis.

Teach Patient/Family:

• Importance of good oral hygiene to prevent soft tissue inflammation

meloxicam

mel-oks′-i-kam
(Mobic)

CATEGORY AND SCHEDULE

Pregnancy Risk Category: C (D if used in third trimester or near delivery)

MECHANISM OF ACTION

An NSAID that produces analgesic and anti-inflammatory effects by inhibiting prostaglandin synthesis. ***Therapeutic Effect:*** Reduces the inflammatory response and intensity of pain.

PHARMACOKINETICS

Route	Onset	Peak	Duration
PO (analgesic)	30 min	4–5 hr	N/A

Well absorbed after PO administration. Protein binding: 99%. Metabolized in the liver. Eliminated in urine and feces. Not removed by hemodialysis. ***Half-life:*** 15–20 hr.

AVAILABILITY

Tablets: 7.5 mg, 15 mg.

INDICATIONS AND DOSAGES

▸ Osteoarthritis, Rheumatoid Arthritis

PO

Adults. Initially, 7.5 mg/day. Maximum: 15 mg/day.

CONTRAINDICATIONS

Aspirin-induced nasal polyps associated with bronchospasm

INTERACTIONS

Drug

Aspirin: May increase the risk of epigastric distress, such as heartburn and indigestion.

Lithium: May increase the plasma concentration and risk of toxicity of lithium.

Herbal

Ginkgo biloba: May increase the risk of bleeding.

Food

None known.

Drug interactions of concern to dentistry

• Increased risk of GI side effects: long-duration NSAIDs, aspirin (except low-dose form), oral glucocorticoids, alcoholism, smoking, older age, and generally poor health

• Increased blood levels: lithium

• Reduced natriuretic effect: furosemide and other loop diuretics

• First-time users of SSRIs also taking NSAIDs may have a higher risk of GI side effects; until more data are available, it may be advisable to avoid use of NSAIDs in these patients (*Br J Clin Pharmacol* 55:591–595, 2003)

DIAGNOSTIC TEST EFFECTS

May increase serum creatinine, AST (SGOT), and ALT (SGPT) levels.

SIDE EFFECTS

Frequent (9%–7%)

Dyspepsia, headache, diarrhea, nausea

Occasional (4%–3%)

Dizziness, insomnia, rash, pruritus, flatulence, constipation, vomiting

Rare (<2%)

Somnolence, urticaria, photosensitivity, tinnitus

SERIOUS REACTIONS

! Rare reactions with long-term use include peptic ulcer disease, GI bleeding, gastritis, severe hepatic reaction (jaundice), nephrotoxicity (hematuria, dysuria, proteinuria), and a severe hypersensitivity reaction (bronchospasm, angioedema).

DENTAL CONSIDERATIONS

General:

- Assess salivary flow as a factor in caries, periodontal disease, and candidiasis.
- Patients on chronic drug therapy may rarely have symptoms of blood dyscrasias, which can include infection, bleeding, and poor healing.
- Consider semisupine chair position for patient comfort if GI side effects occur.

Consultations:

- In a patient with symptoms of blood dyscrasias, request a medical consultation for blood studies and postpone treatment until normal values are reestablished.

Teach Patient/Family:

- Use of electric toothbrush if patient has difficulty holding conventional devices
- Importance of updating health and drug history if physician makes any changes in evaluation or drug regimens
- Importance of good oral hygiene to prevent soft tissue inflammation
- To prevent trauma when using oral hygiene aids
- *When chronic dry mouth occurs, advise patient:*
  - To avoid mouth rinses with high alcohol content because of drying effects
  - To use daily home fluoride products for anticaries effect
  - To use sugarless gum, frequent sips of water, or saliva substitutes

melphalan

mel′-fah-lan

(Alkeran)

Do not confuse Alkeran with Leukeran, or melphalan with Mephyton or Myleran.

CATEGORY AND SCHEDULE

Pregnancy Risk Category: D

MECHANISM OF ACTION

An alkylating agent that inhibits protein synthesis primarily by cross-linking with strands of DNA and RNA, producing cell death. Cell cycle-phase nonspecific.

Therapeutic Effect: Disrupts nucleic acid function.

AVAILABILITY

Tablets: 2 mg.

Powder for Injection: 50 mg.

INDICATIONS AND DOSAGES

▸ Ovarian Carcinoma

PO

Adults, Elderly. 0.2 mg/kg/day for 5 successive days. Repeat at 4- to 6-wk intervals.

▸ Multiple Myeloma

PO

Adults. Initially, 6 mg once a day, adjusted as indicated; or 0.15 mg/kg/day for 7 days or 0.25 mg/kg/day for 4 days. Repeat at 4- to 6-wk intervals.

IV

Adults. 16 mg/m^2/dose every 2 wk for 4 doses, then repeated monthly according to protocol.

▸ Dosage in Renal Impairment

PO, IV

BUN level greater than 30 mg/dl. Decrease melphalan dosage by 50%.

Serum creatinine level greater than 1.5 mg/dl. Decrease the melphalan dosage by 50%.

OFF-LABEL USES
Treatment of breast carcinoma, neuroblastoma, rhabdomyosarcoma, testicular carcinoma

CONTRAINDICATIONS
Pregnancy, severe myelosuppression

INTERACTIONS
Drug
Antigout medications: May decrease the effects of these drugs.
Bone marrow depressants: May increase myelosuppression.
Live-virus vaccines: May potentiate virus replication, increase vaccine side effects, and decrease the patient's antibody response to the vaccine.
Herbal
None known.
Food
None known.
Drug interactions of concern to dentistry
• Increased toxicity: antineoplastics, radiation

DIAGNOSTIC TEST EFFECTS
May increase serum uric acid level and cause a positive direct Coombs' test.

IV INCOMPATIBILITIES
Don't mix melphalan with any other medications.

SIDE EFFECTS
Frequent
Nausea, vomiting (may be severe with large dose)
Occasional
Diarrhea, stomatitis, rash, pruritus, alopecia

SERIOUS REACTIONS
! Myelosuppression may cause hematologic toxicity, manifested principally as leukopenia and thrombocytopenia and, to lesser extent, anemia, pancytopenia, and agranulocytosis. Leukopenia may occur as early as 5 days after drug initiation.
! WBC and platelet counts return to normal levels during the 5th week of therapy, but leukopenia and thrombocytopenia may last more than 6 weeks after the drug is discontinued.
! Hyperuricemia, marked by hematuria, crystalluria, and flank pain, may occur.

DENTAL CONSIDERATIONS
General:
• Patients receiving chemotherapy may be taking chronic opioids for pain. Consider NSAIDs for dental pain management.
• Patients receiving chemotherapy may require palliative therapy for stomatitis.
• Patients on chronic drug therapy may rarely have symptoms of blood dyscrasias, which can include infection, bleeding, and poor healing.
Consultations:
• Medical consultation may be required to assess disease control.
• In a patient with symptoms of blood dyscrasias, request a medical consultation for blood studies and postpone dental treatment until normal values are reestablished.
Teach Patient/Family:
• About the possibility of secondary oral infection; must see dentist immediately if infection occurs
• *When chronic dry mouth occurs, advise patient:*
  • To avoid mouth rinses with high alcohol content because of drying effects
  • To use sugarless gum, frequent sips of water, or saliva substitutes
  • To use daily home fluoride products for anticaries effect

memantine hydrochloride

meh-man′-teen
(Ebixa[AUS], Namenda)

CATEGORY AND SCHEDULE

Pregnancy Risk Category: B

MECHANISM OF ACTION

A neurotransmitter inhibitor that decreases the effects of glutamate, the principle excitatory neurotransmitter in the brain. Persistent CNS excitation by glutamate is thought to cause the symptoms of Alzheimer's disease.
Therapeutic Effect: May reduce clinical deterioration in moderate to severe Alzheimer's disease.

PHARMACOKINETICS

M

Rapidly and completely absorbed after PO administration. Protein binding: 45%. Undergoes little metabolism; most of the dose is excreted unchanged in urine.
Half-life: 60–80 hr.

AVAILABILITY

Tablets: 5 mg, 10 mg.

INDICATIONS AND DOSAGES

▸ Alzheimer's Disease

PO

Adults, Elderly. Initially, 5 mg once a day. May increase dosage at intervals of at least 1 wk in 5-mg increments to 10 mg/day (5 mg twice a day), then 15 mg/day (5 mg and 10 mg as separate doses), and finally 20 mg/day (10 mg twice a day). Target dose: 20 mg/day.

CONTRAINDICATIONS

Severe renal impairment

INTERACTIONS

Drug

Carbonic anhydrase inhibitors, sodium bicarbonate: May decrease the renal elimination of memantine.

Herbal

None known.

Food

None known.

Drug interactions of concern to dentistry

- None reported

DIAGNOSTIC TEST EFFECTS

None known.

SIDE EFFECTS

Occasional (7%–4%)
Dizziness, headache, confusion, constipation, hypertension, cough
Rare (3%–2%)
Back pain, nausea, fatigue, anxiety, peripheral edema, arthralgia, insomnia

SERIOUS REACTIONS

! None known.

DENTAL CONSIDERATIONS

- Monitor vital signs at every appointment because of CV side effects.

General:

- Patients with Alzheimer's disease may be taking other drugs; get a complete drug history.
- Drug may be used late in disease process; ensure caregiver or responsible person understands informed consent.
- Place on frequent recall to evaluate oral health.

Consultations:

- Consultation with physician may be necessary if sedation or general anesthesia is required.

Teach Patient/Family:

- Use of electric toothbrush if patient has difficulty holding conventional devices

- Importance of good oral hygiene to prevent soft tissue inflammation/infection
- To prevent trauma when using oral hygiene aids
- Importance of updating health and drug history and reporting changes in health status, drug regimen, or disease/treatment status

meperidine hydrochloride

me-per′-i-deen

Schedule II

(Demerol, Pethidine Injection[AUS])

Do not confuse with Demulen or Dymelor.

CATEGORY AND SCHEDULE

Pregnancy Risk Category: B (D if used for prolonged periods or at high dosages at term)

Controlled Substance: Schedule II

MECHANISM OF ACTION

An opioid agonist that binds to opioid receptors in the CNS. ***Therapeutic Effect:*** Alters the perception of and emotional response to pain.

PHARMACOKINETICS

Route	Onset	Peak	Duration
PO	15 min	60 min	2–4 hr
IV	less than 5 min	5–7 min	2–3 hr
IM	10–15 min	30–50 min	2–4 hr
subcutaneous	10–15 min	30–50 min	2–4 hr

Variably absorbed from the GI tract; well absorbed after IM administration. Protein binding: 60%–80%. Widely distributed. Metabolized in the liver to active metabolite. Primarily excreted in urine. Not removed by hemodialysis. ***Half-life:*** 2.4–4 hr; metabolite 8–16 hr (increased in hepatic impairment and disease).

AVAILABILITY

Syrup: 50 mg/5 ml.
Tablets: 50 mg, 100 mg.
Injection: 25 mg/ml, 50 mg/ml, 75 mg/ml, 100 mg/ml.

INDICATIONS AND DOSAGES

▸ **Analgesia**

PO, IM, SUBCUTANEOUS

Adults, Elderly. 50–150 mg q3–4h.
Children. 1.1–1.5 mg/kg q3–4h. Don't exceed single dose of 100 mg.

▸ **Patient-Controlled Analgesia (PCA)**

IV

Adults. Loading dose: 50–100 mg. Intermittent bolus: 5–30 mg. Lockout interval: 10–20 min. Continuous infusion: 5–40 mg/hr. Maximum (4-hr): 200–300 mg.

▸ **Dosage in Renal Impairment**

Dosage is based on creatinine clearance.

Creatinine Clearance	Dosage
10–50 ml/min	75% of usual dose
less than 10 ml/min	50% of usual dose

CONTRAINDICATIONS

Delivery of premature infant, diarrhea due to poisoning, use within 14 days of MAOIs

INTERACTIONS

Drug

Alcohol, other CNS depressants: May increase CNS or respiratory depression and hypotension.

MAOIs: May produce a severe, sometimes fatal reaction. Meperidine use is contraindicated.

M

Herbal
Valerian: May increase CNS depression.
Food
None known.
Drug interactions of concern to dentistry
- Increased effects with all CNS depressants, neuromuscular blocking agents
- Contraindication: MAOIs, sibutramine
- Increased effects of anticholinergics
- Suspected increase in normeperidine levels: ritonavir
- Increased risk of hypotension: antihypertensive drugs

DIAGNOSTIC TEST EFFECTS
May increase serum amylase and lipase levels. Therapeutic serum level is 100–550 ng/ml; toxic serum level is greater than 1,000 ng/ml.

IV INCOMPATIBILITIES
Allopurinol (Aloprim), amphotericin B complex (Abelcet, AmBisome, Amphotec), cefepime (Maxipime), cefoperazone (Cefobid), doxorubicin liposomal (Doxil), furosemide (Lasix), idarubicin (Idamycin), nafcillin (Nafcil)
IV COMPATIBILITIES
Atropine, bumetanide (Bumex), diltiazem (Cardizem), diphenhydramine (Benadryl), dobutamine (Dobutrex), dopamine (Intropin), glycopyrrolate (Robinul), heparin, hydroxyzine (Vistaril), insulin, lidocaine, magnesium, midazolam (Versed), oxytocin (Pitocin), potassium

SIDE EFFECTS
Frequent
Sedation, hypotension (including orthostatic hypotension), diaphoresis, facial flushing, dizziness, nausea, vomiting, constipation
Occasional
Confusion, arrhythmias, tremors, urine retention, abdominal pain, dry mouth, headache, irritation at injection site, euphoria, dysphoria
Rare
Allergic reaction (rash, pruritus), insomnia

SERIOUS REACTIONS
! Overdose results in respiratory depression, skeletal muscle flaccidity, cold or clammy skin, cyanosis, and extreme somnolence progressing to seizures, stupor, and coma. The antidote is 0.4 mg naloxone.
! The patient who uses meperidine repeatedly may develop a tolerance to the drug's analgesic effect and physical dependence.

DENTAL CONSIDERATIONS
General:
- After supine positioning, have patient sit upright for at least 2 min before standing to avoid orthostatic hypotension.
- Psychologic and physical dependence may occur with chronic administration.

Teach Patient/Family:
- To avoid mouth rinses with high alcohol content because of drying effects

mephentermine sulfate
meh-**fen**-ter-meen
(Wyamine Sulfate)

CATEGORY AND SCHEDULE
Pregnancy Risk Category: C

MECHANISM OF ACTION
A sympathomimetic amine that acts indirectly by releasing norepinephrine and directly by exerting a slight

effect on α- and β_1-receptors and a moderate effect on β_2-receptors mediating vasodilation. ***Therapeutic Effect:*** Produces cardiac stimulation.

PHARMACOKINETICS

Onset of action occurs immediately and persists 15–30 min. Metabolized in liver. Excreted in urine. ***Half-life:*** 17–18 hr.

AVAILABILITY

Injection: 15 mg/ml, 30 mg/ml (Wyamine Sulfate).

INDICATIONS AND DOSAGES

▸ Hypotension (Secondary to Spinal Anesthesia)

IM/IV

Adults. 30–45 mg as a single injection.

Prophylaxis of hypotension in spinal anesthesia

IM/IV

Adults. 30–45 mg 10–20 min before anesthesia.

UNLABELED USES

Hypotension (due to heart failure), hypotension (due to myocardial infarction)

CONTRAINDICATIONS

Concurrent use or within 14 days of discontinuation of MAOI therapy, hypotension induced by chlorpromazine, hypersensitivity to mephentermine or sympathomimetic amines

INTERACTIONS

Drug

Cyclopropane, halogenated hydrocarbon, general anesthetics: May cause ventricular arrhythmias.
Phenothiazines: May potentiate hypotensive effects of phenothiazines.
MAOIs: May potentiate the pressor effects of mephentermine.
Reserpine, guanethidine: May reduce the pressor response to mephentermine.

Herbal

None known.

Food

None known.

Drug interactions of concern to dentistry

- Increased risk of arrhythmia: halogenated hydrocarbon anesthetics

DIAGNOSTIC TEST EFFECTS

None known.

SIDE EFFECTS

Occasional

Anxiety, nervousness, cardiac arrhythmias, increased BP

SERIOUS REACTIONS

! Mephentermine may produce arrhythmias, including transient extrasystoles, AV block, and hypertension.
! CNS effects, including hyperexcitability, prolonged wakefulness, weeping, incoherence, convulsions, flushing, tremor, and hallucinations, may occur with large doses of mephentermine.

DENTAL CONSIDERATIONS

General:

- For use in hospitals or emergency rooms for selected hypotensive episodes.

mephobarbital

me′-foe-bar′-bi-tal
Schedule IV
(Mebaral)

CATEGORY AND SCHEDULE

Controlled substance: Schedule IV

M

MECHANISM OF ACTION

A barbiturate that increases seizure threshold in the motor cortex.
Therapeutic Effect: Depresses monosynaptic and polysynaptic transmission in the central nervous system (CNS).

PHARMACOKINETICS

PO route onset 20–60 minutes, peak N/A, duration 6–8 hours. Well absorbed after PO administration. Widely distributed. Metabolized in liver to active metabolite, a form of phenobarbital. Minimally excreted in urine. Removed by hemodialysis.
Half-life: 34 hrs.

AVAILABILITY

Tablets: 32 mg, 50 mg, 100 mg (Mebaral).

INDICATIONS AND DOSAGES

▸ Epilepsy

PO
Adults, Elderly. 400–600 mg/day in divided doses or at bedtime.
Children older than 5 yrs. 32–64 mg 3 or 4 times/day.
Children younger than 5 yrs. 16–32 mg 3 or 4 times/day.

▸ Sedation

PO
Adults, Elderly. 32–100 mg/day in 3–4 divided doses.
Children. 16–32 mg in 3–4 divided doses.

CONTRAINDICATIONS

Porphyria, history of hypersensitivity to mephobarbital or other barbituates

INTERACTIONS

Drug

Alcohol, CNS depressants: May increase the effects of mephobarbital.
Carbamazepine: May increase the metabolism of carbamazepine.
Digoxin, glucocorticoids, metronidazole, oral anticoagulants, quinidine, tricyclic antidepressants: May decrease the effects of these medications.
Pyridoxine: May decrease the effectiveness of mephobarbital.
Valproic acid: Decreases the metabolism and increases the concentration and risk of toxicity of mephobarbital.

Herbal

Catnip oil: May increase the CNS effects of mephobarbital.
Eucalyptol: May decrease the effectiveness of mephobarbital.
Evening primrose oil: May decrease the anticonvulsant effectiveness of mephobarbital.
Ginkgo biloba: May decrease the anticonvulsant effectiveness of mephobarbital.
Kava kava: May increase the CNS effects of mephobarbital.
Passion flower: May increase the CNS effects of mephobarbital.
St. John's Wort: May decrease CNS depressive effects of mephobarbital.
Valerian: May increase the CNS effects of mephobarbital.

Food

None known.

Drug interactions of concern to dentistry

- Increased effects: alcohol, all CNS depressants
- Decreased effects of corticosteroids, doxycycline, carbamazepine

DIAGNOSTIC TEST EFFECTS

None known.

SIDE EFFECTS

Frequent

Dizziness, lightheadedness, somnolence

Occasional

Confusion, headache, insomnia, mental depression, nervousness, nightmares, unusual excitement

Rare
Rash, paradoxical CNS hyperactivity or nervousness in children, excitement or restlessness in elderly, generally noted during first 2 weeks of therapy, particularly noted in presence of uncontrolled pain

SERIOUS REACTIONS

! Abrupt withdrawal after prolonged therapy may produce effects including markedly increased dreaming, nightmares or insomnia, tremor, sweating, vomiting, to hallucinations, delirium, seizures, and status epilepticus.
! Skin eruptions appear as hypersensitivity reaction.
! Blood dyscrasias, liver disease, and hypocalcemia occur rarely.
! Overdosage produces cold or clammy skin, hypothermia, severe CNS depression, cyanosis, rapid pulse, and Cheyne-Stokes respirations.
! Toxicity may result in severe renal impairment.

DENTAL CONSIDERATIONS

General:
- Determine type of epilepsy, seizure frequency, and quality of seizure control. A stress reduction protocol may be required.
- Monitor vital signs at every appointment because of CV and respiratory side effects.
- Patients on chronic drug therapy may rarely have symptoms of blood dyscrasias, which can include infection, bleeding, and poor healing.
- Barbiturates induce liver microsomal enzymes, which alters the metabolism of other drugs.
- Avoid drugs that may lower seizure threshold (phenothiazines).
- Be sure patient is regularly taking medication.

Consultations:
- In a patient with symptoms of blood dyscrasias, request a medical consultation for blood studies and postpone dental treatment until normal values are reestablished.
- Medical consultation may be required to assess disease control and patient's ability to tolerate stress.

Teach Patient/Family:
- Importance of good oral hygiene to prevent soft tissue inflammation
- Caution to prevent injury when using oral hygiene aids
- To avoid mouth rinses with high alcohol content because of drying effects

mepivacaine HCl (local) mepivacaine hydrochloride

me-**piv**-a-kane
(Carbocaine Caudal 1.5%[AUS], Carbocaine HCl, Polocaine, Polocaine-MPF)

CATEGORY AND SCHEDULE

Pregnancy Risk Category: C

MECHANISM OF ACTION

An amino amide anesthetic that inhibits conduction of nerve impulses. ***Therapeutic Effect:*** Causes temporary loss of feeling and sensation.

PHARMACOKINETICS

Onset	Peak	Duration
3–20 min	N/A	2–2.5 hr

Protein binding: 75%. Rapidly metabolized in liver. Small amount is excreted in urine. ***Half-life:*** 1.9–3.2 hr; 8.7–9 hr (neonates).

AVAILABILITY

Injectable Solution (Carbocaine, Polocaine, Polocaine-MPF): 1%, 1.5%, 2%.

INDICATIONS AND DOSAGES

Recommended Concentrations and Doses of Mepivacaine

	Total Dose		
Concentration	**ml**	**mg**	**Comments**
Cervical, Brachial, Intercostal, Pudendal Nerve Block			
1%	5–40	50–400	Pudendal block: half of total dose injected each side
2%	5–20	100–400	
Transvaginal Block (paracervical plus pudendal)			
1%	Up to 30 (both sides)	Up to 300 (both sides)	Half of total dose injected each side.
Paracervical Block			
1%	Up to 20 (both sides)	Up to 200 (both sides)	Half of total dose injected each side. This is maximum recommended dose per 90-min period in obstetrical patients. Inject slowly, 5 min between sides.
Caudal and Epidural Block			
1%	15–30	150–300	Use only single-dose vials that do not contain a preservative.
1.5%	10–25	150–375	
2%	10–20	200–400	
Infiltration			
1%	Up to 40	Up to 400	An equivalent amount of a 0.5% solution (prepared by diluting the1% solution with sodium chloride) injection can be used for large areas.
Therapeutic Block (pain management)			
1%	1–5	10–50	
2%	1–5	20–100	

M

▸ **Regional Anesthesia**
Children younger than 3 yr or weighing less than 30 lb. Maximum dose of mepivacaine should not exceed 5–6 mg/kg. Concentrations greater than 1.5% should be avoided.

CONTRAINDICATIONS

Hypersensitivity to any local anesthetic agent of the amide-type or to other components of solutions of mepivacaine

INTERACTIONS

Drug

Ergot-type oxytocic drugs: May cause severe, persistent hypertension or cerebrovascular accidents.
MAOIs, tricyclic antidepressants: May produce severe, prolonged hypertension.

Herbal

None known.

Food

None known.

Drug interactions of concern to dentistry

• CNS depressants: may see increased risk of CNS depression with all CNS depressants, especially in children and when larger doses are used
• Avoid placing dental cartridges in disinfectant solutions with heavy metals or surface-active agents; may see release of metal ions into local anesthetic solutions with tissue irritation following injection
• Avoid excessive exposure of dental cartridges to light or heat, which hastens deterioration of vasoconstrictor; observe for color change in local anesthetic solution
• Risk of CV side effects: rapid intravascular administration of local anesthetic containing vasoconstrictor, either alone or in patients taking tricyclic antidepressants, MAOIs, digitalis drugs, cocaine, phenothiazines, β-blockers, and in the presence of halogenated-hydrocarbon general anesthetics; use lowest effective vasoconstrictor dose and careful aspiration techniques
• Avoid use of vasoconstrictors in patients with uncontrolled hyperthyroidism, diabetes, angina, or hypertension; refer these patients for medical treatment before elective dental procedures

DIAGNOSTIC TEST EFFECTS

None known.

IV COMPATIBILITIES

Do not mix with other medications.

SIDE EFFECTS

CNS and cardiovascular effects are generally dose related and of short duration.

Occasional

Burning, stinging, tenderness

Rare

Generally with high dose: Drowsiness, dizziness, disorientation, light-headedness, tremors, apprehension, euphoria, blurred or double vision, ringing or roaring in ears (tinnitus), nausea, sensation of heat, cold, numbness

SERIOUS REACTIONS

! CNS toxicity may occur, especially with regional anesthesia use, progressing rapidly from mild side effects to tremors, somnolence, seizures, vomiting, and respiratory depression.
! Allergic reactions, bradyarrhythmia, cardiac arrest, fetal bradycardia, heart block, hypotension, seizure, and ventricular arrhythmia have been reported.
! Allergic reactions occur rarely.

DENTAL CONSIDERATIONS

General:

- Drug is often used with a vasoconstrictor for increased duration of action.
- Monitor vital signs at every appointment because of CV and respiratory side effects.
- Lubricate dry lips before injection.

Teach Patient/Family:

- To use care to prevent injury while numbness exists and to refrain from chewing gum and eating following dental anesthesia
- To report any signs of infection, muscle pain, or fever to dentist when feeling returns
- To report any unusual soft tissue reactions

M

meprobamate

me-proe′-ba-mate

Schedule IV

(Miltown, Novo-Mepro[CAN])

CATEGORY AND SCHEDULE

Pregnancy Risk Category: D

MECHANISM OF ACTION

A carbamate derivative that affects the thalamus and limbic system. Appears to inhibit multi-neuronal spinal reflexes. ***Therapeutic Effect:*** Relieves pain or muscle spasms.

PHARMACOKINETICS

Slowly absorbed from the gastrointestinal (GI) tract. Protein binding: 0–30%. Metabolized in liver. Excreted in urine and feces. Moderately dialyzable. ***Half-life:*** 10 hrs.

AVAILABILITY

Tablets: 200 mg, 400 mg, 600 mg (Miltown).

INDICATIONS AND DOSAGES

▸ Anxiety Disorders

PO

Adults, Children 12 yrs and older. 400 mg 3–4 times. Maximum: 2400 mg/day.

Children 6–12 yrs. 100–200 mg 2–3 times/day.

Elderly. Use lowest effective dose. 200 mg 2–3 times/day

▸ Dosage in Renal Impairment

Creatinine Clearance	Dosage Interval
10–50 ml/min	every 9–12 hrs
less than 10 ml/min	every 12–18 hrs

OFF-LABEL USES

Muscle contraction, headache, premenstrual tension, external sphincter spasticity, muscle rigidity, opisthotonos-associated with tetanus

CONTRAINDICATIONS

Acute intermittent porphyria, hypersensitivity to meprobamate or related compounds

INTERACTIONS

Drug

Alcohol, central nervous system (CNS) depressants: May increase CNS depression.

Herbal

Gotu kola, kava kava, St. John's Wort: May increase CNS depression.

Food

None known.

Drug interactions of concern to dentistry

- Increased effects: CNS depressants, alcohol

DIAGNOSTIC TEST EFFECTS

None known.

SIDE EFFECTS

Frequent

Drowsiness, dizziness

Occasional

Tachycardia, palpitations, headache, lightheadedness, dermatitis, diarrhea, nausea, vomiting, dyspnea, rash, weakness, blurred vision, wheezing.

SERIOUS REACTIONS

! Agranulocytosis, aplastic anemia, leucopenia, anaphylaxis, cardiac arrhythmias, hypotensive crisis, syncope, Stevens-Johnson syndrome and bullous dermatitis have been reported.

! Overdose may cause CNS depression, ataxia, coma, shock, hypotension and death.

DENTAL CONSIDERATIONS

General:

- Monitor vital signs at every appointment because of CV side effects.
- Patients on chronic drug therapy may rarely have symptoms of blood dyscrasias, which can include infection, bleeding, and poor healing.
- Assess salivary flow as a factor in caries, periodontal disease, and candidiasis.
- Avoid dental light in patient's eyes; offer dark glasses for patient comfort.
- Determine why the patient is taking the drug.
- Psychologic and physical dependence may occur with chronic administration.

Consultations:

- In a patient with symptoms of blood dyscrasias, request a medical consultation for blood studies and postpone dental treatment until normal values are reestablished.
- Medical consultation may be required to assess disease control.

Teach Patient/Family:

- Importance of good oral hygiene to prevent soft tissue inflammation
- Caution to prevent injury when using oral hygiene aids
- *When chronic dry mouth occurs, advise patient:*
  - To avoid mouth rinses with high alcohol content because of drying effects
  - To use sugarless gum, frequent sips of water, or saliva substitutes
  - To use daily home fluoride products for anticaries effect

mercaptopurine

mur-cap-tow′-pure-een

(Purinethol)

CATEGORY AND SCHEDULE

Pregnancy Risk Category: D

M

MECHANISM OF ACTION

An antimetabolite that is incorporated into RNA and DNA, blocks purine synthesis, and inhibits DNA and RNA synthesis. ***Therapeutic Effect:*** Causes death of cancer cells.

AVAILABILITY

Tablets: 50 mg.

INDICATIONS AND DOSAGES

▸ Acute Lymphoblastic Leukemia

PO

Adults, Elderly, Children. 2.5–5 mg/kg once a day as induction dose. Maintenance: 1.5–2.5 mg/kg/day.

▸ Dosage in Renal Impairment:

Creatinine clearance less than 50 ml/min. Administer usual dose q48h.

CONTRAINDICATIONS

Pregnancy, severe myelosuppression or hepatic disease

INTERACTIONS

Drug

Alcohol: May increase the risk of toxicity of mercaptopurine.
Allopurinol, doxorubicin, hepatotoxic medications: May increase the effects and risk of toxicity of mercaptopurine.
Bone marrow depressants: May increase the risk of myelosuppression.
Live-virus vaccines: May potentiate virus replication, increase vaccine side effects, and decrease the patient's antibody response to the vaccine.
Warfarin: May decrease the effects of this drug.

Herbal

None known.

Food

All foods: Decrease the bioavailability of mercaptopurine.

Drug interactions of concern to dentistry

• Increased risk of hepatotoxicity: hepatotoxic drugs

DIAGNOSTIC TEST EFFECTS

None known.

SIDE EFFECTS

Frequent (>10%)

Myelosuppression (leading to leukopenia, thrombocytopenia, anemia), intrahepatic cholestasis, hepatic necrosis

Occasional (10%–1%)

Drug fever, hyperpigmentation, rash, hyperuricemia, nausea, vomiting, diarrhea, stomatitis, anorexia, abdominal pain, mucositis

SERIOUS REACTIONS

! Myelosuppression, hepatic necrosis, and gastroenteritis may occur.

DENTAL CONSIDERATIONS

General:

• Patients on chronic drug therapy may rarely have symptoms of blood dyscrasias, which can include infection, bleeding, and poor healing.
• Avoid prescribing aspirin-containing products.
• Prophylactic antibiotics may be indicated to prevent infection if surgery or deep scaling is planned.
• Patients receiving chemotherapy may require palliative treatment for stomatitis.

Consultations:

• In a patient with symptoms of blood dyscrasias, request a medical consultation for blood studies and postpone dental treatment until normal values are reestablished.

Teach Patient/Family:

• Importance of good oral hygiene to prevent soft tissue inflammation
• Caution to prevent injury when using oral hygiene aids
• To avoid mouth rinses with high alcohol content

meropenem

murr-oh-peh′-nem
(Merrem IV)

CATEGORY AND SCHEDULE

Pregnancy Risk Category: B

MECHANISM OF ACTION

A carbapenem that binds to penicillin-binding proteins and inhibits bacterial cell wall synthesis.
Therapeutic Effect: Produces bacterial cell death.

PHARMACOKINETICS

After IV administration, widely distributed into tissues and body fluids, including CSF. Protein binding: 2%.

Primarily excreted unchanged in urine. Removed by hemodialysis. ***Half-life:*** 1 hr.

AVAILABILITY

Powder for Injection: 500 mg, 1 g.

INDICATIONS AND DOSAGES

▸ Mild to Moderate Infections

IV

Adults, Elderly. 0.5–1 g q8h.
Children 3 mo and older. 20 mg/kg/dose q8h.
Children younger than 3 mo. 20 mg/kg/dose q8–12h.

▸ Meningitis

IV

Adults, Elderly, Children weighing 50 kg or more. 2 g q8h.
Children 3 mo and older weighing less than 50 kg. 40 mg/kg q8h. Maximum: 2 g/dose.

▸ Dosage in Renal Impairment

Dosage and frequency are modified on the basis of creatinine clearance.

Creatinine Clearance	Dosage	Interval
26–49 ml/min	Recommended dose (1,000 mg)	q12h
10–25 ml/min	1/2 of recommended dose	q12h
less than 10 ml/min	1/2 of recommended dose	q24h

OFF-LABEL USES

Lower respiratory tract infections, febrile neutropenia, gynecologic and obstetric infections, sepsis

CONTRAINDICATIONS

None known.

INTERACTIONS

Drug

Probenecid: Reduces renal excretion of meropenem.

Herbal

None known.

Food

None known.

Drug interactions of concern to dentistry

• Increased or prolonged plasma levels: probenecid

DIAGNOSTIC TEST EFFECTS

May increase BUN level and serum alkaline phosphatase, bilirubin, creatinine, LDH, AST (SGOT), and ALT (SGPT) levels. May decrease blood Hct and Hgb levels and serum potassium levels.

IV INCOMPATIBILITIES

Acyclovir (Zovirax), amphotericin B (Fungizone), diazepam (Valium), doxycycline (Vibramycin), metronidazole (Flagyl), ondansetron (Zofran)

IV COMPATIBILITIES

Dobutamine (Dobutrex), dopamine (Intropin), heparin, magnesium

SIDE EFFECTS

Frequent (5%–3%)

Diarrhea, nausea, vomiting, headache, inflammation at injection site

Occasional (2%)

Oral candidiasis, rash, pruritus

Rare (<2%)

Constipation, glossitis

SERIOUS REACTIONS

! Antibiotic-associated colitis and other superinfections may occur.

! Anaphylactic reactions have been reported.

! Seizures may occur in those with CNS disorders (including brain lesions and a history of seizures), bacterial meningitis, or impaired renal function.

DENTAL CONSIDERATIONS

General:

- For selected infections in the hospital setting: provide emergency dental treatment only.
- Examine for oral manifestation of opportunistic infection.
- Determine why patient is taking the drug.
- Caution regarding allergy to medication.

Consultations:

- Consult patient's physician if an acute dental infection occurs and another antiinfective is required.
- Medical consultation may be required to assess disease control.

Teach Patient/Family:

- Importance of good oral hygiene to prevent soft tissue inflammation
- To report oral lesions, soreness, or bleeding to dentist
- To prevent trauma when using oral hygiene aids

M

mesalamine/5 aminosalicylic acid (5-ASA)

mez-al'-a-meen
(Asacol, Fiv-Canasa, Mesasal[CAN], Pentasa, Rowasa, Salofalk[CAN])
Do not confuse Asacol with Os-Cal.

CATEGORY AND SCHEDULE

Pregnancy Risk Category: B

MECHANISM OF ACTION

A salicylic acid derivative that locally inhibits arachidonic acid metabolite production, which is increased in patients with chronic inflammatory bowel disease. ***Therapeutic Effect:*** Blocks prostaglandin production and diminishes inflammation in the colon.

PHARMACOKINETICS

Poorly absorbed from the colon. Moderately absorbed from the GI tract. Metabolized in the liver to active metabolite. Unabsorbed portion eliminated in feces; absorbed portion excreted in urine. Unknown if removed by hemodialysis. ***Half-life:*** 0.5–1.5 hr; metabolite, 5–10 hr.

AVAILABILITY

Tablets (Delayed-Release [Asacol]): 400 mg.
Capsules (Controlled-Release [Pentasa]): 250 mg.
Rectal Suspension (Rowasa): 4 g/60 ml.
Suppositories (Canasa): 500 mg, 1 g.

INDICATIONS AND DOSAGES

▸ Ulcerative Colitis, Proctosigmoiditis, Proctitis

PO (Asacol)
Adults, Elderly. 800 mg 3 times a day for 6 wk.
Children. 50 mg/kg/day q8–12h.
PO (Pentasa)
Adults, Elderly. 1 g 4 times a day for 8 wk.
Children. 50 mg/kg/day q6–12h.
Rectal (retention enema)
Adults, Elderly. 60 ml (4 g) at bedtime; retain overnight (about 8 hr) for 3–6 wk.
Rectal (suppositories)
Adults, Elderly. 1 suppository (500 mg) twice a day, retain 1–3 hr for 3–6 wk.

▸ To Maintain Remission in Ulcerative Colitis

PO (Asacol)
Adults, Elderly. 1.6 g/day in divided doses.
PO (Pentasa)
Adults, Elderly. 1 g 4 times a day

CONTRAINDICATIONS

None known.

INTERACTIONS

Drug

None known.

Herbal

None known.

Food

None known.

DIAGNOSTIC TEST EFFECTS

May increase BUN, serum alkaline phosphatase, creatinine, AST(SGOT), and ALT(SGPT) levels.

SIDE EFFECTS

Mesalamine is generally well tolerated, with only mild and transient effects.

Frequent (greater than 6%)

PO: Abdominal cramps or pain, diarrhea, dizziness, headache, nausea, vomiting, rhinitis, unusual fatigue
Rectal: Abdominal or stomach cramps, flatulence, headache, nausea

Occasional (6%–2%)

PO: Hair loss, decreased appetite, back or joint pain, flatulence, acne
Rectal: Hair loss

Rare (<2%)

Rectal: Anal irritation

SERIOUS REACTIONS

! Sulfite sensitivity may occur in susceptible patients, manifested by cramping, headache, diarrhea, fever, rash, hives, itching, and wheezing. Discontinue drug immediately.

! Hepatitis, pancreatitis, and pericarditis occur rarely with oral forms.

DENTAL CONSIDERATIONS

General:

- Consider semisupine chair position for patient comfort because of GI effects of disease.

Consultations

- To reduce any potential risk of antibiotic-associated pseudomembranous colitis, a consultation is recommended before selecting an antibiotic for a dental infection.

mesna

mess′-na
(Mesnex, Uromitexan[CAN])

CATEGORY AND SCHEDULE

Pregnancy Risk Category: B

MECHANISM OF ACTION

An antineoplastic adjunct and cytoprotective agent that binds with and detoxifies urotoxic metabolites of ifosfamide and cyclophosphamide. ***Therapeutic Effect:*** Inhibits ifosfamide-and cyclophosphamide-induced hemorrhagic cystitis.

PHARMACOKINETICS

Rapidly metabolized after IV administration to mesna disulfide, which is reduced to mesna in kidney. Excreted in urine. ***Half-life:*** 24 min.

AVAILABILITY

Tablets: 400 mg.
Injection: 100 mg/ml.

INDICATIONS AND DOSAGES

▸ Prevention of Hemorrhagic Cystitis in Patients Receiving Ifosfamide

IV

Adults, Elderly. 20% of ifosfamide dose at time of ifosfamide administration and 4 and 8 hr after each dose of ifosfamide. Total dose: 60% of ifosfamide dosage. Range: 60%–160% of the daily ifosfamide dose.

▸ Prevention of Hemorrhagic Cystitis in Patients Receiving Cyclophosphamide

PO

Adults, Elderly. 40% of cyclophosphamide dose q4h for 3 doses.

IV

Adults, Elderly. 20% of cyclophosphamide dose at time of

M

cyclophosphamide administration and q3h for 3–4 doses.

CONTRAINDICATIONS

None known.

INTERACTIONS

Drug

None known.

Herbal

None known.

Food

None known.

Drug interactions of concern to dentistry

• None reported

DIAGNOSTIC TEST EFFECTS

May produce false-positive test result for urinary ketones.

IV INCOMPATIBILITIES

Amphotericin B complex (Abelcet, AmBisome, Amphotec)

IV COMPATIBILITIES

Allopurinol (Aloprim), docetaxel (Taxotere), doxorubicin (Adriamycin), etoposide (VePesid), gemcitabine (Gemzar), granisetron (Kytril), methotrexate, ondansetron (Zofran), paclitaxel (Taxol), vinorelbine (Navelbine)

SIDE EFFECTS

Frequent (>17%)

Bad taste, soft stools

Large doses: Diarrhea, myalgia, headache, fatigue, nausea, hypotension, allergic reaction

SERIOUS REACTIONS

! Hematuria occurs rarely.

DENTAL CONSIDERATIONS

General:

• Patient will be taking ifosfamide or cyclophosphamide; determine use and disease.

• Question patient about other diseases and medications taken.

• Note side effects and precautions associated with chemotherapeutic drugs.

Consultations:

• Medical consultation should include routine blood counts including platelet counts and bleeding time.

• Consult physician; prophylactic or therapeutic antiinfectives may be indicated if surgery or periodontal treatment is required.

• Medical consultation may be required to assess immunologic status during cancer chemotherapy and determine safety risk, if any, posed by the required dental treatment.

• Medical consultation may be required to assess disease control and patient's ability to tolerate stress.

Teach Patient/Family:

• Importance of good oral hygiene to prevent soft tissue inflammation

• To prevent trauma when using oral hygiene aids

• To report oral lesions, soreness, or bleeding to dentist

• Importance of updating health and medication history if physician makes any changes in evaluation or drug regimens; include OTC, herbal, and nonherbal in the update

mesoridazine besylate

mez-oh-rid′-a-zeen

(Serentil)

Do not confuse Serentil with Proventil, Serevent, or sertraline.

CATEGORY AND SCHEDULE

Pregnancy Risk Category: C

MECHANISM OF ACTION

A phenothiazine that blocks dopamine at postsynaptic receptor sites in the brain. ***Therapeutic Effect:*** Diminishes schizophrenic behavior. Also has anticholinergic and sedative effects.

AVAILABILITY

Oral Solution: 25 mg/ml.
Tablets: 10 mg, 25 mg, 50 mg, 100 mg.
Injection: 25 mg/ml.

INDICATIONS AND DOSAGES

▸ Schizophrenia

PO
Adults, Elderly. 25–50 mg 3 times a day. Maximum: 400 mg/day.
IM
Adults, Elderly. Initially, 25 mg. May repeat in 30–60 min. Range: 25–200 mg.

▸ Severe Behavioral Problems (Combativeness or Explosive, Hyperexcitable Behavior) Associated with Neurologic Diseases

PO
Elderly. Initially, 10 mg once or twice a day. May increase at 4–7 day intervals. Maximum: 250 mg.
IM
Adults, Elderly. Initially, 25 mg. May repeat in 30–60 min. Range: 25–200 mg.

CONTRAINDICATIONS

Coma, myelosuppression, severe cardiovascular disease, severe CNS depression, subcortical brain damage

INTERACTIONS

Drug

Alcohol, other CNS depressants: May increase CNS and respiratory depression and the hypotensive effects of mesoridazine.
Antithyroid agents: May increase the risk of agranulocytosis.
Extrapyramidal symptom-producing medications: May increase extrapyramidal symptoms.
Hypotension-producing medications: May increase hypotension.
Levodopa: May decrease the effects of levodopa.
Lithium: May decrease mesoridazine absorption and produce adverse neurologic effects.
MAOIs, tricyclic antidepressants: May increase the anticholinergic and sedative effects of mesoridazine.

Herbal

None known.

Food

None known.

Drug interactions of concern to dentistry

- Increased sedation: other CNS depressants, alcohol, barbiturate anesthetics, opioid analgesics
- Hypotension, tachycardia: epinephrine
- Increased extrapyramidal effects: phenothiazines and related drugs (haloperidol, droperidol), metoclopramide
- Additive photosensitization: tetracyclines
- Increased anticholinergic effects: anticholinergics

DIAGNOSTIC TEST EFFECTS

May produce false-positive pregnancy and phenylketonuria test results. May produce ECG changes, including prolonged QT and QTc intervals and T-wave depression or inversion.

SIDE EFFECTS

Frequent

Orthostatic hypotension, dizziness, syncope (occur frequently after first injection, occasionally after subsequent injections, and rarely with oral form)

Occasional
Somnolence (during early therapy), dry mouth, blurred vision, lethargy, constipation or diarrhea, nasal congestion, peripheral edema, urine retention
Rare
Ocular changes, altered skin pigmentation (in those taking high doses for prolonged periods), darkening of urine

SERIOUS REACTIONS

! Abrupt withdrawal after long-term therapy may precipitate nausea, vomiting, gastritis, dizziness, and tremors.
! Blood dyscrasias, particularly agranulocytosis and mild leukopenia, may occur.
! Mesoridazine use may lower the seizure threshold.

DENTAL CONSIDERATIONS

General:
- Monitor vital signs at every appointment because of CV side effects.
- Patients on chronic drug therapy may rarely have symptoms of blood dyscrasias, which can include infection, bleeding, and poor healing.
- After supine positioning, have patient sit upright for at least 2 min before standing to avoid orthostatic hypotension.
- Assess salivary flow as a factor in caries, periodontal disease, and candidiasis.
- Avoid dental light in patient's eyes; offer dark glasses for patient comfort.
- Assess for presence of extrapyramidal motor symptoms, such as tardive dyskinesia and akathisia. Extrapyramidal motor activity may complicate dental treatment.
- Geriatric patients are more susceptible to drug effects; use lower dose.
- Use vasoconstrictors with caution, in low doses, and with careful aspiration. Avoid use of gingival retraction cord with epinephrine.

Consultations:
- In a patient with symptoms of blood dyscrasias, request a medical consultation for blood studies and postpone dental treatment until normal values are reestablished.
- Take precautions if dental surgery is anticipated and anesthesia is required.
- Refer to physician if signs of tardive dyskinesia or akathisia are present.
- Physician should be informed if significant xerostomic side effects occur (e.g., increased caries, sore tongue, problems eating or swallowing, difficulty wearing prosthesis) so that a medication change can be considered.

Teach Patient/Family:
- Importance of good oral hygiene to prevent soft tissue inflammation
- Caution to prevent injury when using oral hygiene aids
- To use electric toothbrush if patient has difficulty holding conventional devices
- *When chronic dry mouth occurs, advise patient:*
  - To avoid mouth rinses with high alcohol content because of drying effects
  - To use sugarless gum, frequent sips of water, or saliva substitutes
  - To use daily home fluoride products for anticaries effect

metaproterenol sulfate

met-a-proe-ter′-e-nole
(Alupent)
Do not confuse metaproterenol with metipranolol or metoprolol, or Alupent with Atrovent.

CATEGORY AND SCHEDULE

Pregnancy Risk Category: C

MECHANISM OF ACTION
A sympathomimetic that stimulates beta$_2$-adrenergic receptors, resulting in relaxation of bronchial smooth muscle. ***Therapeutic Effect:*** Relieves bronchospasm and reduces airway resistance.

AVAILABILITY
Syrup: 10 mg/5 ml.
Tablets: 10 mg, 20 mg.
Aerosol Oral Inhalation (Alupent): 0.65 mg/inhalation.
Solution for Oral Inhalation: 0.4%, 0.6%, 5%.

INDICATIONS AND DOSAGES
▸ Treatment of Bronchospasm
PO
Adults, Children 10 yr and older. 20 mg 3–4 times a day.
Elderly. 10 mg 3–4 times a day. May increase to 20 mg/dose.
Children 6–9 yr. 10 mg 3–4 times a day.
Children 2–5 yr. 1.3–2.6 mg/kg/day in 3–4 divided doses.
Children younger than 2 yr. 0.4 mg/kg 3–4 times a day.
INHALATION
Adults, Elderly, Children 12 yr and older. 2–3 inhalations q3–4h. Maximum: 12 inhalations/24 hr.
NEBULIZATION
Adults, Elderly, Children 12 yr and older. 10–15 mg (0.2–0.3 ml) of 5% q4–6h.
Children younger than 12 yr, Infants. 0.5–1 mg/kg (0.01–0.02 ml/kg) of 5% q4–6h.

CONTRAINDICATIONS
Angle-closure glaucoma, preexisting arrhythmias associated with tachycardia

INTERACTIONS
Drug
Beta blockers: May decrease the effects of beta blockers.
Digoxin, other sympathomimetics: May increase the risk of arrhythmias.
MAOIs: May increase the risk of hypertensive crisis.
Tricyclic antidepressants: May increase cardiovascular effects.
Herbal
None known.
Food
None known.
Drug interactions of concern to dentistry
- Increased effects of both drugs: other sympathomimetics, CNS stimulants
- Increased dysrhythmias: halogenated hydrocarbon anesthetics

DIAGNOSTIC TEST EFFECTS
May decrease serum potassium level.

SIDE EFFECTS
Frequent (>10%)
Rigors, tremors, anxiety, nausea, dry mouth
Occasional (9%–1%)
Dizziness, vertigo, asthenia, headache, GI distress, vomiting, cough, dry throat
Rare (<1%)
Somnolence, diarrhea, altered taste

SERIOUS REACTIONS
! Excessive sympathomimetic stimulation may cause palpitations, extrasystoles, tachycardia, chest pain, a slight increase in BP followed by a substantial decrease, chills, diaphoresis, and blanching of skin.
! Too-frequent or excessive use may lead to decreased drug effectiveness and severe, paradoxical bronchoconstriction.

DENTAL CONSIDERATIONS
General:
- Assess salivary flow as a factor in caries, periodontal disease, and candidiasis.

M

• Consider semisupine chair position for patients with respiratory disease.
• Short appointments and a stress reduction protocol may be required for anxious patients.
• Be aware that aspirin or sulfite preservatives in vasoconstrictor-containing products can exacerbate asthma.
• Acute asthmatic episodes may be precipitated in the dental office. Sympathomimetic inhalants should be available for emergency use.

Consultations:
• Medical consultation may be required to assess disease control and patient's ability to tolerate stress.

Teach Patient/Family:
• For inhalation dosage forms: rinse mouth with water after each dose to prevent dryness
• *When chronic dry mouth occurs, advise patient:*
  • To avoid mouth rinses with high alcohol content because of drying effects
  • To use sugarless gum, frequent sips of water, or saliva substitutes
  • To use daily home fluoride products for anticaries effect

M

metaraminol

met-ar-am′-e-nol
(Aramine)

CATEGORY AND SCHEDULE

Pregnancy Risk Category: D

MECHANISM OF ACTION

An alpha-adrenergic receptor agonist that causes vasoconstriction, reflex bradycardia, inhibits GI smooth muscle and vascular smooth muscle supplying skeletal muscle and increases heart rate and force of heart muscle contraction. ***Therapeutic Effect:*** Increases both systolic and diastolic pressure.

PHARMACOKINETICS

Route	Onset	Peak	Duration
IM (pressor effect)	10 min	N/A	20–60 min
IV	1–2 min	N/A	
SC	5–20 min	N/A	

Metabolized in the liver. Excreted in the urine and the bile.

AVAILABILITY

Injection: 10 mg/ml (Aramine).

INDICATIONS AND DOSAGES

▸ Prevention of Hypotension

IM/SC

Adults, Elderly. 2–10 mg as a single dose.

Children. 0.01 mg/kg as a single dose.

▸ Adjunctive Treatment of Hypotension

IV

Adults, Elderly. 15–100 mg IV infusion, administered at a rate to maintain the desired blood pressure.

▸ Severe Shock

IV

Adults, Elderly. 0.5–5 mg direct IV injection followed by 15–100 mg IV infusion in 250–500 ml fluid for control of blood pressure.

CONTRAINDICATIONS

Cyclopropane or halothane anesthesia, use of MAOIs, pregnancy, hypersensitivity to metaraminol

INTERACTIONS

Drug

Cyclopropane, halothane, MAOIs, digoxin, oxytocin, reserpine: May increase the risk of metaraminol toxicity.

Tricyclic antidepressants: May decrease the effect of metaraminol.

Herbal
None known.
Food
None known.
Drug interactions of concern to dentistry
• Increased risk of arrhythmia: halogenated hydrocarbon anesthetics

DIAGNOSTIC TEST EFFECTS
None known.

IV INCOMPATIBILITIES
Amphotericin B, dexamthasone, erythromycin, hydrocortisone, methicillin, peniciilin G, prednisolone, thiopental (Pentothal)

IV COMPATIBILITIES
Amikacin (Amikin), amiodarone (Cordarone), cephalothin (Ceporacin), cephapirin (Cefadyl), chloramphenicol, cimetidine (Tagamet), cyanocobalamin, dexamthasone, dobutamine (Dobutrex), ephedrine, hydrocortisone, inamrinone, lidocaine, oxytocin (Pitocin), potassium, procainamide, promazine (Sparine), secobarbital (Seconal), sodium bicarbonate, sulfisoxazole (Gantrisin), tetracycline, verapamil

SIDE EFFECTS
Occasional
Tachycardia, hypertension, cardiac arrhythmias, flushing, palpitations, hypotension, angina, tremors, nervousness, headache, dizziness, weakness, sloughing of skin, nausea, abscess formation, diaphoresis

SERIOUS REACTIONS
! Overdosage produces hypertension, cerebral hemorrhage, cardiac arrest, and seizures.

DENTAL CONSIDERATIONS
General:
• Acute-use drug for use in hospitals or emergency rooms for selected hypotensive episodes.

metaxalone
me-tax′-a-lone
(Skelaxin)

CATEGORY AND SCHEDULE
Pregnancy Risk Category: C

MECHANISM OF ACTION
A central depressant whose exact mechanism is unknown. Many effects due to its central depressant actions. ***Therapeutic Effect:*** Relieves pain or muscle spasms.

PHARMACOKINETICS
PO route onset 1 hour, peak 3 hours, duration 4–6 hours. Well absorbed from the gastrointestinal (GI) tract. Metabolized in liver. Primarily excreted in urine. ***Half-life:*** 9 hrs.

AVAILABILITY
Tablets: 400 mg, 800 mg (Skelaxin).

INDICATIONS AND DOSAGES
▸ **Muscle Relaxant**
PO
Adults, Elderly, Children older than 12 yrs. 800 mg 3–4 times/day.

CONTRAINDICATIONS
Impaired renal or hepatic function, history of drug-induced hemolytic anemias or other anemias, history of hypersensitivity to metaxalone

INTERACTIONS
Drug
Alcohol, central nervous system (CNS) depression-producing medications, tricyclic antidepressants: May increase CNS depression.
MAOIs: May increase the risk of hypertensive crisis and severe seizures.
Herbal
None known.

M

Food
None known.

Drug interactions of concern to dentistry
• No data reported; however, this drug does cause a nonspecific CNS depression: monitor patients if other CNS depressants are used

DIAGNOSTIC TEST EFFECTS
May give false-positive Benedict's test.

SIDE EFFECTS
Occasional
Drowsiness, headache, lightheadedness, dermatitis, nausea, vomiting, stomach cramps, dyspnea

SERIOUS REACTIONS
! Overdose may cause CNS depression, coma, shock, and respiratory depression.

DENTAL CONSIDERATIONS
General:
• Determine why patient is taking the drug.
• Patients on chronic drug therapy may rarely have symptoms of blood dyscrasias, which can include infection, bleeding, and poor healing.
• Consider semisupine chair position for patient comfort if GI side effects occur.

Consultations:
• In a patient with symptoms of blood dyscrasias, request a medical consultation for blood studies and postpone treatment until normal values are reestablished.

Teach Patient/Family:
• Importance of updating health and drug history if physician makes any changes in evaluation or drug regimens

metformin hydrochloride
met-for′-min
(Diabex[AUS], Diaformin[AUS], Fortamet, Glucohexal[AUS], Glucomet[AUS], Glucophage, Glucophage XL, Glycon[CAN], Novo-Metformin[CAN], Riomet)

CATEGORY AND SCHEDULE
Pregnancy Risk Category: B

MECHANISM OF ACTION
An antihyperglycemic that decreases hepatic production of glucose. Decreases absorption of glucose and improves insulin sensitivity.
Therapeutic Effect: Improves glycemic control, stabilizes or decreases body weight, and improves lipid profile.

PHARMACOKINETICS
Slowly, incompletely absorbed after oral administration. Food delays or decreases the extent of absorption. Protein binding: Negligible. Primarily distributed to intestinal mucosa and salivary glands. Primarily excreted unchanged in urine. Removed by hemodialysis. ***Half-life:*** 3–6 hr.

AVAILABILITY
Oral Solution (Riomet): 100 mg/ml.
Tablets (Glucophage): 500 mg, 850 mg, 1,000 mg.
Tablets (Extended-Release [Glucophage XL]): 500 mg, 750 mg.
Tablets (Extended-Release [Fortamet]): 500 mg, 1000 mg.

INDICATIONS AND DOSAGES
▸ **Diabetes Mellitus**
PO (500-mg, 1000-mg tablet)
Adults, Elderly. Initially, 500 mg twice a day, with morning and evening meals. May increase in

500-mg increments every week, in divided doses. May give twice a day up to 2000 mg/day (e.g., 1000 mg twice a day [with morning and evening meals]). If 2500 mg/day are required, give 3 times a day with meals. Maximum: 2500 mg/day.
Children 10–16 yr. Initially, 500 mg twice a day. May increase by 500 mg/day at weekly intervals. Maximum: 2000 mg/day.
PO (850-mg tablet)
Adults, Elderly. Initially, 850-mg/day, with morning meal. May increase dosage in 850-mg increments every other week, in divided doses. Maintenance: 850 mg twice a day, with morning and evening meals. Maximum: 2550 mg/day (850 mg 3 times a day).
PO (Extended-Release tablets)
Adults, Elderly. Initially, 500 mg once a day. May increase by 500 mg/day at weekly intervals. Maximum: 2000 mg once a day.

Adjunct to Insulin Therapy

PO
Adults, Elderly. Initially, 500 mg/day. May increase by 500 mg at 7-day intervals. Maximum: 2500 mg/day (2000 mg/day for extended-release form).

OFF-LABEL USES

Treatment of metabolic complications of AIDS, prediabetes, weight reduction

CONTRAINDICATIONS

Acute CHF, MI, cardiovascular collapse, renal disease or dysfunction, respiratory failure, septicemia

INTERACTIONS

Drug

Alcohol, amiloride, cimetidine, digoxin, furosemide, morphine, nifedipine, procainamide, quinidine, quinine, ranitidine, triamterene, trimethoprim, vancomycin: Increase metformin blood concentration.
Furosemide, hypoglycemia-causing medications: May require a decrease in metformin dosage.
Iodinated contrast studies: May cause acute renal failure and increased risk of lactic acidosis.

Herbal

None known.

Food

None known.

Drug interactions of concern to dentistry

- None reported

DIAGNOSTIC TEST EFFECTS

None known.

SIDE EFFECTS

Occasional (>3%)

GI disturbances (including diarrhea, nausea, vomiting, abdominal bloating, flatulence, and anorexia) that are transient and resolve spontaneously during therapy.

Rare (3%–1%)

Unpleasant or metallic taste that resolves spontaneously during therapy

SERIOUS REACTIONS

! Lactic acidosis occurs rarely but is a fatal complication in 50% of cases. Lactic acidosis is characterized by an increase in blood lactate levels (>5 mmol/L), a decrease in blood pH, and electrolyte disturbances. Signs and symptoms of lactic acidosis include unexplained hyperventilation, myalgia, malaise, and somnolence, which may advance to cardiovascular collapse (shock), acute CHF, acute MI, and prerenal azotemia.

DENTAL CONSIDERATIONS

General:

- Short appointments and a stress reduction protocol may be required for anxious patients.
- Consider semisupine chair position for patient comfort if GI side effects occur.
- Question patient about self-monitoring of drug's antidiabetic effect, including blood glucose values or finger-stick records.
- Ensure that patient is following prescribed diet and regularly takes medication.
- Diabetics may be more susceptible to infection and have delayed wound healing.
- Place on frequent recall to evaluate healing response.

Consultations:

- Medical consultation may be required to assess disease control and patient's ability to tolerate stress.
- Notify physician immediately if symptoms of lactic acidosis are observed (myalgia, respiratory distress, weakness, diarrhea, malaise, muscle cramps, somnolence).
- Medical consultation may include data from patient's blood glucose monitoring, including glycosylated hemoglobin or HbA_{1c} testing.
- Oral and maxillofacial surgical procedures associated with significantly restricted food intake require a medical consultation and temporary cessation of metformin use.

Teach Patient/Family:

- Importance of good oral hygiene to prevent soft tissue inflammation
- That alteration of taste may be due to drug side effects

methadone hydrochloride

meth′-a-done
Schedule II
(Dolophine, Metadol[CAN], Methadone Intensol, Methadose, Physeptone[AUS])

CATEGORY AND SCHEDULE

Pregnancy Risk Category: B (D if used for prolonged periods or at high dosages at term)
Controlled Substance: Schedule II

MECHANISM OF ACTION

An opioid agonist that binds with opioid receptors in the CNS. ***Therapeutic Effect:*** Alters the perception of and emotional response to pain; reduces withdrawal symptoms from other opioid drugs.

PHARMACOKINETICS

Route	Onset	Peak	Duration
Oral	0.5–1 hr	1.5–2 hr	6–8 hr
IM	10–20 min	1–2 hr	4–5 hr
IV	N/A	15–30 min	3–4 hr

Well absorbed after IM injection. Protein binding: 80%–85%. Metabolized in the liver. Primarily excreted in urine. Not removed by hemodialysis. ***Half-life:*** 15–25 hr.

AVAILABILITY

Oral Concentrate (Methadone Intensol, Methadose): 10 mg/ml.
Oral Solution: 5 mg/5 ml, 10 mg/5 ml.
Tablets (Dolophine, Methadose): 5 mg, 10 mg.
Tablets (Dispersible [Methadose]): 40 mg.
Injection (Dolophine): 10 mg/ml.

INDICATIONS AND DOSAGES

▸ Analgesia

PO

Adults, Elderly. Initially, 5–10 mg q3–4h.

Children. 0.1–0.2 mg/kg q6h as needed. Maximum: 10 mg/dose.

IV, IM, SUBCUTANEOUS

Adults, Elderly. Initially, 2.5–10 mg q3–4h.

▸ Narcotic Addiction

IM, PO

Adults, Elderly. 15–40 mg once daily or as needed. Reduce dose at 1–2 day intervals based on patient response. Maintenance: Individualized.

CONTRAINDICATIONS

Delivery of premature infant, diarrhea due to poisoning, hypersensitivity to narcotics, labor

INTERACTIONS

Drug

Alcohol, other CNS depressants: May increase CNS or respiratory depression and hypotension.

MAOIs: May produce a severe, sometimes fatal reaction; plan to administer one quarter of usual methadone dose.

Herbal

Valerian: May increase CNS depression.

Food

None known.

Drug interactions of concern to dentistry

- Increased CNS depression: alcohol, narcotics, sedative-hypnotics, skeletal muscle relaxants, benzodiazepines, and other CNS depressants
- Increased effects of anticholinergics

DIAGNOSTIC TEST EFFECTS

May increase serum amylase and lipase levels.

SIDE EFFECTS

Frequent

Sedation, decreased BP (including orthostatic hypotension), diaphoresis, facial flushing, constipation, dizziness, nausea, vomiting

Occasional

Confusion, urine retention, palpitations, abdominal cramps, visual changes, dry mouth, headache, decreased appetite, anxiety, insomnia

Rare

Allergic reaction (rash, pruritus)

SERIOUS REACTIONS

! Overdose results in respiratory depression, skeletal muscle flaccidity, cold or clammy skin, cyanosis, and extreme somnolence progressing to seizures, stupor, and coma. The antidote is 0.4 mg naloxone.

! The patient who uses methadone long-term may develop a tolerance to the drug's analgesic effect and physical dependence.

DENTAL CONSIDERATIONS

General:

- Assess salivary flow as a factor in caries, periodontal disease, and candidiasis.
- Psychologic and physical dependence may occur with chronic administration.
- Determine why the patient is taking the drug.
- Be aware of the needs of patients who are in recovery from substance abuse.
- In an opioid-dependent patient, NSAIDs are the drugs of choice for posttreatment pain control.

Consultations:

- Patients in the methadone maintenance program should not receive additional opioids or other controlled substances without a consultation.

Teach Patient/Family:

- *When chronic dry mouth occurs, advise patient:*
  - To avoid mouth rinses with high alcohol content because of drying effects
  - To use sugarless gum, frequent sips of water, or saliva substitutes
  - To use daily home fluoride products for anticaries effect

methamphetamine

meth-am-fet′-a-meen
Schedule II
(Desoxyn, Gradumet)
Do not confuse with Dextran, dextromethorphan, or Excedrin.

CATEGORY AND SCHEDULE

Pregnancy Risk Category: C
Controlled substance: Schedule II

M

MECHANISM OF ACTION

A sympathomimetic amine related to amphetamine and ephedrine that enhances CNS stimulant activity. Peripheral actions include elevation of systolic and diastolic blood pressure and weak bronchodilator and respiratory stimulant action. ***Therapeutic Effect:*** Increases motor activity, mental alertness; decreases drowsiness, fatigue.

PHARMACOKINETICS

Rapidly absorbed from the gastrointestinal (GI) tract. Metabolized in liver. Primarily excreted in the urine. Unknown if removed by hemodialysis. ***Half-life:*** 4–5 hrs.

AVAILABILITY

Tablets: 5 mg.
Tablets (extended-release): 5 mg, 10 mg, 15 mg (Desoxyn, Gradumet).

INDICATIONS AND DOSAGES

▸ Attention Deficit/Hyperactivity Disorder (ADHD)

PO
Adults, Children 6 yrs and older. Initially, 2.5–5 mg 1–2 times/day. Increase by 5 mg/day at weekly intervals until therapeutic response achieved.

▸ Appetite Suppressant

PO
Adults, Children 12 yrs and older. 5 mg daily, given 30 min before meals. Extended-release 10–15 mg in the morning.

OFF-LABEL USES

Narcolepsy

CONTRAINDICATIONS

Advanced arteriosclerosis, agitated states, glaucoma, history of drug abuse, history of hypersensitivity to sympathomimetic amines, hyperthyroidism, moderate to severe hypertension, symptomatic cardiovascular disease, within 14 days following discontinuation of an MAOI

INTERACTIONS

Drug

Beta-blockers: May increase risk of bradycardia, heart block, and hypertension.
Central nervous system (CNS) stimulants: May increase the effects of methamphetamine.
Digoxin: May increase the risk of arrhythmias with this drug.
MAOIs: May prolong and intensify the effects of methamphetamine.
Meperidine: May increase the risk of hypotension, respiratory depression, seizures, and vascular collapse.
Tricyclic antidepressants: May increase cardiovascular effects.

Herbal

Ephedra: May cause arrhythmias and hypertension.

Food
None known.

Drug interactions of concern to dentistry
• Increased effect of methamphetamine: CNS stimulants, sympathomimetics
• Decreased effects of both drugs: haloperidol, sedative-hypnotics
• Ventricular dysrhythmia: inhalation anesthetics

DIAGNOSTIC TEST EFFECTS
May increase plasma corticosteroid concentrations.

SIDE EFFECTS
Frequent
Irregular pulse, increased motor activity, talkativeness, nervousness, mild euphoria, insomnia
Occasional
Headache, chills, dry mouth, gastrointestinal (GI) distress, worsening depression in patients who are clinically depressed, tachycardia, palpitations, chest pain

SERIOUS REACTIONS
! Overdose may produce skin pallor, flushing, arrhythmias, and psychosis.
! Abrupt withdrawal following prolonged administration of high dosage may produce lethargy which may last for weeks.
! Prolonged administration to children with ADHD may produce a temporary suppression of normal weight and height patterns.

DENTAL CONSIDERATIONS
General:
• Assess salivary flow as a factor in caries, periodontal disease, and candidiasis.

Consultations:
• Physician should be informed if significant xerostomic side effects occur (e.g., increased caries, sore tongue, problems eating or swallowing, difficulty wearing prosthesis) so that a medication change can be considered.

Teach Patient/Family:
• *When chronic dry mouth occurs, advise patient:*
  • To avoid mouth rinses with high alcohol content because of drying effects
  • To use sugarless gum, frequent sips of water, or saliva substitutes
  • To use daily home fluoride products for anticaries effect

methazolamide
meth-ah-zole′-ah-mide
(Apo-Methazolamide[CAN], Glauctabs, Neptazane)
Do not confuse with nefazodone.

CATEGORY AND SCHEDULE
Pregnancy Risk Category: C

M

MECHANISM OF ACTION
A noncompetitive inhibitor of carbonic anhydrase that inhibits the enzyme at the luminal border of cells of the proximal tubule. Increases urine volume and changes to an alkaline pH with subsequent decreases in the excretion of titratable acid and ammonia.
Therapeutic Effect: Produces a diuretic and antiglaucoma effect.

PHARMACOKINETICS
PO route onset 2–4 hrs, peak 6–8 hrs, duration10–18 hrs. Well absorbed slowly from the GI tract. Protein binding: 55%. Distributed into the tissues (including CSF). Metabolized slowly from the

gastrointestinal (GI) tract. Partially excreted in urine. Not removed by hemodialysis. ***Half-life:*** 14 hrs.

AVAILABILITY

Tablets: 25 mg, 50 mg.

INDICATIONS AND DOSAGES

▸ Glaucoma

PO

Adults, Elderly. 50–100 mg/day 2–3 times/day.

OFF-LABEL USES

Motion sickness, essential tremor

CONTRAINDICATIONS

Kidney or liver dysfunction, severe pulmonary obstruction, hypersensitivity to methazolamide or any component of the formulation

INTERACTIONS

Drug

Amphetamines, quinidine, procainamide, methenamine, phenobarbital, salicylates: May increase the excretion of these drugs.
Aspirin: May increase the risk for anorexia, tachypnea, lethargy, coma and death have been reported when receiving high-dose aspirin and methazolamide concomitantly.
Diuretics: May increase the risk of hypokalemia.
Lithium: May increase the excretion of lithium.
Memantine: May decrease the clearance of memantine.
Steroids: May increase the risk of hypokalemia.
Topiramate: May increase the risk of nephrolithiasis.

Herbal

None known.

Food

None known.

Drug interactions of concern to dentistry methazolamide (neptazane, gluctabs)

- Toxicity: salicylates (high doses)
- Hypokalemia: corticosteroids (systemic use)

DIAGNOSTIC TEST EFFECTS

None known.

SIDE EFFECTS

Occasional

Paresthesias, hearing dysfunction or tinnitus, fatigue, malaise, loss of appetite, taste alteration, nausea, vomiting, diarrhea, polyuria, drowsiness, confusion, hypokalemia

Rare

Metabolic acidosis, electrolyte imbalance, transient myopia, urticaria, melena, hematuria, glycosuria, hepatic insufficiency, flaccid paralysis, photosensitivity, convulsions, and rarely, crystalluria, renal calculi

SERIOUS REACTIONS

! Malaise and complaints of tiredness and myalgia are signs of excessive dosing and acidosis in the elderly.
! Stevens-Johnson syndrome, toxic epidermal necrolysis, fulminant hepatic necrosis, agranulocytosis, aplastic anemia, and other blood dyscrasias have been reported and have caused fatalities.

DENTAL CONSIDERATIONS

METHAZOLAMIDE (NEPTAZANE, GLUCTABS)

General:

- Protect patient's eyes from accidental spatter during dental treatment.
- Avoid dental light in patient's eyes; offer dark glasses for patient comfort.
- Avoid prescribing aspirin-containing products.

• Consider semisupine chair position for patient comfort if GI side effects occur.
• Question patient about tolerance of NSAIDS or aspirin related to GI disease.
• Patient on chronic drug therapy may rarely present with symptoms of blood dyscrasias, which can include infection, bleeding, and poor healing. If dyscrasia is present.
• Caution patient to prevent oral tissue trauma when using oral hygiene aids.

Consultations:

• In a patient with symptoms of blood dyscrasias, request a medical consultation for blood studies and postpone treatment until normal values are reestablished.

Teach Patient/Family:

• Importance of good oral hygiene to prevent soft tissue inflammation
• To prevent trauma when using oral hygiene aids
• Importance of updating health and medication history if physician makes any changes in evaluation or drug regimens; include OTC, herbal, and nonherbal in the update

methenamine

(Dehydral[CAN], Hiprex, Hip-Rex[CAN], Mandelamine, Urasal[CAN], Urex)

CATEGORY AND SCHEDULE

Pregnancy Risk Category: C

MECHANISM OF ACTION

A hippuric acid salt that hydrolyzes to formaldehyde and ammonia in acidic urine. ***Therapeutic Effect:*** Formaldehyde has antibacterial action. Bacteriocidal.

PHARMACOKINETICS

Readily absorbed from the gastrointestinal (GI) tract. Partially metabolized by hydrolysis (unless protected by enteric coating) and partially by the liver. Primarily excreted in urine. ***Half-life:*** 3-6 hrs.

AVAILABILITY

Oral Suspension, as mandelate: 0.5 g/5 ml.
Tablets, as hippurate: 1 g (Urex, Hiprex).
Tablets, enteric coated, as mandelate: 500 mg, 1 g (Mandelamine).

INDICATIONS AND DOSAGES

▸ Urinary Tract Infection (UTI)

PO

Adults, Elderly. 1 g 2 times/day (as hippurate). 1 g 4 times/day (as mandelate)
Children 6–12 yrs. 25–50 mg/kg/day q12h (as hippurate). 50–75 mg/kg/day q6h (as mandelate).

M

OFF-LABEL USES

Hyperhidrosis

CONTRAINDICATIONS

Moderate to severe renal impairment, hepatic impairment (hippurate salt), tartrazine sensitivity (Hiprex contains tartrazine), hypersensitivity to methenamine or any of its components

INTERACTIONS

Drug

Acetazolamide, sodium bicarbonate: May decrease effect secondary to alkalinization of urine.
Antacids: May decrease the effectivness of methenamine.
Dichlorphenamide: May inhibit the action of methenamine to alkalinize the urine.
Sulfamethizole: May increase the risk of crystalluria.

Herbal
None known.
Food
None known.
Drug interactions of concern to dentistry
- None reported

DIAGNOSTIC TEST EFFECTS
Formaldehyde, the active form of methenamine, interferes with fluorometric procedures for the determination of urinary catecholamines and vanillylmandelic acid (VMA), causing false high results.

SIDE EFFECTS
Occasional
Rash, nausea, dyspepsia, difficulty urinating
Rare
Bladder irritation, increased liver enzymes

SERIOUS REACTIONS
! Crystalluria can occur when methenamine is given in large doses.

DENTAL CONSIDERATIONS
General:
- Determine why the patient is taking the drug.
- Antibiotics for dental infections are not contraindicated, but a physician notification may be advisable.
- Palliative treatment may be required for oral side effects.
- Consider semisupine chair position for patient comfort because of GI effects of drug.

methimazole
meth-im′-a-zole
(Tapazole)

CATEGORY AND SCHEDULE
Pregnancy Risk Category: D

MECHANISM OF ACTION
A thiomidazole derivative that inhibits synthesis of thyroid hormone by interfering with the incorporation of iodine into tyrosyl residues. ***Therapeutic Effect:*** Effectively treats hyperthyroidism by decreasing thyroid hormone levels.

AVAILABILITY
Tablets: 5 mg, 10 mg.

INDICATIONS AND DOSAGES
▸ **Hyperthyroidism**
PO
Adults, Elderly. Initially, 15–60 mg/day in 3 divided doses. Maintenance: 5–15 mg/day.
Children. Initially, 0.4 mg/kg/day in 3 divided doses. Maintenance: One-half the initial dose.

CONTRAINDICATIONS
None known.

INTERACTIONS
Drug
Amiodarone, iodinated glycerol, iodine, potassium iodide: May decrease response to methimazole.
Digoxin: May increase the blood concentration of digoxin as patient becomes euthyroid.
I^{131}: May decrease thyroid uptake of I^{131}.
Oral anticoagulants: May decrease the effects of oral anticoagulants.
Herbal
None known.
Food
None known.
Drug interactions of concern to dentistry
- Increased CV side effects in uncontrolled patients: anticholinergics and sympathomimetics
- Patients with uncontrolled hyperthyroidism are at risk when vasoconstrictors are used

• Patients with uncontrolled hypothyroidism may be more responsive to CNS depressants

DIAGNOSTIC TEST EFFECTS

May increase LDH, serum alkaline phosphatase, bilirubin, AST(SGOT), and ALT(SGPT) levels and prothrombin time. May decrease prothrombin level and WBC count.

SIDE EFFECTS

Frequent (5%–4%)
Fever, rash, pruritus
Occasional (3%–1%)
Dizziness, loss of taste, nausea, vomiting, stomach pain, peripheral neuropathy or numbness in fingers, toes, face
Rare (<1%)
Swollen lymph nodes or salivary glands

SERIOUS REACTIONS

! Agranulocytosis as long as 4 months after therapy, pancytopenia, and hepatitis have occurred.

DENTAL CONSIDERATIONS

General:

• Monitor vital signs at every appointment because of CV effects of disease.
• Patients on chronic drug therapy may rarely have symptoms of blood dyscrasias; examine for evidence of oral manifestations of blood dyscrasias (infection, bleeding, poor healing).
• Evaluate for clotting ability during periodontal instrumentation.
• Evaluate for control of hyperthyroidism. Patients with uncontrolled condition should not be treated in the dental office until thyroid values are normalized.
• Patients with uncontrolled condition should be referred for medical evaluation and treatment.

Consultations:

• Medical consultation may be required to assess disease control.
• Medical consultation for blood studies (CBC); leukopenic or thrombocytopenic side effects may result in infection, delayed healing, and excessive bleeding. Postpone elective dental treatment until normal values are maintained.

Teach Patient/Family:

• Importance of good oral hygiene to prevent soft tissue inflammation
• Caution in use of oral hygiene aids to prevent injury

methocarbamol

meth-oh-kar-′-ba-mole
(Carbacot, Robaxin)

CATEGORY AND SCHEDULE

Pregnancy Risk Category: C

M

MECHANISM OF ACTION

A carbamate derivative of guaifenesin that causes skeletal muscle relaxation by general CNS depression.
Therapeutic Effect: Relieves muscle spasticity.

PHARMACOKINETICS

Rapidly and almost completely absorbed from the gastrointestinal (GI) tract. Protein binding: 46–50%. Metabolized in liver by dealkylation and hydroxylation. Primarily excreted in urine as metabolites.
Half-life: 1–2 hrs.

AVAILABILITY

Injection: 100 mg/ml (Robaxin).
Tablets: 325 mg, 500 mg (Carbacot, Robaxin), 750 mg (Carbacot).

INDICATIONS AND DOSAGES

▸ Musculoskeletal Spasm

IM/IV

Adults, Children 16 yrs and older. 1 g q8h for no more than 3 consecutive days. May repeat course of therapy after a drug-free interval of 48 hrs.

PO

Adults, Children 16 yrs and older. 1.5 g 4 times/day for 2–3 days (up to 8 g/day may be given in severe conditions). Decrease to 4–4.5 g/day in 3–6 divided doses.

Elderly. Initially, 500 mg 4 times a day. May gradually increase dosage.

▸ Tetanus Spasm

IV

Adults. 1–3 g q6h until oral dosing is possible. Injection should be used no more than 3 consecutive days.

Children. 15 mg/kg/dose or 500 mg/m^2/dose q6h as needed. Maximum: 1.8 g/m^2/day for 3 days only.

CONTRAINDICATIONS

Hypersensitivity to methocarbamol or any component of the formulation, renal impairment (injection formulation)

INTERACTIONS

Drug

CNS depressants, including alcohol: May potentiate effects when used with other CNS depressants, including alcohol.

Herbal

Gotu kola, kava, kava, St. John's Wort: May increase CNS depression.

Food

None known.

Drug interactions of concern to dentistry

- Increased CNS depression: alcohol, narcotics, sedative-hypnotics

DIAGNOSTIC TEST EFFECTS

None known.

SIDE EFFECTS

Frequent

Transient drowsiness, weakness, dizziness, lightheadedness, nausea, vomiting.

Occasional

Headache, constipation, anorexia, hypotension, confusion, blurred vision, vertigo, facial flushing, rash

Rare

Paradoxical CNS excitement and restlessness, slurred speech, tremor, dry mouth, diarrhea, nocturia, impotence, bradycardia, hypotension, syncope

SERIOUS REACTIONS

! Anaphylactoid reactions, leukopenia, and seizures (intravenous form) have been reported.

! Methocarbamol overdosage results in cardiac arrhythmias, nausea, vomiting, drowsiness, and coma.

DENTAL CONSIDERATIONS

General:

- Determine why the patient is taking the drug.
- Consider semisupine chair position for patient comfort if back is involved.

Teach Patient/Family:

- Importance of good oral hygiene to prevent soft tissue inflammation
- Caution to prevent injury when using oral hygiene aids
- To avoid mouth rinses with high alcohol content because of drying effects

methotrexate sodium

meth-oh-trex′-ate
(Apo-Methotrexate[CAN], Ledertrexate[AUS], Methoblastin[AUS], Rheumatrex, Trexall)
Do not confuse Trexall with Trexan.

CATEGORY AND SCHEDULE

Pregnancy Risk Category: D (X for patients with psoriasis or rheumatoid arthritis)

MECHANISM OF ACTION

An antimetabolite that competes with enzymes necessary to reduce folic acid to tetrahydrofolic acid, a component essential to DNA, RNA, and protein synthesis. This action inhibits DNA, RNA, and protein synthesis. ***Therapeutic Effect:*** Causes death of cancer cells.

PHARMACOKINETICS

Variably absorbed from the GI tract. Completely absorbed after IM administration. Protein binding: 50%–60%. Widely distributed. Metabolized intracellularly in the liver. Primarily excreted in urine. Removed by hemodialysis but not by peritoneal dialysis. ***Half-life:*** 8–12 hr (large doses, 8–15 hr).

AVAILABILITY

Tablets (Rheumatrex): 2.5 mg.
Tablets (Trexall): 5 mg, 7.5 mg, 10 mg, 15 mg.
Injection Solution: 25 mg/ml.
Injection Powder for Reconstitution: 20 mg, 1 g.

INDICATIONS AND DOSAGES

▸ Trophoblastic Neoplasms
PO, IM
Adults, Elderly. 15–30 mg/day for 5 days; repeat in 7 days for 3–5 courses.

▸ Head and Neck Cancer
PO, IV, IM
Adults, Elderly. 25–50 mg/m^2 once weekly.

▸ Choriocarcinoma, Chorioadenoma Destruens, Hydatidiform Mole
PO, IM
Adults, Elderly. 15–30 mg/day for 5 days; repeat 3–5 times with 1–2 wk between courses.

▸ Breast Cancer
IV
Adults, Elderly. 30–60 mg/m^2 days 1 and 8 q3–4wk.

▸ Acute Lymphocytic Leukemia
PO, IV, IM
Adults, Elderly. Induction: 3.3 mg/m^2/day in combination with other chemotherapeutic agents. Maintenance: 30 mg/m^2/wk PO or IM in divided doses or 2.5 mg/kg IV every 14 days.

▸ Burkitt's Lymphoma
PO
Adults. 10–25 mg/day for 4–8 days; repeat with 7- to 10-day rest between courses.

▸ Lymphosarcoma
PO
Adults, Elderly. 0.625–2.5 mg/kg/day.

▸ Mycosis Fungoides
PO
Adults, Elderly. 2.5–10 mg/day.
IM
Adults, Elderly. 50 mg/wk or 25 mg twice a week.

▸ Rheumatoid Arthritis
PO
Adults, Elderly. 7.5 mg once weekly or 2.5 mg q12h for 3 doses once weekly. Maximum: 20 mg/wk.

▸ Juvenile Rheumatoid Arthritis
PO, IM, Subcutaneous
Children. 5–15 mg/m^2/wk as a single dose or in 3 divided doses given q12h.

Psoriasis
PO
Adults, Elderly. 10–25 mg once weekly or 2.5–5 mg q12h for 3 doses once weekly.
IM
Adults, Elderly. 10–25 mg once weekly.

Antineoplastic Dosage for Children
PO, IM
Children. 7.5–30 mg/m²/wk or q2wk.
IV
Children. 10–33,000 mg/m² bolus or continuous infusion over 6–42 hr.

Dosage in Renal Impairment
Creatinine clearance 61–80 ml/min. Reduce dose by 25%.
Creatinine clearance 51–60 ml/min. Reduce dose by 33%.
Creatinine clearance 10–50 ml/min. Reduce dose by 50%–70%.

M

OFF-LABEL USES

Treatment of acute myelocytic leukemia; bladder, cervical, ovarian, prostatic, renal, and testicular carcinomas; psoriatic arthritis; systemic dermatomyositis

CONTRAINDICATIONS

Pre-existing myelosuppression, severe hepatic or renal impairment

INTERACTIONS

Drug

Acyclovir (parenteral): May increase the risk of neurotoxicity.
Alcohol, hepatotoxic medications: May increase the risk of hepatotoxicity.
Asparaginase: May decrease the effects of methotrexate.
Bone marrow depressants: May increase myelosuppression.
Live-virus vaccines: May potentiate virus replication, increase vaccine side effects, and decrease the patient's antibody response to the vaccine.
NSAIDs: May increase the risk of methotrexate toxicity.
Probenecid, salicylates: May increase blood methotrexate concentration and risk of toxicity.

Herbal

None known.

Food

None known.

Drug interactions of concern to dentistry

- Increased toxicity: aspirin, alcohol, NSAIDs
- Possible fatal interactions: NSAIDs, high-dose IV methotrexate
- Suspected increase in methotrexate toxicity: amoxicillin, tetracycline, doxycycline

DIAGNOSTIC TEST EFFECTS

May increase serum uric acid and AST (SGOT) levels.

IV INCOMPATIBILITIES

Chlorpromazine (Thorazine), droperidol (Inapsine), gemcitabine (Gemzar), idarubicin (Idamycin), midazolam (Versed), nalbuphine (Nubain)

IV COMPATIBILITIES

Cisplatin (Platinol AQ), cyclophosphamide (Cytoxan), daunorubicin (DaunoXome), doxorubicin (Adriamycin), etoposide (VePesed), 5-fluorouracil, granisetron (Kytril), leucovorin, mitomycin (Mutamycin), ondansetron (Zofran), paclitaxel (Taxol), vinblastine (Velban), vincristine (Oncovin), vinorelbine (Navelbine)

SIDE EFFECTS

Frequent (10%–3%)
Nausea, vomiting, stomatitis; burning and erythema at psoriatic site (in patients with psoriasis)

Occasional (3%–1%)
Diarrhea, rash, dermatitis, pruritus, alopecia, dizziness, anorexia, malaise, headache, drowsiness, blurred vision

SERIOUS REACTIONS

! GI toxicity may produce gingivitis, glossitis, pharyngitis, stomatitis, enteritis, and hematemesis.
! Hepatotoxicity is more likely to occur with frequent small doses than with large intermittent doses.
! Pulmonary toxicity may be characterized by interstitial pneumonitis.
! Hematologic toxicity, which may develop rapidly from marked myelosuppression, may be manifested as leukopenia, thrombocytopenia, anemia, and hemorrhage.
! Dermatologic toxicity may produce a rash, pruritus, urticaria, pigmentation, photosensitivity, petechiae, ecchymosis, and pustules.
! Severe nephrotoxicity may produce azotemia, hematuria, and renal failure.

DENTAL CONSIDERATIONS

General:
- Patients on chronic drug therapy may rarely have symptoms of blood dyscrasias, which can include infection, bleeding, and poor healing.
- Avoid prescribing aspirin- or NSAID-containing products.
- Place on frequent recall because of increased risk for infection and to evaluate healing response.
- Determine why the patient is taking the drug.
- Palliative treatment may be necessary if stomatitis or oral desquamative lesions occur.

Consultations:
- In a patient with symptoms of blood dyscrasias, request a medical consultation for blood studies and postpone dental treatment until normal values are reestablished.
- Medical consultation may be required to assess disease control.

Teach Patient/Family:
- Importance of good oral hygiene to prevent soft tissue inflammation
- Caution to prevent injury when using oral hygiene aids
- About palliative therapy for sore mouth
- To avoid mouth rinses with high alcohol content because of drying effects

methsuximide

meth-sux′-i-mide
(Celontin)
Do not confuse with methoxsalen.

CATEGORY AND SCHEDULE

Pregnancy Risk Category: C

MECHANISM OF ACTION

An anticonvulsant agent that increases the seizure threshold, suppresses paroxysmal spike-and-wave pattern in absence seizures and depresses nerve transmission in the motor cortex. ***Therapeutic Effect:*** Controls absence (petit mal) seizures.

PHARMACOKINETICS

Rapidly metabolized in liver to active metabolite, N-desmethylmethsuximide. Primarily excreted in urine. Unknown if removed by hemodialysis. ***Half-life:*** 1.4 hrs.

AVAILABILITY

Capsules: 150 mg, 300 mg (Celontin).

INDICATIONS AND DOSAGES

▸ Absence Seizures

PO

Adults, Elderly. Initially, 300 mg/day for the first week. Increase dosage by 300 mg/day at weekly intervals until response is attained. Maintenance: 1200 mg/day at 2–4 times/day. Do not exceed 1000 mg/day in children 12–15 yrs, 1200 mg/day in patients older than 15 yrs.

Children. Initially, 10–15 mg/kg/day 3–4 times/day. Increase at weekly intervals. Maximum: 30 mg/kg/day.

OFF-LABEL USES

Partial complex (psychomotor) seizures

CONTRAINDICATIONS

Hypersensitivity to succinimides or any component of the formulation

M

INTERACTIONS

Drug

Alcohol, benzodiazepines, barbiturates, and other CNS depressants: May cause increased sedative effects.

Anticonvulsants: May increase plasma concentrations of other anticonvulsants.

Cyclosporine: May decrease cyclosporine blood levels by increasing its metabolism.

Herbal

Evening primrose oil: May decrease the effects of methsuximide.

Ginkgo biloba: May decrease the effects of methsuximide.

Food

None known.

Drug interactions of concern to dentistry

- Enhanced CNS depression: alcohol, CNS depressants
- Decreased effects: phenothiazines, thioxanthenes, barbiturates
- Changes in seizure pattern, frequency: haloperidol

DIAGNOSTIC TEST EFFECTS

None known.

SIDE EFFECTS

Frequent

Drowsiness, dizziness, nausea, vomiting

Occasional

Visual abnormalities, such as spots before eyes, difficulty focusing, blurred vision, dry mouth or pharynx, tongue irritation, nervousness, insomnia, headache, constipation or diarrhea, rash, weight loss, proteinuria, edema

SERIOUS REACTIONS

! Toxic reactions appear as blood dyscrasias, including aplastic anemia, agranulocytosis, thrombocytopenia, leukopenia, leukocytosis, eosinophilia, cardiovascular disturbances, such as congestive heart failure (CHF), hypotension or hypertension, thrombophlebitis, arrhythmias, and dermatologic effects, such as rash, urticaria, pruritus, photosensitivity.

! Abrupt withdrawal may precipitate status epilepticus.

DENTAL CONSIDERATIONS

General:

- Patients on chronic drug therapy may rarely have symptoms of blood dyscrasias, which can include infection, bleeding, and poor healing.
- Avoid dental light in patient's eyes; offer dark glasses for patient comfort.
- Determine type of epilepsy, seizure frequency, and quality of seizure control. A stress reduction protocol may be required.
- Place on frequent recall to monitor gingival condition.

Consultations:
- In a patient with symptoms of blood dyscrasias, request a medical consultation for blood studies and postpone dental treatment until normal values are reestablished.
- Take precautions if dental surgery is anticipated and anesthesia is required.
- Medical consultation may be required to assess disease control.

Teach Patient/Family:
- Importance of good oral hygiene to prevent soft tissue inflammation
- Caution to prevent injury when using oral hygiene aids
- To avoid mouth rinses with high alcohol content if oral side effects occur

methyldopa

meth-ill-doe'-pa
(Aldomet, Apo-Methyldopa[CAN], Hydopa[AUS], Novomedopa[CAN], Nudopa[AUS])
Do not confuse Aldomet with Anzemet.

CATEGORY AND SCHEDULE

Pregnancy Risk Category: B

MECHANISM OF ACTION

An antihypertensive agent that stimulates central inhibitory alpha-adrenergic receptors, lowers arterial pressure, and reduces plasma renin activity. ***Therapeutic Effect:*** Reduces BP.

AVAILABILITY

Tablets: 250 mg, 500 mg.
Injection: 50 mg/ml.

INDICATIONS AND DOSAGES

▸ Moderate to Severe Hypertension

PO

Adults. Initially, 250 mg 2–3 times a day for 2 days. Adjust dosage at intervals of 2 days (minimum).
Elderly. Initially, 125 mg 1–2 times a day. May increase by 125 mg q2–3 days. Maintenance: 500 mg to 2 g/day in 2–4 divided doses.
Children. Initially, 10 mg/kg/day in 2–4 divided doses. Adjust dosage at intervals of 2 days (minimum). Maximum: 65 mg/kg/day or 3 g/day, whichever is less.

IV

Adults. 250–1,000 mg q6–8h. Maximum: 4 g/day.
Children. Initially, 2–4 mg/kg/dose. May increase to 5–10 mg/kg/dose in 4–6h if no response. Maximum: 65 mg/kg/day or 3 g/day, whichever is less.

CONTRAINDICATIONS

Hepatic disease, pheochromocytoma

INTERACTIONS

Drug

Hypotensive-producing medications, such as antihypertensives and diuretics: May increase the effects of methyldopa.
Lithium: May increase the risk of lithium toxicity.
MAOIs: May cause hyperexcitability.
NSAIDs, tricyclic antidepressants: May decrease the effects of methyldopa.
Other sympathomimetics: May decrease the effects of sympathomimetics.

Herbal

None known.

Food

None known.

Drug interactions of concern to dentistry
- Decreased effects: indomethacin and other NSAIDs
- Increased pressor response: epinephrine and other sympathomimetics

M

• Increased sedation: haloperidol, alcohol, CNS depressants
• Increased hypotensive action of general anesthetics

DIAGNOSTIC TEST EFFECTS

May increase BUN and serum prolactin, alkaline phosphatase, bilirubin, creatinine, potassium, sodium, uric acid, AST (SGOT), and ALT (SGPT) levels. May produce false-positive Coombs' test and prolong prothrombin time.

SIDE EFFECTS

Frequent

Peripheral edema, somnolence, headache, dry mouth

Occasional

Mental changes (such as anxiety, depression), decreased sexual function or libido, diarrhea, swelling of breasts, nausea, vomiting, light-headedness, paraesthesia, rhinitis

SERIOUS REACTIONS

! Hepatotoxicity (abnormal liver function test results, jaundice, hepatitis), hemolytic anemia, unexplained fever and flulike symptoms may occur. If these conditions appear, discontinue the medication and contact the physician.

DENTAL CONSIDERATIONS

General:

• Monitor vital signs at every appointment because of CV side effects.
• Patients on chronic drug therapy may rarely have symptoms of blood dyscrasias, which can include infection, bleeding, and poor healing.
• Assess salivary flow as a factor in caries, periodontal disease, and candidiasis.
• Limit use of sodium-containing products, such as saline IV fluids, for patients with a dietary salt restriction.
• After supine positioning, have patient sit upright for at least 2 min before standing to avoid orthostatic hypotension.
• Stress from dental procedures may compromise CV function; determine patient risk.

Consultations:

• In a patient with symptoms of blood dyscrasias, request a medical consultation for blood studies and postpone dental treatment until normal values are reestablished.
• Medical consultation may be required to assess disease control and patient's ability to tolerate stress.

Teach Patient/Family:

• Importance of good oral hygiene to prevent soft tissue inflammation
• Caution to prevent injury when using oral hygiene aids
• *When chronic dry mouth occurs, advise patient:*
  • To avoid mouth rinses with high alcohol content because of drying effects
  • To use sugarless gum, frequent sips of water, or saliva substitutes
  • To use daily home fluoride products for anticaries effect

methylergonovine

meth-ill-er-goe-noe′-veen
(Methergine)

CATEGORY AND SCHEDULE

Pregnancy Risk Category: C

MECHANISM OF ACTION

An ergot alkaloid that stimulates alpha-adrenergic and serotonin receptors, producing arterial vasoconstriction. Causes vasospasm of coronary arteries and directly stimulates uterine muscle. ***Therapeutic Effect:*** Increases strength and frequency of uterine contractions. Decreases uterine bleeding.

PHARMACOKINETICS

Route	Onset	Peak	Duration
PO	5–10 min	N/A	N/A
IV	Immediate	N/A	3 hr
IM	2–5 min	N/A	N/A

Rapidly absorbed from the GI tract after IM administration. Distributed rapidly to plasma, extracellular fluid, and tissues. Metabolized in the liver and undergoes first-pass effect. Primarily excreted in urine. ***Half-life:*** IV (alpha phase), 2–3 min or less; IV (beta phase), 20-30 min or longer.

AVAILABILITY

Tablets: 0.2 mg.
Injection: 0.2 mg/ml.

INDICATIONS AND DOSAGES

▸ Prevention and Treatment of Postpartum and Postabortion Hemorrhage due to Atony or Involution

PO

Adults. 0.2 mg 3–4 times a day. Continue for up to 7 days.

IV, IM

Adults. Initially, 0.2 mg. May repeat q2–4h for no more than a total of 5 doses.

OFF-LABEL USES

Treatment of incomplete abortion

CONTRAINDICATIONS

Hypertension, pregnancy, toxemia, untreated hypocalcemia

INTERACTIONS

Drug

Vasoconstrictors, vasopressors: May increase the effects of methylergonovine.

Herbal

None known.

Food

None known.

Drug interactions of concern to dentistry

- Increased effects: sympathomimetics

DIAGNOSTIC TEST EFFECTS

May decrease serum prolactin concentration.

IV INCOMPATIBILITIES

No information available for Y-site administration.

IV COMPATIBILITIES

Heparin, potassium

SIDE EFFECTS

Frequent

Nausea, uterine cramping, vomiting

Occasional

Abdominal pain, diarrhea, dizziness, diaphoresis, tinnitus, bradycardia, chest pain

Rare

Allergic reaction, such as rash and itching; dyspnea; severe or sudden hypertension

SERIOUS REACTIONS

! Severe hypertensive episodes may result in CVA, serious arrhythmias, and seizures. Hypertensive effects are more frequent with patient susceptibility, rapid IV administration, and concurrent use of regional anesthesia or vasoconstrictors.

! Peripheral ischemia may lead to gangrene.

DENTAL CONSIDERATIONS

General:

- Acute-use drug normally given in the hospital; provide palliative dental care for dental emergencies only.

M

Teach Patient/Family:
- To remind patient to follow up with more definite dental care at an opportune date

methylphenidate hydrochloride

meth-ill-fen′-i-date
Schedule II
(Attenta[AUS], Concerta, Metadate CD, Metadate ER, Methylin, Methylin ER, PMS-Methylphenidate[CAN], Riphenidate[CAN], Ritalin, Ritalin LA, Ritalin SR)
Do not confuse Ritalin with Rifadin.

CATEGORY AND SCHEDULE

Pregnancy Risk Category: C
Controlled Substance: Schedule II

MECHANISM OF ACTION

A CNS stimulant that blocks the reuptake of norepinephrine and dopamine into presynaptic neurons. ***Therapeutic Effect:*** Decreases motor restlessness and fatigue; increases motor activity, attention span, and mental alertness; produces mild euphoria.

PHARMACOKINETICS

Onset	Peak	Duration
Immediate-release	2 hr	3–5 hr
Sustained-release	4–7 hr	3–8 hr
Extended-release	N/A	8–12 hr

Slowly and incompletely absorbed from the GI tract. Protein binding: 15%. Metabolized in the liver. Eliminated in urine and in feces by biliary system. Unknown if removed by hemodialysis. ***Half-life:*** 2–4 hr.

AVAILABILITY

Capsules (Extended-Release [Metadate CD]): 10 mg, 20 mg, 30 mg.
Capsules (Extended-Release [Ritalin LA]): 10 mg, 20 mg, 30 mg, 40 mg.
Tablets (Ritalin): 5 mg, 10 mg, 20 mg.
Tablets (Extended-Release [Mentadate ER, Mehtylin ER]): 10 mg, 20 mg.
Tablets (Extended-Release [Concerta]): 18 mg, 27 mg, 36 mg, 54 mg, 72 mg.
Tablets (Sustained-Release [Ritalin SR]): 20 mg.
Tablets (Chewable [Methylin]): 2.5 mg, 5 mg, 10 mg.
Oral Solution (Methylin): 5 mg/5 ml, 10 mg/5 ml.

INDICATIONS AND DOSAGES

▸ **Attention Deficit Hyperactivity Disorder (ADHD)**

PO
Children 6 yr and older. Immediate release: Initially, 2.5–5 mg before breakfast and lunch. May increase by 5–10 mg/day at weekly intervals. Maximum: 60 mg/day.
PO (Concerta)
Children 6 yr and older. Initially, 18 mg once a day; may increase by 18 mg/day at weekly intervals. Maximum: 72 mg/day.
PO (Metadate CD)
Children 6 yr and older. Initially, 20 mg/day. May increase by 20 mg/day at weekly intervals. Maximum: 60 mg/day.
PO (Ritalin LA)
Children 6 yr and older. Initially, 20 mg/day. May increase by 10 mg/day at weekly intervals. Maximum: 60 mg/day.
PO (Metadate ER, Methylin ER, Ritalin SR)
Children 6 yr and older. May replace regular tablets after daily dose is

titrated and 8-hr dosage corresponds to sustained-release or extended-release tablet size.

▸ **Narcolepsy**

PO

Adults, Elderly. 10 mg 2–3 times a day. Range: 10–60 mg/day.

OFF-LABEL USES

Treatment of disease-related fatigue, secondary mental depression

CONTRAINDICATIONS

Use within 14 days of MAOIs

INTERACTIONS

Drug

MAOIs: May increase the effects of methylphenidate.

Other CNS stimulants: May have an additive effect.

Herbal

None known.

Food

None known.

Drug interactions of concern to dentistry

- Increased effects of CNS stimulants, tricyclic antidepressants, SSRIs, sympathomimetics

DIAGNOSTIC TEST EFFECTS

None known.

SIDE EFFECTS

Frequent

Anxiety, insomnia, anorexia

Occasional

Dizziness, drowsiness, headache, nausea, abdominal pain, fever, rash, arthralgia, vomiting

Rare

Blurred vision, Tourette syndrome (marked by uncontrolled vocal outbursts, repetitive body movements, and tics), palpitations

SERIOUS REACTIONS

! Prolonged administration to children with ADHD may delay growth.

! Overdose may produce tachycardia, palpitations, arrhythmias,chest pain, psychotic episode, seizures, and coma.

! Hypersensitivity reactions and blood dyscrasias occur rarely.

DENTAL CONSIDERATIONS

General:

- Monitor vital signs often because of CV side effects.
- Patients on chronic drug therapy may rarely have symptoms of blood dyscrasias, which can include infection, bleeding, and poor healing.
- Assess salivary flow as a factor in caries, periodontal disease, and candidiasis.
- Use vasoconstrictors with caution, in low doses, and with careful aspiration.
- Determine why the patient is taking the drug.

Consultations:

- In a patient with symptoms of blood dyscrasias, request a medical consultation for blood studies and postpone dental treatment until normal values are reestablished.
- Medical consultation may be required to assess disease control.

Teach Patient/Family:

- Importance of good oral hygiene to prevent soft tissue inflammation
- Caution to prevent injury when using oral hygiene aids
- *When chronic dry mouth occurs, advise patient:*
  - To avoid mouth rinses with high alcohol content because of drying effects
  - To use sugarless gum, frequent sips of water, or saliva substitutes
  - To use daily home fluoride products for anticaries effect

methylprednisolone

meth-il-pred-niss′-oh-lone
(methylprednisolone) Medrol
(methylprednisolone acetate) Depo-Medrol, Depo-Nisolone[AUS]
(methylprednisolone sodium succinate) A-Methapred, Solu-Medrol

Do not confuse methylprednisolone with medroxyprogesterone or Medrol with Mebaral.

CATEGORY AND SCHEDULE

Pregnancy Risk Category: C

MECHANISM OF ACTION

An adrenocortical steroid that suppresses migration of polymorphonuclear leukocytes and reverses increased capillary permeability. ***Therapeutic Effect:*** Decreases inflammation.

M

PHARMACOKINETICS

Route	Onset	Peak	Duration
PO	N/A	1–2 hr	30–36 hr
IM	N/A	4–8 days	1–4 wk

Well absorbed from the GI tract after IM administration. Widely distributed. Metabolized in the liver. Excreted in urine. Removed by hemodialysis. ***Half-life:*** 3.5 hr.

AVAILABILITY

Tablets (Medrol): 2 mg, 4 mg, 8 mg, 16 mg, 32 mg.
Injection Powder for Reconstitution (A-Methapred, Solu-Medrol): 40 mg, 125 mg, 500 mg, 1 g.
Injection Suspension (Depo-Medrol): 20 mg/ml, 40 mg/ml, 80 mg/ml.

INDICATIONS AND DOSAGES

▸ Substitution Therapy for Deficiency States: Acute or Chronic Adrenal Insufficiency, Adrenal Insufficiency Secondary to Pituitary Insufficiency, and Congenital Adrenal Hyperplasia; Nonendocrine Disorders: Allergic, Collagen, Hepatic, Intestinal Tract, Ocular, Renal, and Skin Diseases; Arthritis; Bronchial Asthma; Cerebral Edema; Malignancies; and Rheumatic Carditis

PO
Adults, Elderly. Initially, 4–48 mg/day.
IV (methylprednisolone sodium succinate)
Adults, Elderly. 40–250 mg q4–6h. High dosage: 30 mg/kg over at least 30 min. Repeat q4–6h for 48–72 hr.

▸ Spinal Cord Injury

IV BOLUS
Adults, Elderly. 30 mg/kg over 15 min. Maintenance dose: 5.4 mg/kg/h over 23 hr, to be given within 45 min of bolus dose.
IM (methylprednisolone acetate)
Adults, Elderly. 10–80 mg/day.
Intra-articular, Intralesional
Adults, Elderly. 4–40 mg, up to 80 mg q1–5wk.

▸ Anti-Inflammatory/ Immunosuppressant

PO/IM/IV
Pediatric. 0.5–1.7 mg/kg/day or 5–25 mg/m^2/day in 2–4 divided doses.

CONTRAINDICATIONS

Administration of live virus vaccines, systemic fungal infection

INTERACTIONS

Drug

Amphotericin: May increase hypokalemia.
Digoxin: May increase the risk of digoxin toxicity caused by hypokalemia

Diuretics, insulin, oral hypoglycemics, potassium supplements: May decrease the effects of these drugs.
Hepatic enzyme inducers: May decrease the effects of methylprednisolone.
Live-virus vaccines: May decrease the patient's antibody response to vaccine, increase vaccine side effects, and potentiate virus replication.

Herbal
None known.

Food
None known.

Drug interactions of concern to dentistry
- Decreased action: barbiturates, rifampin, rifabutin
- Increased GI side effects: alcohol, salicylates, NSAIDs
- Increased action: ketoconazole, macrolide antibiotics
- Hepatotoxicity: acetaminophen (chronic, high doses)

DIAGNOSTIC TEST EFFECTS
May increase blood cholesterol, glucose and serum lipid, amylase, and sodium levels. May decrease serum calcium, potassium, and thyroxine levels.

IV INCOMPATIBILITIES
Ciprofloxacin (Cipro), diltiazem (Cardizem), docetaxel (Taxotere), etoposide (VePesid), filgrastim (Neupogen), gemcitabine (Gemzar), paclitaxel (Taxol), potassium chloride, propofol (Diprivan), vinorelbine (Navelbine)

IV COMPATIBILITIES
Dopamine (Intropin), heparin, midazolam (Versed), theophylline

SIDE EFFECTS
Frequent
Insomnia, heartburn, anxiety, abdominal distention, diaphoresis, acne, mood swings, increased appetite, facial flushing, GI distress, delayed wound healing, increased susceptibility to infection, diarrhea or constipation

Occasional
Headache, edema, tachycardia, change in skin color, frequent urination, depression

Rare
Psychosis, increased blood coagulability, hallucinations

SERIOUS REACTIONS
! Long-term therapy may cause hypocalcemia, hypokalemia, muscle wasting (especially in arms and legs), osteoporosis, spontaneous fractures, amenorrhea, cataracts, glaucoma, peptic ulcer disease, and CHF.
! Abruptly withdrawing the drug after long-term therapy may cause anorexia, nausea, fever, headache, sudden severe myalgia, rebound inflammation, fatigue, weakness, lethargy, dizziness, and orthostatic hypotension.

DENTAL CONSIDERATIONS
General:
- Patients on chronic drug therapy may rarely have symptoms of blood dyscrasias, which can include infection, bleeding, and poor healing.
- Assess salivary flow as a factor in caries, periodontal disease, and candidiasis.
- Symptoms of oral infections may be masked.
- Place on frequent recall to evaluate healing response.
- Prophylactic antibiotics may be indicated to prevent infection if surgery or deep scaling is planned.
- Avoid prescribing aspirin-containing products.

• Determine dose and duration of steroid therapy for each patient to assess risk for stress tolerance and immunosuppression.
• Patients who have been or are currently on chronic steroid therapy (>2 wk) may require supplemental steroids for dental treatment.

Consultations:

• In a patient with symptoms of blood dyscrasias, request a medical consultation for blood studies and postpone dental treatment until normal values are reestablished.
• Medical consultation may be required to assess disease control.
• Consultation may be required to confirm steroid dose and duration of use.

Teach Patient/Family:

• Importance of good oral hygiene to prevent soft tissue inflammation
• Caution to prevent injury when using oral hygiene aids because of reduced healing response
• *When chronic dry mouth occurs, advise patient:*
  • To avoid mouth rinses with high alcohol content because of drying effects
  • To use sugarless gum, frequent sips of water, or saliva substitutes
  • To use daily home fluoride products for anticaries effect

M

methyltestosterone

meth-il-tes-tos-′te-rone
Schedule III
(Android, Android-10, Android-25, Oreton Methyl, Testred, Virilon)
Do not confuse with methylprednisolone.

CATEGORY AND SCHEDULE

Pregnancy Risk Category: X
Controlled substance: Schedule III

MECHANISM OF ACTION

A synthetic testosterone derivative with androgen activity that promotes growth and development of male sex organs and maintains secondary sex characteristics in androgen-deficient males. ***Therapeutic Effect:*** Treats hypogonadism and delayed puberty in males.

PHARMACOKINETICS

Well absorbed from the gastrointestinal (GI) tract. Protein binding: 98%. Metabolized in liver. Primarily excreted in urine. Unknown if removed by hemodialysis. ***Half-life:*** 10–100 min.

AVAILABILITY

Capsules: 10 mg (Android, Testred, Virilon).
Tablets: 10 mg (Android-10, Oreton Methyl), 25 mg (Android-25).

INDICATIONS AND DOSAGES

▸ **Breast Cancer**

PO

Adults, Elderly. 50–200 mg/day.

▸ **Delayed Puberty**

PO

Adults. 10–50 mg/day.
Adults, Elderly. 50–200 mg/day.

▸ **Hypogonadism**

PO

Adults. 10–50 mg/day.

OFF-LABEL USES

Hereditary angiodema

CONTRAINDICATIONS

Pregnancy, prostatic or breast cancer in males, hypersensitivity to methyltestosterone or any other component of its formulation

INTERACTIONS

Drug

Bupropion: May increase the risk of seizures by decreasing seizure threshold.

Cyclosporine: May increase risk of cyclosporine toxicity.
Liver toxic medications: May increase liver toxicity
Oral anticoagulants: May increase the effects of oral anticoagulants.

Herbal
None known.

Food
None known.

Drug interactions of concern to dentistry
Edema: ACTH, corticosteroids.

DIAGNOSTIC TEST EFFECTS

May increase blood Hgb and Hct, LDL concentrations, serum alkaline phosphatase, bilirubin, calcium, potassium, SGOT (AST) levels, and sodium levels. May decrease HDL concentrations.

IV INCOMPATIBILITIES

None known.

IV COMPATIBILITIES

None known.

SIDE EFFECTS

Frequent
Gynecomastia, acne, amenorrhea or other menstrual irregularities
Females: Hirsutism, deepening of voice, clitoral enlargement that may not be reversible when drug is discontinued.

Occasional
Edema, nausea, insomnia, oligospermia, priapism, male pattern of baldness, bladder irritability, hypercalcemia in immobilized patients or those with breast cancer, hypercholesterolemia

Rare
Polycythemia

SERIOUS REACTIONS

! Cholestatic jaundice, hepatocellular neoplasms, peliosis hepatitis, edema with or without congestive heart failure and suppression of clotting factors II, V, VII, and X have been reported.

DENTAL CONSIDERATIONS

General:
- Determine why patient is taking the drug.
- Short appointments and a stress reduction protocol may be required for anxious patients.
- Possible risk of bleeding when used concurrently with oral anticoagulants and aspirin.

Consultations:
- Medical consultation may be required to assess disease control.

Teach Patient/Family:
- Importance of good oral hygiene to prevent soft tissue inflammation
- Importance of updating health and medication history if physician makes any changes in evaluation or drug regimens; include OTC, herbal, and nonherbal in the update

M

metipranolol hydrochloride

met-ee-pran′-oh-lol
(OptiPranolol)
Do not confuse with metoprolol or propranolol.

CATEGORY AND SCHEDULE

Pregnancy Risk Category: C

MECHANISM OF ACTION

An antiglaucoma agent that non-selectively blocks beta-adrenergic receptors. Reduces aqueous humor production.

Therapeutic Effect: Reduces intraocular pressure (IOP).

PHARMACOKINETICS

Route	Onset	Peak	Duration
Eye drops	0.5–3 hrs	2–7 hrs	24 hrs or more

Systemic absorption may occur.

AVAILABILITY

Ophthalmic Solution: 0.3% (OptiPranolol).

INDICATIONS AND DOSAGES

▸ **Glaucoma, Ocular Hypertension**

OPHTHALMIC

Adults, Elderly. Instill 1 drop 2 times/day.

CONTRAINDICATIONS

Bronchial asthma or chronic obstructive pulmonary disease, cardiogenic shock, overt cardiac failure, second or third degree heart AV block, severe sinus bradycardia, hypersensitivity to metipranolol or any component of the formulation.

INTERACTIONS

Drug

None known.

Herbal

None known.

Food

None known.

Drug interactions of concern to dentistry

• Avoid or use with caution: drugs with anticholinergic effects

DIAGNOSTIC TEST EFFECTS

None known.

SIDE EFFECTS

Frequent

Eye burning/stinging, hyperemia, blurred vision, headache, fatigue

Occasional

Sensitivity to light, dizziness, hypotension

Rare

Dry eye, conjunctivitis, eye pain, rash, muscle pain

SERIOUS REACTIONS

! Ophthalmic overdosage may produce bradycardia, hypotension, bronchospasm, and acute cardiac failure.

! Arrhythmias and myocardial infarction have been reported.

DENTAL CONSIDERATIONS

General:

• Determine why patient is taking the drug.

• Avoid drugs with anticholinergic activity, such as antihistamines, opioids, benzodiazepines, propantheline, atropine, and scopolamine.

• Avoid dental light in patient's eyes; offer dark glasses for patient comfort.

• Protect patient's eyes from accidental spatter during dental treatment.

• Question glaucoma patient about compliance with prescribed drug regimen.

Consultations:

• Medical consultation may be required to assess disease control.

Teach Patient/Family:

• Importance of updating health and medication history if physician makes any changes in evaluation or drug regimens; include OTC, herbal, and nonherbal in the update

metoclopramide

met′-oh-kloe-pra′-mide
(Apo-Metoclop[CAN], Maxolon [AUS], Pramin[AUS], Reglan)
Do not confuse Reglan with Renagel.

CATEGORY AND SCHEDULE

Pregnancy Risk Category: B

MECHANISM OF ACTION

A dopamine receptor antagonist that stimulates motility of the upper GI tract and decreases reflux into the esophagus. Also raises the threshold of activity in the chemoreceptor trigger zone. ***Therapeutic Effect:*** Accelerates intestinal transit and gastric emptying; relieves nausea and vomiting.

PHARMACOKINETICS

Route	Onset	Peak	Duration
PO	30–60 min	N/A	N/A
IV	1–3 min	N/A	N/A
IM	10–15 min	N/A	N/A

Well absorbed from the GI tract. Metabolized in the liver. Protein binding: 30%. Primarily excreted in urine. Not removed by hemodialysis. ***Half-life:*** 4–6 hr.

AVAILABILITY

Syrup: 5 mg/5 ml.
Tablets: 5 mg, 10 mg.
Injection: 5 mg/ml.

INDICATIONS AND DOSAGES

▸ Prevention of Chemotherapy-Induced Nausea and Vomiting

IV

Adults, Elderly, Children. 1–2 mg/kg 30 min before chemotherapy; repeat q2h for 2 doses, then q3h as needed.

▸ Postoperative Nausea and Vomiting

IV

Adults, Elderly, Children 15 yr and older. 10 mg; repeat q6–8h as needed.
Children 14 yr and younger. 0.1–0.2 mg/kg/dose; repeat q6–8h as needed.

▸ Diabetic Gastroparesis

PO, IV

Adults. 10 mg 30 min before meals and at bedtime for 2–8 wk.

PO

Elderly. Initially, 5 mg 30 min before meals and at bedtime. May increase to 10 mg.

IV

Elderly. 5 mg over 1–2 min. May increase to 10 mg.

▸ Symptomatic Gastroesophageal Reflux

PO

Adults. 10–15 mg up to 4 times a day, or single doses up to 20 mg as needed.
Elderly. Initially, 5 mg 4 times a day. May increase to 10 mg.
Children. 0.4–0.8 mg/kg/day in 4 divided doses.

▸ To Facilitate Small Bowel Intubation (single dose)

IV

Adults, Elderly. 10 mg as a single dose.
Children 6–14 yr. 2.5–5 mg as a single dose.
Children younger than 6 yr. 0.1 mg/kg as a single dose.

▸ Dosage in Renal Impairment

Dosage is modified on the basis of creatinine clearance.

Creatinine Clearance	% of normal dose
40–50 ml/min	75%
10–40 ml/min	50%
less than 10 ml/min	25%–50%

M

OFF-LABEL USES

Prevention of aspiration pneumonia; treatment of drug-related postoperative nausea and vomiting, persistent hiccups, slow gastric emptying, vascular headaches

CONTRAINDICATIONS

Concurrent use of medications likely to produce extrapyramidal reactions, GI hemorrhage, GI obstruction or perforation, history of seizure disorders, pheochromocytoma

INTERACTIONS

Drug

Alcohol, other CNS suppressants: May increase CNS depressant effect.

Herbal

None known.

Food

None known.

Drug interactions of concern to dentistry

- Decreased GI action: anticholinergics, opioids
- Increased sedation: alcohol, other CNS depressants
- Increased effects of succinylcholine

DIAGNOSTIC TEST EFFECTS

May increase serum aldosterone and prolactin concentrations.

IV INCOMPATIBILITIES

Allopurinol (Aloprim), cefepime (Maxipime), doxorubicin liposomal (Doxil), furosemide (Lasix), propofol (Diprivan)

IV COMPATIBILITIES

Dexamethasone, diltiazem (Cardizem), diphenhydramine (Benadryl), fentanyl (Sublimaze), heparin, hydromorphone (Dilaudid), morphine, potassium chloride

SIDE EFFECTS

Frequent (10%)
Somnolence, restlessness, fatigue, lethargy

Occasional (3%)
Dizziness, anxiety, headache, insomnia, breast tenderness, altered menstruation, constipation, rash, dry mouth, galactorrhea, gynecomastia

Rare (<3%)
Hypotension or hypertension, tachycardia

SERIOUS REACTIONS

! Extrapyramidal reactions occur most commonly in children and young adults (18–30 years) receiving large doses (2 mg/kg) during chemotherapy and are usually limited to akathisia (involuntary limb movement and facial grimacing).

DENTAL CONSIDERATIONS

General:

- Assess salivary flow as a factor in caries, periodontal disease, and candidiasis.
- Assess for presence of extrapyramidal motor symptoms, such as tardive dyskinesia and akathisia. Extrapyramidal motor activity may complicate dental treatment.
- Determine why the patient is taking the drug.
- Consider semisupine chair position for patient comfort because of GI effects of disease.

Teach Patient/Family:

- *When chronic dry mouth occurs, advise patient:*
  - To avoid mouth rinses with high alcohol content because of drying effects
  - To use sugarless gum, frequent sips of water, or saliva substitutes
  - To use daily home fluoride products for anticaries effect

metolazone

met-tole′-a-zone

(Mykrox, Zaroxolyn)

Do not confuse metolazone with methazolamide or metoprolol, or Zaroxolyn with Zarontin.

CATEGORY AND SCHEDULE

Pregnancy Risk Category: B
(D if used in pregnancy-induced hypertension)

MECHANISM OF ACTION

A thiazide-like diuretic and antihypertensive. As a diuretic, blocks reabsorption of sodium, potassium, and chloride at the distal convoluted tubule, increasing renal excretion of sodium and water. As an antihypertensive, reduces plasma and extracellular fluid volume and peripheral vascular resistance.
Therapeutic Effect: Promotes diuresis and reduces BP.

PHARMACOKINETICS

Route	Onset	Peak	Duration
PO (diuretic)	1 hr	2 hr	12–24 hr

Incompletely absorbed from the GI tract. Protein binding: 95%. Primarily excreted unchanged in urine. Not removed by hemodialysis.
Half-life: 14 hr.

AVAILABILITY

Tablets (Prompt-Release [Mykrox]): 0.5 mg.
Tablets (Extended-Release [Zaroxolyn]): 2.5 mg, 5 mg, 10 mg.

INDICATIONS AND DOSAGES

▸ Edema

PO (Zaroxolyn)
Adults, Elderly. 5–10 mg/day. May increase to 20 mg/day in edema associated with renal disease or heart failure.
Children. 0.2–0.4 mg/kg/day in 1–2 divided doses.

▸ Hypertension

PO (Zaroxolyn)
Adults, Elderly. 2.5–5 mg/day.
PO (Mydrox)
Adults, Elderly. Initially, 0.5 mg/day. May increase up to 1 mg/day.

CONTRAINDICATIONS

Anuria, hepatic coma or precoma, history of hypersensitivity to sulfonamides or thiazide diuretics, renal decompensation

INTERACTIONS

Drug

Cholestyramine, colestipol: May decrease the absorption and effects of metolazone.
Digoxin: May increase the risk of digoxin toxicity associated with metolazone-induced hypokalemia.
Lithium: May increase the risk of lithium toxicity.

Herbal

None known.

Food

None known.

Drug interactions of concern to dentistry

- Increased photosensitization: tetracycline
- Decreased hypotensive response: indomethacin and other NSAIDs

DIAGNOSTIC TEST EFFECTS

May increase blood glucose and serum cholesterol, LDL, bilirubin, calcium, creatinine, uric acid, and triglyceride levels. May decrease urinary calcium and serum magnesium, potassium, and sodium levels.

M

SIDE EFFECTS

Expected

Increase in urinary frequency and urine volume

Frequent (10%–9%)

Dizziness, light-headedness, headache

Occasional (6%–°4%)

Muscle cramps and spasm, fatigue, lethargy

Rare (<2%)

Asthenia, palpitations, depression, nausea, vomiting, abdominal bloating, constipation, diarrhea, urticaria

SERIOUS REACTIONS

! Vigorous diuresis may lead to profound water and electrolyte depletion, resulting in hypokalemia, hyponatremia, and dehydration.

! Acute hypotensive episodes may occur.

! Hyperglycemia may occur during prolonged therapy.

! Pancreatitis, paresthesia, blood dyscrasias, pulmonary edema, allergic pneumonitis, and dermatologic reactions occur rarely.

! Overdose can lead to lethargy and coma without changes in electrolytes or hydration.

DENTAL CONSIDERATIONS

General:

- Patients on chronic drug therapy may rarely have symptoms of blood dyscrasias, which can include infection, bleeding, and poor healing.
- Assess salivary flow as a factor in caries, periodontal disease, and candidiasis.
- After supine positioning, have patient sit upright for at least 2 min before standing to avoid orthostatic hypotension.
- Short appointments and a stress reduction protocol may be required for anxious patients.
- Limit use of sodium-containing products, such as saline IV fluids, for patients with a dietary salt restriction.
- Stress from dental procedures may compromise CV function; determine patient risk.

Consultations:

- In a patient with symptoms of blood dyscrasias, request a medical consultation for blood studies and postpone dental treatment until normal values are reestablished.
- Medical consultation may be required to assess disease control and patient's ability to tolerate stress.

Teach Patient/Family:

- Importance of good oral hygiene to prevent soft tissue inflammation
- Caution to prevent injury when using oral hygiene aids
- *When chronic dry mouth occurs, advise patient:*
  - To avoid mouth rinses with high alcohol content because of drying effects
  - To use sugarless gum, frequent sips of water, or saliva substitutes
  - To use daily home fluoride products for anticaries effect

metoprolol tartrate

me-toe′-pro-lole

(Apo-Metoprolol[CAN], Betaloc[CAN], Lopresor[AUS], Lopressor, Metohexal[AUS], Metolol[AUS], Minax[AUS], Nu-Metop[CAN], PMS-Metoprolol [CAN], Toprol XL)

Do not confuse metoprolol with metaproterenol or metolazone.

CATEGORY AND SCHEDULE

Pregnancy Risk Category: C (D if used in second or third trimester)

MECHANISM OF ACTION

An antianginal, antihypertensive, and MI adjunct that selectively blocks $beta_1$-adrenergic receptors; high dosages may block $beta_2$-adrenergic receptors. Decreases oxygen requirements. Large doses increase airway resistance. ***Therapeutic Effect:*** Slows sinus node heart rate, decreases cardiac output, and reduces BP. Also decreases myocardial ischemia severity.

PHARMACOKINETICS

Route	Onset	Peak	Duration
PO	10–15 min	N/A	6 hr
PO (extended release)	N/A	6–12 hr	24 hr
IV	Immediate	20 min	5–8 hr

Well absorbed from the GI tract. Protein binding: 12%. Widely distributed. Metabolized in the liver (undergoes significant first-pass metabolism). Primarily excreted in urine. Removed by hemodialysis. ***Half-life:*** 3–7 hr.

AVAILABILITY

Tablets (Lopressor): 25 mg, 50 mg, 100 mg.
Tablets (Extended-Release [Toprol XL]): 25 mg, 50 mg, 100 mg, 200 mg.
Injection (Lopressor): 1 mg/ml.

INDICATIONS AND DOSAGES

▸ Mild to Moderate Hypertension

PO

Adults. Initially, 100 mg/day as single or divided dose. Increase at weekly (or longer) intervals. Maintenance: 100–450 mg/day.
Elderly. Initially, 25 mg/day. Range: 25–300 mg/day.

PO (Extended-Release)

Adults. 50–100 mg/day as single dose. May increase at least at weekly intervals until optimum BP attained. Maximum: 200 mg/day.
Elderly. Initially, 25–50 mg/day as a single dose. May increase at 1–2 week intervals.

▸ Chronic, Stable Angina Pectoris

PO

Adults. Initially, 100 mg/day as single or divided dose. Increase at weekly (or longer) intervals. Maintenance: 100–450 mg/day.

PO (Extended-Release)

Adults. Initially, 100 mg/day as single dose. May increase at least at weekly intervals until optimum clinical response achieved. Maximum: 200 mg/day.

▸ Congestive Heart Failure

PO (Extended-Release)

Adults. Initially, 25 mg/day. May double dose q2wk. Maximum: 200 mg/day.

▸ Early Treatment of MI

IV

Adults. 5 mg q2min for 3 doses, followed by 50 mg orally q6h for 48 hr. Begin oral dose 15 min after last IV dose. Or, in patients who do not tolerate full IV dose, give 25–50 mg orally q6h, 15 min after last IV dose.

▸ Late Treatment and Maintenance after an MI

PO

Adults. 100 mg twice a day for at least 3 mo.

OFF-LABEL USES

To increase survival rate in diabetic patients with coronary artery disease (CAD); treatment or prevention of anxiety; cardiac arrhythmias; hypertrophic cardiomyopathy; mitral valve prolapse syndrome; pheochromocytoma; tremors; thyrotoxicosis; vascular headache

CONTRAINDICATIONS
Cardiogenic shock, MI with a heart rate less than 45 beats/minute or systolic BP less than 100 mm Hg, overt heart failure, second- or third-degree heart block, sinus bradycardia

INTERACTIONS
Drug
Cimetidine: May increase metoprolol blood concentration.
Diuretics, other antihypertensives: May increase hypotensive effect.
Insulin, oral hypoglycemics: May mask symptoms of hypoglycemia and prolong hypoglycemic effect of these drugs.
NSAIDs: May decrease antihypertensive effect.
Sympathomimetics, xanthines: May mutually inhibit effects.
Herbal
None known.
Food
None known.
Drug interactions of concern to dentistry
- Increased hypotension, bradycardia: fentanyl derivatives, inhalation anesthetics
- Decreased antihypertensive effects: indomethacin and possibly other NSAIDs, sympathomimetics
- May slow metabolism of lidocaine
- Decreased β-blocking effects (or decreased β-adrenergic effects) of epinephrine, levonordefrin, isoproterenol, and other sympathomimetics
- Increased plasma concentrations: diphenhydramine
- Decreased effects: didanosine (take 2 hr before didanosine tabs)

DIAGNOSTIC TEST EFFECTS
May increase serum antinuclear antibody titer and BUN, serum lipoprotein, serum LDH, serum alkaline phosphatase, serum bilirubin, serum creatinine, serum potassium, serum uric acid, AST levels, ALT levels, and serum triglyceride levels.

IV INCOMPATIBILITIES
Amphotericin B complex (Abelcet, AmBisome, Amphotec)
IV COMPATIBILITIES
Alteplase (Activase)

SIDE EFFECTS
Metoprolol is generally well tolerated, with transient and mild side effects.
Frequent
Diminished sexual function, drowsiness, insomnia, unusual fatigue or weakness
Occasional
Anxiety, nervousness, diarrhea, constipation, nausea, vomiting, nasal congestion, abdominal discomfort, dizziness, difficulty breathing, cold hands or feet
Rare
Altered taste, dry eyes, nightmares, paraesthesia, allergic reaction (rash, pruritus)

SERIOUS REACTIONS
! Overdose may produce profound bradycardia, hypotension, and bronchospasm.
! Abrupt withdrawal of metoprolol may result in diaphoresis, palpitations, headache, tremulousness, exacerbation of angina, MI, and ventricular arrhythmias.
! Metoprolol administration may precipitate CHF and MI in patients with heart disease; thyroid storm in those with thyrotoxicosis; and peripheral ischemia in those with existing peripheral vascular disease.

! Hypoglycemia may occur in patients with previously controlled diabetes mellitus.

DENTAL CONSIDERATIONS

General:

• Monitor vital signs at every appointment because of CV and respiratory side effects.
• After supine positioning, have patient sit upright for at least 2 min before standing to avoid orthostatic hypotension.
• Patients on chronic drug therapy may rarely have symptoms of blood dyscrasias, which can include infection, bleeding, and poor healing.
• Assess salivary flow as a factor in caries, periodontal disease, and candidiasis.
• Stress from dental procedures may compromise CV function; determine patient risk.
• Short appointments and a stress reduction protocol may be required for anxious patients.
• Use vasoconstrictors with caution, in low doses, and with careful aspiration. Avoid use of gingival retraction cord with epinephrine.
• Determine why patient is taking the drug.

Consultations:

• In a patient with symptoms of blood dyscrasias, request a medical consultation for blood studies and postpone dental treatment until normal values are reestablished.
• Medical consultation may be required to assess disease control and patient's ability to tolerate stress.
• Take precautions if general anesthesia is required for dental surgery.

Teach Patient/Family:

• Importance of good oral hygiene to prevent soft tissue inflammation
• Caution to prevent injury when using oral hygiene aids
• *When chronic dry mouth occurs, advise patient:*
  • To avoid mouth rinses with high alcohol content because of drying effects
  • To use sugarless gum, frequent sips of water, or saliva substitutes
  • To use daily home fluoride products for anticaries effect

metronidazole hydrochloride

me-troe-ni′-da-zole
(Apo-Metronidazole[CAN], Flagyl, Flagyl ER, MetroCream, MetroGel, Metrogyl[AUS], MetroLotion, Metronidazole IV [AUS], Metronide[AUS], NidaGel[CAN], Noritate, Novonidazol[CAN], Rozex[AUS])

CATEGORY AND SCHEDULE

Pregnancy Risk Category: B

MECHANISM OF ACTION

A nitroimidazole derivative that disrupts bacterial and protozoal DNA, inhibiting nucleic acid synthesis. ***Therapeutic Effect:*** Produces bactericidal, antiprotozoal, amebicidal, and trichomonacidal effects. Produces anti-inflammatory and immunosuppressive effects when applied topically.

PHARMACOKINETICS

Well absorbed from the GI tract; minimally absorbed after topical application. Protein binding: less than 20%. Widely distributed; crosses blood-brain barrier. Metabolized in the liver to active metabolite. Primarily excreted in urine; partially eliminated in feces.

Removed by hemodialysis. ***Half-life:*** 8 hr (increased in alcoholic hepatic disease and in neonates).

AVAILABILITY

Capsules (Flagyl): 375 mg.
Tablets (Flagyl): 250 mg, 500 mg.
Tablets (Extended-Release [Flagyl ER]): 750 mg.
Injection (Infusion): 500 mg/100 ml.
Lotion: 0.75%.
Topical Gel (MetroGel): 0.75%.
Topical Cream (MetroCream): 0.75%.
Topical Cream (Noritate): 1%.
Vaginal Gel (MetroGel-Vaginal): 0.75%.

INDICATIONS AND DOSAGES

▸ **Amebiasis**
PO
Adults, Elderly. 500–750 mg q8h.
Children. 35–50 mg/kg/day in divided doses q8h.

▸ **Trichomoniasis**
PO
Adults, Elderly. 250 mg q8h or 2 g as a single dose.
Children. 15–30 mg/kg/day in divided doses q8h.

▸ **Anaerobic Skin and Skin-Structure, CNS, Lower Respiratory Tract, Bone, Joint, Intra-Abdominal, and Gynecologic Infections; Endocarditis; Septicemia**
PO, IV
Adults, Elderly, Children. 30 mg/kg/day in divided doses q6h. Maximum: 4 g/day.

▸ **Antibiotic-Associated Pseudomembranous Colitis**
PO
Adults, Elderly. 250–500 mg 3–4 times a day for 10–14 days.
Children. 30 mg/kg/day in divided doses q6h for 7–10 days.

▸ **Helicobacter Pylori Infections**
PO
Adults, Elderly. 250–500 mg 3 times a day (in combination).
Children. 15–20 mg/kg/day in 2 divided doses.

▸ **Bacterial Vaginosis**
PO
Adults. 750 mg at bedtime for 7 days.

▸ **Intravaginal**
Adults. One applicatorful twice a day or once a day at bedtime for 5 days.

▸ **Rosacea**
TOPICAL
Adults. Apply thin layer of lotion to affected area twice a day or cream once a day.

OFF-LABEL USES

Treatment of bacterial vaginosis, grade III-IV decubitus ulcers with anaerobic infection, *H. pylori*-associated gastritis and duodenal ulcer, inflammatory bowel disease; topical treatment of acne rosacea

CONTRAINDICATIONS

Hypersensitivity to metronidazole or other nitroimidazole derivatives (also parabens with topical application)

INTERACTIONS

Drug

Alcohol: May cause a disulfiram-type reaction.
Disulfiram: May increase the risk of toxicity.
Oral anticoagulants: May increase the effects of these drugs.

Herbal

None known.

Food

None known.

Drug interactions of concern to dentistry

- Antabuse-like reaction: alcohol, alcohol-containing products

M

- Decreased action: phenobarbital
- Possible increase in blood levels of tacrolimus
- Enhanced effects of warfarin, carbamazepine

DIAGNOSTIC TEST EFFECTS

May increase serum LDH, AST (SGOT), and ALT (SGPT) levels.

IV INCOMPATIBILITIES

Amphotericin B complex (Abelcet, AmBisome, Amphotec), filgrastim (Neupogen)

IV COMPATIBILITIES

Diltiazem (Cardizem), dopamine (Intropin), heparin, hydromorphone (Dilaudid), lorazepam (Ativan), magnesium sulfate, midazolam (Versed), morphine

SIDE EFFECTS

Frequent

Systemic: Anorexia, nausea, dry mouth, metallic taste
Vaginal: Symptomatic cervicitis and vaginitis, abdominal cramps, uterine pain

Occasional

Systemic: Diarrhea or constipation, vomiting, dizziness, erythematous rash, urticaria, reddish brown urine
Topical: Transient erythema, mild dryness, burning, irritation, stinging, tearing when applied too close to eyes
Vaginal: Vaginal, perineal, or vulvar itching; vulvar swelling

Rare

Mild, transient leukopenia; thrombophlebitis with IV therapy

SERIOUS REACTIONS

! Oral therapy may result in furry tongue, glossitis, cystitis, dysuria, pancreatitis, and flattening of T waves on ECG readings.
! Peripheral neuropathy, manifested as numbness and tingling in hands or feet, is usually reversible if treatment is stopped immediately after neurologic symptoms appear.
! Seizures occur occasionally.

DENTAL CONSIDERATIONS

General:

- Patients on chronic drug therapy may rarely have symptoms of blood dyscrasias, which can include infection, bleeding, and poor healing.
- Assess salivary flow as a factor in caries, periodontal disease, and candidiasis.
- Determine why the patient is taking the drug.

Consultations:

- In a patient with symptoms of blood dyscrasias, request a medical consultation for blood studies and postpone dental treatment until normal values are reestablished.
- Medical consultation may be required to assess disease control.

Teach Patient/Family:

- To avoid alcoholic beverages
- That taste alterations may occur
- Importance of good oral hygiene to prevent soft tissue inflammation
- Caution to prevent injury when using oral hygiene aids
- *When chronic dry mouth occurs, advise patient:*
  - To avoid mouth rinses with high alcohol content because of drying effects
  - To use sugarless gum, frequent sips of water, or saliva substitutes
  - To use daily home fluoride products for anticaries effect

metyrosine

me-tye′-roe-seen
(Demser)

CATEGORY AND SCHEDULE

Pregnancy Risk Category: C

MECHANISM OF ACTION

A tyrosine hydroxylase inhibitor that blocks conversion of tyrosine to dihydroxyphenylalanine, the rate-limiting step in the biosynthetic pathway of catecholamines.
Therapeutic Effect: Reduces levels of endogenous catecholamines.

PHARMACOKINETICS

Well absorbed from the gastrointestinal (GI) tract. Metabolized in the liver. Excreted primarily in the urine. ***Half-life:*** 7.2 hrs.

AVAILABILITY

Capsule: 250 mg (Demser).

INDICATIONS AND DOSAGES

▸ Pheochromocytoma (preoperative)

PO
Adults, Elderly. Initially, 250 mg 4 times/day. Increase by 250–500 mg/day up to 4 g/day. Maintenance: 2–4 g/day in 4 divided doses for 5–7 days.

OFF-LABEL USES

Tourette syndrome

CONTRAINDICATIONS

Hypertension of unknown etiology, hypersensitivity to metyrosine or any component of the formulation

INTERACTIONS

Drug

Alcohol: May increase CNS depression.
Phenothiazines, haloperidol: May potentiate extrapyramidal symptoms (EPS).

Herbal

None known.

Food

None known.

Drug interactions of concern to dentistry

- Increased CNS depression with CNS depressants

DIAGNOSTIC TEST EFFECTS

None known.

SIDE EFFECTS

Frequent

Drowsiness, extrapyramidal symptoms, diarrhea

Occasional

Galactorrhea, edema of the breasts, nausea, vomiting, dry mouth, impotence, nasal congestion

Rare

Lower extremity edema, urinary problems, urticaria, anemia, depression, disorientation

SERIOUS REACTIONS

! Serious or life-threatening allergic reaction characterized by hallucinations, hematuria, hyperstimulation after withdrawal, severe lower extremity edema, and parkinsonism.

DENTAL CONSIDERATIONS

General:

- Medication may be used in anticipation of surgery to remove the adrenal tumor.
- Hypertension may preclude all dental care except for palliative emergency treatment.
- Question patient about compliance with drug therapy.
- Risk of increased CNS depression when other CNS depressants are used.

• Trismus may be a symptom of excessive doses of this drug.
• Determine why patient is taking the drug.
• Monitor and record vital signs.
• Use vasoconstrictor with caution, in low doses, and with careful aspiration. Avoid using gingival retraction cord containing epinephrine.
• Assess for presence of extrapyramidal motor symptoms, such as tardive dyskinesia and akathisia; extrapyramidal motor activity may complicate dental treatment. Advise seeing physician if tardive dyskinesia or akathisia is present.

Consultations:
• Medical consultation may be required to assess disease control and patient's ability to tolerate stress.

Teach Patient/Family:
• Importance of good oral hygiene to prevent soft tissue inflammation
• Caution patients about driving or performing other tasks requiring mental alertness

mexiletine hydrochloride

mex-il′-e-teen
(Mexitil)

CATEGORY AND SCHEDULE

Pregnancy Risk Category: C

MECHANISM OF ACTION

An antiarrhythmic that shortens duration of action potential and decreases effective refractory period in the His-Purkinje system of the myocardium by blocking sodium transport across myocardial cell membranes. ***Therapeutic Effect:*** Suppresses ventricular arrhythmias.

AVAILABILITY

Capsules: 150 mg, 200 mg, 250 mg.

INDICATIONS AND DOSAGES

▸ Arrhythmia

PO
Adults, Elderly. Initially, 200 mg q8h. Adjust dosage by 50–100 mg at 2- to 3-day intervals. **Maximum:** 1,200 mg/day.

OFF-LABEL USES

Treatment of diabetic neuropathy

CONTRAINDICATIONS

Cardiogenic shock, preexisting second- or third-degree AV block, right bundle-branch block without presence of pacemaker

INTERACTIONS

Drug

Antacids: May reduce mexiletine absorption.
Cimetidine: May increase mexiletine blood concentration.
Metoclopramide: May increase mexiletine absorption.
Phenobarbital, phenytoin, rifampin: May decrease mexiletine blood concentration.

Herbal

None known.

Food

None known.

Drug interactions of concern to dentistry

• No specific interactions are reported with dental drugs; however, any drug that could affect the cardiac action of mexiletine should be used in the least effective dose, such as other local anesthetics, vasoconstrictors, and anticholinergics

DIAGNOSTIC TEST EFFECTS

May increase liver enzymes, such as ALT and AST. May decrease WBCs and thrombocytes.

SIDE EFFECTS

Frequent (>10%)
GI distress, including nausea, vomiting, and heartburn; dizziness; light-headedness; tremor
Occasional (10%–1%)
Nervousness, change in sleep habits, headache, visual disturbances, paresthesia, diarrhea or constipation, palpitations, chest pain, rash, respiratory difficulty, edema

SERIOUS REACTIONS

! Mexiletine has the ability to worsen existing arrhythmias or produce new ones.
! CHF may occur, and existing CHF may worsen.

M

DENTAL CONSIDERATIONS

General:

- Monitor vital signs at every appointment because of CV side effects.
- Patients on chronic drug therapy may rarely have symptoms of blood dyscrasias, which can include infection, bleeding, and poor healing.
- Assess salivary flow as a factor in caries, periodontal disease, and candidiasis.
- Stress from dental procedures may compromise CV function; determine patient risk.

Consultations:

- In a patient with symptoms of blood dyscrasias, request a medical consultation for blood studies and postpone dental treatment until normal values are reestablished.
- Medical consultation should be made to assess disease control.
- Medical consultation may be required to assess patient's ability to tolerate stress.

Teach Patient/Family:

- Importance of good oral hygiene to prevent soft tissue inflammation
- Caution to prevent injury when using oral hygiene aids
- *When chronic dry mouth occurs, advise patient:*
  - To avoid mouth rinses with high alcohol content because of drying effects
  - To use sugarless gum, frequent sips of water, or saliva substitutes
  - To use daily home fluoride products for anticaries effect

miconazole

mih-kon′-ah-zole
(Femizol-M, Micatin, Micozole[CAN], Monistat[CAN], Monistat-3, Monistat-7, Monistat-Derm)

CATEGORY AND SCHEDULE

Pregnancy Risk Category: C

MECHANISM OF ACTION

An imidazole derivative that inhibits synthesis of ergosterol (vital component of fungal cell formation), damaging cell membrane.
Therapeutic Effect: Fungistatic; may be fungicidal, depending on concentration.

PHARMACOKINETICS

Parenteral: Widely distributed in tissues. Metabolized in liver. Primarily excreted in urine. ***Half-life:*** 24 hrs. Topical: No systemic absorption following application to intact skin. Intravaginally: Small amount absorbed systemically.

AVAILABILITY

Injection: 10 mg/ml.
Vaginal Suppository: 100 mg (Monistat-7), 200 mg (Monistat-3).
Topical Cream: 2% (Micatin, Monistat-Derm).
Vaginal Cream: 2% (Femizol-M).
Topical Powder: 2% (Micatin).
Topical Spray: 2% (Lotrimin-AF).

INDICATIONS AND DOSAGES

▸ **Coccidioidomycosis**
IV
Adults, Elderly. 1.8–3.6 g/day for 3–20 wks or longer.

▸ **Cryptococcosis**
IV
Adults, Elderly. 1.2–2.4 g/day for 3–12 wks or longer.

▸ **Petriellidiosis**
IV
Adults, Elderly. 0.6–3.0 g/day for 5–20 wks or longer.

▸ **Candidiasis**
IV
Adults, Elderly. 0.6–1.8 g/day for 1–20 wks or longer.

▸ **Paracoccidioidomycosis**
IV
Adults, Elderly. 0.2–1.2 g/day for 2–16 wks or longer.
Usual dosage for children
IV
20–40 mg/kg/day in 3 divided doses. (Do not exceed 15 mg/kg for any 1 infusion).

▸ **Vulvovaginal Candidiasis**
INTRAVAGINALLY
Adults, Elderly. One 200 mg suppository at bedtime for 3 days; one 100 mg suppository or one applicatorful at bedtime for 7 days.
Topical fungal infections, cutaneous candidiasis
TOPICAL
Adults, Elderly, Children 2 years and older. Apply liberally 2 times/day, morning and evening.

CONTRAINDICATIONS

Children younger than 1 year old, hypersensitivity to miconazole or any component of the formulation
Topically: Children younger than 2 years old

INTERACTIONS

Drug

Oral anticoagulants, oral hypoglycemics: May increase effects of these drugs.
Isoniazid, rifampin: May decrease concentrations.

Herbal

None known.

Food

None known.

DIAGNOSTIC TEST EFFECTS

None known.

IV INCOMPATIBILITIES

Do not administer other medications via Y-site.

M

SIDE EFFECTS

Frequent

Phlebitis, fever, chills, rash, itching, nausea, vomiting

Occasional

Dizziness, drowsiness, headache, flushed face, abdominal pain, constipation, diarrhea, decreased appetite
Topical: Itching, burning, stinging, erythema, urticaria
Vaginal: Vulvovaginal burning, itching, irritation, headache, skin rash

SERIOUS REACTIONS

! Anemia, thrombocytopenia, and liver toxicity occur rarely

DENTAL CONSIDERATIONS

General:

- Examine oral mucous membranes for signs of fungal infection.

• Broad-spectrum antibiotics may evoke vaginal yeast infections.

Teach Patient/Family:

• To prevent reinoculation of *Candida* infection by disposing of toothbrush or other contaminated oral hygiene devices used during period of infection

midazolam hydrochloride

mid-az'-zoe-lam

Schedule IV

(Apo-Midazolam[CAN], Hypnovel[AUS], Versed)

Do not confuse Versed with VePesid.

CATEGORY AND SCHEDULE

Pregnancy Risk Category: D

Controlled substance: Schedule IV

M

MECHANISM OF ACTION

A benzodiazepine that enhances the action of gamma-aminobutyric acid, one of the major inhibitory neurotransmitters in the brain. ***Therapeutic Effect:*** Produces anxiolytic, hypnotic, anticonvulsant, muscle relaxant, and amnestic effects.

PHARMACOKINETICS

Route	Onset	Peak	Duration
PO	10–20 min	N/A	N/A
IV	1–5 min	5–7 min	20–30 min
IM	5–15 min	15–60 min	2–6 hr

Well absorbed after IM administration. Protein binding: 97%. Metabolized in the liver to active metabolite. Primarily excreted in urine. Not removed by hemodialysis. ***Half-life:*** 1–5 hr.

AVAILABILITY

Syrup: 2 mg/ml.

Injection: 1 mg/ml, 5 mg/ml.

INDICATIONS AND DOSAGES

▸ Preoperative Sedation

PO

Children. 0.25–0.5 mg/kg. Maximum: 20 mg.

IV

Children 6–12 yr. 0.025–0.05 mg/kg.

Children 6 mo–5 yr. 0.05–0.1 mg/kg.

IM

Adults, Elderly. 0.07–0.08 mg/kg 30–60 min before surgery.

Children. 0.1–0.15 mg/kg 30–60 min before surgery. Maximum: 10 mg.

▸ Conscious Sedation for Diagnostic, Therapeutic, and Endoscopic Procedures

IV

Adults, Elderly. 1–2.5 mg over 2 min. Titrate as needed. Maximum total dose: 2.5–5 mg.

▸ Conscious Sedation During Mechanical Ventilation

IV

Adults, Elderly. 0.01–0.05 mg/kg; may repeat q10–15min until adequately sedated. Then continuous infusion at initial rate of 0.02–0.1 mg/kg/hr (1–7 mg/hr).

Children older than 32 wk. Initially, 1 mcg/kg/min as continuous infusion.

Children 32 wk and younger. Initially, 0.5 mcg/kg/min as continuous infusion.

▸ Status Epilepticus

IV

Children older than 2 mo. Loading dose of 0.15 mg/kg followed by continuous infusion of 1 mcg/kg/min. Titrate as needed. Range: 1–18 mcg/kg/min.

CONTRAINDICATIONS

Acute alcohol intoxication, acute angle-closure glaucoma, coma, shock

INTERACTIONS

Drug

Alcohol, other CNS depressants: May increase CNS and respiratory depression and hypotensive effects of midazolam.
Hypotension-producing medications: May increase hypotensive effects of midazolam.

Herbal

Kava kava, valerian: May increase CNS depression.

Food

Grapefruit, grapefruit juice: Increases the oral absorption and systemic availability of midazolam.

Drug interactions of concern to dentistry

• Prolonged respiratory depression: all CNS depressants, including alcohol, barbiturates, narcotics. All doses of midazolam must be reduced when used in combination with any CNS depressant. Serious respiratory and CV depression, including death, has occurred when midazolam is used in combination with other CNS depressants or given too rapidly. Medically compromised and elderly patients are at greater risk.
• Increased serum levels and prolonged effect of benzodiazepines: erythromycin, ketoconazole, itraconazole, fluconazole, miconazole (systemic), diltiazem, fluvoxamine
• Contraindicated with nelfinavir, ritonavir, indinavir, saquinavir
• Possible increase in CNS side effects: kava (herb)
• Suspected increase in midazolam effects when used in general anesthesia: atorvastatin (*Anesthesia* 58:899–904, 2003)

DIAGNOSTIC TEST EFFECTS

None known.

IV INCOMPATIBILITIES

Albumin, ampicillin and sulbactam (Unasyn), amphotericin B complex (Abelcet, AmBisome, Amphotec), ampicillin (Polycillin), bumetanide (Bumex), co-trimoxazole (Bactrim), dexamethasone (Decadron), fosphenytoin (Cerebyx), furosemide (Lasix), hydrocortisone (Solu-Cortef), methotrexate, nafcillin (Nafcil), sodium bicarbonate, sodium pentothal (Thiopental)

IV COMPATIBILITIES

Amiodarone (Cordarone), atropine, calcium gluconate, diltiazem (Cardizem), diphenhydramine (Benadryl), dobutamine (Dobutrex), dopamine (Intropin), etomidate (Amidate), fentanyl (Sublimaze), glycopyrrolate (Robinul), heparin, hydromorphone (Dilaudid), hydroxyzine (Vistaril), insulin, lorazepam (Ativan), milrinone (Primacor), morphine, nitroglycerin, norepinephrine (Levophed), potassium chloride, propofol (Diprivan)

SIDE EFFECTS

Frequent (10%–4%)

Decreased respiratory rate, tenderness at IM or IV injection site, pain during injection, oxygen desaturation, hiccups

Occasional (3%–2%)

Hypotension, paradoxical CNS reaction

Rare (<2%)

Nausea, vomiting, headache, coughing

SERIOUS REACTIONS

! Inadequate or excessive dosage or improper administration may result in cerebral hypoxia, agitation, involuntary movements, hyperactivity, and combativeness.
! A too-rapid IV rate, excessive doses, or a single large dose increases the risk of respiratory depression or arrest.
! Respiratory depression or apnea may produce hypoxia and cardiac arrest.

DENTAL CONSIDERATIONS

General:

- Monitor vital signs every 5 min during general anesthesia because of CV and respiratory side effects. Monitor vital signs at regular intervals during recovery.
- Degree of CNS depression is dose dependent; titrate all doses.
- Drug produces amnesia, especially in the elderly patient.
- Longer recovery period could be observed in an obese patient because half-life may be extended.
- Assist patient with ambulation until drowsy period has passed.

Teach Patient/Family:

- That drug may impair reaction time; avoid driving or potentially hazardous activities until drowsiness or weakness subsides
- That amnesia occurs; events may not be remembered
- Treatment of overdose: O_2, vasopressors, flumazenil, resuscitation measures as required

M

midodrine

mid′-o-dreen
(Amatine, ProAmatine)
Do not confuse Amatine or ProAmatine with amantadine or protamine.

CATEGORY AND SCHEDULE

Pregnancy Risk Category: C

MECHANISM OF ACTION

A vasopressor that forms the active metabolite desglymidodrine, an alpha$_1$-agonist, activating alpha receptors of the arteriolar and venous vasculature. ***Therapeutic Effect:*** Increases vascular tone and BP.

AVAILABILITY

Tablets: 2.5 mg, 5 mg, 10 mg.

INDICATIONS AND DOSAGES

▸ Orthostatic Hypotension

PO

Adults, Elderly. 10 mg 3 times a day. Give during the day when patient is upright, such as upon arising, midday, and late afternoon. Do not give later than 6 p.m.

▸ Dosage in Renal Impairment

For adults and elderly patients, give 2.5 mg 3 times a day; increase gradually, as tolerated.

CONTRAINDICATIONS

Acute renal function impairment, persistent hypertension, pheochromocytoma, severe cardiac disease, thyrotoxicosis, urine retention

INTERACTIONS

Drug

Digoxin: May have additive bradycardia effects.

Sodium-retaining steroids (such as fludrocortisone): May increase sodium retention.
Vasoconstrictors: May have an additive vasocontricting effect.

Herbal
None known.

Food
None known.

Drug interactions of concern to dentistry
- Risk of increased pressor effects: α-adrenergic agonists

DIAGNOSTIC TEST EFFECTS
None known.

SIDE EFFECTS
Frequent (20%–7%)
Paresthesia, piloerection, pruritus, dysuria, supine hypertension
Occasional (< 7%–1%)
Pain, rash, chills, headache, facial flushing, confusion, dry mouth, anxiety

SERIOUS REACTIONS
! None known.

DENTAL CONSIDERATIONS

General:
- Carefully review patients medical and drug history.
- Supine hypotension is a serious side effect; a more upright chair position is highly desirable.
- Determine why patient is taking the drug.
- Monitor and record vital signs.
- Use vasoconstrictor with caution, in low doses, and with careful aspiration. Avoid using gingival retraction cord containing epinephrine.
- Examine for oral manifestation of opportunistic infection.
- Assess salivary flow as a factor in caries, periodontal disease, and candidiasis.
- Be aware of patient's disease, its severity, and frequency when known.
- Short appointments and a stress reduction protocol may be required for anxious patients.
- Precaution if dental surgery is anticipated or general anesthesia is required.

Consultations:
- Medical consultation may be required to assess disease control and patient's ability to tolerate stress.

Teach Patient/Family:
- Advise the patient to use OTC medications, such as cough, cold, and diet preparations, cautiously because that may affect blood pressure
- *When chronic dry mouth occurs advise patient:*
  - To avoid mouth rinses with high alcohol content due to drying effects
  - To use daily home fluoride products for anticaries effect
  - To use sugarless gum, frequent sips of water, or saliva substitutes

miglitol
mig-lee′-tall
(Glyset)

CATEGORY AND SCHEDULE
Pregnancy Risk Category: B

MECHANISM OF ACTION
An alpha-glucosidase inhibitor that delays the digestion of ingested carbohydrates into simple sugars such as glucose. ***Therapeutic Effect:*** Produces smaller rise in blood glucose concentration after meals.

AVAILABILITY
Tablets: 25 mg, 50 mg, 100 mg.

INDICATIONS AND DOSAGES

▸ Diabetes Mellitus

PO

Adults, Elderly. Initially, 25 mg 3 times a day with first bite of each main meal. Maintenance: 50 mg 3 times a day. Maximum: 100 mg 3 times a day.

CONTRAINDICATIONS

Colonic ulceration, diabetic ketoacidosis, hypersensitivity to miglitol, inflammatory bowel disease, partial intestinal obstruction

INTERACTIONS

Drug

Digoxin, propranolol, ranitidine: May decrease the blood concentrations and effects of these drugs.

Herbal

None known.

Food

None known.

Drug interactions of concern to dentistry

- None reported

DIAGNOSTIC TEST EFFECTS

None known.

SIDE EFFECTS

Frequent (40%–10%)

Flatulence, loose stools, diarrhea, abdominal pain

Occasional (5%)

Rash

DENTAL CONSIDERATIONS

General:

- Ensure that patient is following prescribed diet and regularly takes medication.
- Type 2 patients may also be using insulin. Should symptomatic hypoglycemia occur while taking this drug, use dextrose rather than sucrose because of interference with sucrose metabolism.
- Place on frequent recall to evaluate healing response.
- Short appointments and a stress reduction protocol may be required for anxious patients.
- Diabetics may be more susceptible to infection and have delayed wound healing.
- Consider semisupine chair position for patient comfort if GI side effects occur.
- Question patient about self-monitoring of drug's antidiabetic effect, including blood glucose values or finger-stick records.
- Examine for oral manifestation of opportunistic infection.

Consultations:

- Medical consultation may be required to assess disease control and patient's ability to tolerate stress.
- Medical consultation may include data from patient's blood glucose monitoring, including glycosylated hemoglobin or HbA_{1c} testing.

Teach Patient/Family:

- Importance of updating health and drug history if physician makes any changes in evaluation or drug regimens
- Importance of good oral hygiene to prevent soft tissue inflammation

miglustat

mig-lew′-stat

(Zavesca)

CATEGORY AND SCHEDULE

Pregnancy Risk Category: X

MECHANISM OF ACTION

A Gaucher disease agent that inhibits the enzyme,

glucosylceramide synthase, reducing the rate of synthesis of most glycosphingolipids. Allows the residual activity of the deficient enzyme, glucocerebrosidase, to be more effective in degrading lysosomal storage within tissues. ***Therapeutic Effect:*** Minimizes conditions associated with Gaucher's disease, such as anemia and bone disease.

AVAILABILITY

Capsules: 100 mg.

INDICATIONS AND DOSAGES

▸ Gaucher's Disease

PO

Adults, Elderly. One 100-mg capsule 3 times a day at regular intervals.

▸ Dosage in Renal Impairment

For patients with creatinine clearance of 50–70 ml/min, dosage is reduced to 100 mg twice a day. For patients with creatinine clearance of 30–49 ml/min dosage is 100 mg once a day.

CONTRAINDICATIONS

Women who are or may become pregnant

INTERACTIONS

Drug

Imiglucerase: May decrease the effects of imiglucerase.

Herbal

None known.

Food

None known.

Drug interactions of concern to dentistry

- None reported

DIAGNOSTIC TEST EFFECTS

None known.

SIDE EFFECTS

Expected (89%–65%)

Diarrhea, weight loss, dry mouth

Frequent (39%–11%)

Hand tremor, flatulence, headache, abdominal pain, nausea

Occasional (7%–4%)

Paresthesia, anorexia, dyspepsia, leg cramps, vomiting

SERIOUS REACTIONS

! Thrombocytopenia occurs in 7% of patients.

! Overdose produces dizziness and neutropenia.

DENTAL CONSIDERATIONS

General:

- Ask patient about disease control.
- Question patient about nosebleeds or other bleeding events.
- Short appointments and a stress reduction protocol may be required for anxious patients.
- Avoid products that affect platelet function, such as aspirin and NSAIDs.
- Patients on chronic drug therapy may rarely have symptoms of blood dyscrasias, which can include infection, bleeding, and poor healing.
- Assess salivary flow as a factor in caries, periodontal disease, and candidiasis.
- Consider semisupine chair position for patient comfort as needed.
- Place on frequent recall to evaluate healing response.

Consultations:

- Medical consultation may be required to assess disease control and patient's ability to tolerate stress.
- Medical consultation should include routine blood counts, including platelet counts and bleeding time.
- In a patient with symptoms of blood dyscrasias, request a medical consultation for blood studies and

postpone treatment until normal values are reestablished.

Teach Patient/Family:

- To inform dentist of unusual bleeding episodes following dental treatment
- Importance of good oral hygiene to prevent soft tissue inflammation/infection
- Use of electric toothbrush if patient has difficulty holding conventional devices

minocycline hydrochloride

mi-noe-sye′-kleen
(Akamin[AUS], Dynacin, Minocin, Minomycin[AUS], Myrac, Novo Minocycline[CAN])
Do not confuse Dynacin with Dynabac or Minocin with Mithracin or niacin.

CATEGORY AND SCHEDULE

Pregnancy Risk Category: D

MECHANISM OF ACTION

A tetracycline antibiotic that inhibits bacterial protein synthesis by binding to ribosomes. ***Therapeutic Effect:*** Bacteriostatic.

AVAILABILITY

Capsules (Dynacin, Minocin): 50 mg, 75 mg, 100 mg.
Capsules (Pellet-filled [Minocin]): 50 mg, 100 mg.
Tablets (Minocin, Myrac): 50 mg, 75 mg, 100 mg.
Powder for Injection (Minocin, Myrac): 100 mg.

INDICATIONS AND DOSAGES

▸ Mild, Moderate, or Severe Prostate, Urinary Tract, and CNS Infections (Excluding Meningitis); Uncomplicated Gonorrhea; Inflammatory Acne; Brucellosis; Skin Granulomas; Cholera; Trachoma; Nocardiasis; Yaws; and Syphilis When Penicillins Are Contraindicated

PO
Adults, Elderly. Initially, 100–200 mg, then 100 mg q12h or 50 mg q6h.
IV
Adults, Elderly. Initially, 200 mg, then 100 mg q12h up to 400 mg/day.
PO, IV
Children older than 8 yr. Initially, 4 mg/kg, then 2 mg/kg q12h.

OFF-LABEL USES

Treatment of atypical mycobacterial infections, rheumatoid arthritis, scleroderma

CONTRAINDICATIONS

Children younger than 8 years, hypersensitivity to tetracyclines, last half of pregnancy

INTERACTIONS

Drug

Carbamazepine, phenytoin: May decrease minocycline blood concentration.
Cholestyramine, colestipol: May decrease minocycline absorption.
Oral contraceptives: May decrease the effects of oral contraceptives.

Herbal

St. John's wort: May increase the risk of photosensitivity.

Food

None known.

Drug interactions of concern to dentistry

- Decreased effect: antacids, milk, or other calcium- and aluminum-containing products
- Decreased effect of penicillins

• Oral contraceptives: advise patient of a potential risk for decreased contraceptive action, to maintain compliance with oral contraceptive use while using antibiotics, and to consider the use of additional nonhormonal contraception
• Contraindicated with isotretinoin (Accutane)

Drug interactions of concern to dentistry minocycline HCl (microspheres)

• No dental drug interactions reported

DIAGNOSTIC TEST EFFECTS

May increase serum alkaline phosphatase, amylase, bilirubin, AST (SGOT), and ALT (SGPT) levels.

IV INCOMPATIBILITIES

Piperacillin and tazobactam (Zosyn)

IV COMPATIBILITIES

Heparin, magnesium, potassium

SIDE EFFECTS

Frequent

Dizziness, light-headedness, diarrhea, nausea, vomiting, abdominal cramps, possibly severe photosensitivity, drowsiness, vertigo

Occasional

Altered pigmentation of skin or mucous membranes, rectal or genital pruritus, stomatitis

SERIOUS REACTIONS

! Superinfection (especially fungal), anaphylaxis, and benign intracranial hypertension may occur.
! Bulging fontanelles occur rarely in infants.

DENTAL CONSIDERATIONS

General:

• This drug is reported to cause intrinsic staining in erupted permanent teeth not associated with the calcification stage.
• The drug readily distributes to gingival crevicular fluid.
• Do not prescribe drug during pregnancy or <8 yr because of tooth discoloration.
• Caution patients about driving or performing other tasks requiring alertness.
• Advise patient if dental drugs prescribed have a potential for photosensitivity.
• Do not use ingestible sodium bicarbonate products, such as the Prophy-Jet air polishing system, at the same time dose is taken; take minocycline 2 hr later.
• Determine why the patient is taking the drug.

Consultations:

Medical consultation may be required to assess disease control.

Teach Patient/Family:

• Importance of good oral hygiene to prevent soft tissue inflammation
• Caution to prevent injury when using oral hygiene aids
• To avoid mouth rinses with high alcohol content because of drying effects
• *When used for dental infection, advise patient:*
  • To report sore throat, oral burning sensation, fever, fatigue, any of which could indicate superinfection
  • To take at prescribed intervals and complete dosage regimen
  • To immediately notify the dentist if signs or symptoms of infection increase

DENTAL CONSIDERATIONS

MINOCYCLINE HCl (MICROSPHERES)

General:

• Follow all general precautions when using tetracyclines.

Teach Patient/Family:

• To avoid eating hard, crunchy foods for 1 wk
• To postpone toothbrushing for 12 hr
• To postpone use of interproximal cleaning devices for 10 days
• To notify dentist immediately if pain, swelling, or other unexpected symptoms occur

M

minoxidil

min-nox′-i-dill
(Apo-Gain[CAN], Loniten, Milnox[CAN], Regaine[AUS], Rogaine, Rogaine Extra Strength)
Do not confuse Loniten with Lotensin.

CATEGORY AND SCHEDULE

Pregnancy Risk Category: C
OTC (topical solution)

MECHANISM OF ACTION

An antihypertensive and hair growth stimulant that has direct action on vascular smooth muscle, producing vasodilation of arterioles.
Therapeutic Effect: Decreases peripheral vascular resistance and BP; increases cutaneous blood flow; stimulates hair follicle epithelium and hair follicle growth.

PHARMACOKINETICS

Route	Onset	Peak	Duration
PO	0.5 hr	2–8 hr	2–5 days

Well absorbed from the GI tract; minimal absorption after topical application. Protein binding: None. Widely distributed. Metabolized in the liver to active metabolite. Primarily excreted in urine. Removed by hemodialysis.
Half-life: 4.2 hr.

AVAILABILITY

Tablets (Loniten): 2.5 mg, 10 mg.
Topical Solution (Rogaine): 2% (20 mg/ml).
Topical Solution (Rogaine ExtraStrength): 5% (50 mg/ml).

INDICATIONS AND DOSAGES

▸ Severe Symptomatic Hypertension, Hypertension Associated with Organ Damage, Hypertension That Has Failed to Respond to Maximal Therapeutic Dosages of a Diuretic or Two Other Antihypertensives

PO

Adults. Initially, 5 mg/day. Increase with at least 3-day intervals to 10 mg, then 20 mg, then up to 40 mg/day in 1–2 doses.
Elderly. Initially, 2.5 mg/day. May increase gradually. Maintenance: 10–40 mg/day. Maximum: 100 mg/day.
Children. Initially, 0.1–0.2 mg/kg (5 mg maximum) daily. Gradually increase at a minimum of 3-day intervals. Maintenance: 0.25–1 mg/kg/day in 1–2 doses. Maximum: 50 mg/day.

▸ Hair Regrowth

TOPICAL

Adults. 1 ml to affected areas of scalp 2 times a day. Total daily dose not to exceed 2 ml.

CONTRAINDICATIONS

Pheochromocytoma

INTERACTIONS

Drug

NSAIDs: May decrease the hypotensive effects of minoxidil.
Parenteral antihypertensives: May increase hypotensive effect.

Herbal

None known.

Food

None known.

Drug interactions of concern to dentistry

• Decreased effects: NSAIDs, indomethacin, sympathomimetics
• Increased hypotension: CNS depressant drug used in conscious sedation technique may also lower blood pressure

DIAGNOSTIC TEST EFFECTS

May increase plasma renin activity and BUN, serum alkaline phosphatase, serum creatinine, and serum sodium levels. May decrease blood Hgb and Hct levels and erythrocyte count.

SIDE EFFECTS

Frequent

PO: Edema with concurrent weight gain, hypertrichosis (elongation, thickening, increased pigmentation of fine body hair; develops in 80% of patients within 3–6 weeks after beginning therapy)

Occasional

PO: T-wave changes (usually revert to pretreatment state with continued therapy or drug withdrawal)
Topical: Pruritus, rash, dry or flaking skin, erythema

Rare

PO: Breast tenderness, headache, photosensitivity reaction
Topical: Allergic reaction, alopecia, burning sensation at scalp, soreness at hair root, headache, visual disturbances

SERIOUS REACTIONS

! Tachycardia and angina pectoris may occur because of increased oxygen demands associated with increased heart rate and cardiac output.
! Fluid and electrolyte imbalance and CHF may occur, especially if a diuretic is not given concurrently with minoxidil.
! Too rapid reduction in BP may result in syncope, CVA, MI, and ocular or vestibular ischemia.
! Pericardial effusion and tamponade may be seen in patients with impaired renal function who are not on dialysis.

DENTAL CONSIDERATIONS

General:

• Monitor vital signs at every appointment because of CV side effects.
• Patients on chronic drug therapy may rarely have symptoms of blood dyscrasias, which can include infection, bleeding, and poor healing.
• Limit use of sodium-containing products, such as saline IV fluids, for patients with a dietary salt restriction.
• Short appointments and a stress reduction protocol may be required for anxious patients.
• After supine positioning, have patient sit upright for at least 2 min before standing to avoid orthostatic hypotension.

Consultations:

• In a patient with symptoms of blood dyscrasias, request a medical consultation for blood studies and postpone dental

treatment until normal values are reestablished.
• Medical consultation may be required to assess disease control and patient's ability to tolerate stress.

mirtazapine

mir-taz′-a-peen
(Avanza[AUS], Mirtazon[AUS], Remeron, Remeron Soltab)
Do not confuse Remeron with Premarin.

CATEGORY AND SCHEDULE

Pregnancy Risk Category: C

MECHANISM OF ACTION

A tetracyclic compound that acts as an antagonist at presynaptic alpha$_2$-adrenergic receptors, increasing both norepinephrine and serotonin neurotransmission. Has low anticholinergic activity. ***Therapeutic Effect:*** Relieves depression and produces sedative effects.

PHARMACOKINETICS

Rapidly and completely absorbed after PO administration; absorption not affected by food. Protein binding: 85%. Metabolized in the liver. Primarily excreted in urine. Unknown if removed by hemodialysis. ***Half-life:*** 20–40 hr (longer in males [37 hr] than females [26 hr]).

AVAILABILITY

Tablets: 7.5 mg, 15 mg, 30 mg, 45 mg.
Tablets (Disintegrating): 15 mg, 30 mg, 45 mg.

INDICATIONS AND DOSAGES

▸ Depression

PO

Adults. Initially, 15 mg at bedtime. May increase by 15 mg/day q1–2wk. Maximum: 45 mg/day.
Elderly. Initially, 7.5 mg at bedtime. May increase by 7.5-15 mg/day q1–2wk. Maximum: 45 mg/day.

CONTRAINDICATIONS

Use within 14 days of MAOIs

INTERACTIONS

Drug

Alcohol, diazepam: May increase impairment of cognition and motor skills.
MAOIs: May increase the risk of neuroleptic malignant syndrome, hypertensive crisis, and severe seizures.

Herbal

None known.

Food

None known.

Drug interactions of concern to dentistry

• Impairment of cognitive and motor performance with diazepam or other drugs used in conscious sedation
• Use opioid analgesics with caution because of impairment of cognitive or motor performance; NSAIDs may be a more appropriate choice

DIAGNOSTIC TEST EFFECTS

May increase serum cholesterol, triglyceride, AST (SGOT), and ALT (SGPT) levels.

SIDE EFFECTS

Frequent

Somnolence (54%), dry mouth (25%), increased appetite (17%), constipation (13%), weight gain (12%)

Occasional
Asthenia (8%), dizziness (7%), flulike symptoms (5%), abnormal dreams (4%)
Rare
Abdominal discomfort, vasodilation, paresthesia, acne, dry skin, thirst, arthralgia

SERIOUS REACTIONS

! Mirtazapine poses a higher risk of seizures than tricyclic antidepressants, especially in those with no previous history of seizures.
! Overdose may produce cardiovascular effects, such as severe orthostatic hypotension, dizziness, tachycardia, palpitations, and arrhythmias.
! Abrupt discontinuation after prolonged therapy may produce headache, malaise, nausea, vomiting, and vivid dreams.
! Agranulocytosis occurs rarely.

DENTAL CONSIDERATIONS

General:
- Patients on chronic drug therapy may rarely have symptoms of blood dyscrasias, which can include infection, bleeding, and poor healing.
- Assess salivary flow as a factor in caries, periodontal disease, and candidiasis.
- Monitor vital signs at every appointment because of CV side effects.
- Consider semisupine chair position for patient comfort of GI or MS side effects occur.
- Place on frequent recall if oral side effects are a problem.

Consultations:
- In a patient with symptoms of blood dyscrasias, request a medical consultation for blood studies and postpone dental treatment until normal values are reestablished.
- Take precaution if dental surgery is anticipated and sedation or general anesthesia is required; risk of hypotensive episode.
- Medical consultation may be required to assess disease control.
- Physician should be informed if significant xerostomic side effects occur (e.g., increased caries, sore tongue, problems eating or swallowing, difficulty wearing prosthesis) so that a medication change can be considered.

Teach Patient/Family:
- Importance of good oral hygiene to prevent soft tissue inflammation
- Caution to prevent soft tissue trauma when using oral hygiene aids
- Importance of updating health history/drug record if physician makes any changes in evaluation or drug regimens
- Caution about driving or performing other tasks requiring alertness
- *When chronic dry mouth occurs, advise patient:*
  - To avoid mouth rinses with high alcohol content because of drying effects
  - To use daily home fluoride products for anticaries effect
  - To use sugarless gum, frequent sips of water, or saliva substitutes

M

misoprostol

mis-oh-pros-toll
(Cytotec)
Do not confuse with Cytomel.

CATEGORY AND SCHEDULE

Pregnancy Risk Category: X

MECHANISM OF ACTION
A prostaglandin that inhibits basal, nocturnal gastric acid secretion via direct action on parietal cells. ***Therapeutic Effect:*** Increases production of protective gastric mucus.

PHARMACOKINETICS
Rapidly absorbed from gastrointestinal (GI) tract. Rapidly converted to active metabolite. Primarily excreted in urine. ***Half-life:*** 20–40 min.

AVAILABILITY
Tablets: 100 mcg, 200 mcg (Cytotec).

INDICATIONS AND DOSAGES
▸ Prevention of NSAID-Induced Gastric Ulcer
PO
Adults. 200 mcg 4 times/day with food (last dose at bedtime). Continue for duration of NSAID therapy. May reduce dosage to 100 mcg if 200 mcg dose is not tolerable.
Elderly: 100–200 mcg 4 times/day with food.

OFF-LABEL USES
Treatment of duodenal ulcer

CONTRAINDICATIONS
Pregnancy (produces uterine contractions), hypersensitivity to misoprostol or any component of the formulation

INTERACTIONS
Drug
Antacids: May decrease misoprostol effectiveness.
Phenylbutazone: May increase neurosensory effects (headache, dizziness, ataxia).
Herbal
None known.
Food
None known.

DIAGNOSTIC TEST EFFECTS
None known.

SIDE EFFECTS
Frequent
Abdominal pain, diarrhea
Occasional
Nausea, flatulence, dyspepsia, headache
Rare
Vomiting, constipation

SERIOUS REACTIONS
! Overdosage may produce sedation, tremor, convulsions, dyspnea, palpitations, hypotension, and bradycardia.

DENTAL CONSIDERATIONS
General:
- Avoid NSAIDs and salicylates in patients with upper active GI disease; acetaminophen/opioids are more appropriate for pain control in these patients.

Consultations:
- Medical consultation may be required to assess disease control.

mitotane
my′-tow-tane
(Lysodren)

CATEGORY AND SCHEDULE
Pregnancy Risk Category: C

MECHANISM OF ACTION
A hormonal agent that inhibits activity of the adrenal cortex. ***Therapeutic Effect:*** Suppresses functional and nonfunctional adrenocortical neoplasms by direct cytoxic effect.

AVAILABILITY

Tablets: 500 mg.

INDICATIONS AND DOSAGES

▸ Adrenocortical Carcinomas

PO

Adults, Elderly. Initially, 2–6 g/day in 3–4 divided doses. Increase by 2–4 g/day every 3–7 days up to 9–10 g/day. Range: 2–16 g/day.

OFF-LABEL USES

Treatment of Cushing's syndrome

CONTRAINDICATIONS

Known hypersensitivity to mitotane

INTERACTIONS

Drug

CNS depressants: May increase CNS depression.

Herbal

None known.

Food

None known.

Drug interactions of concern to dentistry

- Increased CNS depression: all CNS depressants
- Decreased effects of corticosteroids; if glucocorticoid replacement is necessary, use hydrocortisone

DIAGNOSTIC TEST EFFECTS

May decrease levels of plasma cortisol, urinary 17-hydroxycorticosteroids, protein-bound iodine, and serum uric acid.

SIDE EFFECTS

Frequent (>15%)

Anorexia, nausea, vomiting, diarrhea, lethargy, somnolence, adrenocortical insufficiency, dizziness, vertigo, maculopapular rash, hypouricemia

Occasional (<15%)

Blurred or double vision, retinopathy, hearing loss, excessive salivation, urine abnormalities (hematuria, cystitis, albuminuria), hypertension, orthostatic hypotension, flushing, wheezing, dyspnea, generalized aching, fever

SERIOUS REACTIONS

! Brain damage and functional impairment may occur with long-term, high-dosage therapy.

DENTAL CONSIDERATIONS

General:

- Evaluate respiration characteristics and rate.
- Drug may cause adrenal hypofunction, especially under conditions of stress such as surgery, trauma, or acute illness. Patients should be carefully monitored and given hydrocortisone or mineralocorticoid as needed.
- Consider semisupine chair position for patient comfort if GI side effects occur.
- Patients taking opioids for acute or chronic pain should be given alternative analgesics for dental pain.

Consultations:

- Medical consultation may be required to assess disease control and patient's ability to tolerate stress.

Teach Patient/Family:

- That secondary oral infection may occur; must see dentist immediately if infection occurs
- To report oral lesions, soreness, or bleeding to dentist
- Importance of updating medical/drug records if physician makes any changes in evaluation or drug regimens

mitoxantrone

my-toe-zan′-trone
(Novantrone, Onkotrone[AUS])

CATEGORY AND SCHEDULE

Pregnancy Risk Category: D

MECHANISM OF ACTION

An anthracenedione that inhibits B-cell, T-cell, and macrophage proliferation and DNA and RNA synthesis. Active throughout the entire cell cycle. ***Therapeutic Effect:*** Causes cell death.

PHARMACOKINETICS

Protein binding: 78%. Widely distributed. Metabolized in the liver. Primarily eliminated in feces by the biliary system. Not removed by hemodialysis. ***Half-life:*** 2.3–13 days.

M

AVAILABILITY

Injection: 2 mg/ml.

INDICATIONS AND DOSAGES

▸ **Leukemias**

IV

Adults, Elderly, Children 2 yr and older. 12 mg/m² once a day for 2–3 days.

Children younger than 2 yr. 0.4 mg/kg once a day for 3–5 days.

▸ **Acute Leukemia in Relapse**

IV

Adults, Elderly, Children older than 2 yr. 8–12 mg/m² once a day for 4–5 days.

▸ **Acute Nonlymphocytic Leukemia**

IV

Adults, Elderly, Children older than 2 yr. 10 mg/m² once a day for 3–5 days.

▸ **Solid Tumors**

IV

Adults, Elderly. 12–14 mg/m² once q3–4wk.

Children. 18–20 mg/m² once q3–4wk.

▸ **Prostate Cancer**

IV

Adults, Elderly. 12–14 mg/m² every 21 days.

▸ **Multiple Sclerosis**

IV

Adults, Elderly. 12 mg/m²/dose q3mo.

OFF-LABEL USES

Treatment of acute lymphocytic leukemia, breast or hepatic carcinoma, non-Hodgkin's lymphoma

CONTRAINDICATIONS

Baseline left ventricular ejection fraction less than 50%, cumulative lifetime mitoxantrone dose of 140 mg/m² or more, multiple sclerosis with hepatic impairment

INTERACTIONS

Drug

Antigout medications: May decrease the effects of these drugs.

Bone marrow depressants: May increase myelosuppression.

Live-virus vaccines: May potentiate virus replication, increase vaccine side effects, and decrease the patient's antibody response to the vaccine.

Herbal

None known.

Food

None known.

Drug interactions of concern to dentistry

- None reported

DIAGNOSTIC TEST EFFECTS
May increase serum bilirubin and uric acid, AST, and ALT levels.

IV INCOMPATIBILITIES
Aztreonam (Azactam), cefepime (Maxipime), heparin, paclitaxel (Taxol), piperacillin and tazobactam (Zosyn)

IV COMPATIBILITIES
Allopurinol (Aloprim), etoposide (VePesid), gemcitabine (Gemzar), granisetron (Kytril), ondansetron (Zofran), potassium chloride

SIDE EFFECTS
Frequent (>10%)
Nausea, vomiting, diarrhea, cough, headache, stomatitis, abdominal discomfort, fever, alopecia
Occasional (9%–4%)
Ecchymosis, fungal infection, conjunctivitis, UTI
Rare (3%)
Arrhythmias

SERIOUS REACTIONS
! Myelosuppression may be severe, resulting in GI bleeding, hematologic toxicity, sepsis, and pneumonia.
! Renal failure, seizures, jaundice, and CHF may occur.
! Cardiotoxicity has been reported during therapy.

DENTAL CONSIDERATIONS
General:
- Monitor and record vital signs.
- If additional analgesia is required for dental pain, consider alternative analgesics (NSAIDs) in patients taking narcotics for acute or chronic pain.
- Examine for oral manifestation of opportunistic infection.
- Avoid products that affect platelet function, such as aspirin and NSAIDs.
- This drug may be used in the hospital or on an outpatient basis. Confirm the patient's disease and treatment status.
- Chlorhexidine mouth rinse prior to and during chemotherapy may reduce severity of mucositis.
- Patient on chronic drug therapy may rarely present with symptoms of blood dyscrasias, which can include infection, bleeding, and poor healing. If dyscrasia is present, caution patient to prevent oral tissue trauma when using oral hygiene aids.
- Palliative medication may be required for management of oral side effects.

Short appointments and a stress reduction protocol may be required for anxious patients.
- Provide emergency dental care only during drug use.
- Patients may be at risk of bleeding, check for oral signs.
- Oral infections should be eliminated and treated aggressively.
- Patients may have received other chemotherapy or radiation, confirm medical and drug history.
- Place on frequent recall due to oral side effects

Consultations:
- Medical consultation should include routine blood counts including platelet counts and bleeding time.
- Consult physician; prophylactic or therapeutic antiinfectives may be indicated if surgery or periodontal treatment is required.
- Medical consultation may be required to assess immunologic status during cancer chemotherapy and determine safety risk, if any, posed by the required dental treatment.
- Medical consultation may be required to assess disease control and patient's ability to tolerate stress.

Teach Patient/Family:
• Secondary oral infection may occur; need to see dentist immediately if infection occurs
• To be aware of oral side effects
• Importance of good oral hygiene to prevent soft tissue inflammation
• To report oral lesions, soreness, or bleeding to dentist
• To prevent trauma when using oral hygiene aids
• Importance of updating health and medication history if physician makes any changes in evaluation or drug regimens; include OTC, herbal, and nonherbal in the update

modafinil

mode-ah-feen′-awl
(Alertec[CAN], Modavigil[AUS], Provigil)

M

CATEGORY AND SCHEDULE

Pregnancy Risk Category: C

MECHANISM OF ACTION

An $alpha_1$-agonist that may bind to dopamine reuptake carrier sites, increasing alpha activity and decreasing delta, theta, and beta brain wave activity. ***Therapeutic Effect:*** Reduces the number of sleep episodes and total daytime sleep.

PHARMACOKINETICS

Well absorbed. Protein binding: 60%. Widely distributed. Metabolized in the liver. Excreted by the kidneys. Unknown if removed by hemodialysis. ***Half-life:*** 8–10 hr.

AVAILABILITY

Tablets: 100 mg, 200 mg.

INDICATIONS AND DOSAGES

▸ **Narcolepsy, Other Sleep Disorders**
PO
Adults, Elderly. 200–400 mg/day.

OFF-LABEL USES

Treatment of depression

CONTRAINDICATIONS

None known.

INTERACTIONS

Drug

Cyclosporine, oral contraceptives, theophylline: May decrease plasma concentrations of these drugs.
Diazepam, phenytoin, propranolol, tricyclic antidepressants, warfarin: May increase plasma concentrations of these drugs.
Other CNS stimulants: May increase CNS stimulation.

Herbal

None known.

Food

None known.

Drug interactions of concern to dentistry

• No documented dental drug interactions reported; however, because it induces cytochrome P-450 isoenzymes, other P-450 isoenzyme inducers or inhibitors (antifungal agents, erythromycin) could result in a drug interaction

DIAGNOSTIC TEST EFFECTS

None known.

SIDE EFFECTS

Frequent

Anxiety, insomnia, nausea

Occasional

Anorexia, diarrhea, dizziness, dry mouth or skin, muscle stiffness, polydipsia, rhinitis, paraesthesia, tremor, headache, vomiting

SERIOUS REACTIONS

! Agitation, excitation, hypertension, and insomnia may occur.

DENTAL CONSIDERATIONS

General:

- Monitor vital signs at every appointment because of CV side effects.
- Assess salivary flow as a factor in caries, periodontal disease, and candidiasis.
- Consider semisupine chair position for patient comfort because of GI side effects of drug.
- Short appointments and a stress reduction protocol may be required for anxious patients.

Teach Patient/Family:

- To prevent trauma when using oral hygiene aids
- *When chronic dry mouth occurs, advise patient:*
  - To avoid mouth rinses with high alcohol content because of drying effects
  - To use daily home fluoride products for anticaries effect
  - To use sugarless gum, frequent sips of water, or saliva substitutes

moexipril hydrochloride

moe-ex′-a-prile
(Univasc)

CATEGORY AND SCHEDULE

Pregnancy Risk Category: C (D if used in second or third trimesters)

MECHANISM OF ACTION

An ACE inhibitor that suppresses the renin-angiotensin-aldosterone system and prevents conversion of angiotensin I to angiotensin II, a potent vasoconstrictor; may also inhibit angiotensin II at local vascular and renal sites. ***Therapeutic Effect:*** Reduces peripheral arterial resistance and lowers BP.

PHARMACOKINETICS

Route	Onset	Peak	Duration
PO	1 hr	3–6 hr	24 hr

Incompletely absorbed from the GI tract. Food decreases drug absorption. Rapidly converted to active metabolite. Protein binding: 50%. Primarily recovered in feces, partially excreted in urine. Unknown if removed by dialysis. ***Half-life:*** 1 hr, metabolite 2–9 hr.

AVAILABILITY

Tablets: 7.5 mg, 15 mg.

INDICATIONS AND DOSAGES

▸ **Hypertension**

PO

Adults, Elderly. For patients not receiving diuretics, initial dose is 7.5 mg once a day 1 hr before meals. Adjust according to BP effect. Maintenance: 7.5–30 mg a day in 1–2 divided doses 1 hr before meals.

▸ **Hypertension in Patients with Impaired Renal Function**

PO

Adults, Elderly. 3.75 mg once a day in patients with creatinine clearance of 40 ml/min. Maximum: May titrate up to 15 mg/day.

CONTRAINDICATIONS

History of angioedema from previous treatment with ACE inhibitors

INTERACTIONS

Drug

Alcohol, antihypertensives, diuretics: May increase the effects of moexipril.

M

Lithium: May increase lithium blood concentration and risk of lithium toxicity.
NSAIDs: May decrease the effects of moexipril.
Potassium-sparing diuretics, potassium supplements: May cause hyperkalemia.

Herbal

None known.

Food

None known.

Drug interactions of concern to dentistry

- IV fluids containing potassium: risk of hyperkalemia
- Increased hypotension: other hypotensive drugs, alcohol, phenothiazines
- Decreased hypotensive effects: indomethacin, possibly other NSAIDs, sympathomimetics
- Suspected reduction in the antihypertensive and vasodilator effects by salicylates; monitor blood pressure if used concurrently

DIAGNOSTIC TEST EFFECTS

May increase BUN, serum alkaline phosphatase, serum bilirubin, serum creatinine, serum potassium, AST (SGOT), and ALT (SGPT) levels. May decrease serum sodium levels. May cause positive serum antinuclear antibody titer.

SIDE EFFECTS

Occasional

Cough, headache (6%); dizziness (4%); fatigue (3%)

Rare

Flushing, rash, myalgia, nausea, vomiting

SERIOUS REACTIONS

! Excessive hypotension ("first-dose syncope") may occur in patients with CHF and in those who are severely salt or volume depleted.
! Angioedema (swelling of face and lips) and hyperkalemia occur rarely.
! Agranulocytosis and neutropenia may be noted in those with collagen vascular disease, including scleroderma and systemic lupus erythematosus, and impaired renal function.
! Nephrotic syndrome may be noted in those with history of renal disease.

DENTAL CONSIDERATIONS

General:

- Monitor vital signs at every appointment because of CV side effects.
- After supine positioning, have patient sit upright for at least 2 min before standing to avoid orthostatic hypotension.
- Take precautions if dental surgery is anticipated and general anesthesia is required.
- Patients on chronic drug therapy may rarely have symptoms of blood dyscrasias, which can include infection, bleeding, and poor healing.
- Stress from dental procedures may compromise CV function; determine patient risk.
- Assess salivary flow as a factor in caries, periodontal disease, and candidiasis.
- Short appointments and a stress reduction protocol may be required for anxious patients.

Consultations:

- Medical consultation may be required to assess disease control and patient's ability to tolerate stress.
- In a patient with symptoms of blood dyscrasias, request a medical consultation for blood studies and postpone dental treatment until normal values are reestablished.

Teach Patient/Family:

- Importance of good oral hygiene to prevent soft tissue inflammation

- Caution to prevent trauma when using oral hygiene aids
- To report oral lesions, soreness, or bleeding to dentist
- *When chronic dry mouth occurs, advise patient:*
  - To avoid mouth rinses with high alcohol content because of drying effects
  - Of need for daily home fluoride use to prevent caries
  - To use sugarless gum, frequent sips of water, or saliva substitutes

molindone

moe-lin-′-done
(Moban)
Do not confuse with Mobic.

CATEGORY AND SCHEDULE

Pregnancy Risk Category: C

MECHANISM OF ACTION

An indole derivative of dihydroindole compounds that reduces spontaneous locomotion and aggressiveness.
Therapeutic Effect: Suppresses behavioral response in psychosis.

PHARMACOKINETICS

Rapidly absorbed from the gastrointestinal (GI) tract. Metabolized in liver. Excreted feces, and a small amount excreted via lungs as carbon dioxide. Not removed by dialysis.
Half-life: unknown.

AVAILABILITY

Oral Solutions: 20 mg/ml (Moban).
Tablets: 5 mg, 10 mg, 25 mg, 50 mg, 100 mg (Moban).

INDICATIONS AND DOSAGES

▸ **Schizophrenia**

PO

Adults, Children 12 yrs and older. Initially, 50–75 mg/day, increased to 100 mg/day in 3–4 days.
Maintenance: 5–15 mg 3–4 times/day (mild psychosis).
Maintenance: 10–25 mg 3–4 times/day (moderate psychosis).
Maintenance: 225 mg/day maximum in divided doses (severe psychosis).
Elderly. Start at a lower dose.

CONTRAINDICATIONS

Severe central nervous system (CNS) depression, hypersensitivity to molindone or any component of the formulation

INTERACTIONS

Drug

Alcohol, CNS depressants: May increase CNS and respiratory depression of molindone.
Lithium: May decrease the absorption of molindone and produce adverse neurologic effects.
Vitex: May decrease effectiveness of molindone.

Herbal

Betel nut: May increase extrapyramidal side effects of molindone.
Kava kava: May add to dopamine antagonist effects.

Food

None known.

Drug interactions of concern to dentistry

- Increased sedation: alcohol, other CNS depressants
- Increased anticholinergic effect: anticholinergics, antihistamines

DIAGNOSTIC TEST EFFECTS

None known.

IV INCOMPATIBILITIES

None known.

IV COMPATIBILITIES

None known.

M

SIDE EFFECTS

Frequent
Blurred vision, constipation, drowsiness, headache, extrapyramidal symptoms
Occasional
Mental depression
Rare
Skin rash, hot and dry skin, inability to sweat, muscle weakness, confusion, jaundice, convulsions

SERIOUS REACTIONS

! Neuroleptic malignant syndrome or tardive dyskinesia has been reported.

DENTAL CONSIDERATIONS

General:

- Patients on chronic drug therapy may rarely have symptoms of blood dyscrasias, which can include infection, bleeding, and poor healing.
- Assess salivary flow as a factor in caries, periodontal disease, and candidiasis.
- After supine positioning, have patient sit upright for at least 2 min before standing to avoid orthostatic hypotension.
- Assess for presence of extrapyramidal motor symptoms, such as tardive dyskinesia and akathisia. Extrapyramidal motor activity may complicate dental treatment.
- Geriatric patients are more susceptible to drug effects; use lower dose.
- Use vasoconstrictors with caution, in low doses, and with careful aspiration.

Consultations:

- In a patient with symptoms of blood dyscrasias, request a medical consultation for blood studies and postpone dental treatment until normal values are reestablished.
- Medical consultation may be required to assess disease control.

Teach Patient/Family:

- Importance of good oral hygiene to prevent soft tissue inflammation
- Caution to prevent injury when using oral hygiene aids
- *When chronic dry mouth occurs, advise patient:*
  - To avoid mouth rinses with high alcohol content because of drying effects
  - To use sugarless gum, frequent sips of water, or saliva substitutes
  - To use daily home fluoride products for anticaries effect

M

mometasone furoate monohydrate

mo-met′-a-sone
(Allermax Aqueous[AUS], Asmanex Twisthaler, Elocon Cream[AUS], Elocon Ointment [AUS], Nasonex, Nasonex Nasal Spray[AUS], Novasone Cream [AUS], Novasone Lotion[AUS], Novasone Ointment[AUS])

CATEGORY AND SCHEDULE

Pregnancy Risk Category: C

MECHANISM OF ACTION

An adrenocorticosteroid that inhibits the release of inflammatory cells into nasal tissue, preventing early activation of the allergic reaction.
Therapeutic Effect: Decreases response to seasonal and perennial rhinitis.

PHARMACOKINETICS

Undetectable in plasma. Protein binding: 98%–99%. The swallowed portion undergoes extensive metabolism. Excreted primarily through bile and, to a lesser extent, urine. ***Half-life:*** 5.8 hr (nasal).

AVAILABILITY
*Nasal Spray (Nasonex):*50 mcg/spray.
Cream (Elocon): 0.1%.
Lotion (Elocon): 0.1%.
Ointment (Elocon): 0.1%.
Oral inhaler (Asmanex Twisthaler): 220 mcg.

INDICATIONS AND DOSAGES
▶ Allergic Rhinitis
Nasal Spray
Adults, Elderly, Children 12 yr and older. 2 sprays in each nostril once a day.
Children 2–11 yr. 1 spray in each nostril once a day.
▶ Asthma
INHALATION
Adults, Elderly, Children 12 yr and older. Initially, inhale 220 mcg (1 puff) once a day. Maximum: 880 mcg once a day.
▶ Skin Disease
TOPICAL
Adults, Elderly, Children 12 yr and older. Apply cream, lotion, or ointment to affected area once a day.
▶ Nasal Polyp
Nasal spray
Adults, Elderly. 2 sprays in each nostril twice a day.

CONTRAINDICATIONS
Hypersensitivity to any corticosteroid, persistently positive sputum cultures for *Candida albicans*, status asthmaticus (inhalation), systemic fungal infections, untreated localized infection involving nasal mucosa.

INTERACTIONS
Drug
Ketoconazole: May increase mometasone plasma concentrations (inhalation).
Herbal
None known.
Food
None known.
Drug interactions of concern to dentistry
- None reported

DIAGNOSTIC TEST EFFECTS
None known.

SIDE EFFECTS
Occasional
Inhalation: Headache, allergic rhinitis, upper respiratory infection, muscle pain, fatigue
Nasal: Nasal irritation, stinging
Topical: Burning
Rare
Inhalation: Abdominal pain, dyspepsia, nausea
Nasal: Nasal or pharyngeal candidiasis
Topical: Pruritus

SERIOUS REACTIONS
! An acute hypersensitivity reaction, including urticaria, angioedema, and severe bronchospasm, occurs rarely.
! Transfer from systemic to local steroid therapy may unmask previously suppressed bronchial asthma condition.

DENTAL CONSIDERATIONS
General:
- Allergic rhinitis may be a factor in mouth breathing and drying of oral tissues.
- Examine for oral manifestation of opportunistic infection.

Teach Patient/Family:
- Importance of gargling, rinsing mouth with water, and expectorating after each aerosol dose

montelukast

mon-te′-loo-kast
(Singulair)

CATEGORY AND SCHEDULE

Pregnancy Risk Category: B

MECHANISM OF ACTION

An antiasthmatic that binds to cysteinyl leukotriene receptors, inhibiting the effects of leukotrienes on bronchial smooth muscle.
Therapeutic Effect: Decreases bronchoconstriction, vascular permeability, mucosal edema, and mucus production.

PHARMACOKINETICS

Route	Onset	Peak	Duration
PO	N/A	N/A	24 hr
PO (chewable)	N/A	N/A	24 hr

Rapidly absorbed from the GI tract. Protein binding: 99%. Extensively metabolized in the liver. Excreted almost exclusively in feces. ***Half-life:*** 2.7–5.5 hr (slightly longer in the elderly).

AVAILABILITY

Oral Granules: 4 mg.
Tablets: 10 mg.
Tablets (Chewable): 4 mg, 5 mg.

INDICATIONS AND DOSAGES

▸ **Bronchial Asthma**

PO

Adults, Elderly, Adolescents older than 14 yr. One 10-mg tablet a day, taken in the evening.
Children 6–14 yr. One 5-mg chewable tablet a day, taken in the evening.
Children 1–5 yr. One 4-mg chewable tablet a day, taken in the evening.

CONTRAINDICATIONS

None known.

INTERACTIONS

Drug

Phenobarbital, rifampin: May decrease montelukast's duration of action.

Herbal

None known.

Food

None known.

Drug interactions of concern to dentistry

• None reported; however, monitor patients when strong inhibitors of CYP3A4 or CYP2C9 are prescribed

DIAGNOSTIC TEST EFFECTS

May increase AST(SGOT) and ALT(SGPT) levels.

SIDE EFFECTS

Adults, Adolescents 15 years and older

Frequent (18%)

Headache

Occasional (4%)

Influenza

Rare (3%–2%)

Abdominal pain, cough, dyspepsia, dizziness, fatigue, dental pain

Children 6–14 years

Rare (<2%)

Diarrhea, laryngitis, pharyngitis, nausea, otitis media, sinusitis, viral infection

SERIOUS REACTIONS

! None known.

DENTAL CONSIDERATIONS

General:

• Midday appointments and a stress reduction protocol may be required for anxious patients.
• Avoid prescribing aspirin-containing products.

• Acute asthmatic episodes may be precipitated in the dental office. Rapid-acting sympathomimetic inhalants should be available for emergency use. A stress reduction protocol may be required.
• Be aware that aspirin or sulfite preservatives in vasoconstrictor-containing products can exacerbate asthma.
• Consider semisupine chair position for patients with respiratory disease or if GI side effects occur.

Consultations:
• Medical consultation may be required to assess disease control.

Teach Patient/Family:
• Importance of updating health and drug history if physician makes any changes in evaluation or drug regimens

moricizine hydrochloride

mor-iss′-i-zeen
(Ethmozine)

CATEGORY AND SCHEDULE
Pregnancy Risk Category: B

MECHANISM OF ACTION
An antiarrhythmic that prevents sodium current across myocardial cell membranes. Has potent local anesthetic activity and membrane stabilizing effects. Slows AV and His-Purkinje conduction and decreases action potential duration and effective refractory period.
Therapeutic Effect: Suppresses ventricular arrhythmias.

AVAILABILITY
Tablets: 200 mg, 250 mg, 300 mg.

INDICATIONS AND DOSAGES
▸ **Arrhythmias**
PO
Adults, Elderly. 200–300 mg q8h. May increase by 150 mg/day at no less than 3-day intervals.

OFF-LABEL USES
Atrial arrhythmias, complete and non-sustained ventricular arrhythmias, premature ventricular contractions (PVCs)

CONTRAINDICATIONS
Cardiogenic shock, preexisting second- or third-degree AV block or right bundle-branch block without pacemaker

INTERACTIONS
Drug
Cimetidine: May increase blood concentration of moricizine.
Theophylline: May decrease blood concentrations of theophylline.
Herbal
None known.
Food
None known.
Drug interactions of concern to dentistry
• No specific interactions are reported with dental drugs; however, any drug that could affect the cardiac action of moricizine (e.g., other local anesthetics, vasoconstrictors, anticholinergics) should be used in the lowest effective dose

DIAGNOSTIC TEST EFFECTS
May cause ECG changes, such as prolonged PR and QT intervals.

SIDE EFFECTS
Frequent (15%–6%)
Dizziness, nausea, headache, fatigue, dyspnea

M

Occasional (5%–2%)
Nervousness, paraesthesia, sleep disturbances, dyspepsia, vomiting, diarrhea, dry mouth

SERIOUS REACTIONS

! Moricizine may worsen existing arrhythmias or produce new ones.
! Jaundice with hepatitis occurs rarely.
! Overdosage produces vomiting, lethargy, syncope, hypotension, conduction disturbances, exacerbation of CHF, MI, and sinus arrest.

DENTAL CONSIDERATIONS

General:
- Monitor vital signs at every appointment because of CV side effects.
- Assess salivary flow as a factor in caries, periodontal disease, and candidiasis.
- Stress from dental procedures may compromise CV function; determine patient risk.

Consultations:
- Medical consultation should be made to assess disease control and patient's ability to tolerate stress.

Teach Patient/Family:
- Importance of good oral hygiene to prevent soft tissue inflammation
- Caution to prevent injury when using oral hygiene aids
- *When chronic dry mouth occurs, advise patient:*
  - To avoid mouth rinses with high alcohol content because of drying effects
  - To use sugarless gum, frequent sips of water, or saliva substitutes
  - To use daily home fluoride products for anticaries effect

M

morphine sulfate

mor′-feen
Schedule II
(Anamorph[AUS], Astramorph, Avinza, DepoDur, Duramorph, Infumorph, Kadian, Kapanol[AUS], M-Eslon, Morphine Mixtures[AUS], MS Contin, MSIR, MS Mono[AUS], Oramorph SR, RMS, Roxanol, Statex[CAN])
Do not confuse morphine with hydromorphone, or Roxanol with Roxicet.

CATEGORY AND SCHEDULE

Pregnancy Risk Category: C (D if used for prolonged periods or at high dosages at term)
Controlled Substance: Schedule II

MECHANISM OF ACTION

An opioid agonist that binds with opioid receptors in the CNS.
Therapeutic Effect: Alters the perception of and emotional response to pain; produces generalized CNS depression.

PHARMACOKINETICS

Route	Onset	Peak	Duration
Oral Solution	N/A	1 hr	3–5 hr
Tablets	N/A	1 hr	3–5 hr
Tablets (ER)	N/A	3–4 hr	8–12 hr
IV	Rapid	0.3 hr	3–5 hr
IM	5–30 min	0.5–1 hr	3–5 hr
Epidural	N/A	1 hr	12–20 hr
Subcutaneous	N/A	1.1–5 hr	3–5 hr
Rectal	N/A	0.5–1 hr	3–7 hr

Variably absorbed from the GI tract. Readily absorbed after IM or subcutaneous administration. Protein binding: 20%–35%. Widely distributed. Metabolized in the liver. Primarily excreted in urine.

Removed by hemodialysis. ***Half-life:*** 2–3 hr. (increased in patients with hepatic disease)

AVAILABILITY

Capsules (Extended-Release [Kadian]): 20 mg, 30 mg, 50 mg, 60 mg, 100 mg.
Capsules (Extended-Release [Avinza]): 30 mg, 60 mg, 90 mg, 120 mg.
Capsules (MSIR): 15 mg, 30 mg.
Solution for Injection: 2 mg/ml, 4 mg/ml, 5 mg/ml, 8 mg/ml, 10 mg/ml, 15 mg/ml, 25 mg/ml.
Solution for Injection (Preservative-Free): 10 mg/ml, 15 mg/ml, 25 mg/ml, 50 mg/ml.
Epidural and Intrathecal via Infusion Device (Infumorph): 10 mg/ml, 25 mg/ml.
Epidural, Intrathecal, IV Infusion (Astramorph, Duramorph): 0.5 mg/ml, 1 mg/ml.
Oral Solution (MSIR): 10 mg/ml, 20 mg/ml.
Oral Solution (Roxanol): 20 mg/ml, 100 mg/ml.
Suppositories (RMS): 5 mg, 10 mg, 20 mg, 30 mg.
Tablets (MSIR): 15 mg, 30 mg.
Tablets (Extended-Release [MS Contin]): 15 mg, 30 mg, 60 mg, 100 mg, 200 mg.
Tablets (Extended-Release [Oramorph SR]): 15 mg, 30 mg, 60 mg, 100 mg.
Liposomal Injection (DepoDur): 10 mg/ml, 15 mg/1.5 ml, 20 mg/2 ml.

INDICATIONS AND DOSAGES

Alert: Dosage should be titrated to desired effect.

▸ Analgesia

PO (Prompt-release)
Adults, Elderly. 10–30 mg q3–4h as needed.
Children. 0.2–0.5 mg/kg q3–4h as needed.
Alert: For the Avinza dosage below, be aware that this drug is to be administered once a day only.
Alert: For the Kadian dosage information below, be aware that this drug is to be administered q12h or once a day only.
Alert: Be aware that pediatric dosages of extended-release preparations Kadian and Avinza have not been established.
Alert: For the MSContin and Oramorph SR dosage information below, be aware that the daily dosage is divided and given q8h or q12h.
PO (Extended-Release [Avinza])
Adults, Elderly. Dosage requirement should be established using prompt-release formulations and is based on total daily dose. Avinza is given once a day only.
PO (Extended-Release [Kadian])
Adults, Elderly. Dosage requirement should be established using prompt-release formulations and is based on total daily dose. Dose is given once a day or divided and given q12h.
PO (Extended-Release [MSContin, Oramorph SR])
Adults, Elderly. Dosage requirement should be established using prompt-release formulations and is based on total daily dose. Daily dose is divided and given q8h or q12h.
Children. 0.3–0.6 mg/kg/dose q12h.
IV
Adults, Elderly. 2.5–5 mg q3–4h as needed. Note: Repeated doses (e.g. 1–2 mg) may be given more frequently (e.g. every hour) if needed.
Children. 0.05–0.1 mg/kg q3–4h as needed.
IV CONTINUOUS INFUSION
Adults, Elderly. 0.8–10 mg/h. Range: Up to 80 mg/h.
Children. 10–30 mcg/kg/hr.

IM
Adults, Elderly. 5–10 mg q3–4h as needed.
Children. 0.1 mg/kg q3–4h as needed.
EPIDURAL
Adults, Elderly. Initially, 1–6 mg bolus, infusion rate: 0.1–1 mg/h. Maximum: 10 mg/24 h.
INTRATHECAL
Adults, Elderly. One-tenth of the epidural dose: 0.2–1 mg/dose.

▸ **PCA**
IV
Adults, Elderly. Loading dose: 5–10 mg. Intermittent bolus: 0.5–3 mg. Lockout interval: 5–12 min. Continuous infusion: 1–10 mg/hr. 4-hr limit: 20–30 mg.

CONTRAINDICATIONS
Acute or severe asthma, GI obstruction, severe hepatic or renal impairment, severe respiratory depression, asthma, severe liver or renal impairment

M

INTERACTIONS
Drug
Alcohol, other CNS depressants: May increase CNS or respiratory depression and hypotension.
MAOIs: May produce a severe, sometimes fatal reaction; expect to administer one quarter of usual morphine dose.
Herbal
None known.
Food
None known.
Drug interactions of concern to dentistry
- Increased CNS depression: alcohol, all CNS depressants
- Contraindication: MAOIs
- Increased effects of anticholinergics

DIAGNOSTIC TEST EFFECTS
May increase serum amylase and lipase levels.

IV INCOMPATIBILITIES
Amphotericin B complex (Abelcet, AmBisome, Amphotec), cefepime (Maxipime), doxorubicin liposomal (Doxil), thiopental

IV COMPATIBILITIES
Amiodarone (Cordarone), atropine, bumetanide (Bumex), bupivacaine (Marcaine, Sensorcaine), diltiazem (Cardizem), diphenhydramine (Benadryl), dobutamine (Dobutrex), dopamine (Intropin), glycopyrrolate (Robinul), heparin, hydroxyzine (Vistaril), lidocaine, lorazepam (Ativan), magnesium, midazolam (Versed), milrinone (Primacor), nitroglycerin, potassium, propofol (Diprivan)

SIDE EFFECTS
Frequent
Sedation, decreased BP (including orthostatic hypotension), diaphoresis, facial flushing, constipation, dizziness, somnolence, nausea, vomiting
Occasional
Allergic reaction (rash, pruritus), dyspnea, confusion, palpitations, tremors, urine retention, abdominal cramps, vision changes, dry mouth, headache, decreased appetite, pain or burning at injection site
Rare
Paralytic ileus

SERIOUS REACTIONS
! Overdose results in respiratory depression, skeletal muscle flaccidity, cold or clammy skin, cyanosis, and extreme somnolence progressing to seizures, stupor, and coma.
! The patient who uses morphine repeatedly may develop a tolerance to the drug's analgesic effect and physical dependence.
! The drug may have a prolonged duration of action and cumulative effect in those with hepatic and renal impairment.

DENTAL CONSIDERATIONS

General:

- Monitor vital signs at every appointment because of CV and respiratory side effects.
- Assess salivary flow as a factor in caries, periodontal disease, and candidiasis.
- After supine positioning, have patient sit upright for at least 2 min before standing to avoid orthostatic hypotension.
- Psychologic and physical dependence may occur with chronic administration.
- Determine why the patient is taking the drug.
- Consider the use of NSAIDs when additional analgesia is required.

Teach Patient/Family:

- *When chronic dry mouth occurs, advise patient:*
  - To use daily home fluoride products for anticaries effect
  - To avoid mouth rinses with high alcohol content because of drying effects
  - To use sugarless gum, frequent sips of water, or saliva substitutes

moxifloxacin hydrochloride

moks-i-floks′-a-sin
(Avelox, Avelox IV, Vigamox)
Do not confuse Avelox with Avonex.

CATEGORY AND SCHEDULE

Pregnancy Risk Category: C

MECHANISM OF ACTION

A fluoroquinolone that inhibits two enzymes, topoisomerase II and IV, in susceptible microorganisms. ***Therapeutic Effect:*** Interferes with bacterial DNA replication. Prevents or delays emergence of resistant organisms. Bactericidal.

PHARMACOKINETICS

Well absorbed from the GI tract after PO administration. Protein binding: 50%. Widely distributed throughout body with tissue concentration often exceeding plasma concentration. Metabolized in liver. Primarily excreted in urine with a lesser amount in feces. ***Half-life:*** 10.7–13.3 hr.

AVAILABILITY

*Tablets (Avelox) :*400 mg.
Injection (Avelox IV): 400 mg.
Ophthalmic Solution (Vigamox): 0.5%.

INDICATIONS AND DOSAGES

▸ Acute Bacterial Sinusitis, Community-Acquired Pneumonia

PO, IV

Adults, Elderly. 400 mg q24h for 10 days.

▸ Acute Bacterial Exacerbation of Chronic Bronchitis

PO, IV

Adults, Elderly. 400 mg q24h for 5 days.

▸ Skin and Skin-Structure Infection

PO, IV

Adults, Elderly. 400 mg once a day for 7 days.

▸ Topical Treatment of Bacterial Conjunctivitis Due to Susceptible Strains of Bacteria

OPHTHALMIC

Adults, Elderly, Children older than 1 yr. 1 drop 3 times/day for 7 days.

CONTRAINDICATIONS

Hypersensitivity to quinolones

M

INTERACTIONS

Drug

Antacids, didanosine chewable, buffered tablets or pediatric powder for oral solution, iron preparations, sucralfate: May decrease moxifloxacin absorption.

Herbal

None known.

Food

None known.

Drug interactions of concern to dentistry

- Increased risk of CNS stimulation and seizures: NSAIDs
- Decreased absorption: divalent and trivalent antacids, iron and zinc salts
- Caution when using erythromycin, tricyclic antidepressants (no data, risk of QT interval)
- Increased risk of life-threatening arrhythmias: procainamide

Drug interactions of concern to dentistry moxifloxacin HCl (Vigamox)

- None reported

DIAGNOSTIC TEST EFFECTS

None known.

IV INCOMPATIBILITIES

Do not add or infuse other drugs simultaneously through the same IV line. Flush line before and after use if same IV line is used with other medications.

SIDE EFFECTS

Frequent (8%–6%)

Nausea, diarrhea

Occasional (3%–2%)

Dizziness, headache, abdominal pain, vomiting

Ophthalmic (6%–1%): conjunctival irritation, reduced visual acuity, dry eye, keratitis, eye pain, ocular itching, swelling of tissue around cornea, eye discharge, fever, cough, pharyngitis, rash, rhinitis

Rare (1%)

Change in sense of taste, dyspepsia (heartburn, indigestion), photosensitivity

SERIOUS REACTIONS

! Pseudomembranous colitis as evidenced by fever, severe abdominal cramps or pain, and severe watery diarrhea may occur.

! Superinfection manifested as anal or genital pruritus, moderate to severe diarrhea, and stomatitis may occur.

DENTAL CONSIDERATIONS

General:

- Determine why patient is taking the drug.
- Examine for oral manifestation of opportunistic infection.
- Advise patient if dental drugs prescribed have a potential for photosensitivity.
- Ruptures of the shoulder, hand, and Achilles tendons that required surgical repair or resulted in prolonged disability have been reported with the use of fluoroquinolones. Question patient about history of side effects associated with fluoroquinolone use.
- Monitor vital signs at every appointment because of CV side effects.
- Patients on chronic drug therapy may rarely have symptoms of blood dyscrasias, which can include infection, bleeding, and poor healing.
- Consider semisupine chair position for patient comfort if GI side effects occur.

Consultations:

- In a patient with symptoms of blood dyscrasias, request a medical consultation for blood studies and postpone treatment until normal values are reestablished.

• Physician consultation is advised in the presence of an acute dental infection requiring another antibiotic.

Teach Patient/Family:

• *If used for dental infection:*
  • To minimize exposure to sunlight and wear sunscreen if sun exposure is planned
  • To discontinue treatment and inform dentist immediately if patient experiences pain or inflammation of a tendon, and to rest and refrain from exercise

DENTAL CONSIDERATIONS

MOXIFLOXACIN HCl (Vigamox)

General:

• Avoid dental light in patient's eyes.
• Protect patient's eyes from accidental spatter during dental treatment.

mupirocin

mew-peer′-oh-sin
(Bactroban)
Do not confuse with Bactrim or Bacitracin

CATEGORY AND SCHEDULE

Pregnancy Risk Category: B

MECHANISM OF ACTION

An antibacterial agent that inhibits bacterial protein, RNA synthesis. Less effective on DNA synthesis. Nasal: Eradicates nasal colonization of MRSA. ***Therapeutic Effect:*** Prevents bacterial growth and replication. Bacteriostatic.

PHARMACOKINETICS

Metabolized in skin to inactive metabolite. Transported to skin surface; removed by normal skin desquamation.

AVAILABILITY

Ointment: 2% (Bactroban).
Nasal ointment: 2% (Bactroban).

INDICATIONS AND DOSAGES

▸ Impetigo, Infected Traumatic Skin Lesions

TOPICAL

Adults, Elderly, Children. Apply 3 times/day (may cover w/gauze).

Nasal colonization of resistant Staphylococcus aureus

INTRANASAL

Adults, Elderly, Children 12 yrs and older. Apply 2 times/day for 5 days.

OFF-LABEL USES

Treatment of infected eczema, folliculitis, minor bacterial skin infections.

CONTRAINDICATIONS

Hypersensitivity to mupirocin or any component of the formulation

INTERACTIONS

Drug

None known.

Herbal

None known.

Food

None known.

DIAGNOSTIC TEST EFFECTS

None known.

IV INCOMPATIBILITIES

None known.

IV COMPATIBILITIES

None known.

SIDE EFFECTS

Frequent

Nasal: Headache, rhinitis, upper respiratory congestion, pharyngitis, altered taste

Occasional
Nasal: Burning, stinging, cough
Topical: Pain, burning, stinging, itching
Rare
Nasal: Pruritis, diarrhea, dry mouth, epistaxis, nausea, rash
Topical: Rash, nausea, dry skin, contact dermatitis

SERIOUS REACTIONS

! Superinfection may result in bacterial or fungal infections, especially with prolonged or repeated therapy.

DENTAL CONSIDERATIONS

General:

• The dentist may choose to postpone elective dental treatment if the infected site may be affected by dental treatment.

M

mycophenolate mofetil

my-co-fen′-o-late
(CellCept)

CATEGORY AND SCHEDULE

Pregnancy Risk Category: C

MECHANISM OF ACTION

An immunologic agent that suppresses the immunologically mediated inflammatory response by inhibiting inosine monophosphate dehydrogenase, an enzyme that deprives lymphocytes of nucleotides necessary for DNA and RNA synthesis, thus inhibiting the proliferation of T and B lymphocytes. ***Therapeutic Effect:*** Prevents transplant rejection.

PHARMACOKINETICS

Rapidly and extensively absorbed after PO administration (food decreases drug plasma concentration but doesn't affect absorption). Protein binding: 97%. Completely hydrolyzed to active metabolite mycophenolic acid. Primarily excreted in urine. Not removed by hemodialysis. ***Half-life:*** 17.9 hr.

AVAILABILITY

Capsules: 250 mg.
Oral Suspension: 200 mg/ml.
Tablets: 500 mg.
Injection: 500 mg.

INDICATIONS AND DOSAGES

▸ **Prevention of Renal Transplant Rejection**
PO, IV
Adults, Elderly. 1 g twice a day.
▸ **Prevention of Heart Transplant Rejection**
PO, IV
Adults, Elderly. 1.5 g twice a day.
▸ **Prevention of Liver Transplant Rejection**
PO
Adults, Elderly. 1.5 g twice a day.
IV
Adults, Elderly. 1 g twice a day.
▸ **Usual Pediatric Dosage**
PO
Children. 600 mg/m^2/dose twice a day. Maximum: 2 g/day.

OFF-LABEL USES

Treatment of liver transplantation rejection, mild heart transplant rejection, moderate to severe psoriasis

CONTRAINDICATIONS

Hypersensitivity to mycophenolic acid

INTERACTIONS

Drug
Acyclovir, ganciclovir: May increase plasma concentrations

of both drugs in patients with renal impairment.
Antacids (aluminum and magnesium-containing), cholestyramine: May decrease the absorption of mycophenolate.
Live-virus vaccines: May potentiate virus replication, increase vaccine side effects, and decrease the patient's antibody response to the vaccine.
Other immunosuppressants: May increase the risk of infection or lymphomas.
Probenecid: May increase mycophenolate plasma concentration.

Herbal

Echinacea: May decrease the effects of mycophenolate.

Food

All foods: May decrease mycophenolate plasma concentration.

Drug interactions of concern to dentistry

- Increased plasma concentration: acyclovir, ganciclovir
- Decreased availability of MPA: drugs that alter the GI flora

DIAGNOSTIC TEST EFFECTS

May increase serum cholesterol, alkaline phosphatase, creatinine, AST(SGOT), and ALT(SGPT) levels. May increase or decrease blood glucose as well as serum lipid, calcium, potassium, phosphate, and uric acid levels.

IV INCOMPATIBILITIES

Mycophenolate is compatible only with D_5W. Do not infuse it concurrently with other drugs or IV solutions.

SIDE EFFECTS

Frequent (37%–20%)

UTI, hypertension, peripheral edema, diarrhea, constipation, fever, headache, nausea

Occasional (18%–10%)

Dyspepsia; dyspnea; cough; hematuria; asthenia; vomiting; edema; tremors; abdominal, chest, or back pain; oral candidiasis; acne

Rare (9%–6%)

Insomnia, respiratory tract infection, rash, dizziness

SERIOUS REACTIONS

! Significant anemia, leukopenia, thrombocytopenia, neutropenia, and leukocytosis may occur, particularly in those undergoing renal transplant rejection.

! Sepsis and infection occur occasionally.

! GI tract hemorrhage occurs rarely.

! Patients receiving mycophenolate have an increased risk of developing neoplasms.

M

DENTAL CONSIDERATIONS

General:

- Determine why the patient is taking the drug.
- Short appointments and a stress reduction protocol may be required for anxious patients.
- Patients who have been or are currently on chronic steroid therapy (>2 wk) may require supplemental steroids for dental treatment.
- Patients on chronic drug therapy may rarely have symptoms of blood dyscrasias, which can include infection, bleeding, and poor healing.
- Place on frequent recall because of oral side effects.
- Determine dose and duration of steroid for patient to assess risk for stress tolerance and immunosuppression.
- Examine for oral manifestation of opportunistic infections.

- Monitor vital signs at every appointment because of CV and respiratory side effects.
- Consider semisupine chair position for patient comfort if GI side effects occur.
- Antibiotic prophylaxis is usually recommended in patients with organ transplants and immunosuppression.
- Monitor time since organ/tissue transplant; note duration of transplant and status of renal function.
- Place on frequent recall because of possible blood dyscrasias and oral side effects.

Consultations:

- Medical consultation may be required to assess disease control and patient's ability to tolerate stress.
- In a patient with symptoms of blood dyscrasias, request a medical consultation for blood studies and postpone dental treatment until normal values are reestablished.
- Request baseline blood pressure in renal transplant patients for patient evaluation before dental treatment.

Teach Patient/Family:

- That secondary oral infection may occur; must see dentist immediately if infection occurs
- Importance of good oral hygiene to prevent soft tissue inflammation
- Need for frequent recall because of possible blood dyscrasias and oral side effects
- To report oral lesions, soreness, or bleeding to dentist

nabumetone

na-byu′-me-tone
(Apo-Nabumetone, Relafen)

CATEGORY AND SCHEDULE

Pregnancy Risk Category: C
(D if used in third trimester or near delivery)

MECHANISM OF ACTION

An NSAID that produces analgesic and anti-inflammatory effects by inhibiting prostaglandin synthesis.
Therapeutic Effect: Reduces the inflammatory response and intensity of pain.

PHARMACOKINETICS

Readily absorbed from the GI tract. Protein binding: 99%. Widely distributed. Metabolized in the liver to active metabolite. Primarily excreted in urine. Not removed by hemodialysis. ***Half-life:*** 22–30 hr.

AVAILABILITY

Tablets: 500 mg, 750 mg.

INDICATIONS AND DOSAGES

▸ Acute or Chronic Rheumatoid Arthritis and Osteoarthritis

PO

Adults, Elderly. Initially, 1000 mg as a single dose or in 2 divided doses. May increase up to 2000 mg/day as a single or in 2 divided doses.

CONTRAINDICATIONS

Active peptic ulcer disease, chronic inflammation of GI tract, GI bleeding or ulceration, history of hypersensitivity to aspirin or NSAIDs, history of significant renal impairment

INTERACTIONS

Drug

Antihypertensives, diuretics: May decrease the effects of these drugs.
Aspirin, other salicylates: May increase the risk of GI side effects such as bleeding.
Bone marrow depressants: May increase the risk of hematologic reactions.
Heparin, oral anticoagulants, thrombolytics: May increase the effects of these drugs.
Lithium: May increase the blood concentration and risk of toxicity of lithium.
Methotrexate: May increase the risk of methotrexate toxicity.
Probenecid: May increase the nabumetone blood concentration.

Herbal

Feverfew: May decrease the effects of feverfew.
Ginkgo biloba: May increase the risk of bleeding.

Food

None known.

Drug interactions of concern to dentistry

- GI ulceration, bleeding: aspirin, alcohol, corticosteroids
- May decrease effects of nabumetone: salicylates
- Nephrotoxicity: acetaminophen (prolonged use and high doses)
- Possible risk of decreased renal function: cyclosporine
- First-time users of SSRIs also taking NSAIDs may have a higher risk of GI side effects; until more data are available, it may be advisable to avoid use of NSAIDs in these patients (*Br J Clin Pharmacol* 55:591–595, 2003)

DIAGNOSTIC TEST EFFECTS

May increase BUN level; urine protein levels; and serum LDH, alkaline phosphatase, creatinine,

N

potassium, AST (SGOT), and ALT (SGPT) levels. May decrease serum uric acid level.

SIDE EFFECTS

Frequent (14%–12%)
Diarrhea, abdominal cramps or pain, dyspepsia, oral lichenoid reaction
Occasional (9%–4%)
Nausea, constipation, flatulence, dizziness, headache
Rare (3%–1%)
Vomiting, stomatitis, confusion

SERIOUS REACTIONS

! Overdose may result in acute hypotension and tachycardia.
! Rare reactions with long-term use include peptic ulcer disease, GI bleeding, gastritis, nephrotoxicity (dysuria, cystitis, hematuria, proteinuria, nephrotic syndrome), severe hepatic reactions (cholestasis, jaundice), and severe hypersensitivity reactions (bronchospasm, angioedema).

N

DENTAL CONSIDERATIONS

General:
- Patients on chronic drug therapy may rarely have symptoms of blood dyscrasias, which can include infection, bleeding, and poor healing.
- Assess salivary flow as a factor in caries, periodontal disease, and candidiasis.
- Avoid prescribing for dental use in last trimester of pregnancy.
- Avoid prescribing aspirin-containing products.
- Consider semisupine chair position for patients with arthritic disease.

Consultations:
- In a patient with symptoms of blood dyscrasias, request a medical consultation for blood studies and postpone dental treatment until normal values are reestablished.
- Medical consultation may be required to assess disease control.

Teach Patient/Family:
- Importance of good oral hygiene to prevent soft tissue inflammation
- Caution to prevent injury when using oral hygiene aids
- *When chronic dry mouth occurs, advise patient:*
  - To avoid mouth rinses with high alcohol content because of drying effects
  - Of need for daily use of home fluoride
  - To use sugarless gum, frequent sips of water, or saliva substitutes

nadolol

nay-doe′-lole
(Apo-Nadol[CAN], Corgard, Novo-Nadolol[CAN])

CATEGORY AND SCHEDULE

Pregnancy Risk Category: C (D if used in second or third trimester)

MECHANISM OF ACTION

A nonselective beta-blocker that blocks $beta_1$- and $beta_2$-adrenergenic receptors. Large doses increase airway resistance. ***Therapeutic Effect:*** Slows sinus heart rate, decreases cardiac output and BP. Decreases myocardial ischemia severity by decreasing oxygen requirements.

AVAILABILITY

Tablets: 20 mg, 40 mg, 80 mg, 120 mg, 160 mg.

INDICATIONS AND DOSAGES

▸ Mild to Moderate Hypertension, Angina

PO
Adults. Initially, 40 mg/day. May increase by 40–80 mg

at 3–7 day intervals. Maximum: 240–360 mg/day.
Elderly. Initially, 20 mg/day. May increase gradually. Range: 20–240 mg/day.

▸ Dosage in Renal Impairment
Dosage is modified on the basis of creatinine clearance.

Creatinine Clearance	% Usual Dosage
10–50 ml/min	50
less than 10 ml/min	25

OFF-LABEL USES
Treatment of arrhythmias, hypertrophic cardiomyopathy, MI, mitral valve prolapse syndrome, neuroleptic-induced akathisia, pheochromocytoma, tremors, thyrotoxicosis, vascular headaches

CONTRAINDICATIONS
Bronchial asthma, cardiogenic shock, CHF secondary to tachyarrhythmias, COPD, patients receiving MAOI therapy, second- or third-degree heart block, sinus bradycardia, uncontrolled cardiac failure

INTERACTIONS
Drug
Cimetidine: May increase nadolol blood concentration.
Diuretics, other antihypertensives: May increase hypotensive effect.
Insulin, oral hypoglycemics: May mask symptoms of hypoglycemia and prolong the hypoglycemic effect of insulin and oral hypoglycemics.
NSAIDs: May decrease antihypertensive effect.
Sympathomimetics, xanthines: May mutually inhibit effects.
Herbal
None known.
Food
None known.
Drug interactions of concern to dentistry
- Decreased effects: sympathomimetics (epinephrine, norepinephrine, isoproterenol)
- Slows metabolism of nadolol: lidocaine
- Increased hypotension, myocardial depression: fentanyl derivatives, hydrocarbon inhalation anesthetics
- Decreased hypotensive effect: indomethacin and other NSAIDs

DIAGNOSTIC TEST EFFECTS
May increase serum antinuclear antibody titer and BUN, serum LDH, serum lipoprotein, serum alkaline phosphatase, serum bilirubin, serum creatinine, serum potassium, serum uric acid, AST(SGOT), ALT (SGPT), and serum triglyceride levels.

SIDE EFFECTS
Nadolol is generally well tolerated, with transient and mild side effects.
Frequent
Diminished sexual ability, drowsiness, unusual fatigue or weakness
Occasional
Bradycardia, difficulty breathing, depression, cold hands or feet, diarrhea, constipation, anxiety, nasal congestion, nausea, vomiting
Rare
Altered taste, dry eyes, itching

SERIOUS REACTIONS
! Overdose may produce profound bradycardia and hypotension.
! Abrupt withdrawal of nadolol may result in diaphoresis, palpitations, headache, tremors, exacerbation of angina, MI, and ventricular arrhythmias.
! Nadolol administration may precipitate CHF and MI in patients

with cardiac disease; thyroid storm in those with thyrotoxicosis; and peripheral ischemia in those with existing peripheral vascular disease.
! Hypoglycemia may occur in patients with previously controlled diabetes.

DENTAL CONSIDERATIONS

General:

- Monitor vital signs at every appointment because of CV side effects.
- Patients on chronic drug therapy may rarely have symptoms of blood dyscrasias, which can include infection, bleeding, and poor healing.
- After supine positioning, have patient sit upright for at least 2 min before standing to avoid orthostatic hypotension.
- Limit use of sodium-containing products, such as saline IV fluids, for patients with a dietary salt restriction.
- Assess salivary flow as a factor in caries, periodontal disease, and candidiasis.
- Stress from dental procedures may compromise CV function; determine patient risk.
- Short appointments and a stress reduction protocol may be required for anxious patients.
- Consider semisupine chair position for patients with respiratory distress.

Consultations:

- In a patient with symptoms of blood dyscrasias, request a medical consultation for blood studies and postpone dental treatment until normal values are reestablished.
- Take precautions if dental surgery is anticipated and anesthesia is required.
- Medical consultation may be required to assess disease control and patient's ability to tolerate stress.

Teach Patient/Family:

- Importance of good oral hygiene to prevent soft tissue inflammation
- Caution to prevent injury when using oral hygiene aids
- *When chronic dry mouth occurs, advise patient:*
  - To avoid mouth rinses with high alcohol content because of drying effects
  - Of need for daily home fluoride use to prevent caries
  - To use sugarless gum, frequent sips of water, or saliva substitutes

N

nafarelin

naf-ah-rell-in
(Synarel)

CATEGORY AND SCHEDULE

Pregnancy Risk Category: X

MECHANISM OF ACTION

A gonadotropin inhibitor that initially stimulates the release of the pituitary gonadotropins, luteinizing hormone and follicle-stimulating hormone, then decreases secretion of gonadal steroids. ***Therapeutic Effect:*** Temporarily increases ovarian steroidogenesis, abolishes the stimulatory effect on the pituitary gland, decreases secretion of gonadal steroids.

PHARMACOKINETICS

Rapidly absorbed after nasal administration. Protein binding: 78%–84%, binds primarily to albumin. Metabolism: unknown. Excreted in urine. ***Half-life:*** 3 hrs.

AVAILABILITY

Nasal Spray: 2 mg/ml (Synarel).

INDICATIONS AND DOSAGES

▸ Endometriosis

INTRANASAL

Adults. 400 mcg/day: 200 mcg (1 spray) into 1 nostril in morning, 1 spray into other nostril in evening. For patients with persistent regular menstruation after months of treatment, increase dose to 800 mcg/day (1 spray into each nostril in morning and evening).

▸ Central Precocious Puberty

INTRANASAL

Children. 1600 mcg/day: 400 mcg (2 sprays into each nostril in morning and evening; total 8 sprays).

CONTRAINDICATIONS

Pregnancy, other agonist analogues, undiagnosed abnormal vaginal bleeding, hypersensitivity to nafarelin or any component of the formulation

INTERACTIONS

Drug

None known.

Herbal

None known.

Food

None known.

Drug interactions of concern to dentistry

- None reported

DIAGNOSTIC TEST EFFECTS

None known.

SIDE EFFECTS

Frequent

Hot flashes. muscle pain, decreased breast size, myalgia

Occasional

Nasal irritation, decreased libido, vaginal dryness, headache, emotional lability, acne

Rare

Insomnia, edema, weight gain, seborrhea, depression.

SERIOUS REACTIONS

! None reported.

DENTAL CONSIDERATIONS

General:

- Determine why patient is taking the drug.
- Bone density may decrease during medication use.

naftifine

naf-ti-feen

(Naftin)

Do not confuse with nafcillin or nafarelin.

CATEGORY AND SCHEDULE

Pregnancy Risk Category: B

MECHANISM OF ACTION

An antifungal that selectively inhibits the enzyme squalene epoxidase in a dose-dependent manner, which results in the primary sterol, ergosterol, within the fungal membrane not being synthesized. ***Therapeutic Effect:*** Results in fungal cell death. Fungistatic and fungicidal.

PHARMACOKINETICS

Minimal systemic absorption. Metabolized in the liver. Excreted in the urine, as well as the feces and bile. ***Half-life:*** 48–72 hrs.

AVAILABILITY

Gel: 1% (Naftin).

Cream: 1% (Naftin).

INDICATIONS AND DOSAGES

▸ Tinea Pedis, T. Cruris, T. Corporis

TOPICAL

Adults, Elderly, Children 12 yrs and older. Apply cream 1 time a day for 4 weeks or until signs and symptoms significantly improve. Apply gel 2 times a day for 4 weeks or until signs and symptoms significantly improve.

OFF-LABEL USES
Trichomycosis

CONTRAINDICATIONS
Hypersensitivity to naftifine or any of its components

INTERACTIONS
Drug
None known.
Herbal
None known.
Food
None known.
Drug interactions of concern to dentistry
- None reported

DIAGNOSTIC TEST EFFECTS
None known.

N

SIDE EFFECTS
Frequent
Burning, stinging
Occasional
Erythema, itching, dryness, irritation

SERIOUS REACTIONS
! Excessive irritation may indicate hypersensitivity reaction.

DENTAL CONSIDERATIONS
General:
- This drug is intended for acute use only, but listed side effects can sometimes be seen.
- Risk of seizures reported in animal studies; be aware of this potential.
- Serious CV events have been associated with opioid reversal in postoperative patients; doses should be carefully titrated to reduce these events.
- Buprenorphine depression may not be completely reversed.
- In all cases, the establishment of a patent airway, ventilatory assistance, oxygen administration, and circulatory access should complement or precede opioid antagonist use.
- Significant opioid depression occurring in the dental office may require relocation of the patient to a medical facility for comprehensive management.
- Patients discharged from the office/emergency facility should be carefully observed for the return of opioid-induced depression.

nalbuphine hydrochloride
nal′-byoo-feen
(Nubain)
Do not confuse Nubain with Navane.

CATEGORY AND SCHEDULE
Pregnancy Risk Category: B
(D if used for prolonged periods or at high dosages at term)

MECHANISM OF ACTION
A narcotic agonist-antagonist that binds with opioid receptors in the CNS. May displace opioid agonists and competitively inhibit their action; may precipitate withdrawal symptoms. ***Therapeutic Effect:*** Alters the perception of and emotional response to pain.

PHARMACOKINETICS

Route	Onset	Peak	Duration
IV	2–3 min	30 min	3–6 hr
IM	less than 15 min	60 min	3–6 hr
Subcutaneous	less than 15 min	N/A	3–6 hr

Well absorbed after IM or subcutaneous administration. Protein binding: 50%. Metabolized in the liver. Primarily eliminated in feces by biliary secretion. ***Half-life:*** 3.5–5 hr.

AVAILABILITY

Injection: 10 mg/ml, 20 mg/ml.

INDICATIONS AND DOSAGES

▸ Analgesia

IV, IM, Subcutaneous

Adults, Elderly. 10 mg q3–6h as needed. Don't exceed maximum single dose of 20 mg or daily dose of 160 mg. For patients receiving long-term narcotic analgesics of similar duration of action, give 25% of usual dose.

Children. 0.1–0.15 mg/kg q3–6h as needed.

▸ Supplement to Anesthesia

IV

Adults, Elderly. Induction: 0.3–3 mg/kg over 10–15 min. Maintenance: 0.25–0.5 mg/kg as needed.

CONTRAINDICATIONS

Respiratory rate less than 12 breaths/minute

INTERACTIONS

Drug

Alcohol, other CNS depressants: May increase CNS or respiratory depression and hypotension.

Buprenorphine: May decrease the effects of nalbuphine.

MAOIs: May produce a severe, possibly fatal reaction; plan to administer 25% of the usual nalbuphine dose.

Herbal

None known.

Food

None known.

Drug interactions of concern to dentistry

- Increased CNS and respiratory depression: all CNS depressants
- Contraindicated with MAOIs
- Avoid use in narcotic-dependent persons; risk of withdrawal reactions
- Increased risk of constipation: anticholinergics
- Increased risk of orthostatic hypotension: antihypertensive medications

DIAGNOSTIC TEST EFFECTS

May increase serum amylase and lipase levels.

IV INCOMPATIBILITIES

Amphotericin B complex (Abelcet, AmBisome, Amphotec), cefepime (Maxipime), docetaxel (Doxil), methotrexate, nafcillin (Nafcil), piperacillin and tazobactam (Zosyn), sargramostim (Leukine, Prokine), sodium bicarbonate

IV COMPATIBILITIES

Diphenhydramine (Benadryl), droperidol (Inapsine), glycopyrrolate (Robinul), hydroxyzine (Vistaril), ketorolac (Toradol), lidocaine, midazolam (Versed), propofol (Diprivan)

SIDE EFFECTS

Frequent (35%)

Sedation

Occasional (9%–3%)

Diaphoresis, cold and clammy skin, nausea, vomiting, dizziness, vertigo, dry mouth, headache

Rare (<1%)

Restlessness, emotional lability, paresthesia, flushing, paradoxical reaction

SERIOUS REACTIONS

! Abrupt withdrawal after prolonged use may produce symptoms of narcotic withdrawal, such as

abdominal cramping, rhinorrhea, lacrimation, anxiety, fever, and piloerection (goose bumps).
! Overdose results in severe respiratory depression, skeletal muscle flaccidity, cyanosis, and extreme somnolence progressing to seizures, stupor, and coma.
! Repeated use may result in drug tolerance and physical dependence.

DENTAL CONSIDERATIONS

General:

- Avoid use in an opioid-dependent patient.
- Acute-use drug, question patient about use for pain.
- If additional analgesia is required for dental pain, consider alternative analgesics (NSAIDs) in patients taking narcotics for acute or chronic pain.
- Monitor and record vital signs.
- Assess salivary flow as a factor in caries, periodontal disease, and candidiasis.

Consultations:

- Medical consultation may be required to assess disease control.

Teach Patient/Family:

- *When chronic dry mouth occurs advise patient:*
  - To avoid mouth rinses with high alcohol content due to drying effects
  - To use daily home fluoride products for anticaries effect
  - To use sugarless gum, frequent sips of water or saliva substitutes
- Importance of good oral hygiene to prevent soft tissue inflammation
- To prevent trauma when using oral hygiene aids
- To avoid driving or other activities requiring mental alertness
- To avoid alcohol ingestion or CNS depressants; serious CNS depression may result
- To avoid OTC preparations that contain CNS depressants (antihistamine, cold remedies)

naloxone hydrochloride

nal-oks′-one
(Narcan)
Do not confuse naltrexone or Narcan with Norcuron.

CATEGORY AND SCHEDULE

Pregnancy Risk Category: B

MECHANISM OF ACTION

A narcotic antagonist that displaces opioids at opioid-occupied receptor sites in the CNS. ***Therapeutic Effect:*** Reverses opioid-induced sleep or sedation, increases respiratory rate, raises BP to normal range.

PHARMACOKINETICS

Route	Onset	Peak	Duration
IV	1–2 min	N/A	20–60 min
IM	2–5 min	N/A	20–60 min
Subcutaneous	2–5 min	N/A	20–60 min

Well absorbed after IM or subcutaneous administration. Metabolized in the liver. Primarily excreted in urine. ***Half-life:*** 60–100 min.

AVAILABILITY

Injection: 0.02 mg/ml, 0.4 mg/ml, 1 mg/ml.

INDICATIONS AND DOSAGES

▸ **Opioid toxicity**

IV, IM, SUBCUTANEOUS
Adults, Elderly. 0.4–2 mg q2–3min as needed. May repeat q20–60min.

Children 5 yr and older and weighing 22 kg or more. 2 mg/dose; if no response, may repeat q2–3min. May need to repeat q20–60min.
Children younger than 5 yr and weighing less than 22 kg. 0.1 mg/kg; if no response, repeat q2–3min. May need to repeat q20–60min.

▸ **Postanesthesia Narcotic Reversal**
IV
Children. 0.01 mg/kg; may repeat q2–3min.

▸ **Neonatal Opioid-Induced Depression**
IV
Neonates. May repeat q2–3min as needed. May need to repeat q1–2h.

OFF-LABEL USES
Treatment of PCP, ethanol ingestion

CONTRAINDICATIONS
Respiratory depression due to nonopioid drugs

INTERACTIONS
Drug
Butorphanol, nalbuphine, opioid agonist analgesics, pentazocine: Reverses the analgesic and adverse effects of these drugs and may precipitate withdrawal symptoms.
Herbal
None known.
Food
None known.
Drug interactions of concern to dentistry
• Antagonizes effects of opioid agonists and mixed agonists/antagonists

DIAGNOSTIC TEST EFFECTS
None known.

IV INCOMPATIBILITIES
Amphotericin B complex (Abelcet, AmBisome, Amphotec)

IV COMPATIBILITIES
Heparin, ondansetron (Zofran), propofol (Diprivan)

SIDE EFFECTS
None known; little or no pharmacologic effect in absence of narcotics.

SERIOUS REACTIONS
! Too-rapid reversal of narcotic-induced respiratory depression may result in nausea, vomiting, tremors, increased BP, and tachycardia.
! Excessive dosage in postoperative patients may produce significant excitement, tremors, and reversal of analgesia.
! Patients with cardiovascular disease may experience hypotension or hypertension, ventricular tachycardia and fibrillation, and pulmonary edema.

DENTAL CONSIDERATIONS
General:
• This drug is intended for acute use only, but listed side effects can sometimes be seen.
• Risk of seizures reported in animal studies; be aware of this potential.
• Serious CV events have been associated with opioid reversal in postoperative patients; doses should be carefully titrated to reduce these events.
• Buprenorphine depression may not be completely reversed.
• In all cases, the establishment of a patent airway, ventilatory assistance, oxygen administration, and circulatory access should complement or precede opioid antagonist use.
• Significant opioid depression occurring in the dental office may require relocation of the patient to a medical facility for comprehensive management.
• Patients discharged from the office/emergency facility should be carefully observed for the return of opioid-induced depression.

naltrexone hydrochloride

nal-trex′-one
(Revia)

CATEGORY AND SCHEDULE

Pregnancy Risk Category: C

MECHANISM OF ACTION

A narcotic antagonist that displaces opioids at opioid-occupied receptor sites in the CNS. ***Therapeutic Effect:*** Blocks physical effects of opioid analgesics; decreases craving for alcohol and relapse rate in alcoholism.

AVAILABILITY

Tablets: 50 mg.

INDICATIONS AND DOSAGES

▸ Naloxone Challenge Test to Determine if Patient Is Opioid Dependent

Alert. Expect to perform the naloxone challenge test if there is any question that the patient is opioid dependent. Don't administer naltrexone until the naloxone challenge test is negative.

IV

Adults, Elderly. Draw 2 ml (0.8 mg) of naloxone into syringe. Inject 0.5 ml (0.2 mg); while needle is still in vein, observe patient for 30 sec for withdrawal signs or symptoms. If no evidence of withdrawal, inject remaining 1.5 ml (0.6 mg); observe patient for additional 20 min for withdrawal signs or symptoms.

SUBCUTANEOUS

Adults, Elderly. Inject 2 ml (0.8 mg) of naloxone; observe patient for 45 min for withdrawal signs or symptoms.

▸ Treatment of Opioid Dependence in Patients Who Have Been Opioid Free for at Least 7–10 Days

PO

Adults, Elderly. Initially, 25 mg. Observe patient for 1 hr. If no withdrawal signs or symptoms appear, give another 25 mg. May be given as 100 mg every other day or 150 mg every 3 days.

▸ Adjunctive Treatment of Alcohol Dependence

PO

Adults, Elderly. 50 mg once a day.

OFF-LABEL USES

Treatment of eating disorders, postconcussional syndrome unresponsive to other treatments

CONTRAINDICATIONS

Acute hepatitis, acute opioid withdrawal, failed naloxone challenge test, hepatic failure, history of hypersensitivity to naltrexone, opioid dependence, positive urine screen for opioids

INTERACTIONS

Drug

Opioid-containing products (including analgesics, antidiarrheals, and antitussives): Blocks the therapeutic effects of these drugs.

Thioridazine: May produce lethargy and somnolence.

Herbal

None known.

Food

None known.

Drug interactions of concern to dentistry

- Decreased effects of opioid narcotics

DIAGNOSTIC TEST EFFECTS

May increase AST (SGOT) and ALT (SGPT) levels.

SIDE EFFECTS

Frequent

Alcoholism (10%–7%): Nausea, headache, depression

Narcotic addiction (10%–5%): Insomnia, anxiety, nervousness, headache, low energy, abdominal cramps, nausea, vomiting, arthralgia, myalgia

Occasional

Alcoholism (4%–2%): Dizziness, nervousness, fatigue, insomnia, vomiting, anxiety, suicidal ideation

Narcotic addiction (5%–2%): Irritability, increased energy, dizziness, anorexia, diarrhea or constipation, rash, chills, increased thirst

SERIOUS REACTIONS

! Signs and symptoms of opioid withdrawal include stuffy or runny nose, tearing, yawning, diaphoresis, tremor, vomiting, piloerection, feeling of temperature change, bone pain, arthralgia, myalgia, abdominal cramps, and feeling of skin crawling.

! Accidental naltrexone overdose produces withdrawal symptoms within 5 minutes of ingestion that may last for up to 48 hours. Symptoms include confusion, visual hallucinations, somnolence, and significant vomiting and diarrhea.

! Hepatocellular injury may occur with large doses.

DENTAL CONSIDERATIONS

General:

- Monitor vital signs at every appointment because of CV and respiratory side effects.
- Patients on chronic drug therapy may rarely have symptoms of blood dyscrasias, which can include infection, bleeding, and poor healing.
- Patients should not be given opioid analgesics for dental pain management. Substitute with NSAID and long-acting local anesthetics.
- The dental professional must be aware of the patient's disease, and the patient must be active in treatment for chemical dependency.

Consultations:

- In a patient with symptoms of blood dyscrasias, request a medical consultation for blood studies and postpone dental treatment until normal values are reestablished.
- Medical consultation may be required to assess disease control.
- Inform aftercare provider or counselor if sedative medications are required for proper management.

Teach Patient/Family:

- Importance of good oral hygiene to prevent soft tissue inflammation
- Caution to prevent injury when using oral hygiene aids

N

naphazoline

naf-az′-oh-leen

(AK-Con, Albalon Liquifilm[AUS], Clear Eyes[AUS], Naphcon, Naphcon Forte[AUS], Privine, Vasocon)

CATEGORY AND SCHEDULE

Pregnancy Risk Category: C

MECHANISM OF ACTION

A sympathomimetic that directly acts on alpha-adrenergic receptors in conjunctival arterioles and nasal blood vessels. ***Therapeutic Effect:*** Causes vasoconstriction, resulting in decreased congestion.

AVAILABILITY

Ophthalmic Solution: 0.012%, 0.1%.
Nasal Drops: 0.05%.
Nasal Spray: 0.05%.

INDICATIONS AND DOSAGES

▸ **Nasal Congestion Due to Acute or Chronic Rhinitis, Common Cold, Hay Fever, or other Allergies**

INTRANASAL

Adults, Elderly, Children older than 12 yr. 1–2 drops or sprays in each nostril q3–6h.

Children 6–12 yr. 1 spray or drop in each nostril q6h as needed.

▸ **Control of Hyperemia in Patients with Superficial Corneal Vascularity; Relief of Congestion and Inflammation; for Use During Ocular Diagnostic Procedures**

OPHTHALMIC

Adults, Elderly, Children older than 6 yr. 1–2 drops in affected eye q3–4h for 3–4 days.

CONTRAINDICATIONS

Angle-closure glaucoma, before peripheral iridectomy, patients with a narrow angle who do not have glaucoma

INTERACTIONS

Drug

Maprotiline, tricyclic antidepressants: May increase the effects of naphazoline.

Herbal

None known.

Food

None known.

Drug interactions of concern to dentistry

- Increased pressor effects: tricyclic antidepressants

DIAGNOSTIC TEST EFFECTS

None known.

SIDE EFFECTS

Occasional

Nasal: Burning, stinging, or drying of nasal mucosa; sneezing; rebound congestion

Ophthalmic: Blurred vision, dilated pupils, increased eye irritation

SERIOUS REACTIONS

! If naphazoline is systemically absorbed, the patient may experience tachycardia, palpitations, headache, insomnia, light-headedness, nausea, nervousness, and tremor.

! Large doses may produce tachycardia, palpitations, light-headedness, nausea, and vomiting.

! Overdose in patients older than 60 years may produce hallucinations, CNS depression, and seizures.

DENTAL CONSIDERATIONS

General:

- Monitor vital signs at every appointment because of CV side effects.
- Avoid dental light in patient's eyes; offer dark glasses for patient comfort.
- Protect patient's eyes from accidental spatter during dental treatment.

naproxen/naproxen sodium

na-prox'-en

(naproxen) Crysanal[AUS], EC-Naprosyn, Inza[AUS], Naprelan, Naprosyn(naproxen sodium) Aleve, Anaprox, Anaprox DS, Apo-Naprosyn[CAN], Naprogesic[AUS], Novo-Naprox[CAN], Nu-Naprox [CAN], Pamprin

Do not confuse Aleve with Allese or Anaprox with Anaspaz.

CATEGORY AND SCHEDULE

Pregnancy Risk Category: B (D if used in third trimester or near delivery)

OTC (220 mg gelcaps, 220 mg tablets)

MECHANISM OF ACTION

An NSAID that produces analgesic and anti-inflammatory effects by inhibiting prostaglandin synthesis. ***Therapeutic Effect:*** Reduces the inflammatory response and intensity of pain.

PHARMACOKINETICS

Route	Onset	Peak	Duration
PO (analgesic)	less than 1 hr	N/A	7 hr or less
PO (antirheumatic)	less than 14 days	2–4 wk	N/A

Completely absorbed from the GI tract. Protein binding: 99%. Metabolized in the liver. Primarily excreted in urine. Not removed by hemodialysis. ***Half-life:*** 13 hr.

AVAILABILITY

Gelcaps (Aleve): 220 mg naproxen sodium (equivalent to 200 mg naproxen).
Oral Suspension (Naprosyn): 125 mg/5 ml naproxen.
Tablets (Aleve): 220 mg naproxen.
Tablets (Anaprox): 275 mg naproxen sodium (equivalent to 250 mg naproxen).
Tablets (Anaprox DS): 550 mg naproxen sodium (equivalent to 500 mg naproxen).
Tablets (Controlled-Release [EC-Naprosyn]): 375 mg naproxen, 500 mg naproxen.
Tablets (Controlled-Release [Naprelan]): 421 mg naproxen, 550 mg naproxen sodium (equivalent to 500 mg naproxen).

INDICATIONS AND DOSAGES

▸ Rheumatoid Arthritis, Osteoarthritis, Ankylosing Spondylitis

PO

Adults, Elderly. 250–500 mg naproxen (275–550 mg naproxen sodium) twice a day or 250 mg naproxen (275 mg naproxen sodium) in morning and 500 mg naproxen (550 mg naproxen sodium) in evening. Naprelan: 750–1,000 mg once a day.

▸ Acute Gouty Arthritis

PO

Adults, Elderly. Initially, 750 mg naproxen (825 mg naproxen sodium), then 250 mg naproxen (275 mg naproxen sodium) q8h until attack subsides. Naprelan: Initially, 1000–1500 mg, then 1000 mg once a day until attack subsides.

▸ Mild to Moderate Pain, Dysmenorrhea, Bursitis, Tendinitis

PO

Adults, Elderly. Initially, 500 mg naproxen (550 mg naproxen sodium), then 250 mg naparoxen (275 mg naproxen sodium) q6–8h as needed. Maximum: 1.25 g/day naproxen (1.375 g/day naproxen sodium). Naprelan: 1000 mg once a day.

▸ Juvenile Rheumatoid Arthritis

PO (naproxen only)

Children. 10–15 mg/kg/day in 2 divided doses. Maximum: 1000 mg/day.

OFF-LABEL USES

Treatment of vascular headaches

CONTRAINDICATIONS

Hypersensitivity to aspirin, naproxen, or other NSAIDs

INTERACTIONS

Drug

Antihypertensives, diuretics: May decrease the effects of these drugs.
Aspirin, other salicylates: May increase the risk of GI side effects such as bleeding.
Bone marrow depressants: May increase the risk of hematologic reactions.

Heparin, oral anticoagulants, thrombolytics: May increase the effects of these drugs.
Lithium: May increase the blood concentration and risk of toxicity of lithium.
Methotrexate: May increase the risk of methotrexate toxicity.
Probenecid: May increase the naproxen blood concentration.

Herbal

Feverfew: May decrease the effects of feverfew.
Ginkgo biloba: May increase the risk of bleeding.

Food

None known.

Drug interactions of concern to dentistry

- GI ulceration, bleeding: aspirin, alcohol, corticosteroids
- Nephrotoxicity: acetaminophen (chronic use and high doses)
- Possible risk of decreased renal function: cyclosporine
- Increased photosensitization: tetracycline
- Increased plasma levels: probenecid
- First-time users of SSRIs also taking NSAIDs may have a higher risk of GI side effects; until more data are available, it may be advisable to avoid use of NSAIDs in these patients (*Br J Clin Pharmacol* 55:591–595, 2003)
- *When prescribed for dental pain:*
  - Risk of increased effects: oral anticoagulants, oral antidiabetics, thium, methotrexate
  - Decreased antihypertensive effects of diuretics, β-adrenergic blockers, and ACE inhibitors

DIAGNOSTIC TEST EFFECTS

May prolong bleeding time and alter blood glucose level.
May increase serum hepatic function test results. May decrease serum sodium and uric acid levels.

SIDE EFFECTS

Frequent (9%–4%)
Nausea, constipation, abdominal cramps or pain, heartburn, dizziness, headache, somnolence, oral lichenoid reaction

Occasional (3%–1%)
Stomatitis, diarrhea, indigestion

Rare (<1%)
Vomiting, confusion

SERIOUS REACTIONS

! Rare reactions with long-term use include peptic ulcer disease, GI bleeding, gastritis, severe hepatic reactions (cholestasis, jaundice), nephrotoxicity (dysuria, hematuria, proteinuria, nephrotic syndrome), and a severe hypersensitivity reaction (fever, chills, bronchospasm).

DENTAL CONSIDERATIONS

General:

- Patients on chronic drug therapy may rarely have symptoms of blood dyscrasias, which can include infection, bleeding, and poor healing.
- Assess salivary flow as a factor in caries, periodontal disease, and candidiasis.
- Avoid prescribing for dental use in last trimester of pregnancy.
- Avoid prescribing aspirin-containing products.
- Consider semisupine chair position for patients with arthritic disease.

Consultations:

- In a patient with symptoms of blood dyscrasias, request a medical consultation for blood studies and postpone dental treatment until normal values are reestablished.
- Medical consultation may be required to assess disease control.

N

Teach Patient/Family:
- Importance of good oral hygiene to prevent soft tissue inflammation
- Caution to prevent injury when using oral hygiene aids
- *When chronic dry mouth occurs, advise patient:*
  - To avoid mouth rinses with high alcohol content because of drying effects
  - Of need for daily use of home fluoride products to prevent caries
  - To use sugarless gum, frequent sips of water, or saliva substitutes

naproxen sodium

na-prox′-en soe′-dee-um
(Aflaxen, Anaprox, Anaprox-DS, Apo-Napro[CAN], Naprelan '375', Naprelan '500' Naprogesic[AUS], Novonaprox[CAN])

CATEGORY AND SCHEDULE

Pregnancy Risk Category: B (D if used in third trimester or near delivery)

MECHANISM OF ACTION

A nonsteroidal anti-inflammatory that produces analgesic and anti-inflammatory effect by inhibiting prostaglandin synthesis. ***Therapeutic Effect:*** Reduces inflammatory response and intensity of pain stimulus reaching sensory nerve endings.

PHARMACOKINETICS

Route	Onset	Peak	Duration
PO (analgesic)	less than 1 hr	N/A	7 hr or less
PO (antirheumatic)	14 days or less	2–4 wk	N/A

Completely absorbed from the gastrointestinal (GI) tract. Protein binding: 99%. Metabolized in liver. Primarily excreted in urine. Not removed by hemodialysis. ***Half-life:*** 13 hrs.

AVAILABILITY

Tablets: 275 mg (Anaprox), 550 mg (Anaprox DS, Aflaxen).
Tablets (extended-release): 412.5 mg (Naprelan '375'), 550 mg (Napralen '500').
Powder for Compounding: 100%.

INDICATIONS AND DOSAGES

▸ **Rheumatoid Arthritis, Osteoarthritis, Ankylosing Spondylitis**
PO
Adults, Elderly. 250– 500 mg (275– 550 mg) 2 times/day or 250 mg (275 mg) in morning and 500 mg (500 mg) in evening.

▸ **Acute gouty arthritis**
PO
Adults, Elderly. Initially, 750 (825) mg, then 250 (275) mg q8h until attack subsides. Mild to moderate pain, dysmenorrhea, bursitis, tendinitis
PO
Adults, Elderly. Initially, 500 (550) mg, then 250 (275) mg q6–8h as needed. Total daily dose not to exceed 1.25 (1.375) g.

OFF-LABEL USES

Treatment of vascular headaches

CONTRAINDICATIONS

Hypersensitivity to aspirin, naproxen, or other NSAIDs

INTERACTIONS

Drug

Antihypertensives, Diuretics: May decrease the effects of antihypertensives and diuretics.

N

Aspirin, Salicylates: May increase the risk of GI bleeding and side effects.
Bone marrow depressants: May increase risk of hematologic reactions.
Heparin, oral anticoagulants, thrombolytics: May increase the effects of heparin, oral anticoagulants, and thrombolytics.
Lithium: May increase the blood concentration and risk of toxicity of lithium.
Methotrexate: May increase the risk of toxicity of methotrexate.
Probenecid: May increase naproxen blood concentration.

Herbal

Feverfew: May decrease the effects of feverfew.
Ginkgo biloba: May increase the risk of bleeding.

Food

None known.

Drug interactions of concern to dentistry

- GI ulceration, bleeding: aspirin, alcohol, corticosteroids
- Nephrotoxicity: acetaminophen (chronic use and high doses)
- Possible risk of decreased renal function: cyclosporine
- Increased photosensitization: tetracycline
- Increased plasma levels: probenecid
- First-time users of SSRIs also taking NSAIDs may have a higher risk of GI side effects; until more data are available, it may be advisable to avoid use of NSAIDs in these patients (*Br J Clin Pharmacol* 55:591–595, 2003)
- *When prescribed for dental pain:*
  - Risk of increased effects: oral anticoagulants, oral antidiabetics, lithium, methotrexate
  - Decreased antihypertensive effects of diuretics, β-adrenergic blockers, and ACE inhibitors

DIAGNOSTIC TEST EFFECTS

May prolong bleeding time, alter blood glucose levels. May increase liver function tests. May decrease serum sodium and uric acid levels.

SIDE EFFECTS

Frequent (9%–4%)
Nausea, constipation, abdominal cramps/pain, heartburn, dizziness, headache, drowsiness
Occasional (3%–1%)
Stomatitis, diarrhea, indigestion, oral lichenoid reaction
Rare (<1%)
Vomiting, confusion

SERIOUS REACTIONS

! Peptic ulcer disease, GI bleeding, gastritis, and severe hepatic reaction, such as cholestasis and jaundice, occur rarely.
! Nephrotoxicity, including dysuria, hematuria, proteinuria, and nephrotic syndrome, and severe hypersensitivity reaction, marked by fever, chills, and bronchospasm, occur rarely.

DENTAL CONSIDERATIONS

General:

- Patients on chronic drug therapy may rarely have symptoms of blood dyscrasias, which can include infection, bleeding, and poor healing.
- Assess salivary flow as a factor in caries, periodontal disease, and candidiasis.
- Avoid prescribing for dental use in last trimester of pregnancy.
- Avoid prescribing aspirin-containing products.
- Consider semisupine chair position for patients with arthritic disease.

Consultations:

- In a patient with symptoms of blood dyscrasias, request

a medical consultation for blood studies and postpone dental treatment until normal values are reestablished.

• Medical consultation may be required to assess disease control.

Teach Patient/Family:

• Importance of good oral hygiene to prevent soft tissue inflammation
• Caution to prevent injury when using oral hygiene aids
• *When chronic dry mouth occurs, advise patient:*
  • To avoid mouth rinses with high alcohol content because of drying effects
  • Of need for daily use of home fluoride products to prevent caries
  • To use sugarless gum, frequent sips of water, or saliva substitutes

naratriptan

nare-a-trip′-tan

(Amerge, Naramig[AUS])

Do not confuse Amerge with Amaryl.

CATEGORY AND SCHEDULE

Pregnancy Risk Category: C

MECHANISM OF ACTION

A serotonin receptor agonist that binds selectively to vascular receptors producing a vasoconstrictive effect on cranial blood vessels. ***Therapeutic Effect:*** Relieves migraine headache.

PHARMACOKINETICS

Well absorbed after PO administration. Protein binding: 28%–31%. Metabolized by the liver to inactive metabolite. Eliminated primarily in urine and, to a lesser extent, in feces. ***Half-life:*** 6 hr (increased in hepatic or renal impairment).

AVAILABILITY

Tablets: 1 mg, 2.5 mg.

INDICATIONS AND DOSAGES

▸ Acute Migraine Attack

PO

Adults. 1 mg or 2.5 mg. If headache improves but then returns, dose may be repeated after 4 hr. Maximum: 5 mg/24 hr.

▸ Dosage in Mild to Moderate Hepatic or Renal Impairment

A lower starting dose is recommended. Don't exceed 2.5 mg/24 hr.

CONTRAINDICATIONS

Basilar or hemiplegic migraine, cerebrovascular or peripheral vascular disease, coronary artery disease, ischemic heart disease (including angina pectoris, history of MI, silent ischemia, and Prinzmetal's angina), severe hepatic impairment (Child-Pugh grade C), severe renal impairment (serum creatinine less than 15 ml/min), uncontrolled hypertension, use within 24 hours of ergotamine-containing preparations or another serotonin receptor agonist, use within 14 days of MAOIs

INTERACTIONS

Drug

Ergotamine-containing medications: May produce a vasospastic reaction.

Fluoxetine, fluvoxamine, paroxetine, sertraline: May produce hyperreflexia, incoordination, and weakness.

Oral contraceptives: Decrease naratriptan clearance and volume of distribution.

Herbal

None known.

Food

None known.

N

Drug interactions of concern to dentistry

- No specific interactions with dental drugs reported
- Should not be used within 24 hr of another 5-HT_1 agonist

DIAGNOSTIC TEST EFFECTS

None known.

SIDE EFFECTS

Occasional (5%)

Nausea

Rare (2%)

Paresthesia; dizziness; fatigue; somnolence; jaw, neck, or throat pressure

SERIOUS REACTIONS

! Corneal opacities and other ocular defects may occur.

! Cardiac reactions (including ischemia, coronary artery vasospasm, and MI) and noncardiac vasospasm-related reactions (such as hemorrhage and CVA), occur rarely, particularly in patients with hypertension, diabetes, or a strong family history of coronary artery disease; obese patients; smokers; males older than 40 years; and postmenopausal women.

N

DENTAL CONSIDERATIONS

General:

- This is an acute-use drug; it is doubtful that patients will come to the office if acute migraine is present.
- Be aware of patient's disease, its severity, and its frequency when known.

Consultations:

- If treating chronic orofacial pain, consult with physician of record.
- Medical consultation may be required to assess disease control and patient's ability to tolerate stress.

Teach Patient/Family:

- Importance of updating health and drug history if physician makes any changes in evaluation or drug regimens
- That dryness of the mouth may occur when taking this drug; avoid mouth rinses with high alcohol content because of additional drying effects.

nateglinide

na-teg'-lin-ide

(Starlix)

CATEGORY AND SCHEDULE

Pregnancy Risk Category: C

MECHANISM OF ACTION

An antihyperglycemic that stimulates release of insulin from beta cells of the pancreas by depolarizing beta cells, leading to an opening of calcium channels. Resulting calcium influx induces insulin secretion. ***Therapeutic Effect:*** Lowers blood glucose concentration.

AVAILABILITY

Tablets: 60 mg, 120 mg.

INDICATIONS AND DOSAGES

▸ Diabetes Mellitus

PO

Adult, Elderly. 120 mg 3 times a day before meals. Initially, 60 mg may be given.

CONTRAINDICATIONS

Diabetic ketoacidosis, type 1 diabetes mellitus

INTERACTIONS

Drug

Beta blockers, MAOIs, NSAIDs, salicylates: May increase hypoglycemic effect of nateglinide.

Corticosteroids, thiazide diuretics, thyroid medication, sympathomimetics: May decrease hypoglycemic effect of nateglinide.

Herbal

None known.

Food

Liquid meal: Peak plasma levels may be significantly reduced if administered 10 minutes before a liquid meal.

Drug interactions of concern to dentistry

- Most drug interactions not clearly identified; may act as an inhibitor of CYP450 2C9 enzymes but not CYP450 3A4. Does not appear to interact with highly protein-bound drugs
- Potential potentiation of hypoglycemic effects: NSAIDs, salicylates, nonselective β-blockers

DIAGNOSTIC TEST EFFECTS

None known.

SIDE EFFECTS

Frequent (10%)

Upper respiratory tract infection

Occasional (4%–3%)

Back pain, flu symptoms, dizziness, arthropathy, diarrhea

Rare (≤ 3%)

Bronchitis, cough

SERIOUS REACTIONS

! Hypoglycemia occurs in less than 2% of patients.

DENTAL CONSIDERATIONS

General:

- If dentist prescribes any of the drugs listed in the drug interaction section, monitor patient's blood sugar levels.
- Consider semisupine chair position for patient comfort if GI side effects occur.
- Ensure that patient is following prescribed diet and regularly takes medication.
- Place on frequent recall to evaluate healing response.
- Short appointments and a stress reduction protocol may be required.
- Diabetics may be more susceptible to infection and have delayed wound healing.

Consultations:

- Medical consultation may include data from patient's blood glucose monitoring, including glycosylated hemoglobin or HbA_{1c} testing.
- Medical consultation may be required to assess disease control and patient's ability to tolerate stress.

Teach Patient/Family:

- To prevent trauma when using oral hygiene aids
- Importance of updating health and drug history if physician makes any changes in evaluation or drug regimens

N

nedocromil sodium

ned-oh-crow′-mil

(Alocril, Mireze[CAN], Tilade, Tilade CFC Free[AUS])

CATEGORY AND SCHEDULE

Pregnancy Risk Category: B

MECHANISM OF ACTION

A mast cell stabilizer that prevents the activation and release of inflammatory mediators, such as histamine, leukotrienes, mast cells, eosinophils, and monocytes.

Therapeutic Effect: Prevents both early and late asthmatic responses.

AVAILABILITY

Aerosol for Inhalation (Tilade): 1.75 mg/activation.

Ophthalmic Solution (Alocril): 2%.

INDICATIONS AND DOSAGES

▸ Mild to Moderate Asthma

Oral Inhalation

Adults, Elderly, Children 6 yr and older. 2 inhalations 4 times a day. May decrease to 3 times a day then twice a day as asthma becomes controlled.

▸ Allergic Conjunctivitis

OPHTHALMIC

Adults, Elderly, Children 3 yr and older. 1–2 drops in each eye twice a day.

OFF-LABEL USES

Prevention of bronchospasm in patients with reversible obstructive airway disease

CONTRAINDICATIONS

None known.

INTERACTIONS

Drug

None known.

Herbal

None known.

Food

None known.

Drug interactions of concern to dentistry

- None reported

DIAGNOSTIC TEST EFFECTS

None known.

SIDE EFFECTS

Frequent (10%–6%)

Cough, pharyngitis, bronchospasm, headache, altered taste

Occasional (5%–1%)

Rhinitis, upper respiratory tract infection, abdominal pain, fatigue

Rare (<1%)

Diarrhea, dizziness

SERIOUS REACTIONS

! None known.

NEDOCROMIL SODIUM (ALOCRIL)

DENTAL CONSIDERATIONS

General:

- Determine why patient is taking the drug.
- Protect patient's eyes from accidental spatter during dental treatment.
- Avoid dental light in patient's eyes; offer dark glasses for patient comfort.
- Users may report unpleasant taste while using this product.

NEDOCROMIL SODIUM

DENTAL CONSIDERATIONS

General:

- Assess salivary flow as a factor in caries, periodontal disease, and candidiasis.
- Consider semisupine chair position for patients with respiratory disease.
- Short appointments and a stress reduction protocol may be required for anxious patients.
- Be aware that aspirin or sulfite preservatives in vasoconstrictor-containing products can exacerbate asthma.

Consultations:

- Medical consultation may be required to assess disease control.

Teach Patient/Family:

- To avoid mouth rinses with high alcohol content because of drying effects
- For inhalation dosage forms, rinse mouth with water after each dose to prevent dryness

nefazodone hydrochloride
neh-faz′-oh-doan

CATEGORY AND SCHEDULE
Pregnancy Risk Category: C

MECHANISM OF ACTION
Exact mechanism is unknown. Appears to inhibit neuronal uptake of serotonin and norepinephrine and to antagonize $alpha_1$-adrenergic receptors. ***Therapeutic Effect:*** Relieves depression.

PHARMACOKINETICS
Rapidly and completely absorbed from the GI tract; food delays absorption. Protein binding: 99%. Widely distributed in body tissues, including CNS. Extensively metabolized to active metabolites. Excreted in urine and eliminated in feces. Unknown if removed by hemodialysis. ***Half-life:*** 2–4 hr.

AVAILABILITY
Tablets: 50 mg, 100 mg, 150 mg, 200 mg, 250 mg.

INDICATIONS AND DOSAGES
▸ Depression, Prevention of Relapse of Acute Depressive Episode
PO

Adults. Initially, 200 mg/day in 2 divided doses. Gradually increase by 100–200 mg/day at intervals of at least 1 wk. Range: 300–600 mg/day.
Elderly. Initially, 100 mg/day in 2 divided doses. Subsequent dosage titration based on clinical response. Range: 200–400 mg/day.
Children. 300–400 mg/day.

CONTRAINDICATIONS
Use within 14 days of MAOIs

INTERACTIONS
Drug
Alprazolam, triazolam: May increase the blood concentration and risk of toxicity of these drugs.
MAOIs: May produce severe reactions.
Herbal
St. John's wort: May increase the risk of adverse effects.
Food
None known.
Drug interactions of concern to dentistry
- Must *not* be used concurrently with or within 14 days of discontinuing MAOI
- Risk of significant adverse drug interaction with triazolam, alprazolam, alcohol-containing products
- Increased sedation: St. John's wort (herb)
- Acts as an inhibitor of CYP3A4 isoenzymes: risk of interaction with drugs metabolized by CYP3A4
- *Note:* No information on use of this drug in patients who are candidates for conscious sedation or general anesthesia is available.

DIAGNOSTIC TEST EFFECTS
None known.

SIDE EFFECTS
Frequent
Headache (36%); dry mouth, somnolence (25%); nausea (22%); dizziness (17%); constipation (14%); insomnia, asthenia, lightheadedness (10%).
Occasional
Dyspepsia, blurred vision (9%); diarrhea, infection (8%); confusion, abnormal vision (7%); pharyngitis (6%); increased appetite (5%); orthostatic hypotension, flushing, feeling of warmth (4%); peripheral edema, cough, flulike symptoms (3%).

SERIOUS REACTIONS

! Serious reactions, such as hyperthermia, rigidity, myoclonus, extreme agitation, delirium, and coma, will occur if the patient takes an MAOI concurrently or fails to let enough time elapse when switching from an MAOI to nefazodone or vice versa.

DENTAL CONSIDERATIONS

General:

- Assess salivary flow as a factor in caries, periodontal disease, and candidiasis.
- Take vital signs at every appointment because of CV side effects.
- After supine positioning, have patient sit upright for at least 2 min before standing to avoid postural hypotension.
- There is no information concerning the use of vasoconstrictors in patients taking this drug.
- Advise patient if dental drugs prescribed have a potential for photosensitivity.

Consultations:

- Medical consultation may be required to assess disease control.
- Physician should be informed if significant xerostomic side effects occur (e.g., increased caries, sore tongue, problems eating or swallowing, difficulty wearing prosthesis) so that a medication change can be considered.
- Because there is no experience with the use of conscious sedation or general anesthesia in patients taking this drug, a medical consultation is recommended for risk evaluation.
- Patients showing anorexia, jaundice, GI complaints, or malaise should be referred for medical evaluation before treatment.

Teach Patient/Family:

- *When chronic dry mouth occurs, advise patient:*
  - To avoid mouth rinses with high alcohol content because of drying effects
  - Of need for daily use of home fluoride products to prevent caries
  - To use sugarless gum, frequent sips of water, or saliva substitutes

nelfinavir

nel-fin′-eh-veer
(Viracept)

CATEGORY AND SCHEDULE

Pregnancy Risk Category: B

MECHANISM OF ACTION

Inhibits the activity of HIV-1 protease, the enzyme necessary for the formation of infectious HIV. ***Therapeutic Effect:*** Formation of immature noninfectious viral particles rather than HIV replication.

PHARMACOKINETICS

Well absorbed after PO administration (absorption increased with food). Protein binding: 98%. Metabolized in the liver. Highly bound to plasma proteins. Eliminated primarily in feces. Unknown if removed by hemodialysis. ***Half-life:*** 3.5–5 hr.

AVAILABILITY

Powder for Oral Suspension: 50 mg/g.
Tablets: 250 mg, 625 mg.

INDICATIONS AND DOSAGES

▸ **HIV Infection**

PO

Adults. 750 mg (three 250-mg tablets) 3 times a day or 1250 mg

twice a day in combination with nucleoside analogues (enhances antiviral activity).
Children 2–13 yr: 20–30 mg/kg/dose 3 times a day. Maximum: 750 mg q8h.

CONTRAINDICATIONS

Concurrent administration with midazolam, rifampin, or triazolam

INTERACTIONS

Drug

Alcohol, psychoactive drugs: May produce additive CNS effects.
Anticonvulsants, rifabutin, rifampin: Decrease nelfinavir plasma concentration.
Indinavir, saquinavir: Increases plasma concentration of these drugs.
Oral contraceptives: Decreases the effects of these drugs.
Ritonavir: Increases nelfinavir plasma concentration.

Herbal

St. John's wort: May decrease plasma concentration and effects of nelfinavir.

Food

All foods: Increase nelfinavir plasma concentration.

Drug interactions of concern to dentistry

- Contraindicated with triazolam, midazolam, and other drugs dependent on CYP3A4 for metabolism
- Increased plasma levels: azithromycin, ketoconazole
- Increased plasma concentrations of fentanyl

DIAGNOSTIC TEST EFFECTS

May decrease Hgb values and neutrophil and WBC counts. May increase serum CK, AST (SGOT), and ALT (SGPT) levels.

SIDE EFFECTS

Frequent (20%)

Diarrhea

Occasional (7%–3%)

Nausea, rash

Rare (2%–1%)

Flatulence, asthenia

SERIOUS REACTIONS

! None known.

DENTAL CONSIDERATIONS

General:

- Examine for oral manifestation of opportunistic infection.
- Patients on chronic drug therapy may rarely have symptoms of blood dyscrasias, which can include infection, bleeding, and poor healing.
- Palliative medication may be required for management of oral side effects.

Consultations:

- In a patient with symptoms of blood dyscrasias, request a medical consultation for blood studies and postpone treatment until normal values are reestablished.
- Medical consultation may be required to assess disease control.

Teach Patient/Family:

- Importance of good oral hygiene to prevent soft tissue inflammation
- Caution to prevent trauma when using oral hygiene aids
- Importance of updating health and drug history if physician makes any changes in evaluation or drug regimens
- That secondary oral infection may occur; must see dentist immediately if infection occurs

neostigmine

nee-oh-stig′-meen
(Prostigmin)
Do not confuse neostigmine with physostigmine.

CATEGORY AND SCHEDULE

Pregnancy Risk Category: C

MECHANISM OF ACTION

A cholinergic that prevents destruction of acetylcholine by inhibiting the enzyme acetylcholinesterase, thus enhancing impulse transmission across the myoneural junction.
Therapeutic Effect: Improves intestinal and skeletal muscle tone; stimulates salivary and sweat gland secretions.

AVAILABILITY

Tablets: 15 mg.
Injection: 0.5 mg/ml, 1 mg/ml.

N

INDICATIONS AND DOSAGES

▸ **Myasthenia Gravis**
PO
Adults, Elderly. Initially, 15–30 mg 3–4 times a day. Increase as necessary. Maintenance: 150 mg/day (range of 15–375 mg).
Children. 2 mg/kg/day or 60 mg/m^2/day divided q3–4h.
IV, IM, Subcutaneous
Adults. 0.5–2.5 mg as needed.
Children. 0.01–0.04 mg/kg q2–4h.

▸ **Diagnosis of Myasthenia Gravis**
IM
Adults, Elderly. 0.022 mg/kg. If cholinergic reaction occurs, discontinue tests and administer 0.4–0.6 mg or more atropine sulfate IV.
Children. 0.025–0.04 mg/kg preceded by atropine sulfate 0.011 mg/kg subcutaneously.

▸ **Prevention of Postoperative Urinary Retention**
IM, SUBCUTANEOUS
Adults, Elderly. 0.25 mg q4–6h for 2–3 days.

▸ **Postoperative Abdomonial Distention and Urine Retention**
IM, SUBCUTANEOUS
Adults, Elderly. 0.5–1 mg. Catheterize patient if voiding does not occur within 1 hr. After voiding, administer 0.5 mg q3h for 5 injections.

▸ **Reversal of Neuromuscular Blockade**
IV
Adults, Elderly. 0.5–2.5 mg given slowly.
Children. 0.025–0.08 mg/kg/dose.
Infants. 0.025–0.1 mg/kg/dose.

CONTRAINDICATIONS

GI or GU obstruction, peritonitis

INTERACTIONS

Drug

Anticholinergics: Reverse or prevent the effects of neostigmine.
Cholinesterase inhibitors: May increase the risk of toxicity.
Neuromuscular blockers: Antagonizes the effects of these drugs.
Procainamide, quinidine: May antagonize the action of neostigmine.

Herbal

None known.

Food

None known.

Drug interactions of concern to dentistry

- Decreased action: hydrocarbon inhalation anesthetics, corticosteroids
- Decreased action of anticholinergics (may be contraindicated)
- Increased action of succinylcholine
- Increased toxicity of ester-type local anesthetics

DIAGNOSTIC TEST EFFECTS
None known.

IV INCOMPATIBILITIES
None known.

IV COMPATIBILITIES
Glycopyrrolate (Robinul), heparin, ondansetron (Zofran), potassium chloride, thiopental (Pentothal)

SIDE EFFECTS
Frequent
Muscarinic effects (diarrhea, diaphoresis, increased salivation, nausea, vomiting, abdominal cramps or pain)
Occasional
Muscarinic effects (urinary urgency or frequency, increased bronchial secretions, miosis, lacrimation)

SERIOUS REACTIONS
! Overdose produces a cholinergic crisis manifested as abdominal discomfort or cramps, nausea, vomiting, diarrhea, flushing, facial warmth, excessive salivation, diaphoresis, lacrimation, pallor, bradycardia or tachycardia, hypotension, bronchospasm, urinary urgency, blurred vision, miosis, and fasciculation (involuntary muscular contractions visible under the skin).

DENTAL CONSIDERATIONS
General:
- Monitor vital signs at every appointment because of CV and respiratory side effects.
- Use amide-type local anesthetic agent.
- Early-morning and brief appointments are preferred because of effects of disease on oral musculature.

Consultations:
- Take precautions if dental surgery is anticipated and anesthesia is required.
- Medical consultation may be required to assess disease control and patient's tolerance for stress.

nesiritide
neh-sir′-i-tide
(Natrecor)

CATEGORY AND SCHEDULE
Pregnancy Risk Category: C

MECHANISM OF ACTION
A brain natriuretic peptide that facilitates cardiovascular homeostasis and fluid status through counter-regulation of the renin-angiotensin-aldosterone system, stimulating cyclic guanosine monophosphate, thereby leading to smooth-muscle cell relaxation. ***Therapeutic Effect:*** Promotes vasodilation, natriuresis, and diuresis, correcting CHF.

PHARMACOKINETICS
Route	Onset	Peak	Duration
IV	15–30 min	1–2 hr	4 hr

Excreted primarily in the heart by the left ventricle. Metabolized by the natriuretic neutral endopeptidase enzymes on the vascular luminal surface. ***Half-life:*** 18–23 min.

AVAILABILITY
Injection Powder for Reconstitution: 1.5 mg/5-ml vial.

INDICATIONS AND DOSAGES
▸ Treatment of Acutely Decompensated CHF in Patients with Dyspnea at Rest or with Minimal Activity
IV BOLUS
Adults, Elderly. 2 mcg/kg followed by a continuous IV infusion of 0.01 mcg/kg/min. May be

incrementally increased q3h to a maximum of 0.03 mcg/kg/min.

CONTRAINDICATIONS

Cardiogenic shock, systolic BP less than 90 mm Hg

INTERACTIONS

Drug

ACE inhibitors, IV nitroglycerin, milrinone, nitroprusside: May increase risk of hypotension.

Herbal

None known.

Food

None known.

Drug interactions of concern to dentistry

- None reported

DIAGNOSTIC TEST EFFECTS

None known.

IV INCOMPATIBILITIES

Sodium metabisulfite, bumetanide (Bumex), enalapril (Vasotec), ethacrynic acid (Edecrin), furosemide (Lasix), heparin, hydralazine (Apresoline), insulin

SIDE EFFECTS

Frequent (11%)

Hypotension

Occasional (8%–2%)

Headache, nausea, bradycardia

Rare (≤1%)

Confusion, paresthesia, somnolence, tremor

SERIOUS REACTIONS

! Ventricular arrhythmias, including ventricular tachycardia, atrial fibrillation, AV node conduction abnormalities, and angina pectoris occur rarely.

DENTAL CONSIDERATIONS

General:

- Acute-use drug for use in hospitals or emergency rooms.
- Review patient's medical and drug history.
- Only palliative dental care may be possible.

Consultations:

- Medical consultation may be required to assess disease control and patient's ability to tolerate stress.

nevirapine

neh-veer′-a-peen

(Viramune)

CATEGORY AND SCHEDULE

Pregnancy Risk Category: C

MECHANISM OF ACTION

A nonnucleoside reverse transcriptase inhibitor that binds directly to HIV-1 reverse transcriptase, thus changing the shape of this enzyme and blocking RNA- and DNA-dependent polymerase activity. ***Therapeutic Effect:*** Interferes with HIV replication, slowing the progression of HIV infection.

PHARMACOKINETICS

Readily absorbed after PO administration. Protein binding: 60%. Widely distributed. Extensively metabolized in the liver. Excreted primarily in urine. ***Half-life:*** 45 hr (single dose), 25–30 hr (multiple doses).

AVAILABILITY

Tablets: 200 mg.
Oral Suspension: 50 mg/5 ml.

INDICATIONS AND DOSAGES

▸ HIV Infection

PO

Adults. 200 mg once a day for 14 days (to reduce the risk of rash). Maintenance: 200 mg twice a day in combination with nucleoside analogues.
Children older than 8 yr. 4 mg/kg once a day for 14 days; then 4 mg/kg twice a day. Maximum: 400 mg/day.
Children 2 mos–8 yr. 4 mg/kg once a day for 14 days; then 7 mg/kg twice a day.

OFF-LABEL USES

To reduce the risk of transmitting HIV from infected mother to newborn

CONTRAINDICATIONS

None known.

INTERACTIONS

Drug

Ketoconazole, oral contraceptives, protease inhibitors: May decrease the plasma concentrations of these drugs.
Rifabutin, rifampin: May decrease nevirapine blood concentration.

Herbal

St. John's wort: May decrease blood concentration and effects of nevirapine.

Food

None known.

Drug interactions of concern to dentistry

- Should not be given with ketoconazole; monitor patients when other CYP3A4 isoenzyme inhibitors are used

DIAGNOSTIC TEST EFFECTS

May significantly increase serum bilirubin, GGT, AST (SGOT), and ALT (SGPT) levels. May significantly decrease Hgb level and neutrophil and platelet counts.

SIDE EFFECTS

Frequent (8%–3%)

Rash, fever, headache, nausea, granulocytopenia (more common in children)

Occasional (3%–1%)

Stomatitis (burning, erythema, or ulceration of the oral mucosa; dysphagia)

Rare (<1%)

Paresthesia, myalgia, abdominal pain

SERIOUS REACTIONS

! Hepatitis and rash may become severe and life threatening.

DENTAL CONSIDERATIONS

General:

- Determine why patient is taking the drug.
- Examine for oral manifestation of opportunistic infection.

Consultations:

- Medical consultation may be required to assess disease control.

Teach Patient/Family:

- Importance of good oral hygiene to prevent soft tissue inflammation
- To report oral lesions, soreness, or bleeding to dentist
- Importance of updating health history/drug record if physician makes any changes in evaluation or drug regimens
- That secondary oral infection may occur; must see dentist immediately if infection occurs

niacin, nicotinic acid

nye′-a-sin
(Niacor, Niaspan, Nicotinex, Slo-Niacin)
Do not confuse niacin, niacor, or niaspan with minocin or nitro-bid.
OTC

CATEGORY AND SCHEDULE

Pregnancy Risk Category: A (C if used at dosages above the recommended daily allowance)

MECHANISM OF ACTION

An antihyperlipidemic, water-soluble vitamin that is a component of two coenzymes needed for tissue respiration, lipid metabolism, and glycogenolysis. Inhibits synthesis of VLDLs. ***Therapeutic Effect:*** Reduces total, LDL, and VLDL cholesterol levels and triglyceride levels; increases HDL cholesterol concentration.

N

PHARMACOKINETICS

Readily absorbed from the GI tract. Widely distributed. Metabolized in the liver. Primarily excreted in urine. ***Half-life:*** 45 min.

AVAILABILITY

Capsules (Timed-Release): 125 mg, 250 mg, 400 mg, 500 mg.
Tablets (Niacor): 50 mg, 100 mg, 250 mg, 500 mg.
Tablets (Timed-Release [Slo-Niacin]): 250 mg, 500 mg, 750 mg.
Tablets (Timed-Release [Niaspan]): 500 mg, 750 mg, 1,000 mg.
Elixir (Nicotinex): 50 mg/5 ml.

INDICATIONS AND DOSAGES

▸ **Hyperlipidemia**

PO (Immediate-Release)

Adults, Elderly. Initially, 50–100 mg twice a day for 7 days. Increase gradually by doubling dose qwk up to 1–1.5 g/day in 2–3 doses. Maximum: 3 g/day.
Children. Initially, 100–250 mg/day (maximum: 10 mg/kg/day) in 3 divided doses. May increase by 100 mg/wk or 250 mg q2–3wk. Maximum: 2250 mg/day.

PO (Timed-Release)

Adults, Elderly. Initially, 500 mg/day in 2 divided doses for 1 week; then increase to 500 mg twice a day. Maintenance: 2 g/day.

▸ **Nutritional Supplement**

PO

Adults, Elderly. 10–20 mg/day. Maximum: 100 mg/day.

▸ **Pellegra**

PO

Adults, Elderly. 50–100 mg 3–4 times a day. Maximum: 500 mg/day.
Children. 50–100 mg 3 times a day.

CONTRAINDICATIONS

Active peptic ulcer disease, arterial hemorrhaging, hepatic dysfunction, hypersensitivity to niacin or tartrazine (frequently seen in patients sensitive to aspirin), severe hypotension

INTERACTIONS

Drug

Alcohol: May increase risk of niacin side effects, such as flushing.
Lovastatin, pravastatin, simvastatin: May increase the risk of acute renal failure and rhabdomyolysis.

Herbal

None known.

Food

None known.

Drug interactions of concern to dentistry

- None reported

DIAGNOSTIC TEST EFFECTS
May increase serum uric acid level.

SIDE EFFECTS
Frequent
Flushing (especially of the face and neck) occurring within 20 minutes of drug administration and lasting for 30–60 minutes, GI upset, pruritus
Occasional
Dizziness, hypotension, headache, blurred vision, burning or tingling of skin, flatulence, nausea, vomiting, diarrhea
Rare
Hyperglycemia, glycosuria, rash, hyperpigmentation, dry skin

SERIOUS REACTIONS
! Arrhythmias occur rarely.

DENTAL CONSIDERATIONS
General:
- Take vital signs at every appointment because of CV side effects.
- After supine positioning, have patient sit upright for at least 2 min before standing to avoid postural hypotension.
- Assess salivary flow as a factor in caries, periodontal disease, and candidiasis.

Teach Patient/Family:
- *When chronic dry mouth occurs, advise patient:*
  - To avoid mouth rinses with high alcohol content because of drying effects
  - Of need for daily use of home fluoride products to prevent caries
  - To use sugarless gum, frequent sips of water, or saliva substitutes

nicardipine hydrochloride
nye-card′-i-peen
(Cardene, Cardene IV, Cardene SR)
Do not confuse nicardipine with nifedipine, cardene with codeine, or cardene SR with cardizem SR or codeine.

CATEGORY AND SCHEDULE
Pregnancy Risk Category: C

MECHANISM OF ACTION
An antianginal and antihypertensive agent that inhibits calcium ion movement across cell membranes, depressing contraction of cardiac and vascular smooth muscle.
Therapeutic Effect: Increases heart rate and cardiac output. Decreases systemic vascular resistance and BP.

PHARMACOKINETICS

Route	Onset	Peak	Duration
PO	N/A	1–2 hr	8 hr

Rapidly, completely absorbed from the GI tract. Protein binding: 95%. Undergoes first-pass metabolism in the liver. Primarily excreted in urine. Not removed by hemodialysis.
Half-life: 2–4 hr.

AVAILABILITY
Capsules (Cardene): 20 mg, 30 mg.
Capsules, (Sustained-Release [Cardene SR]): 30 mg, 45 mg, 60 mg.
Injection (Cardene IV): 2.5 mg/ml.

INDICATIONS AND DOSAGES
▸ Chronic Stable (Effort-Associated) Angina
PO
Adults, Elderly. Initially, 20 mg 3 times a day. Range: 20–40 mg 3 times a day.

▸ Essential Hypertension
PO
Adults, Elderly. Initially, 20 mg 3 times a day. Range: 20–40 mg 3 times a day.
PO (Sustained-Release)
Adults, Elderly. Initially, 30 mg twice a day. Range: 30–60 mg twice a day.

▸ Short-term Treatment of Hypertension When Oral Therapy Isn't Feasible or Desirable (substitute for oral nicardipine)
IV
Adults, Elderly. 0.5 mg/hr (for patient receiving 20 mg PO q8h); 1.2 mg/hr (for patient receiving 30 mg PO q8h); 2.2 mg/hr (for patient receiving 40 mg PO q8h).

▸ Patients Not Already Receiving Nicardipine
IV
Adults, Elderly (gradual BP decrease). Initially, 5 mg/hr. May increase by 2.5 mg/hr q15min. After BP goal is achieved, decrease rate to 3 mg/hr.
Adults, Elderly (rapid BP decrease). Initially, 5 mg/hr. May increase by 2.5 mg/hr q5min. Maximum: 15 mg/hr until desired BP attained. After BP goal achieved, decrease rate to 3 mg/hr.

▸ Changing from IV to Oral Antihypertensive Therapy
Adults, Elderly. Begin antihypertensives other than nicardipine when IV has been discontinued; for nicardipine, give first dose 1 hr before discontinuing IV.

▸ Dosage in Hepatic Impairment
For adults and elderly patients, initially give 20 mg twice a day; then titrate.

▸ Dosage in Renal Impairment
For adults and elderly patients, initially give 20 mg q8h (30 mg twice a day [sustained-release capsules]); then titrate.

N

OFF-LABEL USES
Treatment of associated neurologic deficits, Raynaud's phenomenon, subarachnoid hemorrhage, vasospastic angina

CONTRAINDICATIONS
Atrial fibrillation or flutter associated with accessory conduction pathways, cardiogenic shock, CHF, second- or third-degree heart block, severe hypotension, sinus bradycardia, ventricular tachycardia, within several hours of IV beta-blocker therapy

INTERACTIONS
Drug
Beta blockers: May have additive effect.
Digoxin: May increase nicardipine blood concentration.
Hypokalemia-producing agents (such as furosemide and certain other diuretics): May increase risk of arrhythmias.
Procainamide, quinidine: May increase risk of QT-interval prolongation.
Herbal
None known.
Food
Grapefruit, grapefruit juice: May alter absorption of nicardipine.
Drug interactions of concern to dentistry
- Decreased effect: indomethacin, possibly other NSAIDs, phenobarbital, St. John's wort (herb)
- Increased effect: parenteral and inhalational general anesthetics or other drugs with hypotensive actions
- Possible risk of increased plasma level, monitor patient: erythromycin, ketoconazole, other CYP3A4 inhibitors
- Increased effects of nondepolarizing muscle relaxants
- Increased effects of carbamazepine

DIAGNOSTIC TEST EFFECTS

None known.

IV INCOMPATIBILITIES

Furosemide (Lasix), heparin, thiopental (Pentothal)

IV COMPATIBILITIES

Diltiazem (Cardizem), dobutamine (Dobutrex), dopamine (Intropin), epinephrine, hydromorphone (Dilaudid), labetalol (Trandate), lorazepam (Ativan), midazolam (Versed), milrinone (Primacor), morphine, nitroglycerin, norepinephrine (Levophed)

SIDE EFFECTS

Frequent (10%–7%)

Headache, facial flushing, peripheral edema, light-headedness, dizziness

Occasional (6%–3%)

Asthenia (loss of strength, energy), palpitations, angina, tachycardia

Rare (< 2%)

Nausea, abdominal cramps, dyspepsia, dry mouth, rash

SERIOUS REACTIONS

! Overdose produces confusion, slurred speech, somnolence, marked hypotension, and bradycardia.

DENTAL CONSIDERATIONS

General:

- Monitor cardiac status; take vital signs at each appointment because of CV side effects. Consider a stress reduction protocol to prevent stress-induced angina during the dental appointment.
- After supine positioning, have patient sit upright for at least 2 min before standing to avoid orthostatic hypotension.
- Place on frequent recall to monitor gingival condition.
- Limit use of sodium-containing products, such as saline IV fluids, for patients with a dietary salt restriction.
- Assess salivary flow as a factor in caries, periodontal disease, and candidiasis.
- Use vasoconstrictors with caution, in low doses, and with careful aspiration. Avoid use of gingival retraction cord with epinephrine.

Consultations:

- Medical consultation may be required to assess disease control and tolerance for stress.

Teach Patient/Family:

- Importance of good oral hygiene to prevent soft tissue inflammation and minimize gingival overgrowth
- Need for frequent oral prophylaxis if hyperplasia occurs
- *When chronic dry mouth occurs, advise patient:*
  - To avoid mouth rinses with high alcohol content because of drying effects
  - Of need for daily use of home fluoride products to prevent caries
  - To use sugarless gum, frequent sips of water, or saliva substitutes

nicotine

nik′-o-teen

(Commit, Habitrol[CAN], Nicabate[AUS], Nicabate CQ Clear[AUS], Nicabate CQ Lozenges[AUS], NicoDerm[CAN], NicoDerm CQ, Nicorette, Nicorette Plus[CAN], Nicotinell [AUS], Nicotrol, Nicotrol NS, Nicotrol Patch[CAN])

Do not confuse Nicoderm with Nitroderm.

CATEGORY AND SCHEDULE

Pregnancy Risk Category: D (transdermal)

OTC (Nicoderm transdermal patch, Nicotrol transdermal patch, Nicorette chewing gum)

MECHANISM OF ACTION

A cholinergic-receptor agonist binds to acetylcholine receptors, producing both stimulating and depressant effects on the peripheral and central nervous systems.
Therapeutic Effect: Provides a source of nicotine during nicotine withdrawal and reduces withdrawal symptoms.

PHARMACOKINETICS

Absorbed slowly after transdermal administration. Protein binding: 5%. Metabolized in the liver. Excreted primarily in urine.
Half-life: 4 hr.

AVAILABILITY

Chewing Gum (Nicorette): 2 mg, 4 mg.
Lozenge (Commit): 2 mg, 4 mg.
Transdermal patch (NicoDerm CQ, Nicotrol): 7 mg, 14 mg, 21 mg.
Nasal Spray (Nicotrol NS): 0.5 mg/spray.
*Inhalation (Nicotrol Inhaler):*10 mg cartridge.

N

INDICATIONS AND DOSAGES

▸ Smoking Cessation Aid to Relieve Nicotine Withdrawal Symptoms

PO (Chewing gum)
Adults, Elderly. Usually, 10–12 pieces/day. Maximum: 30 pieces/day.
PO (Lozenge)
Adults, Elderly. One 4-mg or 2-mg lozenge q1–2h for the first 6 weeks; one lozenge q2–4h for wk 7–9; and one lozenge q4–8h for wk 10–12. Maximum: one lozenge at a time, 5 lozenges/6 hr, 20 lozenges/day.
TRANSDERMAL
Adults, Elderly who smoke 10 cigarettes or more per day. Follow the guidelines below.
Step 1: 21 mg/day for 4–6 wk.
Step 2: 14 mg/day for 2 wk.
Step 3: 7 mg/day for 2 wk.
Adults, Elderly who smoke fewer than 10 cigarettes per day. Follow the guidelines below.
Step 1: 14 mg/day for 6 wk.
Step 2: 7 mg/day for 2 wk.*Patients weighing less than 100 lb, patients with a history of cardiovascular disease.* Initially, 14 mg/day for 4–6 wk, then 7 mg/day for 2–4 wk.
TRANSDERMAL (Nicotrol)
Adults, Elderly. One patch a day for 6 wk.
NASAL
Adults, Elderly. 1–2 doses/hr (1 dose = 2 sprays [1 in each nostril] = 1 mg). Maximum: 5 doses (5 mg)/hr; 40 doses (40 mg) /day.
INHALER (Nicotrol)
Adults, Elderly. Puff on nicotine cartridge mouthpiece for about 20 min as needed.

CONTRAINDICATIONS

Immediate post MI period, life-threatening arrhythmias, severe or worsening angina

INTERACTIONS

Drug

Beta-adrenergic blockers, bronchodilators (such as theophylline), insulin, propoxyphene: May increase the effects of these drugs.

Herbal

None known.

Food

None known.

Drug interactions of concern to dentistry

• Decreased dose at cessation of smoking: acetaminophen, caffeine, oxazepam, pentazocine
• Decreased metabolism of propoxyphene

Drug interactions of concern to dentistry nicotine polacrilex

• Increased blood levels with cessation of smoking: propoxyphene

DIAGNOSTIC TEST EFFECTS

None known.

SIDE EFFECTS

Frequent

All forms: Hiccups, nausea
Gum: Mouth or throat soreness, nausea, hiccups
Transdermal: Erythema, pruritus, or burning at application site

Occasional

All forms: Eructation, GI upset, dry mouth, insomnia, diaphoresis, irritability
Gum: Hiccups, hoarseness
Inhaler: Mouth or throat irritation, cough

Rare

All forms: Dizziness, myalgia, arthralgia

SERIOUS REACTIONS

! Overdose produces palpitations, tachyarrhythmias, seizures, depression, confusion, diaphoresis, hypotension, rapid or weak pulse, and dyspnea. Lethal dose for adults is 40–60 mg. Death results from respiratory paralysis.

DENTAL CONSIDERATIONS

General:

- Assess salivary flow as a factor in caries, periodontal disease, and candidiasis.

Teach Patient/Family:

- *When chronic dry mouth occurs, advise patient:*
  - To avoid mouth rinses with high alcohol content because of drying effects
  - Of need for daily use of home fluoride products to prevent caries
  - To use sugarless gum, frequent sips of water, or saliva substitutes
  - *When used in conjunction with a smoking cessation program in the dental office, teach:*
- All aspects of product drug; give package insert to patient and explain
  - That patch is to be used only to deter smoking
  - Not to use during pregnancy; birth defects may occur
  - To keep used and unused system out of reach of children and pets; potentially toxic if chewed or swallowed
  - To apply once per day to a nonhairy, clean, dry area of skin on upper body or upper outer arm
  - To stop smoking immediately when beginning treatment with patch
  - To apply promptly after removing from protective covering; system may lose strength

DENTAL CONSIDERATIONS

NICOTINE POLACRILEX

General:

- Take vital signs at every appointment because of CV side effects.
- Temporomandibular joint (TMJ) disorder may be aggravated by chewing because of heavier viscosity of gum.

Teach Patient/Family:

- Need for good oral hygiene to prevent periodontal inflammation
- *When chronic dry mouth occurs, advise patient:*
  - To avoid mouth rinses with high alcohol content because of drying effects
  - Of need for daily use of home fluoride products to prevent caries
  - To use sugarless gum, frequent sips of water, or saliva substitutes
- *When used in conjunction with a smoking cessation program in the dental office, teach:*
  - All aspects of product use; give package insert to patient and explain

- That gum is to be used only to deter smoking
- To avoid use in pregnancy; birth defects may occur
- To stop smoking when beginning treatment with gum
- To dispose of gum carefully because nicotine will still be present; to protect from children

nifedipine

nye-fed′-i-peen

(Adalat 5[AUS], Adalat 10[AUS], Adalat 20[AUS], Adalat CC, Adalat Oros[AUS], Apo-Nifed[CAN], Nifecard[AUS], Nifedicol XL, Nifehexal[AUS], Novo-Nifedin[CAN], Nyefax[AUS], Procardia, Procardia XL)

Do not confuse nifedipine with nicardipine or nimodipine.

CATEGORY AND SCHEDULE

Pregnancy Risk Category: C

N

MECHANISM OF ACTION

An antianginal and antihypertensive agent that inhibits calcium ion movement across cell membranes, depressing contraction of cardiac and vascular smooth muscle. ***Therapeutic Effect:*** Increases heart rate and cardiac output. Decreases systemic vascular resistance and BP.

PHARMACOKINETICS

Route	Onset	Peak	Duration
Sublingual	1–5 min	N/A	N/A
PO	20–30 min	N/A	4–8 hr
PO (extended release)	2 hr	N/A	24 hr

Rapidly, completely absorbed from the GI tract. Protein binding: 92%–98%. Undergoes first-pass metabolism in the liver. Primarily excreted in urine. Not removed by hemodialysis. ***Half-life:*** 2–5 hr.

AVAILABILITY

Capsules (Procardia): 10 mg.
Tablets (Extended-Release [Adalat CC, Procardia XL]): 30 mg, 60 mg, 90 mg.
Tablets (Extended-Release [Nifedical XL]): 30 mg, 60 mg.

INDICATIONS AND DOSAGES

▸ Prinzmetal's Variant Angina, Chronic Stable (Effort-Associated) Angina

PO

Adults, Elderly. Initially, 10 mg 3 times a day. Increase at 7- to 14-day intervals. Maintenance: 10 mg 3 times a day up to 30 mg 4 times a day.

PO (Extended-Release)

Adults, Elderly. Initially, 30–60 mg/day. Maintenance: Up to 120 mg/day.

▸ Essential Hypertension

PO (Extended-Release)

Adults, Elderly. Initially, 30–60 mg/day. Maintenance: Up to 120 mg/day.

OFF-LABEL USES

Treatment of Raynaud's phenomenon

CONTRAINDICATIONS

Advanced aortic stenosis, severe hypotension

INTERACTIONS

Drug

Beta blockers: May have additive effect.
Digoxin: May increase digoxin blood concentration.
Hypokalemia-producing agents (such as furosemide and certain other diuretics): May increase risk of arrhythmias.

Herbal
None known.
Food
Grapefruit, grapefruit juice: May increase nifedipine plasma concentration.
Drug interactions of concern to dentistry
• Decreased effect: indomethacin, possibly other NSAIDs, phenobarbital
• Increased effect: parenteral and inhalational general anesthetics or other drugs with hypotensive actions
• Possible increase in effects, monitor patients: inhibitors of CYP3A4 isoenzyme
• Increased effects of nondepolarizing muscle relaxants
• Increased effects of carbamazepine

DIAGNOSTIC TEST EFFECTS

May cause positive ANA and direct Coombs' test.

SIDE EFFECTS

Frequent (30%–11%)
Peripheral edema, headache, flushed skin, dizziness
Occasional (12%–6%)
Nausea, shakiness, muscle cramps and pain, somnolence, palpitations, nasal congestion, cough, dyspnea, wheezing, oral gingival overgrowth
Rare (5%–3%)
Hypotension, rash, pruritus, urticaria, constipation, abdominal discomfort, flatulence, sexual difficulties

SERIOUS REACTIONS

! Nifedipine may precipitate CHF and MI in patients with cardiac disease and peripheral ischemia.
! Overdose produces nausea, somnolence, confusion, and slurred speech.

DENTAL CONSIDERATIONS

General:
• Monitor cardiac status; take vital signs at each appointment because of CV side effects. Consider a stress reduction protocol to prevent stress-induced angina during the dental appointment.
• After supine positioning, have patient sit upright for at least 2 min before standing to avoid orthostatic hypotension at dismissal.
• Place on frequent recall to monitor gingival condition.
• Limit use of sodium-containing products, such as saline IV fluids, for patients with a dietary salt restriction.
• Assess salivary flow as a factor in caries, periodontal disease, and candidiasis.
• Use vasoconstrictors with caution, in low doses, and with careful aspiration. Avoid use of gingival retraction cord with epinephrine.

Consultations:
• Medical consultation may be required to assess disease control and stress tolerance.

Teach Patient/Family:
• Importance of good oral hygiene to prevent soft tissue inflammation and minimize gingival overgrowth
• Need for frequent oral prophylaxis if hyperplasia occurs
• *When chronic dry mouth occurs, advise patient:*
  • To avoid mouth rinses with high alcohol content because of drying effects
  • Of need for daily use of home fluoride products to prevent caries
  • To use sugarless gum, frequent sips of water, or saliva substitutes

nilutamide

nih-lute′-ah-myd
(Anandron[CAN], Nilandron)

CATEGORY AND SCHEDULE

Pregnancy Risk Category: C

MECHANISM OF ACTION

An antiandrogen hormone and antineoplastic agent that competitively inhibits androgen action by binding to androgen receptors in target tissue.
Therapeutic Effect: Decreases growth of abnormal prostate tissue.

AVAILABILITY

Tablets: 150 mg.

INDICATIONS AND DOSAGES

▶ Prostatic Carcinoma

PO

Adults, Elderly. 300 mg once a day for 30 days, then 150 mg once a day. Begin on day of, or day after, surgical castration.

CONTRAINDICATIONS

Severe hepatic impairment, severe respiratory insufficiency

INTERACTIONS

Drug

None known.

Herbal

None known.

Food

None known.

Drug interactions of concern to dentistry

- Avoid drugs that may aggravate urinary retention when symptoms are present
- This is an inhibitor of CYP3A4 isoenzymes; no specific studies have been done, but use caution when prescribing drugs metabolized by this enzyme

DIAGNOSTIC TEST EFFECTS

May increase serum bilirubin, creatinine, AST (SGOT), and ALT (SGPT) levels.

SIDE EFFECTS

Frequent (>10%)

Hot flashes, delay in recovering vision after bright illumination (such as sun, television, bright lights), decreased libido, diminished sexual function, mild nausea, gynecomastia, alcohol intolerance

Occasional (<10%)

Constipation, hypertension, dizziness, dyspnea, UTIs

SERIOUS REACTIONS

! Interstitial pneumonitis occurs rarely.

DENTAL CONSIDERATIONS

General:

- Monitor and record vital signs.
- If additional analgesia is required for dental pain, consider alternative analgesics (NSAIDs) in patients taking narcotics for acute or chronic pain.
- Avoid dental light in patient's eyes; offer dark glasses for patient comfort.
- This drug may be used in the hospital or on an outpatient basis. Confirm the patient's disease and treatment status.
- Short appointments and a stress reduction protocol may be required for anxious patients.

Consultations:

- Medical consultation may be required to assess immunologic status during cancer chemotherapy and determine safety risk, if any, posed by the required dental treatment.

N

• Medical consultation may be required to assess disease control and patient's ability to tolerate stress.

Teach Patient/Family:

• Importance of good oral hygiene to prevent soft tissue inflammation
• To prevent trauma when using oral hygiene aids
• To report oral lesions, soreness, or bleeding to dentist
• Importance of updating health and medication history if physician makes any changes in evaluation or drug regimens; include OTC, herbal, and nonherbal in the update

nimodipine

nye-mode′-i-peen
(Nimotop)
Do not confuse nimodipine with nifedipine.

CATEGORY AND SCHEDULE

Pregnancy Risk Category: C

MECHANISM OF ACTION

A cerebral vasospasm agent that inhibits movement of calcium ions across vascular smooth-muscle cell membranes. ***Therapeutic Effect:*** Produces favorable effect on severity of neurologic deficits due to cerebral vasospasm. Exerts greatest effect on cerebral arteries; may prevent cerebral spasm.

PHARMACOKINETICS

Rapidly absorbed from the GI tract. Protein binding: 95%. Metabolized in the liver. Excreted in urine; eliminated in feces. Not removed by hemodialysis. ***Half-life:*** terminal, 3 hr.

AVAILABILITY

Capsules: 30 mg.

INDICATIONS AND DOSAGES

▸ Improvement Neurologic Deficits after Subarachnoid Hemorrhage from Ruptured Congenital Aneurysms

PO

Adults, Elderly. 60 mg q4h for 21 days. Begin within 96 hr of subarachnoid hemorrhage.

OFF-LABEL USES

Treatment of chronic and classic migraine, chronic cluster headaches

CONTRAINDICATIONS

Atrial fibrillation or flutter, cardiogenic shock, CHF, heart block, sinus bradycardia, ventricular tachycardia, within several hours of IV beta-blocker therapy

INTERACTIONS

Drug

Beta blockers: May prolong SA and AV conduction, which may lead to severe hypotension, bradycardia, and cardiac failure.
Erythromycin, itraconazole, ketoconazole, protease inhibitors: May inhibit the metabolism of nimodipine.
Rifabutin, rifampin: May increase the metabolism of nimodipine.

Herbal

Garlic: May increase antihypertensive effect.
Ginseng, yohimbe: May worsen hypertension.

Food

Grapefruit juice: May increase nimodipine blood concentration and risk of toxicity.

Drug interactions of concern to dentistry

• Hypotension: anesthetics, other antihypertensive medications
• Antagonism of antihypertensive effect: indomethacin and possibly other NSAIDs

• Possible reduction in antihypertensive effects: sympathomimetics

DIAGNOSTIC TEST EFFECTS

None known.

SIDE EFFECTS

Occasional (6%–2%)

Hypotension, peripheral edema, diarrhea, headache

Rare (<2%)

Allergic reaction (rash, hives), tachycardia, flushing of skin

SERIOUS REACTIONS

! Overdose produces nausea, weakness, dizziness, somnolence, confusion, and slurred speech.

DENTAL CONSIDERATIONS

General:

• Patients may have significant neurologic deficit; dental care may not be practical.
• Caution: potential for interactions with drugs used in dentistry.
• Determine why patient is taking the drug.
• Monitor and record vital signs.
• After supine positioning, have patient sit upright for at least 2 min before standing to avoid orthostatic hypotension.

Consultations:

• This drug may be used in the hospital or on an outpatient basis. Confirm the patient's disease and treatment status.
• Medical consultation may be required to assess disease control and patient's ability to tolerate stress.

Teach Patient/Family:

• Importance of good oral hygiene to prevent soft tissue inflammation
• Use of electric toothbrush if patient has difficulty holding conventional devices.
• Importance of updating health and medication history if physician makes any changes in evaluation or drug regimens; include OTC, herbal, and nonherbal in the update

nisoldipine

nye-soul-dih-peen
(Sular)
Do not confuse with nicardipine.

CATEGORY AND SCHEDULE

Pregnancy Risk Category: C

MECHANISM OF ACTION

A calcium channel blocker that inhibits calcium ion movement across cell membrane, depressing contraction of cardiac and vascular smooth muscle. ***Therapeutic Effect:*** Increases heart rate and cardiac output. Decreases systemic vascular resistance and blood pressure (B/P).

PHARMACOKINETICS

Poor absorption from the gastrointestinal (GI) tract. Food increases bioavailability. Protein binding: more than 99%. Metabolism occurs in the gut wall. Primarily excreted in urine. Not removed by hemodialysis. ***Half-life:*** 7–12 hrs.

AVAILABILITY

Tablets (extended-release): 10 mg, 20 mg, 30 mg, 40 mg (Sular).

INDICATIONS AND DOSAGES

▸ Hypertension

PO

Adults. Initially, 20 mg once daily, then increase by 10 mg per week, or longer intervals until therapeutic B/P response is attained.

Elderly. Initially, 10 mg once daily. Increase by 10 mg per week to therapeutic response. Maintenance: 20–40 mg once daily. Maximum: 60 mg once daily.

OFF-LABEL USES
Stable angina pectoris, CHF

CONTRAINDICATIONS
Sick-sinus syndrome/second- or third-degree AV block (except in presence of pacemaker), hypersensitivity to nisoldipine or any component of the formulation

INTERACTIONS
Drug
Amiodarone: May increase risk of bradycardia, atrioventricular block, and/or sinus arrest.
Beta-blockers: May have additive effect.
Delavirdine, ketoconazole, voriconazole: May increase serum nisoldipine concentrations.
Digoxin: May increase digoxin blood concentration.
Epirubicin: May increase risk of heart failure.
Fentanyl: May increase risk of severe hypotension.
Phenytoin, fosphenytoin: May decrease nisoldipine concentrations.
NSAIDs, oral anticoagulants: May increase risk of gastrointestinal hemorrhage and/or antagonism of hypotensive effect.
Quinidine: May increase risk of quinidine toxicity.
Quinupristin/dalfopristin, saquinavir: May increase risk of nisoldipine toxicity.
Rifampin: May decrease nisoldipine efficacy.
Herbal
Licorice, Ma huang, peppermint oil, yohimbine: May decrease effectiveness of nisoldipine.
St. John's Wort: May decrease bioavailability of nisoldipine.
Food
Grapefruit and grapefruit juice: May increase nisoldipine plasma concentration.

Drug interactions of concern to dentistry
- Possible increase in serum levels: fluconazole, ketoconazole, itraconazole, and other CYP3A4 isoenzyme inhibitors
- Decreased antihypertensive effect: indomethacin, possibly other NSAIDs, phenobarbital
- Increased effect: parenteral and inhalational general anesthetics or other drugs with hypotensive actions
- Increased effects of carbamazepine

DIAGNOSTIC TEST EFFECTS
None known.

IV INCOMPATIBILITIES
None known.
IV COMPATIBILITIES
None known.

SIDE EFFECTS
Frequent
Giddiness, dizziness, lightheadedness, peripheral edema, headache, flushing, weakness, nausea, oral gingival overgrowth
Occasional
Transient hypotension, heartburn, muscle cramps, nasal congestion, cough, wheezing, sore throat, palpitations, nervousness, mood changes
Rare
Increase in frequency, intensity, duration of anginal attack during initial therapy

SERIOUS REACTIONS
! May precipitate congestive heart failure (CHF) and myocardial infarction (MI) in patients with cardiac disease and peripheral ischemia.
! Overdose produces nausea, drowsiness, confusion, and slurred speech.

DENTAL CONSIDERATIONS

General:

- Stress from dental procedures may compromise CV function; determine patient risk.
- Monitor vital signs at every appointment because of CV side effects.
- Short appointments and a stress reduction protocol may be required for anxious patients.
- When taken with grapefruit juice may see increased plasma levels.
- Limit use of sodium-containing products, such as saline IV fluids, for patients with a dietary salt restriction.
- After supine positioning, have patient sit upright for at least 2 min before standing to avoid orthostatic hypotension.
- Assess salivary flow as a factor in caries, periodontal disease, and candidiasis.

Consultations:

- Medical consultation may be required to assess disease control and patient's ability to tolerate stress.

Teach Patient/Family:

- Need for frequent oral prophylaxis if gingival overgrowth should occur
- *When chronic dry mouth occurs, advise patient:*
  - To avoid mouth rinses with high alcohol content because of drying effects
  - To use daily home fluoride products for anticaries effect
  - To use sugarless gum, frequent sips of water, or saliva substitutes

N

nitazoxanide

nigh-tazz-oks′-ah-nide
(Alinia)

CATEGORY AND SCHEDULE

Pregnancy Risk Category: B

MECHANISM OF ACTION

An antiparasitic that interferes with the body's reaction to pyruvate ferredoxin oxidoreductase, an enzyme essential for anaerobic energy metabolism. ***Therapeutic Effect:*** Produces antiprotozoal activity, reducing or terminating diarrheal episodes.

PHARMACOKINETICS

Rapidly hydrolyzed to an active metabolite. Protein binding: 99%. Excreted in the urine, bile, and feces. ***Half-life:*** 2–4 hr.

AVAILABILITY

Powder for Oral Suspension: 100 mg/5 ml.

INDICATIONS AND DOSAGES

▸ Diarrhea

PO

Children 12 yr and older. 200 mg q12h.
Children 4–11 yr. 200 mg (10 ml) q12h for 3 days.
Children 12–47 mo. 100 mg (5 ml) q12h for 3 days.

CONTRAINDICATIONS

History of sensitivity to aspirin and salicylates

INTERACTIONS

Drug

None known.

Herbal

None known.

Food
None known.
Drug interactions of concern to dentistry
- None reported

DIAGNOSTIC TEST EFFECTS
May increase serum creatinine and ALT(SGPT) levels.

SIDE EFFECTS
Occasional (8%)
Abdominal pain
Rare (2%–1%)
Diarrhea, vomiting, headache

SERIOUS REACTIONS
! None known.

DENTAL CONSIDERATIONS
General:
- This is a acute-use drug; patients highly unlikely to present for dental care.
- Ensure patients are well hydrated and electrolytes reestablished following recovery if they present for dental treatment.

Consultations:
- Medical consultation may be required to assess disease control.

Teach Patient/Family:
- To maintain or reestablish oral hygiene care

nitrofurantoin sodium
nye-troe-fyoor′-an-toyn
(Apo-Nitrofurantoin[CAN], Furadantin, Macrobid, Macrodantin, Novo-Furan[CAN], Ralodantin[AUS])

CATEGORY AND SCHEDULE
Pregnancy Risk Category: B

MECHANISM OF ACTION
An antibacterial UTI agent that inhibits the synthesis of bacterial DNA, RNA, proteins, and cell walls by altering or inactivating ribosomal proteins. ***Therapeutic Effect:*** Bacteriostatic (bactericidal at high concentrations).

PHARMACOKINETICS
Microcrystalline form rapidly and completely absorbed; macrocrystalline form more slowly absorbed. Food increases absorption. Protein binding: 40%. Primarily concentrated in urine and kidneys. Metabolized in most body tissues. Primarily excreted in urine. Removed by hemodialysis. ***Half-life:*** 20–60 min.

AVAILABILITY
Capsules (Macrocrystalline [Macrobid]): 100 mg.
Capsules (Macrocrystalline [Macrodantin]): 25 mg, 50 mg, 100 mg
Oral Suspension (Microcrystalline [Furadantin]): 25 mg/5 ml.

INDICATIONS AND DOSAGES
▸ **Urinary Tract Infections (UTIs)**
PO (Furadantin, Macrodantin)
Adults, Elderly. 50–100 mg q6h. Maximum: 400 mg/day.
Children. 5–7 mg/kg/day in divided doses q6h. Maximum: 400 mg/day.
PO (Macrobid)
Adults, Elderly. 100 mg twice a day. Maximum: 400 mg/day.
▸ **Long-term Prevention of UTIs**
PO
Adults, Elderly. 50–100 mg at bedtime.
Children. 1–2 mg/kg/day as a single dose. Maximum: 100 mg/day.

OFF-LABEL USES
Prevention of bacterial UTIs

N

CONTRAINDICATIONS
Anuria, oliguria, substantial renal impairment (creatinine clearance less than 40 ml/min); infants younger than 1 mo old because of the risk of hemolytic anemia

INTERACTIONS
Drug
Hemolytics: May increase the risk of nitrofurantoin toxicity.
Neurotoxic medications: May increase the risk of neurotoxicity.
Probenecid: May increase blood concentration and toxicity of nitrofurantoin.
Herbal
None known.
Food
None known.
Drug interactions of concern to dentistry
- Increased effects: anticholinergic drugs

N

DIAGNOSTIC TEST EFFECTS
None known.

SIDE EFFECTS
Frequent
Anorexia, nausea, vomiting, dark urine
Occasional
Abdominal pain, diarrhea, rash, pruritus, urticaria, hypertension, headache, dizziness, drowsiness
Rare
Photosensitivity, transient alopecia, asthmatic exacerbation in those with history of asthma

SERIOUS REACTIONS
! Superinfection, hepatotoxicity, peripheral neuropathy (may be irreversible), Stevens-Johnson syndrome, permanent pulmonary function impairment, and anaphylaxis occur rarely.

DENTAL CONSIDERATIONS
General:
- Determine why the patient is taking the drug.
Consultations:
- Medical consultation may be required to assess disease control and to select an antiinfective if a dental infection is diagnosed.

nitrofurazone
nye-troe-fyoor′-a-zone
(Furacin)
Do not confuse with nitrofurantoin.

CATEGORY AND SCHEDULE
Pregnancy Risk Category: C
OTC (ointment)

MECHANISM OF ACTION
A synthetic nitrofuran that inhibits bacterial enzymes involved in carbohydrate metabolism.
Therapeutic Effect: Inhibits a variety of enzymes. Bactericidal.

PHARMACOKINETICS
Not known.

AVAILABILITY
Cream: 0.2% (Furacin).
Ointment: 0.2% (Furacin).
Solution: 0.2% (Furacin).

INDICATIONS AND DOSAGES
▸ Burns, Catheter-Related Urinary Tract Infection, Skin Grafts
TOPICAL
Adults. Apply directly on lesion with spatula or place on a piece of gauze first. Use of a bandage is optional. Preparation should remain

on lesion for at least 24 hours. Dressing may be changed several times daily or left on the lesion for a longer period.

OFF-LABEL USES

Treatment of fire and ant bites, scabies, urethritis, vaginal malodor, vasectomy, wounds

CONTRAINDICATIONS

Hypersensitivity to nitrofurazone or any of its components

INTERACTIONS

Drug

None known.

Herbal

None known.

Food

None known.

Drug interactions of concern to dentistry

- None reported

DIAGNOSTIC TEST EFFECTS

None known.

SIDE EFFECTS

Occasional

Itching, rash, swelling

SERIOUS REACTIONS

! Use of nitrofurazone may result in bacterial or fungal overgrowth of nonsusceptible pathogens, which may lead to secondary infection.

DENTAL CONSIDERATIONS

General:

- Dental management depends on extent and severity of burns and patients ability to cooperate; use aseptic techniques.
- Provide palliative dental care for dental emergencies only.
- Monitor and record vital signs.

Consultations:

- Medical consultation may be required to assess disease control and patient's ability to tolerate stress.
- Consult patient's physician if an acute dentol infection occurs and another antiinfective is required.

Teach Patient/Family:

- Importance of good oral hygiene to prevent soft tissue inflammation
- To prevent trauma when using oral hygiene aids

nitroglycerin

nye-troe-gli′-ser-in

(Anginine[AUS], Minitran, Nitradisc[AUS], Nitrek, Nitro-Bid, Nitro-Dur, Nitrogard, Nitroject[CAN], Nitrolingual, Nitrolingual Spray[AUS], Nitrong-SR, NitroQuick, Nitrostat, Nitro-Tab, Rectogesic[AUS], Transiderm Nitro[AUS], Trinipatch[CAN])

Do not confuse nitroglycerin with nitroprusside; Nitro-Bid with Nicobid; Nitro-Dur with Nicoderm; Nitrostat with Hyperstat, Nilstat, or Nystatin; or Nitrong-SR with Nizoral.

CATEGORY AND SCHEDULE

Pregnancy Risk Category: B

MECHANISM OF ACTION

A nitrate that decreases myocardial oxygen demand. Reduces left ventricular preload and afterload.

Therapeutic Effect: Dilates coronary arteries and improves collateral blood flow to ischemic areas within myocardium.

IV form produces peripheral vasodilation.

N

PHARMACOKINETICS

Route	Onset	Peak	Duration
Sublingual	1–3 min	4–8 min	30–60 min
Translingual spray	2 min	4–10 min	30–60 min
Buccal Tablet	2–5 min	4–10 min	2 hr
PO (Extended-Release)	20–45 min	45–120 min	4–8 hr
Topical	15–60 min	30–120 min	2–12 hr
Transdermal Patch	40–60 min	60–180 min	18–24 hr
IV	1–2 min	Immediate	3–5 min

Well absorbed after PO, sublingual, and topical administration. Undergoes extensive first-pass metabolism. Metabolized in the liver and by enzymes in the bloodstream. Primarily excreted in urine. Not removed by hemodialysis. ***Half-life:*** 1–4 min.

AVAILABILITY

Capsules (Extended-Release [NitroBid]): 2.5 mg, 6.5 mg, 9 mg.
Tablets (Buccal [Nitrogard]): 2 mg, 3 mg.
Tablets (Sublingual [Nitro Quick, Nitrostat, Nitro-Tab]): 0.4 mg, 0.6 mg.
Spray (Translingual [Nitrolingual]): 0.4 mg/spray.
Infusion Solution: 0.1 mg/ml, 0.2 mg/ml, 0.4 mg/ml.
Topical Ointment (Nitro-Bid, Nitrol): 2%.
Transdermal Patch (Minitran): 0.1 mg/h, 0.2 mg/h, 0.3 mg/h, 0.4 mg/h.
Transdermal Patch (NitroDur): 0.1 mg/h, 0.2 mg/h, 0.3 mg/h, 0.4 mg/h, 0.6 mg/h, 0.8 mg/h.
Transdermal Patch (Nitrek): 0.2 mg/h, 0.4 mg/h, 0.6 mg/h.

INDICATIONS AND DOSAGES

▸ Acute Relief of Angina Pectoris, Acute Prophylaxis

Lingual Spray
Adults, Elderly. 1 spray onto or under tongue q3–5min until relief is noted (no more than 3 sprays in 15-min period).
SUBLINGUAL
Adults, Elderly. 0.4 mg q5min until relief is noted (no more than 3 doses in 15-min period). Use prophylactically 5–10 min before activities that may cause an acute attack.

▸ Long-Term Prophylaxis of Angina

PO (Extended-Release)
Adults, Elderly. 2.5–9 mg q8–12h.
TOPICAL
Adults, Elderly. Initially, ½ inch q8h. Increase by ½ inch with each application. Range: 1–2 inches q8h up to 4–5 inches q4h.
TRANSDERMAL PATCH
Adults, Elderly. Initially, 0.2–0.4 mg/hr. Maintenance: 0.4–0.8 mg/hr. Consider patch on for 12–14 hr, patch off for 10–12 hr (prevents tolerance).

▸ CHF Associated with Acute MI

IV
Adults, Elderly. Initially, 5 mcg/min via infusion pump. Increase in 5-mcg/min increments at 3- to 5-min intervals until BP response is noted or until dosage reaches 20 mcg/min; then increase as needed by 10 mcg/min. Dosage may be further titrated according to clinical, therapeutic response up to 200 mcg/min.
Children. Initially, 0.25–0.5 mcg/kg/min; titrate by 0.5–1 mcg/kg/min up to 20 mcg/kg/min.

CONTRAINDICATIONS

Allergy to adhesives (transdermal), closed-angle glaucoma, constrictive pericarditis (IV), early MI (sublingual), GI hypermotility or malabsorption (extended-release), head trauma, hypotension (IV), inadequate cerebral circulation (IV), increased intracranial pressure, nitrates, orthostatic hypotension, pericardial tamponade (IV), severe anemia, uncorrected hypovolemia (IV)

INTERACTIONS

Drug

Alcohol, other antihypertensives, vasodilators: May increase risk of orthostatic hypotension.
Sildenafil, tadalafil, vardenafil: Concurrent use of these drugs produces significant hypotension.

Herbal

None known.

Food

None known.

Drug interactions of concern to dentistry

• Increased hypotensive effects: alcohol, opioids, benzodiazepines, phenothiazines, and other drugs used in conscious sedation techniques

DIAGNOSTIC TEST EFFECTS

May increase blood methemoglobin, urine catecholamine, and urine vanillylmandelic acid concentrations.

IV INCOMPATIBILITIES

Alteplase (Activase)

IV COMPATIBILITIES

Amiodarone (Cordarone), diltiazem (Cardizem), dobutamine (Dobutrex), dopamine (Intropin), epinephrine, famotidine (Pepcid), fentanyl (Sublimaze), furosemide (Lasix), heparin, hydromorphone (Dilaudid), insulin, labetalol (Trandate), lidocaine, lorazepam (Ativan), midazolam (Versed), milrinone (Primacor), morphine, nicardipine (Cardene), nitroprusside (Nipride), norepinephrine (Levophed), propofol (Diprivan)

SIDE EFFECTS

Frequent

Headache (possibly severe; occurs mostly in early therapy, diminishes rapidly in intensity, and usually disappears during continued treatment), transient flushing of face and neck, dizziness (especially if patient is standing immobile or is in a warm environment), weakness, orthostatic hypotension
Sublingual: Burning, tingling sensation at oral point of dissolution
Ointment: Erythema, pruritus

Occasional

GI upset
Transdermal: Contact dermatitis

SERIOUS REACTIONS

! Nitroglycerin should be discontinued if blurred vision or dry mouth occurs.
! Severe orthostatic hypotension may occur, manifested by fainting, pulselessness, cold or clammy skin, and diaphoresis.
! Tolerance may occur with repeated, prolonged therapy; minor tolerance may occur with intermittent use of sublingual tablets.
! High doses of nitroglycerin tend to produce severe headache.

DENTAL CONSIDERATIONS

General:

• Take vital signs at every appointment because of CV side effects.
• After supine positioning, have patient sit upright for at least 2 min before standing to avoid orthostatic hypotension.

N

- Assess salivary flow as a factor in caries, periodontal disease, and candidiasis.
- Ensure that patient's drug is easily available if angina occurs.
- A benzodiazepine or nitrous oxide/oxygen may be prescribed to allay anxiety.
- Check expiration date on prescription to ensure drug activity. If bottle has been opened, the shelf life is 3 months.
- Stress from dental procedures may compromise CV function; determine patient risk.
- Talk with patient about disease control (frequency of angina episodes).
- Use vasoconstrictors with caution, in low doses, and with careful aspiration. Avoid gingival retraction cord with epinephrine.
- Short appointments and a stress reduction protocol may be required for anxious patients.
- Consider semisupine chair position for patients with CV disease.

Consultations:

- Medical consultation may be required to assess disease control and patient's ability to tolerate stress.

Teach Patient/Family:

- Importance of good oral hygiene to prevent soft tissue inflammation
- Caution to prevent injury when using oral hygiene aids
- *When chronic dry mouth occurs, advise patient:*
  - To avoid mouth rinses with high alcohol content because of drying effects
  - Of need for daily use of home fluoride products to prevent caries
  - To use sugarless gum, frequent sips of water, or saliva substitutes

N

nizatidine

ni-za′-ti-deen

(Apo-Nizatidine[CAN], Axid, Axid AR, Tazac[AUS])

Do not confuse Axid with Ansaid.

CATEGORY AND SCHEDULE

Pregnancy Risk Category: B

OTC (75 mg capsules)

MECHANISM OF ACTION

An antiulcer agent and gastric acid secretion inhibitor that inhibits histamine action at histamine 2 receptors of parietal cells. ***Therapeutic Effect:*** Inhibits basal and nocturnal gastric acid secretion.

PHARMACOKINETICS

Rapidly, well absorbed from the GI tract. Protein binding: 35%. Metabolized in the liver. Primarily excreted in urine. Not removed by hemodialysis. ***Half-life:*** 1–2 hr (increased with impaired renal function).

AVAILABILITY

Capsules: 75 mg (Axid AR), 150 mg (Axid), 300 mg (Axid).
Oral Solution (Axid): 15 mg/ml.

INDICATIONS AND DOSAGES

▸ Active Duodenal Ulcer

PO

Adults, Elderly. 300 mg at bedtime or 150 mg twice a day.

▸ Prevention of Duodenal Ulcer Recurrence

PO

Adults, Elderly. 150 mg at bedtime.

▸ Gastroesophageal Reflux Disease

PO

Adults, Elderly. 150 mg twice a day.

▸ **Active Benign Gastric Ulcer**
PO
Adults, Elderly. 150 mg twice a day or 300 mg at bedtime.
PO, oral solution
Children 12 yr and older. 2 tsp twice a day.

▸ **Dyspepsia**
PO
Adults, Elderly. 75 mg 30–60 min before meals; no more than 2 tablets a day.

▸ **Dosage in Renal Impairment**
Dosage adjustment is based on creatinine clearance.

Creatinine Clearance	Active Ulcer	Maintenance Therapy
20–50 ml/min	150 mg at bedtime	150 mg every other day
less than 20 ml/min	150 mg every other day	150 mg q3 days

OFF-LABEL USES
Gastric hypersecretory conditions, multiple endocrine adenoma, Zollinger-Ellison syndrome, weight gain reduction in patients taking Zyprexa

CONTRAINDICATIONS
Hypersensitivity to other H_2-antagonists

INTERACTIONS
Drug
Antacids: May decrease the absorption of nizatidine.
Ketoconazole: May decrease the absorption of ketoconazole.
Herbal
None known.
Food
None known.
Drug interactions of concern to dentistry
- Increased serum salicylate when administered with high doses of aspirin
- Decreased absorption of ketoconazole (take doses 2 hr apart)

DIAGNOSTIC TEST EFFECTS
Interferes with skin tests using allergen extracts. May increase serum alkaline phosphatase, AST, and ALT levels.

SIDE EFFECTS
Occasional (2%)
Somnolence, fatigue
Rare (1%)
Diaphoresis, rash

SERIOUS REACTIONS
! Asymptomatic ventricular tachycardia, hyperuricemia not associated with gout, and nephrolithiasis occur rarely.

DENTAL CONSIDERATIONS
General:
- Avoid prescribing aspirin-containing products in patients with active GI disease.

Teach Patient/Family:
- To avoid mouth rinses with high alcohol content because of drying effects

N

norepinephrine bitartrate
nor-ep-i-nef′-rin
nor-ep-i-nef′-rin
(Levophed)
Do not confuse Levophed with Levid, or norepinephrine with epinephrine.

CATEGORY AND SCHEDULE
Pregnancy Risk Category: C

MECHANISM OF ACTION
A sympathomimetic that stimulates $beta_1$-adrenergic receptors and

alpha-adrenergic receptors, increasing peripheral resistance. Enhances contractile myocardial force, increases cardiac output. Constricts resistance and capacitance vessels. ***Therapeutic Effect:*** Increases systemic BP and coronary blood flow.

PHARMACOKINETICS

Route	Onset	Peak	Duration
IV	Rapid	1–2 min	N/A

Localized in sympathetic tissue. Metabolized in the liver. Primarily excreted in urine.

AVAILABILITY

Injection: 1-mg/ml ampules.

INDICATIONS AND DOSAGES

▸ Acute Hypotension Unresponsive to Fluid Volume Replacement

IV

Adults, Elderly. Initially, administer at 0.5–1 mcg/min. Adjust rate of flow to establish and maintain desired BP (40 mm Hg below preexisting systolic pressure). Average maintenance dose: 8–12 mcg/min.

Children. Initially, 0.05–0.1 mcg/kg/min; titrate to desired effect. Maximum: 1–2 mcg/kg/min. Range: 0.5–3 mcg/min.

CONTRAINDICATIONS

Hypovolemic states (unless as an emergency measure), mesenteric or peripheral vascular thrombosis, profound hypoxia

INTERACTIONS

Drug

Beta blockers: May have mutually inhibitory effects.

Digoxin: May increase risk of arrhythmias.

Ergonovine, oxytocin: May increase vasoconstriction.

Maprotiline, tricyclic antidepressants: May increase cardiovascular effects.

Methyldopa: May decrease the effects of methyldopa.

Herbal

None known.

Food

None known.

Drug interactions of concern to dentistry

- Risk of arrhythmia: halogenated hydrocarbon anesthetics
- Risk of severe hypertension: tricyclic antidepressants, MAOIs, oxytocin, guanethidine

DIAGNOSTIC TEST EFFECTS

None known.

IV INCOMPATIBILITIES

Regular insulin

IV COMPATIBILITIES

Amiodarone (Cordarone), calcium gluconate, diltiazem (Cardizem), dobutamine (Dobutrex), dopamine (Intropin), epinephrine, esmolol (Brevibloc), fentanyl (Sublimaze), furosemide (Lasix), haloperidol (Haldol), heparin, hydromorphone (Dilaudid), labetalol (Trandate), lorazepam (Ativan), magnesium, midazolam (Versed), milrinone (Primacor), morphine, nicardipine (Cardene), nitroglycerin, potassium chloride, propofol (Diprivan)

SIDE EFFECTS

Norepinephrine produces less pronounced and less frequent side effects than epinephrine.

Occasional (5%–3%)

Anxiety, bradycardia, palpitations

Rare (2%–1%)

Nausea, anginal pain, shortness of breath, fever

SERIOUS REACTIONS

! Extravasation may produce tissue necrosis and sloughing.
! Overdose is manifested as severe hypertension with violent headache (which may be the first clinical sign of overdose), arrhythmias, photophobia, retrosternal or pharyngeal pain, pallor, excessive sweating, and vomiting.
! Prolonged therapy may result in plasma volume depletion. Hypotension may recur if plasma volume is not restored.

DENTAL CONSIDERATIONS

General:

• Acute-use drug for use in hospitals or emergency rooms for selected hypotensive episodes.

norethindrone

nor-eth′-in-drone
(Aygestin, Camila, Errin, Jolivette, Micronor, Nora-BE, Nor-QD, Norlutate[CAN])

CATEGORY AND SCHEDULE

Pregnancy Risk Category: X

MECHANISM OF ACTION

A synthetic progestin that is used as a single agent or in combination with estrogens for the treatment of gynecological disorders. It inhibits secretion of pituitary gonadotropin (LH) which prevents follicular maturation and ovulation.
Therapeutic Effect: Transforms endometrium from proliferative to secretory in an estrogen-primed endometrium, promotes mammary gland development, relaxes uterine smooth muscle.

PHARMACOKINETICS

Rapidly absorbed from the gastrointestinal (GI) tract. Widely distributed. Protein binding: 61%. Metabolized in liver. Excreted in urine and feces. ***Half-life:*** 4–13 hrs.

AVAILABILITY

Tablets: 0.35 mg (Camila, Errin, Jolivette, Micronor, Nora-BE, Nor-QD).
Tablets, as norethindrone acetate: 5 mg (Aygestin).

INDICATIONS AND DOSAGES

▸ **Contraception**

PO

Adults. 1 tablet/day.

▸ **Amenorrhea and Abnormal Uterine Bleeding**

PO

Adults. 5–20 mg/day cyclically (21 days on; 7 days off or continuously) or for acetate salt formulation, 2.5–10 mg cyclically.

▸ **Endometriosis**

PO

Adults. 10 mg/day for 2 weeks increase at increments of 5 mg/day every 2 weeks until 30 mg/day; continue for 6–9 months or until breakthrough bleeding demands temporary termination. For acetate salt formulation, 5 mg/day for 14 days increase at increments of 2.5 mg/day every 2 weeks up to 15 mg/day continue for 6–9 months or until breakthrough bleeding demands temporary termination.

OFF-LABEL USES

Treatment of corpus luteum dysfunction

CONTRAINDICATIONS

Acute liver disease, benign or malignant liver tumors, hypersensitivity to norethindrone and any component of the formulation, known or suspected carcinoma of the breast, known or suspected pregnancy, undiagnosed abnormal genital bleeding

INTERACTIONS

Drug

Antibiotics such as the penicillins and erythromycin: May decrease effectiveness of norethindrone.
Aprepitant: May decrease the effects of both drugs.
Benzodiazepines: May increase risk of benzodiazepine toxicity.
Cyclosporine: May increase risk of cyclosporine toxicity.
CYP3A4 inducers (carbamazepine, phenobarbital, phenytoin, rifampin, rifabutin): May decrease the levels and/or effects of norethindrone.
Atorvastatin, rosuvastatin: May increase concentrations of norethindrone.
Amprenavir, nelfinavir, nevirapine, ritonavir: May decrease norethindrone concentrations.
Corticosteroids: May prolong the effects of cortisones.
Fluconazole: May increase risk of adverse effects of norethindrone.
Griseofulvin, modafinil, primidone: May decrease effectiveness of norethindrone.
Lamotrigine: May increase or decrease plasma lamotrigne concentrations.
Thiazolidinediones: May decrease the effects of norethindrone.
Selegiline: May increase the risk of adverse effects of selegiline.
Theophylline: May increase the risk of theophylline toxicity.
Warfarin: May increase or decrease anticoagulant effects.
Zolmitriptan: May increase risk of adverse effects of zolmitriptan.

Herbal

Licorice: May increase risk of fluid retention and elevated blood pressure.
Red Cover: May alter effectiveness of norethindrone or increase side effects.
St. John's Wort: May decrease plasma concentrations of norethindrone.
Vitamin C (at high doses, more than 1g/day): May increase adverse effects of norethindrone.

Food

Caffeine: May increase CNS stimulation.

Drug interactions of concern to dentistry

- Decreased effectiveness of oral contraceptives: antibiotics, barbiturates

DIAGNOSTIC TEST EFFECTS

May increase LDL concentrations and serum alkaline phosphatase levels. May decrease glucose tolerance and HDL concentrations. May cause abnormal thyroid, metapyrone, liver, and endocrine function tests.

SIDE EFFECTS

Occasional

Breast tenderness, dizziness, headache, breakthrough bleeding, amenorrhea, menstrual irregularity, nausea, weakness

Rare

Mental depression, fever, insomnia, rash, acne, increased breast tenderness, weight gain/loss, changes in cervical erosion and secretions, cholestatic jaundice

SERIOUS REACTIONS

! Thrombophlebitis, cerebrovascular disorders, retinal thrombosis, cholestatic jaundice, and pulmonary embolism occur rarely.

DENTAL CONSIDERATIONS

General:

- Place on frequent recall to evaluate gingival inflammation, if present.

• Increased incidence of dry socket has been reported after extraction.
• Monitor vital signs at each appointment.

Teach Patient/Family:

• Need for good oral hygiene to prevent periodontal inflammation
• That smoking cessation decreases risk of serious adverse CV effects
• Need for additional method of birth control while undergoing antibiotic therapy

norfloxacin

nor-flox′-a-sin
(Apo-Norflox[CAN], Insensye[AUS], Norfloxacine[CAN], Noroxin, Novo-Norfloxacin[CAN], PMS-Norfloxacin[CAN], Roxin[AUS])

CATEGORY AND SCHEDULE

Pregnancy Risk Category: C

MECHANISM OF ACTION

A quinolone that inhibits DNA gyrase in susceptible microorganisms, interfering with bacterial cell replication and repair. ***Therapeutic Effect:*** Bactericidal.

AVAILABILITY

Tablets: 400 mg.

INDICATIONS AND DOSAGES

▸ **Urinary Tract Infections (UTIs)**

PO

Adults, Elderly. 400 mg twice a day for 7–21 days.

▸ **Prostatitis**

PO

Adults. 400 mg twice a day for 28 days.

▸ **Uncomplicated gonococcal infections**

PO

Adults. 800 mg as a single dose.

▸ **Dosage in renal impairment**

Dosage and frequency are modified on the basis of creatinine clearance.

Creatinine Clearance	Dosage
30 ml/min or higher	400 mg twice a day
less than 30 ml/min	400 mg once a day

CONTRAINDICATIONS

Children younger than 18 years because of risk arthropathy; hypersensitivity to norfloxacin, other quinolones, or their components

INTERACTIONS

Drug

Antacids, sucralfate: May decrease norfloxacin absorption.
Oral anticoagulants: May increase effects of oral anticoagulants.
Theophylline: Decreases clearance and may increase blood concentration and risk of toxicity of theophylline.

Herbal

None known.

Food

None known.

Drug interactions of concern to dentistry

• Decreased absorption: sodium bicarbonate

DIAGNOSTIC TEST EFFECTS

May increase BUN level and serum alkaline phosphatase, bilirubin, creatinine, LDH, AST (SGOT), and ALT (SGPT) levels.

SIDE EFFECTS

Frequent

Nausea, headache, dizziness

Rare

Vomiting, diarrhea, dry mouth, bitter taste, nervousness, drowsiness, insomnia, photosensitivity, tinnitus, crystalluria, rash, fever, seizures

SERIOUS REACTIONS

! Superinfection, anaphylaxis, Stevens-Johnson syndrome, and arthropathy occur rarely.
! Hypersensitivity reactions, including photosensitivity (as evidenced by rash, pruritus, blisters, edema, and burning skin), have occurred in patients receiving fluoroquinolones.

DENTAL CONSIDERATIONS

General:

- Assess salivary flow as a factor in caries, periodontal disease, and candidiasis.
- Determine why the patient is taking the drug.
- Because of drug interaction, do not use ingestible sodium bicarbonate products, such as the Prophy-Jet air polishing system, until 2 hr after drug use.
- Avoid dental light in patient's eyes; offer dark glasses for patient comfort.
- Ruptures of the shoulder, hand, and Achilles tendons that required surgical repair or resulted in prolonged disability have been reported with this drug.

Consultations:

- Consult with patient's physician if an acute dental infection occurs and another antiinfective is required.

Teach Patient/Family:

- To avoid mouth rinses with high alcohol content because of drying effects
- To discontinue treatment and inform dentist immediately if patient experiences pain or inflammation of a tendon, and to rest and refrain from exercise

N

norgestrel

nor-jes-′-trel
(Ovrette)

CATEGORY AND SCHEDULE

Pregnancy Risk Category: X

MECHANISM OF ACTION

A progestin that inhibits secretion of pituitary gonadotropin (LH), which prevents follicular maturation and ovulation. ***Therapeutic Effect:*** Transforms endometrium from proliferative to secretory in an estrogen-primed endometrium, promotes mammary gland development, relaxes uterine smooth muscle.

PHARMACOKINETICS

Well absorbed from the gastrointestinal (GI) tract. Widely distributed. Protein binding: 97%. Metabolized in liver via reduction and conjugation. Primarily excreted in urine. ***Half-life:*** 20 hrs.

AVAILABILITY

Tablets: 0.075 mg (Ovrette).

INDICATIONS AND DOSAGES

▸ Contraception, Female

PO
Adults. 0.075 mg/day.

OFF-LABEL USES

Endometrial protection, endometriosis, menorrhagia

CONTRAINDICATIONS

Hypersensitivity to norgestrel or any component of the formulation, hypersensitivity to tartrazine, thromboembolic disorders, severe hepatic disease; breast cancer; undiagnosed vaginal bleeding, pregnancy

INTERACTIONS

Drug

Antibiotics, such as the penicillins: May decrease contraceptive efficacy.
Amprenavir, nevirapine, ritonavir: May decrease contraceptive efficacy.
Bromocriptine: May interfere with the effects of bromocriptine.
Aprepitant: May reduce efficacy of norgestrel.
Caffeine: May increase the effects of caffeine.
Fluconazole: May increase risk of norgestrel adverse effects.
Griseofulvin: May decrease contraceptive effectiveness.
Phenobarbital, phenytoin: May decrease contraceptive effectiveness.
Pioglitazone, troglitazone: May decrease contraceptive effectiveness.
Rifampin: May decrease contraceptive effectiveness
Rosuvastatin: May increase plasma concentrations of norgestrel.
Warfarin: May decrease or increase anticoagulant effects.

Herbal

St. John's Wort: May decrease levels of St. John's Wort.
Dong quai, black cohosh: May add estrogen activity.
Saw palmetto, red clover, ginseng: May alter contraceptive effectiveness or increase side effects.

Food

None known.

Drug interactions of concern to dentistry

- Decreased effectiveness of oral contraceptives: antibiotics, barbiturates

DIAGNOSTIC TEST EFFECTS

None known.

IV INCOMPATIBILITIES

None known.

IV COMPATIBILITIES

None known.

SIDE EFFECTS

Frequent

Breakthrough bleeding or spotting at beginning of therapy, amenorrhea, change in menstrual flow, breast tenderness

Occasional

Edema, weight gain or loss, rash, pruritus, photosensitivity, skin pigmentation

Rare

Pain or swelling at injection site, acne, mental depression, alopecia, hirsutism

SERIOUS REACTIONS

! Thrombophlebitis, cerebrovascular disorders, retinal thrombosis, and pulmonary embolism occur rarely.

DENTAL CONSIDERATIONS

General:

- Place on frequent recall to evaluate gingival inflammation, if present.
- Increased incidence of dry socket has been reported after extraction.
- Monitor vital signs at each appointment.

Teach Patient/Family:

- Need for good oral hygiene to prevent periodontal inflammation
- That smoking cessation decreases risk of serious and adverse CV side effects
- Need for additional method of birth control while undergoing antibiotic therapy

nortriptyline hydrochloride

nor-trip′-ti-leen
(Allegron[AUS], Apo-Nortriptyline [CAN], Aventyl, Norventyl, Novo-Nortriptyline[CAN], Pamelor)
Do not confuse nortriptyline with amitriptyline, or aventyl with ambenyl or bentyl.

CATEGORY AND SCHEDULE

Pregnancy Risk Category: D

MECHANISM OF ACTION

A tricyclic antidepressant that blocks reuptake of the neurotransmitters norepinephrine and serotonin at neuronal presynaptic membranes, increasing their availability at postsynaptic receptor sites. ***Therapeutic Effect:*** Relieves depression.

PHARMACOKINETICS

N

Well absorbed from the GI tract. Protein binding: 86–95%. Metabolized in the liver. Primarily excreted in urine. ***Half-life:*** 17.6 hr.

AVAILABILITY

Capsules (Aventyl): 10 mg, 25 mg.
Capsules (Pamelor): 10 mg, 25 mg, 50 mg, 75 mg.
Oral Solution (Aventyl, Pamelor): 10 mg/5 ml .

INDICATIONS AND DOSAGES

▸ **Depression**

PO

Adults. 75–100 mg/day in 1–4 divided doses until therapeutic response is achieved. Reduce dosage gradually to effective maintenance level.
Elderly. Initially, 10–25 mg at bedtime. May increase by 25 mg every 3–7 days. Maximum: 150 mg/day.
Children 12 yr and older. 30–50 mg/day in 3–4 divided doses. Maximum: 150 mg/day.
Children 6–11 yr. 10–20 mg/day in 3–4 divided doses.

▸ **Enuresis**

PO

Children 12 yr and older. 25–35 mg/day.
Children 8–11 yr. 10–20 mg/day.
Children 6–7 yr. 10 mg/day.

OFF-LABEL USES

Treatment of neurogenic pain, panic disorder; prevention of migraine headache

CONTRAINDICATIONS

Acute recovery period after MI, use within 14 days of MAOIs

INTERACTIONS

Drug

Alcohol, other CNS depressants: May increase CNS and respiratory depression and the hypotensive effects of nortriptyline.
Antithyroid agents: May increase the risk of agranulocytosis.
Cimetidine: May increase the blood concentration and risk of toxicity of nortriptyline.
Clonidine, guanadrel: May decrease the effects of these drugs.
MAOIs: May increase the risk of neuroleptic malignant syndrome, seizures, hyperpyrexia, and hypertensive crisis.
Phenothiazines: May increase the anticholinergic and sedative effects of nortriptyline.
Sympathomimetics: May increase the risk of cardiac effects.

Herbal

None known.

Food

None known.

Drug interactions of concern to dentistry

- Increased anticholinergic effects: muscarinic blockers, antihistamines, phenothiazines
- Increased effects of direct-acting sympathomimetics (epinephrine, levonordefrin)
- Potential risk of increased CNS depression: alcohol, barbiturates, benzodiazepines, and other CNS depressants
- Decreased antihypertensive effect: clonidine, guanadrel, guanethidine
- Avoid concurrent use with St. John's wort (herb)

DIAGNOSTIC TEST EFFECTS

May alter blood glucose level and ECG readings. The therapeutic peak serum level is 6–10 mcg/ml; the therapeutic trough serum level is 0.5–2 mcg/ml. The toxic peak serum level is greater than 12 mcg/ml; the toxic trough serum level is greater than 2 mcg/ml.

SIDE EFFECTS

Frequent

Somnolence, fatigue, dry mouth, blurred vision, constipation, delayed micturition, orthostatic hypotension, diaphoresis, impaired concentration, increased appetite, urine retention

Occasional

GI disturbances (nausea, GI distress, metallic taste), photosensitivity

Rare

Paradoxical reactions (agitation, restlessness, nightmares, insomnia), extrapyramidal symptoms (particularly fine hand tremor)

SERIOUS REACTIONS

! Overdose may produce seizures; cardiovascular effects, such as severe orthostatic hypotension, dizziness, tachycardia, palpitations, and arrhythmias; and altered temperature regulation, such as hyperpyrexia or hypothermia.

! Abrupt discontinuation after prolonged therapy may produce headache, malaise, nausea, vomiting, and vivid dreams.

DENTAL CONSIDERATIONS

General:

- Take vital signs at every appointment because of CV side effects.
- Assess salivary flow as a factor in caries, periodontal disease, and candidiasis.
- Patients on chronic drug therapy may rarely have symptoms of blood dyscrasias, which can include infection, bleeding, and poor healing.
- After supine positioning, have patient sit upright for at least 2 min before standing to avoid orthostatic hypotension.
- Use vasoconstrictors with caution, in low doses, and with careful aspiration. Avoid use of gingival retraction cord with epinephrine.
- Place on frequent recall because of oral side effects.

Consultations:

- In a patient with symptoms of blood dyscrasias, request a medical consultation for blood studies and postpone dental treatment until normal values are reestablished.
- Medical consultation may be required to assess disease control.
- Physician should be informed if significant xerostomic side effects occur (e.g., increased caries, sore tongue, problems eating or swallowing, difficulty wearing prosthesis) so that a medication change can be considered.

Teach Patient/Family:

- Importance of good oral hygiene to prevent soft tissue inflammation
- Caution to prevent injury when using oral hygiene aids

- *When chronic dry mouth occurs, advise patient:*
  - To avoid mouth rinses with high alcohol content because of drying effects
  - Of need for daily use of home fluoride products to prevent caries
  - To use sugarless gum, frequent sips of water, or saliva substitutes

nystatin

nye-stat′-in
(Mycostatin, Nilstat[CAN], Nyaderm, Nystop)
Do not confuse nystatin or mycostatin with nitrostat.

CATEGORY AND SCHEDULE

Pregnancy Risk Category: C

N

MECHANISM OF ACTION

A fungistatic antifungal that binds to sterols in the fungal cell membrane. ***Therapeutic Effect:*** Increases fungal cell-membrane permeability, allowing loss of potassium and other cellular components.

PHARMACOKINETICS

PO: Poorly absorbed from the GI tract. Eliminated unchanged in feces. Topical: Not absorbed systemically from intact skin.

AVAILABILITY

Oral Suspension (Mycostatin): 100,000 units/ml.
Tablets (Mycostatin): 500,000 units.
Vaginal Tablets: 100,000 units.
Cream (Mycostatin): 100,000 units/g.
Ointment: 100,000 units/g.
Topical Powder (Mycostatin, Nystop): 100,000 units/g.

INDICATIONS AND DOSAGES

▸ Intestinal Infections

PO
Adults, Elderly.
500,000–1,000,000 units q8h.

▸ Oral Candidiasis

PO
Adults, Elderly, Children.
400,000–600,000 units 4 times/day.
Infants. 200,000 units 4 times/day.

▸ Vaginal Infections

VAGINAL
Adults, Elderly, Adolescents.
1 tablet/day at bedtime for 14 days.

▸ Cutaneous Candidal Infections

TOPICAL
Adults, Elderly, Children. Apply 2–4 times/day.

OFF-LABEL USES

Prophylaxis and treatment of oropharyngeal candidiasis, tinea barbae, tinea capitis

CONTRAINDICATIONS

None known.

INTERACTIONS

Drug
None known.
Herbal
None known.
Food
None known.

DIAGNOSTIC TEST EFFECTS

None known.

SIDE EFFECTS

Occasional
PO: None known
Topical: Skin irritation
Vaginal: Vaginal irritation

SERIOUS REACTIONS

! High dosages of oral form may produce nausea, vomiting, diarrhea, and GI distress.

DENTAL CONSIDERATIONS

General:

• Determine why the patient is taking the drug.

• Broad-spectrum antibiotic may contribute to oral *Candida* infections.

Teach Patient/Family:

• That long-term therapy may be necessary to clear infection; to complete entire course of medication

• Not to use commercial mouthwashes for mouth infection unless prescribed by dentist

• To soak full or partial dentures in a suitable antifungal solution nightly

• To prevent reinoculation of *Candida* infection by disposing of toothbrush or other contaminated oral hygiene devices used during period of infection

N

octreotide acetate

ok-tree′-oh-tide

(Sandostatin, Sandostatin LAR)

Do not confuse octreotide with OctreoScan, or Sandostatin with Sandimmune or Sandoglobulin.

CATEGORY AND SCHEDULE

Pregnancy Risk Category: B

MECHANISM OF ACTION

An antidiarrheal and growth hormone suppressant that suppresses the secretion of serotonin and gastroenteropancreatic peptides and enhances fluid and electrolyte absorption from the GI tract. ***Therapeutic Effect:*** Prolongs intestinal transit time.

PHARMACOKINETICS

Route	Onset	Peak	Duration
Subcutaneous	N/A	N/A	Up to 12 hr

O

Rapidly and completely absorbed from injection site. Excreted in urine. Removed by hemodialysis. ***Half-life:*** 1.5 hr.

AVAILABILITY

Injection (Sandostatin): 0.05 mg/ml, 0.1 mg/ml, 0.2 mg/ml, 0.5 mg/ml, 1 mg/ml.

Suspension for Injection (Sandostatin LAR): 10-mg, 20-mg, 30-mg vials.

INDICATIONS AND DOSAGES

▸ **Diarrhea**

IV (Sandostatin)

Adults, Elderly. Initially, 50–100 mcg q8h. May increase by 100 mcg/dose q48h. Maximum: 500 mcg q8h.

SUBCUTANEOUS (Sandostatin)

Adults, Elderly. 50 mcg 1–2 times a day.

IV, SUBCUTANEOUS (Sandostatin)

Children. 1–10 mcg/kg q12h.

▸ **Carcinoid Tumors**

IV, SUBCUTANEOUS (Sandostatin)

Adults, Elderly. 100–600 mcg/day in 2–4 divided doses.

IM (Sandostatin LAR)

Adults, Elderly. 20 mg q4wk.

▸ **Vipomas**

IV, SUBCUTANEOUS (Sandostatin)

Adults, Elderly. 200–300 mcg/day in 2–4 divided doses.

IM (Sandostatin LAR)

Adults, Elderly. 20 mg q4wk.

▸ **Esophageal Varices**

IV (Sandostatin)

Adults, Elderly. Bolus of 25–50 mcg followed by IV infusion of 25–50 mcg/hr.

▸ **Acromegaly**

IV, SUBCUTANEOUS (Sandostatin)

Adults, Elderly. 50 mcg 3 times a day. Increase as needed. Maximum: 500 mcg 3 times a day.

▸ **Acromegaly**

IM (Sandostatin LAR)

Adults, Elderly. 20 mg q4wk for 3 mo. Maximum: 40 mg q4wk.

OFF-LABEL USES

Treatment of AIDS-associated secretory diarrhea, chemotherapy-induced diarrhea, insulinomas, small-bowel fistulas, control of bleeding esophageal varices

CONTRAINDICATIONS

None known.

INTERACTIONS

Drug

Glucagon, growth hormone, insulin, oral antidiabetics: May alter glucose concentrations.

Herbal

None known.

Food

None known.

Drug interactions of concern to dentistry

• May cause decrease in vitamin B_{12} levels

DIAGNOSTIC TEST EFFECTS

May decrease serum thyroxine (T_4) concentration.

SIDE EFFECTS

Frequent (10%–6%, 58%–30% in acromegaly patients)

Diarrhea, nausea, abdominal discomfort, headache, injection site pain

Occasional (5%–1%)

Vomiting, flatulence, constipation, alopecia, facial flushing, pruritus, dizziness, fatigue, arrhythmias, ecchymosis, blurred vision

Rare (<1%)

Depression, diminished libido, vertigo, palpitations, dyspnea

SERIOUS REACTIONS

! Patients using octreotide may develop cholelithiasis or, with prolonged high dosages, hypothyroidism.

! GI bleeding, hepatitis, and seizures occur rarely.

DENTAL CONSIDERATIONS

General:

• This drug is administered in several disease states; determine patient's medical and drug history and exact use to accurately plan patient management.

• Monitor and record vital signs.

• Consider semisupine chair position for patient comfort if GI side effects occur.

• Question patient about tolerance of NSAIDS or aspirin related to GI disease.

• This drug may be used in the hospital or on an outpatient basis. Confirm the patient's disease and treatment status.

• Patient may need assistance in getting into and out of dental chair. Adjust chair position for patient comfort.

• Examine for oral manifestation of opportunistic infection.

Consultations:

• Medical consultation may be required to assess disease control and patient's ability to tolerate stress.

Teach Patient/Family:

• Importance of good oral hygiene to prevent soft tissue inflammation

• To prevent trauma when using oral hygiene aids

• Use of electric toothbrush if patient has difficulty holding conventional devices

• Importance of updating health and medication history if physician makes any changes in evaluation or drug regimens; include OTC, herbal, and nonherbal in the update

O

ofloxacin

o-flox′-a-sin

(Apo-Oflox[CAN], Floxin, Floxin Otic, Ocuflox)

Do not confuse Floxin with Flexeril or Flexon, or Ocuflox with Ocufen.

CATEGORY AND SCHEDULE

Pregnancy Risk Category: C

MECHANISM OF ACTION

A fluoroquinolone antibiotic that inhibits DNA gyrase in susceptible microorganisms, interfering with bacterial cell replication and repair. ***Therapeutic Effect:*** Bactericidal.

PHARMACOKINETICS

Rapidly and well absorbed from the GI tract. Protein binding: 20%–25%. Widely distributed (including to CSF). Metabolized in the liver. Primarily excreted in urine. Removed by hemodialysis. ***Half-life:*** 4.7–7 hr (increased in impaired renal function, cirrhosis, and the elderly).

AVAILABILITY

Tablets (Floxin): 200 mg, 300 mg, 400 mg.
Injection Solution (Floxin): 40 mg/ml.
Premixed Infusion Solution (Floxin): 200 mg/50 ml, 400 mg/100 ml.
Ophthalmic Solution (Ocuflox): 0.3%.
Otic Solution (Floxin): 0.3%.

INDICATIONS AND DOSAGES

▸ **UTIs**
PO, IV
Adults. 200 mg q12h.

▸ **Pelvic Inflammatory Disease (PID)**
PO
Adults. 400 mg q12h for 10–14 days.

▸ **Lower Respiratory Tract, Skin and Skin-Structure Infections**
PO, IV
Adults. 400 mg q12h for 10 days.

▸ **Prostatitis, Sexually Transmitted Diseases (Cervicitis, Urethritis)**
PO
Adults. 300 mg q12h.

▸ **Prostatitis**
IV
Adults. 300 mg q12h.

▸ **Sexually Transmitted Diseases**
IV
Adults. 400 mg as a single dose.

▸ **Acute, Uncomplicated Gonorrhea**
PO
Adults. 400 mg 1 time.

▸ **Usual Elderly Dosage**
PO
Elderly. 200–400 mg q12–24h for 7 days up to 6 wk.

▸ **Bacterial Conjunctivitis**
OPHTHALMIC
Adults, Elderly. 1–2 drops q2–4h for 2 days, then 4 times a day for 5 days.

▸ **Corneal Ulcers**
OPHTHALMIC
Adults. 1–2 drops q30min while awake for 2 days, then q60min while awake for 5–7 days, then 4 times a day.

▸ **Acute Otitis Media**
OTIC
Children 1–12 yr. 5 drops into the affected ear 2 times/day for 10 days.

▸ **Otitis Externa**
OTIC
Adults, Elderly, Children 12 yr and older. 10 drops into the affected ear once a day for 7 days.
Children 6 mo–11 yr. 5 drops into the affected ear once a day for 7 days.

▸ **Dosage in Renal Impairment**
After a normal initial dose, dosage and frequency are based on creatinine clearance.

Creatinine Clearance	Adjusted Dose	Dosage Interval
greater than 50 ml/min	None	q12h
10–50 ml/min	None	q24h
less than 10 ml/min	1/2	q24h

CONTRAINDICATIONS

Children younger than 18 years, hypersensitivity to any quinolones

INTERACTIONS

Drug

Antacids, sucralfate: May decrease absorption and effects of ofloxacin.
Caffeine: May increase the effects of caffeine.
Theophylline: May increase theophylline blood concentration and risk of toxicity.

Herbal

None known.

Food

None known.

Drug interactions of concern to dentistry

- Decreased effects: antacids
- Possible increased risk of life-threatening arrhythmias: procainamide

Drug interactions of concern to dentistry

- Studies have not been conducted for this product

DIAGNOSTIC TEST EFFECTS

None known.

IV INCOMPATIBILITIES

Amphotericin B complex (Abelcet, AmBisome, Amphotec), cefepime (Maxipime), doxorubicin liposomal (Doxil)

IV COMPATIBILITIES

Propofol (Diprivan)

SIDE EFFECTS

Frequent (10%–7%)
Nausea, headache, insomnia
Occasional (5%–3%)
Abdominal pain, diarrhea, vomiting, dry mouth, flatulence, dizziness, fatigue, drowsiness, rash, pruritus, fever
Rare (< 1%)
Constipation, paraesthesia

SERIOUS REACTIONS

! Antibiotic-associated colitis and other superinfections may occur from altered bacterial balance.
! Hypersensitivity reactions, including photosensitivity (as evidenced by rash, pruritus, blisters, edema, and burning skin), have occurred in patients receiving fluoroquinolones.
! Arthropathy (swelling, pain, and clubbing of fingers and toes, degeneration of stress-bearing portion of a joint) may occur if the drug is given to children.

DENTAL CONSIDERATIONS

General:

- Because of drug interaction, do not use ingestible sodium bicarbonate products, such as the Prophy-Jet air polishing system, until 2 hr after drug use.
- Examine for oral manifestation of opportunistic infections.
- Avoid dental light in patient's eyes; offer dark glasses for patient comfort.
- Minimize exposure to sunlight and wear sunscreen if sun exposure is planned.
- Ruptures of the shoulder, hand, and Achilles tendons that required surgical repair or resulted in prolonged disability have been reported with this drug.

Consultations:

- Consult with patient's physician if an acute dental infection occurs and another antiinfective is required.

Teach Patient/Family:

- Importance of good oral hygiene to prevent soft tissue inflammation
- To avoid mouth rinses with high alcohol content because of drying effects
- To discontinue treatment and inform dentist immediately if patient experiences pain or inflammation of a tendon, and to rest and refrain from exercise

DENTAL CONSIDERATIONS

OFLOXACIN (OPTIC)

General:

- Avoid dental light in patient's eyes; offer dark glasses for patient comfort and safety protection during dental treatment.

DENTAL CONSIDERATIONS

OFLOXACIN OTIC SOLUTION

General:

- Determine why the patient is taking the drug.
- Severity or discomfort of infection may require postponement of elective dental treatment

Consultations:

- Consult with patient's physician if an acute dental infection occurs and another antiinfective is required.
- Medical consultation may be required to assess disease control in the patient.

Teach Patient/Family:

- *When chronic dry mouth occurs, advise patient:*
  - To avoid mouth rinses with high alcohol content because of drying effects
  - To use daily home fluoride products for anticaries effect
  - To use sugarless gum, frequent sips of water, or saliva substitutes

O

olanzapine

oh-lan′-za-peen
(Zyprexa, Zyprexa Intramuscular, Zyprexa Zydis)
Do not confuse olanzapine with olsalazine, or Zyprexa with Zyrtec.

CATEGORY AND SCHEDULE

Pregnancy Risk Category: C

MECHANISM OF ACTION

A dibenzepin derivative that antagonizes alpha$_1$-adrenergic, dopamine, histamine, muscarinic, and serotonin receptors. Produces anticholinergic, histaminic, and CNS depressant effects. ***Therapeutic Effect:*** Diminishes manifestations of psychotic symptoms.

PHARMACOKINETICS

Well absorbed after PO administration. Protein binding: 93%. Extensively distributed throughout the body. Undergoes extensive first-pass metabolism in the liver. Excreted primarily in urine and, to a lesser extent, in feces. Not removed by dialysis. ***Half-life:*** 21–54 hr.

AVAILABILITY

Tablets (Zyprexa): 2.5 mg, 5 mg, 7.5 mg, 10 mg, 15 mg, 20 mg).
Tablets (Orally-Disintegrating [Zyprexa Zydis]): 5 mg, 10 mg, 15 mg, 20 mg.
Injection (Zyprexa Intramuscular). 10 mg.

INDICATIONS AND DOSAGES

▸ Schizophrenia

PO

Adults. Initially, 5–10 mg once daily. May increase by 10 mg/day at 5–7 day intervals. If further

adjustments are indicated, may increase by 5–10 mg/day at 7-day intervals. Range: 10–30 mg/day.
Elderly. Initially, 2.5 mg/day. May increase as indicated. Range: 2.5–10 mg/day.
Children. Initially, 2.5 mg/day. Titrate as needed up to 20 mg/day.

▸ **Bipolar Mania**
PO
Adults. Initially, 10–15 mg/day. May increase by 5 mg/day at intervals of at least 24 hr. Maximum: 20 mg/day.
Children. Initially, 2.5 mg/day. Titrate as needed up to 20 mg/day.

▸ **Dosage for Elderly or Debilitated Patients and Those Predisposed to Hypotensive Reactions**
The initial dosage for these patients is 5 mg/day.

▸ **Control Agitation in Schizophrenic or Bipolar Patients**
IM
Adults, Elderly. 2.5–10 mg. May repeat 2h after first dose and 4h after 2nd dose. Maximum: 30 mg/day.

OFF-LABEL USES
Treatment of anorexia, maintenance of long-term treatment response in schizophrenic patients, nausea, vomiting

CONTRAINDICATIONS
None known.

INTERACTIONS
Drug
Alcohol, other CNS depressants: May increase CNS depressant effects.
Antihypertensives: May increase the hypotensive effects of these drugs.
Carbamazepine: Increases olanzapine clearance.
Ciprofloxacin, fluvoxamine: May increase the olanzapine blood concentration.
Dopamine agonists, levodopa: May antagonize the effects of these drugs.
Imipramine, theophylline: May inhibit the metabolism of these drugs.
Herbal
None known.
Food
None known.
Drug interactions of concern to dentistry
• Potentiation of orthostatic hypotension: diazepam, alcohol, other CNS depressants
• Increased anticholinergic effects: anticholinergic drugs
• Suspected reduction of plasma levels: carbamazepine

DIAGNOSTIC TEST EFFECTS
May significantly increase serum GGT, prolactin, AST (SGOT), and ALT (SGPT) levels.

SIDE EFFECTS
Frequent
Somnolence (26%), agitation (23%), insomnia (20%), headache (17%), nervousness (16%), hostility (15%), dizziness (11%), rhinitis (10%)
Occasional
Anxiety, constipation (9%); nonaggressive atypical behavior (8%); dry mouth (7%); weight gain (6%); orthostatic hypotension, fever, arthralgia, restlessness, cough, pharyngitis, visual changes (dim vision) (5%)
Rare
Tachycardia; back, chest, abdominal, or extremity pain; tremor

SERIOUS REACTIONS
! Rare reactions include seizures and neuroleptic malignant syndrome, a potentially fatal syndromecharacterized by hyperpyrexia, muscle rigidity, irregular pulse or BP, tachycardia, diaphoresis, and cardiac arrhythmias.

! Extrapyramidal symptoms and dysphagia may also occur.
! Overdose (300 mg) produces drowsiness and slurred speech.

DENTAL CONSIDERATIONS

General:

- Consider semisupine chair position for patient comfort because of GI effects of drug.
- Assess salivary flow as factor in caries, periodontal disease, and candidiasis.
- Monitor vital signs at every appointment because of CV side effects.
- After supine positioning, have patient sit upright for at least 2 min before standing to avoid orthostatic hypotension.
- Patients on chronic drug therapy may rarely have symptoms of blood dyscrasias, which can include infection, bleeding, and poor healing.
- Assess for presence of extrapyramidal motor symptoms, such as tardive dyskinesia and akathisia. Extrapyramidal motor activity may complicate dental treatment.

Consultations:

- In a patient with symptoms of blood dyscrasias, request a medical consultation for blood studies and postpone dental treatment until normal values are reestablished.
- Medical consultation may be required to assess disease control.
- Physician should be informed if significant xerostomic side effects occur (e.g., increased caries, sore tongue, problems eating or swallowing, difficulty wearing prosthesis) so that a medication change can be considered.

Teach Patient/Family:

- Importance of good oral hygiene to prevent soft tissue inflammation
- Use of electric toothbrush if patient has difficulty holding conventional devices
- Use caution when driving or performing other tasks requiring alertness
- *When chronic dry mouth occurs, advise patient:*
  - To avoid mouth rinses with high alcohol content because of drying effects
  - To use daily home fluoride products for anticaries effect
  - To use sugarless gum, frequent sips of water, or saliva substitutes

O

olmesartan medoxomil

ol-mess′-er-tan
(Benicar)

CATEGORY AND SCHEDULE

Pregnancy Risk Category: C (D if used in second or third trimester)

MECHANISM OF ACTION

An angiotensin II receptor, type AT_1, antagonist that blocks the vasoconstrictor and aldosterone-secreting effects of angiotensin II, inhibiting the binding of angiotensin II to the AT_1 receptors. ***Therapeutic Effect:*** Causes vasodilation, decreases peripheral resistance, and decreases BP.

PHARMACOKINETICS

Rapidly and completely absorbed after PO administration. Metabolized in the liver. Recovered primarily in feces and, to a lesser extent, in urine. Not removed by hemodialysis. ***Half-life:*** 13 hr.

AVAILABILITY

Tablets: 5 mg, 20 mg, 40 mg.

INDICATIONS AND DOSAGES

▸ Hypertension

PO

Adults, Elderly, Patients with mildly impaired hepatic or renal function. 20 mg once a day in patients who are not volume depleted. After 2 weeks of therapy, if further reduction in BP is necessary, may increase dosage to 40 mg/day.

CONTRAINDICATIONS

Bilateral renal artery stenosis

INTERACTIONS

Drug

Diuretics: Further reduces BP.

Herbal

None known.

Food

None known.

Drug interactions of concern to dentistry

- No significant drug interactions have been reported, but increased hypotensive effects always are possible when used with other antihypertensives or sedatives

DIAGNOSTIC TEST EFFECTS

May increase blood Hgb and Hct levels.

SIDE EFFECTS

Occasional (3%)

Dizziness

Rare (< 2%)

Headache, diarrhea, upper respiratory tract infection

SERIOUS REACTIONS

! Overdosage may manifest as hypotension and tachycardia. Bradycardia occurs less often.

DENTAL CONSIDERATIONS

General:

- Monitor vital signs at every appointment because of CV side effects.
- Consider semisupine chair position for patient comfort if GI side effects occur.
- Limit use of sodium-containing products, such as saline IV fluids, for patients with a dietary salt restriction.
- Stress from dental procedures may compromise CV function, determine patient risk.
- Patients with hypertensive disease may be taking more than one drug to control blood pressure; although not specifically noted for this drug, postural hypotension is always a possibility.
- After supine positioning, have patient sit upright for at least 2 min before standing to avoid orthostatic hypotension.
- Short appointments and a stress reduction protocol may be required for anxious patients.
- Use precaution if sedation or general anesthesia is required; risk of hypotensive episode.

Consultations:

- Medical consultation may be required to assess disease control and patient's ability to tolerate stress.

Teach Patient/Family:

- Importance of updating health and drug history if physician makes any changes in evaluation or drug regimens

olopatadine

oh-loe-pa-ta′-deen
(Patanol)

CATEGORY AND SCHEDULE

Pregnancy Risk Category: C

MECHANISM OF ACTION

An antihistamine that inhibits histamine release from the mast cell. ***Therapeutic Effect:*** Inhibits symptoms associated with allergic conjunctivitis.

PHARMACOKINETICS

The time to peak concentration is less than 2 hours and duration of action is 8 hours. Minimal absorption after topical administration. Metabolized to inactive metabolites. Primarily excreted in urine. ***Half-life:*** 3 hrs.

AVAILABILITY

Ophthalmic Solution: 0.1% (Patanol).

INDICATIONS AND DOSAGES

▸ **Allergic Conjunctivitis**

OPHTHALMIC

Adults, Elderly, Children 3 yrs and older. 1–2 drops in affected eye(s) twice daily q6–8h.

CONTRAINDICATIONS

Hypersensitivity to olopatadine hydrochloride or any other component of the formulation

INTERACTIONS

Drug

None known.

Herbal

None known.

Food

None known.

Drug interactions of concern to dentistry

- None reported

DIAGNOSTIC TEST EFFECTS

None known.

SIDE EFFECTS

Occasional

Headache, weakness, cold syndrome, taste perversion, burning, stinging, dry eyes, foreign body sensation, hyperemia, keratitis, eyelid edema, itching, pharyngitis, rhinitis, sinusitis

SERIOUS REACTIONS

! None reported.

DENTAL CONSIDERATIONS

General:

- Protect patient's eyes from accidental spatter during dental treatment.

olsalazine sodium

ohl-sal′-ah-zeen
(Dipentum)

Do not confuse olsalazine with olanzapine.

CATEGORY AND SCHEDULE

Pregnancy Risk Category: C

MECHANISM OF ACTION

A salicylic acid derivative that is converted to mesalamine in the colon by bacterial action. Blocks prostaglandin production in bowel mucosa. ***Therapeutic Effect:*** Reduces colonic inflammation in inflammatory bowel disease.

AVAILABILITY

Capsules: 250 mg.

INDICATIONS AND DOSAGES

▸ Maintenance of Controlled Ulcerative Colitis

PO

Adults, Elderly. 1 g/day in 2 divided doses, preferably q12h.

OFF-LABEL USES

Treatment of inflammatory bowel disease

CONTRAINDICATIONS

History of hypersensitivity to salicylates

INTERACTIONS

Drug

None known.

Herbal

None known.

Food

None known.

DIAGNOSTIC TEST EFFECTS

May increase AST(SGOT) and ALT(SGPT) levels.

SIDE EFFECTS

Frequent (10%–5%)

Headache, diarrhea, abdominal pain or cramps, nausea

Occasional (5%–1%)

Depression, fatigue, dyspepsia, upper respiratory tract infection, decreased appetite, rash, itching, arthralgia

Rare (1%)

Dizziness, vomiting, stomatitis

SERIOUS REACTIONS

! Sulfite sensitivity may occur in susceptible patients manifested by cramping, headache, diarrhea, fever, rash, hives, itching, and wheezing may occur. Discontinue drug immediately.

! Excessive diarrhea associated with extreme fatigue is noted rarely.

DENTAL CONSIDERATIONS

General:

• Consider semisupine chair position for patient comfort because of GI effects of disease.

Consultations:

• Avoid drugs that could aggravate an inflammatory colon disease; consultation is recommended before selection of an antibiotic.

Teach Patient/Family:

• Importance of good oral hygiene to prevent soft tissue inflammation

• Caution to prevent injury when using oral hygiene aids

• To avoid mouth rinses with high alcohol content because of drying effects

omalizumab

oh-mah-liz′-uw-mab

(Xolair)

CATEGORY AND SCHEDULE

Pregnancy Risk Category: B

O

MECHANISM OF ACTION

A monoclonal antibody that selectively binds to human immunoglobulin E (IgE), preventing it from binding to the surface of mast cells and basophiles.

Therapeutic Effect: Prevents or reduces the number of asthmatic attacks.

PHARMACOKINETICS

Absorbed slowly after subcutaneous administration, with peak concentration in 7–8 days. Excreted in the liver, reticuloendothelial system, and endothelial cells. ***Half-life:*** 26 days.

AVAILABILITY

Powder for Injection: 202.5 mg/1.2 ml or 150 mg/1.2 ml after reconstitution.

INDICATIONS AND DOSAGES

▸ Moderate to Severe Persistent Asthma in Patients Who Are Reactive to a Perennial Allergen and Whose Asthma Symptoms Have Been Inadequately Controlled with Inhaled Corticosteroids

SUBCUTANEOUS

Adults, Elderly, Children 12 yr and older. 150–375 mg every 2 or 4 wk; dose and dosing frequency are individualized on the basis of weight and pretreatment immunoglobulin E (IgE) level (as shown below).

▸ 4-week Dosing Table

Pretreatment serum IgE levels (units/ml)	Weight 30–60 kg	Weight 61–70 kg	Weight 71–90 kg	Weight 91–150 kg
30 to 100	150 mg	150 mg	150 mg	300 mg
101–200	300 mg	300 mg	300 mg	See next table
201–300	300 mg	See next table	See next table	See next table

▸ 2-week Dosing Table

Pretreatment serum IgE levels (units/ml)	Weight 30–60 kg	Weight 61–70 kg	Weight 71–90 kg	Weight 91–150 kg
101–200	see preceding table	see preceding table	see preceding table	225 mg
201–300	see previous table	225 mg	225 mg	300 mg
301–400	225 mg	225 mg	300 mg	Do not dose
401–500	300 mg	300 mg	375 mg	Do not dose
501–600	300 mg	375 mg	Do not dose	Do not dose
601–700	375 mg	Do not dose	Do not dose	Do not dose

OFF-LABEL USES

Treatment of seasonal allergic rhinitis

CONTRAINDICATIONS

None known.

INTERACTIONS

Drug

None known.

Herbal

None known.

Food

None known.

Drug interactions of concern to dentistry

- None reported

DIAGNOSTIC TEST EFFECTS

May increase serum IgE levels.

SIDE EFFECTS

Frequent (45%–11%)

Injection site ecchymosis, redness, warmth, stinging, and urticaria; viral infections; sinusitis; headache; pharyngitis

Occasional (8%–3%)

Arthralgia, leg pain, fatigue, dizziness

Rare (2%)

Arm pain, earache, dermatitis, pruritus

SERIOUS REACTIONS

! Anaphylaxis occurs within 2 hours of the first dose or subsequent doses in 0.1% of patients.

! Malignant neoplasms occur in 0.5% of patients.

DENTAL CONSIDERATIONS

General:

- Determine why patient is taking the drug.
- Be aware of patient's disease, its severity, and its frequency, when known.

• Question patient about other medications used for asthma or to prevent bronchoconstriction.
• Avoid drugs that may aggravate asthma.
• Short appointments and a stress reduction protocol may be required for anxious patients.
• Have patient bring personal short-acting bronchodilator to appointment for use in emergency.
• Acute asthmatic episodes may be precipitated in the dental office. Rapid-acting sympathomimetic inhalants should be available for emergency use. A stress reduction protocol may be required.

Consultations:
• Consultation with physician may be necessary if sedation or general anesthesia is required.
• Medical consultation may be required to assess disease control and patient's ability to tolerate stress.

Teach Patient/Family:
• Importance of good oral hygiene to prevent soft tissue inflammation/infection
• Importance of updating health and drug history and reporting changes in health status, drug regimen, or disease/treatment status

omeprazole

oh-mep′-rah-zole
(Losec[CAN], Maxor[AUS], Prilosec, Prilosec OTC, Probitor[AUS], Zegerid)
Do not confuse Prilosec with prilocaine, Prinivil, or Prozac.

CATEGORY AND SCHEDULE

Pregnancy Risk Category: C

MECHANISM OF ACTION

A benzimidazole that is converted to active metabolites that irreversibly bind to and inhibit hydrogen-potassium adenosine triphosphatase, an enzyme on the surface of gastric parietal cells. Inhibits hydrogen ion transport into gastric lumen.
Therapeutic Effect: Increases gastric pH, reduces gastric acid production.

PHARMACOKINETICS

Route	Onset	Peak	Duration
PO	1 hr	2 hr	72 hr

Rapidly absorbed from the GI tract. Protein binding: 99%. Primarily distributed into gastric parietal cells. Metabolized extensively in the liver. Primarily excreted in urine. Unknown if removed by hemodialysis. ***Half-life:*** 0.5–1 hr (increased in patients with hepatic impairment).

AVAILABILITY

Capsules (Delayed-Release [Prilosec]): 10 mg, 20 mg, 40 mg.
Oral Suspension (Zegerid): 20 mg.

INDICATIONS AND DOSAGES

▸ **Erosive Esophagitis, Poorly Responsive Gastroesophageal Reflux Disease, Active Duodenal Ulcer, Prevention and Treatment of NSAID-Induced Ulcers**
PO
Adults, Elderly. 20 mg/day.

▸ **To Maintain Healing of Erosive Esophagitis**
PO
Adults, Elderly. 20 mg/day.

▸ **Pathologic Hypersecretory Conditions**
PO
Adults, Elderly. Initially, 60 mg/day up to 120 mg 3 times a day.

O

▸ **Duodenal Ulcer Caused by *Helibacter Pylori***
PO
Adults, Elderly. 20 mg twice a day for 10 days.

▸ **Active Benign Gastric Ulcer**
PO
Adults, Elderly. 40 mg/day for 4–8 wk.

▸ **Usual Pediatric Dosage**
Children older than 2 yr, weighing 20 kg and more. 20 mg/day.
Children older than 2 yr, weighing less than 20 kg. 10 mg/day.

OFF-LABEL USES

H. pylori–associated duodenal ulcer (with amoxicillin and clarithromycin), prevention and treatment of NSAID-induced ulcers, treatment of active benign gastric ulcers

CONTRAINDICATIONS

None known.

INTERACTIONS

Drug

Diazepam, oral anticoagulants, phenytoin: May increase the blood concentration of diazepam, oral anticoagulants, and phenytoin.

Herbal

None known.

Food

None known.

Drug interactions of concern to dentistry

- Increased serum levels: diazepam

DIAGNOSTIC TEST EFFECTS

May increase serum alkaline phosphatase, AST(SGOT), and ALT(SGPT) levels.

SIDE EFFECTS

Frequent (7%)

Headache

Occasional (3%–2%)

Diarrhea, abdominal pain, nausea

Rare (2%)

Dizziness, asthenia or loss of strength, vomiting, constipation, upper respiratory tract infection, back pain, rash, cough

SERIOUS REACTIONS

! None known.

DENTAL CONSIDERATIONS

General:

- Question the patient about tolerance of NSAIDs or aspirin related to GI problem.
- Consider semisupine chair position for patient comfort because of GI effects of disease.
- Assess salivary flow as a factor in caries, periodontal disease, and candidiasis.

Teach Patient/Family:

- Caution to prevent injury when using oral hygiene aids
- *When chronic dry mouth occurs, advise patient:*
  - To avoid mouth rinses with high alcohol content because of drying effects
  - Of need for daily use of home fluoride products to prevent caries
  - To use sugarless gum, frequent sips of water, or saliva substitutes

oprelvekin (interleukin-2, IL-2)

oh-prel′-vee-kinn
Schedule IV
(Neumega)
Do not confuse Neumega with Neupogen.

CATEGORY AND SCHEDULE

Pregnancy Risk Category: C

MECHANISM OF ACTION

A hematopoietic that stimulates production of blood platelets, essential to the blood-clotting process. ***Therapeutic Effect:*** Increases platelet production.

AVAILABILITY

Injection: 5 mg.

INDICATIONS AND DOSAGES

▸ **Prevention of Thrombocytopenia**

SUBCUTANEOUS

Adults. 50 mcg/kg once a day.
Children. 75–100 mcg/kg once a day. Continue for 14–28 days or until platelet count reaches 50,000 cells/mcl after its nadir.

CONTRAINDICATIONS

None known.

INTERACTIONS

Drug

None known.

Herbal

None known.

Food

None known.

Drug interactions of concern to dentistry

• No data available

DIAGNOSTIC TEST EFFECTS

May decrease Hgb and Hct, usually within 3–5 days of initiation of therapy; reverses about 1 week after discontinuance of therapy.

SIDE EFFECTS

Frequent

Nausea or vomiting (77%); fluid retention (59%); neutropenic fever (48%); diarrhea (43%); rhinitis (42%); headache (41%); dizziness (38%); fever (36%); insomnia (33%); cough (29%); rash, pharyngitis (25%); tachycardia (20%); vasodilation (19%)

SERIOUS REACTIONS

! Transient atrial fibrillation or flutter occurs in 10% of patients and may be caused by increased plasma volume; oprelvekin is not directly arrhythmogenic. Arrhythmias are usually brief in duration and convert spontaneously to normal sinus rhythm.
! Papilledema may occur in children.

DENTAL CONSIDERATIONS

General:

• If bleeding problem has not been diagnosed; refer for evaluation prior to any dental treatment.
• Question patient about medical and drug history in relationship to bleeding problems.
• Provide dental treatment in conjunction with hematologist.
• Patients may present with localized gingival bleeding with incomplete clotting.
• Avoid elective dental procedures if severe neutropenia (<500 cells/mm^3) or thrombocytopenia (<50,000 cells/mm^3) is present.
• Avoid products that affect platelet function, such as aspirin and NSAIDs.
• Monitor and record vital signs.
• Consider local hemostasis measures to prevent excessive bleeding.

O

• Short appointments and a stress reduction protocol may be required for anxious patients.
• Place on frequent recall to evaluate healing response

Consultations:

• Consultation with hematologist or physician of record required.
• Medical consultation should include routine blood counts including platelet counts and bleeding time.
• Consultation with physician may be necessary if sedation or general anesthesia is required.
• In a patient with symptoms of blood dyscrasias, request a medical consultation for blood studies and postpone treatment until normal values are reestablished.
• Medical consultation should include partial prothrombin time, prothrombin time, or INR

Teach Patient/Family:

• Use of soft tooth brush to prevent trauma to oral tissues and risk of bleeding
• Importance of good oral hygiene to prevent soft tissue inflammation
• To report oral lesions, soreness, or bleeding to dentist
• Importance of updating health and medication history if physician makes any changes in evaluation or drug regimens; include OTC, herbal, and nonherbal in the update
• To prevent trauma when using oral hygiene aids

orlistat

ohr′-lih-stat
(Xenical)
Do not confuse Xenical with Xeloda.

CATEGORY AND SCHEDULE

Pregnancy Risk Category: B

MECHANISM OF ACTION

A gastric and pancreatic lipase inhibitor that inhibits absorption of dietary fats by inactivating gastric and pancreatic enzymes.
Therapeutic Effect: Resulting caloric deficit may positively affect weight control.

PHARMACOKINETICS

Minimal absorption after administration. Protein binding: 99%. Primarily eliminated unchanged in feces. Unknown if removed by hemodialysis. ***Half-life:*** 1–2 hr.

AVAILABILITY

Capsules: 120 mg.

INDICATIONS AND DOSAGES

▸ Weight Reduction

PO
Adults, Elderly, Children 12–16 yr. 120 mg 3 times a day.

CONTRAINDICATIONS

Cholestasis, chronic malabsorption syndrome

INTERACTIONS

Drug

Pravastatin: May increase the blood concentration of pravastatin and risk of rhabdomyolysis.

Herbal

None known.

Food
None known.
Drug interactions of concern to dentistry
• None reported

DIAGNOSTIC TEST EFFECTS
Decreases blood glucose, total serum cholesterol, and serum LDL levels. Decreases absorption and levels of vitamins A and E.

SIDE EFFECTS
Frequent (30%–20%)
Headache, abdominal discomfort, flatulence, fecal urgency, fatty or oily stool
Occasional (14%–5%)
Back pain, menstrual irregularity, nausea, fatigue, diarrhea, dizziness
Rare (< 4%)
Anxiety, rash, myalgia, dry skin, vomiting

SERIOUS REACTIONS
! None known.

DENTAL CONSIDERATIONS
General:
• Although no dental drug interactions are reported, observe expected outcomes of systemically administered drugs.
• Severely obese patients may have type 2 diabetes or CV diseases.
• Consider semisupine chair position for patient comfort if GI side effects occur.
• Ensure that patient is following prescribed diet and regularly takes medication.
Consultations:
• Medical consultation may be required to assess disease control.
Teach Patient/Family:
• Importance of updating health and drug history if physician makes any changes in evaluation or drug regimens

orphenadrine
or-fen′-a-dreen
(Norflex, Orphenace[CAN], Rhoxal-orphenadrine[CAN])

CATEGORY AND SCHEDULE
Pregnancy Risk Category: C

MECHANISM OF ACTION
A skeletal muscle relaxant that is structurally related to diphenhydramine and is thought to indirectly affect skeletal muscle by central atropine-like effects.
Therapeutic Effect: Relieves musculoskeletal pain.

PHARMACOKINETICS
Well absorbed after PO and IM absorption. Protein binding: low. Metabolized in liver. Primarily excreted in urine and feces.
Half-life: 14 hrs.

AVAILABILITY
Injection: 30 mg/ml (Norflex).
Tablets, extended-release: 100 mg (Norflex).

INDICATIONS AND DOSAGES
▸ **Musculoskeletal Pain**
IM/IV
Adults, Elderly. 60 mg 2 times/day. Switch to oral form for maintenance.
PO
Adults, Elderly. 100 mg 2 times/day.

OFF-LABEL USES
Drug-induced extrapyramidal reactions

CONTRAINDICATIONS

Angle-closure glaucoma, myasthenia gravis, pyloric or duodenal obstruction, stenosing peptic ulcer, prostatic hypertrophy, obstruction of the bladder neck, achalasia, cardiospasm (megaesophagus), hypersensitivity to orphenadrine or any component of the formulation

INTERACTIONS

Drug

Alcohol, CNS depressants: May increase sedative effects.
Anticholinergics: May increase anticholinergic effects
Cisapride: May decrease effectiveness of cisapride
Levodopa: May decrease effects of orphenadrine.

Herbal

St. John's Wort, kava kava, gotu kola: May increase CNS depression.

Food

None known.

Drug interactions of concern to dentistry

- Increased CNS effects: propoxyphene, CNS depressants, alcohol
- Increased anticholinergic effect: other anticholinergics

DIAGNOSTIC TEST EFFECTS

None known.

IV INCOMPATIBILITIES

None known.

IV COMPATIBILITIES

None known.

SIDE EFFECTS

Frequent

Drowsiness, dizziness, muscular weakness, hypotension, dry mouth, nose, throat, and lips, urinary retention, thickening of bronchial secretions

Elderly

Frequent

Sedation, dizziness, hypotension

Occasional

Flushing, visual or hearing disturbances, paresthesia, diaphoresis, chill

SERIOUS REACTIONS

! Hypersensitivity reaction, such as eczema, pruritus, rash, cardiac disturbances, and photosensitivity, may occur.

! Overdosage may vary from CNS depression, including sedation, apnea, hypotension, cardiovascular collapse, or death to severe paradoxical reaction, such as hallucinations, tremor, and seizures.

DENTAL CONSIDERATIONS

General:

- Consider semisupine chair position for patients with back pain.
- Patients on chronic drug therapy may rarely have symptoms of blood dyscrasias, which can include infection, bleeding, and poor healing.
- Assess salivary flow as a factor in caries, periodontal disease, and candidiasis.

Consultations:

- In a patient with symptoms of blood dyscrasias, request a medical consultation for blood studies and postpone dental treatment until normal values are reestablished.
- Medical consultation may be required to assess disease control.

Teach Patient/Family:

- Importance of good oral hygiene to prevent soft tissue inflammation
- Caution to prevent injury when using oral hygiene aids
- Caution when driving or operating equipment because of risk of dizziness

O

- *When chronic dry mouth occurs, advise patient:*
  - To avoid mouth rinses with high alcohol content because of drying effects
  - Of need for daily use of home fluoride products to prevent caries
  - To use sugarless gum, frequent sips of water, or saliva substitutes

oseltamivir

ah-suhl-tahm′-ah-veer
(Tamiflu)

CATEGORY AND SCHEDULE

Pregnancy Risk Category: C

MECHANISM OF ACTION

A selective inhibitor of influenza virus neuraminidase, an enzyme essential for viral replication. Acts against both influenza A and B viruses. ***Therapeutic Effect:*** Suppresses the spread of infection within the respiratory system and reduces the duration of clinical symptoms.

PHARMACOKINETICS

Readily absorbed. Protein binding: 3%. Extensively converted to active drug in the liver. Primarily excreted in urine. ***Half-life:*** 6–10 hr.

AVAILABILITY

Capsules: 75 mg.
Oral Suspension: 12 mg/ml.

INDICATIONS AND DOSAGES

▸ **Influenza**

PO

Adults, Elderly. 75 mg 2 times a day for 5 days.
Children weighing more than 40 kg 75 mg twice a day.
Children weighing 24–40 kg. 60 mg twice a day.
Children weighing 15–23 kg. 45 mg twice a day.
Children weighing less than 15 kg. 30 mg twice a day.

▸ **Prevention of Influenza**

PO

Adults, Elderly. 75 mg once a day.

▸ **Dosage in Renal Impairment**

PO

For adult and elderly patients, dosage is decreased to 75 mg once a day for at least 7 days and possibly up to 6 wk.

CONTRAINDICATIONS

None known.

INTERACTIONS

Drug

None known.

Herbal

None known.

Food

None known.

Drug interactions of concern to dentistry

- None reported

DIAGNOSTIC TEST EFFECTS

None known.

SIDE EFFECTS

Frequent (5%)

Nausea, vomiting, diarrhea

Occasional (4%–1%)

Abdominal pain, bronchitis, dizziness, headache, cough, insomnia, fatigue, vertigo

SERIOUS REACTIONS

! Colitis, pneumonia, and pyrexia occur rarely.

O

DENTAL CONSIDERATIONS

General:

- Acute influenza patients are unlikely to be seen in the dental office except for dental emergencies.
- Consider semisupine chair position for patient comfort because of respiratory effects of disease.

oxacillin

ox-a-sill′-in

CATEGORY AND SCHEDULE

Pregnancy Risk Category: B

MECHANISM OF ACTION

A penicillin that binds to bacterial membranes. ***Therapeutic Effect:*** Bactericidal.

AVAILABILITY

Powder for Injection: 1-g vials, 2-g vials.

INDICATIONS AND DOSAGES

▸ **Upper Respiratory Tract, Skin, and Skin-Structure Infections**

IV, IM

Adults, Elderly, Children weighing 40 kg or more. 250–500 mg q4–6h.

Children weighing less than 40 kg. 50 mg/kg/day in divided doses q6h. Maximum: 12 g/day.

▸ **Lower Respiratory Tract and Other Serious Infections**

IV, IM

Adults, Elderly, Children weighing 40 kg or more. 1 g q4–6h. Maximum: 12 g/day.

Children weighing less than 40 kg. 100 mg/kg/day in divided doses q4–6h.

CONTRAINDICATIONS

Hypersensitivity to any penicillin

INTERACTIONS

Drug

Probenecid: May increase oxacillin blood concentration and risk of toxicity.

Herbal

None known.

Food

None known.

Drug interactions of concern to dentistry

- Increased or prolonged plasma levels: probenecid
- Aminoglycosides: injections must be separated by 1 hr
- Possible decrease in antimicrobial effectiveness: tetracyclines, erythromycins, lincomycins
- Suspected increase in methotrexate toxicity
- *When used for dental infection:*
  - Oral contraceptives: advise patient of a potential risk for decreased contraceptive action, to maintain compliance with oral contraceptive while using antibiotics, and to consider the use of nonhormonal contraception

DIAGNOSTIC TEST EFFECTS

May increase AST (SGOT) levels. May cause a positive Coombs' test.

SIDE EFFECTS

Frequent

Mild hypersensitivity reaction (fever, rash, pruritus), GI effects (nausea, vomiting, diarrhea)

Occasional

Phlebitis, thrombophlebitis (more common in elderly), hepatotoxicity (with high IV dosage)

SERIOUS REACTIONS

! Antibiotic-associated colitis and other superinfections may result from altered bacterial balance.
! A mild to severe hypersensitivity reaction may occur in those allergic to penicillins.

DENTAL CONSIDERATIONS

General:
- Determine why patient is taking the drug.
- Caution regarding allergy to medication.

Consultations:
- Consult patient's physician if an acute dental infection occurs and another antiinfective is required.
- Medical consultation may be required to assess disease control.

Teach Patient/Family:
- Importance of good oral hygiene to prevent soft tissue inflammation
- To prevent trauma when using oral hygiene aids
- *When antibiotics are used for dental infection:*
  - Oral contraceptives: advise patient of a potential risk for decreased contraceptive action, to maintain compliance with oral contraceptive use while using antibiotics, and to consider the use of additional nonhormonal contraception
- DENIF
- To report sore throat, oral burning sensation, fever, or fatigue, any of which could indicate presence of a superinfection

oxaliplatin

ahks-al-eh-plah′-tin
(Eloxatin)

CATEGORY AND SCHEDULE

Pregnancy Risk Category: D

MECHANISM OF ACTION

A platinum-containing complex that cross-links with DNA strands, preventing cell division. Cell cycle-phase nonspecific. ***Therapeutic Effect:*** Inhibits DNA replication.

PHARMACOKINETICS

Rapidly distributed. Protein binding: 90%. Undergoes rapid, extensive nonenzymatic biotransformation. Excreted in urine. ***Half-life:*** 70 hr.

AVAILABILITY

Powder for Injection: 50-mg, 100-mg vials.

INDICATIONS AND DOSAGES

▸ **Metastatic Colon or Rectal Cancer in Patients Whose Disease Has Recurred or Progressed During or Within 6 Months of Completing First-Line Therapy with Bolus 5-Fluorouracil (5-FU), Leucovorin, and Irinotecan.**

IV

Adults. Day 1: Oxaliplatin 85 mg/m2 in 250–500 ml D_5W and leucovorin 200 mg/m^2, both given simultaneously over more than 2 hr in separate bags using a Y-line, followed by 5-FU 400 mg/m2 IV bolus given over 2–4 min, followed by 5-FU 600 mg/m2 in 500 ml D_5W as a 22-hr continuous IV infusion. Day 2: Leucovorin 200 mg/m2 IV infusion given over more than 2 hr, followed by 5-FU 400 mg/m^2 IV bolus given over 2–4 min, followed by 5-FU 600 mg/m^2 in 500 ml D_5W as a 22-hr continuous IV infusion.

▸ **Ovarian Cancer**

IV

Adults. Cisplatin 100 mg/m^2 and oxaliplatin 130 mg/m^{2}every 3 wk.

OFF-LABEL USES

Treatment of ovarian cancer

CONTRAINDICATIONS
History of allergy to platinum compounds

INTERACTIONS
Drug
Live-virus vaccines: May potentiate virus replication, increase vaccine side effects, and decrease the patient's antibody response to the vaccine.
Nephrotic medications: May decrease the clearance of oxaliplatin.
Herbal
None known.
Food
None known.
Drug interactions of concern to dentistry
- None reported

DIAGNOSTIC TEST EFFECTS
May alter serum bilirubin, AST (SGOT), and ALT (SGPT) levels. May decrease blood Hgb and Hct levels and platelet count.

IV INCOMPATIBILITIES
Don't infuse oxaliplatin with alkaline medications.

SIDE EFFECTS
Frequent (76%–20%)
Peripheral or sensory neuropathy (usually occurs in hands, feet, perioral area, and throat but may present as jaw spasm, abnormal tongue sensation, eye pain, chest pressure, or difficulty walking, swallowing, or writing), nausea (64%), fatigue, diarrhea, vomiting, constipation, abdominal pain, fever, anorexia
Occasional (14%–10%)
Stomatitis, earache, insomnia, cough, difficulty breathing, backache, edema
Rare (7%–3%)
Dyspepsia, dizziness, rhinitis, flushing, alopecia

SERIOUS REACTIONS
! Peripheral or sensory neuropathy can occur, sometimes precipitated or exacerbated by drinking or holding a glass of cold liquid during the IV infusion.
! Pulmonary fibrosis, characterized by a nonproductive cough, dyspnea, crackles, and radiologic pulmonary infiltrates, may require drug discontinuation.
! Hypersensitivity reaction (rash, urticaria, pruritus) occurs rarely.

DENTAL CONSIDERATIONS
General:
- If additional analgesia is required for dental pain, consider alternative analgesics (NSAIDs) in patients taking narcotics for acute or chronic pain.
- Examine for oral manifestation of opportunistic infection.
- Avoid products that affect platelet function, such as aspirin and NSAIDs.
- This drug may be used in the hospital or on an outpatient basis. Confirm the patient's disease and treatment status.
- Chlorhexidine mouth rinse prior to and during chemotherapy may reduce severity of mucositis.
- Patient on chronic drug therapy may rarely present with symptoms of blood dyscrasias, which can include infection, bleeding, and poor healing. If dyscrasia is present, caution patient to prevent oral tissue trauma when using oral hygiene aids.
- Palliative medication may be required for management of oral side effects.

• Short appointments and a stress reduction protocol may be required for anxious patients.
• Provide palliative emergency dental care during drug use.
• Patients may be at risk of bleeding, check for oral signs.
• Oral infections should be eliminated and treated aggressively.
• Monitor vital signs.

Consultations:
• Medical consultation should include routine blood counts including platelet counts and bleeding time.
• Consult physician; prophylactic or therapeutic antiinfectives may be indicated if surgery or periodontal treatment is required.
• Medical consultation may be required to assess immunologic status during cancer chemotherapy and determine safety risk, if any, posed by the required dental treatment.
• Medical consultation may be required to assess disease control and patient's ability to tolerate stress.

Teach Patient/Family:
• Secondary oral infection may occur; need to see dentist immediately if infection occurs
• To be aware of oral side effects
• Importance of good oral hygiene to prevent soft tissue inflammation
• To report oral lesions, soreness, or bleeding to dentist
• To prevent trauma when using oral hygiene aids
• Importance of updating health and medication history if physician makes any changes in evaluation or drug regimens; include OTC, herbal, and nonherbal in the update
• Avoid ice water rinses and exposure to cold to prevent exacerbation of neuropathy symptoms

oxandrolone

ox-an′-droe-lone
Schedule III
(Lonavar[AUS], Oxandrin)
Do not confuse with testolactone.

CATEGORY AND SCHEDULE

Pregnancy Risk Category: X
Controlled substance: Schedule III

MECHANISM OF ACTION

A synthetic testosterone derivative that promotes growth and development of male sex organs, maintains secondary sex characteristics in androgen-deficient males. ***Therapeutic Effect:*** Androgenic and anabolic actions.

PHARMACOKINETICS

Well absorbed from the gastrointestinal (GI) tract. Protein binding: 94–97%. Metabolized in liver. Primarily excreted in urine. Unknown if removed by hemodialysis. ***Half-life:*** 5–13 hrs.

AVAILABILITY

Tablets: 2.5 mg, 10 mg (Oxandrin).

INDICATIONS AND DOSAGES

▸ Weight Gain

Adults, Elderly. 2.5–20 mg in divided doses 2–4 times/day usually for 2–4 weeks. Course of therapy is based on individual response. Repeat intermittently as needed.
Children. Total daily dose is 0.1 mg/kg. Repeat intermittently as needed.

OFF-LABEL USES

AIDS wasting syndrome, alcoholic hepatitis, athletic performance enhancement, burns, growth hormone deficiency, hyperlipidemia, Turner syndrome

CONTRAINDICATIONS

Nephrosis, carcinoma of breast or prostate hypercalcemia, pregnancy, hypersensitivity to oxandrolone or any component of the formulation

INTERACTIONS

Drug

ACTH: May increase the risk of edema and acne.
Adrenal steroids: May increase the risk of edema and acne.
Bupropion: May lower seizure threshold.
Oral anticoagulants: May increase the effects of oral anticoagulants.

Herbal

Chaparral: May increase liver enzymes.
Comfrey: May increase liver enzymes.
Eucalyptus: May increase risk of hepatoxicity.
Germander: May increase liver enzymes.
Jin bu huan: May increase liver enzymes.
Kava kava: May increase liver enzymes.
Pennyroyal: May increase liver enzymes.
Skullcap: May increase the risk of liver damage.
Velerian: May increase risk of hepatotoxicity.

Food

None known.

Drug interactions of concern to dentistry

- Increased risk of bleeding: aspirin
- Edema: adrenocorticotropic hormone (ACTH), adrenal steroids

DIAGNOSTIC TEST EFFECTS

May decrease levels of thyroxine-binding globulin, resulting in decreased total T_4 serum levels and increased resin uptake of T_3 and T_4. May increase PBI and radioactive iodine uptake.

SIDE EFFECTS

Frequent

Gynecomastia, acne, amenorrhea, other menstrual irregularities
Females: Hirsutism, deepening of voice, clitoral enlargement that may not be reversible when drug is discontinued

Occasional

Edema, nausea, insomnia, oligospermia, priapism, male pattern of baldness, bladder irritability, hypercalcemia in immobilized patients or those with breast cancer, hypercholesterolemia

Rare

Polycythemia with high dosage

SERIOUS REACTIONS

! Peliosis hepatitis of the liver, spleen replaced with blood-filled cysts, hepatic neoplasms and hepatocellular carcinoma have been associated with prolonged high-dosage, anaphylactic reactions.

DENTAL CONSIDERATIONS

General:

- Monitor vital signs at every appointment because of CV side effects.
- Determine why the patient is taking the drug.
- Consider local hemostasis measures to prevent excessive bleeding.
- Short appointments and a stress reduction protocol may be required for anxious patients.
- Avoid prescribing aspirin-containing products.

Consultations:

- If signs of anemia are observed in oral tissues, physician consultation may be required.

• Medical consultation may be required to assess disease control and patient's ability to tolerate stress.
• Medical consultation should include partial prothrombin time or prothrombin time.

Teach Patient/Family:

• Importance of good oral hygiene to prevent soft tissue inflammation
• That secondary oral infection may occur; must see dentist immediately if infection occurs

oxaprozin

ox-a-pro′-zin
(Daypro)
Do not confuse oxaprozin with oxazepam.

CATEGORY AND SCHEDULE

Pregnancy Risk Category: C
(D if used in third trimester or near delivery)

MECHANISM OF ACTION

An NSAID that produces analgesic and anti-inflammatory effects by inhibiting prostaglandin synthesis. ***Therapeutic Effect:*** Reduces the inflammatory response and intensity of pain.

PHARMACOKINETICS

Well absorbed from the GI tract. Protein binding: 99%. Widely distributed. Metabolized in the liver. Primarily excreted in urine; partially eliminated in feces. Not removed by hemodialysis. ***Half-life:*** 42–50 hr.

AVAILABILITY

Tablets: 600 mg.

INDICATIONS AND DOSAGES

▸ Osteoarthritis

PO

Adults, Elderly. 1200 mg once a day (600 mg in patients with low body weight or mild disease). Maximum: 1800 mg/day.

▸ Rheumatoid Arthritis

PO

Adults, Elderly. 1200 mg once a day. Range: 600–1800 mg/day.

▸ Juvenile Rheumatoid Arthritis

Children weighing more than 54 kg. 1200 mg/day.
Children weighing 32–54 kg. 900 mg/day.
Children weighing 22–31 kg. 600 mg/day.

▸ Dosage in Renal Impairment

For adults and elderly patients with renal impairment, the recommended initial dose is 600 mg/day; may be increased up to 1200 mg/day.

CONTRAINDICATIONS

Active peptic ulcer disease, chronic inflammation of GI tract, GI bleeding or ulceration, history of hypersensitivity to aspirin or NSAIDs

INTERACTIONS

Drug

Antihypertensives, diuretics: May decrease the effects of these drugs.
Aspirin, other salicylates: May increase the risk of GI side effects, such as bleeding.
Bone marrow depressants: May increase the risk of hematologic reactions.
Heparin, oral anticoagulants, thrombolytics: May increase the effects of these drugs.
Lithium: May increase the blood concentration and risk of toxicity of lithium.
Methotrexate: May increase the risk of methotrexate toxicity.

Probenecid: May increase the oxaprozin blood concentration.

Herbal

Feverfew: May decrease the effects of feverfew.

Ginkgo biloba: May increase the risk of bleeding.

Food

None known.

Drug interactions of concern to dentistry

- GI ulceration, bleeding: aspirin, alcohol, corticosteroids
- Decreased action: salicylates
- Nephrotoxicity: acetaminophen (prolonged use and high doses)
- Possible risk of decreased renal function: cyclosporine
- First-time users of SSRIs also taking NSAIDs may have a higher risk of GI side effects; until more data are available, it may be advisable to avoid use of NSAIDs in these patients (*Br J Clin Pharmacol* 55:591–595, 2003)
- *When prescribed for dental pain:*
  - Risk of increased effects: oral anticoagulants, oral antidiabetics, lithium, methotrexate
  - Decreased antihypertensive effects of diuretics, β-adrenergic blockers, and ACE inhibitors

DIAGNOSTIC TEST EFFECTS

May increase BUN, serum creatinine, AST (SGOT), and ALT (SGPT) levels.

SIDE EFFECTS

Occasional (9%–3%)

Nausea, diarrhea, constipation, dyspepsia, edema

Rare (<3%)

Vomiting, abdominal cramps or pain, flatulence, anorexia, confusion, tinnitus, insomnia, somnolence

SERIOUS REACTIONS

! Hypertension, acute renal failure, respiratory depression, GI bleeding, and coma occur rarely.

DENTAL CONSIDERATIONS

General:

- Patients on chronic drug therapy may rarely have symptoms of blood dyscrasias, which can include infection, bleeding, and poor healing.
- Assess salivary flow as a factor in caries, periodontal disease, and candidiasis.
- Avoid prescribing for dental use in pregnancy.
- Consider semisupine chair position for patients with arthritic disease.

Consultations:

- Medical consultation may be required to assess disease control.
- In a patient with symptoms of blood dyscrasias, request a medical consultation for blood studies and postpone dental treatment until normal values are reestablished.

Teach Patient/Family:

- Importance of good oral hygiene to prevent soft tissue inflammation
- Caution to prevent injury when using oral hygiene aids
- *When chronic dry mouth occurs, advise patient:*
  - To avoid mouth rinses with high alcohol content because of drying effects
  - Of need for daily use of home fluoride products to prevent caries
  - To use sugarless gum, frequent sips of water, or saliva substitutes

oxazepam

ox-a′-ze-pam
Schedule IV
(Alepam[AUS], Apo-Oxazepam[CAN], Murelax[AUS], Serax, Serepax[AUS])
Do not confuse oxazepam with oxaprozin, or Serax with Eurax or Xerac.

CATEGORY AND SCHEDULE

Pregnancy Risk Category: D
Controlled Substance Schedule IV

MECHANISM OF ACTION

A benzodiazepine that potentiates the effects of gamma-aminobutyric acid and other inhibitory neurotransmitters by binding to specific receptors in the CNS. ***Therapeutic Effect:*** Produces anxiolytic effect and skeletal muscle relaxation.

PHARMACOKINETICS

Well absorbed from the GI tract. Protein binding: 97%. Metabolized in the liver. Primarily excreted in urine. Not removed by hemodialysis. ***Half-life:*** 5–20 hr.

AVAILABILITY

Capsules: 10 mg, 15 mg, 30 mg.
Tablet: 15 mg.

INDICATIONS AND DOSAGES

▸ Mild to Moderate Anxiety

PO

Adults. 10–15 mg 3–4 times a day.

▸ Severe Anxiety

PO

Adults. 15–30 mg 3–4 times a day.

▸ Alcohol Withdrawal

PO

Adults. 15–30 mg 3–4 times a day.
Elderly. Initially, 10–20 mg 3 times a day. May gradually increase up to 30–45 mg/day.

CONTRAINDICATIONS

Angle-closure glaucoma; preexisting CNS depression; severe, uncontrolled pain

INTERACTIONS

Drug

Alcohol, other CNS depressants: May potentiate CNS depression.

Herbal

Kava kava, valerian: May increase CNS depression.

Food

None known.

Drug interactions of concern to dentistry

- Increased effects: CNS depressants, alcohol, and anticonvulsant medications
- Possible increase in CNS side effects of kava (herb)

DIAGNOSTIC TEST EFFECTS

May elevate serum alkaline phosphatase, bilirubin, LDH, AST (SGOT), and ALT (SGPT) levels. May produce abnormal renal function test results. Therapeutic serum drug level is 0.2–1.4 mcg/ml; toxic serum drug level has not been established.

SIDE EFFECTS

Frequent

Mild, transient somnolence at beginning of therapy

Occasional

Dizziness, headache

Rare

Paradoxical CNS reactions, such as hyperactivity or nervousness in children and excitement or restlessness in the elderly or debilitated (generally noted during the first 2 weeks of therapy)

SERIOUS REACTIONS

! Abrupt or too-rapid withdrawal may result in pronounced restlessness, irritability, insomnia, hand tremor, abdominal or muscle cramps, diaphoresis, vomiting, and seizures.
! Overdose results in somnolence, confusion, diminished reflexes, and coma.

DENTAL CONSIDERATIONS

General:

- Monitor vital signs at every appointment because of CV side effects.
- Psychologic and physical dependence may occur with chronic administration.
- Geriatric patients are more susceptible to drug effects; use lower dose.
- Assess salivary flow as a factor in caries, periodontal disease, and candidiasis.

Consultations:

- Medical consultation may be required to assess disease control.

Teach Patient/Family:

- To avoid mouth rinses with high alcohol content because of drying effects

oxcarbazepine

oks-kar-bays′-uh-peen
(Trileptal)

CATEGORY AND SCHEDULE

Pregnancy Risk Category: C

MECHANISM OF ACTION

An anticonvulsant that blocks sodium channels, resulting in stabilization of hyperexcited neural membranes, inhibition of repetitive neuronal firing, and diminishing synaptic impulses. ***Therapeutic Effect:*** Prevents seizures.

PHARMACOKINETICS

Completely absorbed from GI tract and extensively metabolized in the liver to active metabolite. Protein binding: 40%. Primarily excreted in urine. ***Half-life:*** 2 hr; metabolite, 6–10 hr.

AVAILABILITY

Oral Suspension: 300 mg/5 ml.
Tablets: 150 mg, 300 mg, 600 mg.

INDICATIONS AND DOSAGES

▸ Adjunctive Treatment of Seizures

PO
Adults, Elderly. Initially, 600 mg/day in 2 divided doses.
May increase by up to 600 mg/day at weekly intervals.
Maximum: 2400 mg/day.
Children 4–16 yr. 8–10 mg/kg.
Maximum: 600 mg/day.
Maintenance (based on weight): 1800 mg/day for children weighing more than 39 kg; 1200 mg/day for children weighing 29.1–39 kg; and 900 mg/day for children weighing 20–29 kg.

▸ Conversion to Monotherapy

PO
Adults, Elderly. 600 mg/day in 2 divided doses (while decreasing concomitant anticonvulsant over 3–6 wk). May increase by 600 mg/day at weekly intervals up to 2400 mg/day.
Children. Initially, 8–10 mg/kg/day in 2 divided doses with simultaneous initial reduction of dose of concomitant antiepileptic.

▸ Initiation of Monotherapy

PO
Adults, Elderly. 600 mg/day in 2 divided doses. May increase by

300 mg/day every 3 days up to 1200 mg/day.
Children. Initially, 8–10 mg/kg/day in 2 divided doses. Increase at 3 day intervals by 5 mg/kg/day to achieve maintenance dose by weight;
(70 kg): 1500–2100 mg/day;
(60–69 kg): 1200–2100 mg/day;
(50–59 kg): 1200–1800 mg/day;
(41–49 kg): 1200–1500 mg/day;
(35–40 kg): 900–1500 mg/day;
(25–34 kg): 900–1200 mg/day;
(20–24 kg): 600–900 mg/day.

▸ Dosage in Renal Impairment
For patients with creatinine clearance less than 30 ml/min, give 50% of normal starting dose, then titrate slowly to desired dose.

OFF-LABEL USES
Atypical panic disorder

CONTRAINDICATIONS
None known.

INTERACTIONS
Drug
Carbamazepine, phenobarbital, phenytoin, valproic acid, verapamil: May decrease the blood concentration and effects of oxcarbazepine.
Felodipine, oral contraceptives: May decrease the effectiveness of these drugs.
Phenobarbital, phenytoin: May increase the blood concentration and risk of toxicity of these drugs.
Herbal
None known.
Food
None known.
Drug interactions of concern to dentistry
- No dental drug interactions reported; CYP450 3A4/5 enzyme inducers may decrease plasma levels
- Possible increase in CNS depression: all CNS depressants, alcohol

DIAGNOSTIC TEST EFFECTS
May increase GGT level and other hepatic function test results. May increase or decrease blood glucose level. May decrease serum calcium, potassium, and sodium levels.

SIDE EFFECTS
Frequent (22%–13%)
Dizziness, nausea, headache
Occasional (7%–5%)
Vomiting, diarrhea, ataxia, nervousness, heartburn, indigestion, epigastric pain, constipation
Rare (4%)
Tremor, rash, back pain, epistaxis, sinusitis, diplopia

SERIOUS REACTIONS
! Clinically significant hyponatremia may occur.

DENTAL CONSIDERATIONS
General:
- Monitor vital signs at every appointment because of CV side effects.
- Patients on chronic drug therapy may rarely have symptoms of blood dyscrasias, which can include infection, bleeding, and poor healing.
- Assess salivary flow as a factor in caries, periodontal disease, and candidiasis
- Consider semisupine chair position for patient comfort if GI side effects occur.
- Short appointments and a stress reduction protocol may be required for anxious patients.

• Determine type of epilepsy, seizure frequency, and quality of seizure control.

Consultations:

• In a patient with symptoms of blood dyscrasias, request a medical consultation for blood studies and postpone treatment until normal values are reestablished.
• Medical consultation may be required to assess disease control and patient's ability to tolerate stress.

Teach Patient/Family:

• Importance of good oral hygiene to prevent soft tissue inflammation
• To prevent trauma when using oral hygiene aids
• *When chronic dry mouth occurs, advise patient:*
  • To avoid mouth rinses with high alcohol content because of drying effects
  • To use daily home fluoride products for anticaries effect
  • To use sugarless gum, frequent sips of water, or saliva substitutes

oxiconazole

ox-i-con′-a-zole
(Oxistat, Oxizole[CAN])
Do not confuse with Nitrostat.

CATEGORY AND SCHEDULE

Pregnancy Risk Category: B

MECHANISM OF ACTION

An antifungal agent that inhibits ergosterol synthesis. ***Therapeutic Effect:*** Destroys cytoplasmic membrane integrity of fungi. Fungicidal.

PHARMACOKINETICS

Low systemic absorption. Absorbed and distributed in each layer of the dermis. Excreted in the urine.

AVAILABILITY

Cream: 1% (Oxistat).
Lotion: 1% (Oxistat).

INDICATIONS AND DOSAGES

▸ Tinea Pedis

TOPICAL

Adults, Elderly, Children 12 yrs and older. Apply 1–2 times daily for one month or until signs and symptoms significantly improve.

▸ Tinea Cruris, Tinea Corporis

TOPICAL

Adults, Elderly, Children 12 yrs and older. Apply 1–2 times daily for two weeks or until signs and symptoms significantly improve.

CONTRAINDICATIONS

Not for ophthalmic use, hypersensitivity to oxiconazole or any other azole fungals

INTERACTIONS

Drug

None known.

Herbal

None known.

Food

None known.

Drug interactions of concern to dentistry

• None reported

DIAGNOSTIC TEST EFFECTS

None known.

SIDE EFFECTS

Occasional

Itching, local irritation, stinging, dryness

SERIOUS REACTIONS

! Hypersensitivity reactions characterized by rash, swelling, pruritus, maceration, and a sensation of warmth may occur.

DENTAL CONSIDERATIONS

General:

• No specific dental considerations other than determining why the patient is using this medication.

oxidized cellulose

oks-i-dyzed **cell**-you-lose
(Interceed, Surgicel)

CATEGORY AND SCHEDULE

Pregnancy Risk Category: Not reported

MECHANISM OF ACTION

Oxidized cellulose is saturated with blood at the bleeding site and swells into a brownish or black gelatinous mass that aids in clot formation. When used in small amounts, it is absorbed from the sites of implantation with minimal tissue reaction. ***Therapeutic Effect:*** Stops blood flow. Weak bactericidal action.

PHARMACOKINETICS

Absorption occurs in 7–14 days. ***Half-life:*** Unknown.

AVAILABILITY

Absorbable Hemostats: Various sizes

INDICATIONS AND DOSAGES

▸ **Surgical Procedures to Assist in the Control of Capillary, Venous, and Small Arterial Hemorrhage When Ligation or Other Conventional Methods of Control are Impractical or Ineffective**

TOPICAL

Adults. Minimal amounts of an appropriate size are laid on the bleeding site or held firmly against the tissues until hemostasis is obtained.

CONTRAINDICATIONS

Use for packing or implantation in fractures or laminectomies, hemorrhage from large arteries, and nonhemorrhagic oozing surfaces; use as a wrap; use around the optic nerve and chiasm; applied as wadding or packing as a hemostatic agent; hypersensitivity to oxidized cellulose or any component of the formulation

INTERACTIONS

Drug

None known.

Herbal

None known.

Food

None known.

DIAGNOSTIC TEST EFFECTS

None known.

SIDE EFFECTS

Frequency not defined

Headache, nasal burning or stinging, sneezing, encapsulation of fluid

SERIOUS REACTIONS

Pain, numbness, and paralysis have been reported.

DENTAL CONSIDERATIONS

General:

• Apply dry; use only amount needed to control bleeding.

• Place loosely and avoid packing; remove excess before closure in surgery; irrigate first, then remove using sterile technique.

• Ensure therapeutic response: decreased bleeding in surgery.
• Can be left in situ when necessary but should be removed once bleeding is controlled.
• Application of topical thrombin solution to the cellulose gauze will inactivate thrombin because of acidity.

oxybutynin

ox-i-byoo′-ti-nin
(Ditropan, Ditropan XL, Oxytrol)
Do not confuse oxybutynin with Oxycontin, or Ditropan with diazepam.

CATEGORY AND SCHEDULE

Pregnancy Risk Category: B

MECHANISM OF ACTION

An anticholinergic that exerts antispasmodic (papaverine-like) and antimuscarinic (atropine-like) action on the detrusor smooth muscle of the bladder. ***Therapeutic Effect:*** Increases bladder capacity and delays desire to void.

PHARMACOKINETICS

Route	Onset	Peak	Duration
PO	0.5–1 hr	3–6 hr	6–10 hr

Rapidly absorbed from the GI tract. Metabolized in the liver. Primarily excreted in urine. Unknown if removed by hemodialysis. ***Half-life:*** 1–2.3 hr.

AVAILABILITY

Syrup (Ditropan): 5 mg/5 ml.
Tablets (Ditropan): 5 mg.
Tablets (Extended-Release [Ditropan XL]): 5 mg, 10 mg, 15 mg.
Transdermal (Oxytrol): 3.9 mg.

INDICATIONS AND DOSAGES

▸ Neurogenic Bladder

PO
Adults. 5 mg 2–3 times a day up to 5 mg 4 times a day.
Elderly. 2.5–5 mg twice a day. May increase by 2.5 mg/day every 1–2 days.
Children 5 yr and older. 5 mg twice a day up to 5 mg 4 times a day.
Children 1–4 yr. 0.2 mg/kg/dose 2–4 times a day.
PO (Extended-Release)
Adults. 5–10 mg/day up to 30 mg/day.
TRANSDERMAL
Adults. 3.9 mg applied twice a week. Apply every 3–4 days.

CONTRAINDICATIONS

GI or GU obstruction, glaucoma, myasthenia gravis, toxic megacolon, ulcerative colitis

INTERACTIONS

Drug

Medications with anticholinergic effects (such as antihistamines): May increase the anticholinergic effects of oxybutynin.

Herbal

None known.

Food

None known.

Drug interactions of concern to dentistry

• Increased anticholinergic effect: anticholinergic drugs
• Increased depressant effect of both drugs: CNS depressants, alcohol

DIAGNOSTIC TEST EFFECTS

None known.

SIDE EFFECTS

Frequent

Constipation, dry mouth, somnolence, decreased perspiration

Occasional

Decreased lacrimation or salivation, impotence, urinary hesitancy and retention, suppressed lactation, blurred vision, mydriasis, nausea or vomiting, insomnia

SERIOUS REACTIONS

! Overdose produces CNS excitation (including nervousness, restlessness, hallucinations, and irritability), hypotension or hypertension, confusion, tachycardia, facial flushing, and respiratory depression.

DENTAL CONSIDERATIONS

General:

- Assess salivary flow as a factor in caries, periodontal disease, and candidiasis.
- Monitor vital signs at every appointment because of CV side effects.
- Avoid dental light in patient's eyes; offer dark glasses for patient comfort.
- Consider semisupine chair position for patient comfort if GI side effects occur.

Consultations:

- Physician should be informed if significant xerostomic side effects occur (e.g., increased caries, sore tongue, problems eating or swallowing, difficulty wearing prosthesis) so that a medication change can be considered.

Teach Patient/Family:

- Importance of good oral hygiene to prevent soft tissue inflammation
- *When chronic dry mouth occurs, advise patient:*
  - To avoid mouth rinses with high alcohol content because of drying effects
  - Of need for daily use of home fluoride products to prevent caries
  - To use sugarless gum, frequent sips of water, or saliva substitutes

oxycodone

ox-ee-koe'-done

Schedule II

(Endone[AUS], OxyContin, Oxydose, OxyFast, OxyIR, Oxynorm[AUS], Roxicodone, Roxicodone Intensol)

Do not confuse oxycodone with oxybutynin.

CATEGORY AND SCHEDULE

Pregnancy Risk Category: B (D if used for prolonged periods or at high dosages at term)

Controlled Substance: Schedule II

MECHANISM OF ACTION

An opioid analgesic that binds with opioid receptors in the CNS.

Therapeutic Effect: Alters the perception of and emotional response to pain.

PHARMACOKINETICS

Route	Onset	Peak	Duration
PO, Immediate-release	N/A	N/A	4–5 hr
PO, Controlled-release	N/A	N/A	12 hr

Moderately absorbed from the GI tract. Protein binding: 38%–45%. Widely distributed. Metabolized in the liver. Excreted in urine. Unknown if removed by hemodialysis. ***Half-life:*** 2–3 hr (3.2 hr controlled-release).

O

AVAILABILITY

Capsules (Immediate-Release [OxyIR]): 5 mg.
Oral Concentrate (Oxydose, OxyFast, Roxicodone Intensol): 20 mg/ml.
Oral Solution (Roxicodone): 5 mg/5ml.
Tablets (Roxicodone): 5 mg, 15 mg, 30 mg.
Tablets (Extended-Release [OxyContin]): 10 mg, 20 mg, 40 mg, 80 mg, 160 mg.

INDICATIONS AND DOSAGES

▸ Analgesia

PO (Controlled-Release)
Adults, Elderly. Initially, 10 mg q12h. May increase every 1–2 days by 25%–50%. Usual: 40 mg/day (100 mg/day for cancer pain).
PO (Immediate-Release)
Adults, Elderly. Initially, 5 mg q6h as needed. May increase up to 30 mg q4h. Usual: 10–30 mg q4h as needed.
Children. 0.05–0.15 mg/kg/dose q4–6h.

CONTRAINDICATIONS

None known.

INTERACTIONS

Drug

Alcohol, other CNS depressants: May increase CNS or respiratory depression and hypotension.
MAOIs: May produce a severe, sometimes fatal reaction; expect to administer one quarter of usual oxycodone dose.

Herbal

None known.

Food

None known.

Drug interactions of concern to dentistry

- Increased effects with other CNS depressants: alcohol, other narcotics, sedative-hypnotics, skeletal muscle relaxants, phenothiazines, benzodiazepines
- Contraindication: MAOIs
- Increased effects of anticholinergics

DIAGNOSTIC TEST EFFECTS

May increase serum amylase and lipase levels.

SIDE EFFECTS

Frequent

Somnolence, dizziness, hypotension (including orthostatic hypotension), anorexia

Occasional

Confusion, diaphoresis, facial flushing, urine retention, constipation, dry mouth, nausea, vomiting, headache

Rare

Allergic reaction, depression, paradoxical CNS hyperactivity or nervousness in children, paradoxical excitement and restlessness in elderly or debilitated patients

SERIOUS REACTIONS

! Overdose results in respiratory depression, skeletal muscle flaccidity, cold or clammy skin, cyanosis, and extreme somnolence progressing to seizures, stupor, and coma.
! Hepatotoxicity may occur with overdose of the acetaminophen component of fixed-combination products.
! The patient who uses oxycodone repeatedly may develop a tolerance to the drug's analgesic effect and physical dependence.

DENTAL CONSIDERATIONS

General:

- Monitor vital signs at every appointment because of CV and respiratory side effects.

- Assess salivary flow as a factor in caries, periodontal disease, and candidiasis.
- Psychologic and physical dependence may occur with chronic administration.
- Determine why the patient is taking the drug.

Teach Patient/Family:

- To avoid mouth rinses with high alcohol content because of drying effects

oxymetazoline

ox-ee-met-az′-oh-leen
(Afrin, Afrin 12-Hour, Afrin Children's Strength Nose Drops, Ocuclear, Sinex 12 Hour Long-Acting)

CATEGORY AND SCHEDULE

Pregnancy Risk Category: C
OTC

MECHANISM OF ACTION

A direct-acting sympathomimetic amine that acts on alpha-adrenergic receptors in arterioles of the nasal mucosa to produce constriction. ***Therapeutic Effect:*** Causes vasoconstriction resulting in decreased blood flow and decreased nasal congestion.

PHARMACOKINETICS

Onset of action is about 10 min., and a duration of action is 7 hrs or more. Absorption occurs from the nasal mucosa and can produce systemic effects, primarily following overdose or excessive use. Excreted mostly in the urine, as well as the feces. ***Half-life:*** 5–8 hrs.

AVAILABILITY

Eye Drops: 0.025% (Ocuclear).
Nasal Drops: 0.025% (Afrin Children's Strength Nose Drops), 0.05% (Afrin).
Nasal Spray: 0.05% (Afrin, Afrin 1 2-Hour, Sinex 12 Hour Long-Acting).

INDICATIONS AND DOSAGES

▸ Rhinitis

INTRANASAL

Adults, Elderly, Children older than 6 yrs. 2–3 drops/sprays (0.05% nasal solution) in each nostril q12h.
Children (2–5 yrs). 2–4 drops/sprays (0.025% nasal solution) in each nostril q12h for up to 3 days.

▸ Conjunctivitis

OPHTHALMIC

Adults, Elderly, Children older than 6 yrs. 1–2 drops (0.025% ophthalmic solution) q6h for 3–4 days.

OFF-LABEL USES

Otitis media surgical procedures

CONTRAINDICATIONS

Narrow-angle glaucoma or hypersensitivity to oxymetazoline or other adrenergic agents

O

INTERACTIONS

Drug

Maprotiline, tricyclic antidepressants: May increase the effects of oxymetazoline.

Herbal

None known.

Food

None known.

Drug interactions of concern to dentistry

- Increased risk of hypertension: tricyclic antidepressants, but it requires adequate systemic absorption of oxymetazoline

DIAGNOSTIC TEST EFFECTS

None known.

SIDE EFFECTS

Occasional

Burning, stinging, drying nasal mucosa, sneezing, rebound congestion, insomnia, nervousness

SERIOUS REACTIONS

! Large doses may produce tachycardia, hypertension, arrhythmias, palpitations, lightheadedness, nausea, and vomiting.

DENTAL CONSIDERATIONS

General:

- Excessive use can lead to rebound congestion and CV side effects; follow recommended dosing intervals.
- Extensive nasal swelling and congestion may interfere with optimal use of nitrous oxide/oxygen sedation.

oxymetholone

ox-ee-meth′-oh-lone

Schedule III

(Anadrol, Anapolon[CAN])

Do not confuse with oxycodone.

CATEGORY AND SCHEDULE

Pregnancy Risk Category: X

Controlled substance: Schedule III

MECHANISM OF ACTION

An androgenic-anabolic steroid that is a synthetic derivative of testosterone synthesized to accentuate anabolic as opposed to androgenic effects. ***Therapeutic Effect:*** Improves nitrogen balance in conditions of unfavorable protein metabolism with adequate caloric and protein intake, stimulates erythropoiesis, suppresses gonadotropic functions of pituitary, and may exert a direct effect upon the testes.

PHARMACOKINETICS

The pharmacokinetics of oxymetholone has been studied. Metabolized in the liver via reduction and oxidation. Unchanged oxymetholone and its metabolites are excreted in urine.

Half-life: Unknown.

AVAILABILITY

Tablets: 50 mg (Anadrol).

INDICATIONS AND DOSAGES

▸ **Anemia, Chronic Renal Failure, Acqured Aplastic Anemia, Chemotherapy-Induced Myelosuppresion, Fanconi's Anemia, Red Cell Aplasia**

PO

Adults, Elderly, Children.

1–5 mg/kg/day. Response is not immediate, and a minimum of 3–6 months should be given.

OFF-LABEL USES

Amegakaryocytic thrombocytopenia, familial antithrombin III deficiency, hereditary angioedema, HIV wasting, metastatic breast cancer in women, relief of bone pain associated with osteoporosis, neutropenia, Turner's syndrome, xeroderma pigmentosum

CONTRAINDICATIONS

Cardiac impairment, hypercalcemia, pregnancy/lactation, prostatic or breast cancer in males, metastatic breast cancer in women with active hypercalcemia, nephrosis or nephritic phase nephritis, severe liver disease, hypersensitivity to oxymetholone or any of its components

INTERACTIONS

Drug

Bupropion: May lower seizure threshold.
Liver toxic medications: May increase liver toxicity.
Oral anticoagulants: May increase effects of oral anticoagulants.

Herbal

Chaparral: May increase liver enzymes.
Comfrey: May increase liver enzymes.
Eucalyptus: May increase risk of heptotoxicity.
Germander: May increase liver enzymes.
Jin bu huan: May increase liver enzymes.
Kava kava: May increase risk of liver damage.
Pennyroyal: May increase liver enzymes.
Skullcap: May increase risk of liver damage.
Valerian: May increase risk of heptotoxicity.

Food

None known.

Drug interactions of concern to dentistry

- Increased risk of bleeding: aspirin
- Edema: ACTH, adrenal steroids

DIAGNOSTIC TEST EFFECTS

May increase blood Hgb and Hct, LDL concentrations, serum alkaline phosphatase, bilirubin, calcium, potassium, SGOT (AST) levels and sodium levels. May decrease HDL concentrations.

SIDE EFFECTS

Frequent

Gynecomastia, acne, amenorrhea, menstrual irregularities
Females: Hirsutism, deepening of voice, clitoral enlargement that may not be reversible when drug is discontinued

Occasional

Edema, nausea, insomnia, oligospermia, priapism, male pattern of baldness, bladder irritability, hypercalcemia in immobilized patients or those with breast cancer, hypercholesterolemia, inflammation and pain at IM injection site
Transdermal: Itching, erythema, skin irritation

Rare

Liver damage, hypersensitivity

SERIOUS REACTIONS

! Cholestatic jaundice, hepatic necrosis and death occur rarely but have been reported in association with long-term androgenic-anabolic steroid use.

DENTAL CONSIDERATIONS

General:

- Monitor vital signs at every appointment because of CV side effects.
- Determine why the patient is taking the drug.
- Consider local hemostasis measures to prevent excessive bleeding.
- Short appointments and a stress reduction protocol may be required for anxious patients.
- Avoid prescribing aspirin-containing products.

Consultations:

- Physician consultation may be required if signs of anemia are observed in oral tissues.

• Medical consultation may be required to assess disease control and patient's ability to tolerate stress.
• Medical consultation should include partial prothrombin time or prothrombin time.

Teach Patient/Family:
• Importance of good oral hygiene to prevent soft tissue inflammation
• That secondary oral infection may occur; must see dentist immediately if infection occurs

paclitaxel

pass-leh-tax′-ell
(Abraxane, Anzatax[AUS], Onxol, Taxol)
Do not confuse paclitaxel with Paxil, or Taxol with Taxotere.

CATEGORY AND SCHEDULE

Pregnancy Risk Category: D

MECHANISM OF ACTION

An antimitotic agent in the taxoid family that disrupts the microtubular cell network, which is essential for cellular function. Blocks cells in the late G_2 phase and M phase of the cell cycle. ***Therapeutic Effect:*** Inhibits cellular mitosis and replication.

PHARMACOKINETICS

Does not readily cross the blood-brain barrier. Protein binding: 89%–98%. Metabolized in the liver to active metabolites; eliminated by bile. Not removed by hemodialysis. ***Half-life:*** 1.3–8.6 hr.

AVAILABILITY

Injection (Abraxane): 100-mg vial.
Injection (Onxol, Taxol): 6 mg/ml.

INDICATIONS AND DOSAGES

▸ Ovarian Cancer
IV
Adults. 135–175 mg/m²/dose over 1–24 hr q3wk.

▸ Breast Carcinoma
IV (Onxol, Taxol)
Adults, Elderly. 175 mg/m² over 3 hr q3wk.
PO (Abraxane)
Adults, Elderly. 260 mg/m² over 30 minutes q3wk.

▸ Non–Small-Cell Lung Carcinoma
IV
Adults, Elderly. 135 mg/m² over 24 hr, followed by cisplatin 75 mg/m² q3wk.

▸ Kaposi's Sarcoma
IV
Adults, Elderly. 135 mg/m²/dose over 3 hr q3wk or 100 mg/m²/dose over 3 hr q2wk.

▸ Dosage in Hepatic Impairment

Total Bilirubin	Total Dose
more than 3 mg/dl	less than 50 mg/m²
1.6–3 mg/dl	less than 75 mg/m²
1.5 mg/dl or less	less than 135 mg/m²

OFF-LABEL USES

Treatment of upper GI tract adenocarcinoma, head and neck cancer, hormone-refractory prostate cancer, metastic breast cancer, non-Hodgkin's lymphoma, small-cell lung cancer, transitional cell cancer of urothelium

CONTRAINDICATIONS

Baseline neutropenia (neutrophil count 1500 cells/mm³), hypersensitivity to drugs developed with Cremophor EL (polyoxyethylated castor oil)

INTERACTIONS

Drug

Bone marrow depressants: May increase myelosuppression.
Live-virus vaccines: May potentiate virus replication, increase vaccine side effects, and decrease the patient's antibody response to the vaccine.

Herbal

None known.

Food

None known.

Drug interactions of concern to dentistry

- Possible (not demonstrated) increase in action by strong inhibitors of CYP2C8 and CYP3A4 isoenzymes: diazepam, ketoconazole, midazolam (monitor patient if prescribed)

DIAGNOSTIC TEST EFFECTS

May elevate serum alkaline phosphatase, bilirubin, AST, and ALT levels. Decreases blood Hgb and Hct levels and platelet, RBC, and WBC counts.

IV INCOMPATIBILITIES

Amphotericin B complex (Abelcet, AmBisome, Amphotec), chlorpromazine (Thorazine), doxorubicin liposomal (Doxil), hydroxyzine (Vistaril), methylprednisolone (Solu-Medrol), mitoxantrone (Novantrone)

IV COMPATIBILITIES

Carboplatin (Paraplatin), cisplatin (Platinol AQ), cyclophosphamide (Cytoxan), cytarabine (Cytosar), dacarbazine (DTIC-Dome), dexamethasone (Decadron), diphenhydramine (Benadryl), doxorubicin (Adriamycin), etoposide (VePesid), gemcitabine (Gemzar), granisetron (Kytril), hydromorphone (Dilaudid), magnesium sulfate, mannitol, methotrexate, morphine, ondansetron (Zofran), potassium chloride, vinblastine (Velban), vincristine (Oncovin)

P

SIDE EFFECTS

Expected (90%–70%)
Diarrhea, alopecia, nausea, vomiting

Frequent (48%–46%)
Myalgia or arthralgia, peripheral neuropathy

Occasional (20%–13%)
Mucositis, hypotension during infusion, pain or redness at injection site

Rare (3%)
Bradycardia

SERIOUS REACTIONS

! Neutropenic nadir occurs at approximately day 11 of paclitaxel therapy.

! Anemia and leukopenia are common reactions. Thrombocytopenia occurs occasionally.

! A severe hypersensitivity reaction, including dyspnea, severe hypotension, angioedema, and generalized urticaria, occurs rarely.

DENTAL CONSIDERATIONS

General:

- Consider semisupine chair position for patient comfort if GI side effects occur.
- Patients receiving chemotherapy may require palliative therapy for stomatitis.
- Patients on chronic drug therapy may rarely have symptoms of blood dyscrasias, which can include infection, bleeding, and poor healing.

Consultations:

- Medical consultation may be required to assess disease control.

Teach Patient/Family:

- Importance of good oral hygiene to prevent soft tissue inflammation
- Caution to prevent trauma when using oral hygiene aids

palonosetron hydrochloride

pal-oh-noe′-seh-tron
(Aloxi)

CATEGORY AND SCHEDULE

Pregnancy Risk Category: B

MECHANISM OF ACTION

A 5-HT_3 receptor antagonist that acts centrally in the chemoreceptor trigger zone and peripherally at the vagal nerve terminals. ***Therapeutic Effect:*** Prevents nausea and vomiting associated with chemotherapy.

PHARMACOKINETICS
Protein binding: 52%. Eliminated in urine. ***Half-life:*** 40 hr.

AVAILABILITY
Injection: 0.25 mg/5 ml.

INDICATIONS AND DOSAGES
▸ Chemotherapy-Induced Nausea and Vomiting
IV
Adults, Elderly. 0.25 mg as a single dose 30 min before starting chemotherapy.

CONTRAINDICATIONS
None known.

INTERACTIONS
Drug
None known.
Herbal
None known.
Food
None known.
Drug interactions of concern to dentistry
• None reported

DIAGNOSTIC TEST EFFECTS
May transiently increase serum bilirubin, AST (SGOT), and ALT (SGPT) levels.

IV INCOMPATIBILITIES
Don't mix palonosetron with any other drugs.

SIDE EFFECTS
Occasional (9%–5%)
Headache, constipation
Rare (< 1%)
Diarrhea, dizziness, fatigue, abdominal pain, insomnia

SERIOUS REACTIONS
! Overdose may produce a combination of CNS stimulant and depressant effects.

DENTAL CONSIDERATIONS
General:
• For acute use in hospitals or cancer treatment centers.
Teach Patient/Family:
• To be aware of possible oral side effects from concurrent chemotherapy

pamidronate disodium
pam-id′-drow-nate
(Aredia, Pamisol[AUS])
Do not confuse Aredia with Adriamcyin.

CATEGORY AND SCHEDULE
Pregnancy Risk Category: D

MECHANISM OF ACTION
A bisphosphate that binds to bone and inhibits osteoclast-mediated calcium resorption. ***Therapeutic Effect:*** Lowers serum calcium concentrations.

PHARMACOKINETICS

Route	Onset	Peak	Duration
IV	24–48 hr	5–7 days	N/A

After IV administration, rapidly absorbed by bone. Slowly excreted unchanged in urine. Unknown if removed by hemodialysis. ***Half-life:*** bone, 300 days; unmetabolized, 2.5 hr.

AVAILABILITY
Powder for Injection: 30 mg, 90 mg. *Injection Solution:* 3 mg/ml, 6 mg/ml, 9 mg/ml.

INDICATIONS AND DOSAGES
▸ Hypercalcemia
IV INFUSION
Adults, Elderly. Moderate hypercalcemia (corrected serum calcium level 12–13.5 mg/dl): 60–90 mg.

P

Severe hypercalcemia (corrected serum calcium level > 13.5 mg/dl): 90 mg.

▸ **Paget's Disease**

IV INFUSION

Adults, Elderly. 30 mg/day for 3 days.

▸ **Osteolytic Bone Lesion**

IV INFUSION

Adults, Elderly. 90 mg over 2–4 hr once a month.

CONTRAINDICATIONS

Hypersensitivity to other bisphosphonates, such as etidronate, tiludronate, risedronate, and alendronate. Dental implants are contraindicated for patients taking this drug.

INTERACTIONS

Drug

Calcium-containing medications, vitamin D: May antagonize effects of pamidronate in treatment of hypercalcemia.

Herbal

None known.

Food

None known.

P

Drug interactions of concern to dentistry

- None reported

DIAGNOSTIC TEST EFFECTS

May decrease serum phosphate, magnesium, calcium, and potassium levels.

IV INCOMPATIBILITIES

Calcium-containing IV fluids

SIDE EFFECTS

Frequent (> 10%)

Temperature elevation (at least 1°C) 24–48 hr after administration (27%); redness, swelling, induration, pain at catheter site with in patients receiving 90 mg (18%); anorexia, nausea, fatigue

Occasional (10%–1%)

Constipation, rhinitis

SERIOUS REACTIONS

! Hypophosphatemia, hypokalemia, hypomagnesemia, and hypocalcemia occur more frequently with higher dosages.

! Anemia, hypertension, tachycardia, atrial fibrillation, and somnolence occur more frequently with 90-mg doses.

! GI hemorrhage occurs rarely.

DENTAL CONSIDERATIONS

General:

- Determine why patient is taking the drug.
- This drug may be used in the hospital or on an outpatient basis. Confirm the patient's disease and treatment status.
- Examine for oral manifestation of opportunistic infection.
- Monitor and record vital signs.
- Consider semisupine chair position for patient comfort if GI side effects occur.
- Question patient about tolerance of NSAIDS or aspirin related to GI disease.
- Be aware of the oral manifestations of Paget's disease (macrognathia, alveolar pain).
- Patients may have received other chemotherapy or radiation; confirm medical and drug history.
- Recent reports indicate osteonecrosis of the jaw may occur with the use of this drug.

Consultations:

- Medical consultation may be required to assess disease control and patient's ability to tolerate stress.

Teach Patient/Family:

- To avoid drugs containing calcium, vitamin D, and antacids; possible antagonism of pamidronate

pancreatin/ pancrelipase

pan-kree-ah′-tin/pan-kree-lie′-pace (pancreatin) Ku-Zyme, Pancreatin (pancrelipase) Cotazym-S[AUS], Cotazym-S Forte[AUS], Creon, Pancrease[CAN], Pancrease MT, Ultrase, Viokase

CATEGORY AND SCHEDULE

Pregnancy Risk Category: C

MECHANISM OF ACTION

Digestive enzymes that replace endogenous pancreatic enzymes. ***Therapeutic Effect:*** Assist in digestion of protein, starch, and fats.

AVAILABILITY

Capsules.
Tablets.

INDICATIONS AND DOSAGES

▸ **Pancreatic Enzyme Replacement or Supplement when Enzymes Are Absent or Deficient, Such as with Chronic Pancreatitis, Cystic Fibrosis, or Ductal Obstruction from Cancer of the Pancreas or Common Bile Duct; to Reduce Malabsorption; Treatment of Steatorrhea Associated with Bowel Resection or Postgastrectomy Syndrome**

PO

Adults, Elderly. 1–3 capsules or tablets before or with meals or snacks. May increase to 8 tablets/dose.
Children. 1–2 tablets with meals or snacks.

CONTRAINDICATIONS

Acute pancreatitis, exacerbation of chronic pancreatitis, hypersensitivity to pork protein

INTERACTIONS

Drug

Antacids: May decrease the effects of pancreatin and pancrelipase.
Iron supplements: May decrease the absorption of iron supplements.

Herbal

None known.

Food

None known.

DIAGNOSTIC TEST EFFECTS

May increase serum uric acid level.

SIDE EFFECTS

Rare

Allergic reaction, mouth irritation, shortness of breath, wheezing

SERIOUS REACTIONS

! Excessive dosage may produce nausea, cramping, and diarrhea.
! Hyperuricosuria and hyperuricemia have occurred with extremely high dosages.

DENTAL CONSIDERATIONS

General:

- Consider semisupine chair position for patient comfort because of GI effects of disease.
- To avoid oral irritation, mouth should be rinsed or drug taken with liquid.

papaverine HCl papaverine

pa-**pav**-er-een
(Papacon, Para-Time SR, Pavabid Plateau, Pavacot, Pavagen)

CATEGORY AND SCHEDULE

Pregnancy Risk Category: C

MECHANISM OF ACTION
A vasodilating agent that acts directly on the heart muscle to depress conduction and prolong the refractory period. ***Therapeutic Effect:*** Relaxes smooth muscle.

PHARMACOKINETICS
Protein binding: 90%. Primarily excreted in urine as inactive metabolites. ***Half-life:*** Unknown.

AVAILABILITY
Tablets (Papacon, Para-Time SR, Pavabid, Pavacot, Pavagen): 150 mg
Injectable Solution: 30 mg/ml.

INDICATIONS AND DOSAGES
▸ **Vascular Spasm**
IV/IM
Adults, Elderly. Inject 1–4 ml slowly and repeat q3h as indicated.
▸ **Vascular Spasm**
PO
Adults, Elderly. One capsule q12h. In difficult cases, administration may be increased to one capsule q8h or two capsules q12h.

UNLABELED USES
Erectile dysfunction

CONTRAINDICATIONS
Complete atrioventricular heart block, impotence by intracorporeal injection, hypersensitivity to papaverine or any component of the formulation

INTERACTIONS
Drug
None known.
Herbal
None known.
Food
None known.
Drug interactions of concern to dentistry
- Increased hypotension: alcohol, other drugs that may also lower blood pressure

DIAGNOSTIC TEST EFFECTS
None known.

SIDE EFFECTS
Frequency not defined
Capsules: Nausea, abdominal distress, anorexia, constipation, malaise, drowsiness, vertigo, perspiration, headache, diarrhea, skin rash
Injection: General discomfort, nausea, abdominal discomfort, anorexia, constipation, diarrhea, skin rash, malaise, vertigo, headache, intensive flushing of the face, perspiration, increased depth of respiration, increased heart rate, slight rise in BP, excessive sedation

SERIOUS REACTIONS
! Hepatotoxicity has been reported.
! Priapism has been reported.

DENTAL CONSIDERATIONS
General:
- Monitor vital signs at every appointment because of CV and respiratory side effects.
- Short appointments and a stress reduction protocol may be required for anxious patients.

Consultations:
- Stress from dental procedures may compromise CV function; determine patient risk.
- Medical consultation may be required to assess disease control.

Teach Patient/Family:
- To avoid mouth rinses with high alcohol content
- Importance of good oral hygiene to prevent soft tissue inflammation

paregoric

par-e-gor′-ik
Schedule III
Do not confuse with opium tincture.

CATEGORY AND SCHEDULE

Pregnancy Risk Category: B, D if used for prolonged periods, high dosages at term
Controlled substance: Schedule III

MECHANISM OF ACTION

An opioid agonist that contains many narcotic alkaloids including morphine. It inhibits gastric motility due to its morphine content. ***Therapeutic Effect:*** Decreases digestive secretions, increases in gastrointestinal (GI) muscle tone, and reduces GI propulsion.

PHARMACOKINETICS

Variably absorbed from the gastrointestinal (GI) tract. Protein binding: low. Metabolized in liver. Primarily excreted in urine primarily as morphine glucuronide conjugates and unchanged drug-morphine, codeine, papaverine, etc. Unknown if removed by hemodialysis.
Half-life: 2–3 hrs.

AVAILABILITY

Tincture: 2 mg/5 ml (Paregoric).

INDICATIONS AND DOSAGES

▸ Antidiarrheal

PO
Adults, Elderly. 5–10 ml 1–4 times/day.
Children. 0.25–0.5 ml/kg/dose 1–4 times/day.

OFF-LABEL USES

Narcotic withdrawal symptoms in neonates

CONTRAINDICATIONS

Diarrhea caused by poisoning until the toxic material is removed, hypersensitivity to morphine sulfate or any component of the formulation, pregnancy (prolonged use or high dosages near term)

INTERACTIONS

Drug

Alcohol, central nervous system (CNS) depressants: May increase CNS or respiratory depression, and hypotension.
MAOIs, tricyclic antidepressants: May produce severe, fatal reaction unless dosage reduced by one quarter.

Herbal

None known.

Food

None known.

Drug interactions of concern to dentistry

- Increased action of both drugs: alcohol, all other CNS depressants
- Decreased peristalsis: anticholinergic drugs

P

DIAGNOSTIC TEST EFFECTS

None known.

SIDE EFFECTS

Frequent

Constipation, drowsiness, nausea, vomiting

Occasional

Paradoxical excitement, confusion, pounding heartbeat, facial flushing, decreased urination, blurred vision, dizziness, dry mouth, headache, hypotension, decreased appetite, redness, burning, pain at injection site

Rare

Hallucinations, depression, stomach pain, insomnia

SERIOUS REACTIONS

! Overdosage results in cold or clammy skin, confusion, convulsions, decreased blood pressure (B/P), restlessness, pinpoint pupils, bradycardia, respiratory depression, decreased level of consciousness (LOC), and severe weakness.
! Tolerance to analgesic effect and physical dependence may occur with repeated use.

DENTAL CONSIDERATIONS

General:

• Psychologic and physical dependence may occur with chronic administration.
• Determine why the patient is taking the drug.

Teach Patient/Family:

• To avoid mouth rinses with high alcohol content because of drying effects

paromomycin

par-oh-moe-mye′-sin
(Humatin)
Do not confuse with Humira.

CATEGORY AND SCHEDULE

Pregnancy Risk Category: C

MECHANISM OF ACTION

An antibacterial agent that acts directly on amoebas and against normal and pathogenic organisms in the GI tract. Interferes with bacterial protein synthesis by binding to 30S ribosomal subunits. ***Therapeutic Effect:*** Produces amoebicidal effects.

PHARMACOKINETICS

Poorly absorbed from the gastrointestinal (GI) tract and most of the dose is eliminated unchanged in feces.

AVAILABILITY

Capsules: 250 mg (Humantin).

INDICATIONS AND DOSAGES

▸ Intestinal Amebiasis

PO

Adults, Elderly, Children.
25–35 mg/kg/day q8h for 5–10 days.

▸ Hepatic Coma

PO

Adults, Elderly. 4 g/day q6–12h for 5–6 days.

OFF-LABEL USES

Cryptosporidiosis, giardiasis, leishmaniasis, microsporidiosis, mycobacterial infections, tapeworm infestation, trichomoniasis, typhoid carriers.

CONTRAINDICATIONS

Intestinal obstruction, renal failure, hypersensitivity to paromomycin or any of its components

INTERACTIONS

Drug

Digoxin: May decrease digoxin serum concentrations and efficacy.

Herbal

None known.

Food

Xylose, sucrose, fats: May cause decreased absorption of xylose, sucrose and fats.

Drug interactions of concern to dentistry

• Possible degradation by penicillins and cephalosporins

DIAGNOSTIC TEST EFFECTS

May increase LDH concentrations, SGOT (AST) and SGPT (ALT) levels.

SIDE EFFECTS

Occasional

Diarrhea, abdominal cramps, nausea, vomiting, heartburn

Rare
Rash, pruritus, vertigo

SERIOUS REACTIONS

! Overdosage may result in nausea, vomiting and diarrhea.

DENTAL CONSIDERATIONS

General:

- Determine why patient is taking the drug.
- Consider semisupine chair position for patient comfort due to GI effects of disease.
- Question patient about tolerance of NSAIDS or aspirin related to GI disease.
- Postpone elective dental treatment until symptoms are controlled.

Consultations:

- Medical consultation may be required to assess disease control.

Teach patient/family:

- Importance of updating health and medication history if physician makes any changes in evaluation or drug regimens; include OTC, herbal, and nonherbal in the update
- To report sore throat, oral burning sensation, fever, or fatigue, any of which could indicate presence of a superinfection

paroxetine hydrochloride

par-ox′-e-teen
(Aropax 20[AUS], Paxeva, Paxil, Paxil CR, Paxtine[AUS])
Do not confuse paroxetine with pyridoxine, or Paxil with Doxil or Taxol.

CATEGORY AND SCHEDULE

Pregnancy Risk Category: C

MECHANISM OF ACTION

An antidepressant, anxiolytic, and antiobsessional agent that selectively blocks uptake of the neurotransmitter serotonin at neuronal presynaptic membranes, thereby increasing its availability at postsynaptic receptor sites. ***Therapeutic Effect:*** Relieves depression, reduces obsessive-compulsive behavior, decreases anxiety.

PHARMACOKINETICS

Well absorbed from the GI tract. Protein binding: 95%. Widely distributed. Metabolized in the liver. Excreted in urine. Not removed by hemodialysis. ***Half-life:*** 24 hr.

AVAILABILITY

Oral Suspension (Paxil): 10 mg/5 ml.
Tablets (Paxil, Pexeva): 10 mg, 20 mg, 30 mg, 40 mg.
Tablets (Controlled-Release [Paxil CR]): 12.5 mg, 25 mg, 37.5 mg.

INDICATIONS AND DOSAGES

▸ **Depression**

PO
Adults. Initially, 20 mg/day. May increase by 10 mg/day at intervals of more than 1 wk.
Maximum: 50 mg/day.
PO (Controlled-Release)
Adults. Initially, 25 mg/day. May increase by 12.5 mg/day at intervals of more than 1 wk.
Maximum: 62.5 mg/day.

▸ **Generalized Anxiety Disorder**

PO
Adults. Initially, 20 mg/day. May increase by 10 mg/day at intervals of more than 1 wk. Range: 20–50 mg/day.

▸ **Obsessive Compulsive Disorder**

PO
Adults. Initially, 20 mg/day. May increase by 10 mg/day at intervals of more than 1 wk.
Range: 20–60 mg/day.

▸ **Panic Disorder**
PO
Adults. Initially, 10–20 mg/day. May increase by 10 mg/day at intervals of more than 1 wk. Range: 10–60 mg/day.

▸ **Social Anxiety Disorder**
PO
Adults. Initially 20 mg/day. Range: 20–60 mg/day.

▸ **Post Traumatic Stress Disorder**
PO
Adults. Initially, 20 mg/day. May increase by 10 mg/day at intervals of more than 1 wk. Range: 20–50 mg/day.

▸ **Premenstrual Dysphoric Disorder**
PO (Paxil CR)
Adults. Initially, 12.5 mg/day. May increase by 12.5 mg at weekly intervals to a maximum of 25 mg/day.

▸ **Usual Elderly Dosage**
PO: Initially, 10 mg/day. May increase by 10 mg/day at intervals of more than 1 wk. Maximum: 40 mg/day.
PO (Controlled-Release): Initially, 12.5 mg/day. May increase by 12.5 mg/day at intervals of more than 1 wk. Maximum: 50 mg/day.

P

OFF-LABEL USES

Eating disorders, impulse disorders, menopause symptoms, premenstrual disorders, treatment of depression and OCD in children

CONTRAINDICATIONS

Use within 14 days of MAOIs

INTERACTIONS

Drug

Cimetidine: May increase paroxetine blood concentration.
MAOIs: May cause serotonin syndrome, marked by excitement, diaphoresis, rigidity, hyperthermia, autonomic hyperactivity, and coma, and neuroleptic malignant syndrome.
Phenytoin: May decrease paroxetine blood concentration.
Risperidone: May increase risperidone blood concentration and cause extrapyramidal symptoms.

Herbal

St. John's wort: May increase paroxetine's pharmacologic effects and risk of toxicity.

Food

None known.

Drug interactions of concern to dentistry

- Possible increased side effects: highly protein-bound drugs (aspirin), other antidepressants, alcohol
- Possible inhibition of fluoxetine metabolism: erythromycin, clarithromycin
- Increased half-life of diazepam
- First-time users of SSRIs also taking NSAIDs may have a higher risk of GI side effects; until more data are available, it may be advisable to avoid use of NSAIDs in these patients (*Br J Clin Pharmacol* 55:591–595, 2003)

DIAGNOSTIC TEST EFFECTS

May increase serum hepatic enzyme levels. May decrease blood Hgb level, Hct, and WBC count.

SIDE EFFECTS

Frequent

Nausea (26%); somnolence (23%); headache, dry mouth (18%); asthenia (15%); constipation (15%); dizziness, insomnia (13%); diarrhea (12%); diaphoresis (11%); tremor (8%)

Occasional

Decreased appetite, respiratory disturbance (such as increased cough) (6%); anxiety, nervousness (5%); flatulence, paresthesia, yawning (4%); decreased libido, sexual dysfunction, abdominal discomfort (3%)

Rare
Palpitations, vomiting, blurred vision, altered taste, confusion

SERIOUS REACTIONS

! Abnormal bleeding, hyponatremia, seizures, hypomania, and suicidal thoughts have been reported.

DENTAL CONSIDERATIONS

General:

- After supine positioning, have patient sit upright for at least 2 min before standing to avoid orthostatic hypotension.
- Assess salivary flow as a factor in caries, periodontal disease, and candidiasis.
- Avoid dental light in patient's eyes; offer dark glasses for patient comfort.

Consultations:

- Medical consultation may be required to assess disease control and patient's ability to tolerate stress.
- Physician should be informed if significant xerostomic side effects occur (e.g., increased caries, sore tongue, problems eating or swallowing, difficulty wearing prosthesis) so that a medication change can be considered.

Teach Patient/Family:

- *When chronic dry mouth occurs, advise patient:*
  - To avoid mouth rinses with high alcohol content because of drying effects
  - Of need for daily use of home fluoride products to prevent caries
  - To use sugarless gum, frequent sips of water, or saliva substitutes

pegfilgrastim

pehg-phil-gras′-tim
(Neulasta)
Do not confuse Neulasta with Neumega.

CATEGORY AND SCHEDULE

Pregnancy Risk Category: C

MECHANISM OF ACTION

A colony-stimulating factor that regulates production of neutrophils within bone marrow. Also a glycoprotein that primarily affects neutrophil progenitor proliferation, differentiation, and selected end-cell functional activation. ***Therapeutic Effect:*** Increases phagocytic ability and antibody-dependent destruction; decreases incidence of infection.

PHARMACOKINETICS

Readily absorbed after subcutaneous administration. ***Half-life:*** 15–80 hr.

AVAILABILITY

Solution for Injection: 10 mg/ml.

INDICATIONS AND DOSAGES

▸ **Myelosuppression**

SUBCUTANEOUS

Adults, Elderly. Give as a single 6-mg injection once per chemotherapy cycle.

CONTRAINDICATIONS

Hypersensitivity to *Escherichia coli*–derived proteins, within 14 days before and 24 hours after cytotoxic chemotherapy

INTERACTIONS

Drug

Lithium: May potentiate the release of neutrophils.

Herbal

None known.

Food
None known.

Drug interactions of concern to dentistry
- None reported

DIAGNOSTIC TEST EFFECTS
May increase LDH concentrations, leukocyte alkaline phosphatase scores, and serum alkaline phosphatase and uric acid levels.

SIDE EFFECTS
Frequent (72%–15%)
Bone pain, nausea, fatigue, alopecia, diarrhea, vomiting, constipation, anorexia, abdominal pain, arthralgia, generalized weakness, peripheral edema, dizziness, stomatitis, mucositis, neutropenic fever

SERIOUS REACTIONS
! Allergic reactions, such as anaphylaxis, rash, and urticaria, occur rarely.
! Cytopenia resulting from an antibody response to growth factors occurs rarely.
! Splenomegaly occurs rarely; assess for left upper abdominal or shoulder pain.
! Adult respiratory distress syndrome (ARDS) may occur in patients with sepsis.

DENTAL CONSIDERATIONS

General:
- Patients may have a history of chemotherapy or radiation; confirm medical and drug history.
- Determine type of chemotherapeutic agents used and related oral side effects.
- Monitor and record vital signs.
- Examine for oral manifestation of opportunistic infection.

Consultations:
- Medical consultation may be required to assess disease control and patient's ability to tolerate stress.

Teach Patient/Family:
- Importance of good oral hygiene to prevent soft tissue inflammation
- To prevent trauma when using oral hygiene aids
- To report oral lesions, soreness, or bleeding to dentist

peginterferon alfa-2a
peg-inn-ter-fear′-on
(Pegasys)

CATEGORY AND SCHEDULE
Pregnancy Risk Category: C

MECHANISM OF ACTION
An immunomodulator that binds to specific membrane receptors on the cell surface, inhibiting viral replication in virus-infected cells, suppressing cell proliferation, and producing reversible decreases in leukocyte and platelet counts. ***Therapeutic Effect:*** Inhibits hepatitis C virus.

PHARMACOKINETICS
Readily absorbed after subcutaneous administration. Excreted by the kidneys. ***Half-life:*** 80 hr.

AVAILABILITY
Injection: 180 mcg/ml.

INDICATIONS AND DOSAGES
▸ **Hepatitis C**
SUBCUTANEOUS
Adults 18 yr and older, Elderly. 180 mcg (1 ml) injected in abdomen or thigh once weekly for 48 wk.

▸ **Dosage in Renal Impairment**
For patients who require hemodialysis, dosage is 135 mg injected in abdomen or thigh once weekly for 48 wk.

▸ **Dosage in Hepatic Impairment**
For patients with progressive ALT(SGPT) increases above baseline values, dosage is 90 mcg injected in abdomen or thigh once weekly for 48 wk.

CONTRAINDICATIONS

Autoimmune hepatitis, decompensated hepatic disease, infants, neonates

INTERACTIONS

Drug

Bone marrow depressants: May increase myelosuppression.
Theophylline: May increase the serum level of theophylline.

Herbal

None known.

Food

None known.

Drug interactions of concern to dentistry

• Risk of hepatotoxicity in severe liver disease: acetaminophen

DIAGNOSTIC TEST EFFECTS

May increase ALT(SGPT) level. May decrease the absolute neutrophil, platelet, and WBC counts. May cause a slight decrease in blood Hgb level and Hct.

SIDE EFFECTS

Frequent (54%)

Headache

Occasional (23%–13%)

Alopecia, nausea, insomnia, anorexia, dizziness, diarrhea, abdominal pain, flulike symptoms, psychiatric reactions (depression, irritability, anxiety), injection site reaction

Rare (8%–5%)

Impaired concentration, diaphoresis, dry mouth, nausea, vomiting

SERIOUS REACTIONS

! Serious, acute hypersensitivity reactions, such as urticaria, angioedema, bronchoconstriction, and anaphylaxis, may occur. Other rare reactions include pancreatitis, colitis, endocrine disorders (e.g. diabetes mellitus), hyperthyroidism or hypothyroidism, ophthalmologic disorders, and pulmonary disorders.

DENTAL CONSIDERATIONS

General:

• Determine why patient is taking the drug.
• Assess salivary flow as a factor in caries, periodontal disease, and candidiasis.
• Consider semisupine chair position for patient comfort if GI side effects occur.
• Question patient about tolerance of NSAIDs or aspirin related to GI disease.
• Patients on chronic drug therapy may rarely have symptoms of blood dyscrasias, which can include infection, bleeding, and poor healing.
• Avoid elective dental procedures if severe neutropenia (<500 cells/mm^3) or thrombocytopenia (<50,000 cell/mm^3) is present.
• Severe side effects may require postponing elective dental procedures until drug therapy is completed.

Consultations:

• Medical consultation may be required to assess disease control in the patient.
• In a patient with symptoms of blood dyscrasias, request a medical consultation for blood studies and postpone treatment

P

until normal values are reestablished
• Liver function tests may be required to determine chronic liver disease.

Teach Patient/Family:

• Importance of good oral hygiene to prevent soft tissue inflammation/infection
• To evaluate efficacy of oral hygiene home care; preventive appointments may be necessary
• To prevent trauma when using oral hygiene aids
• *When chronic dry mouth occurs, advise patient:*
  • To avoid mouth rinses with high alcohol content because of drying effects
  • To use daily home fluoride products for anticaries effect
  • To use sugarless gum, frequent sips of water, or saliva substitutes

P

peginterferon alfa-2b

peg-inn-ter-fear′-on
(PEG-Intron)

CATEGORY AND SCHEDULE

Pregnancy Risk Category: C

MECHANISM OF ACTION

An immunomodulator that inhibits viral replication in virus-infected cells, suppresses cell proliferation, increases phagocytic action of macrophages, and augments specific cytotoxicity of lymphocytes for target cells. ***Therapeutic Effect:*** Inhibits hepatitis C virus.

AVAILABILITY

Injection Powder for Reconstitution: 50 mcg, 80 mcg, 120 mcg, 150 mcg.

INDICATIONS AND DOSAGES

▸ Chronic Hepatitis C, Monotherapy

SUBCUTANEOUS

Adults 18 yr and older, Elderly. Administer appropriate dosage (see chart below) once weekly for 1 yr on the same day each wk.

Vial Strength	Weight (kg)	mcg*	ml*
100 mcg/ml	37–45	40	0.4
	46–56	50	0.5
160 mcg/ml	57–72	64	0.4
	73–88	80	0.5
240 mcg/ml	89–106	96	0.4
	107–136	120	0.5
300 mcg/ml	137–160	150	0.5

*Of peginterferon alpha-2b to administer

▸ Chronic Hepatitis C

SUBCUTANEOUS

Combination therapy with ribavirin (400 mg twice a day). Initially, 1.5 mcg/kg/wk.

CONTRAINDICATIONS

Autoimmune hepatitis, decompensated hepatic disease, history of psychiatric disorders

INTERACTIONS

Drug

Bone marrow depressants: May increase myelosuppression.

Herbal

None known.

Food

None known.

Drug interactions of concern to dentistry

• Risk of hepatotoxicity in severe liver disease: acetaminophen

DIAGNOSTIC TEST EFFECTS

May increase blood glucose and ALT(SGPT) levels. May decrease blood neutrophil and platelet counts.

SIDE EFFECTS

Frequent (50%–47%)
Flulike symptoms; inflammation, bruising, pruritus, and irritation at injection site

Occasional (29%–18%)
Psychiatric reactions (depression, anxiety, emotional lability, irritability), insomnia, alopecia, diarrhea

Rare
Rash, diaphoresis, dry skin, dizziness, flushing, vomiting, dyspepsia

SERIOUS REACTIONS

! Serious, acute hypersensitivity reactions (such as urticaria, angioedema, bronchoconstriction, and anaphylaxis), pulmonary disorders, endocrine disorders (e.g. diabetes mellitus), hypothyroidism, hyperthyroidism, and pancreatitis occur rarely.

! Ulcerative colitis may occur within 12 weeks of starting treatment.

DENTAL CONSIDERATIONS

General:

- Determine why patient is taking the drug.
- Assess salivary flow as a factor in caries, periodontal disease, and candidiasis.
- Consider semisupine chair position for patient comfort if GI side effects occur.
- Question patient about tolerance of NSAIDs or aspirin related to GI disease.
- Patients on chronic drug therapy may rarely have symptoms of blood dyscrasias, which can include infection, bleeding, and poor healing.
- Avoid elective dental procedures if severe neutropenia (<500 cells/mm^3) or thrombocytopenia (<50,000 cell/mm^3) is present.
- Severe side effects may require postponing elective dental procedures until drug therapy is completed.

Consultations:

- Medical consultation may be required to assess disease control in the patient.
- In a patient with symptoms of blood dyscrasias, request a medical consultation for blood studies and postpone treatment until normal values are reestablished
- Liver function tests may be required to determine chronic liver disease.

Teach Patient/Family:

- Importance of good oral hygiene to prevent soft tissue inflammation/infection
- To evaluate efficacy of oral hygiene home care; preventive appointments may be necessary
- To prevent trauma when using oral hygiene aids
- *When chronic dry mouth occurs, advise patient:*
  - To avoid mouth rinses with high alcohol content because of drying effects
  - To use daily home fluoride products for anticaries effect
  - To use sugarless gum, frequent sips of water, or saliva substitutes

pegvisomant

peg-vis′-oh-mant
(Somavert)
Do not confuse Somavert with somatrem or somatropin.

CATEGORY AND SCHEDULE

Pregnancy Risk Category: B

MECHANISM OF ACTION

A protein that selectively binds to growth hormone (GH) receptors on cell surfaces, blocking the binding of endogenous growth hormones

P

and interfering with growth hormone signal transduction. ***Therapeutic Effect:*** Decreases serum concentrations of insulin-like growth factor 1 (IGF-1) and other GH-responsive serum proteins.

PHARMACOKINETICS

Not distributed extensively into tissues after subcutaneous administration. Less than 1% excreted in urine.
Half-life: 6 days.

AVAILABILITY

Powder for Injection: 10-mg, 15-mg, 20-mg vials.

INDICATIONS AND DOSAGES

▸ Acromegaly

SUBCUTANEOUS

Adults, Elderly. Initially, 40 mg, as a loading dose, then 10 mg daily. After 4–6 wk, adjust dosage in 5-mg increments if serum IGF-1 level is still elevated, or in 5-mg decrements if IGF-1 level has decreased below the normal range. Maximum: 30 mg daily.

CONTRAINDICATIONS

Latex allergy (stopper on vial contains latex)

INTERACTIONS

Drug

Insulin, oral antidiabetics: May enhance effects of these drugs, possibly resulting in hypoglycemia. Dosage should be decreased when initiating pegvisomant therapy.
Opioids: Decrease serum pegvisomant level.

Herbal

None known.

Food

None known.

Drug interactions of concern to dentistry

- Opioids: decreased serum levels

DIAGNOSTIC TEST EFFECTS

Interferes with measurement of serum growth hormone concentration. May increase AST(SGOT), ALT(SGPT), and transaminase levels. Decreases effect of insulin on carbohydrate metabolism.

SIDE EFFECTS

Frequent (23%)

Infection (cold symptoms, upper respiratory tract infection, blister, ear infection)

Occasional (8%–5%)

Back pain, dizziness, injection site reaction, peripheral edema, sinusitis, nausea

Rare (< 4%)

Diarrhea, paresthesia

SERIOUS REACTIONS

! Pegvisomant use may markedly elevate liver function test results, including serum transaminase levels.
! Substantial weight gain occurs rarely.

DENTAL CONSIDERATIONS

General:

- Confirm history of previous medical, surgical, or radiation treatment for this disease.
- Monitor vital signs.
- Patient may complain of TMD due to disease.
- Place on frequent recall to evaluate healing response

Consultations:

- Physician consultation should include liver function tests.

Teach Patient/Family:

- Importance of good oral hygiene to prevent soft tissue inflammation
- To prevent trauma when using oral hygiene aids

• Importance of updating health and medication history if physician makes any changes in evaluation or drug regimens; include OTC, herbal, and nonherbal in the update

pemirolast potassium

pe-meer′-oh-last poe-tass′-ee-um
(Alamast)

CATEGORY AND SCHEDULE

Pregnancy Risk Category: C

MECHANISM OF ACTION

An antiallergic agent that prevents activation and release of mediators of inflammation (e.g., mast cells). ***Therapeutic Effect:*** Reduces symptoms of allergic conjunctivitis.

PHARMACOKINETICS

Detected in plasma. Excreted in urine. ***Half-life:*** 4.5 hrs.

AVAILABILITY

Ophthalmic Solution: 0.1% (Alamast).

INDICATIONS AND DOSAGES

▸ **Allergic Conjunctivitis**

OPHTHALMIC

Adults, Elderly, Children 3 yrs and older. 1–2 drops in affected eye(s) 4 times/day.

CONTRAINDICATIONS

Hypersensitivity to pemirolast potassium or any other component of the formulation

INTERACTIONS

Drug

None known.

Herbal

None known.

Food

None known.

Drug interactions of concern to dentistry

• None reported

DIAGNOSTIC TEST EFFECTS

None known.

SIDE EFFECTS

Frequent

Headache, rhinitis, cold and flu symptoms

Occasional

Transient ocular stinging, burning, itching, dry eye, foreign body sensation, tearing

Rare

Sinusitis, sneezing/nasal congestion

SERIOUS REACTIONS

! None reported.

DENTAL CONSIDERATIONS

General:

• Question patient about history of allergies to avoid using other potential allergens.
• Avoid dental light in patient's eyes; offer dark glasses for patient comfort.
• Protect patient's eyes from accidental spatter during dental treatment.

P

pemoline

pem′-oh-leen
Schedule IV
(Cylert, PemADD, PemADD CT)

CATEGORY AND SCHEDULE

Pregnancy Risk Category: B
Controlled Substance: Schedule IV

MECHANISM OF ACTION
A CNS stimulant that blocks the reuptake mechanism present in dopaminergic neurons in the cerebral cortex and subcortical structures. ***Therapeutic Effect:*** Reduces motor restlessness and fatigue, increases alertness, elevates mood.

AVAILABILITY
Tablets (Cylert, PemADD): 18.75 mg, 37.5 mg, 75 mg.
Tablets (Chewable [PemADD CT]): 37.5 mg.

INDICATIONS AND DOSAGES
▸ ADHD
PO
Children 6 yr and older. Initially, 37.5 mg/day as a single dose in morning. May increase by 18.75 mg at weekly intervals until therapeutic response is achieved. Range: 56.25–75 mg/day. Maximum: 112.5 mg/day.

CONTRAINDICATIONS
Family history of Tourette syndrome, hepatic impairment, motor tics

P

INTERACTIONS
Drug
Other CNS stimulants: May increase CNS stimulation.
Herbal
None known.
Food
None known.
Drug interactions of concern to dentistry
- Increased irritability, stimulation: caffeine-containing products and food

DIAGNOSTIC TEST EFFECTS
May increase serum LDH, AST (SGOT), and ALT (SGPT) levels.

SIDE EFFECTS
Frequent
Anorexia, insomnia
Occasional
Nausea, abdominal discomfort, diarrhea, headache, dizziness, somnolence

SERIOUS REACTIONS
! Visual disturbances, rash, and dyskinetic movements of the tongue, lips, face, and extremities have occurred.
! Large doses of pemoline may produce extreme nervousness and tachycardia.
! Hepatic effects, such as hepatitis and jaundice, appear to be reversible when the drug is discontinued.
! Prolonged administration to children with ADHD may temporarily delay growth.

DENTAL CONSIDERATIONS
General:
- Keep dental appointments short because of effects of disease.
Teach Patient/Family:
- Use of electric toothbrush for effective plaque control

penbutolol
pen-beaut-oh-lol
(Levatol)
Do not confuse with pindolol

CATEGORY AND SCHEDULE
Pregnancy Risk Category: C (D if used in the second or third trimester)

MECHANISM OF ACTION
An antihypertensive that possesses nonselective beta-blocking. Has moderate intrinsic sympathomimetic activity. ***Therapeutic Effect:*** Reduces cardiac output, decreases blood pressure (B/P), increases

airway resistance and decreases myocardial ischemia severity.

PHARMACOKINETICS

Rapidly and extensively absorbed from the gastrointestinal (GI) tract. Protein binding: 80%–90%. Metabolized in liver. Excreted primarily via urine. ***Half-life:*** 17–26 hrs.

AVAILABILITY

Tablets: 20 mg (Levatol).

INDICATIONS AND DOSAGES

▸ Hypertension

PO

Adults. Initially, 20 mg/day as a single dose. May increase to 40–80 mg/day.
Elderly. Initially, 10 mg/day.

CONTRAINDICATIONS

Bronchial asthma or related bronchospastic conditions, cardiogenic shock, pulmonary edema, second- or third-degree atrioventricular (AV) block, severe bradycardia, overt cardiac failure, hypersensitivity to penbutolol or any component of the formulation

INTERACTIONS

Drug

Calcium blockers: Increase risk of conduction disturbances.
Clonidine: May potentiate blood pressure (B/P) effects.
Cimetidine: May increase penbutolol concentrations.
Digoxin: Increases concentrations of this drug.
Diuretics, other hypotensives: May increase hypotensive effect.
Fentanyl: May cause severe hypotension.
Insulin, oral hypoglycemics: May mask symptoms of hypoglycemia and prolong hypoglycemic effect of these drugs.
Lidocaine: May prolong the elimination of lidocaine
NSAIDs: May decrease antihypertensive effect.
Verapamil: May increase risk of hypotension and bradycardia.
Sympathomimetics, xanthines: May mutually inhibit effects.

Herbal

Dong quai: May decrease blood pressure.
St. John's Wort, yohimbine: May decrease effectiveness of penbutolol.

Food

None known.

Drug interactions of concern to dentistry

- Decreased hypotensive effect: indomethacin, NSAIDs
- Increased hypotension, myocardial depression: hydrocarbon inhalation anesthetics
- Hypertension, bradycardia: sympathomimetics (epinephrine, ephedrine)
- Slow metabolism of lidocaine

DIAGNOSTIC TEST EFFECTS

May increase ANA titer, SGOT (AST), SGPT (ALT), alkaline phosphatase, LDH, bilirubin, BUN, creatinine, potassium, uric acid, lipoproteins, triglycerides

SIDE EFFECTS

Frequent

Decreased sexual ability, drowsiness, trouble sleeping, unusual tiredness/weakness

Occasional

Diarrhea, bradycardia, depression, cold hands/feet, constipation, anxiety, nasal congestion, nausea, vomiting

Rare

Altered taste, dry eyes, itching, numbness of fingers, toes, scalp

SERIOUS REACTIONS

! Abrupt withdrawal may result in sweating, palpitations, headache, and tremulousness.

! Hypoglycemia may occur in patients with previously controlled diabetes.

DENTAL CONSIDERATIONS

General:

- Monitor vital signs at every appointment because of CV side effects.
- Patients on chronic drug therapy may rarely have symptoms of blood dyscrasias, which can include infection, bleeding, and poor healing.
- Limit use of sodium-containing products, such as saline IV fluids, for patients with a dietary salt restriction.
- Assess salivary flow as a factor in caries, periodontal disease, and candidiasis.
- After supine positioning, have patient sit upright for at least 2 min before standing to avoid orthostatic hypotension.
- Stress from dental procedures may compromise CV function; determine patient risk.
- Short appointments and a stress reduction protocol may be required for anxious patients.
- Use vasoconstrictor with caution, in low doses, and with careful aspiration.
- Avoid using gingival retraction cord containing epinephrine.

Consultations:

- In a patient with symptoms of blood dyscrasias, request a medical consultation for blood studies and postpone dental treatment until normal values are reestablished.
- Medical consultation may be required to assess disease control and patient's ability to tolerate stress.

Teach Patient/Family:

- Caution to prevent injury when using oral hygiene aids
- Importance of good oral hygiene to prevent soft tissue inflammation
- If taste alterations occur, consider drug effects
- *When chronic dry mouth occurs, advise patient:*
  - To avoid mouth rinses with high alcohol content because of drying effects
  - Of need for daily use of home fluoride products to prevent caries
  - To use sugarless gum, frequent sips of water, or saliva substitutes

penciclovir

pen-sye′-kloe-veer

(Denavir, Vectavir[South Africa, Costa Rica, Dominican Republic, El Salvador, Germany, Guatemala, Honduras, Israel, Nicaragua, Panama])

Do not confuse with acyclovir

CATEGORY AND SCHEDULE

Pregnancy Risk Category: B

MECHANISM OF ACTION

Penciclovir triphosphate inhibits HSV polymerase competitively with deoxyguanosine triphosphate. Consequently, herpes viral DNA synthesis and, therefore, replication are selectively inhibited.

Therapeutic Effect: An antiviral compound that has inhibitory activity against herpes simplex virus types 1 (HSV-1) and 2 (HSV-2).

PHARMACOKINETICS

Measurable penciclovir concentrations were not detected in plasma or urine. The systemic absorption of penciclovir following topical administration has not been evaluated.

AVAILABILITY

Cream: 10 mg/g

INDICATIONS AND DOSAGES

▸ Herpes Labialis (cold sores)

TOPICAL

Adolescents, Adults. Penciclovir should be applied every 2 hours during waking hours for a period of 4 days. Treatment should be started as early as possible (i.e., during the prodrome or when lesions appear).

OFF-LABEL USES

Varicella-zoster virus

CONTRAINDICATIONS

Hypersensitivity to penciclovir or any of its components.

INTERACTIONS

Drug

None known.

Herbal

None known.

Food

None known.

DIAGNOSTIC TEST EFFECTS

None known.

SIDE EFFECTS

Frequent

Headache

Occasional

Change in sense of taste; decreased sensitivity of skin, particularly to touch; redness of the skin; skin rash (maculopapular, erythematous) local edema, skin discoloration; pruritis; hypoesthesia; parathesias; parosmia; urticaria; oral/ pharyngeal edema

Rare

Mild pain, burning, or stinging

DENTAL CONSIDERATIONS

General:

- Use in immunocompromised patients not established.
- Postpone dental treatment when oral herpetic lesions are present.

Teach Patient/Family:

- To dispose of toothbrush or other contaminated oral hygiene devices used during period of infection to prevent reinoculation of herpetic infection
- To apply with a finger cot or latex glove to prevent herpes infection on fingers

penicillin G benzathine

pen-ih-sil′-lin G benz′-ah-thene

(Bicillin LA, Permapen)

Do not confuse penicillin G benzathine with penicillin G potassium or penicillin G procaine.

CATEGORY AND SCHEDULE

Pregnancy Risk Category: B

MECHANISM OF ACTION

A penicillin that inhibits bacterial cell wall synthesis by binding to one or more of the penicillin-binding proteins of bacteria. ***Therapeutic Effect:*** Bactericidal.

AVAILABILITY

Injection (Prefilled Syringe [Bicillin LA, Permapen]): 600,000 units/ml.

INDICATIONS AND DOSAGES

▸ Group A Streptococcal Infections

IM

Adults, Elderly. 1.2 million units as a single dose.

Children. 25,000–50,000 units/kg as a single dose.

▸ Prevention of Rheumatic Fever

IM

Adults, Elderly. 1.2 million units every 3–4 wk or 600,000 units twice monthly.

Children. 25,000–50,000 units/kg every 3–4 wk.

▸ Early Syphilis

IM

Adults, Elderly. 2.4 million units divided and administered in two separate injection sites.

▸ Congenital Syphilis

IM

Children. 50,000 units/kg weekly for 3 wk.

▸ Syphilis of More Than 1 Year's Duration

IM

Adults, Elderly. 2.4 million units divided and administered in two separate injection sites weekly for 3 wk.

Children. 50,000 units/kg weekly for 3 wk.

CONTRAINDICATIONS

Hypersensitivity to any penicillin

INTERACTIONS

Drug

Erythromycin: May antagonize effects of penicillin.

Probenecid: Increases serum concentration of penicillin.

Herbal

None known.

Food

None known.

Drug interactions of concern to dentistry

- Decreased antimicrobial effect of penicillin: tetracyclines, erythromycins, lincomycins
- Increased penicillin concentrations: aspirin, probenecid
- Suspected increased risk of methotrexate toxicity
- Oral contraceptives: advise patient of a potential risk for decreased contraceptive action, to maintain compliance with oral contraceptive use while using antibiotics, and to consider the use of additional nonhormonal contraception

DIAGNOSTIC TEST EFFECTS

May cause a positive Coombs' test.

SIDE EFFECTS

Occasional

Lethargy, fever, dizziness, rash, pain at injection site

Rare

Seizures, interstitial nephritis

SERIOUS REACTIONS

! Hypersensitivity reactions, ranging from chills, fever, and rash to anaphylaxis, may occur.

DENTAL CONSIDERATIONS

General:

- Take precautions regarding allergy to medication.
- Determine why the patient is taking the drug.
- Place on frequent recall to evaluate healing response.

Consultations:

- Medical consultation may be required to assess disease control.

Teach Patient/Family:

- *When used for dental infection, advise patient:*
  - To report sore throat, oral burning sensation, fever, fatigue, any of which could indicate superinfection
  - To take at prescribed intervals and complete dosage regimen
  - To immediately notify the dentist if signs or symptoms of infection increase

penicillin G potassium

pen-ih-sil'-lin G
(Megacillin[CAN], Novepen-G[CAN], Pfizerpen)

Do not confuse penicillin G potassium with penicillin G benzathine or penicillin G procaine.

CATEGORY AND SCHEDULE

Pregnancy Risk Category: B

MECHANISM OF ACTION

A penicillin that inhibits bacterial cell wall synthesis by binding to one or more of the penicillin-binding proteins of bacteria. ***Therapeutic Effect:*** Bactericidal.

AVAILABILITY

Injection: 5 million units.
Premixed Dextrose Solution: 1 million units, 2 million units, 3 million units.

INDICATIONS AND DOSAGES

▸ **Sepsis, Meningitis, Pericarditis, Endocarditis, Pneumonia Due to Susceptible Gram-Positive Organisms (not Staphylococcus aureus) and Some Gram-Negative Organisms**

IV, IM

Adults, Elderly. 2–24 million units/day in divided doses q4–6h.
Children. 100,000–400,000 units/kg/day in divided doses q4–6h.

▸ **Dosage in Renal Impairment**

Dosage interval is modified on the basis of creatinine clearance.

Creatinine Clearance	Dosage Interval
10–30 ml/min	Usual dose q8–12h
less than 10 ml/min	Usual dose q12–18h

CONTRAINDICATIONS

Hypersensitivity to any penicillin

INTERACTIONS

Drug

Erythromycin: May antagonize effects of penicillin.
Probenecid: Increases serum concentration of penicillin.

Herbal

None known.

Food

Food, milk: Decrease penicillin absorption.

Drug interactions of concern to dentistry

- Increased or prolonged plasma levels: probenecid
- Possible decrease in antimicrobial effectiveness: tetracyclines, erythromycins, lincomycins
- *When used for dental infection:*
  - Oral contraceptives: advise patient of a potential risk for decreased contraceptive action, to maintain compliance with oral contraceptive while using antibiotics, and to consider the use of nonhormonal contraception

DIAGNOSTIC TEST EFFECTS

May cause a positive Coombs' test.

IV INCOMPATIBILITIES

Amikacin (Amikin), aminophylline, amphotericin B, dopamine (Intropin)

IV COMPATIBILITIES

Amiodarone (Cordarone), calcium gluconate, diltiazem (Cardizem), diphenhydramine (Benadryl), furosemide (Lasix), heparin, hydromorphone (Dilaudid), lidocaine, magnesium sulfate, methylprednisolone (Solu-Medrol), morphine, potassium chloride

SIDE EFFECTS

Occasional
Lethargy, fever, dizziness, rash, electrolyte imbalance, diarrhea, thrombophlebitis
Rare
Seizures, interstitial nephritis

SERIOUS REACTIONS

! Hypersensitivity reactions ranging from rash, fever, and chills to anaphylaxis occur.

DENTAL CONSIDERATIONS

General:
- Determine why patient is taking the drug.
- Caution regarding allergy to medication.
- Use with caution in patients with a history of antibiotic-associated colitis.

Consultations:
- Consult patient's physician if an acute dental infection occurs and another antiinfective is required.
- Medical consultation may be required to assess disease control.

P

Teach Patient/Family:
- Importance of good oral hygiene to prevent soft tissue inflammation
- To prevent trauma when using oral hygiene aids
- *When antibiotics are used for dental infection:*
  - Oral contraceptives: advise patient of a potential risk for decreased contraceptive action, to maintain compliance with oral contraceptive use while using antibiotics, and to consider the use of additional nonhormonal contraception.
  - DENIF
  - To report sore throat, oral burning sensation, fever, or fatigue, any of which could indicate presence of a superinfection

penicillin

pen-i-sil′-in
amoxicillin, ampicillin, bacampicillin, carbenicillin, cloxacillin, dicloxacillin, flucloxacillin, methicillin, mezlocillin, nafcillin, oxacillin, penicillin G benzathine, penicillin G potassium, penicillin V potassium, piperacillin, pivampicillin, pivmecillinam, ticarcillin; Penicillin and beta-lactamase inhibitors; amoxicillin/clavulanate potassium, ampicillin/sulbactam sodium, piperacillin sodium/tazobactam sodium, ticarcillin disodium/clavulanate potassium

CATEGORY AND SCHEDULE

Pregnancy Risk Category: B

MECHANISM OF ACTION

Penicillins bind to bacterial cell wall, inhibiting bacterial cell wall synthesis. ***Therapeutic Effect:*** Inhibits bacterial cell wall synthesis. Beta-lactamase inhibitors: inhibit the action of bacterial beta-lactamase. ***Therapeutic Effect:*** Protects the penicillin from enzymatic degradation.

PHARMACOKINETICS

Penicillins are generally well absorbed from the gastrointestinal (GI) tract after oral administration. Widely distributed to most tissues and body fluids. Protein binding: 20%. Partially metabolized in liver. Primarily excreted in urine. ***Half-life:*** varies (half-life increased in reduced renal function).

AVAILABILITY

Penicillins are available in tablets, chewable tablets, capsules, powder for oral suspension, powder for injection, prefilled syringes for injection, premixed dextrose solutions for injection, and solutions for infusion.

INDICATIONS AND DOSAGES

Penicillins may be used to treat a large number of infections, including pneumonia and other respiratory diseases, urinary tract infections, septicemia, meningitis, intra-abdominal infections, gonorrhea, syphilis, and bone and joint infections.

Doses vary depending on the drug used. In general, penicillins should be taken on an empty stomach. Patients with impaired renal function may require dose adjustment.

OFF-LABEL USES

Some penicillins, such as amoxicillin, have been used in the treatment of Lyme disease and typhoid fever.

CONTRAINDICATIONS

Hypersensitivity to any penicillin, infectious mononucleosis

INTERACTIONS

Drug

Allopurinol: May increase incidence of rash.
Oral contraceptives: May decrease effects of oral contraceptives.
Probenecid: May increase penicillin blood concentration and risk for penicillin toxicity.

Herbal

None known.

Food

None known.

Drug interactions of concern to dentistry

- Decreased antimicrobial effect of penicillin: tetracyclines, erythromycins, lincomycins
- Increased penicillin concentrations: aspirin, probenecid
- Suspected increased risk of methotrexate toxicity
- Oral contraceptives: advise patient of a potential risk for decreased contraceptive action, to maintain compliance with oral contraceptive use while using antibiotics, and to consider the use of additional nonhormonal contraception

Drug interactions of concern to dentistry penicillin V potassium/penicillin V

- Decreased antimicrobial effectiveness of penicillin: tetracyclines, erythromycins, lincomycins
- Increased penicillin concentrations: probenecid
- Oral contraceptives: advise patient of a potential risk for decreased contraceptive action, to maintain compliance with oral contraceptive use while using antibiotics, and to consider the use of additional nonhormonal contraception

Drug interactions of concern to dentistry penicillin G potassium, aqueous (Pfizerpen)

- Increased or prolonged plasma levels: probenecid
- Possible decrease in antimicrobial effectiveness: tetracyclines, erythromycins, lincomycins
- *When used for dental infection:*
  - Oral contraceptives: advise patient of a potential risk for decreased contraceptive action, to maintain compliance with oral contraceptive while using antibiotics, and to consider the use of nonhormonal contraception

DIAGNOSTIC TEST EFFECTS

May increase BUN, LDH, serum bilirubin, serum creatinine, SGOT (AST), and SGPT (ALT) levels. May cause positive Coombs' test.

SIDE EFFECTS

Frequent

Gastrointestinal (GI) disturbances (mild diarrhea, nausea, or vomiting), headache, oral or vaginal candidiasis

Occasional

Generalized rash, urticaria

SERIOUS REACTIONS

! Altered bacterial balance may result in potentially fatal superinfections and antibiotic-associated colitis as evidenced by abdominal cramps, watery or severe diarrhea, and fever.

! Severe hypersensitivity reactions, including anaphylaxis and acute interstitial nephritis occur rarely.

DENTAL CONSIDERATIONS

PENICILLIN G BENZATHINE

General:

- Take precautions regarding allergy to medication.
- Determine why the patient is taking the drug.
- Place on frequent recall to evaluate healing response.

Consultations:

- Medical consultation may be required to assess disease control.

Teach Patient/Family:

- *When used for dental infection, advise patient:*
  - To report sore throat, oral burning sensation, fever, fatigue, any of which could indicate superinfection
  - To take at prescribed intervals and complete dosage regimen
  - To immediately notify the dentist if signs or symptoms of infection increase

P

DENTAL CONSIDERATIONS

PENICILLIN V POTASSIUM/ PENICILLIN V

General:

- Take precautions regarding allergy to medication.
- Determine why the patient is taking the drug.
- If used for dental infection, place on frequent recall to evaluate healing response.

Consultations:

- Medical consultation may be required to assess disease control.

Teach Patient/Family:

- *When used for dental infection, advise patient:*
  - To report sore throat, oral burning sensation, fever, fatigue, any of which could indicate superinfection
  - To take at prescribed intervals and complete dosage regimen
  - To immediately notify the dentist if signs or symptoms of infection increase

PENICILLIN G POTASSIUM, AQUEOUS (PFIZERPEN)

General:

- Determine why patient is taking the drug.
- Caution regarding allergy to medication.
- Use with caution in patients with a history of antibiotic associated colitis.

Consultations:

- CONIF
- Medical consultation may be required to assess disease control.

Teach Patient/Family:

- Importance of good oral hygiene to prevent soft tissue inflammation
- To prevent trauma when using oral hygiene aids

- *When antibiotics are used for dental infection:*
  - Oral contraceptives: advise patient of a potential risk for decreased contraceptive action, to maintain compliance with oral contraceptive use while using antibiotics, and to consider the use of additional nonhormonal contraception.
- DENIF
- To report sore throat, oral burning sensation, fever, or fatigue, any of which could indicate presence of a superinfection

penicillin V potassium

pen-ih-sil′-in V
(Abbocillin VK[AUS], Apo-Pen-VK[CAN], Cilicaine VK[AUS], L.P.V.[AUS], Novo-Pen-VK[CAN], Veetids)

CATEGORY AND SCHEDULE

Pregnancy Risk Category: B

MECHANISM OF ACTION

A penicillin that inhibits cell wall synthesis by binding to bacterial cell membranes. ***Therapeutic Effect:*** Bactericidal.

PHARMACOKINETICS

Moderately absorbed from the GI tract. Protein binding: 80%. Widely distributed. Metabolized in the liver. Primarily excreted in urine. ***Half-life:*** 1 hr (increased in impaired renal function).

AVAILABILITY

Tablets: 250 mg, 500 mg.
Powder for Oral Solution: 125 mg/5 ml, 250 mg/5 ml.

INDICATIONS AND DOSAGES

▸ Mild to Moderate Respiratory Tract or Skin or Skin-Structure Infections, Otitis Media, Necrotizing Ulcerative Gingivitis

PO

Adults, Elderly, Children 12 yr and older. 125–500 mg q6–8h.
Children younger than 12 yr. 25–50 mg/kg/day in divided doses q6–8h. Maximum: 3 g/day.

▸ Primary Prevention of Rheumatic Fever

PO

Adults, Elderly. 500 mg 2–3 times/day for 10 days.
Children. 250 mg 2–3 times/day for 10 days.

CONTRAINDICATIONS

Hypersensitivity to any penicillin

INTERACTIONS

Drug

Probenecid: May increase penicillin blood concentration and risk of toxicity.

Herbal

None known.

Food

None known.

Drug interactions of concern to dentistry

- Decreased antimicrobial effectiveness of penicillin: tetracyclines, erythromycins, lincomycins
- Increased penicillin concentrations: probenecid
- Oral contraceptives: advise patient of a potential risk for decreased contraceptive action, to maintain compliance with oral contraceptive use while using antibiotics, and to consider the use of additional nonhormonal contraception

DIAGNOSTIC TEST EFFECTS

May cause positive a Coombs' test.

SIDE EFFECTS

Frequent

Mild hypersensitivity reaction (chills, fever, rash), nausea, vomiting, diarrhea

Rare

Bleeding, allergic reaction

SERIOUS REACTIONS

! Severe hypersensitivity reactions, including anaphylaxis, may occur.

! Nephrotoxicity, antibiotic-associated colitis, and other superinfections may result from high dosages or prolonged therapy.

DENTAL CONSIDERATIONS

General:

- Take precautions regarding allergy to medication.
- Determine why the patient is taking the drug.
- If used for dental infection, place on frequent recall to evaluate healing response.

Consultations:

- Medical consultation may be required to assess disease control.

Teach Patient/Family:

- *When used for dental infection, advise patient:*
  - To report sore throat, oral burning sensation, fever, fatigue, any of which could indicate superinfection
  - To take at prescribed intervals and complete dosage regimen
  - To immediately notify the dentist if signs or symptoms of infection increase

pentamidine isethionate

pen-tam′-i-deen

(NebuPent, Pentacarinat[CAN], Pentam-300)

CATEGORY AND SCHEDULE

Pregnancy Risk Category: C

MECHANISM OF ACTION

An antiinfective that interferes with nuclear metabolism and incorporation of nucleotides, inhibiting DNA, RNA, phospholipid, and protein synthesis. ***Therapeutic Effect:*** Produces antibacterial and antiprotozoal effects.

PHARMACOKINETICS

Well absorbed after IM administration; minimally absorbed after inhalation.Widely distributed. Primarily excreted in urine. Minimally removed by hemodialysis. ***Half-life:*** 6.5 hr (increased in impaired renal function).

AVAILABILITY

Injection (Pentam-300): 300 mg.
Powder for Nebulization (Nebupent): 300 mg.

INDICATIONS AND DOSAGES

▸ ***Pneumocystis Carinii*** **Pneumonia (PCP)**

IV, IM

Adults, Elderly. 4 mg/kg/day once a day for 14–21 days.

Children. 4 mg/kg/day once a day for 10–14 days.

▸ **Prevention of PCP**

INHALATION

Adults, Elderly. 300 mg once q4wk.

Children 5 yr and older. 300 mg q3–4wks.

Children younger than 5 yr. 8 mg/kg/dose once q3–4wk.

OFF-LABEL USES
Treatment of African trypanosomiasis, cutaneous or visceral leishmaniasis

CONTRAINDICATIONS
Concurrent use with didanosine

INTERACTIONS
Drug
Blood dyscrasia-producing medications, bone marrow depressants: May increase the abnormal hematologic effects of pentamidine.
Didanosine: May increase the risk of pancreatitis.
Foscarnet: May increase the risk of hypocalcemia, hypomagnesemia, and nephrotoxicity of pentamidine.
Nephrotoxic medications: May increase the risk of nephrotoxicity.
Herbal
None known.
Food
None known.
Drug interactions of concern to dentistry
- None reported

DIAGNOSTIC TEST EFFECTS
May increase BUN and serum alkaline phosphatase, bilirubin, creatinine, AST (SGOT), and ALT (SGPT) levels. May decrease serum calcium and magnesium levels. May alter blood glucose levels.

IV INCOMPATIBILITIES
Cefazolin (Ancef), cefotaxime (Claforan), ceftazidime (Fortaz), ceftriaxone (Rocephin), fluconazole (Diflucan), foscarnet (Foscavir), interleukin (Proleukin)
IV COMPATIBILITIES
Diltiazem (Cardizem), zidovudine (Retrovir)

SIDE EFFECTS
Frequent
Injection (> 10%): Abscess, pain at injection site
Inhalation (> 5%): Fatigue, metallic taste, shortness of breath, decreased appetite, dizziness, rash, cough, nausea, vomiting, chills
Occasional
Injection (10%–1%): Nausea, decreased appetite, hypotension, fever, rash, altered taste, confusion
Inhalation (5%–1%): Diarrhea, headache, anemia, muscle pain
Rare
Injection (< 1%): Neuralgia, thrombocytopenia, phlebitis, dizziness

SERIOUS REACTIONS
! Rare reactions include life-threatening or fatal hypotension, arrhythmias, hypoglycemia, leukopenia, nephrotoxicity or renal failure, anaphylactic shock, Stevens-Johnson syndrome, and toxic epidural necrolysis.
! Hyperglycemia and insulin-dependent diabetes mellitus (often permanent) may occur even months after therapy has stopped.

DENTAL CONSIDERATIONS
General:
- Monitor vital signs at every appointment because of CV side effects.
- Patients on chronic drug therapy may rarely have symptoms of blood dyscrasias, which can include infection, bleeding, and poor healing.
- Place on frequent recall to evaluate healing response.
- Assess salivary flow as a factor in caries, periodontal disease, and candidiasis.
- Consider semisupine chair position for patients with respiratory disease.

• For inhalation dosage forms, rinse mouth with water after each dose to prevent dryness.
• Place on frequent recall because of oral side effects.

Consultations:

• In a patient with symptoms of blood dyscrasias, request a medical consultation for blood studies and postpone dental treatment until normal values are reestablished.
• Medical consultation may be required to assess disease control.

Teach Patient/Family:

• That secondary oral infection may occur; must see dentist immediately if infection occurs
• Importance of good oral hygiene to prevent soft tissue inflammation
• Caution to prevent injury when using oral hygiene aids
• Importance of dietary suggestions to maintain oral and systemic health
• *When chronic dry mouth occurs, advise patient:*
  • To avoid mouth rinses with high alcohol content because of drying effects
  • Of need for daily use of home fluoride products to prevent caries
  • To use sugarless gum, frequent sips of water, or saliva substitutes

P

pentazocine hydrochloride; naloxone hydrochloride

Schedule IV
(Talwin Nx)

CATEGORY AND SCHEDULE

Pregnancy Risk Category: NR

MECHANISM OF ACTION

Naloxone is a narcotic antagonist that displaces opiates at opiate-occupied receptor sites in the central nervous system (CNS). Pentazocine is both a narcotic agonist and antagonist that induces analgesia by stimulating the kappa and sigma opioid receptors. ***Therapeutic Effect:*** Naloxone: blocks narcotic effects; reverses opiate-induced sleep or sedation; increases respiratory rate, returns depressed blood pressure (B/P) to normal rate. Pentazocine: induces analgesia.

PHARMACOKINETICS

Well absorbed. Metabolized in liver. Primarily excreted in urine. Minimal excretion in bile and feces. ***Half-life:*** 2–3 hrs.

AVAILABILITY

Tablets: 50 mg pentazocine hydrochloride/0.5 mg naloxone hydrochloride (Talwin Nx).

INDICATIONS AND DOSAGES

▸ Pain, Moderate to Severe

PO

Adults, Elderly, Children 12 yrs and older. 1 tablet every 3–4 hrs. May be increased to 2 tablets when needed. Maximum: 12 tablets/day.

CONTRAINDICATIONS

Hypersensitivity to pentazocine or naloxone or any component on the formulation

INTERACTIONS

Drug

Alcohol: May increase sedation.
Clonidine: May cause hypertension.
Fluoxetine, sibutramine: May increase risk of serotonin syndrome.
Methohexital, thiopental: May increase the risk of CNS depression.

Opioid analgesics: May cause precipitation of withdrawal symptoms.
Tobacco: May decrease pentazocine concentrations.

Herbal

Yohimbine: May increase adverse effects, such as nervousness, anxiety, palpitations, nausea, and hot and cold flashes.

Food

None known.

Drug interactions of concern to dentistry

- Increased effects: all CNS depressants, alcohol
- Contraindication: MAOIs
- Do not mix in solutions or syringe with barbiturates
- Additive side effects of opioid agonists
- Increased effects of anticholinergics
- Decreased effects of opioid agonists

DIAGNOSTIC TEST EFFECTS

None known.

SIDE EFFECTS

Occasional

Confusion, dizziness, fatigue, lightheadedness, drowsiness, mood changes, headache, GI upset, vomiting, constipation, stomach pain, rash, difficulty urinating

SERIOUS REACTIONS

! Respiratory depression and serious skin reactions, such as Stevens-Johnson Syndrome, have been reported but occur rarely.

DENTAL CONSIDERATIONS

General:

- Monitor vital signs at every appointment because of CV and respiratory side effects.
- Assess salivary flow as a factor in caries, periodontal disease, and candidiasis.
- Consider semisupine chair position for patient comfort if GI side effects occur.
- Psychologic and physical dependence may occur with chronic administration.

Teach Patient/Family:

- *When chronic dry mouth occurs, advise patient:*
  - To avoid mouth rinses with high alcohol content because of drying effects
  - Of need for daily use of home fluoride products to prevent caries
  - To use sugarless gum, frequent sips of water, or saliva substitutes

pentazocine

pen-tah-zoe-seen
Schedule IV
(Talwin)

Combination Products

With naloxone, a narcotic antagonist (oral) (Talwin NX); with aspirin (oral) (Talwin Compound); w/acetaminophen (oral) (Talacen)

CATEGORY AND SCHEDULE

With naloxone, a narcotic antagonist (oral) (Talwin NX); with aspirin (oral) (Talwin Compound); w/acetaminophen (oral) (Talacen)

MECHANISM OF ACTION

An opioid antagonist that binds with opioid receptors within CNS.
Therapeutic Effect: Alters processes affecting pain perception, emotional response to pain.

PHARMACOKINETICS

Well absorbed after administration. Widely distributed including CSF. Metabolized in liver via oxidative and glucuronide conjugation pathways, extensive first-pass effect. Excreted in small amounts as unchanged drug. ***Half-life:*** 2–3 hrs, prolonged with hepatic impairment.

AVAILABILITY

Tablets: 12.5 mg and 325 mg aspirin (Talwin Compound), 25 mg and 650 mg acetaminophen (Talacen), 50 mg pentazocine and 0.5 mg naloxone (Talwin NX), 50 mg (Talwin).
Injection: 30 mg (Talwin).

INDICATIONS AND DOSAGES

▸ Analgesia

PO
Adults. 50 mg q3–4h. May increase to 100 mg q3–4h, if needed. Maximum: 600 mg/day.
Elderly. 50 mg q4h.
SUBCUTANEOUS/IM/IV
Adults. 30 mg q3–4h. Do not exceed 30 mg IV or 60 mg subcutaneous/IM per dose. Maximum: 360 mg/day.
IM
Elderly. 25 mg q4h.

▸ Obstetric labor

IM
Adults. 30 mg as a single dose.
IV
Adults. 20 mg when contractions are regular. May repeat 2–3 times q2–3h.

CONTRAINDICATIONS

Hypersensitivity to pentazocine or any component of the formulation

INTERACTIONS

Drug

Alcohol, CNS depressants: May increase CNS or respiratory depression and hypotension.
Fluoxetine: May cause hypertension, diaphoresis, ataxia, flushing, nausea, dizziness, and anxiety.
MAOIs: May produce severe, fatal reaction.
Opioid analgesics: May increase withdrawal symptoms.
Sibutramine: May increase risk of serotonin syndrome.

Herbal

None known.

Food

None known.

Drug interactions of concern to dentistry

- Increased effects: all CNS depressants, alcohol
- Contraindication: MAOIs
- Do not mix in solutions or syringe with barbiturates
- Additive side effects of opioid agonists
- Increased effects of anticholinergics
- Decreased effects of opioid agonists

DIAGNOSTIC TEST EFFECTS

May increase amylase and lipase.

SIDE EFFECTS

Frequent

Drowsiness, euphoria, nausea, vomiting

Occasional

Allergic reaction, histamine reaction (decreased B/P, increased sweating, flushing, wheezing), decreased urination, altered vision, constipation, dizziness, dry mouth, headache, hypotension, pain/burning at injection site

SERIOUS REACTIONS

! Overdosage results in severe respiratory depression, skeletal muscle flaccidity, cyanosis, extreme somnolence progressing to convulsions, stupor, and coma.
! Abrupt withdrawal after prolonged use may produce symptoms of narcotic withdrawal (abdominal cramps, rhinorrhea, lacrimation, nausea, vomiting, restlessness, anxiety, increased temperature, piloerection).

P

DENTAL CONSIDERATIONS

General:

- Monitor vital signs at every appointment because of CV and respiratory side effects.
- Assess salivary flow as a factor in caries, periodontal disease, and candidiasis.
- Consider semisupine chair position for patient comfort if GI side effects occur.
- Psychologic and physical dependence may occur with chronic administration.

Teach Patient/Family:

- *When chronic dry mouth occurs, advise patient:*
  - To avoid mouth rinses with high alcohol content because of drying effects
  - Of need for daily use of home fluoride products to prevent caries
  - To use sugarless gum, frequent sips of water, or saliva substitutes

pentobarbital

pen-toe-bar′-bi-tal
Schedule II, Schedule III
(Nembutal, Phenobarbitone[AUS])
Do not confuse with phenobarbital.

CATEGORY AND SCHEDULE

Pregnancy Risk Category: D
Controlled substance: Schedule II (capsules, injection), Schedule III (suppositories)

MECHANISM OF ACTION

A barbiturate that binds at the GABA receptor complex, enhancing GABA activity. ***Therapeutic Effect:*** Depresses central nervous system (CNS) activity and reticular activating system.

PHARMACOKINETICS

Well absorbed after PO, parenteral administration. Protein binding: 35%–55%. Rapidly, widely distributed. Metabolized in liver. Primarily excreted in urine. Removed by hemodialysis. ***Half-life:*** 15–48 hrs.

AVAILABILITY

Capsules: 50 mg, 100 mg.
Injection: 50 mg/ml.
Suppositories: 30 mg, 120 mg, 200 mg.

INDICATIONS AND DOSAGES

▸ **Preanesthetic**

PO

Adults, Elderly. 100 mg.
Children. 2–6 mg/kg. Maximum: 100 mg/dose.

IM

Adults, Elderly. 150–200 mg.
Children. 2–6 mg/kg. Maximum: 100 mg/dose.

RECTAL

Children 12–14 yrs. 60 or 120 mg.
Children 5–12 yrs. 60 mg.
Children 1–4 yrs. 30–60 mg.
Children 1 yr–2 mos. 30 mg.

▸ **Hypnotic**

PO

Adults, Elderly. 100 mg at bedtime.

IM

Adults, Elderly. 150–200 mg at bedtime.
Children. 2–6 mg/kg. Maximum: 100 mg/dose at bedtime.

IV

Adults, Elderly. 100 mg initially then, after 1 minute, may give additional small doses at 1 minute intervals, up to 500 mg total.
Children. 50 mg initially then, after 1 minute, may give additional small doses at 1 minute intervals, up to desired effect.

RECTAL
Adults, Elderly. 120–200 mg at bedtime.
Children 12–14 yrs. 60 or 120 mg at bedtime.
Children 5–12 yrs. 60 mg at bedtime.
Children 1–4 yrs. 30–60 mg at bedtime.
Children 2 mos–1 yr. 30 mg at bedtime.

▸ **Anticonvulsant**
IV
Adults, Elderly. 2–15 mg/kg loading dose given slowly over 1–2 hours. Maintenance infusion: 0.5–5 mg/kg/hr.
Children. 5–15 mg/kg loading dose given slowly over 1–2 hours. Maintenance infusion: 0.5–3 mg/kg/hr.

OFF-LABEL USES
Intracranial hypertension, psychiatric interviews, sedative withdrawal, drug abuse withdrawal

CONTRAINDICATIONS
Porphyria, hypersensitivity to barbiturates

P

INTERACTIONS
Drug
Alcohol, CNS depressants: May increase the effects of pentobarbital.
Alprenolol, metoprolol: May decrease alprenolol and metoprolol effectiveness.
Barbituates: May increase the risk of respiratory depression.
Chloral hydrate: May increase the risk of respiratory depression.
Dicumarol: May decrease the anticoagulant effectiveness.
Opioid analgesics: May increase the risk of respiratory depression.
Prednisolone, prednisone: May decrease therapeutic effect of prednisolone and prednisone.
Procarbazine: May increase the risk of CNS depression.
Quetiapine: May decrease serum quetiapine concentrations.
Theophylline: May decrease theophylline effectiveness.

Herbal
Catnip oil: May increase risk of CNS depression.
Eucalyptol: May decrease effectiveness of barbiturates.
Kava kava: May increase CNS depression.
St. John's Wort: May decrease CNS depressive effect of barbiturates.
Valerian: May increase CNS depression.

Food
None known.

Drug interactions of concern to dentistry
- Hepatotoxicity: halogenated-hydrocarbon anesthetics
- Increased CNS depression: alcohol, all other CNS depressants
- Increased metabolism of carbamazepine, tricyclic antidepressants, corticosteroids
- Decreased half-life of doxycycline

DIAGNOSTIC TEST EFFECTS
None known.

IV INCOMPATIBILITIES
Anileridine, atracurium (Tacrium), benzquinamide, butorphanol, cefazolin (Ancef), chlordiazepoxide (Librium), chlorpheniramine, clindamycin (Cleocin), codeine, cyclizine, diphenhydramine (Benadryl), droperidol (Inapsine), fenoldopam (Corlopam), fentanyl, glycopyrrolate (Robinul), hydrocortisone (Solu-Cortef), insulin, kanamycin (Kantrex), levorphanol (Levo-Dromoran), meperidine (Demerol), metaraminol (Aramin), methadone, methyldopa (Aldomet), metocurine (Metubine), midazolam (Versed), nalbuphine

(Nubain), opium alkaloids, oxytetracycline, pancuronium (Pavulon), penicillin G (Pfizerpen), pentazocine (Talwin), perphenazine (Trilafon), phytonadione (Aqua-Mephyton), prochlorperazine (Compazine), promazine (Sparine), protein hydrolysate (Nembutal), sodium bicarbonate, streptomycin, thiamine, triflupromazine (Stelazine), tripelennamine (PBZ), vancomycin (Vancocin)

IV COMPATIBILITIES

Acyclovir (Zovirax), amikacin (Amikin), aminophylline, calcium chloride, cephapirin (Cefadyl), chloramphenicol, hyaluronidase (Wydase), hydromorphone (Dilaudid), lidocaine, neostigmine (Prostigmin), propofol (Diprivan), ranitidine (Zantac), scopolamine, sodium iodide, thiopental (Pentothal), verapamil

SIDE EFFECTS

Occasional

Agitation, confusion, dizziness, somnolence

Rare

Confusion, paradoxical CNS hyperactivity or nervousness in children, excitement or restlessness in elderly

SERIOUS REACTIONS

! Agranulocytosis, megaloblastic anemia, apnea, hypoventilation, bradycardia, hypotension, syncope, hepatic damage, and Stevens-Johnson syndrome occur rarely.

! Abrupt withdrawal after prolonged therapy may produce effects ranging from markedly increased dreaming, nightmares or insomnia, tremor, sweating and vomiting, to hallucinations, delirium, seizures, and status epilepticus.

! Skin eruptions appear as hypersensitivity reactions.

! Overdosage produces cold or clammy skin, hypothermia, severe CNS depression, cyanosis, and rapid pulse.

DENTAL CONSIDERATIONS

General:

- Determine why the patient is taking the drug.
- Monitor vital signs at every appointment because of CV side effects. Evaluate respiration characteristics and rate.
- Patients on chronic drug therapy may rarely have symptoms of blood dyscrasias, which can include infection, bleeding, and poor healing.
- *When used for sedation in dentistry:*
  - Assess vital signs before use and q30min after use as sedative.
  - Observe respiratory dysfunction: respiratory depression, character, rate, rhythm; hold drug if respirations are <10/min or if pupils are dilated.
- After supine positioning, have patient sit upright for at least 2 min before standing to avoid orthostatic hypotension.
- Have someone drive patient to and from dental office when drug used for conscious sedation.
- Barbiturates induce liver microsomal enzymes, which alter the metabolism of other drugs.
- Geriatric patients are more susceptible to drug effects; use lower dose.

Consultations:

- In a patient with symptoms of blood dyscrasias, request a medical consultation for blood studies and postpone dental treatment until normal values are reestablished.

Teach Patient/Family:

- To avoid driving or other activities requiring alertness

• To avoid alcohol ingestion or CNS depressants; serious CNS depression may result
• To avoid OTC preparations (antihistamines, cold remedies) that contain CNS depressants

pentosan polysulfate

pen-toe-san
(Elmiron)
Do not confuse with pentostatin.

CATEGORY AND SCHEDULE

Pregnancy Risk Category: B

MECHANISM OF ACTION

A negatively charged synthetic sulfated polysaccharide with heparin-like properties that appear to adhere to bladder wall mucosal membrane, may act as a buffering agent to control cell permeability, preventing irritating solutes in the urine. Has anticoagulant/fibrinolytic effects. ***Therapeutic Effect:*** Relieves bladder pain.

P

PHARMACOKINETICS

Poorly and erratically absorbed from the gastrointestinal tract. Distributed in uroepithelium of GU tract with lesser amount found in the liver, spleen, lung, skin, periosteum and bone marrow. Metabolized in liver and kidney (secondary). Eliminated in the urine. ***Half-life:*** 4.8 hrs.

AVAILABILITY

Capsules: 100 mg (Elmiron).

INDICATIONS AND DOSAGES

▸ Interstitial Cystitis

PO
Adults, Elderly. 100 mg 3 times/day.

OFF-LABEL USES

Urolithiasis

CONTRAINDICATIONS

Hypersensitivity to pentosan polysulfate sodium or structurally related compounds

INTERACTIONS

Drug

Anticoagulants: May increase risk of bleeding.

Herbal

Chondroitin, ginseng: May increase INR serum values and increase anticoagulant effects.
Alfalfa, coenzyme Q, green tea: May decrease anticoagulant effectiveness.
Arnica, bilberry, black currant, bromelain, cat's claw, chamomile, clove oil, curcumin, dong quai, primrose oil, fenugreek, garlic, ginger, kava kava, licorice, red clover, skullcap, tan-shen, vitamin A: May increase risk of bleeding.

Food

Avocado: May decrease anticoagulant effectiveness.
Rhubarb: May increase risk of bleeding.

Drug interactions of concern to dentistry

• Potential risk of bleeding: high-dose aspirin

DIAGNOSTIC TEST EFFECTS

May increase transaminase, alkaline phosphatase, PTT, PT. May decrease WBC count, thrombocytes.

IV INCOMPATIBILITIES

None known.

IV COMPATIBILITIES

None known.

SIDE EFFECTS

Frequent

Alopecia areata (a single area on the scalp), diarrhea, nausea, headache, rash, abdominal pain, dyspepsia.

Occasional
Dizziness, depression, increased liver function tests.

SERIOUS REACTIONS

! Ecchymosis, epistaxis, gum hemorrhage have been reported (drug produces weak anticoagulant effect).
! Overdose may produce liver function abnormalities.

DENTAL CONSIDERATIONS

General:
- Possesses weak anticoagulant activity; question patient about bleeding or bruising.
- Consider semisupine chair position for patient comfort if GI side effects occur.
- Question patient about tolerance of NSAIDS or aspirin related to GI disease.
- Avoid products that affect platelet function, such as aspirin and NSAIDs.
- Consider local hemostasis measures to prevent excessive bleeding.

Consultations:
- Confer with physician if bleeding is a problem; epistaxis, spontaneous gingival bleeding.
- Medical consultation should include routine blood counts including platelet counts and bleeding time.

Teach Patient/Family:
- Importance of good oral hygiene to prevent soft tissue inflammation
- To prevent trauma when using oral hygiene aids
- To report oral lesions, soreness, or bleeding to dentist
- Importance of updating health and medication history if physician makes any changes in evaluation or drug regimens; include OTC, herbal, and nonherbal in the update

pentostatin

pen-toe-**stat**-inn
(Nipent)
Do not confuse with pravastatin.

CATEGORY AND SCHEDULE

Pregnancy Risk Category: D

MECHANISM OF ACTION

An antimetabolite that inhibits the enzyme adenosine deaminase (ADA) (increases intracellular levels of adenine deoxynucleotide). Greatest activity in T cells of lymphoid system. Inhibits ADA and RNA synthesis. Produces DNA damage. ***Therapeutic Effect:*** Leads to cell death.

PHARMACOKINETICS

After IV administration, rapidly distributed to body tissues (poorly distributed to cerebrospinal fluid). Protein binding: 4%. Excreted primarily in urine unchanged or as active metabolite. ***Half-life:*** 5.7 hr (half-life increased with renal impairment).

AVAILABILITY

Powder for Injection: 10 mg (Nipent).

INDICATIONS AND DOSAGES

▸ Hairy Cell Leukemia
IV
Adults, Elderly. 4 mg/m^2 q2wk until complete response attained (without any major toxicity). Discontinue if no response in 6 months; partial response in 12 months.

▸ Dosage in Renal Impairment
Only when benefits justify risks, give 2–3 mg/m^2 in patients with creatinine clearance 50–60 ml/min.

P

UNLABELED USES
Treatment of Hodgkin's lymphoma, myelodysplastic syndrome

CONTRAINDICATIONS
Hypersensitivity to pentostatin

INTERACTIONS
Drug
Bone marrow depressants: May increase bone marrow depression.
Fludarabine: May increase pulmonary toxicity.
Live virus vaccines: May potentiate virus replication, increase vaccine side effects, and decrease the patient's antibody response to vaccine.
Vidarabine: May increase effects and toxicity of vidarabine.
Herbal
None known.
Food
None known.

DIAGNOSTIC TEST EFFECTS
May increase serum glutamate oxaloacetate (SGOT) (aspartate aminotransferase [AST]), serum glutamate pyruvate transaminase (SGPT) (alanine aminotransferase [ALT]), alkaline phosphatase, lactate dehydrogenase (LDH), uric acid, and creatinine levels.

SIDE EFFECTS
Frequent
Nausea, vomiting (53%), fever (42%), rash (26%), fatigue (29%), pain (20%), cough (17%), upper respiratory tract infection, anorexia (16%), diarrhea (15%)
Occasional (13%–10%)
Headache, pharyngitis, sinusitis, myalgia, chills, arthralgia, peripheral edema, anorexia, blurred vision, conjunctivitis, skin discoloration, sweating, anxiety, depression, dizziness, confusion

SERIOUS REACTIONS
! Bone marrow depression is manifested as hematologic toxicity (principally leukopenia, anemia, thrombocytopenia).
! Doses higher than recommended (20–50 mg/m^2 in divided doses for more than 5 days) may produce severe renal, hepatic, pulmonary, or CNS toxicity.

pentoxifylline
pen-tox-if′-ih-lin
(Albert[CAN], Apo-Pentoxifylline SR[CAN], Pentoxifylline[CAN], Pentoxyl, Trental)
Do not confuse Trental with Tegretol or Trandate.

CATEGORY AND SCHEDULE
Pregnancy Risk Category: C

MECHANISM OF ACTION
A blood viscosity-reducing agent that alters the flexibility of RBCs; inhibits production of tumor necrosis factor, neutrophil activation, and platelet aggregation. ***Therapeutic Effect:*** Reduces blood viscosity and improves blood flow.

PHARMACOKINETICS
Well absorbed after oral administration. Undergoes first-pass metabolism in the liver. Primarily excreted in urine. Unknown if removed by hemodialysis. ***Half-life:*** 24–48 min; metabolite, 60–90 min.

AVAILABILITY
Tablets (Controlled-Release [Pentoxil, Trental]): 400 mg.

INDICATIONS AND DOSAGES

▸ Intermittent Claudication

PO

Adults, Elderly. 400 mg 3 times a day. Decrease to 400 mg twice a day if GI or CNS adverse effects occur. Continue for at least 8 wk.

CONTRAINDICATIONS

History of intolerance to xanthine derivatives, such as caffeine, theophylline, or theobromine; recent cerebral or retinal hemorrhage

INTERACTIONS

Drug

Antihypertensives: May increase the effects of antihypertensives.

Herbal

None known.

Food

None known.

DIAGNOSTIC TEST EFFECTS

None known.

SIDE EFFECTS

Occasional (5%–2%)

Dizziness, nausea, altered taste, dyspepsia, marked by heartburn, epigastric pain, and indigestion

Rare (< 2%)

Rash, pruritus, anorexia, constipation, dry mouth, blurred vision, edema, nasal congestion, anxiety

SERIOUS REACTIONS

! Angina and chest pain occur rarely and may be accompanied by palpitations, tachycardia, and arrhythmias.

! Signs and symptoms of overdose, such as flushing, hypotension, nervousness, agitation, hand tremor, fever, and somnolence, appear 4–5 hours after ingestion and last for 12 hours.

DENTAL CONSIDERATIONS

General:

- Monitor vital signs at every appointment because of CV side effects.
- Assess salivary flow as a factor in caries, periodontal disease, and candidiasis.
- Stress from dental procedures may compromise CV function; determine patient risk.
- Short appointments and a stress reduction protocol may be required for anxious patients.
- Talk with patient about potential systemic diseases (e.g., diabetes, CV disease) that may be associated with claudication.

Consultations:

- Medical consultation may be required to assess disease control and patient's ability to tolerate stress.

Teach Patient/Family:

- Importance of good oral hygiene to prevent soft tissue inflammation
- Caution to prevent injury when using oral hygiene aids
- *When chronic dry mouth occurs, advise patient:*
  - To avoid mouth rinses with high alcohol content because of drying effects
  - Of need for daily use of home fluoride products to prevent caries
  - To use sugarless gum, frequent sips of water, or saliva substitutes

pergolide mesylate

per′-go-lide

(Permax)

Do not confuse Permax with Pentrax or Pernox.

CATEGORY AND SCHEDULE

Pregnancy Risk Category: B

MECHANISM OF ACTION

A centrally active dopamine agonist that directly stimulates dopamine receptors. ***Therapeutic Effect:*** Decreases signs and symptoms of Parkinson's disease.

PHARMACOKINETICS

Well absorbed from the GI tract. Protein binding: 90%. Undergoes extensive first-pass metabolism in the liver. Primarily excreted in urine. Unknown if removed by hemodialysis.

AVAILABILITY

Tablets: 0.05 mg, 0.25 mg, 1 mg.

INDICATIONS AND DOSAGES

▸ Parkinsonism

PO

Adults, Elderly. Initially, 0.05 mg/day for 2 days. May increase by 0.1–0.15 mg/day every 3 days over the next 12 days; afterward may increase by 0.25 mg/day every 3 days. Range: 2–3 mg/day in 3 divided doses. Maximum: 5 mg/day.

CONTRAINDICATIONS

Hypersensitivity to pergolide or other ergot derivatives

INTERACTIONS

Drug

Haloperidol, loxapine, methyldopa, metoclopramide, phenothiazines: May decrease the effectiveness of pergolide.

Hypotension-producing medications: May increase the hypotensive effect.

Herbal

None known.

Food

None known.

Drug interactions of concern to dentistry

- Decreased action: phenothiazines, haloperidol, droperidol, thiothixenes, and metoclopramide

DIAGNOSTIC TEST EFFECTS

May increase the serum growth hormone level.

SIDE EFFECTS

Frequent (24%–10%)

Nausea, dizziness, hallucinations, constipation, rhinitis, dystonia, confusion, somnolence

Occasional (9%–3%)

Orthostatic hypotension, insomnia, dry mouth, peripheral edema, anxiety, diarrhea, dyspepsia, abdominal pain, headache, abnormal vision, anorexia, tremor, depression, rash

Rare (< 2%)

Urinary frequency, vivid dreams, neck pain, hypotension, vomiting

SERIOUS REACTIONS

! Symptoms of overdose may vary from CNS depression, characterized by sedation, apnea, cardiovascular collapse, and death, to severe paradoxical reactions, such as hallucinations, tremor, and seizures.

DENTAL CONSIDERATIONS

General:

- Monitor vital signs at every appointment because of CV side effects.
- Short appointments may be required because of disease effects on musculature.
- Use precaution if sedation or general anesthesia is required; risk of hypotensive episode.
- After supine positioning, have patient sit upright for at least 2 min before standing to avoid orthostatic hypotension.
- Assess salivary flow as a factor in caries, periodontal disease, and candidiasis.
- Assess for presence of extrapyramidal motor symptoms, such as tardive dyskinesia and akathisia.

P

Extrapyramidal motor activity may complicate dental treatment.
• Consider semisupine chair position for patient comfort because of GI effects of drug.

Consultations:
• Medical consultation may be required to assess disease control.

Teach Patient/Family:
• Use of electric toothbrush if patient has difficulty holding conventional devices
• Importance of updating health history/drug record if physician makes any changes in evaluation or drug regimens
• *When chronic dry mouth occurs, advise patient:*
  • To avoid mouth rinses with high alcohol content because of drying effects
  • Of need for daily use of home fluoride products to prevent caries
  • To use sugarless gum, frequent sips of water, or saliva substitutes

perindopril erbumine

per-in′-doh-pril
(Aceon)

CATEGORY AND SCHEDULE

Pregnancy Risk Category: C (D if used in second or third trimester)

MECHANISM OF ACTION

An ACE inhibitor that suppresses the renin-angiotensin-aldosterone system and prevents conversion of angiotensin I to angiotensin II, a potent vasoconstrictor; may also inhibit angiotensin II at local vascular and renal sites. ***Therapeutic Effect:*** Reduces peripheral arterial resistance and BP.

AVAILABILITY

Tablets: 2 mg, 4 mg, 8 mg.

INDICATIONS AND DOSAGES

▸ Hypertension

PO

Adults, Elderly. 2–8 mg/day as single dose or in 2 divided doses. Maximum: 16 mg/day.

OFF-LABEL USES

Management of heart failure

CONTRAINDICATIONS

History of angioedema from previous treatment with ACE inhibitors

INTERACTIONS

Drug

Alcohol, antihypertensives, diuretics: May increase the effects of perindopril.
Lithium: May increase lithium blood concentration and risk of lithium toxicity.
NSAIDs: May decrease the effects of perindopril.
Potassium-sparing diuretics, potassium supplements: May cause hyperkalemia.

Herbal

None known.

Food

None known.

Drug interactions of concern to dentistry

• Decreased hypotensive effects: NSAIDs, aspirin
• Increased hypotension: caution in use of other drugs that have hypotensive effects
• Suspected reduction in the antihypertensive and vasodilator effects by salicylates; monitor blood pressure if used concurrently

DIAGNOSTIC TEST EFFECTS

May increase BUN, serum alkaline phosphatase, serum bilirubin, serum creatinine, serum potassium, AST (SGOT), and ALT (SGPT) levels. May decrease serum sodium levels. May cause positive antinuclear antibody titer.

SIDE EFFECTS

Occasional (5%–1%)

Cough, back pain, sinusitis, upper extremity pain, dyspepsia, fever, palpitations, hypotension, dizziness, fatigue, syncope

SERIOUS REACTIONS

! Excessive hypotension ("first-dose syncope") may occur in patients with CHF and in those who are severely salt or volume depleted.
! Angioedema (swelling of face and lips) and hyperkalemia occur rarely.
! Agranulocytosis and neutropenia may be noted in those with collagen vascular disease, including scleroderma and systemic lupus erythematosus, and impaired renal function.
! Nephrotic syndrome may be noted in those with history of renal disease.

P

DENTAL CONSIDERATIONS

General:

- Monitor vital signs at every appointment because of CV side effects.
- Limit use of sodium-containing products, such as saline IV fluids, for patients with a dietary salt restriction.
- Short appointments and a stress reduction protocol may be required for anxious patients.
- Stress from dental procedures may compromise CV function; determine patient risk.
- After supine positioning, have patient sit upright for at least 2 min before standing to avoid orthostatic hypotension.
- Use precaution if sedation or general anesthesia is required; risk of hypotensive episode.
- Assess salivary flow as a factor in caries, periodontal disease, and candidiasis.
- Consider semisupine chair position for patient comfort if GI or respiratory side effects occur.
- Patients on chronic drug therapy may rarely have symptoms of blood dyscrasias, which can include infection, bleeding, and poor healing.

Consultations:

- In a patient with symptoms of blood dyscrasias, request a medical consultation for blood studies and postpone treatment until normal values are reestablished.
- Medical consultation may be required to assess disease control and patient's ability to tolerate stress.

Teach Patient/Family:

- Importance of updating health and drug history if physician makes any changes in evaluation or drug regimens
- Importance of good oral hygiene to prevent soft tissue inflammation
- To prevent trauma when using oral hygiene aids
- *When chronic dry mouth occurs, advise patient:*
  - To avoid mouth rinses with high alcohol content because of drying effects
  - To use daily home fluoride products for anticaries effect
  - To use sugarless gum, frequent sips of water, or saliva substitutes

perphenazine

per-fen′-ah-zeen
(Trilafon)
Do not confuse perphenazine with promazine.

CATEGORY AND SCHEDULE

Pregnancy Risk Category: C

MECHANISM OF ACTION

An antipsychotic agent and antiemetic that blocks postsynaptic dopamine receptor sites in the brain. ***Therapeutic Effect:*** Suppresses behavioral response in psychosis, and relieves nausea and vomiting.

AVAILABILITY

Oral Concentrate: 15 mg/5 ml.
Tablets: 2 mg, 4 mg, 8 mg, 16 mg.

INDICATIONS AND DOSAGES

▸ Severe Schizophrenia

PO
Adults. 4–16 mg 2–4 times/day. Maximum: 64 mg/day.
Elderly. Initially, 2–4 mg/day. May increase at 4–7 day intervals by 2–4 mg/day up to 32 mg/day.

▸ Severe Nausea and Vomiting

PO
Adults. 8–16 mg/day in divided doses up to 24 mg/day.

CONTRAINDICATIONS

Coma, myelosuppression, severe cardiovascular disease, severe CNS depression, subcortical brain damage

INTERACTIONS

Drug

Alcohol, other CNS depressants: May increase hypotensive effects and CNS and respiratory depression.
Antihypotensives: May increase the risk of hypotension.
Antithyroid agents: May increase the risk of agranulocytosis.
Extrapyramidal symptom–producing medications: May increase the severity and frequency of extrapyramidal symptoms.
Levodopa: May decrease the effects of this drug.
Lithium: May decrease perphenazine absorption and produce adverse neurologic effects.
MAOIs, tricyclic antidepressants: May increase anticholinergic and sedative effects.

Herbal

None known.

Food

Apple juice, caffeine- or tannic-containing beverages (such as tea): Don't mix oral concentrate with these beverages.

Drug interactions of concern to dentistry

- Increased sedation: other CNS depressants, alcohol, barbiturate anesthetics, opioid analgesics
- Hypotension, tachycardia: epinephrine
- Increased extrapyramidal effects: phenothiazines and related drugs (haloperidol, droperidol), metoclopramide
- Additive photosensitization: tetracyclines, fluoroquinolones
- Increased anticholinergic effects: anticholinergics

DIAGNOSTIC TEST EFFECTS

May produce false-positive pregnancy and phenylketonuria test results. May produce ECG changes, including prolonged QT and QTc intervals and T-wave depression or inversion.

IV INCOMPATIBILITIES

Aminophylline, cefoperazone (Cefobid), midazolam (Versed), opium alkaloids, oxytocin, pentobarbital (Nembutal), secobarbital (Seconal), thiopental (Pentothal)

IV COMPATIBILITIES

Atropine, chlorpromazine (Librium), dimenhydrinate (Dramamine), diphenhydramine (Benadryl), droperidol (Inapsine), fentanyl (Sublimaze), hydroxyzine (Vistaril), meperidine (Demerol), morphine, pentazocine (Talwin), prochlorperazine (Compazine), promethazine (Phenergan), ranitidine (Zantac), scopolamine (Transderm)

SIDE EFFECTS

Occasional

Marked photosensitivity, somnolence, dry mouth, blurred vision, lethargy, constipation or diarrhea, nasal congestion, peripheral edema, urine retention

Rare

Ocular changes, altered skin pigmentation, hypotension, dizziness, syncope

SERIOUS REACTIONS

! Extrapyramidal symptoms appear to be dose related and are divided into 3 categories: akathisia (characterized by inability to sit still, tapping of feet), parkinsonian symptoms (including masklike face, tremors, shuffling gait, hypersalivation), and acute dystonias (such as torticollis, opisthotonos, and oculogyric crisis).

! Tardive dyskinesia occurs rarely.

! Abrupt withdrawal after long-term therapy may precipitate nausea, vomiting, gastritis, dizziness, and tremors.

DENTAL CONSIDERATIONS

General:

- Monitor vital signs at every appointment because of CV side effects.
- Patients on chronic drug therapy may rarely have symptoms of blood dyscrasias, which can include infection, bleeding, and poor healing.
- After supine positioning, have patient sit upright for at least 2 min before standing to avoid orthostatic hypotension.
- Assess salivary flow as a factor in caries, periodontal disease, and candidiasis.
- Avoid dental light in patient's eyes; offer dark glasses for patient comfort.
- Assess for presence of extrapyramidal motor symptoms, such as tardive dyskinesia and akathisia. Extrapyramidal motor activity may complicate dental treatment.
- Geriatric patients are more susceptible to drug effects; use lower dose.
- Use vasoconstrictors with caution, in low doses, and with careful aspiration. Avoid use of gingival retraction cord with epinephrine.

Consultations:

- In a patient with symptoms of blood dyscrasias, request a medical consultation for blood studies and postpone dental treatment until normal values are reestablished.
- Take precautions if dental surgery is anticipated and anesthesia is required.
- If signs of tardive dyskinesia or akathisia are present, refer to physician.
- Physician should be informed if significant xerostomic side effects occur (e.g., increased caries, sore tongue, problems eating or swallowing, difficulty wearing prosthesis) so that a medication change can be considered.

Teach Patient/Family:

- Importance of good oral hygiene to prevent soft tissue inflammation
- Caution to prevent injury when using oral hygiene aids

P

- To use electric toothbrush if patient has difficulty holding conventional devices
- *When chronic dry mouth occurs, advise patient:*
  - To avoid mouth rinses with high alcohol content because of drying effects
  - Of need for daily use of home fluoride products to prevent caries
  - To use sugarless gum, frequent sips of water, or saliva substitutes

phenazopyridine hydrochloride

fen-az′-o-peer′-i-deen
(Azo-Gesic, Azo-Standard, Phenazo[CAN], Prodium, Pyridium, Uristat)
Do not confuse phenazopyridine with pyridoxine, or Prodium with Perdiem.

CATEGORY AND SCHEDULE

Pregnancy Risk Category: B

MECHANISM OF ACTION

An interstitial cystitis agent that exerts topical analgesic effect on urinary tract mucosa. ***Therapeutic Effect:*** Relieves urinary pain, burning, urgency, and frequency.

PHARMACOKINETICS

Well absorbed from the GI tract. Partially metabolized in the liver. Primarily excreted in urine.

AVAILABILITY

Tablets (Azo-Gesic, Azo-Standard, Prodium, Uristat): 100 mg, 200 mg.
Tablets (Pyridium): 95 mg.

INDICATIONS AND DOSAGES

▸ Urinary Analgesic

PO

Adults. 100–200 mg 3–4 times a day.
Children 6 yr and older. 12 mg/kg/day in 3 divided doses for 2 days.

▸ Dosage in Renal Impairment

Dosage interval is modified on the basis of creatinine clearance.

Creatinine Clearance	Interval
50–80 ml/min	Usual dose q8–16h
less than 50 ml/min	Avoid use.

CONTRAINDICATIONS

Hepatic or renal insufficiency

INTERACTIONS

Drug

None known.

Herbal

None known.

Food

None known.

DIAGNOSTIC TEST EFFECTS

May interfere with urinalysis tests based on color reactions, such as urinary glucose, ketones, protein, and 17-ketosteroids.

SIDE EFFECTS

Occasional

Headache, GI disturbance, rash, pruritus

SERIOUS REACTIONS

! Overdose may lead to hemolytic anemia, nephrotoxicity, or hepatotoxicity. Patients with renal impairment or severe hypersensitivity to the drug may also develop these reactions.

! A massive and acute overdose may result in methemoglobinemia.

DENTAL CONSIDERATIONS

General:

- Consider semisupine chair position for patient comfort if GI side effects occur.

• Patients on chronic drug therapy may rarely have symptoms of blood dyscrasias, which can include infection, bleeding, and poor healing.
• Be aware that patient might have UTI; question if antiinfectives are also being used.

phendimetrazine

fen-dye-me′-tra-zeen
Schedule IIISchedule IV
(Adipost, Bontril PDM, Bontril Slow-Release, Melfiat, Obezine, Phendiet, Phendiet-105, Plegine, Prelu-2)

CATEGORY AND SCHEDULE

Pregnancy Risk Category: C

MECHANISM OF ACTION

A phenylalkylamine sympathomimetic with activity similar to amphetamines that stimulates the central nervous system (CNS) and elevates blood pressure (B/P) most likely mediated via norepinephrine and dopamine metabolism. Causes stimulation of the hypothalamus. ***Therapeutic Effect:*** Decreases appetite.

PHARMACOKINETICS

The pharmacokinetics of phendimetrazine tartrate has not been well established. Metabolized to active metabolite, phendimetrazine. Excreted in urine. ***Half-life:*** 2-4 hrs.

AVAILABILITY

Tablets:. 35 mg (Bontril PDM, Obezine, Phendiet, Plegine)
Capsules (extended-release): 105 mg (Adipost, Bontril Slow-Release, Melfiat, Phendiet-105, Prelu-2).

INDICATIONS AND DOSAGES

▸ **Obesity**

PO

Adults, Elderly. 105 mg/day in the morning or before the morning meal (sustained-release); 35 mg 2–3 times/day (immediate-release). Maximum: 70 mg 3 times/day.

CONTRAINDICATIONS

Advanced arteriosclerosis, agitated states, glaucoma, history of drug abuse, history of hypersensitivity to sympathomimetic amines, hyperthyroidism, moderate to severe hypertension, symptomatic cardiovascular disease, use within 14 days of discontinuation MAOI, hypersensitivity to phendimetrazine or sympathomimetics

INTERACTIONS

Drug

Guanethidine: May decrease hypotensive effect of guanethidine.
MAOIs: May increase risk of hypertensive crisis.
Sibutramine: May increase risk of hypertension and tachycardia.
Tricyclic antidepressants: May increase cardiovascular effects.

Herbal

None known.

Food

None known.

Drug interactions of concern to dentistry

• Hypertensive crisis: MAOIs or within 14 days of MAOIs
• Increased risk of dysrhythmia: hydrocarbon inhalation general anesthetics
• Decreased effect: tricyclic antidepressants, ascorbic acid, phenothiazines
• Caffeine or caffeine-containing products: may increase risk of insomnia and dry mouth

DIAGNOSTIC TEST EFFECTS

None known.

SIDE EFFECTS

Occasional

Constipation, nausea, diarrhea, dry mouth, dysuria, libido changes, flushing, hypertension, insomnia, nervousness, headache, dizziness, irritability, agitation, restlessness, palpitations, increased heart rate, sweating, tremor, urticaria

SERIOUS REACTIONS

! Multivalvular heart disease, primary pulmonary hypertension, and arrhythmias occur rarely.
! Overdose may produce flushing, arrhythmias, and psychosis.
! Abrupt withdrawal following prolonged administration of high doses may produce extreme fatigue and depression.

DENTAL CONSIDERATIONS

General:

- Monitor vital signs at every appointment because of CV side effects.
- Assess salivary flow as a factor in caries, periodontal disease, and candidiasis.
- Determine why the patient is taking the drug.
- Psychologic and physical dependence may occur with chronic administration.
- Patients on chronic drug therapy may rarely have symptoms of blood dyscrasias, which can include infection, bleeding, and poor healing.

Consultations:

- In a patient with symptoms of blood dyscrasias, request a medical consultation for blood studies and postpone dental treatment until normal values are reestablished.

Teach Patient/Family:

- Importance of good oral hygiene to prevent soft tissue inflammation
- To report oral lesions, soreness, or bleeding to dentist
- Caution to prevent injury when using oral hygiene aids
- *When chronic dry mouth occurs, advise patient:*
  - To avoid mouth rinses with high alcohol content because of drying effects
  - Of need for daily use of home fluoride products to prevent caries
  - To use sugarless gum, frequent sips of water, or saliva substitutes

phenelzine sulfate

fen-az-o-peer′-i-deen
(Nardil)

CATEGORY AND SCHEDULE

Pregnancy Risk Category: C

P

MECHANISM OF ACTION

An MAOI that inhibits the activity of the enzyme monoamine oxidase at CNS storage sites, leading to increased levels of the neurotransmitters epinephrine, norepinephrine, serotonin, and dopamine at neuronal receptor sites. ***Therapeutic Effect:*** Relieves depression.

PHARMACOKINETICS

Well absorbed from GI tract. Metabolized in the liver. Primarily excreted in urine. ***Half-life:*** 1.2 hr.

AVAILABILITY

Tablets: 15 mg.

INDICATIONS AND DOSAGES

▸ Depression Refractory to Other Antidepressants or Electroconvulsive Therapy

PO

Adults. 15 mg 3 times a day. May increase to 60–90 mg/day.
Elderly. Initially, 7.5 mg/day. May increase by 7.5–15 mg/day q3–4wk up to 60 mg/day in divided doses.

OFF-LABEL USES

Treatment of panic disorder, selective mutism, vascular or tension headaches

CONTRAINDICATIONS

Cardiovascular or cerebrovascular disease, hepatic or renal impairment, pheochromocytoma

INTERACTIONS

Drug

Alcohol, other CNS depressants: May increase CNS depression.
Buspirone: May increase BP.
Caffeine-containing medications: May increase the risk of cardiac arrhythmias and hypertension.
Carbamazepine, cyclobenzaprine, maprotiline, other MAOIs: May precipitate hypertensive crisis.
Dopamine, tryptophan: May cause sudden, severe hypertension.
Fluoxetine, trazodone, tricyclic antidepressants: May cause serotonin syndrome.
Insulin, oral antidiabetics: May increase the effects of these drugs.
Meperidine, other opioid analgesics: May produce diaphoresis, immediate excitation, rigidity, and severe hypertension or hypotension, sometimes leading to severe respiratory distress, vascular collapse, seizures, coma, and death.
Methylphenidate: May increase the CNS stimulant effects of methylphenidate.
Sympathomimetics: May increase the cardiac stimulant and vasopressor effects of phenelzine.

Herbal

None known.

Food

Caffeine, chocolate, tyramine-containing foods (such as aged cheese): May cause sudden, severe hypertension.

Drug interactions of concern to dentistry

- Increased anticholinergic effect: anticholinergics, haloperidol, phenothiazines, antihistamines
- Hyperpyretic crisis, convulsions, hypertensive episode: meperidine, carbamazepine, cyclobenzaprine
- Cardiac dysrhythmia: caffeine-containing medications
- Increased risk of serotonin syndrome: tricyclic antidepressants, other serotonin reuptake inhibitors
- Increased sedative effects of alcohol, barbiturates, benzodiazepines, CNS depressants
- Increased pressor effects: indirect-acting sympathomimetics, such as ephedrine, amphetamine

DIAGNOSTIC TEST EFFECTS

None known.

SIDE EFFECTS

Frequent

Orthostatic hypotension, restlessness, GI upset, insomnia, dizziness, headache, lethargy, asthenia, dry mouth, peripheral edema

Occasional

Flushing, diaphoresis, rash, urinary frequency, increased appetite, transient impotence

Rare

Visual disturbances

SERIOUS REACTIONS

! Hypertensive crisis occurs rarely and is marked by severe hypertension,

P

occipital headache radiating frontally, neck stiffness or soreness, nausea, vomiting, diaphoresis, fever or chilliness, clammy skin, dilated pupils, palpitations, tachycardia or bradycardia, and constricting chest pain.

! Intracranial bleeding has been reported in association with severe hypertension.

DENTAL CONSIDERATIONS

General:

- Monitor vital signs at every appointment because of CV side effects.
- Assess salivary flow as a factor in caries, periodontal disease, and candidiasis.
- After supine positioning, have patient sit upright for at least 2 min before standing to avoid orthostatic hypotension.
- Hypertensive episodes are possible even though there are no specific contraindications to vasoconstrictor use in local anesthetics.
- Avoid prescribing caffeine-containing products.
- Take precautions if dental surgery is anticipated and general anesthesia is required.

Consultations:

- Medical consultation may be required to assess disease control and patient's ability to tolerate stress.

Teach Patient/Family:

- To use electric toothbrush if patient has difficulty holding conventional devices
- *When chronic dry mouth occurs, advise patient:*
  - To avoid mouth rinses with high alcohol content because of drying effects
  - Of need for daily use of home fluoride products to prevent caries
  - To use sugarless gum, frequent sips of water, or saliva substitutes

phenobarbital

fee-noe-bar′-bi-tal

Schedule IV

(Luminal, Phenobarbitone[AUS])

Do not confuse phenobarbital with pentobarbital, or Luminal with Tuinal.

CATEGORY AND SCHEDULE

Pregnancy Risk Category: D

Controlled Substance Schedule IV

MECHANISM OF ACTION

A barbiturate that enhances the activity of gamma-aminobutyric acid (GABA) by binding to the GABA receptor complex. ***Therapeutic Effect:*** Depresses CNS activity.

PHARMACOKINETICS

Route	Onset	Peak	Duration
PO	20–60 min	N/A	6–10 hr
IV	5 min	30 min	4–10 hr

Well absorbed after PO or parenteral administration. Protein binding: 35%–50%. Rapidly and widely distributed. Metabolized in the liver. Primarily excreted in urine. Removed by hemodialysis. ***Half-life:*** 53–118 hr.

AVAILABILITY

Elixir: 20 mg/5 ml.

Tablets: 30 mg, 100 mg.

Injection: 60 mg/ml, 130 mg/ml.

INDICATIONS AND DOSAGES

▸ Status Epilepticus

IV

Adults, Elderly, Children, Neonates. Loading dose of 15–20 mg/kg as a single dose or in divided doses.

▸ **Seizure Control**
PO, IV
Adults, Elderly, Children older than 12 yr. 1–3 mg/kg/day.
Children 6–12 yr. 4–6 mg/kg/day.
Children 1–5 yr. 6–8 mg/kg/day.
Children younger than 1 yr. 5–6 mg/kg/day.
Neonates. 3–4 mg/kg/day.
▸ **Sedation**
PO, IM
Adults, Elderly. 30–120 mg/day in 2–3 divided doses.
Children. 2 mg/kg 3 times a day.
▸ **Hypnotic**
PO, IV, IM, Subcutaneous
Adults, Elderly. 100–320 mg at bedtime.
Children. 3–5 mg/kg at bedtime.

OFF-LABEL USES

Prevention and treatment of hyperbilirubinemia

CONTRAINDICATIONS

Porphyria, preexisting CNS depression, severe pain, severe respiratory disease

P

INTERACTIONS

Drug

Alcohol, other CNS depressants: May increase the effects of phenobarbital.
Carbamazepine: May increase the metabolism of carbamazepine.
Digoxin, glucocorticoids, metronidazole, oral anticoagulants, quinidine, tricyclic antidepressants: May decrease the effects of these drugs.
Valproic acid: Increases the blood concentration and risk of toxicity of phenobarbital.

Herbal

None known.

Food

None known.

Drug interactions of concern to dentistry

- Increased effects: alcohol, all CNS depressants, saquinavir
- Decreased effects of corticosteroids, doxycycline, carbamazepine

DIAGNOSTIC TEST EFFECTS

May decrease serum bilirubin level. Therapeutic serum level is 10–40 mcg/ml; toxic serum level is greater than 40 mcg/ml.

IV INCOMPATIBILITIES

Amphotericin B complex (Abelcet, AmBisome, Amphotec), hydrocortisone (Solu-Cortef), hydromorphone (Dilaudid), insulin

IV COMPATIBILITIES

Calcium gluconate, enalapril (Vasotec), fentanyl (Sublimaze), fosphenytoin (Cerebyx), morphine, propofol (Diprivan)

SIDE EFFECTS

Occasional (3%–1%)
Somnolence
Rare (< 1%)
Confusion; paradoxical CNS reactions, such as hyperactivity or nervousness in children and excitement or restlessness in the elderly (generally noted during first 2 weeks of therapy, particularly in presence of uncontrolled pain)

SERIOUS REACTIONS

! Abrupt withdrawal after prolonged therapy may produce increased dreaming, nightmares, insomnia, tremor, diaphoresis, and vomiting, hallucinations, delirium, seizures, and status epilepticus.
! Skin eruptions may be a sign of a hypersensitivity reaction.
! Blood dyscrasias, hepatic disease, and hypocalcemia occur rarely.

! Overdose produces cold or clammy skin, hypothermia, severe CNS depression, cyanosis, tachycardia, and Cheyne-Stokes respirations.
! Toxicity may result in severe renal impairment.

DENTAL CONSIDERATIONS

General:

- Determine why the patient is taking the drug.
- Monitor vital signs at every appointment because of CV side effects. Evaluate respiration characteristics and rate.
- Patients on chronic drug therapy may rarely have symptoms of blood dyscrasias, which can include infection, bleeding, and poor healing.
- *When used for sedation in dentistry:*
  - Assess vital signs before use and q30min after use as sedative.
  - Observe respiratory dysfunction: respiratory depression, character, rate, rhythm; hold drug if respirations are <10/min or if pupils are dilated.
- After supine positioning, have patient sit upright for at least 2 min before standing to avoid orthostatic hypotension.
- Have someone drive patient to and from dental office when drug used for conscious sedation.
- Barbiturates induce liver microsomal enzymes, which alter the metabolism of other drugs.
- Geriatric patients are more susceptible to drug effects; use lower dose.

Consultations:

- In a patient with symptoms of blood dyscrasias, request a medical consultation for blood studies and postpone dental treatment until normal values are reestablished.

Teach Patient/Family:

- To avoid driving or other activities requiring alertness
- To avoid alcohol ingestion or CNS depressants; serious CNS depression may result
- To use OTC preparations with caution because they may contain other CNS depressants (e.g., antihistamines, cold remedies)

phenoxybenzamine

fen-ox-ee-ben′-za-meen
(Dibenzyline)

CATEGORY AND SCHEDULE

Pregnancy Risk Category: C

MECHANISM OF ACTION

An antihypertensive that produces long-lasting noncompetitive alpha-adrenergic blockade of postganglionic synapses in exocrine glands and smooth muscles. Relaxes urethra and increases opening of the bladder.
Therapeutic Effect: Controls hypertension.

PHARMACOKINETICS

Well absorbed from the gastrointestinal (GI) tract. Distributed into fatty tissue. Metabolized in liver. Eliminated in urine and feces. Not removed by hemodialysis. ***Half-life:*** 24 hours.

AVAILABILITY

Tablets: 10 mg (Dibenzyline).

INDICATIONS AND DOSAGES

▸ **Pheochromocytoma**

PO

Adults. Initially, 10 mg twice daily. May increase dose every other day to 20–40 mg 2–3 times/day

P

Children. 1–2 mg/kg/day in divided doses.

OFF-LABEL USES

Bladder instability, complex regional pain syndrome (CRPS), contraception, prostatic obstruction, Raynaud's disease

CONTRAINDICATIONS

Any condition compromised by hypotension, hypersensitivity to phenoxybenzamine or any component of the formulation

INTERACTIONS

Drug

Beta-blockers (used concurrently): May increase risk of toxicity (hypotension, tachycardia.

Hypotensive-producing medications: May increase the effects of phenoxybenzamine.

Alpha-adrenergic agonists: May decrease the effects of phenoxybenzamine.

Herbal

Licorice, Ma huang, yohimbine: May decrease the effects of phenoxybenzamine.

Food

None known.

Drug interactions of concern to dentistry

- Exaggerated hypotension, tachycardia: epinephrine, other β-adrenergic agonists

DIAGNOSTIC TEST EFFECTS

None known.

SIDE EFFECTS

Frequent

Headache, lethargy, confusion, fatigue

Occasional

Nausea, postural hypotension, syncope, dry mouth

Rare

Palpitations, diarrhea, constipation, inhibition of ejaculation, weakness, altered vision, dizziness

SERIOUS REACTIONS

! Overdosage produces severe hypotension, irritability, lethargy, tachycardia, dizziness and shock.

DENTAL CONSIDERATIONS

General:

- Medication may be used in anticipation of surgery to remove the adrenal tumor.
- Hypertension may preclude all dental care except for palliative emergency treatment.
- Question patient about compliance with drug therapy.
- Risk of increased CNS depression when other CNS depressants are used.
- Determine why patient is taking the drug.
- Monitor and record vital signs.
- Use vasoconstrictor with caution, in low doses, and with careful aspiration. Avoid using gingival retraction cord containing epinephrine.
- After supine positioning, have patient sit upright for at least 2 min before standing to avoid orthostatic hypotension.

Consultations:

- Medical consultation may be required to assess disease control and patient's ability to tolerate stress.

Teach Patient/Family:

- Importance of good oral hygiene to prevent soft tissue inflammation
- Caution patients about driving or performing other tasks requiring mental alertness

phentermine

Schedule IV
(Adipex-P, Fastin, Ionamin, Oby-Cap, Phentercot, Pro-Fast HS, Pro-Fast SA, Pro-Fast SR, T-Diet, Teramine, Zantryl)

CATEGORY AND SCHEDULE

Pregnancy Risk Category: B
Controlled substance: Schedule IV

MECHANISM OF ACTION

A sympathomimetic amine structurally similar to dextroamphetamine and is most likely mediated via norephinephrine and dopamine metabolism. Causes stimulation of the hypothalamus.
Therapeutic Effect: Decreased appetite.

PHARMACOKINETICS

Well absorbed from the gastrointestinal (GI) tract; resin absorbed slower. Excreted unchanged in urine.
Half-life: 20 hrs.

AVAILABILITY

Capsules (as hydrochloride): 15 mg, 18.75 mg, 30 mg (Fastin), 37.5 mg (Adipex-P).
Capsules (as resin complex): 15 mg (Ionamin), 30 mg (Ionamin).
Tablets (as hydrochloride): 8 mg, 37.5 mg (Adipex-P).

INDICATIONS AND DOSAGES

▸ Obesity

PO

Adults, Children older than 16 yrs.
Adipex-P: 37.5 mg as a single daily dose or in divided doses.
Ionamin: 15–37.5 mg/day before breakfast or 1–2 hrs. after breakfast.
Fastin: 30 mg/day taken in the morning.

CONTRAINDICATIONS

Advanced arteriosclerosis, agitated states, cardiovascular disease, concurrent use or within 14 days of discontinuation of MAOI therapy, glaucoma, history of drug abuse, hypertension (moderate-to-severe), hyperthyroidism, hypersensitivity to phentermine or sympathomimetic amines

INTERACTIONS

Drug

Fenfluramine: May increase risk of pulmonary hypertension and valvular heart disease.
MAOIs: May increase risk of hypertensive crisis (headache, hyperpyrexia, hypertension).
Sibutramine: May increase risk of hypertension and tachycardia.

Herbal

None known.

Food

None known.

Drug interactions of concern to dentistry

- Hypertensive crisis: MAOIs or within 14 days of MAOIs
- Increased risk of dysrhythmia: hydrocarbon inhalation general anesthetics
- Decreased effect: tricyclic antidepressants, ascorbic acid, phenothiazines
- Caffeine or caffeine-containing products may increase risk of insomnia

DIAGNOSTIC TEST EFFECTS

May interfere and give false-positive amphetamine EMIT assay result.

SIDE EFFECTS

Occasional

Restlessness, insomnia, tremor, palpitations, tachycardia, elevation in blood pressure, headache, dizziness, dry mouth, unpleasant taste, diarrhea or constipation, changes in libido

SERIOUS REACTIONS

! Primary pulmonary hypertension (PPH), psychotic episodes, and valvular heart disease rarely occur.
! Anorectic agents have been associated with regurgitant multivalvular heart disease involving mitral, aortic, and/or tricuspid valves.
! Prolonged use may cause physical or psychological dependence.

DENTAL CONSIDERATIONS

General:

- Monitor vital signs at every appointment because of CV side effects.
- Assess salivary flow as a factor in caries, periodontal disease, and candidiasis.
- Determine why the patient is taking the drug.
- Psychologic and physical dependence may occur with chronic administration.
- Patients on chronic drug therapy may rarely have symptoms of blood dyscrasias, which can include infection, bleeding, and poor healing.

P

Consultations:

- In a patient with symptoms of blood dyscrasias, request a medical consultation for blood studies and postpone dental treatment until normal values are reestablished.

Teach Patient/Family:

- Importance of good oral hygiene to prevent soft tissue inflammation
- To prevent injury when using oral hygiene aids
- To report oral lesions, soreness, or bleeding to dentist
- *When chronic dry mouth occurs, advise patient:*
  - To avoid mouth rinses with high alcohol content because of drying effects
  - Of need for daily use of home fluoride products to prevent caries
  - To use sugarless gum, frequent sips of water, or saliva substitutes

phentolamine

fen-tole′-a-meen
(Regitine)

CATEGORY AND SCHEDULE

Pregnancy Risk Category: C

MECHANISM OF ACTION

An alpha-adrenergic blocking agent which produces peripheral vasodilation and cardiac stimulation.
Therapeutic Effect: Decreases blood pressure (B/P).

PHARMACOKINETICS

Poorly absorbed from the gastrointestinal (GI) tract. Protein binding: 72%. Metabolized in liver. Eliminated in urine and feces. Not removed by hemodialysis. ***Half-life:*** 19 min.

AVAILABILITY

Injection: 5 mg/ml (Regitine).

INDICATIONS AND DOSAGES

▸ Extravasation - Norepinephrine

SC

Adults, Elderly. Infiltrate area with a small amount (1 ml) of solution (made by diluting 5–10 mg in 10 ml of NS) within 12 hours of extravasation. Do not exceed 0.1–0.2 mg/kg or 5 mg total. If dose is effective, normal skin color should return to the blanched area within 1 hour.

Children. Infiltrate area with a small amount (1 ml) of solution (made by diluting 5–10 mg in 10 ml of NS) within 12 hours of extravasation.

Do not exceed 0.1–0.2 mg/kg or 5 mg total.

▸ **Diagnosis of Pheochromocytoma**

IM/IV

Adults, Elderly. 5 mg as a single dose.

Children. 0.05–0.1 mg/kg/dose. Maximum single dose: 5 mg.

▸ **Surgery for Pheochromocytoma: Hypertension**

IM/IV

Adults, Elderly. 5 mg given 1–2 hours before procedure and repeated as needed every 2-4 hours.

Children. 0.05–0.1 mg/kg/dose given 1–2 hours before procedure. Repeat as needed every 2-4 hours until hypertension is controlled. Maximum single dose: 5 mg.

▸ **Hypertensive Crisis**

IV

Adults, Elderly. 5–20 mg as a single dose.

OFF-LABEL USES

Treatment of pralidoxime-induced hypertension, arrhythmias, asthma, bladder instability, cardiac diseases, diabetes mellitus, erectile dysfunction, extravasation (dopamine and epinephrine), hyperhidrosis, myocardial infarction, Raynaud's phenomenon, surgery, sympathetic pain

CONTRAINDICATIONS

Renal impairment, coronary or cerebral arteriosclerosis, concurrent use with phosphodiesterase-5 (PDE-5) inhibitors including sildenafil (>25 mg), tadalafil, or vardenafil, hypersensitivity to phentolamine or related compounds.

INTERACTIONS

Drug

Alcohol: May increase the risk of disulfiram-type reactions.

Beta-blockers: May exaggerate hypotensive effects.

Epinephrine, ephedrine: May decrease the effects of phentolamine

Sildenafil, tadalafil, vardenafil: May increase blood pressure-lowering effects.

Herbal

None known.

Food

None known.

Drug interactions of concern to dentistry

- Hypotension, tachycardia: epinephrine
- Decreased pressor effects of epinephrine, ephedrine

DIAGNOSTIC TEST EFFECTS

May increase liver function tests.

IV INCOMPATIBILITIES

Iron

IV COMPATIBILITIES

Amiodarone (Cordarone), dobutamine (Dobutrex), norepinephrine (Levophed), papaverine (Papacon), verapamil

SIDE EFFECTS

Occasional

Hypotension, tachycardia, arrhythmia, flushing, orthostatic hypotension, weakness, dizziness, nausea, vomiting, diarrhea, nasal congestion, pulmonary hypertension

SERIOUS REACTIONS

! Symptoms of overdosage include tachycardia, shock, vomiting, and dizziness.

! Mixed agents, such as epinephrine, may cause more hypotension.

DENTAL CONSIDERATIONS

General:

- This is an acute-use drug; hypertension and pheochromocytoma are the immediate concerns.

P

- Patients with untreated pheochromocytoma or with extreme, uncontrolled hypertension are not candidates for elective dental treatment. Physician consultation is required.
- Short appointments and a stress reduction protocol may be required for anxious patients.
- Stress from dental procedures may compromise CV function; determine patient risk.
- Use vasoconstrictors with caution, in low doses, and with careful aspiration. Avoid use of gingival retraction cord with epinephrine.
- Assess vital signs at each appointment because of nature of disease.

Consultations:

- Medical consultation may be required to assess disease control and patient's ability to tolerate stress

phenylephrine hydrochloride

fen-ill-eh′-frin

(AK-Dilate, AD-Nephrin, Isopto Frin[AUS], Mydfrin, Neo-Synephrine, Neo-Synephrine Ophthalmic Viscous 10%[AUS], Prefrin)

CATEGORY AND SCHEDULE

Pregnancy Risk Category: C

OTC (nasal solution, nasal spray, ophthalmic solution)

MECHANISM OF ACTION

A sympathomimetic, alpha receptor stimulant that acts on the alpha-adrenergic receptors of vascular smooth muscle. Causes vasoconstriction of arterioles of nasal mucosa or conjunctiva, activates dilator muscle of the pupil to cause contraction, produces systemic arterial vasoconstriction. ***Therapeutic Effect:*** Decreases mucosal blood flow and relieves congestion and increases systolic BP.

PHARMACOKINETICS

Route	Onset	Peak	Duration
IV	Immediate	N/A	15–20 min
IM	10–15 min	N/A	0.5–2 hr
Subcutaneous	10–15 min	N/A	1 hr

Minimal absorption after intranasal and ophthalmic administration. Metabolized in the liver and GI tract. Primarily excreted in urine. ***Half-life:*** 2.5 hr.

AVAILABILITY

Injection: 1% (10 mg/ml).
Nasal Solution Drops (Neosynephrine): 0.5%, 1%.
Nasal Spray (Neosynephrine): 0.25%, 0.5%, 1%.
Ophthalmic Solution (Ak-Nephrin): 0.12%.
Ophthalmic Solution (AK-Dilate): 2.5%, 10%.
Ophthalmic Solution (Mydfrin, Neosynephrine): 2.5%.

INDICATIONS AND DOSAGES

▸ **Nasal Decongestant**

Nasal Spray, Nasal Solution

Adults, Elderly, Children 12 yr and older. 2–3 drops or 1–2 sprays of 0.25%–0.5% solution into each nostril.

Children 6–11 yr. 2–3 drops or 1–2 sprays of 0.25% solution into each nostril.

Children younger than 6 yr. 2–3 drops of 0.125% solution (dilute 0.5% solution with 0.9% NaCl to achieve 0.125%) in each nostril. Repeat q4h as needed. Do not use for more than 3 days.

▸ Conjunctival Congestion, Itching, and Minor Irritation; Whitening of Sclera
OPHTHALMIC
Adults, Elderly, Children 12 yr and older. 1–2 drops of 0.12% solution q3–4h.
▸ Hypotension, Shock
IM, SUBCUTANEOUS
Adults, Elderly. 2–5 mg/dose q1–2h.
Children. 0.1 mg/kg/dose q1–2h.
IV BOLUS
Adults, Elderly. 0.1–0.5 mg/dose q10–15min as needed.
Children. 5–20 mcg/kg/dose q10–15min.
IV INFUSION
Adults, Elderly. 100–180 mcg/min.
Children. 0.1–0.5 mcg/kg/min. Titrate to desired effect.

CONTRAINDICATIONS

Acute pancreatitis, heart disease, hepatitis, narrow-angle glaucoma, pheochromocytoma, severe hypertension, thrombosis, ventricular tachycardia

INTERACTIONS

Drug

Beta blockers: May have mutually inhibitory effects.
Digoxin: May increase risk of arrhythmias.
Ergonovine, oxytocin: May increase vasoconstriction.
MAOIs: May increase vasopressor effects.
Maprotiline, tricyclic antidepressants: May increase cardiovascular effects.
Methyldopa: May decrease effects of methyldopa.

Herbal

None known.

Food

None known.

Drug interactions of concern to dentistry

- None reported with normal topical use
- *With systemic absorption, risk of:*
  - Bradycardia: β-adrenergic blockers
  - Increased dysrhythmias and hypertension: tricyclic antidepressants

DIAGNOSTIC TEST EFFECTS

None known.

IV INCOMPATIBILITIES

Thiopentothal (Pentothal)

IV COMPATIBILITIES

Amiodarone (Cordarone), dobutamine (Dobutrex), lidocaine, potassium chloride, propofol (Diprivan)

SIDE EFFECTS

Frequent

Nasal: Rebound nasal congestion due to overuse, especially when used longer than 3 days

Occasional

Mild CNS stimulation (restlessness, nervousness, tremors, headache, insomnia, particularly in those hypersensitive to sympathomimetics, such as elderly patients)
Nasal: Stinging, burning, drying of nasal mucosa
Ophthalmic: Transient burning or stinging, brow ache, blurred vision

SERIOUS REACTIONS

! Large doses may produce tachycardia and palpitations (particularly in those with cardiac disease), light-headedness, nausea, and vomiting.
! Overdose in those older than 60 years may result in hallucinations, CNS depression, and seizures.

! Prolonged nasal use may produce chronic swelling of nasal mucosa and rhinitis.

DENTAL CONSIDERATIONS

General:

- Consider semisupine chair position for patient comfort because of respiratory effects of disease.
- Assess salivary flow as a factor in caries, periodontal disease, and candidiasis.
- Patients with significant nasal congestion may complicate nasal administration of nitrous oxide/oxygen sedation.

Teach Patient/Family:

- That this product is not indicated for prolonged use because of congestion rebound; however, this may not always be the case

phenylephrine hydrochloride; sulfacetamide sodium

fen-ill-eh′-frin hye-droh-klor′-ide; sul-fa-see′-ta-mide soe′-dee-um
(Vasosulf)

CATEGORY AND SCHEDULE

Pregnancy Risk Category: C

MECHANISM OF ACTION

Phenylephrine is a sympathomimetic that acts on alpha-adrenergic receptors of vascular smooth muscle. Sulfacetamide is a sulfonamide that interferes with synthesis of folic acid that bacteria require for growth.
Therapeutic Effect: Increases systolic/diastolic blood pressure (B/P), produces constriction of blood vessels, conjunctival arterioles, nasal arterioles. Prevents bacterial growth.

PHARMACOKINETICS

Minimal absorption following ophthalmic administration.

AVAILABILITY

Ophthalmic Solution: 0.125% phenylephrine hydrochloride and 15% sulfacetamide sodium (Vasosulf).

INDICATIONS AND DOSAGES

▸ **Topical Application to Conjunctiva That Relieves Congestion, Itching, Minor Irritation; Whitens Sclera of Eye**

OPHTHALMIC

Adults, Elderly, Children 12 yrs and older. Instill 1–2 drops of q3–4h.

CONTRAINDICATIONS

Angle-closure glaucoma, those with soft contact lenses, hypersensitivity to phenylephrine, sulfacetamide, or any component of the formulation

INTERACTIONS

Drug

None known.

Herbal

None known.

Food

None known.

Drug interactions of concern to dentistry

- None reported with normal topical use
- *With systemic absorption, risk of:*
  - Bradycardia: β-adrenergic blockers
  - Increased dysrhythmias and hypertension: tricyclic antidepressants

DIAGNOSTIC TEST EFFECTS

None known.

SIDE EFFECTS

Occasional

Transient burning/stinging, brow ache, blurred vision

SERIOUS REACTIONS

! None reported.

DENTAL CONSIDERATIONS

General:

- Consider semisupine chair position for patient comfort because of respiratory effects of disease.
- Assess salivary flow as a factor in caries, periodontal disease, and candidiasis.
- Patients with significant nasal congestion may complicate nasal administration of nitrous oxide/oxygen sedation.

Teach Patient/Family:

- That this product is not indicated for prolonged use because of congestion rebound; however, this may not always be the case

physostigmine

fi-zoe-stig′-meen

(Antilirium)

Do not confuse physostigmine with Prostigmin or pyridostigmine.

CATEGORY AND SCHEDULE

Pregnancy Risk Category: C

MECHANISM OF ACTION

A cholinergic that inhibits destruction of acetylcholine by enzyme acetylcholinesterase, thus enhancing impulse transmission across the myoneural junction. ***Therapeutic Effect:*** Improves skeletal muscle tone, stimulates salivary and sweat gland secretions.

AVAILABILITY

Injection: 1 mg/ml.

INDICATIONS AND DOSAGES

▸ To Reverse CNS Effects of Anticholinergic Drugs and Tricyclic Antidepressants

IV, IM

Adults, Elderly. Initially, 0.5–2 mg. If no response, repeat q20min until response or adverse cholinergic effects occur. If initial response occurs, may give additional doses of 1–4 mg q30–60min as life-threatening signs, such as arrhythmias, seizures, and deep coma, recur.

Children. 0.01–0.03 mg/kg. May give additional doses q5–10min until response or adverse cholinergic effects occur or total dose of 2 mg given.

OFF-LABEL USES

Treatment of hereditary ataxia

CONTRAINDICATIONS

Active uveal inflammation, angle-closure glaucoma before iridectomy, asthma, cardiovascular disease, concurrent use of ganglionic-blocking agents, diabetes, gangrene, glaucoma associated with iridocyclitis, hypersensitivity to cholinesterase inhibitors or their components, mechanical obstruction of intestinal or urogenital tract, vagotonic state

INTERACTIONS

Drug

Cholinesterase agents, including bethanechol and carbachol: May increase the effects of these drugs.

Succinylcholine: May prolong the action of succinylcholine.

Herbal

None known.

Food

None known.

Drug interactions of concern to dentistry

- Contraindicated: succinylcholine

DIAGNOSTIC TEST EFFECTS

None known.

SIDE EFFECTS

Expected

Miosis, increased GI and skeletal muscle tone, bradycardia

Occasional

Marked drop in BP (hypertensive patients)

Rare

Allergic reaction

SERIOUS REACTIONS

! Parenteral overdose produces a cholinergic crisis manifested as abdominal discomfort or cramps, nausea, vomiting, diarrhea, flushing, facial warmth, excessive salivation, diaphoresis, urinary urgency, and blurred vision. If overdose occurs, stop all anticholinergic drugs and immediately administer 0.6–1.2 mg atropine sulfate IM or IV for adults, or 0.01 mg/kg for infants and children younger than 12 years.

DENTAL CONSIDERATIONS

General:

- For acute use in hospitals and emergency rooms

Teach Patient/Family:

- To avoid driving at night or participating in activities requiring visual acuity in the presence of dim lighting

P

pilocarpine hydrochloride

pye-loe-kar′-peen

(Isopto Carpin[AUS], Ocusert Pilo-20[AUS], Ocusert Pilo-40 [AUS], Pilopt Eye Drops[AUS], P.V. Carpine Liquifilm Ophthalmic Solution[AUS], Salagen)

CATEGORY AND SCHEDULE

Pregnancy Risk Category: C

MECHANISM OF ACTION

A cholinergic that increases exocrine gland secretions by stimulating cholinergic receptors.

Therapeutic Effect: Improves symptoms of dry mouth in patients with salivary gland hypofunction.

PHARMACOKINETICS

Route	Onset	Peak	Duration
PO	20 min	1 hr	3–5 hrs

Absorption decreased if taken with a high-fat meal. Inactivation of pilocarpine thought to occur at neuronal synapses and probably in plasma. Excreted in urine. ***Half-life:*** 4–12 hr.

AVAILABILITY

Tablets: 5 mg.

INDICATIONS AND DOSAGES

▸ **Dry Mouth Associated with Radiation Treatment for Head and Neck Cancer**

PO

Adults, Elderly. 5 mg three times a day. Range: 15–30 mg/day. Maximum: 2 tablets/dose.

▸ **Dry Mouth Associated with Sjögren's Syndrome**

PO

Adults, Elderly. 5 mg four times a day. Range: 20–40 mg/day.

▸ **Dosage in Hepatic Impairment**

Dosage decreased to 5 mg twice a day for adults and elderly with hepatic impairment.

CONTRAINDICATIONS

Conditions in which miosis is undesirable, such as acute iritis and angle-closure glaucoma; uncontrolled asthma

INTERACTIONS

Drug

Anticholinergics: May antagonize the effects of anticholinergics.
Beta blockers: May produce conduction disturbances.

Herbal

None known.

Food

High-fat meals: May decrease the absorption rate of pilocarpine.

DIAGNOSTIC TEST EFFECTS

None known.

SIDE EFFECTS

Frequent (29%)

Diaphoresis

Occasional (11%–05%)

Headache, dizziness, urinary frequency, flushing, dyspepsia, nausea, asthenia, lacrimation, visual disturbances

Rare (< 4%)

Diarrhea, abdominal pain, peripheral edema, chills

SERIOUS REACTIONS

! Patients with diaphoresis who don't drink enough fluids may develop dehydration.

DENTAL CONSIDERATIONS

General:

- Avoid drugs with anticholinergic activity, such as antihistamines, opioids, benzodiazepines, propantheline, atropine, and scopolamine.
- Avoid dental light in patient's eyes; offer dark glasses for patient comfort.
- Monitor vital signs at every appointment because of CV and respiratory side effects.

Consultations:

- Medical consultation may be required to assess disease control.

DENTAL CONSIDERATIONS

PILOCARPINE HCL (ORAL)

General:

- Patients receiving chemotherapy may require palliative treatment for stomatitis.
- Assess salivary flow as a factor in caries, periodontal disease, and candidiasis.
- Monitor vital signs at every appointment because of CV side effects.
- Place on frequent recall because of oral effects of head and neck radiation.

Consultations:

- Medical consultation may be required to assess disease control.
- Medical consultation may be necessary before prescribing for patients with CV, retinal, or respiratory disease.

Teach Patient/Family:

- To use caution when driving at night or performing hazardous activities in reduced lighting (visual blurring)
- That sweating can become extensive with high dose; have patient take plenty of fluids, observe for dehydration, or discontinue drug
- *When chronic dry mouth occurs, advise patient:*
  - To avoid mouth rinses with high alcohol content because of drying effects
  - Of need for daily use of home fluoride products to prevent caries
  - To use sugarless gum, frequent sips of water, or saliva substitutes

pimecrolimus

pim-eh-crow-leh-mus
(Elidel)

CATEGORY AND SCHEDULE

Pregnancy Risk Category: C

P

MECHANISM OF ACTION

An immunomodulator that inhibits release of cytokine, an enzyme that produces an inflammatory reaction. ***Therapeutic Effect:*** Produces anti-inflammatory activity.

PHARMACOKINETICS

Minimal systemic absorption with topical application. Metabolized in liver. Excreted in feces.

AVAILABILITY

Cream: 1% (Elidel).

INDICATIONS AND DOSAGES

▸ Atopic Dermatitis (eczema)

TOPICAL

Adults, Elderly, Children 2–17 yrs. Apply to affected area twice daily for up to 3 weeks (up to 6 weeks in adolescents, children 2–17 yrs). Rub in gently and completely.

OFF-LABEL USES

Allergic contact dermatitis, irritant contact dermatitis, psoriasis

CONTRAINDICATIONS

Hypersensitivity to pimecrolimus or any component of the formulation, Netherton's syndrome (potential for increased systemic absorption), application to active cutaneous viral infections.

INTERACTIONS

Drug

None known.

Herbal

None known.

Food

None known.

Drug interactions of concern to dentistry

• Drug interactions have not been evaluated. Low blood levels were measured in some patients. Use drugs that inhibit CYP3A4 isoenzymes with caution in patients with widespread and erythrodermic disease.

DIAGNOSTIC TEST EFFECTS

None known.

IV INCOMPATIBILITIES

None known.

IV COMPATIBILITIES

None known.

SIDE EFFECTS

Rare

Transient application-site sensation of burning or feeling of heat

SERIOUS REACTIONS

! Lymphadenopathy and phototoxicity occur rarely.

DENTAL CONSIDERATIONS

General:

• Determine why the patient is taking this drug.

pimozide

pi'-moe-zide

(Orap)

CATEGORY AND SCHEDULE

Pregnancy Risk Category: C

MECHANISM OF ACTION

A diphenylbutylpiperidine that blocks dopamine at postsynaptic receptor sites in the brain. ***Therapeutic Effect:*** Suppresses behavioral response in psychosis.

AVAILABILITY

Tablets: 1 mg, 2 mg (Orap).

INDICATIONS AND DOSAGES

▸ Tourette's Disorder

PO

Adults, Elderly. 1–2 mg/day in divided doses 3 times/day. Maximum: 10 mg/day.

Children older than 12 yrs. Initially, 0.5 mg/kg/day. Maximum: 10 mg/day.

CONTRAINDICATIONS

Aggressive schizophrenics when sedation is required, concurrent administration of pemoline, methylphenidate or amphetamines, concurrent administration with dofetilide, sotalol, quinidine, other Class IA and III anti-arrhythmics, mesoridazine, thioridazine, chlorpromazine, droperidol, sparfloxacin, gatifloxacin, moxifloxacin, halofantrine, mefloquine, pentamidine, arsenic trioxide, levomethadyl acetate, dolasetron mesylate, probucol, tacrolimus, ziprasidone, sertraline, macrolide antibiotics, drugs that cause QT prolongation, and less potent inhibitors of CYP3A, congenital or drug-induced long QT syndrome, doses greater than 10 mg daily, history of cardiac arrhythmias, Parkinson's disease, patients with known hypokalemia or hypomagnesemia, severe central nervous system depression, simple tics or tics not associated with Tourette's syndrome, hypersensitivity to pimozide or any of its components

INTERACTIONS

Drug

Alcohol, CNS depressants: May increase CNS and respiratory depression.

Aprepitant: May increase pimozide plasma concentrations.

Drugs that prolong QT interval: May increase risk for QT prolongation and cardiotoxicity.

Belladonna alkaloids: May increase anticholinergic effects.

Lithium: May increase extrapyramidal symptoms.

Phenylalanine: May increase incidence of tardive dyskinesia.

Sertraline: May increase plasma pimozide levels.

Tramadol: May increase risk of seizures.

Vitex: May decrease effectiveness of dopamine antagonists.

Herbal

Betel nut: May increase extrapyramidal side effects of pimozide

Kava kava: May increase dopamine antagonist effects.

Food

Grapefruit juice: May inhibit metabolism of pimozide.

Drug interactions of concern to dentistry

- Increased CNS depression: alcohol, CNS depressants
- Increased effects of both drugs: phenothiazines
- Increased effects of anticholinergic drugs
- Prolonged QT interval, fatal cardiac arrhythmia, contraindicated: clarithromycin, erythromycin, azithromycin, dirithromycin, itraconazole

DIAGNOSTIC TEST EFFECTS

None known.

SIDE EFFECTS

Occasional

Akathisia, dystonic extrapyramidal effects, parkinsonian extrapyramidal effects, tardive dyskinesia, blurred vision, ocular changes, constipation, decreased sweating, dry mouth, nasal congestion, dizziness, drowsiness, orthostatic hypotension, urinary retention, somnolence

Rare

Rash, cholestatic jaundice, priapism

SERIOUS REACTIONS

! Serious reactions such as blood dyscrasias, agranulocytosis, leukocytopenia, thrombocytopenia, cholestatic jaundice, neuroleptic malignant syndrome (NMS), constipation or paralytic ileus, priapism, QT prolongation and torsades de pointes, seizure, systemic lupus erythematosus-like syndrome, and temperature regulation dysfunction (heatstroke or hypothermia) occur rarely.

! Abrupt withdrawal following long-term therapy may precipitate nausea, vomiting, gastritis, dizziness, and tremors.

DENTAL CONSIDERATIONS

General:

- Assess salivary flow as a factor in caries, periodontal disease, and candidiasis.
- Monitor vital signs at every appointment because of CV side effects.
- Assess for presence of extrapyramidal motor symptoms, such as tardive dyskinesia and akathisia. Extrapyramidal motor activity may complicate dental treatment.
- After supine positioning, have patient sit upright for at least 2 min before standing to avoid orthostatic hypotension.
- Consider action of drug in assessment of altered taste.

Consultations:

- Medical consultation may be required to assess disease control.
- If signs of tardive dyskinesia or akathisia are present, refer to physician.

Teach Patient/Family:

- Importance of good oral hygiene to prevent soft tissue inflammation
- Caution to prevent injury when using oral hygiene aids
- *When chronic dry mouth occurs, advise patient:*
  - To avoid mouth rinses with high alcohol content because of drying effects
  - Of need for daily use of home fluoride products to prevent caries
  - To use sugarless gum, frequent sips of water, or saliva substitutes

pindolol

pin′-doe-loll

(Apo-Pindol[CAN], Visken)

CATEGORY AND SCHEDULE

Pregnancy Risk Category: B (D if used in second or third trimester)

MECHANISM OF ACTION

A nonselective beta blocker that blocks $beta_1$- and $beta_2$-adrenergic receptors. ***Therapeutic Effect:*** Slows heart rate, decreases cardiac output, decreases blood pressure (B/P), and exhibits antiarrhythmic activity. Decreases myocardial ischemia severity by decreasing oxygen requirements.

PHARMACOKINETICS

Completely absorbed from GI tract. Metabolized in liver. Primarily excreted in urine. ***Half-life:*** 3–4 hrs (half-life increased with impaired renal function, elderly).

AVAILABILITY

Capsules: 5 mg, 10 mg (Visken).

INDICATIONS AND DOSAGES

▸ Mild to Moderate Hypertension

PO

Adults. Initially, 5 mg 2 times/day. Gradually increase dose by 10 mg/day at 2–4 week intervals. Maintenance: 10–30 mg/day in 2–3 divided doses. Maximum: 60 mg/day.

Usual elderly dosage:

PO

Initially, 5 mg/day. May increase by 5 mg q3–4 wks.

OFF-LABEL USES

Treatment of chronic angina pectoris, hypertrophic cardiomyopathy, tremors, and mitral valve prolapse syndrome. Increases antidepressant effect with fluoxetine and other SSRIs.

CONTRAINDICATIONS

Bronchial asthma, COPD, uncontrolled cardiac failure, sinus bradycardia, heart block greater than first degree, cardiogenic shock, CHF, unless secondary to tachyarrhythmias

INTERACTIONS

Drug

Diuretics, other hypotensives: May increase hypotensive effect of pindolol.

Sympathomimetics, xanthines: May mutually inhibit effects of pindolol.

Insulin and oral hypoglycemics: May mask symptoms of hypoglycemia and/or prolong hypoglycemic effect.

Herbal

None known.

Food

None known.

Drug interactions of concern to dentistry

- Increased hypotension, bradycardia: anticholinergics, hydrocarbon inhalation anesthetics, fentanyl derivatives
- Decreased antihypertensive effects: indomethacin, sympathomimetics
- Increased effect of both drugs: phenothiazines, xanthines
- Decreased bronchodilation: theophyllines
- Hypertension, bradycardia: epinephrine, ephedrine
- Slow metabolism of drug: lidocaine

DIAGNOSTIC TEST EFFECTS

May increase ANA titer, SGOT (AST), SGPT (ALT), alkaline phosphatase, LDH, bilirubin, BUN, creatinine, potassium, uric acid, lipoproteins, and triglycerides.

SIDE EFFECTS

Frequent

Decreased sexual ability, drowsiness, trouble sleeping, unusual tiredness/weakness

Occasional

Bradycardia, depression, cold hands/feet, diarrhea, constipation, anxiety, nasal congestion, nausea, vomiting

Rare

Altered taste, dry eyes, itching, numbness of fingers, toes and scalp

SERIOUS REACTIONS

! Overdosage may produce profound bradycardia and hypotension.

! Abrupt withdrawal may result in sweating, palpitations, headache, and tremulousness.

! May precipitate congestive heart failure (CHF) or myocardial infarction (MI) in patients with heart disease; thyroid storm in those with thyrotoxicosis; or peripheral ischemia in those with existing peripheral vascular disease.

! Hypoglycemia may occur in previously controlled diabetics.

! Signs of thrombocytopenia, such as unusual bleeding or bruising, occur rarely.

DENTAL CONSIDERATIONS

General:

- Monitor vital signs at every appointment because of CV side effects.
- Patients on chronic drug therapy may rarely have symptoms of blood dyscrasias, which can include infection, bleeding, and poor healing.
- Stress from dental procedures may compromise CV function; determine patient risk.
- Use vasoconstrictors with caution, in low doses, and with careful aspiration. Avoid use of gingival retraction cord with epinephrine.
- Consider semisupine chair position for patient comfort if GI side effects occur.
- Assess salivary flow as a factor in caries, periodontal disease, and candidiasis.
- Consider drug effects if taste alteration occurs.

Consultations:

- In a patient with symptoms of blood dyscrasias, request a medical consultation for blood studies and postpone dental treatment until normal values are reestablished.
- Medical consultation may be required to assess disease control and patient's ability to tolerate stress.

Teach Patient/Family:

- Of need for good oral hygiene to prevent soft tissue inflammation
- Caution to prevent injury when using oral hygiene aids
- *When chronic dry mouth occurs, advise patient:*
    - To avoid mouth rinses with high alcohol content because of drying effects
    - Of need for daily use of home fluoride products to prevent caries
    - To use sugarless gum, frequent sips of water, or saliva substitutes

pioglitazone

pye-oh-gli′-ta-zone
(Actos)

CATEGORY AND SCHEDULE

Pregnancy Risk Category: C

MECHANISM OF ACTION

An antidiabetic that improves target-cell response to insulin without increasing pancreatic insulin secretion. Decreases hepatic glucose output and increases insulin-dependent glucose utilization in skeletal muscle. ***Therapeutic Effect:*** Lowers blood glucose concentration.

PHARMACOKINETICS

Rapidly absorbed. Highly protein bound (99%), primarily to albumin. Metabolized in the liver. Excreted in urine. Unknown if removed by hemodialysis. ***Half-life:*** 16–24 hr.

AVAILABILITY

Tablets: 15 mg, 30 mg, 45 mg.

INDICATIONS AND DOSAGES

▸ **Diabetes Mellitus, Combination Therapy**

PO

Adult, Elderly. With insulin: Initially, 15–30 mg once a day. Initially continue current insulin dosage; then decrease insulin dosage by 10% to 25% if hypoglycemia occurs or plasma glucose level decreases to less than 100 mg/dl. Maximum: 45 mg/day. With sulfonylureas: Initially, 15–30 mg/day. Decrease sulfonylurea dosage if hypoglycemia occurs. With metformin: Initially, 15–30 mg/day. As monotherapy: Monotherapy is not to be used if patient is well controlled with diet and exercise alone. Initially, 15–30 mg/day. May increase dosage in increments until 45 mg/day is reached.

CONTRAINDICATIONS

Active hepatic disease; diabetic ketoacidosis; increased serum transaminase levels, including ALT(SGPT) greater than 2.5 times normal serum level; type 1 diabetes mellitus

INTERACTIONS

Drug

Gemfibrizol: May increase the effect and toxicity of pioglitazone.
Ketoconazole: May significantly inhibit metabolism of pioglitazone.
Oral contraceptives: May alter the effects of oral contraceptives.

Herbal

None known.

Food

None known.

Drug interactions of concern to dentistry

- None reported

DIAGNOSTIC TEST EFFECTS

May increase creatine kinase (CK) level. May decrease Hgb levels by 2% to 4% and serum alkaline phosphatase, bilirubin, and ALT(SGOT) levels. Less than 1% of patients experience ALT values 3 times the normal level.

SIDE EFFECTS

Frequent (13%–9%)
Headache, upper respiratory tract infection
Occasional (6%–5%)
Sinusitis, myalgia, pharyngitis, aggravated diabetes mellitus

SERIOUS REACTIONS

! None known.

DENTAL CONSIDERATIONS

General:

- Ensure that patient is following prescribed diet and regularly takes medication.
- Place on frequent recall to evaluate healing response.
- Short appointments and a stress reduction protocol may be required for anxious patients.
- Diabetics may be more susceptible to infection and have delayed wound healing.
- Question patient about self-monitoring of drug's antidiabetic effect, including blood glucose values or finger-stick records.
- Consider semisupine chair position for patient comfort if GI side effects occur.

Consultations:

- Medical consultation may be required to assess disease control and patient's ability to tolerate stress.
- Medical consultation may include data from patient's blood glucose monitoring, including glycosylated hemoglobin or HbA_{1c} testing.

Teach Patient/Family:

- To prevent trauma when using oral hygiene aids
- Importance of updating health and drug history if physician makes any changes in evaluation or drug regimens

P

pirbuterol

peer-beut-er-all
(Maxair, Maxair Autohaler)

CATEGORY AND SCHEDULE

Pregnancy Risk Category: C

MECHANISM OF ACTION

A sympathomimetic, adrenergic agonist, that stimulates beta2-adrenergic receptors in the lungs, resulting in relaxation of bronchial smooth muscle. ***Therapeutic Effect:*** Relieves bronchospasm, reduces airway resistance.

PHARMACOKINETICS

Absorbed from bronchi following inhalation. Metabolized in liver. Primarily excreted in urine. Unknown if removed by hemodialysis. ***Half-life:*** 2–3 hrs.

AVAILABILITY

Oral Inhalation: 0.2 mg/actuation (Autohaler).

INDICATIONS AND DOSAGES

▸ Prevention of Bronchospasm

INHALATION

Adults, Elderly, Children 12 yrs and older. 2 inhalations q4–6h. Maximum: 12 inhalations daily.

▸ Treatment of Bronchospasm

INHALATION

Adults, Elderly, Children 12 yrs and older. 2 inhalations separated by at least 1–3 minutes, followed by a third inhalation. Maximum: 12 inhalations daily.

CONTRAINDICATIONS

History of hypersensitivity to pirbuterol, albuterol or any of its components

INTERACTIONS

Drug

Beta-adrenergic blocking agents: Antagonizes effects of pirbuterol.
MAOIs, tricyclic antidepressants: May potentiate cardiovascular effects.

Herbal

None known.

Food

None known.

DIAGNOSTIC TEST EFFECTS

May decrease serum potassium levels.

SIDE EFFECTS

Occasional (7%–1%)

Nervousness, tremor, headache, palpitations, nausea, dizziness, tachycardia, cough

SERIOUS REACTIONS

! Excessive sympathomimetic stimulation may produce palpitations, extrasystoles, tachycardia, chest pain, slight increases in B/P followed by a substantial decrease, chills, sweating and blanching of skin.

! Too frequent or excessive use may lead to loss of bronchodilating effectiveness and severe, paradoxical bronchoconstriction.

DENTAL CONSIDERATIONS

General:

- Acute asthmatic episodes may be precipitated in the dental office. Sympathomimetic inhalants should be available for emergency use.
- Be aware that aspirin or sulfite preservatives in vasoconstrictor-containing products can exacerbate asthma.
- Monitor vital signs at every appointment because of CV and respiratory side effects.
- Assess salivary flow as a factor in caries, periodontal disease, and candidiasis.
- Consider semisupine chair position for patients with respiratory disease.
- Short appointments and a stress reduction protocol may be required for anxious patients.

Consultations:

- Medical consultation may be required to assess disease control and patient's ability to tolerate stress.

Teach Patient/Family:

- To rinse mouth with water after each dose to prevent dryness (for inhalation dosage forms)
- *When chronic dry mouth occurs, advise patient:*
  - To avoid mouth rinses with high alcohol content because of drying effects
  - Of need for daily use of home fluoride products to prevent caries
  - To use sugarless gum, frequent sips of water, or saliva substitutes

piroxicam

peer-ox′-i-kam

(Apo-Piroxicam[CAN], Candyl-D[AUS], Feldene, Fexicam[CAN], Mobilis[AUS], Novopirocam[CAN], Pirohexal-D[AUS], Rosig[AUS], Rosig-D[AUS])

Do not confuse Feldene with Seldane.

CATEGORY AND SCHEDULE

Pregnancy Risk Category: C (D if used in third trimester or near delivery)

MECHANISM OF ACTION

An NSAID that produces analgesic and anti-inflammatory effects by inhibiting prostaglandin synthesis. ***Therapeutic Effect:*** Reduces inflammatory response and intensity of pain.

AVAILABILITY

Capsules: 10 mg, 20 mg.

INDICATIONS AND DOSAGES

▸ Acute or Chronic Rheumatoid Arthritis and Osteoarthritis

PO

Adults, Elderly. Initially, 10–20 mg/day as a single dose or in divided doses. Some patients may require up to 30–40 mg/day.

Children. 0.2–0.3 mg/kg/day. Maximum: 15 mg/day.

OFF-LABEL USES

Treatment of acute gouty arthritis, ankylosing spondylitis, dysmenorrhea

CONTRAINDICATIONS

Active peptic ulcer disease, chronic inflammation of the GI tract, GI bleeding or ulceration, history of hypersensitivity to aspirin or NSAIDs

INTERACTIONS

Drug

Antihypertensives, diuretics: May decrease the effects of these drugs.

Aspirin, other salicylates: May increase the risk of GI side effects, such as bleeding.

Bone marrow depressants: May increase the risk of hematologic reactions.

Heparin, oral anticoagulants, thrombolytics: May increase the effects of these drugs.

Lithium: May increase the blood concentration and risk of toxicity of lithium.

Methotrexate: May increase the risk of methotrexate toxicity.

Probenecid: May increase the piroxicam blood concentration.

Herbal

Feverfew: May decrease the effects of feverfew.

Ginkgo biloba: May increase the risk of bleeding.

St. John's wort: May increase the risk of phototoxicity.

Food
None known.

Drug interactions of concern to dentistry

- GI ulceration, bleeding: aspirin, alcohol, corticosteroids
- Nephrotoxicity: acetaminophen (prolonged use and high doses)
- Possible risk of decreased renal function: cyclosporine
- Decreased action: salicylates
- First-time users of SSRIs also taking NSAIDs may have a higher risk of GI side effects; until more data are available, it may be advisable to avoid use of NSAIDs in these patients (*Br J Clin Pharmacol* 55:591–595, 2003)
- *When prescribed for dental pain:*
  - Risk of increased effects of oral anticoagulants, oral antidiabetics, lithium, methotrexate
  - Decreased antihypertensive effects of diuretics, β-adrenergic blockers, ACE inhibitors

DIAGNOSTIC TEST EFFECTS

May increase AST (SGOT) and ALT (SGPT) levels. May decrease serum uric acid levels.

P

SIDE EFFECTS

Frequent (9%–4%)
Dyspepsia, nausea, dizziness
Occasional (3%–1%)
Diarrhea, constipation, abdominal cramps or pain, flatulence, stomatitis
Rare (< 1%)
Hypertension, urticaria, dysuria, ecchymosis, blurred vision, insomnia, phototoxicity

SERIOUS REACTIONS

! Rare reactions with long-term use include peptic ulcer disease, GI bleeding, gastritis, severe hepatic reaction (cholestasis, jaundice), nephrotoxicity (dysuria, hematuria, proteinuria, nephrotic syndrome), hematologic sensitivity (anemia, leukopenia, eosinophilia, thrombocytopenia), and a severe hypersensitivity reaction (fever, chills, bronchospasm).

DENTAL CONSIDERATIONS

General:

- Patients on chronic drug therapy may rarely have symptoms of blood dyscrasias, which can include infection, bleeding, and poor healing.
- Assess salivary flow as a factor in caries, periodontal disease, and candidiasis.
- Avoid prescribing for dental use during pregnancy.
- Minimize use of aspirin-containing products.
- Consider semisupine chair position for patients with arthritic disease or if GI side effects occur.

Consultations:

- In a patient with symptoms of blood dyscrasias, request a medical consultation for blood studies and postpone dental treatment until normal values are reestablished.
- Medical consultation may be required to assess disease control.

Teach Patient/Family:

- Importance of good oral hygiene to prevent soft tissue inflammation
- Caution to prevent injury when using oral hygiene aids
- To report oral lesions, soreness, or bleeding to dentist
- *When chronic dry mouth occurs, advise patient:*
  - To avoid mouth rinses with high alcohol content because of drying effects
  - Of need for daily use of home fluoride products to prevent caries
  - To use sugarless gum, frequent sips of water, or saliva substitutes

podofilox

po-doe-fil′-ox
(Condyline[CAN], Condyline Paint[AUS], Condylox)

CATEGORY AND SCHEDULE

Pregnancy Risk Category: C

MECHANISM OF ACTION

An active component of podophyllin resin that binds to tubulin to prevent formation of microtubules resulting in mitotic arrest. Exercises many biological effects, such as damages endothelium of small blood vessels, attenuates nucleoside transport, suppresses immune responses, inhibits macrophage metabolism, induces interleukin-1 and interleukin-2, decreases lymphocytes response to mitogens, and enhances macrophage growth. ***Therapeutic Effect:*** Removes genital warts.

PHARMACOKINETICS

Time to peak occurs in 1 to 2 hours. Some degree of absorption. ***Half-life:*** 1–4.5 hrs.

AVAILABILITY

Gel: 0.5% (Condylox).
Solution: 0.5% (Condylox).

INDICATIONS AND DOSAGES

▸ **Anogenital Warts**

TOPICAL

Adults. Apply 0.5% gel for 3 days, then withhold for 4 days. Repeat cycle up to 4 times.

▸ **Genital Warts (condylomata acuminate)**

TOPICAL

Adults. Apply 0.5% solution or gel q12h in the morning and evening for 3 days, then withhold for 4 days. Repeat cycle up to 4 times.

OFF-LABEL USES

Systemic: Treatment of fungal pneumonia, prostate cancer, septicemia

CONTRAINDICATIONS

Bleeding warts, moles, birthmarks or unusual warts with hair, diabetes, poor blood circulation, pregnancy, steroid use, hypersensitivity to podofilox or any component of its formulation

INTERACTIONS

Drug

None known.

Herbal

None known.

Food

None known.

Drug interactions of concern to dentistry

- None reported

DIAGNOSTIC TEST EFFECTS

None known.

SIDE EFFECTS

Occasional

Erosion, inflammation, itching, pain, burning

Rare

Nausea, vomiting

SERIOUS REACTIONS

! Nausea and vomiting occur rarely and usually after cumulative doses.

DENTAL CONSIDERATIONS

General:

- Determine why patient is taking the drug.
- Exam oral mucous membranes for lesions; overuse may be associated with oral ulcers.
- Tactful questions related to STD may be appropriate.
- Explore medical and drug history.
- Not for use on mucous membranes.

Consultations:

- Medical consultation may be required to assess disease control.

Teach Patient/Family:

- Importance of good oral hygiene to prevent soft tissue inflammation
- To prevent trauma when using oral hygiene aids
- Importance of updating health and medication history if physician makes any changes in evaluation or drug regimens; include OTC, herbal, and nonherbal in the update

podophyllum

po-dof-fil-um rez-in
(Podocon-25, Pododerm)

CATEGORY AND SCHEDULE

Pregnancy Risk Category: X

MECHANISM OF ACTION

A cytotoxic agent that directly affects epithelial cell metabolism by arresting mitosis through binding to a protein subunit of spindle microtubules. ***Therapeutic Effect:*** Removes soft genital warts.

PHARMACOKINETICS

Topical podophyllum is systemically absorbed. Absorption may be increased if applied to bleeding, friable, or recently biopsied warts.

AVAILABILITY

Liquid: 25% (Podocon-25, Pododerm).

INDICATIONS AND DOSAGES

▸ Genital Warts (condylomata acuminate)

TOPICAL

Adults, Elderly, Children. Apply 10%–25% solution in compound benzoin tincture to dry surface. Use 1 drop at a time allowing drying between drops until area is covered. Total volume should be limited to less than 0.5 ml per treatment session.

OFF-LABEL USES

Epitheliomatosis, laryngeal papilloma

CONTRAINDICATIONS

Diabetes mellitus, concomitant steroids therapy, circulation disorders, bleeding warts, moles, birthmarks or unusual warts with hair growing from them, pregnancy, hypersensitivity to podophyllum resin preparations

INTERACTIONS

Drug

None known.

Herbal

None known.

Food

None known.

Drug interactions of concern to dentistry

- None reported

DIAGNOSTIC TEST EFFECTS

May increase BUN, serum alkaline phosphatase, serum creatinine, SGOT (AST), and SGPT (ALT) levels.

IV INCOMPATIBILITIES

None known.

IV COMPATIBILITIES

None known.

SIDE EFFECTS

Occasional (10%–1%)

Pruritus, nausea, vomiting, abdominal pain, diarrhea

SERIOUS REACTIONS

! Paresthesia, polyneuritis, paralytic ileus, pyrexia, leukopenia, thrombocytopenia, coma and death have been reported with podophyllum resin use.

DENTAL CONSIDERATIONS

General:

- Determine why patient is taking the drug.
- This medication is applied in physician's office.
- Tactful questions related to STD may be appropriate.
- Explore medical and drug history.

Consultations:

- Medical consultation may be required to assess disease control.

Teach Patient/Family:

- Importance of good oral hygiene to prevent soft tissue inflammation
- Prevent trauma when using oral hygiene aids
- Importance of updating health and medication history if physician makes any changes in evaluation or drug regimens; include OTC, herbal, and nonherbal in the update

polymyxin B

polly-mix-in

(Aerosporin)

CATEGORY AND SCHEDULE

Pregnancy Risk Category: B

MECHANISM OF ACTION

An antibiotic that alters cell membrane permeability in susceptible microorganisms. ***Therapeutic Effect:*** Bactericidal activity.

PHARMACOKINETICS

Negligible absorption. Protein binding: low. Excreted in urine. Poor removal in hemodialysis. ***Half-life:*** 6 hrs.

AVAILABILITY

Powder: 500,000 (Aerosporin).

INDICATIONS AND DOSAGES

▸ Mild to Moderate Infections

IV

Adults, Elderly, Children 2 yrs and older. 15,000–25,000 units/kg/day in divided doses q12h.

Infants. Up to 40,000 units/kg/day.

IM

Adults, Elderly, Children 2 yrs and older. 25,000–30,000 units/kg/day in divided doses q4–6h.

Infants. Up to 40,000 units/kg/day.

▸ Usual Irrigation Dosage

Continuous Bladder Irrigation

Adults, Elderly. 1 ml urogenital concentrate (contains 200,000 units polymyxin B, 57 mg neomycin) added to 1000 ml 0.9% NaCl. Give each 1000 ml >24 hrs for up to 10 days (may increase to 2000 ml/day when urine output >2 L/day).

▸ Usual Ophthalmic Dosage

OPHTHALMIC

Adults, Elderly, Children. 1 drop q3–4h.

CONTRAINDICATIONS

Hypersensitivity to polymyxin B or any component of the formulation

INTERACTIONS

Drug

Neuromuscular blocking agents or anesthetics: May produce muscle paralysis and prolonged or increased skeletal muscle relaxation.

Aminoglycosides, other nephrotoxic drugs: May increase nephrotoxicity.

SIDE EFFECTS

Frequent

Severe pain, irritation at IM injection sites, phlebitis, thrombophlebitis with IV administration

Occasional

Fever, urticaria

SERIOUS REACTIONS

! Nephrotoxicity, especially with concurrent/sequential use of other nephrotoxic drugs, renal impairment, concurrent/sequential use of muscle relaxants.

! Superinfection, especially with fungi, may occur.

DENTAL CONSIDERATIONS

General:

- Avoid dental light in patient's eyes; offer dark glasses for patient comfort and safety during dental treatment.

P

polymyxin B sulfate; trimethoprim sulfate

pol-ee-mix′-in bee sul′-fate; trye-meth′-oh-prim sul′-fate (Polytrim)

CATEGORY AND SCHEDULE

Pregnancy Risk Category: C

MECHANISM OF ACTION

Polymyxin B damages bacterial cytoplasmic membrane which causes leakage of intracellular components. Trimethoprim is a folate antagonist that blocks bacterial biosynthesis of nucleic acids and proteins by interfering with metabolism of folinic acid *Therapeutic Effect:* Prevents inflammatory process. Interferes with bacterial protein synthesis. Produces antibacterial activity.

PHARMACOKINETICS

Absorption through intact skin and mucous membranes is insignificant.

AVAILABILITY

Solution, ophthalmic: 1 mg trimethoprim sulfate and 10,000 units polymyxin B sulfate per ml (Polytrim).

INDICATIONS AND DOSAGES

▸ **Treatment of Surface Ocular Bacterial Conjunctivitis and Blepharoconjunctivitis**

OPHTHALMIC

Adults, Elderly, Children. Instill 1–2 drops in eye(s) every 3 hours for 7–10 days. Maximum: 6 doses/day.

CONTRAINDICATIONS

Hypersensitivity to polymyxin B, trimethoprim sulfate, or any component of the formulation

INTERACTIONS

Drug

None known.

Herbal

None known.

Food

None known.

DIAGNOSTIC TEST EFFECTS

None known.

SIDE EFFECTS

Occasional

Local irritation, redness, burning, stinging, itching

SERIOUS REACTIONS

! Prolonged use may result in overgrowth of nonsusceptible organisms, including superinfection.

! Hypersensitivity reactions consisting of lid edema, itching, increased redness, tearing, and/or circumocular rash have been reported.
! Photosensitivity has been reported in patients taking oral trimethoprim.

DENTAL CONSIDERATIONS

General:
• Avoid dental light in patient's eyes; offer dark glasses for patient comfort and safety during dental treatment.

potassium chloride

poe-tass′-ee-um klor′-ide
(Apo-K[CAN], Cena K; Ed K+10, K+Care; K-10, K-8, Kaochlor, Kaochlor S-F, Kaon-CI, Kaon-CL 10, Kaon-CL 20%, Kato, Kay Ciel, KCl-20, KCl-40, K-Dur 10, K-Dur 20, K-Lor; Klor-Con, Klor-Con/25, Klor-Con 10, Klor-Con 8, Klor-Con M10, Klor-Con M15, Klor-Con M20, Klotrix, K-Lyte CI, K-Norm, K-Sol, K-Tab, Micro-K, Micro-K 10, Rum-K)
Do not confuse with Cardura or Slow-FE.

CATEGORY AND SCHEDULE

Pregnancy Risk Category: C

MECHANISM OF ACTION

An electrolyte that is necessary for multiple cellular metabolic processes. Primary action is intracellular. ***Therapeutic Effect:*** Necessary for nerve impulse conduction, contraction of cardiac, skeletal, and smooth muscle; maintains normal renal function and acid-base balance.

PHARMACOKINETICS

Well absorbed from the gastrointestinal (GI) tract. Enters cells via active transport from extracellular fluid. Primarily excreted in urine.

AVAILABILITY

Capsules, extended-release: 8 mEq (Micro-K), 10 mEq (K-Norm).
Intravenous solution: 2 mEq/ml, 30 mEq/100 ml, 40 mEq/100 ml, 10 mEq/100 ml, 20 mEq/100 ml.
Liquid: 20 mEq/15 ml (Cena-K, KCl-20, Kay Ciel, Kaochlor S-F), 30 mEq/ 15 ml (Rum-K), 40 mEq/15 ml (Cena K, Kaon-CL 20%, KCl-40).
Powder for compounding: 100%.
Powder for reconstitution: 15 mEq (K+Care), 20 mEq (K+ Care, K-Sol, Kay Ciel, Kato, K-Lor, Klor-Con), 25 mEq (Klor-Con/25).
Tablets: 500 mg, 595 mg.
Tablets, effervescent: 25 mEq (K-Lyte CI), 50 mEq (K-Lyte CI)
Tablets, extended-release: 8 mEq (Kaon-CI, K-8, Klor-Con 8), 10 mEq (Ed K+10, K-10, K-Dur 10, Kaon-CL 10, Klor-Con M10, K-Tab, Klotrix), 15 mEq (Klor-Con M15) 20 mEq (K-Dur 20, Klor-Con M20).

INDICATIONS AND DOSAGES

▸ Prevention of Hypokalemia (on Diuretic Therapy)

PO
Adults, Elderly. 20–40 mEq/day in 1–2 divided doses.
Children. 1–2 mEq/kg in 1–2 divided doses.

▸ Treatment of Hypokalemia

IV
Adults, Elderly. 5–10 mEq/hr. Maximum: 400 mEq/day.
Children. 1 mEq/kg over 1–2 hrs.

P

PO
Adults, Elderly. 40–80 mEq/day further doses based on laboratory values.
Children. 1–2 mEq/day, further doses based on laboratory values.

CONTRAINDICATIONS

Digitalis toxicity, heat cramps, hyperkalemia, patients receiving potassium-sparing diuretics, postoperative oliguria, severe burns, severe renal impairment, shock with dehydration or hemolytic reaction, untreated Addison's disease, hypersensitivity to any component of the formulation.

INTERACTIONS

Drug

Anticholinergics: May increase the risk of gastrointestinal (GI) lesions.
Angiotensin-converting enzyme inhibitors (ACE) inhibitors, beta-adrenergic blockers, heparin, NSAIDs, potassium-containing medications, potassium-sparing diuretics, salt substitutes: May increase potassium blood concentration.

Herbal

None known.

Food

None known.

Drug interactions of concern to dentistry

- Decreased potassium requirement: corticosteroids
- Increased GI side effects: anticholinergic drugs, NSAIDs
- Increased serum potassium: NSAIDs, cyclosporine

DIAGNOSTIC TEST EFFECTS

None known.

SIDE EFFECTS

Occasional

Nausea, vomiting, diarrhea, flatulence, abdominal discomfort with distention, phlebitis with IV administration (particularly when potassium concentration of greater than 40 mEq/L is infused).

Rare

Rash

SERIOUS REACTIONS

! Hyperkalemia (observed particularly in elderly or in patients with impaired renal function) manifested as paresthesia of extremities, heaviness of legs, cold skin, grayish pallor, hypotension, mental confusion, irritability, flaccid paralysis, and cardiac arrhythmias.

DENTAL CONSIDERATIONS

General:

- Patients taking potassium supplements will normally be taking a diuretic. Compliance with potassium supplements can be a problem. Verify serum potassium levels as required.
- Consider semisupine chair position for patient comfort if GI side effects occur.

potassium acetate/potassium bicarbonate-citrate/potassium chloride/potassium gluconate

poe-tah'-see-um

(potassium bicarbonate-citrate) K-Lyte, Klor-Con EF, Effer K, K-Lyte DS(potassium chloride) Apo-K[CAN], Kaochlor, K-Dur, K-Lor, K-Lor-Con M 15, Kaon-Cl, KSR[AUS], KSR-600 [AUS], Micro-K, Slow-K[AUS], Span-K[AUS](potassium gluconate) Kaon

Do not confuse K-dur with Cardura.

CATEGORY AND SCHEDULE

Pregnancy Risk Category: C (A for potassium chloride)

MECHANISM OF ACTION

An electrolyte that is necessary for multiple cellular metabolic processes. Primary action is intracellular. ***Therapeutic Effect:*** Is necessary for nerve impulse conduction and contraction of cardiac, skeletal, and smooth muscle; maintains normal renal function and acid-base balance.

PHARMACOKINETICS

Well absorbed from the GI tract. Enters cells by active transport from extracellular fluid. Primarily excreted in urine.

AVAILABILITY

Potassium Acetate
Injection: 2 mEq/ml.
Potassium Bicarbonate and Potassium Citrate
Tablet for Solution (Klor-Con EF, Effer-K, K-Lyte): 25 mEq.
Tablet for Solution (K-Lyte DS): 50 mEq.
Potassium Chloride
Capsules (Controlled-Release [Micro-K]): 8 mEq, 10 mEq.
Liquid (Kaochlor): 20 mEq/15 ml.
Liquid (Kaon-Cl): 40 mEq/15 ml.
Powder for Oral Solution (K-Lor): 20 mEq.
Injection: 2 mEq/ml.
Tablets (Extended-Release [Klor-Con, Micro-K]): 8 mEq, 10 mEq.
Tablets (Extended-Release [Kaon-Cl, K-Tab]): 10 mEq.
Tablets (Extended-Release [K-Dur]): 10 mEq, 20 mEq.
Potassium Gluconate
Elixir (Kaon): 20 mEq/15 ml.

INDICATIONS AND DOSAGES

▸ Prevention of Hypokalemia (in patients on diuretic therapy)

PO

Adults, Elderly. 20–40 mEq/day in 1–2 divided doses.
Children. 1–2 mEq/kg/day in 1–2 divided doses.

▸ Treatment of Hypokalemia

PO

Adults, Elderly. 40–80 mEq/day; further doses based on laboratory values.
Children. 2–5 mEq/day; further doses based on laboratory values.

IV

Adults, Elderly. 5–10 mEq/hr. Maximum: 400 mEq/day.
Children. 1 mEq/kg over 1–2 hr.

CONTRAINDICATIONS

Concurrent use of potassium-sparing diuretics, digitalis toxicity, heat cramps, hyperkalemia, postoperative oliguria, severe burns, severe renal impairment, shock with dehydration or hemolytic reaction, untreated Addison's disease

INTERACTIONS

Drug

ACE inhibitors, beta-adrenergic blockers, heparin, NSAIDs, potassium-containing medications, potassium-sparing diuretics, salt substitutes: May increase potassium blood concentration.
Anticholinergics: May increase the risk of GI lesions.

Herbal

None known.

Food

None known.

Drug interactions of concern to dentistry

- Decreased potassium requirement: corticosteroids
- Increased GI side effects: anticholinergic drugs, NSAIDs
- Increased serum potassium: NSAIDs, cyclosporine

DIAGNOSTIC TEST EFFECTS

None known.

IV INCOMPATIBILITIES

Amphotericin B complex (Abelcet, AmBisome, Amphotec), methylprednisolone (Solu-Medrol), phenytoin (Dilantin)

IV COMPATIBILITIES

Aminophylline, amiodarone (Cordarone), atropine, aztreonam (Azactam), calcium gluconate, cefepime (Maxipime), ciprofloxacin (Cipro), clindamycin (Cleocin), dexamethasone (Decadron), digoxin (Lanoxin), diltiazem (Cardizem), diphenhydramine (Benadryl), dobutamine (Dobutrex), dopamine (Intropin), enalapril (Vasotec), famotidine (Pepcid), fluconazole (Diflucan), furosemide (Lasix), granisetron (Kytril), heparin, hydrocortisone (Solu-Cortef), insulin, lidocaine, lorazepam (Ativan), magnesium sulfate, methylprednisolone (Solu-Medrol), metoclopramide (Reglan), midazolam (Versed), milrinone (Primacor), morphine, norepinephrine (Levophed), ondansetron (Zofran), oxytocin (Pitocin), piperacillin and tazobactam (Zosyn), procainamide (Pronestyl), propofol (Diprivan), propranolol (Inderal)

SIDE EFFECTS

Occasional

Nausea, vomiting, diarrhea, flatulence, abdominal discomfort with distention, phlebitis with IV administration (particularly when potassium concentration of > 40 mEq/L is infused)

Rare

Rash

SERIOUS REACTIONS

! Hyperkalemia (more common in elderly patients and those with impaired renal function) may be manifested as paresthesia, feeling of heaviness in the lower extremities, cold skin, grayish pallor, hypotension, confusion, irritability, flaccid paralysis, and cardiac arrhythmias.

DENTAL CONSIDERATIONS

General:

- Patients taking potassium supplements will normally be taking a diuretic. Compliance with potassium supplements can be a problem. Verify serum potassium levels as required.
- Consider semisupine chair position for patient comfort if GI side effects occur.

pramipexole

pram-eh-pex′-ol
(Mirapex)
Do not confuse Mirapex with Mifeprex or MiraLax.

CATEGORY AND SCHEDULE

Pregnancy Risk Category: C

MECHANISM OF ACTION

An antiparkinson agent that stimulates dopamine receptors in the striatum. ***Therapeutic Effect:*** Relieves signs and symptoms of Parkinson's disease.

PHARMACOKINETICS

Rapidly and extensively absorbed after PO administration. Protein binding: 15%. Widely distributed. Steady-state concentrations achieved within 2 days. Primarily eliminated in urine. Not removed by hemodialysis. ***Half-life:*** 8 hr (12 hr in patients older than 65 yr).

AVAILABILITY

Tablets: 0.125 mg, 0.25 mg, 0.5 mg, 1 mg, 1.5 mg.

INDICATIONS AND DOSAGES

▸ Parkinson's Disease

PO

Adults, Elderly. Initially, 0.375 mg/day in 3 divided doses. Don't increase dosage more frequently than every 5–7 days. Maintenance: 1.5–4.5 mg/day in 3 equally divided doses.

▸ Dosage in Renal Impairment

Dosage and frequency are modified on the basis of creatinine clearance.

Creatinine clearance	Initial Dose	Maximum Dose
Greater than 60 ml/min	0.125 mg 3 times a day	1.5 mg 3 times a day
35–59 ml/min	0.125 mg twice a day	1.5 mg twice a day
15–34 ml/min	0.125 mg once a day	1.5 mg once a day

CONTRAINDICATIONS

History of hypersensitivity to pramipexole

INTERACTIONS

Drug

Carbidopa and levodopa, levodopa: May increase plasma level of levodopa.
Cimetidine: Increases pramipexole plasma concentration and half-life.
Cimetidine, diltiazem, quinidine, quinine, ranitidine, triamterene, verapamil: May decrease pramipexole clearance.

Herbal

None known.

Food

All foods: Delay peak drug plasma levels by 1 hour but don't affect drug absorption.

Drug interactions of concern to dentistry

- Increased CNS depression: all CNS depressants
- Possible decreased effects: dopamine antagonists (phenothiazines, butyrophenones, or thioxanthenes) and metoclopramide

DIAGNOSTIC TEST EFFECTS

None known.

SIDE EFFECTS

Frequent

Early Parkinson's disease (28%–10%): Nausea, asthenia, dizziness, somnolence, insomnia, constipation
Advanced Parkinson's disease (53%–17%): Orthostatic hypotension,

extrapyramidal reactions, insomnia, dizziness, hallucinations

Occasional

Early Parkinson's disease (5%–2%): Edema, malaise, confusion, amnesia, akathisia, anorexia, dysphagia, peripheral edema, vision changes, impotence

Advanced Parkinson's disease (10%–7%): Asthenia, somnolence, confusion, constipation, abnormal gait, dry mouth

Rare

Advanced Parkinson's disease (6%–2%): General edema, malaise, chest pain, amnesia, tremor, urinary frequency or incontinence, dyspnea, rhinitis, vision changes

SERIOUS REACTIONS

! None known.

DENTAL CONSIDERATIONS

General:

- Monitor vital signs at every appointment because of CV side effects.
- Assess salivary flow as factor in caries, periodontal disease, and candidiasis.
- Consider semisupine chair position for patient comfort if GI side effects occur.
- After supine positioning, have patient sit upright for at least 2 min before standing to avoid orthostatic hypotension.

Consultations:

- Medical consultation may be required to assess disease control and patient's ability to tolerate stress.

Teach Patient/Family:

- Importance of good oral hygiene to prevent soft tissue inflammation
- Caution to prevent trauma when using oral hygiene aids
- Use of electric toothbrush if patient has difficulty holding conventional devices
- Importance of updating health and drug history if physician makes any changes in evaluation or drug regimens
- *When chronic dry mouth occurs, advise patient:*
  - To avoid mouth rinses with high alcohol content because of drying effects
  - To use daily home fluoride products for anticaries effect
  - To use sugarless gum, frequent sips of water, or saliva substitutes

pravastatin

prav-i-sta′-tin

(Pravachol)

Do not confuse pravastatin with Prevacid, or Pravachol with propranolol.

CATEGORY AND SCHEDULE

Pregnancy Risk Category: X

MECHANISM OF ACTION

An HMG-CoA reductase inhibitor that interferes with cholesterol biosynthesis by preventing the conversion of HMG-CoA reductase to mevalonate, a precursor to cholesterol. ***Therapeutic Effect:*** Lowers serum LDL and VLDL cholesterol and plasma triglyceride levels; increases serum HDL concentration.

PHARMACOKINETICS

Poorly absorbed from the GI tract. Protein binding: 50%. Metabolized in the liver (minimal active metabolites). Primarily excreted in feces via the biliary system. Not removed by hemodialysis. ***Half-life:*** 2.7 hr.

AVAILABILITY

Tablets: 10 mg, 20 mg, 40 mg, 80 mg.

P

INDICATIONS AND DOSAGES

▸ **Hyperlipidemia, Primary and Secondary Prevention of Cardiovascular Events in Patient with Elevated Cholesterol Levels**

PO

Adults, Elderly. Initially, 40 mg/day. Titrate to desired response. Range: 10–80 mg/day.

Children 14–18 yr. 40 mg/day.

Children 8–13 yr. 20 mg/day.

▸ **Dosage in Hepatic and Renal Impairment**

For adults, give 10 mg/day initially. Titrate to desired response.

CONTRAINDICATIONS

Active hepatic disease or unexplained, persistent elevations of liver function test results

INTERACTIONS

Drug

Cyclosporine, erythromycin, gemfibrozil, immunosuppressants, niacin: Increases the risk of acute renal failure and rhabdomyolysis.

Herbal

None known.

Food

None known.

Drug interactions of concern to dentistry

- Increased risk of myopathy or rhabdomyolysis: erythromycin, itraconazole

DIAGNOSTIC TEST EFFECTS

May increase serum CK and transaminase concentrations.

SIDE EFFECTS

Pravastatin is generally well tolerated. Side effects are usually mild and transient.

Occasional (7%–4%)

Nausea, vomiting, diarrhea, constipation, abdominal pain, headache, rhinitis, rash, pruritus

Rare (3%–2%)

Heartburn, myalgia, dizziness, cough, fatigue, flu-like symptoms

SERIOUS REACTIONS

! Malignancy and cataracts may occur.

! Hypersensitivity occurs rarely.

DENTAL CONSIDERATIONS

General:

- Monitor vital signs at every appointment because of possible CV disease.
- Consider semisupine chair position for patient comfort if GI side effects occur.

prazosin hydrochloride

pra′-zoe-sin

(Minipress, Prasig[AUS], Pratisol[AUS], Pressin[AUS])

CATEGORY AND SCHEDULE

Pregnancy Risk Category: C

MECHANISM OF ACTION

An antidote, antihypertensive, and vasodilator that selectively blocks alpha$_1$-adrenergic receptors, decreasing peripheral vascular resistance. ***Therapeutic Effect:*** Produces vasodilation of veins and arterioles, decreases total peripheral resistance, and relaxes smooth muscle in bladder neck and prostate.

AVAILABILITY

Capsules: 1 mg, 2 mg, 5 mg.

INDICATIONS AND DOSAGES

▸ **Mild to Moderate Hypertension**

PO

Adults, Elderly. Initially, 1 mg 2–3 times a day.

Maintenance: 3–15 mg/day in divided doses.
Maximum: 20 mg/day.
Children. 5 mcg/kg/dose q6h. Gradually increase up to 25 mcg/kg/dose.

OFF-LABEL USES

Treatment of benign prostate hyperplasia, CHF, ergot alkaloid toxicity, pheochromocytoma, Raynaud's phenomenon

CONTRAINDICATIONS

None known.

INTERACTIONS

Drug

Estrogen, NSAIDs, other sympathomimetics: May decrease the effects of prazosin.
Hypotension-producing medications, such as antihypertensives and diuretics: May increase the effects of prazosin.

Herbal

Licorice: Causes sodium and water retention and potassium loss.

Food

None known.

Drug interactions of concern to dentistry

- Increased effects: epinephrine
- Decreased effect: indomethacin, NSAIDs

DIAGNOSTIC TEST EFFECTS

None known.

SIDE EFFECTS

Frequent (10%–7%)
Dizziness, somnolence, headache, asthenia (loss of strength, energy)
Occasional (5%–4%)
Palpitations, nausea, dry mouth, nervousness
Rare (< 1%)
Angina, urinary urgency

P

SERIOUS REACTIONS

! First-dose syncope (hypotension with sudden loss of consciousness) may occur 30 to 90 minutes following initial dose of more than 2 mg, a too-rapid increase in dosage, or addition of another antihypertensive agent to therapy. First-dose syncope may be preceded by tachycardia (pulse rate of 120–160 beats/minute).

DENTAL CONSIDERATIONS

General:

- Monitor vital signs at every appointment because of CV side effects.
- After supine positioning, have patient sit upright for at least 2 min before standing to avoid orthostatic hypotension.
- Assess salivary flow as a factor in caries, periodontal disease, and candidiasis.
- Limit use of sodium-containing products, such as saline IV fluids, for patients with a dietary salt restriction.
- Stress from dental procedures may compromise CV function; determine patient risk.
- Short appointments and a stress reduction protocol may be required for anxious patients.

Consultations:

- Medical consultation may be required to assess disease control.

Teach Patient/Family:

- *When chronic dry mouth occurs, advise patient:*
  - To avoid mouth rinses with high alcohol content because of drying effects
  - Of need for daily use of home fluoride products to prevent caries
  - To use sugarless gum, frequent sips of water, or saliva substitutes

prednisolone

pred-niss′-oh-lone
(AK-Pred, AK-Tate[CAN], Inflamase Forte, Inflamase Mild, Minims-Prednisolone[CAN], Novo-Prednisolone[CAN], Orapred, Pediapred, Pred Forte, Pred Mild, Prelone, Solone[AUS])
Do not confuse prednisolone with prednisone or primidone.

CATEGORY AND SCHEDULE

Pregnancy Risk Category: C (D if used in first trimester)

MECHANISM OF ACTION

An adrenocortical steroid that inhibits accumulation of inflammatory cells at inflammation sites, phagocytosis, lysosomal enzyme release and synthesis, and release of mediators of inflammation. ***Therapeutic Effect:*** Prevents or suppresses cell-mediated immune reactions. Decreases or prevents tissue response to inflammatory process.

AVAILABILITY

Oral Solution (Pediapred): 6.7 mg/5 ml.
Oral Solution (Orapred): 20 mg/5 ml.
Tablets: 5 mg.
Syrup (Prelone): 5 mg/5 ml.
Ophthalmic Solution (Inflamase Mild): 0.125%.
Ophthalmic Solution (AK-Pred, Inflamase Forte): 1%.
Ophthalmic Suspension (Pred Mild): 0.12%.
*Ophthalmic Suspension (Pred Forte):*1%.

INDICATIONS AND DOSAGES

▸ **Substitution Therapy for Deficiency States: Acute or Chronic Adrenal Insufficiency, Congenital Adrenal Hyperplasia, and Adrenal Insufficiency Secondary to Pituitary Insufficiency; Nonendocrine Disorders: Arthritis; Rheumatic Carditis; Allergic, Collagen, Intestinal Tract, Liver, Ocular, Renal, Skin Diseases; Bronchial Asthma; Cerebral Edema; Malignancies**

PO
Adults, Elderly. 5–60 mg/day in divided doses.
Children. 0.1–2 mg/kg/day in 1–4 divided doses.

▸ **Treatment of Conjuctivitis and Corneal Injury**

OPHTHALMIC
Adults, Elderly. 1–2 drops every hr during day and q2h during night. After response, decrease dosage to 1 drop q4h, then 1 drop 3–4 times a day.

CONTRAINDICATIONS

Acute superficial herpes simplex keratitis, systemic fungal infections, varicella

INTERACTIONS

Drug

Amphotericin: May increase hypokalemia.
Digoxin: May increase the risk of digoxin toxicity caused by hypokalemia
Diuretics, insulin, oral hypoglycemics, potassium supplements: May decrease the effects of these drugs.
Hepatic enzyme inducers: May decrease the effects of prednisolone.
Live-virus vaccines: May decrease the patient's antibody response to vaccine, increase vaccine side effects, and potentiate virus replication.

Herbal

None known.

Food
None known.

Drug interactions of concern to dentistry
- Decreased action: barbiturates, rifampin, rifabutin
- Increased side effects: alcohol, salicylates, NSAIDs
- Increased action: ketoconazole, macrolide antibiotics (erythromycin, clarithromycin, azithromycin)
- Hepatotoxicity: acetaminophen (chronic use, high doses)

DIAGNOSTIC TEST EFFECTS

May increase blood glucose and serum lipid, amylase, and sodium levels. May decrease serum calcium, potassium, and thyroxine levels.

SIDE EFFECTS

Frequent
Insomnia, heartburn, nervousness, abdominal distention, increased sweating, acne, mood swings, increased appetite, facial flushing, delayed wound healing, increased susceptibility to infection, diarrhea or constipation

P

Occasional
Headache, edema, change in skin color, frequent urination

Rare
Tachycardia, allergic reaction (such as rash and hives), psychological changes, hallucinations, depression
Ophthalmic: stinging or burning, posterior subcapsular cataracts

SERIOUS REACTIONS

! Long-term therapy may cause hypocalcemia, hypokalemia, muscle wasting (especially in the arms and legs), osteoporosis, spontaneous fractures, amenorrhea, cataracts, glaucoma, peptic ulcer disease, and CHF.

! Abruptly withdrawing the drug after long-term therapy may cause anorexia, nausea, fever, headache, severe or sudden joint pain, rebound inflammation, fatigue, weakness, lethargy, dizziness, and orthostatic hypotension.

! Suddenly discontinuing prednisolone may be fatal.

DENTAL CONSIDERATIONS

General:
- Monitor vital signs at every appointment because of CV side effects.
- Patients on chronic drug therapy may rarely have symptoms of blood dyscrasias, which can include infection, bleeding, and poor healing.
- Assess salivary flow as a factor in caries, periodontal disease, and candidiasis.
- Avoid prescribing aspirin-containing products.
- Place on frequent recall to evaluate healing response.
- Prophylactic antibiotics may be indicated to prevent infection if surgery or deep scaling is planned.
- Symptoms of oral infections may be masked.
- Determine dose and duration of steroid therapy for each patient to assess risk for stress tolerance and immunosuppression.
- Patients who have been or are currently on chronic steroid therapy (>2 wk) require supplemental steroids for dental treatment.
- Determine why the patient is taking the drug.

Consultations:
- In a patient with symptoms of blood dyscrasias, request a medical consultation for blood studies and postpone dental treatment until normal values are reestablished.
- Medical consultation may be required to assess disease control.

- Consultation may be required to confirm steroid dose and duration of use.

Teach Patient/Family:

- Importance of good oral hygiene to prevent soft tissue inflammation
- Caution to prevent injury when using oral hygiene aids
- *When chronic dry mouth occurs, advise patient:*
  - To avoid mouth rinses with high alcohol content because of drying effects
  - Of need for daily use of home fluoride products to prevent caries
  - To use sugarless gum, frequent sips of water, or saliva substitutes

prednisolone acetate

pred-niss′-oh-lone as′-i-tate
(AK-Pred, Econopred Plus, Inflamase Forte, Inflamase Mild, Ocu-Pred, Ocu-Pred-A, Ocu-Pred Forte, Pred Forte, Pred Mild, Prednisol)

CATEGORY AND SCHEDULE

Pregnancy Risk Category: C

MECHANISM OF ACTION

An adrenal corticosteroid that inhibits accumulation of inflammatory cells at inflammation sites, phagocytosis, lysosomal enzyme release and synthesis, and release of mediators of inflammation. ***Therapeutic Effect:*** Prevents or suppresses cell-mediated immune reactions. Decreases or prevents tissue response to inflammatory process.

PHARMACOKINETICS

Absorbed into aqueous humor, cornea, iris, choroids, ciliary body, and retina. Systemic absorption may occur, but significant only at high dosages.

AVAILABILITY

Ophthalmic solution: 0.125% (AK-Pred, Inflamase Mild, Ocu-Pred), 1% (AK-Pred, Inflamase Forte, Ocu-Pred Forte, Prednisol).
Ophthalmic suspension: 0.12% (Pred Mild), 0.125%, 1% (Econopred Plus, Ocu-Pred-A, Pred Forte).

INDICATIONS AND DOSAGES

▸ **Conjunctivitis**

OPHTHALMIC

Adults, Elderly, Children. 1–2 drops 2–4 times/day.

CONTRAINDICATIONS

Fungal, mycobacterial, or viral infections of the eye, hypersensitivity to prednisolone acetate or any component of the formulation

INTERACTIONS

Drug

None known.

Herbal

None known.

Food

None known.

Drug interactions of concern to dentistry

- Decreased action: barbiturates, rifampin, rifabutin
- Increased side effects: alcohol, salicylates, NSAIDs
- Increased action: ketoconazole, macrolide antibiotics (erythromycin, clarithromycin, azithromycin)
- Hepatotoxicity: acetaminophen (chronic use, high doses)

DIAGNOSTIC TEST EFFECTS

None known.

SIDE EFFECTS

Occasional

Stinging or burning

SERIOUS REACTIONS

! Prolonged use of corticosteroids may result in glaucoma with damage to the optic nerve, defects in visual acuity and fields of vision, posterior subcapsular cataract formation, and delayed wound healing.
! Long-term use may cause corneal and scleral thinning.
! Systemic effects are uncommon, but systemic hypercorticoidism have been reported.
! Acute anterior uveitis and perforation of the globe, keratitis, conjunctivitis, corneal ulcers, mydriasis, conjunctival hyperemia, loss of accommodation, and ptosis have occasionally been reported.
! The development of secondary ocular infection has occurred. Fungal and viral infections of the cornea may develop with long-term applications of steroid.

DENTAL CONSIDERATIONS

General:

- Monitor vital signs at every appointment because of CV side effects.
- Patients on chronic drug therapy may rarely have symptoms of blood dyscrasias, which can include infection, bleeding, and poor healing.
- Assess salivary flow as a factor in caries, periodontal disease, and candidiasis.
- Avoid prescribing aspirin-containing products.
- Place on frequent recall to evaluate healing response.
- Prophylactic antibiotics may be indicated to prevent infection if surgery or deep scaling is planned.
- Symptoms of oral infections may be masked.
- Determine dose and duration of steroid therapy for each patient to assess risk for stress tolerance and immunosuppression.
- Patients who have been or are currently on chronic steroid therapy (>2 wk) require supplemental steroids for dental treatment.
- Determine why the patient is taking the drug.

Consultations:

- In a patient with symptoms of blood dyscrasias, request a medical consultation for blood studies and postpone dental treatment until normal values are reestablished.
- Medical consultation may be required to assess disease control.
- Consultation may be required to confirm steroid dose and duration of use.

Teach Patient/Family:

- Importance of good oral hygiene to prevent soft tissue inflammation
- Caution to prevent injury when using oral hygiene aids
- *When chronic dry mouth occurs, advise patient:*
  - To avoid mouth rinses with high alcohol content because of drying effects
  - Of need for daily use of home fluoride products to prevent caries
  - To use sugarless gum, frequent sips of water, or saliva substitutes

prednisolone acetate; sulfacetamide sodium

pred-niss′-oh-lone ass′-eh-tate; sul-fa-see′-ta-mide soe′-dee-um
(AK-Cide; Blephamide; Blephamide S.O.P.; Medasulf; Metimyd; Ocu-Lone C; Vasocidin)

CATEGORY AND SCHEDULE

Pregnancy Risk Category: C

MECHANISM OF ACTION

Prednisolone is an adrenal corticosteroid that inhibits accumulation of inflammatory cells at inflammation sites, phagocytosis, lysosomal enzyme release and synthesis, and release of mediators of inflammation. Sulfacetamide is a sulfonamide that interferes with synthesis of folic acid that bacteria require for growth. ***Therapeutic Effect:*** Prevents or suppresses cell-mediated immune reactions. Decreases or prevents tissue response to inflammatory process. Prevents further bacterial growth; bacteriostatic.

PHARMACOKINETICS

None reported.

AVAILABILITY

Ophthalmic ointment: 0.2% prednisolone acetate and 10% sulfacetamide sodium (Blephamide, Blephamide S.O.P.), 0.5% prednisolone acetate and 10% sulfacetamide sodium (AK-Cide, Ocu-Lone C, Medasulf, Metimyd). *Ophthalmic solution:* 0.25% prednisolone acetate and 10% sulfacetamide sodium (Vasocidin). *Ophthalmic suspension:* 0.2% prednisolone acetate and 10% sulfacetamide sodium (Blephamide), 0.5% prednisolone acetate and 10% sulfacetamide sodium (AK-Cide, Metimyd, Ocu-Lone C, Vasocidin).

INDICATIONS AND DOSAGES

▸ Steroid-Responsive Inflammatory Ocular Conditions for Which a Corticosteroid Is Indicated and Where Superficial Bacterial Ocular Infection or a Risk of Bacterial Ocular Infection Exists

OPHTHALMIC OINTMENT

Adults, Elderly, Children. Apply 3 or 4 times/day and once at bedtime.

OPHTHALMIC SUSPENSION

Adults, Elderly, Children. Instill 2-3 drops every 1–2 hours while awake.

CONTRAINDICATIONS

Epithelial herpes simplex keratitis (dendritic keratitis), vaccinia, varicella, and other viral diseases of the cornea or conjunctiva, mycobacterial infection of the eye, and fungal diseases of ocular structure, known or suspected hypersensitivity to other sulfonamides or other corticosteroids or any component of the formulation.

INTERACTIONS

Drug

Silver preparations: This drug is incompatible with silver preparations.

Local anesthetics (related to p-amino benzoic acid): May antagonize the action of sulfonamides.

Herbal

None known.

Food

None known.

Drug interactions of concern to dentistry

- Decreased action: barbiturates, rifampin, rifabutin
- Increased side effects: alcohol, salicylates, NSAIDs
- Increased action: ketoconazole, macrolide antibiotics (erythromycin, clarithromycin, azithromycin)
- Hepatotoxicity: acetaminophen (chronic use, high doses)

DIAGNOSTIC TEST EFFECTS

None known.

SIDE EFFECTS

Occasional

Local irritation

Rare

Elevation of intraocular pressure

SERIOUS REACTIONS

! Prolonged use of corticosteroids may result in glaucoma with damage to the optic nerve, defects in visual acuity and fields of vision, posterior subcapsular cataract formation, and delayed wound healing.

! Long-term use may cause corneal and scleral thinning.

! Systemic effects are uncommon, but systemic hypercorticoidism has been reported.

! Acute anterior uveitis and perforation of the globe, keratitis, conjunctivitis, corneal ulcers, mydriasis, conjunctival hyperemia, loss of accommodation and ptosis have occasionally been reported.

! The development of secondary ocular infection has occurred. Fungal and viral infections of the cornea may develop with long-term applications of steroid.

! Fatalities due to reactions to sulfonamides including Stevens-Johnson syndrome, toxic epidermal necrolysis, fulminant hepatic necrosis, agranulocytosis, aplastic anemia, and other blood dyscrasias have occurred.

P

DENTAL CONSIDERATIONS

General:

- Monitor vital signs at every appointment because of CV side effects.
- Patients on chronic drug therapy may rarely have symptoms of blood dyscrasias, which can include infection, bleeding, and poor healing.
- Assess salivary flow as a factor in caries, periodontal disease, and candidiasis.
- Avoid prescribing aspirin-containing products.
- Place on frequent recall to evaluate healing response.
- Prophylactic antibiotics may be indicated to prevent infection if surgery or deep scaling is planned.
- Symptoms of oral infections may be masked.
- Determine dose and duration of steroid therapy for each patient to assess risk for stress tolerance and immunosuppression.
- Patients who have been or are currently on chronic steroid therapy (>2 wk) require supplemental steroids for dental treatment.
- Determine why the patient is taking the drug.

Consultations:

- In a patient with symptoms of blood dyscrasias, request a medical consultation for blood studies and postpone dental treatment until normal values are reestablished.
- Medical consultation may be required to assess disease control.
- Consultation may be required to confirm steroid dose and duration of use.

Teach Patient/Family:

- Importance of good oral hygiene to prevent soft tissue inflammation
- Caution to prevent injury when using oral hygiene aids
- *When chronic dry mouth occurs, advise patient:*
  - To avoid mouth rinses with high alcohol content because of drying effects
  - Of need for daily use of home fluoride products to prevent caries
  - To use sugarless gum, frequent sips of water, or saliva substitutes

Drug interactions of concern to dentistry

- Decreased action: barbiturates, rifampin, rifabutin
- Increased side effects: alcohol, salicylates, NSAIDs

- Increased action: ketoconazole, macrolide antibiotics
- Hepatotoxicity: acetaminophen (chronic, high doses)

prednisolone sodium phosphate

pred-nis'-oh-lone soe'-dee-um foss'-fate
(AK-Pred, Inflamase Forte, Inflamase Mild, Orapred, Pediapred)

CATEGORY AND SCHEDULE

Pregnancy Risk Category: C

MECHANISM OF ACTION

An adrenal corticosteroid that inhibits accumulation of inflammatory cells at inflammation sites, phagocytosis, lysosomal enzyme release and synthesis, and release of mediators of inflammation. ***Therapeutic Effect:*** Prevents or suppresses cell-mediated immune reactions. Decreases or prevents tissue response to inflammatory process.

PHARMACOKINETICS

Rapidly and well absorbed from the gastrointestinal (GI tract) following oral administration. Protein binding: 90%–95%. Widely distributed. Metabolized in the liver. Excreted in the urine as sulfate and glucuronide conjugates. ***Half-life:*** 2–4 hrs. Absorbed into aqueous humor, cornea, iris, choroid, ciliary body, and retina following ocular administration. Systemic absorption occurs, but may be significant only at higher dosages or in extended pediatric therapy.

AVAILABILITY

Ophthalmic solution: 1% (AK-Pred, Inflamase Forte), 0.125% (Inflamase Mild).
Oral solution: 20 mg/5ml (Orapred), 6.7 mg/5ml (Pediapred).

INDICATIONS AND DOSAGES

▸ **Asthma**
PO
Children. 1–2 mg/kg/day in single or divided doses for 3–10 days.

▸ **Endocrine Disorders, Hematologic and Neoplastic Disorders, Inflammatory Conditions**
PO
Adults, Elderly. 5–60 mg/day.
Children. 0.14–2 mg/kg/day divided into 3 or 4 doses.

▸ **Multiple Sclerosis Exacerbations**
PO
Adults, Elderly. 200 mg/day for 1 week, followed by 80 mg every other day for 1 month.

▸ **Nephrotic Syndrome**
PO
Children. 60 mg/m^2 daily. Maximum: 80 mg/day divided 3 times/day for 4 weeks, then 40 mg/m^2 every other day for 4 weeks.

▸ **Ophthalmic Disorders**
OPHTHALMIC SUSPENSION
Adults, Elderly, Children. Instill 1 or 2 drops up to 6 times/day.

CONTRAINDICATIONS

Systemic fungal infections, live or live attenuated vaccines, hypersensitivity to prednisolone sodium phosphate or any component of the formulation

INTERACTIONS

Drug

Amphotericin: May increase hypokalemia.
Digoxin: May increase the risk of toxicity of this drug caused by hypokalemia.

P

Diuretics, insulin, oral hypoglycemics, potassium supplements: May decrease the effects of diuretics, insulin, oral hypoglycemics, and potassium supplements.
Liver enzyme inducers: May decrease the effects of prednisolone.
Live virus vaccines: May decrease the patient's antibody response to vaccine, increase vaccine side effects, and potentiate virus replication.

Herbal

None known.

Food

None known.

Drug interactions of concern to dentistry

• Decreased action: barbiturates, rifampin, rifabutin
• Increased side effects: alcohol, salicylates, NSAIDs
• Increased action: ketoconazole, macrolide antibiotics (erythromycin, clarithromycin, azithromycin)
• Hepatotoxicity: acetaminophen (chronic use, high doses)

DIAGNOSTIC TEST EFFECTS

None known.

P

SIDE EFFECTS

Frequent

Insomnia, heartburn, nervousness, abdominal distention, increased sweating, acne, mood swings, increased appetite, facial flushing, delayed wound healing, increased susceptibility to infection, diarrhea or constipation

Occasional

Headache, edema, change in skin color, frequent urination

Rare

Tachycardia, allergic reaction, such as rash and hives, psychic changes, hallucinations, depression
Ophthalmic: stinging or burning, posterior subcapsular cataracts

SERIOUS REACTIONS

! Prolonged use of corticosteroids may result in glaucoma with damage to the optic nerve, defects in visual acuity and fields of vision, posterior subcapsular cataract formation, and delayed wound healing.
! Long-term use may cause corneal and scleral thinning.
! Systemic effects are uncommon, but systemic hypercorticoidism has been reported.
! Acute anterior uveitis and perforation of the globe, keratitis, conjunctivitis, corneal ulcers, mydriasis, conjunctival hyperemia, loss of accommodation and ptosis have occasionally been reported.
! The development of secondary ocular infection has occurred. Fungal and viral infections of the cornea may develop with long-term applications of steroid.

DENTAL CONSIDERATIONS

General:

• Monitor vital signs at every appointment because of CV side effects.
• Patients on chronic drug therapy may rarely have symptoms of blood dyscrasias, which can include infection, bleeding, and poor healing.
• Assess salivary flow as a factor in caries, periodontal disease, and candidiasis.
• Avoid prescribing aspirin-containing products.
• Place on frequent recall to evaluate healing response.
• Prophylactic antibiotics may be indicated to prevent infection if surgery or deep scaling is planned.
• Symptoms of oral infections may be masked.
• Determine dose and duration of steroid therapy for each patient to

assess risk for stress tolerance and immunosuppression.
- Patients who have been or are currently on chronic steroid therapy (>2 wk) require supplemental steroids for dental treatment.
- Determine why the patient is taking the drug.

Consultations:
- In a patient with symptoms of blood dyscrasias, request a medical consultation for blood studies and postpone dental treatment until normal values are reestablished.
- Medical consultation may be required to assess disease control.
- Consultation may be required to confirm steroid dose and duration of use.

Teach Patient/Family:
- Importance of good oral hygiene to prevent soft tissue inflammation
- Caution to prevent injury when using oral hygiene aids
- *When chronic dry mouth occurs, advise patient:*
  - To avoid mouth rinses with high alcohol content because of drying effects
  - Of need for daily use of home fluoride products to prevent caries
  - To use sugarless gum, frequent sips of water, or saliva substitutes

prednisolone sodium phosphate; sulfacetamide sodium

pred-nis′-oh-lone soe′-dee-um foss′-ate; sul-fa-see′-ta-mide soe′-dee-um

CATEGORY AND SCHEDULE
Pregnancy Risk Category: C

MECHANISM OF ACTION
Prednisolone is an adrenal corticosteroid that inhibits accumulation of inflammatory cells at inflammation sites, phagocytosis, lysosomal enzyme release and synthesis, and release of mediators of inflammation. Sulfacetamide is a sulfonamide that interferes with synthesis of folic acid that bacteria require for growth. ***Therapeutic Effect:*** Prevents or suppresses cell-mediated immune reactions. Decreases or prevents tissue response to inflammatory process. Prevents further bacterial growth; bacteriostatic.

PHARMACOKINETICS
None reported.

AVAILABILITY
Ophthalmic suspension: 0.25% prednisolone sodium phosphate and 10% sulfacetamide sodium.

INDICATIONS AND DOSAGES
▸ Steroid-Responsive Inflammatory Ocular Conditions for Which a Corticosteroid Is Indicated and Where Superficial Bacterial Ocular Infection or a Risk of Bacterial Ocular Infection Exists

OPHTHALMIC

Adults, Elderly, Children. Instill 1–3 drops every 2–3 hours while awake.

CONTRAINDICATIONS
Viral diseases of the cornea and conjunctiva including epithelial herpes simplex keratitis (dendritic keratitis), vaccinia, and varicella, mycobacterial infection of the eye, fungal diseases of ocular structures, hypersensitivity to prednisolone sodium phosphate, sulfacetamide sodium, or any component of the formulation.

INTERACTIONS

Drug

Silver preparations: This drug is not compatible with silver preparations.
Local anesthetics (related to p-amino benzoic acid): May antagonize the action of sulfonamides.

Herbal

None known.

Food

None known.

Drug interactions of concern to dentistry

- Decreased action: barbiturates, rifampin, rifabutin
- Increased side effects: alcohol, salicylates, NSAIDs
- Increased action: ketoconazole, macrolide antibiotics (erythromycin, clarithromycin, azithromycin)
- Hepatotoxicity: acetaminophen (chronic use, high doses)

DIAGNOSTIC TEST EFFECTS

None known.

SIDE EFFECTS

Occasional

Local irritation

Rare

Elevation of intraocular pressure

SERIOUS REACTIONS

! Prolonged use of corticosteroids may result in glaucoma with damage to the optic nerve, defects in visual acuity and fields of vision, posterior subcapsular cataract formation, and delayed wound healing.
! Long-term use may cause corneal and scleral thinning.
! Systemic effects are uncommon, but systemic hypercorticoidism have been reported.
! Acute anterior uveitis and perforation of the globe, keratitis, conjunctivitis, corneal ulcers, mydriasis, conjunctival hyperemia, loss of accommodation, and ptosis have occasionally been reported.
! The development of secondary ocular infection has occurred. Fungal and viral infections of the cornea may develop with long-term applications of steroid.
! Fatalities due to reactions to sulfonamides including Stevens-Johnson syndrome, toxic epidermal necrolysis, fulminant hepatic necrosis, agranulocytosis, aplastic anemia, and other blood dyscrasias have occurred.

DENTAL CONSIDERATIONS

General:

- Monitor vital signs at every appointment because of CV side effects.
- Patients on chronic drug therapy may rarely have symptoms of blood dyscrasias, which can include infection, bleeding, and poor healing.
- Assess salivary flow as a factor in caries, periodontal disease, and candidiasis.
- Avoid prescribing aspirin-containing products.
- Place on frequent recall to evaluate healing response.
- Prophylactic antibiotics may be indicated to prevent infection if surgery or deep scaling is planned.
- Symptoms of oral infections may be masked.
- Determine dose and duration of steroid therapy for each patient to assess risk for stress tolerance and immunosuppression.
- Patients who have been or are currently on chronic steroid therapy (>2 wk) require supplemental steroids for dental treatment.
- Determine why the patient is taking the drug.

Consultations:

- In a patient with symptoms of blood dyscrasias, request a

medical consultation for blood studies and postpone dental treatment until normal values are reestablished.
- Medical consultation may be required to assess disease control.
- Consultation may be required to confirm steroid dose and duration of use.

Teach Patient/Family:
- Importance of good oral hygiene to prevent soft tissue inflammation
- Caution to prevent injury when using oral hygiene aids
- *When chronic dry mouth occurs, advise patient:*
  - To avoid mouth rinses with high alcohol content because of drying effects
  - Of need for daily use of home fluoride products to prevent caries
  - To use sugarless gum, frequent sips of water, or saliva substitutes

prednisone

pred′-ni-sone
(Apo-Prednisone[CAN], Deltasone, Panafcort[AUS], Prednisone Intensol, Sone[AUS], Sterapred, Sterapred DS, Winpred[CAN])
Do not confuse prednisone with prednisolone or primidone.

CATEGORY AND SCHEDULE
Pregnancy Risk Category: C (D if used in first trimester)

MECHANISM OF ACTION
An adrenocortical steroid that inhibits accumulation of inflammatory cells at inflammation sites, phagocytosis, lysosomal enzyme release and synthesis, and release of mediators of inflammation. ***Therapeutic Effect:*** Prevents or suppresses cell-mediated immune reactions. Decreases or prevents tissue response to inflammatory process.

PHARMACOKINETICS
Well absorbed from the GI tract. Protein binding: 70%–90%. Widely distributed. Metabolized in the liver and converted to prednisolone. Primarily excreted in urine.
Not removed by hemodialysis.
Half-life: 3.4–3.8 hr.

AVAILABILITY
*Oral Concentrate (Prednisone Intensol):*5 mg/ml .
Oral Solution: 5 mg/5 ml.
Tablets (Deltasone): 2.5 mg, 5 mg, 10 mg, 20 mg, 50 mg.
Tablets (Sterapred): 5 mg, 10 mg.

INDICATIONS AND DOSAGES
▸ **Substitution Therapy in Deficiency States: Acute or Chronic Adrenal Insufficiency, Congenital Adrenal Hyperplasia, and Adrenal Insufficiency Secondary to Pituitary Insufficiency; Nonendocrine Disorders: Arthritis; Rheumatic Carditis; Allergic, Collagen, Intestinal Tract, Liver, Ocular, Renal, Skin Diseases; Bronchial Asthma; Cerebral Edema; Malignancies**
PO
Adults, Elderly. 5–60 mg/day in divided doses.
Children. 0.05–2 mg/kg/day in 1–4 divided doses.

CONTRAINDICATIONS
Acute superficial herpes simplex keratitis, systemic fungal infections, varicella

INTERACTIONS
Drug
Amphotericin: May increase hypokalemia.

Digoxin: May increase the risk of digoxin toxicity caused by hypokalemia
Diuretics, insulin, oral hypoglycemics, potassium supplements: May decrease the effects of these drugs.
Hepatic enzyme inducers: May decrease the effects of prednisone.
Live-virus vaccines: May decrease the patient's antibody response to vaccine, increase vaccine side effects, and potentiate virus replication.

Herbal
None known.

Food
None known.

Drug interactions of concern to dentistry
- Decreased action: barbiturates, rifampin, rifabutin
- Increased side effects: alcohol, salicylates, NSAIDs
- Increased action: ketoconazole, macrolide antibiotics
- Hepatotoxicity: acetaminophen (chronic, high doses)

P

DIAGNOSTIC TEST EFFECTS

May increase blood glucose and serum lipid, amylase, and sodium levels. May decrease serum calcium, potassium, and thyroxine levels.

SIDE EFFECTS

Frequent
Insomnia, heartburn, nervousness, abdominal distention, increased sweating, acne, mood swings, increased appetite, facial flushing, delayed wound healing, increased susceptibility to infection, diarrhea or constipation

Occasional
Headache, edema, change in skin color, frequent urination

Rare
Tachycardia, allergic reaction (including rash and hives), psychological changes, hallucinations, depression

SERIOUS REACTIONS

! Long-term therapy may cause muscle wasting in the arms and legs, osteoporosis, spontaneous fractures, amenorrhea, cataracts, glaucoma, peptic ulcer disease, and CHF.
! Abruptly withdrawing the drug following long-term therapy may cause anorexia, nausea, fever, headache, sudden or severe joint pain, rebound inflammation, fatigue, weakness, lethargy, dizziness, and orthostatic hypotension.
! Suddenly discontinuing prednisone may be fatal.

DENTAL CONSIDERATIONS

General:
- Monitor vital signs at every appointment because of CV side effects.
- Patients on chronic drug therapy may rarely have symptoms of blood dyscrasias, which can include infection, bleeding, and poor healing.
- Avoid aspirin-containing products.
- Assess salivary flow as a factor in caries, periodontal disease, and candidiasis.
- Symptoms of oral infections may be masked.
- Place on frequent recall to evaluate healing response.
- Prophylactic antibiotics may be indicated to prevent infection if surgery or deep scaling is planned.
- Determine dose and duration of steroid therapy for each patient to assess risk for stress tolerance and immunosuppression.
- Patients who have been or are currently on chronic steroid therapy

(>2 wk) may require supplemental steroids for dental treatment.
• Determine why the patient is taking the drug.

Consultations:
• In a patient with symptoms of blood dyscrasias, request a medical consultation for blood studies and postpone dental treatment until normal values are reestablished.
• Medical consultation may be required to assess disease control.
• Consultation may be required to confirm steroid dose and duration of use.

Teach Patient/Family:
• Importance of good oral hygiene to prevent soft tissue inflammation
• Caution to prevent injury when using oral hygiene aids
• *When chronic dry mouth occurs, advise patient:*
  • To avoid mouth rinses with high alcohol content because of drying effects
  • Of need for daily use of home fluoride products to prevent caries
  • To use sugarless gum, frequent sips of water, or saliva substitutes

primaquine
prim-a-kween
(Primacin[AUS])
Do not confuse with primidone.

CATEGORY AND SCHEDULE
Pregnancy Risk Category: C

MECHANISM OF ACTION
An antimalarial and antirheumatic that eliminates tissue exoerythrocytic forms of *Plasmodium falciparum.* Disrupts mitochondria and binds to DNA. ***Therapeutic Effect:*** Inhibits parasite growth.

PHARMACOKINETICS
Well absorbed. Metabolized in the liver to the active metabolite, carboxyprimaquine. Excreted in the urine in small amounts as unchanged drug. ***Half-life:*** 4–6 hrs

AVAILABILITY
Tablets: 26.3 mg (Primaquine phosphate).

INDICATIONS AND DOSAGES
▸ Treatment of Malaria
PO
Adults, Elderly. 15 mg base daily for 14 days.
Children. 0.3 mg base/kg/wk once daily for 14 days.
Malaria prophylaxis
Adults, Elderly. 30 mg base daily. Begin 1 day before departure and continue for 7 days after leaving malarious area.

CONTRAINDICATIONS
Concomitant medications that cause bone marrow suppression, rheumatoid arthritis, lupus erythematosus, glucose-6-phosphate dehydrogenase (G-6-PD) deficiency, pregnancy, hypersensitivity to primaquine or any of its components

INTERACTIONS
Drug
Aurothioglucose: May increase risk of blood dyscrasias.
Levomethadyl: May increase risk of cardiotoxicity (QT prolongation, torsades de pointes, cardiac arrest).
Herbal
None known.
Food
None known.

Drug interactions of concern to dentistry
- None reported

DIAGNOSTIC TEST EFFECTS
None known.

SIDE EFFECTS
Frequent
Abdominal pain, nausea, vomiting
Rare
Leukopenia, hemolytic anemia, methemoglobinemia

SERIOUS REACTIONS
! Leukopenia, hemolytic anemia, methemoglobinemia occur rarely.
! Overdosage include symptoms of abdominal cramps, vomiting, burning epigastric distress, central nervous system and cardiovascular disturbances, cyanosis, methemoglobinemia, moderate leukocytosis or leukopenia, and anemia.
! Acute hemolysis occurs, but patients recover completely if the dosage is discontinued.

P

DENTAL CONSIDERATIONS
General:
- Patients on chronic drug therapy may rarely have symptoms of blood dyscrasias, which can include infection, bleeding, and poor healing.
- Avoid dental light in patient's eyes; offer dark glasses for patient comfort.

Consultations:
- In a patient with symptoms of blood dyscrasias, request a medical consultation for blood studies and postpone dental treatment until normal values are reestablished.

Teach Patient/Family:
- Importance of good oral hygiene to prevent soft tissue inflammation
- Caution to prevent injury when using oral hygiene aids

primidone
pri′-mi-done
Schedule IV
(Apo-Primidone[CAN], Mysoline)
Do not confuse primidone with prednisone.

CATEGORY AND SCHEDULE
Pregnancy Risk Category: D

MECHANISM OF ACTION
A barbiturate that decreases motor activity from electrical and chemical stimulation and stabilizes the seizure threshold against hyperexcitability.
Therapeutic Effect: Reduces seizure activity.

AVAILABILITY
Tablets: 50 mg, 250 mg.

INDICATIONS AND DOSAGES
▸ Seizure Control
PO
Adults, Elderly, Children 8 yr and older. 125–150 mg/day at bedtime. May increase by 125–250 mg/day every 3–7 days. Maximum: 2 g/day.
Children younger than 8 yr. Initially, 50–125 mg/day at bedtime. May increase by 50–125 mg/day every 3–7 days. Usual dose: 10–25 mg/kg/day in divided doses.
Neonates. 12–20 mg/kg/day in divided doses.

OFF-LABEL USES
Treatment of essential tremor

CONTRAINDICATIONS
History of bronchopneumonia, porphyria

INTERACTIONS
Drug
Alcohol, other CNS depressants: May increase the effects of primidone.

Carbamazepine: May increase the metabolism of carbamazepine.
Digoxin, glucocorticoids, metronidazole, oral anticoagulants, quinidine, tricyclic antidepressants: May decrease the effects of these drugs.
Valproic acid: Increases the blood concentration and risk of toxicity of primidone.

Herbal

None known.

Food

None known.

Drug interactions of concern to dentistry

- Increased CNS depression: alcohol, other CNS depressants
- Increased metabolism/hepatotoxicity: halothane, halogenated-hydrocarbon inhalation anesthetics
- Increased seizure threshold: haloperidol, phenothiazines
- Decreased effects of acetaminophen, corticosteroids, doxycycline, fenoprofen
- Lower blood concentrations: carbamazepine

DIAGNOSTIC TEST EFFECTS

May decrease serum bilirubin level. Therapeutic serum level is 4–12 mcg/ml; toxic serum level is greater than 12 mcg/ml.

SIDE EFFECTS

Frequent

Ataxia, dizziness

Occasional

Anorexia, drowsiness, mental changes, nausea, vomiting, paradoxical excitement

Rare

Rash

SERIOUS REACTIONS

! Abrupt withdrawal after prolonged therapy may produce effects ranging from increased dreaming, nightmares, insomnia, tremor, diaphoresis, and vomiting to hallucinations, delirium, seizures, and status epilepticus.

! Skin eruptions may may be a sign of a hypersensitivity reaction.

! Blood dyscrasias, hepatic disease, and hypocalcemia occur rarely.

! Overdose produces cold or clammy skin, hypothermia, and severe CNS depression, followed by high fever and coma.

DENTAL CONSIDERATIONS

General:

- Ask about type of epilepsy, seizure frequency, and quality of seizure control.
- After supine positioning, have patient sit upright for at least 2 min before standing to avoid orthostatic hypotension.
- Patients on chronic drug therapy may rarely have symptoms of blood dyscrasias, which can include infection, bleeding, and poor healing.
- Short appointments and a stress reduction protocol may be required for anxious patients.

Consultations:

- Medical consultation may be required to assess disease control and patient's ability to tolerate stress.
- In a patient with symptoms of blood dyscrasias, request a medical consultation for blood studies and postpone dental treatment until normal values are reestablished.

Teach Patient/Family:

- Importance of good oral hygiene to prevent soft tissue inflammation
- Caution to prevent injury when using oral hygiene aids
- To avoid mouth rinses with high alcohol content because of drying effects

probenecid

proe-ben′-e-sid
(Benuryl[CAN], Pro-Cid[AUS])
Do not confuse probenecid with procainamide.

CATEGORY AND SCHEDULE

Pregnancy Risk Category: C

MECHANISM OF ACTION

A uricosuric that competitively inhibits reabsorption of uric acid at the proximal convoluted tubule. Also, inhibits renal tubular secretion of weak organic acids, such as penicillins.
Therapeutic Effect: Promotes uric acid excretion, reduces serum uric acid level, and increases plasma levels of penicillins and cephalosporins.

AVAILABILITY

Tablets: 500 mg.

INDICATIONS AND DOSAGES

▸ **Gout**

PO

Adults, Elderly. Initially, 250 mg twice a day for 1 wk; then 500 mg twice a day. May increase by 500 mg q4wk. Maximum: 2–3 g/day. Maintenance: Dosage that maintains normal uric acid level.

▸ **As Adjunct to Penicillin or Cephalosporin Therapy to Prolong Antibiotic Plasma Levels**

PO

Adults, Elderly. 2 g/day in divided doses.
Children weighing more than 50 kg. Receive adult dosage.
Children 2–14 yr. Initially, 25 mg/kg. Maintenance: 40 mg/kg/day in 4 divided doses.

▸ **Gonorrhea**

PO

Adults, Elderly. 1 g 30 min before penicillin, ampicillin, or amoxicillin.

CONTRAINDICATIONS

Blood dyscrasias, children younger than 2 years, concurrent high-dose aspirin therapy, severe renal impairment, uric acid calculi

INTERACTIONS

Drug

Alcohol: May increase serum urate level.
Antineoplastics: May increase the risk of uric acid nephropathy.
Cephalosporins, methotrexate, nitrofurantoin, NSAIDs, penicillins, zidovudine: May increase blood concentrations of these drugs.
Heparin: May increase and prolong the effects of heparin.
Salicylates: May decrease uricosuric effect.

Herbal

None known.

Food

None known.

Drug interactions of concern to dentistry

- Increased toxicity: dapsone, indomethacin, other NSAIDs, acyclovir
- Increased sedation: benzodiazepines
- Decreased action: alcohol, salicylates
- Increased duration of action: penicillins, cephalosporins
- Contraindicated: ketorolac

DIAGNOSTIC TEST EFFECTS

May inhibit renal excretion of serum PSP (phenolsulfonphthalein), 17-ketosteroids, and BSP (sulfobromophthalein).

SIDE EFFECTS

Frequent (10%–6%)
Headache, anorexia, nausea, vomiting
Occasional (5%–1%)
Lower back or side pain, rash, hives, itching, dizziness, flushed face, frequent urge to urinate, gingivitis

SERIOUS REACTIONS

! Severe hypersensitivity reactions, including anaphylaxis, occur rarely and usually within a few hours after administration following previous use. If severe hypersensitivity reactions develop, discontinue the drug immediately and contact the physician.
! Pruritic maculopapular rash, possibly accompanied by malaise, fever, chills, arthralgia, nausea, vomiting, leukopenia, and aplastic anemias should be considered a toxic reaction.

DENTAL CONSIDERATIONS

General:

- Avoid prescribing aspirin-containing products.

Teach Patient/Family:

- Importance of good oral hygiene to prevent soft tissue inflammation
- Caution to prevent injury when using oral hygiene aids
- To avoid mouth rinses with high alcohol content because of drying effects

procaine

proe′-kane
(Novocain, Mericaine)

CATEGORY AND SCHEDULE

Pregnancy Risk Category: C

MECHANISM OF ACTION

Procaine causes a reversible blockade of nerve conduction by decreasing nerve membrance permeability to sodium. ***Therapeutic effect:*** Local anesthesia.

PHARMACOKINETICS

Highly plasma protein-bound and distributed to all body tissues. Excreted in the urine (80%). ***Half-life:*** 40 ± 9 seconds in adults, 84 ± 30 seconds in neonates.

AVAILABILITY

Solution: 0.25%, 0.5%, 10% (Novocaine)

INDICATIONS AND DOSAGES

▸ Spinal Anesthesia

INTRATHECAL

Adults. 0.5–1 ml of a 10% solution (50–100 mg) mixed with an equal volume of diluent injected into the third or fourth lumber interspace (perineum and lower extremeties). 2 ml of a 10% solution (200 mg) mixed with 1 ml of diluent injected into the second, third, or fourth interspace.

▸ Infiltration Anesthesia, Dental Anesthesia, Control of Severe Pain (post-herpatic neuralgia, cancer pain, or burns)

TOPICAL

Adults. A single dose of 350–600 mg using a 0.25 or 0.5% solution. Use 0.9% sodium chloride for dilution.
Children. 15 mg/kg of a 0.5% solution is the maximum recommended dose.

▸ Peripheral or Sympathetic Nerve Block (regional anesthesia)

TOPICAL

Adults. Up to 200 ml of a 0.5% solution (1 g), 100 ml of a 1% solution (1 g), or 50 ml of a 2% solution (1 g). The 2% solution should only be used when a small volume of anesthetic is required.

OFF-LABEL USES

Severe pain

CONTRAINDICATIONS

Hypersensitivity to ester local anesthetics, sulfites, PABA, patients on anticoagulant therapy, and in patients with coagulopathy, infection, thrombocytopenia. Should not be given intraarterial, intrathecal, or intravenous.

INTERACTIONS

Drug

Local anesthetics: May cause a toxic additive effect.
Medications that cause QT prolongation: May cause additive cardiotoxic effects.
Cholinesterase inhibitors: Procaine may antagonize the effect of these medication.
Antihypertensives, nitrates: May experience additive hypotensive effects.
MAOIs: Increased risk of hypotension.
CNS depressants: May cause additive suppression.

Herbal

None known.

Food

None known.

Drug interactions of concern to dentistry

- Possible prolonged effects of succinylcholine
- Increased CNS depression with all CNS depressants, especially in children and when larger doses are used
- Risk of CV side effects: rapid intravascular injection
- Suspected interference with antimicrobial activity of sulfonamides

DIAGNOSTIC TEST EFFECTS

None known.

SIDE EFFECTS

Frequent

Numbness or tingling of the face or mouth, pain at the injection site, dizziness, drowsiness, lightheadedness, nausea, vomiting, back pain, headache

Rare

Anxiety, restlessness, difficulty breathing, shortness of breath, seizures (convulsions), skin rash, itching (hives), slow, irregular heartbeat (palpitations), swelling of the face or mouth, tremors, QT prolongation, PR prolongation, atrial fibrillation, sinus bradycardia, hypotension, angina, cardiovascular collapse, fecal or urinary incontinence, loss of perineal sensation and sexual function, persistent motor, sensory, and/or autonomic (sphincter control) deficit

SERIOUS REACTIONS

! Procaine-induced CNS toxicity usually presents with symptoms of stimulation, such as anxiety, apprehension, restlessness, nervousness, disorientation, confusion, dizziness, blurred vision, tremor, nausea/vomiting, shivering, or seizures. Subsequently, depressive symptoms can occur including drowsiness, unconsciousness, and respiratory arrest.

! If higher concentrations are introduced into the bloodstream, depression of cardiac excitability and contractility may cause AV block, ventricular arrhythmias, or cardiac arrest. CNS toxicity including dizziness, tongue numbness, visual impairment and disturbances, and muscular twitching appear to occur before cardiotoxic effects.

Alert

! Procaine should be used with caution in patients that have asthma because there is the increased risk of anaphylactoid reactions including bronchospasm and status asthmaticus.

Alert

! Local anesthetics can cause varying degrees of maternal, fetal, and neonatal toxicities during labor and obstetric delivery. Fetal heart rate should be monitored, as well as the presence of symptoms indicating fetal bradycardia, fetal acidosis, and

P

maternal hypotension. Epidural procaine may cause decreased uterine contractility or maternal expulsion efforts and alter the forces of parturition.

Alert

! Unintentional fetal intracranial injection of procaine occurring during pudenal or paracervical block has been shown to lead to neonatal depression at birth and can lead to seizures within 6 hours as a result of high serum concentrations.

DENTAL CONSIDERATIONS

General:

- Not available for use in dental local anesthesia.

procarbazine hydrochloride

pro-car′-bah-zeen

(Matulane, Natulan[CAN])

Do not confuse procarbazine with dacarbazine.

CATEGORY AND SCHEDULE

Pregnancy Risk Category: D

MECHANISM OF ACTION

A methylhydrazine derivative that inhibits DNA, RNA, and protein synthesis. May also directly damage DNA. Cell cycle-phase specific for S phase of cell division. ***Therapeutic Effect:*** Causes cell death.

AVAILABILITY

Capsules: 50 mg.

INDICATIONS AND DOSAGES

▸ Advanced Hodgkin's Disease

PO

Adults, Elderly. Initially, 2–4 mg/kg/day as a single dose or in divided doses for 1 wk, then 4–6 mg/kg/day. Maintenance: 1–2 mg/kg/day.

Children. 50–100 $mg/m^2/day$ for 10–14 days of a 28-day cycle. Continue until maximum response occurs, leukocyte count falls below 4000/mm3, or platelet count falls below 100,000/mm3. Maintenance: 50 $mg/m^2/day$.

OFF-LABEL USES

Treatment of lung carcinoma, malignant melanoma, multiple myeloma, non-Hodgkin's lymphoma, polycythemia vera, primary brain tumors

CONTRAINDICATIONS

Myelosuppression

INTERACTIONS

Drug

Alcohol: May cause a disulfiram-like reaction.

Anticholinergics, antihistamines: May increase the anticholinergic effects of these drugs.

Bone marrow depressants: May increase myelosuppression.

Buspirone, caffeine-containing medications: May increase BP.

Carbamazepine, cyclobenzaprine, MAOIs, maprotiline: May cause hyperpyretic crisis, seizures, or death.

CNS depressants: May increase CNS depression.

Insulin, oral antidiabetics: May increase the effects of these drugs.

Meperidine: May produce coma, seizures, immediate excitation, rigidity, severe hypertension or hypotension, severe respiratory distress, diaphoresis, and vascular collapse.

Sympathomimetics: May increase cardiac stimulant and vasopressor effects.

Tricyclic antidepressants: May increase anticholinergic effects; may cause seizures and hyperpyretic crisis.

Herbal

None known.

Food

Caffeine-containing beverages: May increase BP.

Drug interactions of concern to dentistry

- Increased CNS depression: barbiturates, antihistamines, narcotics
- Disulfiram-like reaction: ethyl alcohol
- Hypertension: indirect-acting sympathomimetics
- Increased anticholinergic effect: anticholinergic drugs, antihistamines
- Increased risk of severe toxic reactions: tricyclic antidepressants, meperidine and other opioids, tyramine-containing foods and other MAOIs; may include cyclobenzaprine and carbamazepine

DIAGNOSTIC TEST EFFECTS

None known.

SIDE EFFECTS

Frequent

Severe nausea, vomiting, respiratory disorders (cough, effusion), myalgia, arthralgia, drowsiness, nervousness, insomnia, nightmares, diaphoresis, hallucinations, seizures

Occasional

Hoarseness, tachycardia, nystagmus, retinal hemorrhage, photophobia, photosensitivity, urinary frequency, nocturia, hypotension, diarrhea, stomatitis, paraesthesia, unsteadiness, confusion, decreased reflexes, foot drop

Rare

Hypersensitivity reaction (dermatitis, pruritus, rash, urticaria), hyperpigmentation, alopecia

SERIOUS REACTIONS

! Procarbazine's major toxic effects are myelosuppression manifested as hematologic toxicity (mainly leukopenia, thrombo-cytopenia, and anemia) and hepatotoxicity manifested as jaundice and ascites.

! UTIs may occur secondary to leukopenia.

DENTAL CONSIDERATIONS

General:

- Patients on chronic drug therapy may rarely have symptoms of blood dyscrasias, which can include infection, bleeding, and poor healing.
- Monitor vital signs at every appointment because of CV side effects.
- Consider semisupine chair position for patient comfort if GI side effects occur.
- Assess salivary flow as a factor in caries, periodontal disease, and candidiasis.
- After supine positioning, have patient sit upright for at least 2 min before standing to avoid orthostatic hypotension.
- Avoid dental light in patient's eyes; offer dark glasses for patient comfort.
- Avoid aspirin-containing products because of bleeding risk.
- Avoid use of gingival retraction cord with epinephrine.
- Patients receiving chemotherapy may require palliative treatment for stomatitis.

Consultations:

- In a patient with symptoms of blood dyscrasias, request a medical consultation for blood studies and postpone dental treatment until normal values are reestablished.
- Take precautions if dental surgery is anticipated and sedation or general anesthesia is required; there is risk of hypotensive episode.

Teach Patient/Family:
- Importance of good oral hygiene to prevent soft tissue inflammation
- Caution to prevent injury when using oral hygiene aids
- To report oral lesions, soreness, or bleeding to dentist
- *When chronic dry mouth occurs, advise patient:*
  - To avoid mouth rinses with high alcohol content because of drying effects
  - Of need for daily use of home fluoride products to prevent caries
  - To use sugarless gum, frequent sips of water, or saliva substitutes

prochlorperazine

proe-klor-per′-a-zeen
(Compazine, Stemetil[CAN], Stemzine[AUS])
Do not confuse prochlorperazine with chlorpromazine, or Compazine with Copaxone.

CATEGORY AND SCHEDULE

Pregnancy Risk Category: C

MECHANISM OF ACTION

A phenothiazine that acts centrally to inhibit or block dopamine receptors in the chemoreceptor trigger zone and peripherally to block the vagus nerve in the GI tract. ***Therapeutic Effect:*** Relieves nausea and vomiting and improves psychotic conditions.

PHARMACOKINETICS

Route	Onset *	Peak	Duration
Tablets, oral solution	30–40 min	N/A	3–4 hr
Capsules (Extended-Release)	30–40 min	N/A	10–12 hr
Rectal	60 min	N/A	3–4 hr

*As an antiemetic

Variably absorbed after PO administration. Widely distributed. Metabolized in the liver and GI mucosa. Primarily excreted in urine. Unknown if removed by hemodialysis. ***Half-life:*** 23 hr.

AVAILABILITY

Capsules (Extended-Release): 10 mg, 15 mg.
Oral solution: 5 mg/5ml.
Tablets: 5 mg, 10 mg.
Suppositories: 2.5 mg, 5 mg, 25 mg.
Injection (Compazine): 5 mg/ml.

INDICATIONS AND DOSAGES

▸ Nausea and Vomiting

PO
Adults, Elderly. 5–10 mg 3–4 times a day.
Children. 0.4 mg/kg/day in 3–4 divided doses.
PO (Extended-Release)
Adults, Elderly. 10 mg twice a day or 15 mg once a day.
IV
Adults, Elderly. 2.5–10 mg. May repeat q3–4h.
Children. 0.1–0.15 mg/kg/dose q8–12h. Maximum: 40 mg/day.
IM
Adults, Elderly. 5–10 mg q3–4h.
Children. 0.1–0.15 mg/kg/dose q8–12h. Maximum: 40 mg/day.
RECTAL
Adults, Elderly. 25 mg twice a day.
Children. 0.4 mg/kg/day in 3–4 divided doses.

▸ Psychosis

PO
Adults, Elderly. 5–10 mg 3–4 times a day. Maximum: 150 mg/day.
Children. 2.5 mg 2-3 times a day. Maximum: 25 mg for children 6–12 yr; 20 mg for children 2–5 yr.
IM
Adults, Elderly. 10–20 mg q4h.
Children. 0.13 mg/kg/dose.

CONTRAINDICATIONS

Angle-closure glaucoma, CNS depression, coma, myelosuppression, severe cardiac or hepatic impairment, severe hypotension or hypertension

INTERACTIONS

Drug

Alcohol, other CNS depressants: May increase CNS and respiratory depression and the hypotensive effects of prochlorperazine.
Antihypertensives: May increase hypotension.
Antithyroid agents: May increase the risk of agranulocytosis.
Extrapyramidal symptom-producing medications: May increase extrapyramidal symptoms.
Levodopa: May decrease the effects of levodopa.
Lithium: May decrease the absorption of prochlorperazine and produce adverse neurologic effects.
MAOIs, tricyclic antidepressants: May increase the anticholinergic and sedative effects of prochlorperazine.

Herbal

None known.

P

Food

None known.

Drug interactions of concern to dentistry

- Increased sedation: other CNS depressants, alcohol, barbiturate anesthetics, opioid analgesics
- Hypotension, tachycardia: epinephrine
- Increased extrapyramidal effects: phenothiazines and related drugs (haloperidol, droperidol), metoclopramide
- Additive photosensitization: tetracyclines
- Increased anticholinergic effects: anticholinergics

DIAGNOSTIC TEST EFFECTS

None known.

IV INCOMPATIBILITIES

Atropine, furosemide (Lasix), midazolam (Versed)

IV COMPATIBILITIES

Calcium gluconate, diphenhydramine (Benadryl), fentanyl, glycopyrrolate (Robinul), heparin, hydromorphone (Dilaudid), morphine, metoclopramide (Reglan), nalbuphine (Nubain), potassium chloride, promethazine (Phenergan), propofol (Diprivan)

SIDE EFFECTS

Frequent

Somnolence, hypotension, dizziness, fainting (commonly occurring after first dose, occasionally after subsequent doses, and rarely with oral form)

Occasional

Dry mouth, blurred vision, lethargy, constipation, diarrhea, myalgia, nasal congestion, peripheral edema, urine retention

SERIOUS REACTIONS

! Extrapyramidal symptoms appear to be dose related and are divided into three categories: akathisia (marked by inability to sit still, tapping of feet), parkinsonian symptoms (including mask-like face, tremors, shuffling gait, hypersalivation), and acute dystonias (such as torticollis, opisthotonos, and oculogyric crisis). A dystonic reaction may also produce diaphoresis or pallor.
! Tardive dyskinesia, manifested as tongue protrusion, puffing of the cheeks, and puckering of the mouth, is a rare reaction that may be irreversible.
! Abrupt withdrawal after long-term therapy may precipitate nausea, vomiting, gastritis, dizziness, and tremors.
! Blood dyscrasias, particularly agranulocytosis and mild leukopenia, may occur.

! Prochlorperazine use may lower the seizure threshold.

DENTAL CONSIDERATIONS

General:

- Monitor vital signs at every appointment because of CV side effects.
- Patients on chronic drug therapy may rarely have symptoms of blood dyscrasias, which can include infection, bleeding, and poor healing.
- After supine positioning, have patient sit upright for at least 2 min before standing to avoid orthostatic hypotension.
- Assess salivary flow as a factor in caries, periodontal disease, and candidiasis.
- Avoid dental light in patient's eyes; offer dark glasses for patient comfort.
- Assess for presence of extrapyramidal motor symptoms, such as tardive dyskinesia and akathisia. Extrapyramidal motor activity may complicate dental treatment.
- Geriatric patients are more susceptible to drug effects; use lower dose.
- Use vasoconstrictors with caution, in low doses, and with careful aspiration.

Consultations:

- In a patient with symptoms of blood dyscrasias, request a medical consultation for blood studies and postpone dental treatment until normal values are reestablished.
- Take precautions if dental surgery is anticipated and anesthesia is required.
- If signs of tardive dyskinesia or akathisia are present, refer to physician.

Teach Patient/Family:

- Importance of good oral hygiene to prevent soft tissue inflammation
- Caution to prevent injury when using oral hygiene aids
- To use electric toothbrush if patient has difficulty holding conventional devices
- *When chronic dry mouth occurs, advise patient:*
  - To avoid mouth rinses with high alcohol content because of drying effects
  - Of need for daily use of home fluoride products to prevent caries
  - To use sugarless gum, frequent sips of water, or saliva substitutes

procyclidine

proe-sye-kli-deen

(Kemadrin)

CATEGORY AND SCHEDULE

Pregnancy Risk Category: C

MECHANISM OF ACTION

An anticholinergic agent that exerts an atropine-like action and produces an antispasmodic effect on smooth muscle, is a potent mydriatic, and inhibits salivation. ***Therapeutic Effect:*** Relieves symptoms of Parkinson's disease and drug-induced extrapyramidal symptoms.

PHARMACOKINETICS

Well absorbed from the gastrointestinal (GI) tract. Protein binding: extensive. Metabolized in liver—undergoes extensive first-pass effect. Primarily excreted in urine. Unknown if removed by hemodialysis. ***Half-life:*** 7.7–16.1 hrs.

AVAILABILITY

Tablets: 5 mg (Kemadrin).

INDICATIONS AND DOSAGES

▸ Drug-Induced Extrapyramidal Reactions

PO

Adults, Elderly. Initially, 2.5 mg 3 times/day. May increase by 2.5 mg

P

daily as needed. Maintenance: 10–20 mg/day in divided doses 3 times/day.

▸ Parkinson's Disease

PO

Adults, Elderly. Initially, 2.5 mg 3 times/day after meals. Maintenance: 2.5–5 mg mg/day in divided doses 3 times/day after meals.

▸ Hepatic Function Impairment

PO

Adults, Elderly. 2.5–5 mg mg/day in divided doses twice a day after meals

CONTRAINDICATIONS

Angle-closure glaucoma

INTERACTIONS

Drug

Alcohol: May increase sedation.
Amantadine, narcotic analgesics, phenothiazines, tricyclic antidepressants, quinidine, antihistamines: May increase anticholinergic effects.
Levodopa: May increase gastric degradation of levodopa and decrease the amount of levodopa absorbed by gastric emptying.
Paroxetine: May increase anticholinergic effects.

P

Herbal

Betel nut: May decrease anticholinergic effect of procyclidine.

Food

None known.

Drug interactions of concern to dentistry

- Increased anticholinergic effect: antihistamines, anticholinergics, meperidine
- Increased CNS depression: alcohol, CNS depressants

DIAGNOSTIC TEST EFFECTS

None known.

IV INCOMPATIBILITIES

None known.

IV COMPATIBILITIES

None known.

SIDE EFFECTS

Frequent

Blurred vision, mydriasis, disorientation, lightheadedness, nausea, vomiting dry mouth, nose, throat, and lips

SERIOUS REACTIONS

! Overdosage may vary from severe anticholinergic effects, such as unsteadiness, severe drowsiness, severe dryness of mouth, nose, or throat, tachycardia, shortness of breath, and skin flushing.
! Also produces severe paradoxical reaction, marked by hallucinations, tremor, seizures, and toxic psychosis.

DENTAL CONSIDERATIONS

General:

- Monitor vital signs at every appointment because of CV side effects.
- Assess salivary flow as a factor in caries, periodontal disease, and candidiasis.
- After supine positioning, have patient sit upright for at least 2 min before standing to avoid orthostatic hypotension.
- Avoid dental light in patient's eyes; offer dark glasses for patient comfort.
- Do not ingest sodium bicarbonate products, such as the Prophy-Jet air polishing system, until 1 hr after drug use.
- Place on frequent recall because of oral side effects.

Consultations:

- Medical consultation may be required to assess disease control.
- Medical consultation may be required to assess patient's ability to tolerate stress.

Teach Patient/Family:

- Use of electric toothbrush if patient has difficulty holding conventional devices
- Importance of good oral hygiene to prevent soft tissue inflammation
- Caution to prevent injury when using oral hygiene aids
- *When chronic dry mouth occurs, advise patient:*
  - To avoid mouth rinses with high alcohol content because of drying effects
  - To use daily home fluoride products for anticaries effect
  - To use sugarless gum, frequent sips of water, or saliva substitutes

progesterone

proe-jess′-ter-one
(Crinone, Prochieve, Prometrium)

CATEGORY AND SCHEDULE

Pregnancy Risk Category: D

MECHANISM OF ACTION

A natural steroid hormone that promotes mammary gland development and relaxes uterine smooth muscle. ***Therapeutic Effect:*** Decreases abnormal uterine bleeding; transforms endometrium from proliferative to secretory in an estrogen-primed endometrium.

AVAILABILITY

Capsules (Prometrium): 100 mg, 200 mg.
Injection: 50 mg/ml.
Vaginal Gel (Crinone, Prochieve): 4% (45 mg), 8% (90 mg).

INDICATIONS AND DOSAGES

▸ Amenorrhea

PO

Adults. 400 mg daily in evening for 10 days.

IM

Adults. 5–10 mg for 6–8 days. Withdrawal bleeding expected in 48–72 hr if ovarian activity produced proliferative endometrium.

VAGINAL

Adults. Apply 45 mg (4% gel) every other day for 6 or fewer doses.

▸ Abnormal Uterine Bleeding

IM

Adults. 5–10 mg for 6 days. When estrogen given concomitantly, begin progesterone after 2 wk of estrogen therapy; discontinue when menstrual flow begins.

▸ Prevention of Endometrial Hyperplasia

PO

Adults. 200 mg in evening for 12 days per 28-day cycle in combination with daily conjugated estrogen.

▸ Infertility

VAGINAL

Adults. 90 mg (8% gel) once a day (2 twice a day in women with partial or complete ovarian failure).

OFF-LABEL USES

Treatment of corpus luteum dysfunction

CONTRAINDICATIONS

Breast cancer; history of active cerebral apoplexy; thromboembolic disorders or thrombophlebitis; missed abortion; severe hepatic dysfunction; undiagnosed vaginal bleeding; use as a pregnancy test

INTERACTIONS

Drug

Bromocriptine: May interfere with the effects of bromocriptine.

Herbal

None known.

Food

None known.

Drug interactions of concern to dentistry
- None reported

DIAGNOSTIC TEST EFFECTS
May increase serum LDL and serum alkaline phosphatase levels. May decrease glucose tolerance and HDL concentrations. May cause abnormal serum thyroid, metapyrone, hepatic, and endocrine function test results.

SIDE EFFECTS
Frequent
Breakthrough bleeding or spotting at beginning of therapy, amenorrhea, change in menstrual flow, breast tenderness
Gel: drowsiness
Occasional
Edema, weight gain or loss, rash, pruritus, photosensitivity, skin pigmentation
Rare
Pain or swelling at injection site, acne, depression, alopecia, hirsutism

SERIOUS REACTIONS
! Thrombophlebitis, cerebrovascular disorders, retinal thrombosis, and pulmonary embolism occur rarely.

DENTAL CONSIDERATIONS
General:
- Determine why patient is taking the drug.
- Advise patient if dental drugs prescribed have a potential for photosensitivity.
- Monitor vital signs.
- Some patients may experience drowsiness; inquire before using CNS depressants.

Teach Patient/Family:
- Caution patients about driving or performing other tasks requiring mental alertness
- Importance of good oral hygiene to prevent soft tissue inflammation
- To prevent trauma when using oral hygiene aids
- Importance of updating health and medication history if physician makes any changes in evaluation or drug regimens; include OTC, herbal, and nonherbal in the update

promethazine hydrochloride
proe-meth′-a-zeen
Schedule V
(Insomn-Eze[AUS], Phenadoz, Phenergan)
Do not confuse promethazine with promazine.

CATEGORY AND SCHEDULE
Pregnancy Risk Category: C

MECHANISM OF ACTION
A phenothiazine that acts as an antihistamine, antiemetic, and sedative-hypnotic. As an antihistamine, inhibits histamine at histamine receptor sites. As an antiemetic, diminishes vestibular stimulation, depresses labyrinthine function, and acts on the chemoreceptor trigger zone. As a sedative-hypnotic, produces CNS depression by decreasing stimulation to the brainstem reticular formation. ***Therapeutic Effect:*** Prevents allergic responses mediated by histamine, such as rhinitis, urticaria, and pruritus. Prevents and relieves nausea and vomiting.

PHARMACOKINETICS

Route	Onset	Peak	Duration
PO	20 min	N/A	2–8 hr
IV	3–5 min	N/A	2–8 hr
IM	20 min	N/A	2–8 hr
Rectal	20 min	N/A	2–8 hr

P

Well absorbed from the GI tract after IM administration. Widely distributed. Metabolized in the liver. Primarily excreted in urine. Not removed by hemodialysis. ***Half-life:*** 16–19 hr.

AVAILABILITY

Syrup (Phenergan): 6.25 mg/ml.
Tablets (Phenergan): 12.5 mg, 25 mg, 50 mg.
Injection (Phenergan): 25 mg/ml, 50 mg/ml.
Suppositories (Phenergan): 12.5 mg, 25 mg, 50 mg.
Suppositories (Phenadoz): 25 mg.

INDICATIONS AND DOSAGES

▸ Allergic Symptoms

PO
Adults, Elderly. 6.25–12.5 mg 3 times a day plus 25 mg at bedtime.
Children. 0.1 mg/kg/dose (maximum: 12.5 mg) 3 times a day plus 0.5 mg/kg/dose (maximum: 25 mg) at bedtime.
IV, IM
Adults, Elderly. 25 mg. May repeat in 2 hr.

▸ Motion Sickness

PO
Adults, Elderly. 25 mg 30–60 min before departure; may repeat in 8–12 hr, then every morning on rising and before evening meal.
Children. 0.5 mg/kg 30–60 min before departure; may repeat in 8–12 hr, then every morning on rising and before evening meal.

▸ Prevention of Nausea and Vomiting

PO, IV, IM, RECTAL
Adults, Elderly. 12.5–25 mg q4–6h as needed.
Children. 0.25–1 mg/kg q4–6h as needed.

▸ Preoperative and Postoperative Sedation; Adjunct to Analgesics

IV, IM
Adults, Elderly. 25–50 mg.
Children. 12.5–25 mg.

▸ Sedative

PO, IV, IM, RECTAL
Adults, Elderly. 25–50 mg/dose. May repeat q4–6h as needed.
Children. 0.5–1 mg/kg/dose q6h as needed. Maximum: 50 mg/dose.

CONTRAINDICATIONS

Angle-closure glaucoma, GI or GU obstruction, severe CNS depression or coma

INTERACTIONS

Drug

Alcohol, other CNS depressants: May increase CNS depressant effects.
Anticholinergics: May increase anticholinergic effects.
MAOIs: May intensify and prolong the anticholinergic and CNS depressant effects of promethazine.

Herbal

None known.

Food

None known.

Drug interactions of concern to dentistry

- Increased CNS depression: alcohol, all CNS depressants
- Hypotension: general anesthetics
- Increased effect of anticholinergic drugs

DIAGNOSTIC TEST EFFECTS

May suppress wheal and flare reactions to antigen skin testing unless the drug is discontinued 4 days before testing.

IV INCOMPATIBILITIES

Allopurinol (Aloprim), amphotericin B complex (Abelcet, AmBisome, Amphotec), heparin, ketorolac (Toradol), nalbuphine (Nubain), piperacillin and tazobactam (Zosyn)

IV COMPATIBILITIES
Atropine, diphenhydramine (Benadryl), glycopyrrolate (Robinul), hydromorphone (Dilaudid), hydroxyzine (Vistaril), meperidine (Demerol), midazolam (Versed), morphine, prochlorperazine (Compazine)

SIDE EFFECTS
Expected
Somnolence, disorientation; in elderly, hypotension, confusion, syncope
Frequent
Dry mouth, nose, or throat; urine retention; thickening of bronchial secretions
Occasional
Epigastric distress, flushing, visual disturbances, hearing disturbances, wheezing, paresthesia, diaphoresis, chills
Rare
Dizziness, urticaria, photosensitivity, nightmares

SERIOUS REACTIONS
! Children may experience paradoxical reactions, such as excitation, nervousness, tremor, hyperactive reflexes, and seizures.
! Infants and young children have experienced CNS depression manifested as respiratory depression, sleep apnea, and sudden infant death syndrome.
! Long-term therapy may produce extrapyramidal symptoms, such as dystonia (abnormal movements), pronounced motor restlessness (most frequently in children), and parkinsonian (most frequently in elderly patients).
! Blood dyscrasias, particularly agranulocytosis, occur rarely.

DENTAL CONSIDERATIONS
General:
- Determine why the patient is taking the drug.
- Patients on chronic drug therapy may rarely have symptoms of blood dyscrasias, which can include infection, bleeding, and poor healing.
- Monitor vital signs at every appointment because of CV side effects.
- Assess salivary flow as a factor in caries, periodontal disease, and candidiasis.
- Assess vital signs q30min after use as sedative.

Teach Patient/Family:
- *When chronic dry mouth occurs, advise patient:*
  - To avoid mouth rinses with high alcohol content because of drying effects
  - Of need for daily use of home fluoride products to prevent caries
  - To use sugarless gum, frequent sips of water, or saliva substitutes

P

propafenone hydrochloride
proe-pa-fen′-one
(Rythmol, Rythmol SR)

CATEGORY AND SCHEDULE
Pregnancy Risk Category: C

MECHANISM OF ACTION
An antiarrhythmic that decreases the fast sodium current in Purkinje or myocardial cells. Decreases excitability and automaticity; prolongs conduction velocity and the refractory period. ***Therapeutic Effect:*** Suppresses arrhythmias.

AVAILABILITY

Tablets (Rythmol): 150 mg, 225 mg, 300 mg).
Capsules (Extended-Release [Rythmol SR]): 225 mg, 325 mg, 425 mg.

INDICATIONS AND DOSAGES

▸ Documented, Life-Threatening Ventricular Arrhythmias, Such as Sustained Ventricular Tachycardia

PO (Prompt-Release)
Adults, Elderly. Initially, 150 mg q8h; may increase at 3-to 4-day intervals to 225 mg q8h, then to 300 mg q8h. Maximum: 900 mg/day.
PO (Extended-Release)
Adults, Elderly. Initially, 225 mg q12h. May increase at 5 day intervals. Maximum: 425 mg q12h.

OFF-LABEL USES

Treatment of supraventricular arrhythmias

CONTRAINDICATIONS

Bradycardia; bronchospastic disorders; cardiogenic shock; electrolyte imbalance; sinoatrial, AV, and intraventricular impulse generation or conduction disorders, such as sick sinus syndrome or AV block, without the presence of a pacemaker; uncontrolled CHF

INTERACTIONS

Drug

Digoxin, propranolol: May increase concentrations of these drugs.
Warfarin: May increase warfarin effects.

Herbal

None known.

Food

None known.

Drug interactions of concern to dentistry

• No specific interactions are reported; however, any drug that could affect the cardiac action of propafenone (other local anesthetics, vasoconstrictors, anticholinergics) should be used in the lowest effective dose

DIAGNOSTIC TEST EFFECTS

May cause ECG changes, such as QRS widening and PR interval prolongation, and positive ANA titers.

SIDE EFFECTS

Frequent (13%–7%)
Dizziness, nausea, vomiting, altered taste, constipation
Occasional (6%–3%)
Headache, dyspnea, blurred vision, dyspepsia (heartburn, indigestion, epigastric pain)
Rare (< 2%)
Rash, weakness, dry mouth, diarrhea, edema, hot flashes

SERIOUS REACTIONS

! Propafenone may produce or worsen existing arrhythmias.
! Overdose may produce hypotension, somnolence, bradycardia, and atrioventricular conduction disturbances.

DENTAL CONSIDERATIONS

General:

• Monitor vital signs at every appointment because of CV side effects.
• Patients on chronic drug therapy may rarely have symptoms of blood dyscrasias, which can include infection, bleeding, and poor healing.
• Assess salivary flow as a factor in caries, periodontal disease, and candidiasis.
• Stress from dental procedures may compromise CV function; determine patient risk.
• Consider semisupine chair position for patients with respiratory distress.

Consultations:

• In a patient with symptoms of blood dyscrasias, request a medical consultation for blood studies and postpone dental treatment until normal values are reestablished.

- Medical consultation may be required to assess disease control and patient's ability to tolerate stress.

Teach Patient/Family:

- Importance of good oral hygiene to prevent soft tissue inflammation
- Caution to prevent injury when using oral hygiene aids
- *When chronic dry mouth occurs, advise patient:*
  - To avoid mouth rinses with high alcohol content because of drying effects
  - Of need for daily use of home fluoride products to prevent caries
  - To use sugarless gum, frequent sips of water, or saliva substitutes

propantheline

proe-pan-the-leen
(Pro-Banthine, Propanthl[CAN])

CATEGORY AND SCHEDULE

Pregnancy Risk Category: C

P

MECHANISM OF ACTION

A quaternary ammonium compound which has anticholinergic properties and that inhibits action of acetylcholine at postganglionic parasympathetic sites. ***Therapeutic Effect:*** Reduces gastric secretions and urinary frequency, urgency and urge incontinence.

PHARMACOKINETICS

Onset occurs within 90 min. but less than 50% is absorbed from gastrointestinal (GI) tract. Extensive hepatic metabolism. Excreted in the urine and feces. ***Half-life:*** 2.9 hrs.

AVAILABILITY

Tablets: 7.5 mg, 15 mg (Pro-Banthine).

INDICATIONS AND DOSAGES

▸ Peptic Ulcer

PO

Adults, Elderly. 15 mg 3 times/day 30 min. before meals and 30 mg at bedtime.

Children. 1–2 mg/kg/day, divided q4–6h and at bedtime.

CONTRAINDICATIONS

GI or genitourinary (GU) obstruction, myasthenia gravis, narrow-angle glaucoma, toxic megacolon, severe ulcerative colitis, unstable cardiovascular adjustment in acute hemorrhage, hypersensitivity to propantheline or other anticholinergics

INTERACTIONS

Drug

Digoxin: May increase serum digoxin levels by increasing absorption due to decreased gastrointestinal motility.

Herbal

None known.

Food

None known.

Drug interactions of concern to dentistry

- Increased anticholinergic effect: other anticholinergic drugs
- Constipation, urinary retention: opioid analgesics
- Decreased absorption of ketoconazole; take doses 2 hr apart

DIAGNOSTIC TEST EFFECTS

SIDE EFFECTS

Frequent

Dry mouth, decreased sweating, constipation

Occasional
Blurred vision, intolerance to light, urinary hesitancy, drowsiness, agitation, excitement
Rare
Confusion, increased intraocular pressure, orthostatic hypotension, tachycardia

SERIOUS REACTIONS

! Overdosage may produce temporary paralysis of ciliary muscle, pupillary dilation, tachycardia, palpitations, hot, dry, or flushed skin, absence of bowel sounds, hyperthermia, increased respiratory rate, ECG abnormalities, nausea, vomiting, rash over face or upper trunk, CNS stimulation, and psychosis, marked by agitation, restlessness, rambling speech, visual hallucinations, paranoid behavior, and delusions, followed by depression.

DENTAL CONSIDERATIONS

General:
- Assess salivary flow as a factor in caries, periodontal disease, and candidiasis.
- Avoid dental light in patient's eyes; offer dark glasses for patient comfort.
- Place on frequent recall because of oral side effects.
- Avoid prescribing aspirin-containing products.
- Consider semisupine chair position for patient comfort because of GI effects of disease.

Consultations:
- Physician should be informed if significant xerostomic side effects occur (e.g., increased caries, sore tongue, problems eating or swallowing, difficulty wearing prosthesis) so that a medication change can be considered.

Teach Patient/Family:
- *When chronic dry mouth occurs, advise patient:*
  - To avoid mouth rinses with high alcohol content because of drying effects
  - Of need for daily use of home fluoride products to prevent caries
  - To use sugarless gum, frequent sips of water, or saliva substitutes

propofol

pro-poe-fall′-
(Diprivan, Recofol[AUS])

CATEGORY AND SCHEDULE

Pregnancy Risk Category: B

MECHANISM OF ACTION

A rapidly acting general anesthetic that inhibits sympathetic vasoconstrictor nerve activity and decreases vascular resistance. ***Therapeutic Effect:*** Produces hypnosis rapidly.

PHARMACOKINETICS

Route	Onset	Peak	Duration
IV	40 sec	N/A	3–10 min

Rapidly and extensively distributed. Protein binding: 97%–99%. Metabolized in the liver. Primarily excreted in urine. Unknown if removed by hemodialysis.
Half-life: 3–12 hr.

AVAILABILITY

Injection: 10 mg/ml.

INDICATIONS AND DOSAGES

▸ **Intensive Care Unit Sedation**
IV
Adults, Elderly. Initially, 0.3 mg/kg/hr. May increase by

P

0.3–0.6 mg/kg/hr q5–10min until desired effect is obtained. Maintenance: 0.3–3 mg/kg/h.

▸ Anesthesia

IV

Adults, American Society of Anesthesiologists (ASA) I and II patients. 2–2.5 mg/kg (about 40 mg q10sec until onset of anesthesia). Maintenance: 0.1–0.2 mg/kg/min.

Elderly, Debilitated, Hypovolemic, ASA III or IV patients. 1–1.5 mg/kg (about 20 mg q10sec until onset of anesthesia). Maintenance: 0.05–0.1 mg/kg/min.

Children 3 yr and older, ASA I or II patients. 2.5–3.5 mg/kg (lower dosage for ASA III or IV patients).

Children 2 mo–16 yr. Maintenance dose: 0.125–0.15 mg/kg/min.

CONTRAINDICATIONS

Impaired cerebral circulation, increased ICP

INTERACTIONS

Drug

Alcohol, other CNS depressants: May increase hypotensive and CNS and respiratory depressant effects of propofol.

Herbal

None known.

Food

None known.

Drug interactions of concern to dentistry

- Increased CNS depression: alcohol, narcotics, sedative-hypnotics, antipsychotics, skeletal muscle relaxants, inhalational anesthetics

DIAGNOSTIC TEST EFFECTS

None known.

IV INCOMPATIBILITIES

Amikacin (Amikin), amphotericin B complex (Abelcet, AmBisome, Amphotec), bretylium (Bretylol), calcium chloride, ciprofloxacin (Cipro), diazepam (Valium), digoxin (Lanoxin), doxorubicin (Adriamycin), gentamicin (Garamycin), methylprednisolone (Solu-Medrol), minocycline (Minocin), phenytoin (Dilantin), tobramycin (Nebcin), verapamil (Isoptin)

IV COMPATIBILITIES

Acyclovir (Zovirax), bumetanide (Bumex), calcium gluconate, ceftazidime (Fortaz), dobutamine (Dobutrex), dopamine (Intropin), enalapril (Vasotec), fentanyl, heparin, insulin, labetalol (Normodyne, Trandate), lidocaine, lorazepam (Ativan), magnesium, milrinone (Primacor), nitroglycerin, norepinephrine (Levophed), potassium chloride, vancomycin (Vancocin)

SIDE EFFECTS

Frequent

Involuntary muscle movements, apnea (common during induction; lasts longer than 60 seconds), hypotension, nausea, vomiting, IV site burning or stinging

Occasional

Twitching, bucking, jerking, thrashing, headache, dizziness, bradycardia, hypertension, fever, abdominal cramps, paresthesia, coldness, cough, hiccups, facial flushing, greenish-colored urine

Rare

Rash, dry mouth, agitation, confusion, myalgia, thrombophlebitis

SERIOUS REACTIONS

! A continuous infusion or repeated intermittent infusions of propofol may result in extreme somnolence, respiratory depression, and circulatory depression.

! Too-rapid IV administration may produce severe hypotension, respiratory depression, and involuntary muscle movements.

P

! The patient may experience an acute allergic reaction, characterized by abdominal pain, anxiety, restlessness, dyspnea, erythema, hypotension, pruritus, rhinitis, and urticaria.

DENTAL CONSIDERATIONS

General:

- Monitor vital signs at regular intervals during recovery after use as anesthetic.
- Have someone drive patient to and from dental office if used for general anesthesia.
- Geriatric patients are more susceptible to drug effects; use lower dose.
- Use only with resuscitative equipment available and only by qualified persons trained in anesthesia.
- Monitor:
  - Injection site: phlebitis, burning/stinging
  - ECG for changes: PVC, PAC, ST-segment changes
  - Allergic reactions: hives
- Administer:
  - After diluting with D_5W, use only glass containers when mixing; not stable in plastic
  - By IV injection only
  - Alone; do not mix with other agents before using
- Perform/provide:
  - Storage in light-resistant area at room temperature
  - Coughing, turning, deep breathing for postoperative patients
  - Safety measures: side rails, night light, call bell within reach
- Evaluate:
  - CNS changes: movement, jerking, tremors, dizziness, LOC, pupil reaction
  - Respiratory dysfunction: respiratory depression, character, rate, rhythm; notify physician if respirations are <10/min
- Treatment of overdose:
  - Discontinue drug, artificial ventilation, administer vasopressor agents or anticholinergics

propoxyphene hydrochloride/propoxyphene napsylate

pro-pox′-ih-feen
Schedule IV
(propoxyphene hydrochloride)
Darvon(propoxyphene napsylate)
Darvon-N[CAN], Doloxene[AUS]
Do not confuse Darvon with Diovan.

CATEGORY AND SCHEDULE

Pregnancy Risk Category: C
(D if used for prolonged periods)
Controlled Substance: Schedule IV

MECHANISM OF ACTION

An opioid agonist that binds with opioid receptors in the CNS. ***Therapeutic Effect:*** Alters the perception of and emotional response to pain.

PHARMACOKINETICS

Route	Onset	Peak	Duration
PO	15–60 min	N/A	4–6 hr

Well absorbed from the GI tract. Protein binding: High. Widely distributed. Metabolized in the liver. Primarily excreted in urine. Not removed by hemodialysis. ***Half-life:*** 6–12 hr; metabolite: 30–36 hr.

AVAILABILITY

Capsules (Hydrochloride): 65 mg.
Tablets (Napsylate): 100 mg.

INDICATIONS AND DOSAGES

▸ **Mild to Moderate Pain**

PO (propoxyphene hydrochloride)

Adults, Elderly. 65 mg q4h as needed. Maximum: 390 mg/day.
PO (propoxyphene napsylate)
Adults, Elderly. 100 mg q4h as needed. Maximum: 600 mg/day.

CONTRAINDICATIONS

None known.

INTERACTIONS

Drug

Alcohol, other CNS depressants: May increase CNS or respiratory depression and risk of hypotension.
Buprenorphine: May decrease the effects of propoxyphene.
Carbamazepine: May increase the blood concentration and risk of toxicity of carbamazepine.
MAOIs: May produce a severe, sometimes fatal reaction; plan to administer 25% of usual propoxyphene dose.

Herbal

None known.

Food

None known.

Drug interactions of concern to dentistry

P

- Increased effects with other CNS depressants: alcohol, narcotics, sedative-hypnotics, skeletal muscle relaxants
- Contraindication: MAOIs
- Increased effects of anticholinergics, antihypertensives, carbamazepine

DIAGNOSTIC TEST EFFECTS

May increase serum alkaline phosphatase, lipase, amylase, bilirubin, LDH, AST (SGOT), and ALT (SGPT) levels. Therapeutic serum drug level is 100–400 ng/ml; toxic serum drug level is greater than 500 ng/ml.

SIDE EFFECTS

Frequent

Dizziness, somnolence, dry mouth, euphoria, hypotension (including orthostatic hypotension), nausea, vomiting, fatigue

Occasional

Allergic reaction (including decreased BP), diaphoresis, flushing, and wheezing), trembling, urine retention, vision changes, constipation, headache

Rare

Confusion, increased BP, depression, abdominal cramps, anorexia

SERIOUS REACTIONS

! Overdose results in respiratory depression, skeletal muscle flaccidity, cold or clammy skin, cyanosis, and extreme somnolence progressing to seizures, stupor, and coma.
! Hepatotoxicity may occur with overdose of the acetaminophen component of fixed-combination products.
! The patient who uses propoxyphene repeatedly may develop a tolerance to the drug's analgesic effect and physical dependence.

DENTAL CONSIDERATIONS

General:

- Monitor vital signs because of CV and respiratory side effects.
- Consider semisupine chair position for patient comfort if GI side effects occur.
- Assess salivary flow as a factor in caries, periodontal disease, and candidiasis.
- Psychologic and physical dependence may occur with chronic administration.
- When combined with nonopioid analgesics (aspirin, NSAIDs, acetaminophen), permits better-quality pain relief.

Teach Patient/Family:

- *When chronic dry mouth occurs, advise patient:*

• To avoid mouth rinses with high alcohol content because of drying effects
• Of need for daily use of home fluoride products to prevent caries
• To use sugarless gum, frequent sips of water, or artificial saliva substitutes

propoxyphene napsylate

proe-pox′-i-feen nap′-seh-late
Schedule IV
(Darvon-N)

CATEGORY AND SCHEDULE

Pregnancy Risk Category: C (D if used for prolonged periods)
Controlled Substance: Schedule IV

MECHANISM OF ACTION

An opioid agonist that binds with opioid receptors within the central nervous system (CNS). ***Therapeutic Effect:*** Alters processes affecting pain perception, emotional response to pain.

PHARMACOKINETICS

Route	Onset	Peak	Duration
PO	15–60 min	N/A	4–6 hrs

Well absorbed from the gastrointestinal (GI) tract. Protein binding: High. Widely distributed. Metabolized in liver. Primarily excreted in urine. Not removed by hemodialysis. ***Half-life:*** 6–12 hrs.

AVAILABILITY

Tablets: 100 mg (Darvon-N).

INDICATIONS AND DOSAGES

▸ Relief of Mild to Moderate Pain

PO

Adults, Elderly. 100 mg q4h, as needed. Maximum: 600 mg/day.

CONTRAINDICATIONS

Hypersensitivity to propoxyphene napsylate or any component of the formulation

INTERACTIONS

Drug

Alcohol, CNS depressants: May increase CNS or respiratory depression and risk of hypotension.
Buprenorphine: Effects may be decreased with buprenorphine.
Carbamazepine: May increase the blood concentration and risk of toxicity of carbamazepine.
MAOIs: May produce severe, fatal reaction; plan to reduce to one quarter usual dose.

Herbal

None known.

Food

None known.

Drug interactions of concern to dentistry

• Increased effects with other CNS depressants: alcohol, narcotics, sedative-hypnotics, skeletal muscle relaxants
• Contraindication: MAOIs
• Increased effects of anticholinergics, antihypertensives, carbamazepine

P

DIAGNOSTIC TEST EFFECTS

May increase serum alkaline phosphatase, amylase, bilirubin, LDH, lipase, SGOT (AST), and SGPT (ALT) levels. Therapeutic blood serum level is 100–400 ng/ml; toxic blood serum level is greater than 500 ng/ml.

SIDE EFFECTS

Frequent

Dizziness, drowsiness, dry mouth, euphoria, hypotension, nausea, vomiting, unusual tiredness

Occasional

Histamine reaction, including decreased blood pressure (B/P), increased sweating, flushing, and

wheezing, trembling, decreased urination, altered vision, constipation, headache
Rare
Confusion, increased B/P, depression, stomach cramps, anorexia

SERIOUS REACTIONS

! Overdosage results in respiratory depression, skeletal muscle flaccidity, cold or clammy skin, cyanosis, extreme somnolence progressing to convulsions, stupor, and coma.
! Liver toxicity may occur with overdosage of acetaminophen component of fixed-combination.
! Tolerance to propoxyphene's analgesic effect and physical dependence may occur with repeated use.

DENTAL CONSIDERATIONS

General:
- Monitor vital signs because of CV and respiratory side effects.
- Consider semisupine chair position for patient comfort if GI side effects occur.
- Assess salivary flow as a factor in caries, periodontal disease, and candidiasis.
- Psychologic and physical dependence may occur with chronic administration.
- When combined with nonopioid analgesics (aspirin, NSAIDs, acetaminophen), permits better-quality pain relief.

Teach Patient/Family:
- *When chronic dry mouth occurs, advise patient:*
  - To avoid mouth rinses with high alcohol content because of drying effects
  - Of need for daily use of home fluoride products to prevent caries
  - To use sugarless gum, frequent sips of water, or artificial saliva substitutes

P

propranolol hydrochloride

proe-pran′-oh-lole
(Apo-Propranolol[CAN], Deralin[AUS], Inderal, Inderal LA, InnoPran XL, Nu-Propranolol [CAN], Propranolol Intensol)
Do not confuse Inderal with Adderall or Isordil, or propranolol with Pravachol.

CATEGORY AND SCHEDULE

Pregnancy Risk Category: C (D if used in second or third trimester)

MECHANISM OF ACTION

An antihypertensive, antianginal, antiarrhythmic, and antimigraine agent that blocks $beta_1$- and $beta_2$-adrenergic receptors. Decreases oxygen requirements. Slows AV conduction and increases refractory period in AV node. Large doses increase airway resistance.
Therapeutic Effect: Slows sinus heart rate; decreases cardiac output, BP, and myocardial ischemia severity. Exhibits antiarrhythmic activity.

PHARMACOKINETICS

Route	Onset	Peak	Duration
PO	1–2 hr	N/A	6 hr

Well absorbed from the GI tract. Protein binding: 93%. Widely distributed. Metabolized in the liver. Primarily excreted in urine. Not removed by hemodialysis. ***Half-life:*** 3–5 hr.

AVAILABILITY

Tablets (Inderal): 10 mg, 20 mg, 40 mg, 60 mg, 80 mg.
Capsules (Extended-Release [Inderal LA]): 60 mg, 80 mg, 120 mg, 160 mg.

Capsules (Extended-Release [InnoPran XL]): 80 mg, 120 mg.
Oral Solution (Inderal): 4 mg/ml.
Oral Concentrate (Propranolol Intensol): 80 mg/ml.
Injection (Inderal): 1 mg/ml.

INDICATIONS AND DOSAGES

▸ Hypertension

PO

Adults, Elderly. Initially, 40 mg twice a day. May increase dose q3–7 days. Range: Up to 320 mg/day in divided doses. Maximum: 640 mg/day.

Children. Initially, 0.5–1 mg/kg/day in divided doses q6–12h. May increase at 3– to 5–day intervals. Usual dose: 1–5 mg/kg/day. Maximum: 16 mg/kg/day.

▸ Angina

PO

Adults, Elderly. 80–320 mg/day in divided doses. (long acting): Initially, 80 mg/day. Maximum: 320 mg/day.

▸ Arrhythmias

IV

Adults, Elderly. 1 mg/dose. May repeat q5min. Maximum: 5 mg total dose.

Children. 0.01–0.1 mg/kg. Maximum: infants, 1 mg; children, 3 mg.

PO

Adults, Elderly. Initially, 10–20 mg q6–8h. May gradually increase dose. Range: 40–320 mg/day.

Children. Initially, 0.5–1 mg/kg/day in divided doses q6–8h. May increase q3–5 days. Usual dosage: 2–4 mg/kg/day. Maximum: 16 mg/kg/day or 60 mg/day.

▸ Life-Threatening Arrhythmias

IV

Adults, Elderly. 0.5–3 mg. Repeat once in 2 min. Give additional doses at intervals of at least 4 hr.

Children. 0.01–0.1 mg/kg.

▸ Hypertrophic Subaortic Stenosis

PO

Adults, Elderly. 20–40 mg in 3–4 divided doses. Or 80–160 mg/day as extended-release capsule.

▸ Adjunct to Alpha-Blocking Agents to Treat Pheochromocytoma

PO

Adults, Elderly. 60 mg/day in divided doses with alpha-blocker for 3 days before surgery. Maintenance (inoperable tumor): 30 mg/day with alpha-blocker.

▸ Migraine Headache

PO

Adults, Elderly. 80 mg/day in divided doses. Or 80 mg once daily as extended-release capsule. Increase up to 160–240 mg/day in divided doses.

Children. 0.6–1.5 mg/kg/day in divided doses q8h. Maximum: 4 mg/kg/day.

▸ Reduction of Cardiovascular Mortality and Reinfarction in Patients with Previous MI

PO

Adults, Elderly. 180–240 mg/day in divided doses.

▸ Essential Tremor

PO

Adults, Elderly. Initially, 40 mg twice a day increased up to 120–320 mg/day in 3 divided doses.

OFF-LABEL USES

Treatment adjunct for anxiety, mitral valve prolapse syndrome, thyrotoxicosis

CONTRAINDICATIONS

Asthma, bradycardia, cardiogenic shock, COPD, heart block, Raynaud's syndrome, uncompensated CHF

INTERACTIONS

Drug

Diuretics, other antihypertensives: May increase hypotensive effect.

Insulin, oral hypoglycemics: May mask symptoms of hypoglycemia and prolong the hypoglycemic effect of insulin and oral hypoglycemics.
IV phenytoin: May increase cardiac depressant effect.
NSAIDs: May decrease antihypertensive effect.
Sympathomimetics, xanthines: May mutually inhibit effects.

Herbal
None known.

Food
None known.

Drug interactions of concern to dentistry
- Decreased hypotensive effect: indomethacin, NSAIDs
- Increased hypotension, myocardial depression: hydrocarbon inhalation anesthetics
- Hypertension, bradycardia: sympathomimetics (epinephrine, ephedrine)
- Suspected increase in plasma levels: diphenhydramine
- Slow metabolism of lidocaine
- Decreased effects: didanosine (take 2 hr before didanosine tabs)

P

DIAGNOSTIC TEST EFFECTS
May increase serum antinuclear antibody titer and BUN, serum LDH, serum lipoprotein, serum alkaline phosphatase, serum bilirubin, serum creatinine, serum potassium, serum uric acid, AST(SGOT), ALT (SGPT), and serum triglyceride levels.

IV INCOMPATIBILITIES
Amphotericin B complex (Abelcet, AmBisome, Amphotec)

IV COMPATIBILITIES
Alteplase (Activase), heparin, milrinone (Primacor), potassium chloride, propofol (Diprivan)

SIDE EFFECTS
Frequent
Diminished sexual ability, drowsiness, difficulty sleeping, unusual fatigue or weakness

Occasional
Bradycardia, depression, sensation of coldness in extremities, diarrhea, constipation, anxiety, nasal congestion, nausea, vomiting

Rare
Altered taste, dry eyes, pruritus, paraesthesia

SERIOUS REACTIONS
! Overdose may produce profound bradycardia and hypotension.
! Abrupt withdrawal may result in sweating, palpitations, headache, and tremors.
! Propranolol administration may precipitate CHF and MI in patients with cardiac disease; thyroid storm in those with thyrotoxicosis; and peripheral ischemia in those with existing peripheral vascular disease.
! Hypoglycemia may occur in patients with previously controlled diabetes.

DENTAL CONSIDERATIONS
General:
- Monitor vital signs at every appointment because of CV side effects.
- Patients on chronic drug therapy may rarely have symptoms of blood dyscrasias, which can include infection, bleeding, and poor healing.
- Limit use of sodium-containing products, such as saline IV fluids, for patients with a dietary salt restriction.
- Assess salivary flow as a factor in caries, periodontal disease, and candidiasis.
- After supine positioning, have patient sit upright for at least 2 min

before standing to avoid orthostatic hypotension.

• Stress from dental procedures may compromise CV function; determine patient risk.

• Short appointments and a stress reduction protocol may be required for anxious patients.

• Consider semisupine chair position for patients with respiratory distress.

• Use vasoconstrictors with caution, in low doses, and with careful aspiration. Avoid use of gingival retraction cord with epinephrine.

Consultations:

• In a patient with symptoms of blood dyscrasias, request a medical consultation for blood studies and postpone dental treatment until normal values are reestablished.

• Medical consultation may be required to assess disease control and patient's ability to tolerate stress.

Teach Patient/Family:

• Caution to prevent injury when using oral hygiene aids

• Importance of good oral hygiene to prevent soft tissue inflammation

• *When chronic dry mouth occurs, advise patient:*

  • To avoid mouth rinses with high alcohol content because of drying effects

  • Of need for daily use of home fluoride products to prevent caries

  • To use sugarless gum, frequent sips of water, or saliva substitutes

propylthiouracil

proe-pill-thye-oh-yoor′-a-sill (Propylthiouracil, Propyl-Thyracil[CAN])

CATEGORY AND SCHEDULE

Pregnancy Risk Category: D

MECHANISM OF ACTION

A thiourea derivative that blocks oxidation of iodine in the thyroid gland and blocks synthesis of thyroxine and triiodothyronine. ***Therapeutic Effect:*** Inhibits synthesis of thyroid hormone.

AVAILABILITY

Tablets: 50 mg.

INDICATIONS AND DOSAGES

▸ Hyperthyroidism

PO

Adults, Elderly. Initially: 300–450 mg/day in divided doses q8h. Maintenance: 100–150 mg/day in divided doses q8–12h.

Children. Initially: 5–7 mg/kg/day in divided doses q8h. Maintenance: 33%–66% of initial dose in divided doses q8–12h.

Neonates. 5–10 mg/kg/day in divided doses q8h.

CONTRAINDICATIONS

None known.

INTERACTIONS

Drug

Amiodarone, iodinated glycerol, iodine, potassium iodide: May decrease response of propylthiouracil.

Digoxin: May increase digoxin blood concentration as patient becomes euthyroid.

I^{131}: May decrease thyroid uptake of I^{131}.

Oral anticoagulants: May decrease the effects of oral anticoagulants.

Herbal

None known.

Food

None known.

Drug interactions of concern to dentistry

- Increased CV side effects in uncontrolled patients: anticholinergics and sympathomimetics
- Patients with uncontrolled hyperthyroidism are at risk when vasoconstrictors are used
- Patients with uncontrolled hypothyroidism may be more responsive to CNS depressants

DIAGNOSTIC TEST EFFECTS

May increase LDH, serum alkaline phosphatase, bilirubin, AST(SGOT), and ALT(SGPT) levels and prothrombin time.

SIDE EFFECTS

Frequent

Urticaria, rash, pruritus, nausea, skin pigmentation, hair loss, headache, paraesthesia

Occasional

Somnolence, lymphadenopathy, vertigo

Rare

Drug fever, lupus-like syndrome

SERIOUS REACTIONS

! Agranulocytosis as long as 4 months after therapy, pancytopenia, and fatal hepatitis have occurred.

DENTAL CONSIDERATIONS

General:

- Patients on chronic drug therapy may rarely have symptoms of blood dyscrasias, which can include infection, bleeding, and poor healing.
- Patients with uncontrolled hyperthyroidism should not be treated in the dental office until thyroid values are normalized.
- Uncontrolled patients should be referred for medical evaluation and treatment.
- Monitor vital signs at every appointment because of CV side effects.
- Consider semisupine chair position for patient comfort if GI side effects occur.

Consultations:

- Medical consultation may be required to assess disease control and patient's ability to tolerate stress.

protamine sulfate

proe'-ta-meen

(Protamine[CAN], Protamine sulfate)

Do not confuse protamine with ProAmatine, Protopam, or Protropin.

CATEGORY AND SCHEDULE

Pregnancy Risk Category: C

MECHANISM OF ACTION

A protein that complexes with heparin to form a stable salt. ***Therapeutic Effect:*** Reduces anticoagulant activity of heparin.

AVAILABILITY

Injection: 10 mg/ml.

INDICATIONS AND DOSAGES

▸ Heparin Overdose (antidote and treatment)

IV

Adults, Elderly. 1 mg protamine sulfate neutralizes 90–115 units of heparin. Heparin disappears rapidly

P

from circulation, reducing the dosage demand for protamine as time elapses.

OFF-LABEL USES
Treatment of enoxaparin toxicity

CONTRAINDICATIONS
None known.

INTERACTIONS
Drug
None known.
Herbal
None known.
Food
None known.
Drug interactions of concern to dentistry
- None reported

DIAGNOSTIC TEST EFFECTS
None known.

SIDE EFFECTS
Frequent
Decreased BP, dyspnea
Occasional
Hypersensitivity reaction (urticaria, angioedema); nausea and vomiting, which generally occur in those sensitive to fish and seafood, vasectomized men, infertile men, those on isophane (NPH) insulin, or those previously on protamine therapy
Rare
Back pain

SERIOUS REACTIONS
! Too rapid IV administration may produce acute hypotension, bradycardia, pulmonary hypertension, dyspnea, transient flushing, and feeling of warmth.
! Heparin rebound may occur several hours after heparin has been neutralized (usually 8–9 hours after protamine administration). Heparin rebound occurs most often after arterial or cardiac surgery.

DENTAL CONSIDERATIONS
General
- Acute-use drug for use in hospitals and emergency rooms; delay any dental treatment until normal clotting mechanism is restored.
- Question patient about use of oral anticoagulants.
- Avoid products that affect platelet function, such as aspirin and NSAIDs.
- Determine why patient is taking the drug.
- Consider local hemostasis measures to prevent excessive bleeding.

Consultations:
- Medical consultation may be required to assess disease control and patient's ability to tolerate stress.
- Medical consultation should include routine blood counts including platelet counts and bleeding time.
- Medical consultation should include partial prothrombin time, prothrombin time, or INR.

Teach Patient/Family:
- To inform dentist of unusual bleeding episodes following dental treatment
- Advise patient to use soft tooth brush to help prevent irritation of oral tissues that could evoke bleeding

protriptyline

proe-trip′-ti-leen
(Vivactil, Triptil[CAN])

CATEGORY AND SCHEDULE

Pregnancy Risk Category: C

MECHANISM OF ACTION

A tricyclic antidepressant that increases synaptic concentration of norepinephrine and/or serotonin by inhibiting their reuptake by presynaptic membranes.
Therapeutic Effect: Produces antidepressant effect.

PHARMACOKINETICS

Well absorbed from the gastrointestinal (GI) tract. Protein binding: 92%. Widely distributed. Extensively metabolized in liver. Excreted in urine. Not removed by hemodialysis. ***Half-life:*** 54–92 hrs.

AVAILABILITY

Tablets: 5 mg, 10 mg (Vivactil).

INDICATIONS AND DOSAGES

▸ Depression

PO

Adults. 15–40 mg/day divided into 3–4 doses/day. Maximum: 600 mg/day.
Elderly. 5 mg 3 times/day. May increase gradually.

OFF-LABEL USES

Narcolepsy, sleep apnea, sleep hypoxemia

CONTRAINDICATIONS

Acute recovery period after myocardial infarction, coadministration with cisapride, use of MAOIs within 14 days, hypersensitivity to protriptyline or any component of the formulation

INTERACTIONS

Drug

Alcohol, central nervous system (CNS) depressants: May increase CNS and respiratory depression and the hypotensive effects of protriptyline.
Antithyroid agents: May increase risk of agranulocytosis.
Cimetidine: May increase protriptyline blood concentration and risk of toxicity.
Clonidine, guanadrel: May decrease the effects of clonidine and guanadrel.
MAOIs: May increase the risk of hyperpyrexia, hypertensive crisis, and seizures.
Phenothiazines: May increase the anticholinergic and sedative effects of protriptyline.
Phenytoin: May decrease protriptyline blood concentration.
Sympathomimetics: May increase the cardiac effects.

Herbal

St. John's Wort: May have additive effects.

Food

None known.

Drug interactions of concern to dentistry

- Increased anticholinergic effects: muscarinic blockers, antihistamines, phenothiazines
- Increased effects of direct-acting sympathomimetics (epinephrine, levonordefrin)
- Possible risk of increased CNS depression: alcohol, barbiturates, benzodiazepines, and other CNS depressants
- Decreased antihypertensive effects of: clonidine, guanadrel, guanethidine
- Avoid concurrent use with St. John's wort (herb)

DIAGNOSTIC TEST EFFECTS

None known.

IV INCOMPATIBILITIES
None known.
IV COMPATIBILITIES
None known.

SIDE EFFECTS
Frequent
Drowsiness, weight gain, fatigue, dry mouth, blurred vision, constipation, delayed micturition, postural hypotension, diaphoresis, disturbed concentration, increased appetite, urinary retention
Occasional
Gastrointestinal (GI) disturbances, such as nausea, diarrhea, GI distress, metallic taste sensation
Rare
Paradoxical reaction, marked by agitation, restlessness, nightmares, insomnia, extrapyramidal symptoms, particularly fine hand tremor

SERIOUS REACTIONS
! High dosage may produce confusion, seizures, severe drowsiness, arrhythmias, fever, hallucinations, agitation, shortness of breath, vomiting, and unusual tiredness or weakness.
! Abrupt withdrawal from prolonged therapy may produce severe headache, malaise, nausea, vomiting, and vivid dreams.

DENTAL CONSIDERATIONS
General:
- Monitor vital signs at every appointment because of CV side effects.
- Assess salivary flow as a factor in caries, periodontal disease, and candidiasis.
- Patients on chronic drug therapy may rarely have symptoms of blood dyscrasias, which can include infection, bleeding, and poor healing.
- After supine positioning, have patient sit upright for at least 2 min before standing to avoid orthostatic hypotension.
- Use vasoconstrictors with caution, in low doses, and with careful aspiration. Avoid use of gingival retraction cord with epinephrine.
- Place on frequent recall because of oral side effects.

Consultations:
- In a patient with symptoms of blood dyscrasias, request a medical consultation for blood studies and postpone dental treatment until normal values are reestablished.
- Medical consultation may be required to assess disease control.
- Physician should be informed if significant xerostomic side effects occur (e.g., increased caries, sore tongue, problems eating or swallowing, difficulty wearing prosthesis) so that a medication change can be considered.

Teach Patient/Family:
- Importance of good oral hygiene to prevent soft tissue inflammation
- Caution to prevent injury when using oral hygiene aids
- *When chronic dry mouth occurs, advise patient:*
  - To avoid mouth rinses with high alcohol content because of drying effects
  - Of need for daily use of home fluoride products to prevent caries
  - To use sugarless gum, frequent sips of water, or saliva substitutes

pseudoephedrine

soo-doe-e-fed′-rin
(Balminil Decongestant[CAN], BioContac Cold 12 Hour Relief Non Drowsy[CAN], Decofed, Dimetapp 12 Hour Non Drowsy Extentabs, Dimetapp Decongestant, Dimetapp sinus liquid caps[AUS], Genaphed, PMS-Pseudoephedrine[CAN], Robidrine [CAN], Sudafed, Sudafed 12h[AUS], Sudafed 12 Hour, Sudafed 24 Hour)

CATEGORY AND SCHEDULE

Pregnancy Risk Category: C
OTC

MECHANISM OF ACTION

A sympathomimetic that directly stimulates alpha-adrenergic and beta-adrenergic receptors. ***Therapeutic Effect:*** Produces vasoconstriction of respiratory tract mucosa; shrinks nasal mucous membranes; reduces edema and nasal congestion.

P

PHARMACOKINETICS

Route	Onset	Peak	Duration
PO (tablets, syrup)	15–30 min	N/A	4–6 hr
PO (extended-release)	N/A	N/A	8–12 hr

Well absorbed from the GI tract. Partially metabolized in the liver. Primarily excreted in urine. Not removed by hemodialysis. ***Half-life:*** 9–16 hr (children, 3.1 hr).

AVAILABILITY

Gelcaps (Dimetapp Decongestant): 30 mg.
Liquid (Sudafed): 15 mg/5 ml.
Oral Drops (Dimetapp Infant Drops): 7.5 mg/0.8 ml.
Syrup (Biofed, Decofed): 30 mg/5 ml.
Tablets (Genaphed, Sudafed): 30 mg.
Tablets (Chewable [Sudafed]): 15 mg.
Tablets (Extended-Release [Dimetapp 12 Hour Non Drowsy Extentabs, Sudafed 12 Hour]): 120 mg.
Tablets (Extended-Release [Sudafed 24 Hour]): 240 mg.

INDICATIONS AND DOSAGES

▸ Decongestant

PO

Adults, Children 12 yr and older. 60 mg q4–6h. Maximum: 240 mg/day.
Children 6–11 yr. 30 mg q6h. Maximum: 120 mg/day.
Children 2–5 yr. 15 mg q6h. Maximum: 60 mg/day.
Children younger than 2 yr. 4 mg/kg/day in divided doses q6h.
Elderly. 30–60 mg q6h as needed.

PO (Extended-Release)

Adults, Children 12 yr and older. 120 mg q12h.

CONTRAINDICATIONS

Breast-feeding women, coronary artery disease, severe hypertension, use within 14 days of MAOIs

INTERACTIONS

Drug

Antihypertensive, beta blockers, diuretics: May decrease the effects of these drugs.
MAOIs: May increase cardiac stimulant and vasopressor effects.

Herbal

None known.

Food

None known.

Drug interactions of concern to dentistry

• Dysrhythmia: hydrocarbon inhalation anesthetics

• Increased CNS, CV effects: sympathomimetics

DIAGNOSTIC TEST EFFECTS

None known.

SIDE EFFECTS

Occasional (10%–5%)
Nervousness, restlessness, insomnia, tremor, headache
Rare (4%–1%)
Diaphoresis, weakness

SERIOUS REACTIONS

! Large doses may produce tachycardia, palpitations (particularly in patients with cardiac disease), light-headedness, nausea, and vomiting.
! Overdose in patients older than 60 years may result in hallucinations, CNS depression, and seizures.

DENTAL CONSIDERATIONS

General:

• Assess salivary flow as a factor in caries, periodontal disease, and candidiasis.
• Monitor vital signs at every appointment because of CV side effects.
• Consider semisupine chair position for patient comfort if GI side effects occur.

Teach Patient/Family:

• Use of electric toothbrush if patient has difficulty holding conventional devices
• *When chronic dry mouth occurs, advise patient:*
  • To avoid mouth rinses with high alcohol content because of drying effects
  • Of need for daily use of home fluoride products to prevent caries
  • To use sugarless gum, frequent sips of water, or saliva substitutes

pyrazinamide

pye-ra-zin′-a-mide
(Pyrazinamide, Tebrazid[CAN], Zinamide[AUS])

CATEGORY AND SCHEDULE

Pregnancy Risk Category: C

MECHANISM OF ACTION

An antitubercular whose exact mechanism of action is unknown.
Therapeutic Effect: Either bacteriostatic or bactericidal, depending on the drug's concentration at the infection site and the susceptibility of infecting bacteria.

AVAILABILITY

Tablets: 500 mg.

INDICATIONS AND DOSAGES

▸ **Tuberculosis (in combination with other antituberculars)**
PO
Adults. 15–30 mg/kg/day in 1–4 doses. Maximum: 3 g/day.
Children. 20–40 mg/kg/day in 1 or 2 doses. Maximum: 2 g/day.

CONTRAINDICATIONS

Severe hepatic dysfunction

INTERACTIONS

Drug
Allopurinol, colchicine, probenecid, sulfinpyrazone: May decrease the effects of these drugs.
Herbal
None known.
Food
None known.

DIAGNOSTIC TEST EFFECTS

May increase AST (SGOT), ALT (SGPT), and serum uric acid concentrations.

SIDE EFFECTS

Frequent

Arthralgia, myalgia (usually mild and self-limiting)

Rare

Hypersensitivity reaction (rash, pruritus, urticaria), photosensitivity, gouty arthritis

SERIOUS REACTIONS

! Hepatotoxicity, gouty arthritis, thrombocytopenia, and anemia occur rarely.

DENTAL CONSIDERATIONS

General:

- Determine why the patient is taking the drug (for prophylaxis or active therapy).
- Determine that noninfectious status exists by ensuring that (1) anti-TB drugs have been taken >3 wk, (2) culture has confirmed TB susceptibility to antiinfectives, (3) patient has had three consecutive negative sputum smears, and (4) patient is not in the coughing stage.

Consultations:

- Medical consultation may be required to assess disease control.

Teach Patient/Family:

- Importance of taking medications for full length of regimen to ensure effectiveness of treatment and to prevent the emergence of resistant strains

P

pyridostigmine bromide

peer-id-oh-stig'-meen

(Mestinon, Mestinon SR[CAN], Mestinon Timespan)

Do not confuse pyridostigmine with physostigmine or Mesitonin with Mesantoin or Metatensin.

CATEGORY AND SCHEDULE

Pregnancy Risk Category: C

MECHANISM OF ACTION

A cholinergic that prevents destruction of acetylcholine by inhibiting the enzyme acetylcholinesterase, thus enhancing impulse transmission across the myoneural junction. ***Therapeutic Effect:*** Produces miosis; increases tone of intestinal, skeletal muscle tone; stimulates salivary and sweat gland secretions.

AVAILABILITY

Syrup (Mestinon): 60 mg/5 ml.
Tablets (Mestinon): 60 mg.
Tablets (Extended-Release [Mestinon Timespan]): 180 mg.
Injection (Mestinon): 5 mg/ml.

INDICATIONS AND DOSAGES

▸ **Myasthenia Gravis**

PO

Adults, Elderly. Initially, 60 mg 3 times a day. Dosage increased at 48 hr intervals. Maintenance: 60 mg–1.5 g a day.

PO (Extended-Release)

Adults, Elderly. 180–540 mg once or twice a day with at least a 6 hr interval between doses.

IV, IM

Adults, Elderly. 2 mg q2–3h.

Children, Neonates. 0.05–0.15 mg/kg/dose. Maximum single dose: 10 mg.

▸ **Reversal of Nondepolarizing Neuromuscular Blockade**

IV

Adults, Elderly. 10–20 mg with, or shortly after, 0.6–1.2 mg atropine sulfate or 0.3–0.6 mg glycopyrrolate.

Children. 0.1–0.25 mg/kg/dose preceded by atropine or glycopyrrolate.

CONTRAINDICATIONS

Mechanical GI or urinary tract obstruction

INTERACTIONS

Drug

Anticholinergics: Prevent or reverse the effects of pyridostigmine.
Cholinesterase inhibitors: May increase the risk of toxicity.
Neuromuscular blockers: Antagonizes the effects of these drugs.
Procainamide, quinidine: May antagonize the action of pyridostigmine.

Herbal

None known.

Food

None known.

Drug interactions of concern to dentistry

- Decreased effects: atropine, scopolamine, and other anticholinergic drugs; methocarbamol
- Reduced rate of metabolism of ester local anesthetics
- Avoid anticholinergic drugs to control excessive salivation

DIAGNOSTIC TEST EFFECTS

None known.

IV INCOMPATIBILITIES

Don't mix pyridostigmine with any other medications.

SIDE EFFECTS

Frequent

Miosis, increased GI and skeletal muscle tone, bradycardia, constriction of bronchi and ureters, diaphoresis, increased salivation

Occasional

Headache, rash, temporary decrease in diastolic BP with mild reflex tachycardia, short periods of atrial fibrillation (in hyperthyroid patients), marked drop in BP (in hypertensive patients)

SERIOUS REACTIONS

! Overdose may produce a cholinergic crisis, manifested as increasingly severe muscle weakness that appears first in muscles involving chewing and swallowing and is followed by muscle weakness of the shoulder girdle and upper extremities, respiratory muscle paralysis, and pelvis girdle and leg muscle paralysis. If overdose occurs, stop all cholinergic drugs and immediately administer 1–4 mg atropine sulfate IV for adults or 0.01 mg/kg for infants and children younger than 12 years.

DENTAL CONSIDERATIONS

General:

- Monitor vital signs at every appointment because of CV and respiratory side effects.
- After supine positioning, have patient sit upright for at least 2 min before standing to avoid orthostatic hypotension.
- Schedule short appointments because of effects of disease on oral musculature.
- Avoid dental light in patient's eyes; offer dark glasses for patient comfort.
- Place on frequent recall because of oral side effects.
- Consider semisupine chair position for patient comfort if GI side effects occur.

Consultations:

- Medical consultation may be required to assess disease control.
- Consult with physician about adjusting dose if excessive salivation becomes a problem.

Teach Patient/Family:

- Use of electric toothbrush or other oral hygiene aids if patient has difficulty in maintaining oral hygiene
- Importance of good oral hygiene to prevent soft tissue inflammation
- To prevent injury when using oral hygiene aids

pyridoxine hydrochloride (vitamin B_6)

peer-i-dox'-een
(Aminoxin, Beesix, Doxine, Nestrex, Pryi, Pyroxin[AUS], Rodex, Vitabee 6)
Do not confuse pyridoxine with paroxetine, pralidoxime, or Pyridium.

CATEGORY AND SCHEDULE

Pregnancy Risk Category: A
OTC

MECHANISM OF ACTION

Acts as a coenzyme for various metabolic functions, including metabolism of proteins, carbohydrates, and fats. Aids in the breakdown of glycogen and in the synthesis of gamma-aminobutyric acid in the CNS. ***Therapeutic Effect:*** Prevents pyridoxine deficiency. Increases the excretion of certain drugs, such as isoniazid, that are pyridoxine antagonists.

P

PHARMACOKINETICS

Readily absorbed primarily in jejunum. Stored in the liver, muscle, and brain. Metabolized in the liver. Primarily excreted in urine. Removed by hemodialysis. ***Half-life:*** 15–20 days.

AVAILABILITY

Capsules: 250 mg.
Tablets: 20 mg, 25 mg, 50 mg, 100 mg, 250 mg, 500 mg.
Injection: 100 mg/ml.

INDICATIONS AND DOSAGES

▸ **Pyridoxine Deficiency**

PO
Adults, Elderly. Initially, 2.5–10 mg/day; then 2.5 mg/day when clinical signs are corrected.
Children. Initially, 5–25 mg/day for 3 wk, then 1.5–2.5 mg/day.

▸ **Pyridoxine Dependent Seizures**

PO, IV, IM
Infants. Initially,10–100 mg/day. Maintenance: PO: 50–100 mg/day.

▸ **Drug-Induced Neuritis**

PO (treatment)
Adults, Elderly. 100–300 mg/day in divided doses
Children. 10–50 mg/day.
PO (prophylaxis)
Adults, Elderly. 25–100 mg/day.
Children. 1–2 mg/kg/day.

CONTRAINDICATIONS

None known.

INTERACTIONS

Drug

Immunosuppressants, isoniazid, penicillamine: May antagonize pyridoxine, causing anemia or peripheral neuritis.
Levodopa: Reverses the effects of levodopa.

Herbal

None known.

Food

None known.

Drug interactions of concern to dentistry

- Decreased effectiveness: levodopa
- Decreased serum levels of phenytoin, phenobarbital

DIAGNOSTIC TEST EFFECTS

None known.

IV INCOMPATIBILITIES

Don't mix pyridoxine with any other medications.

SIDE EFFECTS

Occasional

Stinging at IM injection site

Rare

Headache, nausea, somnolence; sensory neuropathy (paresthesia, unstable gait, clumsiness of hands) with high doses

SERIOUS REACTIONS

! Long-term megadoses (2–6 g over more than 2 mo) may produce sensory neuropathy (reduced deep tendon reflexes, profound impairment of sense of position in distal limbs, gradual sensory ataxia). Toxic symptoms subside when drug is discontinued.

! Seizures have occurred after IV megadoses.

DENTAL CONSIDERATIONS

General:

- Vitamin B deficiency and peripheral neuropathy may manifest with oral symptoms of glossitis and cheilosis.

pyrimethamine

pye-ri-meth′-a-meen

(Daraprim, Malocide[FRANCE])

Do not confuse with Dantrium, Daranide.

CATEGORY AND SCHEDULE

Pregnancy Risk Category: C

MECHANISM OF ACTION

An antiprotozoal with blood and some tissue schizonticidal activity against malaria parasites of humans. Highly selective activity against plasmodia and *Toxoplasma gondii.* ***Therapeutic Effect:*** Inhibition of tetrahydrofolic acid synthesis.

PHARMACOKINETICS

Well absorbed, peak levels occurring between 2 and 6 hours following administration. Protein binding: 87%. Eliminated slowly. ***Half-life:*** approximately 96 hours.

AVAILABILITY

Tablets: 25 mg (Daraprim)

INDICATIONS AND DOSAGES

▸ **Toxoplasmosis**

PO

Adults. Initially, 50–75 mg daily, with 1–4 g daily of a sulfonamide of the sulfapyrimidine type (e.g., sulfadoxine). Continue for 1–3 weeks, depending on response of patient and tolerance to therapy then reduce dose to one-half that previously given for each drug and continue for additional 4–5 weeks.

Children. 1 mg/kg/day divided into 2 equal daily doses; after 2–4 days reduce to one-half and continue for approximately 1 month. The usual pediatric sulfonamide dosage is used in conjunction with pyrimethamine.

▸ **Acute Malaria**

PO

Adults (in combination with sulfonamide). 25 mg daily for 2 days with a sulfonamide

Adults (without concomitant sulfonamide). 50 mg for 2 days

Children 4–10 yrs. 25 mg daily for 2 days.

▸ **Chemoprophylaxis of Malaria**

PO

Adults and pediatric patients over 10 years: 25 mg once weekly.

Children 4–10 years: 12.5 mg once weekly.

Infants and children under 4 years: 6.25 mg once weekly.

OFF-LABEL USES

Prophylaxis for first episode and recurrence of *Pneumocystis carinii* pneumonia and *Toxoplasma gondii* in HIV-infected patients.

CONTRAINDICATIONS
Hypersensitivity to pyrimethamine, megaloblastic anemia due to folate deficiency, monotherapy for treatment of acute malaria.

INTERACTIONS
Drug
Antifolic drugs: Pyrimethamine may be used with sulfonamides, quinine, and other antimalarials and antibiotics. However, the concomitant use of other antifolic drugs, such as sulfonamides or trimethoprim-sulfamethoxazole combinations, while the patient is receiving pyrimethamine, may increase the risk of bone marrow suppression. If signs of folate deficiency develop, pyrimethamine should be discontinued. Folinic acid (leucovorin) should be administered until normal hematopoiesis is restored.
Benzodiazepines: Mild hepatotoxicity has been reported in some patients when lorazepam and pyrimethamine were administered concomitantly.
Herbal
None known.
Food
None known.
Drug interactions of concern to dentistry
- Possible mild hepatoxicity: lorazepam

DIAGNOSTIC TEST EFFECTS
None known.

SIDE EFFECTS
Frequent
Anorexia, vomiting
Occasional
Hypersensitivity reactions, Stevens-Johnson syndrome, toxic epidermal necrolysis, erythema multiforme, anaphylaxis, hyperphenylalaninemia, megaloblastic anemia, leukopenia, thrombocytopenia, pancytopenia, atrophic glossitis, hematuria, and disorders of cardiac rhythm
Rare
Pulmonary eosinophilia

SERIOUS REACTIONS
! None known.

DENTAL CONSIDERATIONS
General:
- Determine why patient is taking the drug.
- Consider semisupine chair position for patient comfort if GI side effects occur.
- Question patient about tolerance of NSAIDS or aspirin related to GI disease.
- Patient on chronic drug therapy may rarely present with symptoms of blood dyscrasias, which can include infection, bleeding, and poor healing. If dyscrasia is present, caution patient to prevent oral tissue trauma when using oral hygiene aids.
- Determine why patient is taking drug (prophylaxis or active therapy).
Consultations:
- Medical consultation may be required to assess disease control and patient's ability to tolerate stress.
Teach Patient/Family:
- To report sore throat, pallor, purpura, or glossitis, which may be symptoms of serious effects
- Importance of good oral hygiene to prevent soft tissue inflammation
- To prevent trauma when using oral hygiene aids
- Importance of updating health and medication history if physician makes any changes in evaluation or drug regimens; include OTC, herbal, and nonherbal in the update

quazepam

kwaz-′-ze-pam

SCHEDULE IV

(Doral)

CATEGORY AND SCHEDULE

Pregnancy Risk Category: X
Controlled Substance: Schedule IV

MECHANISM OF ACTION

A BZ-1 receptor selective benzodiazepine with sedative properties. ***Therapeutic Effect:*** Produces sedative effect from its central nervous system (CNS) depressant action.

PHARMACOKINETICS

Rapidly absorbed from gastrointestinal (GI) tract. Food increases absorption. Protein binding: 95%. Extensively metabolized in liver. Excreted in urine and feces. Unknown if removed by hemodialysis. ***Half-life:*** 25–41 hrs.

AVAILABILITY

Tablets: 7.5 mg, 15 mg (Doral).

INDICATIONS AND DOSAGES

▸ Insomnia

PO

Adults (older than 18 yrs). Initially, 15 mg at bedtime. Adjust dose up or down from 7.5 mg to 30 mg at bedtime depending on initial response.

Elderly, debilitated, liver disease. Initially, 7.5–15 mg at bedtime. Adjust dose depending on initial response.

CONTRAINDICATIONS

Pregnancy, sleep apnea, hypersensitivity to quazepam or any component of the formulation

INTERACTIONS

Drug

Alcohol, central nervous system (CNS) depressants: Potentiates effects of quazepam.
Azole antifungals: May inhibit liver metabolism and increase quazepam blood serum concentrations.
Theophylline: May decrease quazepam effectiveness.

Herbal

Dong quai, kava kava, magnolia, passionflower, skullcap, tan-shen, valerian: May increase CNS depressant effect of quazepam

Food

Caffeine: May decrease sedative and anxiolytic effects of quazepam.

Drug interactions of concern to dentistry

- Increased effects: CNS depressants, alcohol
- Delayed elimination: erythromycin
- Contraindicated with saquinavir, ritonavir
- Possible increase in CNS side effects: kava (herb)
- Increased serum levels and prolonged effect of benzodiazepines: erythromycin, ketoconazole, itraconazole, fluconazole, miconazole (systemic)

DIAGNOSTIC TEST EFFECTS

None known.

IV INCOMPATIBILITIES

None known

IV COMPATIBILITIES

None known

SIDE EFFECTS

Frequent

Muscular incoordination (ataxia), lightheadedness, transient mild drowsiness, slurred speech (particularly in elderly or debilitated patients)

Q

Occasional
Confusion, depression, blurred vision, constipation, diarrhea, dry mouth, headache, nausea
Rare
Behavioral problems such as anger, impaired memory, paradoxical reactions, such as insomnia, nervousness, or irritability

SERIOUS REACTIONS

! Abrupt or too rapid withdrawal may result in pronounced restlessness, irritability, insomnia, hand tremors, abdominal and muscle cramps, sweating, vomiting, and seizures.
! Overdosage results in somnolence, confusion, diminished reflexes, and coma.
! Blood dyscrasias have been reported rarely.

DENTAL CONSIDERATIONS

General:
- Assess salivary flow as a factor in caries, periodontal disease, and candidiasis.
- Psychologic and physical dependence may occur with chronic administration.
- Geriatric patients are more susceptible to drug effects; use a lower dose.
- Avoid using this drug in a patient with a history of drug abuse or alcoholism.

Consultations:
- Medical consultation may be required to assess disease control.

Teach Patient/Family:
- *When chronic dry mouth occurs, advise patient:*
  - To avoid mouth rinses with high alcohol content because of drying effects
  - Of need for daily use of home fluoride products to prevent caries
  - To use sugarless gum, frequent sips of water, or saliva substitutes

quetiapine

kwe-tye′-a-peen
(Seroquel)

CATEGORY AND SCHEDULE

Pregnancy Risk Category: C

MECHANISM OF ACTION

A dibenzepin derivative that antagonizes dopamine, serotonin, histamine, and alpha1-adrenergic receptors. ***Therapeutic Effect:*** Diminishes manifestations of psychotic disorders. Produces moderate sedation, few extrapyramidal effects, and no anticholinergic effects.

PHARMACOKINETICS

Well absorbed after PO administration. Protein binding: 83%. Widely distributed in tissues; CNS concentration exceeds plasma concentration. Undergoes extensive first-pass metabolism in the liver. Primarily excreted in urine. ***Half-life:*** 6 hr.

AVAILABILITY

Tablets: 25 mg, 100 mg, 200 mg, 300 mg.

INDICATIONS AND DOSAGES

▸ To Manage Manifestations of Psychotic Disorders, Bipolar Disorder

PO

Adults, Elderly. Initially, 25 mg twice a day, then 25–50 mg 2–3 times a day on the second and third days, up to 300–400 mg/day in divided doses 2–3 times a day by the fourth day. Further adjustments of 25–50 mg twice a day may be made at intervals of 2 days or longer. Maintenance: 300–800 mg/day (adults); 50–200 mg/day (elderly).

▸ **Dosage in Hepatic Impairment, Elderly or Debilitated Patients, and Those Predisposed to Hypotensive Reactions**

These patients should receive a lower initial dose and lower dosage increases.

CONTRAINDICATIONS

None known.

INTERACTIONS

Drug

Alcohol, other CNS depressants: May increase CNS depression.
Antihypertensives: May increase the hypotensive effects of these drugs.
Hepatic enzyme inducers (such as phenytoin): May increase quetiapine clearance.

Herbal

None known.

Food

None known.

Drug interactions of concern to dentistry

- Risk of increased CNS depression: CNS depressants

DIAGNOSTIC TEST EFFECTS

May decrease serum total and free thyroxine (T_4) serum levels. May increase serum cholesterol, triglyceride, AST (SGOT), and ALT (SGPT) levels. May produce a false-positive pregnancy test result.

SIDE EFFECTS

Frequent (19%–10%)
Headache, somnolence, dizziness
Occasional (9%–3%)
Constipation, orthostatic hypotension, tachycardia, dry mouth, dyspepsia, rash, asthenia, abdominal pain, rhinitis
Rare (2%)
Back pain, fever, weight gain

SERIOUS REACTIONS

! Overdose may produce heart block hypotension, hypokalemia, and tachycardia.

DENTAL CONSIDERATIONS

General:

- Monitor vital signs at every appointment because of CV and respiratory side effects
- Assess salivary flow as factor in caries, periodontal disease, and candidiasis.
- Assess for presence of extrapyramidal motor symptoms, such as tardive dyskinesia and akathisia. Extrapyramidal motor activity may complicate dental treatment.
- After supine positioning, have patient sit upright for at least 2 min before standing to avoid orthostatic hypotension.
- Consider semisupine chair position for patient comfort if GI side effects occur.
- Patients on chronic drug therapy may rarely have symptoms of blood dyscrasias, which can include infection, bleeding, and poor healing.
- Place on frequent recall because of oral side effects.

Consultations:

- In a patient with symptoms of blood dyscrasias, request a medical consultation for blood studies and postpone treatment until normal values are reestablished.
- Medical consultation may be required to assess disease control and patient's ability to tolerate stress.
- If signs of tardive dyskinesia or akathisia are present, refer to physician.
- Consultation with physician may be necessary if sedation or general anesthesia is required.
- Physician should be informed if significant xerostomic side effects

Q

occur (e.g., increased caries, sore tongue, problems eating or swallowing, difficulty wearing prosthesis) so that a medication change can be considered.

Teach Patient/Family:

- Caution to prevent trauma when using oral hygiene aids
- Use of electric toothbrush if patient has difficulty holding conventional devices
- Importance of good oral hygiene to prevent soft tissue inflammation
- Importance of updating health and drug history if physician makes any changes in evaluation or drug regimens
- To be aware of oral side effects and potential sequelae
- *When chronic dry mouth occurs, advise patient:*
  - To avoid mouth rinses with high alcohol content because of drying effects
  - To use daily home fluoride products for anticaries effect
  - To use sugarless gum, frequent sips of water, or saliva substitutes

Q

quinapril

kwin′-na-pril

(Accupril, Asig[AUS])

Do not confuse Accupril with Accolate or Accutane.

CATEGORY AND SCHEDULE

Pregnancy Risk Category: C (D if used in second or third trimester)

MECHANISM OF ACTION

An ACE inhibitor that suppresses the renin-angiotensin-aldosterone system and prevents the conversion of angiotensin I to angiotensin II, a potent vasoconstrictor; may also inhibit angiotensin II at local vascular and renal sites. ***Therapeutic Effect:*** Reduces peripheral arterial resistance, BP, and pulmonary capillary wedge pressure; improves cardiac output.

PHARMACOKINETICS

Route	Onset	Peak	Duration
PO	1 hr	N/A	24 hr

Readily absorbed from the GI tract. Protein binding: 97%. Metabolized in the liver, GI tract, and extravascular tissue to active metabolite. Primarily excreted in urine. Minimal removal by hemodialysis. ***Half-life:*** 1–2 hr; metabolite, 3 hr (increased in those with impaired renal function).

AVAILABILITY

Tablets: 5 mg, 10 mg, 20 mg, 40 mg.

INDICATIONS AND DOSAGES

▸ **Hypertension (monotherapy)**

PO

Adults. Initially, 10–20 mg/day. May adjust dosage at intervals of at least 2 wk or longer. Maintenance: 20–80 mg/day as single dose or 2 divided doses.
Maximum: 80 mg/day.

Elderly. Initially, 2.5–5 mg/day. May increase by 2.5–5 mg q1–2wk.

▸ **Hypertension (combination therapy)**

PO

Adults. Initially, 5 mg/day titrated to patient's needs.

Elderly. Initially, 2.5–5 mg/day. May increase by 2.5–5 mg q1–2wk.

▸ **Adjunct to Manage Heart Failure**

PO

Adults, Elderly. Initially, 5 mg twice a day. Range: 20–40 mg/day.

Dosage in Renal Impairment

Dosage is titrated to the patient's needs after the following initial doses:

Creatinine Clearance	Initial Dose
more than 60 ml/min	10 mg
30–60 ml/min	5 mg
10–29 ml/min	2.5 mg

OFF-LABEL USES

Treatment of hypertension and renal crisis in scleroderma

CONTRAINDICATIONS

Bilateral renal artery stenosis

INTERACTIONS

Drug

Alcohol, antihypertensives, diuretics: May increase the effects of quinapril.
Lithium: May increase lithium blood concentration and risk of lithium toxicity.
NSAIDs: May decrease the effects of quinapril.
Potassium-sparing diuretics, potassium supplements: May cause hyperkalemia.

Herbal

Garlic: May increase antihypertensive effect.
Ginseng, yohimbe: May worsen hypertension.

Food

None known.

Drug interactions of concern to dentistry

- Increased hypotension: alcohol, phenothiazines
- Decreased hypotensive effects: indomethacin and possibly other NSAIDs, sympathomimetics
- Suspected reduction in the antihypertensive and vasodilator effects by salicylates; monitor blood pressure if used concurrently

DIAGNOSTIC TEST EFFECTS

May increase BUN, serum alkaline phosphatase, serum bilirubin, serum creatinine, serum potassium, AST (SGOT), and ALT (SGPT) levels. May decrease serum sodium levels. May cause positive antinuclear antibody titer.

SIDE EFFECTS

Frequent (7%–5%)
Headache, dizziness
Occasional (4%–2%)
Fatigue, vomiting, nausea, hypotension, chest pain, cough, syncope
Rare (< 2%)
Diarrhea, cough, dyspnea, rash, palpitations, impotence, insomnia, drowsiness, malaise

SERIOUS REACTIONS

! Excessive hypotension ("first-dose syncope") may occur in patients with CHF and in those who are severely salt or volume depleted.
! Angioedema and hyperkalemia occur rarely.
! Agranulocytosis and neutropenia may be noted in those with collagen vascular disease, including scleroderma and systemic lupus erythematosus, and impaired renal function.
! Nephrotic syndrome may be noted in those with history of renal disease.

DENTAL CONSIDERATIONS

General:

- Monitor vital signs at every appointment because of CV side effects.
- After supine positioning, have patient sit upright for at least 2 min before standing to avoid orthostatic hypotension.
- Patients on chronic drug therapy may rarely have symptoms of blood dyscrasias, which can include infection, bleeding, and poor healing.

• Assess salivary flow as a factor in caries, periodontal disease, and candidiasis.
• Limit use of sodium-containing products, such as saline IV fluids, for patients with a dietary salt restriction.
• Use vasoconstrictors with caution, in low doses, and with careful aspiration.
• Stress from dental procedures may compromise CV function; determine patient risk.
• Short appointments and a stress reduction protocol may be required for anxious patients.

Consultations:

• Medical consultation may be required to assess disease control and patient's ability to tolerate stress.
• In a patient with symptoms of blood dyscrasias, request a medical consultation for blood studies and postpone dental treatment until normal values are reestablished.
• Take precautions if dental surgery is anticipated and sedation or general anesthesia is required; risk of hypotensive episode.

Teach Patient/Family:

• Importance of good oral hygiene to prevent soft tissue inflammation
• Caution to prevent injury when using oral hygiene aids
• *When chronic dry mouth occurs, advise patient:*
  • To avoid mouth rinses with high alcohol content because of drying effects
  • Of need for daily use of home fluoride products to prevent caries
  • To use sugarless gum, frequent sips of water, or saliva substitutes

Q

quinidine

kwin'-ih-deen
(Apo-Quin-G[CAN], Apo-Quinidine[CAN], BioQuin Durules[CAN], Kinidin Durules[AUS], Quinaglute Dura-Tabs, Quinate[CAN], Quinidex Extentabs)
Do not confuse quinidine with clonidine or quinine.

CATEGORY AND SCHEDULE

Pregnancy Risk Category: C

MECHANISM OF ACTION

An antiarrhythmic that decreases sodium influx during depolarization, potassium efflux during repolarization, and reduces calcium transport across the myocardial cell membrane. Decreases myocardial excitability, conduction velocity, and contractility.
Therapeutic Effect: Suppresses arrhythmias.

AVAILABILITY

Injection: 80 mg/ml.
Tablets: 200 mg, 300 mg.
Tablets (Extended-Release [Quinidex Extentabs]): 300 mg.
Tablets (Extended-Release [Quinaglute Dura-Tabs]): 324 mg.

INDICATIONS AND DOSAGES

▸ **Maintenance of Normal Sinus Rhythm After Conversion of Atrial Fibrillation or Flutter; Prevention of Premature Atrial, AV, and Ventricular Contractions; Paroxysmal Atrial Tachycardia; Paroxysmal AV Junctional Rhythm; Atrial Fibrillation; Atrial Flutter; Paroxysmal Ventricular Tachycardia not Associated with Complete Heart Block**

PO

Adults, Elderly. 100–600 mg q4–6h. (Long-acting): 324–972 mg q8–12h.

Children: 30 mg/kg/day in divided doses q4–6h.
IV
Adults, Elderly. 200–400 mg.
Children. 2–10 mg/kg.

OFF-LABEL USES

Treatment of malaria (IV only)

CONTRAINDICATIONS

Complete AV block, intraventricular conduction defects (widening of QRS complex)

INTERACTIONS

Drug

Antimyasthenics: May decrease effects of these drugs on skeletal muscle.
Digoxin: May increase digoxin serum concentration.
Other antiarrhythmics, pimozide: May increase cardiac effects.
Neuromuscular blockers, oral anticoagulants: May increase effects of these drugs.
Urinary alkalizers, such as antacids: May decrease quinidine renal excretion.

Herbal

None known.

Food

None known.

Drug interactions of concern to dentistry

- May decrease effects of quinidine: barbiturates
- Increased anticholinergic effect: anticholinergic drugs
- Increased effects of neuromuscular blockers, tricyclic antidepressants
- Contraindicated with itraconazole
- Prevention of action: cholinergics

DIAGNOSTIC TEST EFFECTS

None known. Therapeutic serum level is 2 to 5 mcg/ml; toxic serum level is greater than 5 mcg/ml.

IV INCOMPATIBILITIES

Furosemide (Lasix), heparin

IV COMPATIBILITIES

Milrinone (Primacor)

SIDE EFFECTS

Frequent

Abdominal pain and cramps, nausea, diarrhea, vomiting (can be immediate, intense)

Occasional

Mild cinchonism (ringing in ears, blurred vision, hearing loss) or severe cinchonism (headache, vertigo, diaphoresis, light-headedness, photophobia, confusion, delirium)

Rare

Hypotension (particularly with IV administration), hypersensitivity reaction (fever, anaphylaxis, photosensitivity reaction)

SERIOUS REACTIONS

! Cardiotoxic effects occur most commonly with IV administration, particularly at high concentrations, and are observed as conduction changes (50% widening of QRS complex, prolonged QT interval, flattened T waves, and disappearance of P wave), ventricular tachycardia or flutter, frequent premature ventricular contractions (PVCs), or complete AV block.
! Quinidine-induced syncope may occur with the usual dosage.
! Severe hypotension may result from high dosages.
! Patients with atrial flutter and fibrillation may experience a paradoxical, exremely rapid ventricular rate that may be prevented by prior digitalization.
! Hepatotoxicity with jaundice due to drug hypersensitivity may occur.

DENTAL CONSIDERATIONS

General:

- Monitor vital signs at every appointment because of CV and respiratory side effects.
- Patients on chronic drug therapy may rarely have symptoms of blood dyscrasias, which can include infection, bleeding, and poor healing.
- After supine positioning, have patient sit upright for at least 2 min before standing to avoid orthostatic hypotension.
- Use vasoconstrictors with caution, in low doses, and with careful aspiration. Avoid use of gingival retraction cord with epinephrine.
- Consider semisupine chair position for patient comfort if GI side effects occur.

Consultations:

- In a patient with symptoms of blood dyscrasias, request a medical consultation for blood studies and postpone dental treatment until normal values are reestablished.
- Medical consultation may be required to assess patient's ability to tolerate stress.

Teach Patient/Family:

- Importance of good oral hygiene to prevent soft tissue inflammation

Q

quinine

kwye′-nine

(Quinine)

Do not confuse with quinidine.

CATEGORY AND SCHEDULE

Pregnancy Risk Category: X

MECHANISM OF ACTION

A cinchone alkaloid that relaxes skeletal muscle by increasing the refractory period, decreasing excitability of motor end plates (curarelike), and affecting distribution of calcium with muscle fiber. Antimalaria: Depresses oxygen uptake, carbohydrate metabolism, elevates pH in intracellular organelles of parasites. ***Therapeutic Effect:*** Relaxes skeletal muscle; produces parasite death.

PHARMACOKINETICS

Rapidly absorbed mainly from upper small intestine. Protein binding: 70%–95%. Metabolized in liver. Excreted in feces, saliva, and urine. ***Half-life:*** 8–14 hrs (adults), 6–12 hrs (children).

AVAILABILITY

Capsules: 200 mg, 325 mg (Quinine).
Tablets: 260 mg (Quinine).

INDICATIONS AND DOSAGES

▸ Nocturnal Leg Cramps

PO

Adults, Elderly. 260–300 mg at bedtime as needed.

▸ Treatment of Malaria

PO

Adults, Elderly. 260–650 mg 3 times a day for 6–12 days.
Children. 10 mg/kg q8h for 5–7 days.

Dosage in renal impairment

Creatinine Clearance	Dosage Interval
10–50 ml/min	75% of normal dose or q12h
Less than 10 ml/min	30%–50% of normal dose or q24h

CONTRAINDICATIONS

Hypersensitivity to quinine (possible cross-sensitivity to quinidine), G-6-PD deficiency, tinnitus, optic neuritis, history of thrombocytopenia during previous quinine therapy, blackwater fever

INTERACTIONS

Drug

Amiodarone, alkalinizing agents, cimetidine, verapamil: May increase quinine serum concentrations.
Beta blockers: May increase bradycardia.
Digoxin: May increase blood concentration of digoxin.
Mefloquine: May increase risk of seizures and ECG abnormalities.
Phenobarbital, phenytoin, rifampin: May decrease quinine serum concentrations.
Warfarin: May increase anticoagulant effect.

Herbal

St. John's Wort: May decrease quinine levels.

Food

None known.

Drug interactions of concern to dentistry

- Decreased absorption: magnesium or aluminum salts
- Prolonged duration of neuromuscular blocking drugs

DIAGNOSTIC TEST EFFECTS

May interfere with 17-OH steroid determinations. May result in positive Coombs' test.

SIDE EFFECTS

Frequent

Nausea, headache, tinnitus, slight visual disturbances (mild cinchonism)

Occasional

Extreme flushing of skin with intense generalized pruritus is most typical hypersensitivity reaction; also rash, wheezing, dyspnea, angioedema.
Prolonged therapy: cardiac conduction disturbances, decreased hearing

SERIOUS REACTIONS

! Overdosage (severe cinchonism) may result in cardiovascular effects, severe headache, intestinal cramps w/vomiting and diarrhea, apprehension, confusion, seizures, blindness, and respiratory depression.
! Hypoprothrombinemia, thrombocytopenic purpura, hemoglobinuria, asthma, agranulocytosis, hypoglycemia, deafness, and optic atrophy occur rarely.

DENTAL CONSIDERATIONS

General:

- Patients on chronic drug therapy may rarely have symptoms of blood dyscrasias, which can include infection, bleeding, and poor healing.
- Avoid dental light in patient's eyes; offer dark glasses for patient comfort.
- Monitor vital signs at every appointment because of CV side effects.
- Consider semisupine chair position for patient comfort if GI side effects occur.

Consultations:

- Medical consultation may be required to assess disease control.
- In a patient with symptoms of blood dyscrasias, request a medical consultation for blood studies and postpone dental treatment until normal values are reestablished.

Teach Patient/Family:

- Importance of good oral hygiene to prevent soft tissue inflammation

rabeprazole sodium

rah-bep′-rah-zole
(Aciphex, Pariet[CAN])
Do not confuse Aciphex with Accupril or Aricept.

CATEGORY AND SCHEDULE

Pregnancy Risk Category: B

MECHANISM OF ACTION

A proton pump inhibitor that converts to active metabolites that irreversibly binds to and inhibit hydrogen-potassium adenosine triphosphate, an enzyme on the surface of gastric parietal cells. Actively secretes hydrogen ions for potassium ions, resulting in an accumulation of hydrogen ions in gastric lumen.
Therapeutic Effect: Increases gastric pH, reducing gastric acid production.

PHARMACOKINETICS

Rapidly absorbed from the GI tract after passing through the stomach relatively intact. Protein binding: 96%. Metabolized extensively in the liver. Primarily excreted in urine. Unknown if removed by hemodialysis. ***Half-life:*** 1–2 hr (increased with hepatic impairment).

AVAILABILITY

Tablets (Delayed-Release): 20 mg.

INDICATIONS AND DOSAGES

▸ **Gastroesophageal Reflux Disease**
PO
Adults, Elderly. 20 mg/day for 4–8 wk. Maintenance: 20 mg/day.
▸ **Duodenal Ulcer**
PO
Adults, Elderly. 20 mg/day after morning meal for 4 wk.
▸ **Non-Steroidal Antiinflammatory Drug (NSAID)-Induced Ulcer**
PO
Adults, Elderly. 20 mg/day.
▸ **Pathologic Hypersecretory Conditions**
PO
Adults, Elderly. Initially, 60 mg once a day. May increase to 60 mg twice a day.
▸ ***Helibacter Pylori*** **Infection**
PO
Adults, Elderly. 20 mg 2 times a day for 7 days (given with amoxicillin 1,000 mg and clarithromycin 500 mg)

CONTRAINDICATIONS

None known.

INTERACTIONS

Drug
Digoxin: May increase the plasma concentration of digoxin.
Ketoconazole: May decrease the blood concentration of ketoconazole.
Herbal
None known.
Food
None known.
Drug interactions of concern to dentistry
- None reported

DIAGNOSTIC TEST EFFECTS

May increase serum alkaline phosphatase, AST(SGOT), and ALT(SGPT) levels.

SIDE EFFECTS

Rare (< 2%)
Headache, nausea, dizziness, rash, diarrhea, malaise

SERIOUS REACTIONS

! Hyperglycemia, hypokalemia, hyponatremia, and hyperlipemia occur rarely.

DENTAL CONSIDERATIONS

General:
- Assess salivary flow as a factor in caries, periodontal disease, and candidiasis.

Consider semisupine chair position for patient comfort because of GI side effects of disease.
- Patients with gastroesophageal reflux may have oral symptoms, including burning mouth, secondary candidiasis, and signs of tooth erosion.
- Question the patient about tolerance of NSAIDs or aspirin related to GI problems.

Teach Patient/Family:
- To prevent trauma when using oral hygiene aids
- *When chronic dry mouth occurs, advise patient:*
  - To avoid mouth rinses with high alcohol content because of drying effects
  - To use daily home fluoride products for anticaries effect
  - To use sugarless gum, frequent sips of water, or saliva substitutes

raloxifene

ra-lox′-i-feen
(Evista)
Do not confuse raloxifene with propoxyphene.

CATEGORY AND SCHEDULE

Pregnancy Risk Category: X

MECHANISM OF ACTION

A selective estrogen receptor modulator that affects some receptors like estrogen. ***Therapeutic Effect:*** Like estrogen, prevents bone loss and improves lipid profiles.

PHARMACOKINETICS

Rapidly absorbed after PO administration. Highly bound to plasma proteins (> 95%) and albumin. Undergoes extensive first-pass metabolism in liver. Excreted mainly in feces and, to a lesser extent, in urine. Unknown if removed by hemodialysis. ***Half-life:*** 27.7 hr.

AVAILABILITY

Tablets: 60 mg.

INDICATIONS AND DOSAGES

▸ Prevention or Treatment of Osteoporosis

PO

Adults, Elderly. 60 mg a day.

OFF-LABEL USES

Treatment of breast cancer in postmenopausal women, prevention of fractures

CONTRAINDICATIONS

Active or history of venous thromboembolic events, such as deep vein thrombosis, pulmonary embolism, and retinal vein thrombosis; women who are or may become pregnant

INTERACTIONS

Drug

Ampicillin, cholestyramine: Reduce raloxifene absorption.
Hormone replacement therapy, systemic estrogen: Don't use raloxifene concurrently with these drugs.
Warfarin: May decrease PT and the effects of warfarin.

Herbal

None known.

Food

None known.

Drug interactions of concern to dentistry
- Reduced absorption: ampicillin
- Risk of potential drug interactions with other highly plasma protein-bound drugs, such as NSAIDs, aspirin, and diazepam, is unknown

DIAGNOSTIC TEST EFFECTS

Lowers serum total cholesterol and LDL levels, but does not affect HDL or triglyceride levels. Slightly decreases platelet count and serum inorganic phosphate, albumin, calcium, and protein levels.

SIDE EFFECTS

Frequent (25%–10%)
Hot flashes, flulike symptoms, arthralgia, sinusitis
Occasional (9%–5%)
Weight gain, nausea, myalgia, pharyngitis, cough, dyspepsia, leg cramps, rash, depression
Rare (4%–3%)
Vaginitis, UTI, peripheral edema, flatulence, vomiting, fever, migraine, diaphoresis

SERIOUS REACTIONS

! Pneumonia, gastroenteritis, chest pain, vaginal bleeding, and breast pain occur rarely.

DENTAL CONSIDERATIONS

General:

- Drug should be discontinued 72 hr before prolonged immobilization, such as hospitalization, postsurgical recovery, and bed rest.
- Consider short appointments and dental chair position if needed for patient comfort.

Consultations:

- Medical consultation may be required to assess disease control and patient's ability to tolerate stress.

ramipril

ram′-i-pril
(Altace, Ramace[AUS], Tritace[AUS])
Do not confuse Altace with Alteplase or Artane.

CATEGORY AND SCHEDULE

Pregnancy Risk Category: C (D if used in second or third trimester)

MECHANISM OF ACTION

An ACE inhibitor that suppresses the renin-angiotensin-aldosterone system. Decreases plasma angiotensin II, increases plasma renin activity, and decreases aldosterone secretion. ***Therapeutic Effect:*** Reduces peripheral arterial resistance and BP.

PHARMACOKINETICS

Route	Onset	Peak	Duration
PO	1–2 hr	3–6 hr	24 hr

Well absorbed from the GI tract. Protein binding: 73%. Metabolized in the liver to active metabolite. Primarily excreted in urine. Not removed by hemodialysis. ***Half-life:*** 5.1 hr.

AVAILABILITY

Capsules: 1.25 mg, 2.5 mg, 5 mg, 10 mg.

INDICATIONS AND DOSAGES

▸ **Hypertension (monotherapy)**
PO
Adults, Elderly. Initially, 2.5 mg/day. Maintenance: 2.5–20 mg/day as single dose or in 2 divided doses.

▸ Hypertension (in combination with Other Antihypertensives)
PO
Adults, Elderly. Initially, 1.25 mg/day titrated to patient's needs.
▸ CHF
PO
Adults, Elderly. Initially, 1.25–2.5 mg twice a day. Maximum: 5 mg twice a day.
▸ Risk Reduction for Myocardial Infarction Stroke
PO
Adults, Elderly. Initially, 2.5 mg/day for 7 days, then 5 mg/day for 21 days, then 10 mg/day as a single dose or in divided doses.
▸ Dosage in Renal Impairment
Creatinine clearance equal to or less than 40 ml/min. 25% of normal dose.
Hypertension. Initially, 1.25 mg/day titrated upward.
CHF. Initially, 1.25 mg/day, titrated up to 2.5 mg twice a day.

OFF-LABEL USES
Treatment of hypertension and renal crisis in scleroderma

CONTRAINDICATIONS
Bilateral renal artery stenosis

INTERACTIONS
Drug
Alcohol, antihypertensives, diuretics: May increase the effects of ramipril.
Lithium: May increase lithium blood concentration and risk of lithium toxicity.
NSAIDs: May decrease the effects of ramipril.
Potassium-sparing diuretics, potassium supplements: May cause hyperkalemia.
Herbal
Garlic: May increase antihypertensive effect.
Ginseng, yohimbe: May worsen hypertension.
Food
None known.
Drug interactions of concern to dentistry
- Increased hypotension: alcohol, phenothiazines
- Decreased hypotensive effects: indomethacin and possibly other NSAIDs, sympathomimetics
- Suspected reduction in the antihypertensive and vasodilator effects by salicylates; monitor blood pressure if used concurrently

DIAGNOSTIC TEST EFFECTS
May increase BUN, serum alkaline phosphatase, serum bilirubin, serum creatinine, serum potassium, AST (SGOT), and ALT (SGPT) levels. May decrease serum sodium levels. May cause positive antinuclear antibody titer.

SIDE EFFECTS
Frequent (12%–5%)
Cough, headache
Occasional (4%–2%)
Dizziness, fatigue, nausea, asthenia (loss of strength)
Rare (<2%)
Palpitations, insomnia, nervousness, malaise, abdominal pain, myalgia

SERIOUS REACTIONS
! Excessive hypotension ("first-dose syncope") may occur in patients with CHF and and in those who are severely salt or volume depleted.
! Angioedema and hyperkalemia occur rarely.
! Agranulocytosis and neutropenia may be noted in those with collagen vascular disease, including scleroderma and systemic lupus erythematosus, and impaired renal function.

! Nephrotic syndrome may be noted in those with history of renal disease.

DENTAL CONSIDERATIONS

General:

- Monitor vital signs at every appointment because of CV and respiratory side effects.
- After supine positioning, have patient sit upright for at least 2 min before standing to avoid orthostatic hypotension.
- Patients on chronic drug therapy may rarely have symptoms of blood dyscrasias, which can include infection, bleeding, and poor healing.
- Assess salivary flow as a factor in caries, periodontal disease, and candidiasis.
- Limit use of sodium-containing products, such as saline IV fluids, for patients with a dietary salt restriction.
- Use vasoconstrictors with caution, in low doses, and with careful aspiration.
- Stress from dental procedures may compromise CV function; determine patient risk.
- Short appointments and a stress reduction protocol may be required for anxious patients.

R

Consultations:

- Medical consultation may be required to assess patient's ability to tolerate stress.
- In a patient with symptoms of blood dyscrasias, request a medical consultation for blood studies and postpone dental treatment until normal values are reestablished.
- Take precautions if dental surgery is anticipated and sedation or general anesthesia is required; risk of hypotensive episode.

Teach Patient/Family:

- Importance of good oral hygiene to prevent soft tissue inflammation
- Caution to prevent injury when using oral hygiene aids
- *When chronic dry mouth occurs, advise patient:*
  - To avoid mouth rinses with high alcohol content because of drying effects
  - Of need for daily use of home fluoride products to prevent caries
  - To use sugarless gum, frequent sips of water, or saliva substitutes

ranitidine hydrochloride/ ranitidine bismuth citrate

ra-ni′-ti-deen

(ranitidine hydrochloride) Apo-Ranitidine[CAN], Ausran [AUS], Novo-Ranitidine[CAN], Rani-2[AUS], Ranihexal[AUS], Zantac, Zantac-75, Zantac-150, Zantac-300, Zantac EFFERdose, Zantac-25 EFFERdose, Zantac-150 EFFERdose, Zantac-150 Maximum Strength (ranitidine bismuth citrate) Pylorid[AUS], Tritec

Do not confuse Zantac with Xanax, Ziac, or Zyrtec.

CATEGORY AND SCHEDULE

Pregnancy Risk Category: B

OTC (75 mg tablets)

MECHANISM OF ACTION

An antiulcer agent that inhibits histamine action at histamine 2 receptors of gastric parietal cells. ***Therapeutic Effect:*** Inhibits gastric acid secretion when fasting, at night, or when stimulated by food, caffeine, or insulin. Reduces volume and hydrogen ion concentration of gastric juice.

PHARMACOKINETICS

Rapidly absorbed from the GI tract. Protein binding: 15%.

Widely distributed. Metabolized in the liver. Primarily excreted in urine. Not removed by hemodialysis. ***Half-life:*** PO, 2.5 hr; IV, 2–2.5 hr (increased with impaired renal function).

AVAILABILITY

Tablets (Effervescent): 25 mg (Zantac-25 EFFERdose), 150 mg (Zantac-150 EFFERdose).
Capsules (Zantac): 150 mg, 300 mg.
Granules (Zantac EFFERdose): 150 mg.
Syrup (Zantac): 15 mg/ml.
Tablets: 75 mg (Zantac-75), 150 mg (Zantac-150, Zantac-150 Maximum Strength), 300 mg (Zantac-300).
Tablets (bisumuth citrate [Tritec]): 400 mg.
Injection (Zantac): 25 mg/ml.

INDICATIONS AND DOSAGES

▸ Duodenal Ulcers, Gastric Ulcers, Gastroesophageal Reflux Disease

PO
Adults, Elderly. 150 mg twice a day or 300 mg at bedtime. Maintenance: 150 mg at bedtime.
Children. 2–4 mg/kg/day in divided doses twice a day.
Maximum: 300 mg/day.

▸ Duodenal Ulcers Associated with *H. Pylori* Infection

PO
Adults, Elderly. 400 mg twice a day for 4 weeks in combination with clarithromycin 500 mg 2–3 times a day for the first 2 weeks.

▸ Erosive Esophagitis

PO
Adults, Elderly. 150 mg 4 times a day. Maintenance: 150 mg twice a day or 300 mg at bedtime.
Children. 4–10 mg/kg/day in 2 divided doses. Maximum: 600 mg/day.

▸ Hypersecretory Conditions

PO
Adults, Elderly. 150 mg twice a day. May increase up to 6 g/day.

▸ OTC Use

PO
Adults, Elderly. 75 mg 30–60 minutes before eating food or drinking beverages that cause heartburn. Maximum: 150 mg per 24 hr period and/or longer than 14 days.

▸ Usual Parenteral Dosage

IV, IM
Adults, Elderly. 50 mg/dose q6–8h. Maximum: 400 mg/day.
Children. 2–4 mg/kg/day in divided doses q6–8h. Maximum: 200 mg/day.

▸ Usual Neonatal Dosage

PO
Neonates. 2 mg/kg/day in divided doses q12h.
IV
Neonates. Initially, 1.5 mg/kg/dose; then 1.5–2 mg/kg/day in divided doses q12h.

▸ Dosage in Renal Impairment

For patients with creatinine clearance less than 50 ml/min, give 150 mg PO q24h or 50 mg IV or IM q18–24h.

OFF-LABEL USES

Prevention of aspiration pneumonia, treatment of recurrent post-operative ulcer, upper GI bleeding, prevention of acid aspiration pneumonitis during surgery, prevention of stress-induced ulcers.

CONTRAINDICATIONS

History of acute porphyria

INTERACTIONS

Drug

Antacids: May decrease the absorption of ranitidine.
Ketoconazole: May decrease the absorption of ketoconazole.

Herbal

None known.

Food

None known.

Drug interactions of concern to dentistry

- Decreased absorption of diazepam, anticholinergics, ketoconazole (take doses 2 hr apart)

DIAGNOSTIC TEST EFFECTS

Interferes with skin tests using allergen extracts. May increase hepatic function enzyme, gamma-glutamyl transpeptidase, and serum creatinine levels.

IV INCOMPATIBILITIES

Amphotericin B complex (Abelcet, AmBisome, Amphotec)

IV COMPATIBILITIES

Diltiazem (Cardizem), dobutamine (Dobutrex), dopamine (Intropin), heparin, hydromorphone (Dilaudid), insulin, lidocaine, lorazepam (Ativan), morphine, norepinephrine (Levophed), potassium chloride, propofol (Diprivan)

SIDE EFFECTS

Occasional (2%)
Diarrhea

Rare (1%)
Constipation, headache (may be severe)

SERIOUS REACTIONS

! Reversible hepatitis and blood dyscrasias occur rarely.

DENTAL CONSIDERATIONS

General:

- Avoid prescribing aspirin-containing products in patients with active GI disease.
- Consider semisupine chair position for patient comfort because of GI effects of disease.

repaglinide

re-pag′-lih-nide
(GlucoNorm[CAN], NovoNorm[AUS], Prandin)

CATEGORY AND SCHEDULE

Pregnancy Risk Category: C

MECHANISM OF ACTION

An antihyperglycemic that stimulates release of insulin from beta cells of the pancreas by depolarizing beta cells, leading to an opening of calcium channels. Resulting calcium influx induces insulin secretion. ***Therapeutic Effect:*** Lowers blood glucose concentration.

PHARMACOKINETICS

Rapidly, completely absorbed from the GI tract. Protein binding: 98%. Metabolized in the liver to inactive metabolites. Excreted primarily in feces with a lesser amount in urine. Unknown if removed by hemodialysis. ***Half-life:*** 1 hr.

AVAILABILITY

Tablets: 0.5 mg, 1 mg, 2 mg.

INDICATIONS AND DOSAGES

▸ Diabetes Mellitus

PO

Adults, Elderly. 0.5–4 mg 2–4 times a day. Maximum: 16 mg/day.

CONTRAINDICATIONS

Diabetic ketoacidosis, type 1 diabetes mellitus

INTERACTIONS

Drug

Beta blockers, chloramphenicol, gemfibrozil, MAOIs, NSAIDs, probenecid, salicylates, sulfonamides, warfarin: May increase the effects of repaglinide.

Herbal
None known.
Food
Food: Decreases repaglinide plasma concentration.
Drug interactions of concern to dentistry
- Clinical studies have not been completed; metabolism may be inhibited by ketoconazole, miconazole, erythromycin
- Risk of increased hypoglycemia: NSAIDs, salicylates
- Suspected increase in plasma levels: clarithromycin, erythromycin

DIAGNOSTIC TEST EFFECTS
None known.

SIDE EFFECTS
Frequent (10%–6%)
Upper respiratory tract infection, headache, rhinitis, bronchitis, back pain
Occasional (5%–3%)
Diarrhea, dyspepsia, sinusitis, nausea, arthralgia, urinary tract infection
Rare (2%)
Constipation, vomiting, paresthesia, allergy

SERIOUS REACTIONS
! Hypoglycemia occurs in 16% of patients.
! Chest pain occurs rarely.

DENTAL CONSIDERATIONS
General:
- If dentist prescribes any of the drugs listed in the drug interactions section, monitor patient blood sugar levels.
- Consider semisupine chair position for patient comfort because of GI side effects of drug.
- Ensure that patient is following prescribed diet and regularly takes medication.
- Place on frequent recall to evaluate healing response.
- Short appointments and a stress reduction protocol may be required.
- Diabetics may be more susceptible to infection and have delayed wound healing.

Consultations:
- Medical consultation may include data from patient's blood glucose monitoring, including glycosylated hemoglobin or HbA_{1c} testing.
- Medical consultation may be required to assess disease control and patient's ability to tolerate stress.

Teach Patient/Family:
- To prevent trauma when using oral hygiene aids
- Importance of updating health and drug history if physician makes any changes in evaluation or drug regimens

reserpine
reh-zer′-peen
Serpalan, Maviserpin[MEX], Novoreserpine[CAN], Rauserpine [TAIWAN], Rauverid[PHILIPPINES], Reserfia[CAN], Serpasil[CAN, INDONESIA], Serpasol[SPAIN]
Do not confuse with Risperdal, risperidone

CATEGORY AND SCHEDULE
Pregnancy Risk Category: C

MECHANISM OF ACTION
An antihypertensive that depletes stores of catecholamines and 5-hydroxytryptamine in many organs, including the brain and adrenal medulla. Depression of sympathetic nerve function results in a decreased heart rate and a lowering of arterial blood pressure. Depletion of catecholamines and

R

5-hydroxytryptamine from the brain is thought to be the mechanism of the sedative and tranquilizing properties. ***Therapeutic Effects:*** Decrease blood pressure and heart rate; sedation.

PHARMACOKINETICS

Characterized by slow onset of action and sustained effects. Both cardiovascular and central nervous system effects may persist for a period of time following withdrawal of the drug. Mean maximum plasma levels were attained after a median of 3.5 hours. Bioavailability was approximately 50% of that of a corresponding intravenous dose. Protein binding: 96%. ***Half life:*** 33 hrs.

AVAILABILITY

Tablets: 0.25 mg, 0.1 mg (reserpine)

INDICATIONS AND DOSAGES

▸ Hypertension

PO

Adults: Usual initial dosage 0.5 mg daily for 1 or 2 weeks. For maintenance, reduce to 0.1 to 0.25 mg daily.

Children: Reserpine is not recommended for use in children. If it is to be used in treating a child, the usual recommended starting dose is 20 µg/kg daily. The maximum recommended dose is 0.25 mg (total) daily.

R

▸ Psychiatric Disorders

PO

Adults: Initial dosage 0.5 mg daily, may range from 0.1–1.0 mg. Adjust dosage upward or downward according to response.

OFF-LABEL USES

Cerebral vasospasm, migraines, Raynaud's syndrome, reflex sympathetic dystrophy, refractory depression, tardive dyskinesia, thyrotoxic crisis.

CONTRAINDICATIONS

Hypersensitivity, mental depression or history of mental depression (especially with suicidal tendencies), active peptic ulcer, ulcerative colitis, patients receiving electroconvulsive therapy.

INTERACTIONS

Drug

MAO inhibitors: May cause hypertensive reactions.
Beta-blockers: Reserpine may increase effect.
CNS depressants/ethanol: Reserpine may increase effects.
Levodopa, quinidine, procainamide, digitalis glycosides: Reserpine may increase effects/toxicity.
Tricyclic antidepressants: May increase antihypertensive effects.

Herbal

Dong quai: Has estrogenic activity
Ephedra/yohimbe: May worsen hypertension
Valerian, St John's wort, kava kava, gotu kola: May increase CNS depression
Garlic: May have increased antihypertensive effects

Food

Ethanol: May increase CNS depression.

Drug interactions of concern to dentistry

- Increased CNS depression: barbiturates, alcohol, opioids
- Increased pressor effects: epinephrine
- Decreased pressor effects: ephedrine, tricyclic antidepressants
- Decreased hypotensive effect: indomethacin and possibly other NSAIDs

DIAGNOSTIC TEST EFFECTS
None known.

SIDE EFFECTS
Occasional
Burning in the stomach, nausea, vomiting, diarrhea, dry mouth, nosebleed, stuffy nose, dizziness, headache, nervousness, nightmares, drowsiness, muscle aches, weight gain, redness of the eyes
Rare
Irregular heart beat, difficulty breathing, heart problems, feeling faint, swelling, gynecomastia, decreased libido

SERIOUS REACTIONS
! None known.

DENTAL CONSIDERATIONS
General:
• Monitor vital signs at every appointment because of CV side effects.
• Patients on chronic drug therapy may rarely have symptoms of blood dyscrasias, which can include infection, bleeding, and poor healing.
• Assess salivary flow as a factor in caries, periodontal disease, and candidiasis.
• After supine positioning, have patient sit upright for at least 2 min before standing to avoid orthostatic hypotension.
• Limit use of sodium-containing products, such as saline IV fluids, for patients with a dietary salt restriction.

Consultations:
• Medical consultation may be required to assess disease control.

Teach Patient/Family:
• Importance of good oral hygiene to prevent soft tissue inflammation
• *When chronic dry mouth occurs, advise patient:*
  • To avoid mouth rinses with high alcohol content because of drying effects
  • Of need for daily use of home fluoride products to prevent caries
  • To use sugarless gum, frequent sips of water, or saliva substitutes

reteplase, recombinant
reh′-te-place
(Rapilysin[AUS], Retavase)
Do not confuse reteplase or Retavase with Restasis.

CATEGORY AND SCHEDULE
Pregnancy Risk Category: C

MECHANISM OF ACTION
A tissue plasminogen activator that activates the fibrinolytic system by directly cleaving plasminogen to generate plasmin, an enzyme that degrades the fibrin of the thrombus. ***Therapeutic Effect:*** Exerts thrombolytic action.

PHARMACOKINETICS
Rapidly cleared from plasma. Eliminated primarily by the liver and kidney. ***Half-life:*** 13–16 min.

AVAILABILITY
Powder for Injection: 10.4 units (18.1 mg).

INDICATIONS AND DOSAGES
▸ **Acute MI, CHF**
IV BOLUS
Adults, Elderly. 10 units over 2 min; repeat in 30 min.

CONTRAINDICATIONS
Active internal bleeding, AV malformation or aneurysm, bleeding

R

diathesis, history of cerebrovascular accident, intracranial neoplasm, recent intracranial or intraspinal surgery or trauma, severe uncontrolled hypertension

INTERACTIONS

Drug

Heparin, platelet aggregation antagonists (such as abciximab, aspirin, dipyridamole), warfarin: Increase the risk of bleeding.

Herbal

Ginkgo biloba: May increase the risk of bleeding.

Food

None known.

Drug interactions of concern to dentistry

- Increased risk of bleeding: drugs that interfere with coagulation or platelet function, such as NSAIDs or aspirin

DIAGNOSTIC TEST EFFECTS

May decrease fibrinogen and serum plasminogen levels.

IV INCOMPATIBILITIES

Do not mix with other medications.

SIDE EFFECTS

Frequent

Bleeding at superficial sites, such as venous injection sites, catheter insertion sites, venous cutdowns, arterial punctures, and sites of recent surgical procedures, gingival bleeding

SERIOUS REACTIONS

! Bleeding at internal sites may occur, including intracranial, retroperitoneal, GI, GU, and respiratory sites.

! Lysis or coronary thrombi may produce atrial or ventricular arrhythmias and stroke.

DENTAL CONSIDERATIONS

General:

- Acute-use drug for use in hospitals or emergency rooms.
- Patients are at risk for bleeding, check for oral signs.
- Monitor and record vital signs.
- Avoid products that affect platelet function, such as aspirin and NSAIDs.
- Patients who have been treated with this drug may present with cardiovascular disease or stoke, review medical and drug history.

Consultations:

- Medical consultation should include routine blood counts including platelet counts and bleeding time.
- In a patient with symptoms of blood dyscrasias, request a medical consultation for blood studies and postpone treatment until normal values are reestablished.
- Medical consultation may be required to assess disease control and patient's ability to tolerate stress.

Teach Patient/Family:

- Use soft tooth brush to reduce risk of bleeding
- Importance of good oral hygiene to prevent soft tissue inflammation
- To report oral lesions, soreness, or bleeding to dentist
- To prevent trauma when using oral hygiene aids
- Importance of updating health and medication history if physician makes any changes in evaluation or drug regimens; include OTC, herbal, and nonherbal remedies in the update

R

ribavirin

rye-ba-vye′-rin
(Copegus, Rebetol, Rebetron, Virazole)
Do not confuse ribavirin with riboflavin.

CATEGORY AND SCHEDULE

Pregnancy Risk Category: X

MECHANISM OF ACTION

A synthetic nucleoside that inhibits influenza virus RNA polymerase activity and interferes with expression of messenger RNA. ***Therapeutic Effect:*** Inhibits viral protein synthesis and replication of viral RNA and DNA.

PHARMACOKINETICS

Rapidly absorbed from the GI tract following oral administration. A small amount is systemically absorbed following inhalation. Primarily excreted in urine. ***Half-life:*** 298 hr (oral); 9.5 hr (inhalation).

AVAILABILITY

Capsules (Rebetol, Rebetron Combination Therapy with alfa-2b injection): 200 mg.
Tablets (Cepegus): 200 mg.
Powder for Reconstitution (Aerosol [Virazole]): 6 g.
Oral Solution (Rebetol): 40 mg/ml.

INDICATIONS AND DOSAGES

▸ Chronic Hepatitis C

PO (capsule or oral solution in combination with interferon alfa-2b)
Adults, Elderly. 1,000–1,200 mg/day in 2 divided doses.
Children weighing 60 kg or more. Use adult dosage. *(51–60 kg):* 400 mg 2 times/day. *(37–50 kg):* 200 mg in morning, 400 mg in evening. *(24–36 kg):* 200 mg 2 times/day.
PO (capsules in combination with peginterferon alfa-2b)
Adults, Elderly. 800 mg/day in 2 divided doses.
PO (tablets in combination with peginterferon alfa-2b)
Adults, Elderly. 800–1200 mg/day in 2 divided doses.

▸ Severe Lower Respiratory Tract Infection Caused by Respiratory Syncytial Virus (RSV)

INHALATION
Children, Infants. Use with Viratek small-particle aerosol generator at a concentration of 20 mg/ml (6 g reconstituted with 300 ml sterile water) over 12–18 hr/day for 3–7 days.

OFF-LABEL USES

Treatment of influenza A or B and west Nile virus

CONTRAINDICATIONS

Autoimmune hepatitis, creatinine clearance less than 50 ml/min, hemoglobinopathies, hepatic decompensation, hypersensitivity to ribavirin products, pregnancy, significant or unstable cardiac disease, women of childbearing age who won't use contraception reliably

R

INTERACTIONS

Drug

Didanosine: May increase the risk of pancreatitis and peripheral neuropathy and decrease the effects of didanosine.
Nucleoside analogues (including adefovir, didanosine, lamivudine, stavudine, zalcitabine, zidovudine): May increase the risk of lactic acidosis.

Herbal

None known.

Food

None known.

Drug interactions of concern to dentistry
• None reported

DIAGNOSTIC TEST EFFECTS
None known.

SIDE EFFECTS
Frequent (>10%)
Dizziness, headache, fatigue, fever, insomnia, irritability, depression, emotional lability, impaired concentration, alopecia, rash, pruritus, nausea, anorexia, dyspepsia, vomiting, decreased hemoglobin, hemolysis, arthralgia, musculoskeletal pain, dyspnea, sinusitis, flu-like symptoms
Occasional (1%–10%)
Nervousness, altered taste, weakness

SERIOUS REACTIONS
! Cardiac arrest, apnea and ventilator dependence, bacterial pneumonia, pneumonia, and pneumothorax occur rarely.
! Anemia may occur if ribavirin therapy exceeds 7 days.

DENTAL CONSIDERATIONS
General:
• Patients taking this drug will also be taking an interferon drug; be sure to conduct a thorough drug history.
• Assess salivary flow as a factor in caries, periodontal disease, and candidiasis.
• Patients on chronic drug therapy may rarely have symptoms of blood dyscrasias, which can include infection, bleeding, and poor healing.
• Consider semisupine chair position for patient comfort if GI side effects occur.
• Examine for oral manifestation of opportunistic infection.
• Take precautions if dental surgery is anticipated and general anesthesia is required.
• Monitor vital signs at every appointment because of CV side effects.

Consultations:
• In a patient with symptoms of blood dyscrasias, request a medical consultation for blood studies and postpone treatment until normal values are reestablished.
• Medical consultation may be required to assess disease control and patient's ability to tolerate stress.
• Consultation with physician may be necessary if sedation or general anesthesia is required.

Teach Patient/Family:
• Importance of updating health and drug history if physician makes any changes in evaluation or drug regimens
• Importance of good oral hygiene to prevent soft tissue inflammation
• To prevent trauma when using oral hygiene aids
• *When chronic dry mouth occurs, advise patient:*
  • To avoid mouth rinses with high alcohol content because of drying effects
  • To use daily home fluoride products for anticaries effect
  • To use sugarless gum, frequent sips of water, or saliva substitutes

rifabutin
rif′-a-byoo-ten
(Mycobutin)
Do not confuse rifabutin with rifampin.

CATEGORY AND SCHEDULE
Pregnancy Risk Category: B

MECHANISM OF ACTION
An antitubercular that inhibits DNA-dependent RNA polymerase,

an enzyme in susceptible strains of *Escherichia coli* and *Bacillus subtilis*. Rifabutin has a broad spectrum of antimicrobial activity, including against mycobacteria such as *Mycobacterium avium* complex (MAC). ***Therapeutic Effect:*** Prevents MAC disease.

PHARMACOKINETICS

Readily absorbed from the GI tract (high-fat meals delay absorption). Protein binding: 85%. Widely distributed. Crosses the blood-brain barrier. Extensive intracellular tissue uptake. Metabolized in the liver to active metabolite. Excreted in urine; eliminated in feces. Unknown if removed by hemodialysis.
Half-life: 16–69 hr.

AVAILABILITY

Capsules: 150 mg.

INDICATIONS AND DOSAGES

▸ Prevention of MAC Disease (first episode)

PO
Adults, Elderly. 300 mg as a single dose or in 2 divided doses if GI upset occurs.

▸ Prevention of Recurrent MAC Disease

PO
Adults, Elderly. 300 mg/day (in combination)

▸ Dosage in Renal Impairment

Dosage is modified on the basis of creatinine clearance. If creatinine clearance is less than 30 ml/min, reduce dosage by 50%.

CONTRAINDICATIONS

Active tuberculosis; hypersensitivity to other rifamycins, including rifampin

INTERACTIONS

Drug

Oral contraceptives: May decrease contraceptive effectiveness.
Zidovudine: May decrease blood concentration of zidovudine, but does not affect the drug's inhibition of HIV.

Herbal

None known.

Food

None known.

Drug interactions of concern to dentistry

• Decreases plasma concentrations of corticosteroids; may be significant
• May induce CYP3A4 isoenzymes, possible reduction in action of ketoconazole, itraconazole, benzodiazepines, doxycycline, erythromycin, clarithromycin

DIAGNOSTIC TEST EFFECTS

May increase serum alkaline phosphatase, AST (SGOT), and ALT (SGPT) levels.

SIDE EFFECTS

Frequent (30%)

Red-orange or red-brown discoloration of urine, feces, saliva, skin, sputum, sweat, or tears

Occasional (11%–3%)

Rash, nausea, abdominal pain, diarrhea, dyspepsia, belching, headache, altered taste, uveitis, corneal deposits

Rare (<2%)

Anorexia, flatulence, fever, myalgia, vomiting, insomnia

SERIOUS REACTIONS

! Hepatitis and thrombocytopenia occur rarely. Anemia and neutropenia may also occur.

DENTAL CONSIDERATIONS

General:

• Examine for evidence of oral signs of opportunistic disease.
• Determine why the patient is taking the drug.

• Patients on chronic drug therapy may rarely have symptoms of blood dyscrasias, which can include infection, bleeding, and poor healing.

Consultations:

• Medical consultation may be required to assess patient's ability to tolerate stress.

• In a patient with symptoms of blood dyscrasias, request a medical consultation for blood studies and postpone dental treatment until normal values are reestablished.

Teach Patient/Family:

• To avoid mouth rinses with high alcohol content because of drying effects

• Importance of good oral hygiene to prevent soft tissue inflammation

rifampin

rye′-fam-pin

(Rifadin, Rimactane, Rimycin[AUS], Rofact[CAN])

Do not confuse rifampin with rifabutin, Rifamate, rifapentine, or Ritalin.

CATEGORY AND SCHEDULE

Pregnancy Risk Category: C

R

MECHANISM OF ACTION

An antitubercular that interferes with bacterial RNA synthesis by binding to DNA-dependent RNA polymerase, thus preventing its attachment to DNA and blocking RNA transcription. ***Therapeutic Effect:*** Bactericidal in susceptible microorganisms.

PHARMACOKINETICS

Well absorbed from the GI tract (food delays absorption). Protein binding: 80%. Widely distributed. Metabolized in the liver to active metabolite. Primarily eliminated by the biliary system. Not removed by hemodialysis. ***Half-life:*** 3–5 hr (increased in hepatic impairment).

AVAILABILITY

Capsules (Rifadin): 150 mg, 300 mg.
Capsules (Rimactane): 300 mg.
Injection, Powder for Reconstitution (Rifadin): 600 mg.

INDICATIONS AND DOSAGES

▸ Tuberculosis

PO, IV

Adults, Elderly. 10 mg/kg/day. Maximum: 600 mg/day.

Children. 10–20 mg/kg/day in divided doses q12–24h.

▸ Prevention of Meningococcal Infections

PO, IV

Adults, Elderly. 600 mg q12h for 2 days.

Children 1 month and older. 20 mg/kg/day in divided doses q12–24h. Maximum: 600 mg/dose.

Infants younger than 1 mo. 10 mg/kg/day in divided doses q12h for 2 days.

▸ Staphylococcal Infections

PO, IV

Adults, Elderly. 600 mg once a day.

Children. 15 mg/kg/day in divided doses q12h.

▸ *Staphylococcus Aureus* Infections (in combination with other Anti-Infectives)

PO

Adults, Elderly. 300–600 mg twice a day.

Neonates. 5–20 mg/kg/day in divided doses q12h.

▸ Prevention of *Haemophilus influenzae* Infection

PO

Adults, Elderly. 600 mg/day for 4 days.

Children 1 mo and older.
20 mg/kg/day in divided doses q12h for 5–10 days.
Children younger than 1 mo.
10 mg/kg/day in divided doses q12h for 2 days.

OFF-LABEL USES

Prophylaxis of *H. influenzae* type b infection; treatment of atypical mycobacterial infection and serious infections caused by *Staphylococcus* species

CONTRAINDICATIONS

Concomitant therapy with amprenavir, hypersensitivity to rifampin or any other rifamycins

INTERACTIONS

Drug

Alcohol, hepatotoxic medications, ritonavir, saquinavir: May increase the risk of hepatotoxicity.
Aminophylline, theophylline: May increase clearance of these drugs.
Chloramphenicol, digoxin, disopyramide, fluconazole, methadone, mexiletine, oral anticoagulants, oral antidiabetics, phenytoin, quinidine, tocainide, verapamil: May decrease the effects of these drugs.
Oral contraceptives: May decrease oral contraceptive effectiveness.

Herbal

None known.

Food

None known.

Drug interactions of concern to dentistry

- Increased risk of hepatotoxicity: acetaminophen (chronic use and high doses), alcohol, hydrocarbon inhalation anesthetics (except isoflurane)
- Decreased effects of corticosteroids, dapsone, ketoconazole, fluconazole, itraconazole, oral contraceptives, benzodiazepines, doxycycline, erythromycin, clarithromycin, opioid analgesics
- Suspected decrease in fexofenadine effects
- Induces CYP450 isoenzymes

DIAGNOSTIC TEST EFFECTS

May increase serum alkaline phosphatase, bilirubin, uric acid, AST (SGOT), and ALT (SGPT) levels.

IV INCOMPATIBILITIES

Diltiazem (Cardizem)

SIDE EFFECTS

Expected

Red-orange or red-brown discoloration of urine, feces, saliva, skin, sputum, sweat, or tears

Occasional (5%–2%)

Hypersensitivity reaction (such as flushing, pruritus, or rash)

Rare (2%–1%)

Diarrhea, dyspepsia, nausea, candida as evidenced by sore mouth or tongue

SERIOUS REACTIONS

! Rare reactions include hepatotoxicity (risk is increased when rifampin is taken with isoniazid), hepatitis, blood dyscrasias, Stevens-Johnson syndrome, and antibiotic-associated colitis.

R

DENTAL CONSIDERATIONS

General:

- Examine for oral manifestation of opportunistic infections.
- Patients on chronic drug therapy may rarely have symptoms of blood dyscrasias, which can include infection, bleeding, and poor healing.
- Determine why the patient is taking the drug (prophylaxis or active therapy).

• Determine that noninfectious status exists by ensuring that (1) anti-TB drugs have been taken >3 wk, (2) culture has confirmed TB susceptibility to antiinfectives, (3) patient has had three consecutive negative sputum smears, and (4) patient is not in the coughing stage.

Consultations:

• Medical consultation may be required to assess patient's ability to tolerate stress.

• In a patient with symptoms of blood dyscrasias, request a medical consultation for blood studies and postpone dental treatment until normal values are reestablished.

Teach Patient/Family:

• To avoid mouth rinses with high alcohol content because of drying effects

• Importance of good oral hygiene to prevent soft tissue inflammation

• Importance of taking medications for full length of regimen to ensure effectiveness of treatment and to prevent the emergence of resistant strains

rifapentine

rif-a-pen′-teen

(Priftin)

Do not confuse rifapentine with rifampin.

R

CATEGORY AND SCHEDULE

Pregnancy Risk Category: C

MECHANISM OF ACTION

An antitubercular that inhibits bacterial RNA synthesis by binding to DNA-dependent RNA polymerase in *Mycobacterium tuberculosis*. This action prevents the enzyme from attaching to DNA, thereby blocking RNA transcription. ***Therapeutic Effect:*** Bactericidal.

AVAILABILITY

Tablets: 150 mg.

INDICATIONS AND DOSAGES

▸ Tuberculosis

PO

Adults, Elderly. Intensive phase: 600 mg twice weekly for 2 mo (interval between doses no less than 3 days). Continuation phase: 600 mg weekly for 4 mo.

CONTRAINDICATIONS

None known.

INTERACTIONS

Drug

Alcohol: May increase the risk of hepatotoxicity.

Oral contraceptives, warfarin: May decrease the effects of these drugs.

Herbal

None known.

Food

None known.

Drug interactions of concern to dentistry

• May accelerate metabolism of clarithromycin, doxycycline, ciprofloxacin, fluconazole, ketoconazole, itraconazole, diazepam, barbiturates, corticosteroids, opioids, zolpidem, sildenafil, tricyclic antidepressants

• Inducer of CYP3A4 and CYP2C8/9 isoenzymes may cause drug interactions

DIAGNOSTIC TEST EFFECTS

May increase serum AST (SGOT), ALT (SGPT), and bilirubin levels.

SIDE EFFECTS

Rare (less than 4%)

Red-orange or red-brown discoloration of urine, feces, saliva, skin, sputum, sweat, or tears; arthralgia, pain, nausea, vomiting, headache, dyspepsia, hypertension, dizziness, diarrhea

SERIOUS REACTIONS

! Hyperuricemia, neutropenia, proteinuria, hematuria, and hepatitis occur rarely.

DENTAL CONSIDERATIONS

General:

- Determine why patient is taking the drug (prophylaxis or active therapy).
- Examine for oral manifestation of opportunistic infections.
- Patients on chronic drug therapy may rarely have symptoms of blood dyscrasias, which can include infection, bleeding, and poor healing.
- Determine that noninfectious status exists by ensuring that (1) anti-TB drugs have been taken >3 wk, (2) culture has confirmed TB susceptibility to antiinfectives, (3) patient has had three consecutive negative sputum smears, and (4) patient is not in the coughing stage.
- Consider semisupine chair position for patient comfort because of GI side effects of drug.

Consultations:

- Medical consultation may be required to assess disease control and patient's ability to tolerate stress.
- In a patient with symptoms of blood dyscrasias, request a medical consultation for blood studies and postpone treatment until normal values are reestablished.

Teach Patient/Family:

- To avoid mouth rinses with high alcohol content because of drying effects
- To prevent trauma when using oral hygiene aids
- Importance of good oral hygiene to prevent soft tissue inflammation
- Importance of taking medication for full length of regimen to ensure effectiveness of treatment and prevent emergence of resistant strains
- Of potential for extrinsic oral staining side effect

riluzole

rye′-loo-zole

(Rilutek)

CATEGORY AND SCHEDULE

Pregnancy Risk Category: C

MECHANISM OF ACTION

An amyotrophic lateral sclerosis (ALS) agent that inhibits presynaptic glutamate release in the CNS and intereferes postsynaptically with the effects of excitatory amino acids.

Therapeutic Effect: Extends survival of ALS patients.

AVAILABILITY

Tablets: 50 mg.

INDICATIONS AND DOSAGES

▸ ALS

PO

Adults, Elderly. 50 mg q12h.

CONTRAINDICATIONS

None significant.

INTERACTIONS

Drug

Alcohol: May increase CNS depression.

Amitriptyline, quinolones, theophylline: May increase the effects and risk of toxicity of riluzole.

Omeprazole, rifampin: May decrease the effects of riluzole.

Herbal

None known.

Food

Caffeine: May increase the effects and risk of toxicity of riluzole.

High-fat meals: May decrease the absorption and effects of riluzole.

Drug interactions of concern to dentistry

- No data reported with dental drugs, but use with caution when given with inducers or inhibitors of CYP1A2 isoenzymes

DIAGNOSTIC TEST EFFECTS

May increase liver function test results.

SIDE EFFECTS

Frequent (>10%)

Nausea, asthenia, reduced respiratory function

Occasional (10%–1%)

Edema, tachycardia, headache, dizziness, somnolence, depression, vertigo, tremor, pruritus, alopecia, abdominal pain, diarrhea, anorexia, dyspepsia, vomiting, stomatitis, increased cough

SERIOUS REACTIONS

! None known.

DENTAL CONSIDERATIONS

General:

- Short appointments may be required because of nature of disease process.
- Monitor vital signs at every appointment because of CV and respiratory side effects.
- Consider semisupine chair position for patient comfort.
- Assess salivary flow as factor in caries, periodontal disease, and candidiasis.
- Examine for oral manifestation of opportunistic infection.
- Patients on chronic drug therapy may rarely have symptoms of blood dyscrasias, which can include infection, bleeding, and poor healing.
- After supine positioning, have patient sit upright for at least 2 min before standing to avoid orthostatic hypotension.

Consultations:

- Medical consultation may be required to assess disease control.
- In a patient with symptoms of blood dyscrasias, request a medical consultation for blood studies and postpone treatment until normal values are reestablished.

Teach Patient/Family:

- Instructions for management of oral hygiene, including use of electric toothbrush if patient has difficulty holding conventional devices or directions for caregiver
- That professional oral hygiene home care may be necessary
- Caution to prevent trauma when using oral hygiene aids
- *When chronic dry mouth occurs, advise patient:*
  - To avoid mouth rinses with high alcohol content because of drying effects
  - To use daily home fluoride products for anticaries effect
  - To use sugarless gum, frequent sips of water, or saliva substitutes

rimantadine hydrochloride

ri-man′-ti-deen

(Flumadine)

Do not confuse rimantadine with ranitidine, or Flumadine with flunisolide or flutamide.

CATEGORY AND SCHEDULE

Pregnancy Risk Category: C

MECHANISM OF ACTION

An antiviral that appears to exert an inhibitory effect early in the viral replication cycle. May inhibit uncoating of the virus.

R

Therapeutic Effect: Prevents replication of influenza A virus.

AVAILABILITY

Syrup: 50 mg/5 ml.
Tablets: 100 mg.

INDICATIONS AND DOSAGES

▸ Influenza A Virus

PO

Adults, Elderly. 100 mg twice a day for 7 days.
Elderly nursing home patients, patients with severe hepatic or renal impairment. 100 mg once a day for 7 days.

▸ Prevention of Influenza A Virus

PO

Adults, Elderly, Children 10 yr and older. 100 mg twice a day for at least 10 days after known exposure (usually for 6–8 wk).
Children younger than 10 yr. 5 mg/kg once a day. Maximum: 150 mg.
Elderly nursing home patients, patients with severe hepatic or renal impairment. 100 mg once a day.

CONTRAINDICATIONS

Hypersensitivity to amantadine or rimantadine

INTERACTIONS

Drug

Acetaminophen, aspirin: May decrease rimantadine blood concentration.
Anticholinergics, CNS stimulants: May increase side effects of rimantadine.
Cimetidine: May increase rimantadine blood concentration.

Herbal

None known.

Food

None known.

Drug interactions of concern to dentistry

- Reduced peak plasma levels: aspirin, acetaminophen

DIAGNOSTIC TEST EFFECTS

None known.

SIDE EFFECTS

Occasional (3%–2%)

Insomnia, nausea, nervousness, impaired concentration, dizziness

Rare (< 2%)

Vomiting, anorexia, dry mouth, abdominal pain, asthenia, fatigue

SERIOUS REACTIONS

! None known.

DENTAL CONSIDERATIONS

General:

- Monitor vital signs at every appointment because of CV side effects.
- Determine why the patient is taking the drug (probably will be used only during peak seasons for influenza).
- Assess salivary flow as a factor in caries, periodontal disease, and candidiasis.

Teach Patient/Family:

- Importance of good oral hygiene to prevent soft tissue inflammation
- *When chronic dry mouth occurs, advise patient:*
  - To avoid mouth rinses with high alcohol content because of drying effects
  - Of need for daily use of home fluoride products to prevent caries
  - To use sugarless gum, frequent sips of water, or saliva substitutes

rimexolone

rye-mex′-o-lone
(Vexol)
Do not confuse with riluzole.

CATEGORY AND SCHEDULE

Pregnancy Risk Category: C

MECHANISM OF ACTION
An ophthalmic agent that suppresses migration of polymorphoneclear leukocytes and reverses increased capillary permeability. ***Therapeutic Effect:*** Decreases inflammation.

PHARMACOKINETICS
Absorbed through aqueous humor. Metabolized in liver. Excreted in urine and feces.

AVAILABILITY
Ophthalmic Suspension: 1% (Vexol).

INDICATIONS AND DOSAGES
▸ **Inflammation After Ocular Surgery, Treatment of Anterior Uveitis**

OPHTHALMIC

Adults, Elderly. Instill 1 drop 2–4 times/day up to q4h. May use q1–2h during the first 1–2 days.

CONTRAINDICATIONS
Fungal, viral, or untreated pus-forming bacterial ocular infections, hypersensitivity to rimexolone or any component of the formulation

INTERACTIONS
Drug

None known.

Herbal

None known.

Food

None known.

Drug interactions of concern to dentistry

• None reported

DIAGNOSTIC TEST EFFECTS
None known.

SIDE EFFECTS
Occasional

Temporary mild blurred vision

Rare

Burning/stinging eyes

SERIOUS REACTIONS
! Prolonged has been associated with the development of corneal or scleral perforation and posterior subcapsular cataracts.

! Cataracts, corneal thinning, glaucoma, increased intraocular pressure, optic nerve damage, secondary ocular infection, and visual acuity defects occur rarely.

DENTAL CONSIDERATIONS
General:

• Determine why the patient is taking the drug.

• Protect patient's eyes from accidental spatter during dental treatment.

• Avoid dental light in patient's eyes; offer dark glasses for patient comfort.

risedronate sodium
rye-se-droe′-nate

(Actonel)

CATEGORY AND SCHEDULE
Pregnancy Risk Category: C

MECHANISM OF ACTION
A bisphosphonate that binds to bone hydroxyapatite and inhibits osteoclasts. ***Therapeutic Effect:*** Reduces bone turnover (the number of sites at which bone is remodeled) and bone resorption.

AVAILABILITY
Tablets: 5 mg, 30 mg, 35 mg.

INDICATIONS AND DOSAGES
▸ **Paget's Disease**

PO

Adults, Elderly. 30 mg/day for 2 mo. Retreatment may occur after 2-mo post-treatment observation period.

▸ **Prevention and Treatment of Postmenopausal Osteoporosis**
PO
Adults, Elderly. 5 mg/day or 35 mg once weekly.
▸ **Glucocorticoid-Induced Osteoporosis**
PO
Adults, Elderly. 5 mg/day.

CONTRAINDICATIONS
Hypersensitivity to other bisphosphonates, including etidronate, tiludronate, risedronate, and alendronate; hypocalcemia; inability to stand or sit upright for at least 20 minutes; renal impairment when serum creatinine clearance is greater than 5 mg/dl

INTERACTIONS
Drug
Antacids containing aluminum, calcium, magnesium; vitamin D: May decrease the absorption of risedronate.
Herbal
None known.
Food
None known.
Drug interactions of concern to dentistry
- Retarded absorption: calcium, antacids, medications with divalent cations
- Increased GI side effects: NSAIDs, aspirin

DIAGNOSTIC TEST EFFECTS
None known.

SIDE EFFECTS
Frequent (30%)
Arthralgia
Occasional (12%–8%)
Rash, flulike symptoms, peripheral edema
Rare (5%–3%)
Bone pain, sinusitis, asthenia, dry eye, tinnitus

SERIOUS REACTIONS
! Overdose causes hypocalcemia, hypophosphatemia, and significant GI disturbances.

DENTAL CONSIDERATIONS
General:
- Be aware of the oral manifestations of Paget's disease (macrognathia, alveolar pain).
- Consider semisupine chair position for patient comfort because of GI side effects of drug.
- Short appointments may be required for patient comfort.

Consultations:
- Medical consultation may be required to assess disease control.

Teach Patient/Family:
- Use of electric toothbrush if patient has difficulty holding conventional devices

risperidone
ris-per′-i-done
(Risperdal, Risperdal Consta, Risperdol M-Tabs)
Do not confuse risperidone with reserpine.

CATEGORY AND SCHEDULE
Pregnancy Risk Category: C

MECHANISM OF ACTION
A benzisoxazole derivative that may antagonize dopamine and serotonin receptors. ***Therapeutic Effect:*** Suppresses psychotic behavior.

PHARMACOKINETICS
Well absorbed from the GI tract; unaffected by food. Protein

binding: 90%. Extensively metabolized in the liver to active metabolite. Primarily excreted in urine. ***Half-life:*** 3–20 hr; metabolite: 21–30 hr (increased in elderly).

AVAILABILITY

Oral Solution (Risperdal): 1 mg/ml.
Tablets (Risperdal): 0.25 mg, 0.5 mg, 1 mg, 2 mg, 3 mg, 4 mg.
Tablets (Orally Disintegrating [Risperdal M-Tabs]): 0.5 mg, 1 mg, 2 mg.
Injection (Risperdal Consta): 25 mg, 37.5 mg, 50 mg.

INDICATIONS AND DOSAGES

▸ Psychotic Disorder

PO
Adults. 0.5–1 mg twice a day. May increase dosage slowly. Range: 2–6 mg/day.
Elderly. Initially, 0.25–2 mg/day in 2 divided doses. May increase dosage slowly. Range: 2–6 mg/day.
IM
Adults, Elderly. 25 mg q2wk. Maximum: 50 mg q2wk.

▸ Mania

PO
Adults, Elderly. Initially, 2–3 mg as a single daily dose.
May increase at 24 hour intervals of 1 mg/day.
Range: 2–6 mg/day.

▸ Dosage in Renal Impairment

Initial dosage for adults and elderly patients is 0.25–0.5 mg twice a day. Dosage is titrated slowly to desired effect.

OFF-LABEL USES

Autism in children, behavioral symptoms associated with dementia, Tourette's disorder

CONTRAINDICATIONS

None known.

INTERACTIONS

Drug

Alcohol, other CNS depressants: May increase CNS depression.
Carbamazepine: May decrease the risperidone blood concentration.
Clozapine: May increase the risperidone blood concentration.
Dopamine agonists, levodopa: May decrease the effects of these drugs.
Paroxetine: May increase the risperidone blood concentration and the risk of extrapyramidal symptoms.

Herbal

None known.

Food

None known.

Drug interactions of concern to dentistry

- Increased excretion: chronic use of carbamazepine
- Increased sedation: other CNS depressants, alcohol, barbiturate anesthesia, opioid analgesics
- Increased extrapyramidal effects: phenothiazines and related drugs (haloperidol, droperidol), metoclopramide
- Additive photosensitization: tetracyclines
- Increased anticholinergic effects: anticholinergics, such as atropine and scopolamine

DIAGNOSTIC TEST EFFECTS

May increase serum prolactin, creatinine, alkaline phosphatase, uric acid, AST (SGOT), ALT (SGPT), and triglyceride levels. May decrease blood glucose and serum potassium, protein, and sodium levels. May cause ECG changes.

SIDE EFFECTS

Frequent (26%–13%)
Agitation, anxiety, insomnia, headache, constipation

R

Occasional (10%–4%)
Dyspepsia, rhinitis, somnolence, dizziness, nausea, vomiting, rash, abdominal pain, dry skin, tachycardia
Rare (3%–2%)
Visual disturbances, fever, back pain, pharyngitis, cough, arthralgia, angina, aggressive behavior, orthostatic hypotension, breast swelling

SERIOUS REACTIONS

! Rare reactions include tardive dyskinesia (characterized by tongue protrusion, puffing of the cheeks, and chewing or puckering of the mouth) and neuroleptic malignant syndrome (marked by hyperpyrexia, muscle rigidity, change in mental status, irregular pulse or BP, tachycardia, diaphoresis, cardiac arrhythmias, rhabdomyolysis, and acute renal failure).

DENTAL CONSIDERATIONS

General:
- Monitor vital signs at every appointment because of CV side effects.
- Patients on chronic drug therapy may rarely have symptoms of blood dyscrasias, which can include infection, bleeding, and poor healing.
- After supine positioning, have patient sit upright for at least 2 min before standing to avoid orthostatic hypotension.
- Assess salivary flow as a factor in caries, periodontal disease, and candidiasis.
- Consider semisupine chair position for patient comfort because of GI effects of drug.
- Assess for presence of extrapyramidal motor symptoms, such as tardive dyskinesia and akathisia. Extrapyramidal motor activity may complicate dental treatment.
- Use vasoconstrictors with caution, in low doses, and with careful aspiration; avoid use of gingival retraction cord with epinephrine.

Consultations:
- In a patient with symptoms of blood dyscrasias, request a medical consultation for blood studies and postpone dental treatment until normal values are reestablished.
- Take precautions if dental surgery is anticipated and anesthesia is required.
- If signs of tardive dyskinesia or other extrapyramidal symptoms are present, refer to physician.
- Physician should be informed if significant xerostomic side effects occur (e.g., increased caries, sore tongue, problems eating or swallowing, difficulty wearing prosthesis) so that a medication change can be considered.

Teach Patient/Family:
- Importance of good oral hygiene to prevent soft tissue inflammation
- Caution to prevent injury when using oral hygiene aids
- Use of electric toothbrush if patient has difficulty holding conventional devices
- *When chronic dry mouth occurs, advise patient:*
  - To avoid mouth rinses with high alcohol content because of drying effects
  - To use daily home fluoride products for anticaries effect
  - To use sugarless gum, frequent sips of water, or saliva substitutes

ritonavir

ri-tone′-a-veer
(Norvir, Norvisec[CAN])
Do not confuse ritonavir with Retrovir.

CATEGORY AND SCHEDULE

Pregnancy Risk Category: B

MECHANISM OF ACTION

Inhibits HIV-1 and HIV-2 proteases, rendering these enzymes incapable of processing the polypeptide precursors; this results in the production of noninfectious, immature HIV particles.
Therapeutic Effect: Impedes HIV replication, slowing the progression of HIV infection.

PHARMACOKINETICS

Well absorbed after PO administration (absorption increased with food). Protein binding: 98%–99%. Extensively metabolized in the liver to active metabolite. Primarily eliminated in feces. Unknown if removed by hemodialysis. ***Half-life:*** 2.7–5 hr.

AVAILABILITY

R

Oral Solution: 80 mg/ml.
Soft Gelatin Capsules: 100 mg.

INDICATIONS AND DOSAGES

▸ HIV Infection

PO

Adults, Children 12 yr and older. 600 mg twice a day. If nausea occurs at this dosage, give 300 mg twice a day for 1 day, 400 mg twice a day for 2 days, 500 mg twice a day for 1 day, then 600 mg twice a day thereafter.
Children younger than 12 yr. Initially, 250 mg/m^2/dose twice a day. Increase by 50 mg/m^2/dose up to 400 mg/m^2/dose. Maximum: 600 mg/dose twice a day.

CONTRAINDICATIONS

Concurrent use of amiodarone, astemizole, bepridil, bupropion, cisapride, clozapine, encainide, flecainide, meperidine, piroxicam, propafenone, propoxyphene, quinidine, rifabutin, or terfenadine (increased risk of serious or life-threatening drug interactions, such as arrhythmias, hematologic abnormalities, and seizures); concurrent use of alprazolam, clorazepate, diazepam, estazolam, flurazepam, midazolam, triazolam, or zolpidem (may produce extreme sedation and respiratory depression)

INTERACTIONS

Drug

Desipramine, fluoxetine, other antidepressants: May increase the blood concentration of these drugs.
Disulfiram, drugs causing disulfiram-like reaction (such as metronidazole): May produce a disulfiram-like reaction.
Enzyme inducers (including carbamazepine, dexamethasone, nevirapine, phenobarbital, phenytoin, rifabutin, rifampin): May increase the metabolism and decrease the efficacy of ritonavir.
Oral contraceptives, theophylline: May decrease the effectiveness of these drugs.

Herbal

St. John's wort: May decrease the blood concentration and effect of ritonavir.

Food

None known.

Drug interactions of concern to dentistry

- Contraindicated with alprazolam, clorazepate, diazepam, bupropion, estazolam, flurazepam, midazolam,

triazolam, zolpidem, meperidine, piroxicam, propoxyphene, chlordiazepoxide, halazepam, quazepam
• Increased plasma levels: clarithromycin, fluconazole, fluoxetine, desipramine, theophylline
• Possible alcohol-disulfiram reaction: metronidazole, disulfiram
• Decreased plasma levels with carbamazepine, dexamethasone, phenobarbital, St. John's wort (herb)
• Increased plasma levels of fentanyl
• *Note:* Multiple drug interactions are reported; check before prescribing dental drugs. This drug is a potent inhibitor of CYP3A4, CYP2D6 isoenzymes.

DIAGNOSTIC TEST EFFECTS

May alter serum CK, GGT, triglyceride, uric acid, AST (SGOT), and ALT (SGPT) levels, as well as creatinine clearance.

SIDE EFFECTS

Frequent

GI disturbances (abdominal pain, anorexia, diarrhea, nausea, vomiting), circumoral and peripheral paresthesias, altered taste, headache, dizziness, fatigue, asthenia

Occasional

Allergic reaction, flulike symptoms, hypotension

Rare

Diabetes mellitus, hyperglycemia

SERIOUS REACTIONS

! None known.

DENTAL CONSIDERATIONS

General:

• Monitor vital signs at every appointment because of CV side effects.
• Examine for oral manifestation of opportunistic infection.
• Place on frequent recall to evaluate healing response.
• Assess salivary flow as a factor in caries, periodontal disease, and candidiasis.
• Consider semisupine chair position for patient comfort because of GI effects of drug.

Consultations:

• Medical consultation may be required to assess disease control.

Teach Patient/Family:

• Importance of good oral hygiene to prevent soft tissue inflammation
• That secondary oral infection may occur; must see dentist immediately if infection occurs
• *When chronic dry mouth occurs, advise patient:*
  • To avoid mouth rinses with high alcohol content because of drying effects
  • To use daily home fluoride products for anticaries effect
  • To use sugarless gum, frequent sips of water, or saliva substitutes

rituximab

rye-tucks′-ih-mab
(Mabthera[AUS], Rituxan)

CATEGORY AND SCHEDULE

Pregnancy Risk Category: C

MECHANISM OF ACTION

Binds to CD20, the antigen found on the surface of B lymphocytes and B-cell non-Hodgkin's lymphomas. ***Therapeutic Effect:*** Produces cytotoxicity, reducing tumor size.

PHARMACOKINETICS

Rapidly depletes B cells. ***Half-life:*** 59.8 hr after first infusion and 174 hr after fourth infusion.

AVAILABILITY

Injection: 10 mg/ml.

INDICATIONS AND DOSAGES

▸ Non-Hodgkin's Lymphoma

IV

Adults. 375 mg/m^2 once weekly for 4–8 wk. May administer a second 4-wk course.

CONTRAINDICATIONS

Hypersensitivity to murine proteins

INTERACTIONS

Drug

None known.

Herbal

None known.

Food

None known.

Drug interactions of concern to dentistry

- None reported

DIAGNOSTIC TEST EFFECTS

None known.

IV INCOMPATIBILITIES

Don't mix rituximab with any other medications.

SIDE EFFECTS

Frequent

Fever (49%), chills (32%), asthenia (16%), headache (14%), angioedema (13%), hypotension (10%), nausea (18%), rash or pruritus (10%)

Occasional (< 10%)

Myalgia, dizziness, abdominal pain, throat irritation, vomiting, neutropenia, rhinitis, bronchospasm, urticaria

SERIOUS REACTIONS

! A hypersensitivity reaction marked by hypotension, bronchospasm, and angioedema may occur.

! Arrhythmias may occur, particularly in those with a history of preexisting cardiac conditions.

DENTAL CONSIDERATIONS

General:

- Monitor and record vital signs.
- If additional analgesia is required for dental pain, consider alternative analgesics (NSAIDs) in patients taking narcotics for acute or chronic pain.
- After supine positioning, have patient sit upright for at least 2 min before standing to avoid orthostatic hypotension.
- Patient on chronic drug therapy may rarely present with symptoms of blood dyscrasias, which can include infection, bleeding, and poor healing. If dyscrasia is present, caution patient to prevent oral tissue trauma when using oral hygiene aids.
- Provide emergency dental care only during drug use.
- Hypersensitivity reactions may occur.
- Oral infections should be eliminated and treated aggressively.

Consultations:

- Medical consultation should include routine blood counts including platelet counts and bleeding time.
- Consult physician; prophylactic or therapeutic antiinfectives may be indicated if surgery or periodontal treatment is required.
- Medical consultation may be required to assess immunologic status during cancer chemotherapy and determine safety risk, if any, posed by the required dental treatment.
- Medical consultation may be required to assess disease control and patient's ability to tolerate stress.

Teach Patient/Family:

- Importance of good oral hygiene to prevent soft tissue inflammation
- To report oral lesions, soreness, or bleeding to dentist
- To prevent trauma when using oral hygiene aids

- Importance of updating health and medication history if physician makes any changes in evaluation or drug regimens; include OTC, herbal, and nonherbal remedies in the update

rivastigmine tartrate

riv-a-stig′-meen
(Exelon)

CATEGORY AND SCHEDULE

Pregnancy Risk Category: B

MECHANISM OF ACTION

A cholinesterase inhibitor that inhibits the enzyme acetylcholinesterase, thus increasing the concentration of acetylcholine at cholinergic synapses and enhancing cholinergic function in the CNS. ***Therapeutic Effect:*** Slows the progression of symptoms of Alzheimer's disease.

PHARMACOKINETICS

Rapidly and completely absorbed. Protein binding: 60%. Widely distributed throughout the body. Rapidly and extensively metabolized. Primarily excreted in urine. ***Half-life:*** 1.5 hr.

AVAILABILITY

Capsules: 1.5 mg, 3 mg, 4.5 mg, 6 mg.
Oral Solution: 2 mg/ml.

INDICATIONS AND DOSAGES

▸ Alzheimer's Disease

PO

Adults, Elderly. Initially, 1.5 mg twice a day. May increase at intervals of least 2 wk to 3 mg twice a day, then 4.5 mg twice a day, and finally 6 mg twice a day. Maximum: 6 mg twice a day.

CONTRAINDICATIONS

None known.

INTERACTIONS

Drug

Anticholinergics: May decrease the effects of rivastigmine or anticholinergics.
Bethanecol: May increase the effects of rivastigmine or bethanecol.

Herbal

None known.

Food

None known.

Drug interactions of concern to dentistry

- Caution in use of NSAIDs if GI side effects are significant
- Decreased response to neuromuscular blocking agents used in general anesthesia
- Increased cholinergic response: other cholinergic drugs
- Decreased cholinergic response: anticholinergics or other drugs with anticholinergic actions

DIAGNOSTIC TEST EFFECTS

None known.

SIDE EFFECTS

Frequent (47%–17%)
Nausea, vomiting, dizziness, diarrhea, headache, anorexia

Occasional (13%–6%)
Abdominal pain, insomnia, dyspepsia (heartburn, indigestion, epigastric pain), confusion, UTI, depression

Rare (5%–3%)
Anxiety, somnolence, constipation, malaise, hallucinations, tremor, flatulence, rhinitis, hypertension, flu-like symptoms, weight loss, syncope

SERIOUS REACTIONS

! Overdose may result in cholinergic crisis, characterized by severe nausea and vomiting, increased salivation, diaphoresis, bradycardia, hypotension, respiratory depression, and seizures.

DENTAL CONSIDERATIONS

General:

- Determine why patient is taking the drug.
- Monitor vital signs at every appointment because of CV side effects.
- Drug is used early in the disease; ensure that patient or caregiver understands informed consent.
- Place on frequent recall because early attention to dental health is important for Alzheimer's patients.
- Assess salivary flow as a factor in caries, periodontal disease, and candidiasis.
- Use precaution if sedation or general anesthesia is required; risk of hypotensive episode.
- Consider semisupine chair position for patient comfort if GI side effects occur.
- Patients on chronic drug therapy may rarely have symptoms of blood dyscrasias, which can include infection, bleeding, and poor healing.

Consultations:

- Consultation with physician may be necessary if sedation or general anesthesia is required.
- In a patient with symptoms of blood dyscrasias, request a medical consultation for blood studies and postpone treatment until normal values are reestablished.
- Medical consultation may be required to assess disease control and patient's ability to tolerate stress.

Teach Patient/Family:

- Use of electric toothbrush if patient has difficulty holding conventional devices
- To prevent trauma when using oral hygiene aids
- Importance of good oral hygiene to prevent soft tissue inflammation

R

rizatriptan benzoate

rize-a-trip′-tan
(Maxalt, Maxalt-MLT)

CATEGORY AND SCHEDULE

Pregnancy Risk Category: C

MECHANISM OF ACTION

A serotonin receptor agonist that binds selectively to vascular receptors, producing a vasoconstrictive effect on cranial blood vessels. ***Therapeutic Effect:*** Relieves migraine headache.

PHARMACOKINETICS

Well absorbed after PO administration. Protein binding: 14%. Crosses the blood-brain barrier. Metabolized by the liver to inactive metabolite. Eliminated primarily in urine and, to a lesser extent, in feces. ***Half-life:*** 2–3 hr.

AVAILABILITY

Tablets (Maxalt): 5 mg, 10 mg.
Tablets (Orally-Disintegrating [Maxalt-MLT]): 5 mg, 10 mg.

INDICATIONS AND DOSAGES

▸ Acute Migraine Attack

PO

Adults older than 18 yr, Elderly. 5–10 mg. If headache improves, but then returns, dose may be repeated after 2 hr. Maximum: 30 mg/24 hr.

CONTRAINDICATIONS

Basilar or hemiplegic migraine, coronary artery disease, ischemic heart disease (including angina pectoris, history of MI, silent ischemia, and Prinzmetal's angina), uncontrolled hypertension, use within 24 hours of ergotamine-containing preparations or another serotonin receptor agonist, use within 14 days of MAOIs.

INTERACTIONS

Drug

Ergotamine-containing medications: May produce a vasospastic reaction.
Fluoxetine, fluvoxamine, paroxetine, sertraline: May produce hyperreflexia, incoordination, and weakness.
MAOIs, propranolol: May dramatically increase plasma concentration of rizatriptan.

Herbal

None known.

Food

All foods: Delay peak drug concentration by 1 hour.

Drug interactions of concern to dentistry

- No specific interactions with dental drugs reported
- Increased plasma levels: propranolol
- Should not be used within 24 hr of another 5–HT agonist

DIAGNOSTIC TEST EFFECTS

None known.

SIDE EFFECTS

Frequent (9%–7%)
Dizziness, somnolence, paraesthesia, fatigue
Occasional (6%–3%)
Nausea, chest pressure, dry mouth
Rare (2%)
Headache; neck, throat, or jaw pressure; photosensitivity

SERIOUS REACTIONS

! Cardiac reactions (such as ischemia, coronary artery vasospasm, and MI) and noncardiac vasospasm-related reactions (including hemorrhage and CVA) occur rarely, particularly in patients with hypertension, diabetes, or a strong family history of coronary artery disease; obese patients; smokers; males older than 40 years; and postmenopausal women.

DENTAL CONSIDERATIONS

General:

- This is an acute-use drug; it is doubtful that patients will be treated in the office if acute migraine is present.
- Be aware of patient's disease, its severity, and its frequency, when known.
- Avoid dental light in patient's eyes; offer dark glasses for patient comfort.
- Short appointments and a stress reduction protocol may be required for anxious patients.
- After supine positioning, have patient sit upright for at least 2 min before standing to avoid orthostatic hypotension.

Consultations:

- If treating chronic orofacial pain, consult with physician of record.
- Medical consultation may be required to assess disease control and patient's ability to tolerate stress.

Teach Patient/Family:

- Importance of updating health and drug history if physician makes any changes in evaluation or drug regimens

rofecoxib

ro-fe-coks′-ib
(Vioxx)

ALERT

Rofecoxib has been withdrawn from the market.
Do not confuse with Zyvox.

CATEGORY AND SCHEDULE

Pregnancy Risk Category: C, D if used in third trimester or near delivery

MECHANISM OF ACTION

A nonsteroidal anti-inflammatory that produces analgesic and anti-inflammatory effect by inhibiting prostaglandin synthesis.
Therapeutic Effect: Reduces inflammatory response and intensity of pain stimulus reaching sensory nerve endings.

PHARMACOKINETICS

Rapid, complete absorption from the gastrointestinal (GI) tract. Protein binding: 87%. Primarily metabolized in liver. Primarily eliminated in urine with a lesser amount excreted in feces. Not removed by hemodialysis.
Half-life: 17 hr.

AVAILABILITY

Tablets: 12.5 mg, 25 mg, 50 mg.
Suspension: 12.5 mg/5 ml, 25 mg/5 ml.

INDICATIONS AND DOSAGES

▸ Osteoarthritis

PO
Adults. Initially, 12.5 mg/day. May increase dosage to 25 mg/day. Maximum is 25 mg/day.

▸ Rheumatoid Arthritis

PO
Adults, Elderly. 25 mg/day.

▸ Acute Pain, Dysmenorrhea

PO
Adults. Initially, 50 mg/day.

R

CONTRAINDICATIONS

Hypersensitivity to aspirin and NSAIDs

INTERACTIONS

Drug

Anticoagulants: May increase the effects of anticoagulants.
Aspirin: May increase the risk of GI bleeding and side effects.

Herbal

Feverfew: May decrease the effects of this herb.
Ginkgo biloba: May increase the risk of bleeding.

Food

None known.

Drug interactions of concern to dentistry

- Possible increased GI symptoms: aspirin
- As with other NSAIDs: reduced effectiveness of diuretics, ACE inhibitors
- Decreased plasma levels: rifampin
- Increased plasma levels of lithium, methotrexate, warfarin
- Monitor INR, small risk of bleeding: warfarin
- First-time users of SSRIs also taking NSAIDs may have a higher risk of GI side effects; until more data are available, it may be advisable to avoid use of NSAIDs in these patients (*Br J Clin Pharmacol* 55:591–595, 2003)

DIAGNOSTIC TEST EFFECTS

May prolong bleeding time. May increase LDH, liver function tests, and serum alkaline phosphatase. May decrease blood Hgb, Hct, and serum sodium levels.

SIDE EFFECTS

Frequent (6%–5%)

Nausea (with or without vomiting), diarrhea, abdominal distress

Occasional (3%)

Dyspepsia, including heartburn, indigestion, epigastric pain

Rare (< 2%)

Constipation, flatulence

SERIOUS REACTIONS

! None known.

DENTAL CONSIDERATIONS

General:

- Assess salivary flow as a factor in caries, periodontal disease, and candidiasis.

• Update health and drug history if physician makes changes in evaluation or drug regimens.
• Monitor vital signs at every appointment because of CV side effects.
• Consider semisupine chair position for patient comfort if GI side effects occur.

Teach Patient/Family:

• Importance of good oral hygiene to prevent soft tissue inflammation
• Use of electric toothbrush if patient has difficulty holding conventional devices
• *When chronic dry mouth occurs, advise patient:*
  • To avoid mouth rinses with high alcohol content because of drying effects
  • To use daily home fluoride products for anticaries effect
  • To use sugarless gum, frequent sips of water, or saliva substitutes

ropinirole hydrochloride

ro-pin′-i-role
(Requip)

CATEGORY AND SCHEDULE

Pregnancy Risk Category: C

MECHANISM OF ACTION

An antiparkinson agent that stimulates dopamine receptors in the striatum. ***Therapeutic Effect:*** Relieves signs and symptoms of Parkinson's disease.

PHARMACOKINETICS

Rapidly absorbed after PO administration. Protein binding: 40%. Extensively distributed throughout the body. Extensively metabolized. Steady-state concentrations achieved within 2 days. Eliminated in urine. Unknown if removed by hemodialysis. ***Half-life:*** 6 hr.

AVAILABILITY

Tablets: 0.25 mg, 0.5 mg, 1 mg, 2 mg, 3 mg, 4 mg, 5 mg.

INDICATIONS AND DOSAGES

▸ Parkinson's Disease

PO

Adults, Elderly. Initially, 0.25 mg 3 times a day. May increase dosage every 7 days.

CONTRAINDICATIONS

None known.

INTERACTIONS

Drug

Butyrophenones, metoclopramide, phenothiazines, thioxanthenes: Decrease the effectiveness of ropinirole.
Cimetidine, diltiazem, enoxacin, erythromycin, fluvoxamine, mexiletine, norfloxacin, tacrine: Alter ropinirole blood concentration.
Ciprofloxacin: Increases ropinirole blood concentration.
CNS depressants: May increase CNS depressant effects.
Estrogens: Reduce the clearance of ropinirole.
Levodopa: Increases the blood concentration of levodopa.

Herbal

None known.

Food

All foods: Delay peak plasma levels by 1 hour but don't affect drug absorption.

Drug interactions of concern to dentistry

• Possible increase in sedation with all CNS depressants
• Possible diminished effects: dopamine antagonists, phenothiazines, haloperidol, droperidol, and metoclopramide

R

DIAGNOSTIC TEST EFFECTS

May increase serum alkaline phosphatase level.

SIDE EFFECTS

Frequent (60%–40%)
Nausea, dizziness, somnolence
Occasional (12%–5%)
Syncope, vomiting, fatigue, viral infection, dyspepsia, diaphoresis, asthenia, orthostatic hypotension, abdominal discomfort, pharyngitis, abnormal vision, dry mouth, hypertension, hallucinations, confusion
Rare (< 4%)
Anorexia, peripheral edema, memory loss, rhinitis, sinusitis, palpitations, impotence

SERIOUS REACTIONS

! None known.

DENTAL CONSIDERATIONS

General:
- Monitor vital signs at every appointment because of CV side effects.
- Assess salivary flow as factor in caries, periodontal disease, and candidiasis.
- After supine positioning, have patient sit upright for at least 2 min before standing to avoid orthostatic hypotension.
- Patients on chronic drug therapy may rarely have symptoms of blood dyscrasias, which can include infection, bleeding, and poor healing.
- Consider semisupine chair position for patient comfort if GI side effects occur.

Consultations:
- In a patient with symptoms of blood dyscrasias, request a medical consultation for blood studies and postpone treatment until normal values are reestablished.
- Medical consultation may be required to assess disease control and patient's ability to tolerate stress.

Teach Patient/Family:
- Caution to prevent trauma when using oral hygiene aids
- Use of electric toothbrush if patient has difficulty holding conventional devices
- Importance of good oral hygiene to prevent soft tissue inflammation
- Importance of updating health and drug history if physician makes any changes in evaluation or drug regimens
- *When chronic dry mouth occurs, advise patient:*
  - To avoid mouth rinses with high alcohol content because of drying effects
  - To use daily home fluoride products for anticaries effect
  - To use sugarless gum, frequent sips of water, or saliva substitutes

rosiglitazone maleate

roz-ih-gli′-ta-zone
(Avandia)
Do not confuse Avandia with Avalide, Avinza, or Prandin.

CATEGORY AND SCHEDULE

Pregnancy Risk Category: C

MECHANISM OF ACTION

An antidiabetic that improves target-cell response to insulin without increasing pancreatic insulin secretion. Decreases hepatic glucose output and increases insulin-dependent glucose utilization in skeletal muscle. ***Therapeutic Effect:*** Lowers blood glucose concentration.

PHARMACOKINETICS

Rapidly absorbed. Protein binding: 99%. Metabolized in the liver. Excreted primarily in urine, with a lesser amount in feces. Not removed by hemodialysis. ***Half-life:*** 3–4 hr.

AVAILABILITY

Tablets: 2 mg, 4 mg, 8 mg.

INDICATIONS AND DOSAGES

▸ **Diabetes Mellitus, Combination Therapy**

PO

Adults, Elderly. Initially, 4 mg as a single daily dose or in divided doses twice a day. May increase to 8 mg/day after 12 wk of therapy if fasting glucose level is not adequately controlled.

▸ **Diabetes Mellitus, Monotherapy**

Adults, Elderly. Initially, 4 mg as single daily dose or in divided doses twice a day. May increase to 8 mg/day after 12 wk of therapy.

CONTRAINDICATIONS

Active hepatic disease, diabetic ketoacidosis, increased serum transaminase levels, including ALT(SGPT) greater than 2.5 times the normal serum level, type 1 diabetes mellitus

INTERACTIONS

Drug

None known.

Herbal

None known.

Food

None known.

Drug interactions of concern to dentistry

- None reported

DIAGNOSTIC TEST EFFECTS

May decrease Hct and Hgb and serum alkaline phosphatase, bilirubin, and AST(SGOT) levels. Less than 1% of patients experience ALT values that are 3 times the normal level.

SIDE EFFECTS

Frequent (9%)

Upper respiratory tract infection

Occasional (4%–2%)

Headache, edema, back pain, fatigue, sinusitis, diarrhea

SERIOUS REACTIONS

! None known.

DENTAL CONSIDERATIONS

General:

- Ensure that patient is following prescribed diet and regularly takes medication.
- Place on frequent recall to evaluate healing response.
- Short appointments and a stress reduction protocol may be required for anxious patients.
- Diabetics may be more susceptible to infection and have delayed wound healing.
- Question patient about self-monitoring of drug's antidiabetic effect, including blood glucose values or finger-stick records.

Consultations:

- Medical consultation may include data from patient's blood glucose monitoring, including glycosylated hemoglobin or HbA_{1c} testing.
- Medical consultation may be required to assess disease control and patient's ability to tolerate stress.

Teach Patient/Family:

- To prevent trauma when using oral hygiene aids
- Importance of updating health and drug history if physician makes any changes in evaluation or drug regimens

rosuvastatin calcium

ross-uh-vah-stah′-tin
(Crestor)

CATEGORY AND SCHEDULE

Pregnancy Risk Category: X

MECHANISM OF ACTION

An antihyperlipidemic that interferes with cholesterol biosynthesis by inhibiting the conversion of the enzyme HMG-CoA to mevalonate, a precursor to cholesterol. ***Therapeutic Effect:*** Decreases LDL cholesterol, VLDL, and plasma triglyceride levels, increases HDL concentration.

PHARMACOKINETICS

Protein binding: 88%.
Minimal hepatic metabolism.
Primarily eliminated in the feces.
Half-life: 19 hr (increased in patients with severe renal dysfunction).

AVAILABILITY

Tablets: 5 mg, 10 mg, 20 mg, 40 mg.

INDICATIONS AND DOSAGES

R

▸ **Hyperlipidemia, Dyslipidemia**

PO

Adults, Elderly. 5 to 40 mg/day. Usual starting dosage is 10 mg/day, with adjustments based on lipid levels; monitor q2–4wk until desired level is achieved.

▸ **Renal Impairment (creatinine clearance < 30 ml/min)**

PO

Adults, Elderly. 5 mg/day; do not exceed 10 mg/day.

▸ **Concurrent Cyclosporine Use**

PO

Adults, Elderly. 5 mg/day.

▸ **Concurrent Lipid-Lowering Therapy**

PO

Adults, Elderly. 10 mg/day.

CONTRAINDICATIONS

Active hepatic disease, breast-feeding, pregnancy, unexplained, persistent elevations of serum transaminase levels

INTERACTIONS

Drug

Cyclosporine, gemfibrozil, niacin: Increases the risk of myopathy with cyclosporine, gemfibrozil, and niacin.
Erythromycin: Reduces the plasma concentration of erythromycin.
Ethinylestradiol, norgestrel: Increases the plasma concentrations of ethinylestradiol and norgestrel.
Warfarin: Enhances anticoagulant effect.

Herbal

None known.

Food

None known.

Drug interactions of concern to dentistry

- No dental drug interactions reported; however, interactions with cyclosporine, warfarin, and gemfibrozil are noted
- Does not inhibit CYP3A4

DIAGNOSTIC TEST EFFECTS

May increase serum CK and transaminase concentrations. May produce hematuria and proteinuria.

SIDE EFFECTS

Rosuvastatin is generally well tolerated. Side effects are usually mild and transient.

Occasional (9%–3%)

Pharyngitis, headache, diarrhea, dyspepsia, including heartburn and epigastric distress, nausea

Rare (< 3%)
Myalgia, asthenia or unusual fatigue and weakness, back pain

SERIOUS REACTIONS

! Lens opacities may occur.
! Hypersensitivity reaction and hepatitis occur rarely.

DENTAL CONSIDERATIONS

General:

- Monitor vital signs because patients with high cholesterol levels are predisposed to CV disease.
- Consider semisupine chair position for patient comfort if GI side effects occur.

salmeterol

sal-me′-te-rol

(Serevent Diskus, Serevent Inhaler and Disks[AUS])

Do not confuse Serevent with Serentil.

CATEGORY AND SCHEDULE

Pregnancy Risk Category: C

MECHANISM OF ACTION

An adrenergic agonist that stimulates $beta_2$-adrenergic receptors in the lungs, resulting in relaxation of bronchial smooth muscle.
Therapeutic Effect: Relieves bronchospasm and reduces airway resistance.

PHARMACOKINETICS

Route	Onset	Peak	Duration
Inhalation	10–20 min	3 hr	12 hr

Low systemic absorption; acts primarily in the lungs. Protein binding: 95%. Metabolized by hydroxylation. Primarily eliminated in feces. ***Half-life:*** 3–4 hr.

AVAILABILITY

Powder for Oral Inhalation (Serevent Diskus): 50 mcg.

S

INDICATIONS AND DOSAGES

▸ **Prevention and Maintenance Treatment of Asthma**

INHALATION (Diskus)

Adults, Elderly, Children 4 yr and older. 1 inhalation (50 mcg) q12h.

▸ **Prevention of Exercise-Induced Bronchospasm**

INHALATION

Adults, Elderly, Children 4 yr and older. 1 inhalation at least 30 min before exercise.

▸ **COPD**

INHALATION

Adults, Elderly. 1 inhalation q12h.

CONTRAINDICATIONS

History of hypersensitivity to sympathomimetics

INTERACTIONS

Drug

Beta blockers: May decrease the effects of beta blockers.

Herbal

None known.

Food

None known.

Drug interactions of concern to dentistry

• Increased CV effects: tricyclic antidepressants

DIAGNOSTIC TEST EFFECTS

May decrease serum potassium level.

SIDE EFFECTS

Frequent (28%)

Headache

Occasional (7%–3%)

Cough, tremor, dizziness, vertigo, throat dryness or irritation, pharyngitis

Rare (3%)

Palpitations, tachycardia, nausea, heartburn, GI distress, diarrhea

SERIOUS REACTIONS

! Salmeterol may prolong the QT interval, which may precipitate ventricular arrhythmias.

! Hypokalemia and hyperglycemia may occur.

DENTAL CONSIDERATIONS

General:

• Monitor vital signs at every appointment because of CV and respiratory side effects.

• Be aware that aspirin or sulfite preservatives in vasoconstrictor-containing products can exacerbate asthma.
• Acute asthmatic episodes may be precipitated in the dental office. Rapid-acting sympathomimetic inhalants should be available for emergency use. Salmeterol is not a rapid-acting drug and is not intended for use in acute asthmatic attacks.
• Consider semisupine chair position for patients with respiratory disease.
• Midmorning appointments and a stress reduction protocol may be required for anxious patients.

Consultations:

• Medical consultation may be required to assess disease control and patient's ability to tolerate stress.

Teach Patient/Family:

• Importance of good oral hygiene to prevent soft tissue inflammation

salsalate

sal′-sa-late
(Amigesic, Disalcid, Mono-Gesic, Salflex)

CATEGORY AND SCHEDULE

Pregnancy Risk Category: C

MECHANISM OF ACTION

An NSAID that inhibits prostaglandin synthesis, reducing the inflammatory response and the intensity of pain stimuli reaching the sensory nerve endings. ***Therapeutic Effect:*** Produces analgesic and anti-inflammatory effects.

AVAILABILITY

Tablets (Amigesic, Disalcid): 500 mg, 750 mg.
Tablets (Mono-Gesic, Slaflex): 750 mg.

INDICATIONS AND DOSAGES

▸ Rheumatoid Arthritis, Osteoarthritis Pain

PO

Adults, Elderly. Initially, 3 g/day in 2–3 divided doses. Maintenance: 2–4 g/day.

CONTRAINDICATIONS

Bleeding disorders, hypersensitivity to salicylates or NSAIDs

INTERACTIONS

Drug

Alcohol, NSAIDs: May increase the risk of GI effects, such as ulceration.
Antacids, urinary alkalinizers: Increase the excretion of salsalate.
Anticoagulants, heparin, thrombolytics: Increase the risk of bleeding.
Insulin, oral antidiabetics: May increase the effects of these drugs (with large doses of salsalate).
Methotrexate, zidovudine: May increase the toxicity of these drugs.
Ototoxic medications, vancomycin: May increase the risk of ototoxicity.
Platelet aggregation inhibitors, valproic acid: May increase the risk of bleeding.
Probenecid, sulfinpyrazone: May decrease the effects of these drugs.

Herbal

Ginkgo biloba: May increase the risk of bleeding.

Food

None known.

Drug interactions of concern to dentistry

• Increased risk of GI complaints and occult blood loss: alcohol, NSAIDs, corticosteroids
• Increased risk of bleeding: oral anticoagulants, valproic acid, dipyridamole

• Avoid prolonged or concurrent use with NSAIDs, corticosteroids, acetaminophen
• Increased risk of hypoglycemia: oral antidiabetics
• Increased risk of toxicity: methotrexate, lithium, zidovudine
• Decreased effects of probenecid, sulfinpyrazone
• Suspected reduction in the antihypertensive and vasodilator effects of ACE inhibitors; monitor blood pressure if used concurrently

DIAGNOSTIC TEST EFFECTS

May alter serum alkaline phosphatase, uric acid, AST (SGOT), and ALT (SGPT) levels. May prolong PT and bleeding time. May decrease serum cholesterol, potassium, T_3, and T_4 levels.

SIDE EFFECTS

Occasional

Nausea, dyspepsia (including heartburn, indigestion, and epigastric pain)

SERIOUS REACTIONS

! Tinnitus may be the first indication that the serum salicylic acid concentration is reaching or exceeding the upper therapeutic range.
! Salsalate use may also produce vertigo, headache, confusion, drowsiness, diaphoresis, hyperventilation, vomiting, and diarrhea.
! Reye's syndrome may occur in children with chickenpox or the flu.
! Severe overdose may result in electrolyte imbalance, hyperthermia, dehydration, and blood pH imbalance.
! GI bleeding, peptic ulcer, and Reye's syndrome rarely occur.

DENTAL CONSIDERATIONS

General:

• Patients on chronic drug therapy rarely have symptoms of blood dyscrasias, which can include infection, bleeding, and poor healing.
• Potential cross-allergies with other salicylates such as aspirin.
• Consider semisupine chair position for patients with inflammatory joint diseases.
• Avoid prescribing aspirin-containing products because this drug is a salicylate.
• If used for dental patients, take with food or milk to decrease GI complaints; give 30 min before meals or 2 hr after meals; take with a full glass of water.

Consultations:

• In a patient with symptoms of blood dyscrasias, request a medical consultation for blood studies and postpone dental treatment until normal values are reestablished.
• Medical consultation may be required to assess disease control.

Teach Patient/Family:

• That salicylates should not be placed directly on a tooth or oral mucosa because of risk of chemical burns
• Not to exceed recommended dosage; acute toxicity may result
• To read label on other OTC drugs; many contain aspirin
• To avoid alcohol ingestion; GI bleeding may occur
• Importance of good oral hygiene to prevent soft tissue inflammation
• Caution to prevent injury when using oral hygiene aids

saquinavir

sa-kwin′-a-veer
(Fortovase, Invirase)
Do not confuse saquinavir with Sinequan.

CATEGORY AND SCHEDULE

Pregnancy Risk Category: B

MECHANISM OF ACTION

Inhibits HIV protease, rendering the enzyme incapable of processing the polyprotein precursors needed to generate functional proteins in HIV-infected cells.
Therapeutic Effect: Intereferes with HIV replication, slowing the progression of HIV infection.

PHARMACOKINETICS

Poorly absorbed after PO administration (absorption increased with high-calorie and high-fat meals). Protein binding: 99%. Metabolized in the liver to inactive metabolite. Primarily eliminated in feces. Unknown if removed by hemodialysis. ***Half-life:*** 13 hr.

AVAILABILITY

Capsules (Invirase): 200 mg.
Capsules, Gelatin (Fortovase): 200 mg.
Tablets: 500 mg.

INDICATIONS AND DOSAGES

▸ HIV Infection in Combination with Other Antiretrovirals

PO

Adults, Elderly. 1,200 mg Fortovase 3 times a day or 600 mg Invirase 3 times a day within 2 hr after a full meal.
Dosage adjustments when given in combination therapy:
Delavirdine: Fortovase 800 mg 3 times/day.
Lopinavir/ritonavir: Fortovase 800 mg 2 times/day.
Nelfinavir: Fortovase 800 mg 3 times/day or 1200 mg 2 times/day.
Ritonavir: Fortovase or Invirase 1000 mg 2 times/day.

CONTRAINDICATIONS

Clinically significant hypersensitivity to saquinavir; concurrent use with ergot medications, lovastatin, midazolam, simvastatin, or triazolam

INTERACTIONS

Drug

Calcium channel blockers, clindamycin, dapsone, quinidine, triazolam: May increase the plasma concentrations of these drugs.
Carbamazepine, dexamethasone, phenobarbital, phenytoin, rifampin: May reduce saquinavir plasma concentration.
Ketoconazole: Increases saquinavir plasma concentration.

Herbal

Garlic, St. John's wort: May decrease the plasma concentration and effect of saquinavir.

Food

Grapefruit, grapefruit juice: May increase saquinavir plasma concentration.

Drug interactions of concern to dentistry

- Increased plasma levels of clindamycin, troleandomycin, ketoconazole, itraconazole, fentanyl, clarithromycin, midazolam, triazolam
- Increased metabolism of carbamazepine, dexamethasone, phenobarbital
- Inhibits CYP3A4 isoenzymes: use with caution or avoid use with drugs metabolized by these enzymes

DIAGNOSTIC TEST EFFECTS

May alter serum CK levels, elevate liver function test results, and lower blood glucose levels.

SIDE EFFECTS

Occasional

Diarrhea, abdominal discomfort and pain, nausea, photosensitivity, stomatitis

Rare

Confusion, ataxia, asthenia, headache, rash

SERIOUS REACTIONS

! Ketoacidosis occurs rarely.

DENTAL CONSIDERATIONS

General:

- Examine for oral manifestations of opportunistic infections.
- Patients on chronic drug therapy may rarely have symptoms of blood dyscrasias, which can include infection, bleeding, and poor healing.
- Palliative medication may be required for management of oral side effects.

Consultations:

- Medical consultation may be required to assess disease control.
- In a patient with symptoms of blood dyscrasias, request a medical consultation for blood studies and postpone dental treatment until normal values are reestablished.

Teach Patient/Family:

- Importance of good oral hygiene to prevent soft tissue inflammation
- Caution to prevent trauma when using oral hygiene aids
- That secondary oral infection may occur; must see dentist immediately if infection occurs
- Importance of updating medical/drug history if physician makes any changes in evaluation or drug regimen

sargramostim (granulocyte macrophage colony-stimulating factor, GM-CSF)

sar-gra-moh′-stim

(Leukine)

Do not confuse Leukine with Leukeran.

CATEGORY AND SCHEDULE

Pregnancy Risk Category: C

MECHANISM OF ACTION

A colony-stimulating factor that stimulates proliferation and differentiation of hematopoietic cells to activate mature granulocytes and macrophages. ***Therapeutic Effect:*** Assists bone marrow in making new WBCs and increases their chemotactic, antifungal, and antiparasitic activity. Increases cytoneoplastic cells and activates neutrophils to inhibit tumor cell growth.

PHARMACOKINETICS

Effect	Onset	Peak	Duration
Increase WBCs	7–14 days	N/A	1 wk

Detected in serum within 5 min after subcutaneous administration.
Half-life: IV, 1 hr; subcutaneous, 3 hr.

AVAILABILITY

Injection Solution: 500 mcg/ml.
Injection Powder for Reconstitution: 250 mcg.

INDICATIONS AND DOSAGES

▸ Myeloid Recovery Following Bone Marrow Transplant (BMT)

IV INFUSION

Adults, Elderly. Usual parenteral dosage: 250 mcg/m²/day for 21 days (as 2-hr infusion). Begin 2–4 hr after autologous bone marrow infusion and not less than 24 hr after last dose of chemotherapy or not less than 12 hr after last radiation treatment. Discontinue if blast cells appear or underlying disease progresses.

▸ **Bone Marrow Transplant Failure, Engraftment Delay**

IV INFUSION

Adults, Elderly. 250 mcg/m^2/day for 14 days. Infuse over 2 hr. May repeat after 7 days off therapy if engraftment has not occurred with 500 mcg/m^2/day for 14 days.

▸ **Stem Cell Transplant**

IV, SUBCUTANEOUS

Adults. 250 mcg/m^2/day.

OFF-LABEL USES

Treatment of AIDS-related neutropenia; chronic, severe neutropenia; drug-induced neutropenia; myelodysplastic syndrome

CONTRAINDICATIONS

Twelve hours before or after radiation therapy; 24 hours before or after chemotherapy; excessive leukemic myeloid blasts in bone marrow or peripheral blood (>10%); known hypersensitivity to GM-CSF, yeast-derived products, or components of drug

INTERACTIONS

Drug

Lithium, steroids: May increase the effects of sargramostim.

Herbal

None known.

Food

None known.

Drug interactions of concern to dentistry

• Potentiation of myeloproliferative effects: corticosteroids

DIAGNOSTIC TEST EFFECTS

May increase serum bilirubin, creatinine, and hepatic enzyme levels. May decrease serum albumin level.

IV INCOMPATIBILITIES

Amphotericin B complex (Abelcet, AmBisome, Amphotec), hydromorphone (Dilaudid), lorazepam (Ativan), morphine

IV COMPATIBILITIES

Calcium gluconate, dopamine (Intropin), heparin, magnesium, potassium chloride

SIDE EFFECTS

Frequent

GI disturbances, including nausea, diarrhea, vomiting, stomatitis, anorexia, and abdominal pain; arthralgia or myalgia; headache; malaise; rash; pruritus

Occasional

Peripheral edema, weight gain, dyspnea, asthenia, fever, leukocytosis, capillary leak syndrome (such as fluid retention, irritation at local injection site, and peripheral edema)

Rare

Rapid or irregular heartbeat, thrombophlebitis

SERIOUS REACTIONS

! Pleural or pericardial effusion occurs rarely after infusion.

DENTAL CONSIDERATIONS

General:

• Caution: graft patients or myelosuppressed patients may be at high risk for infection.

• Provide palliative care for dental emergencies only.

• Oral infections should be eliminated and/or treated aggressively.

- If additional analgesia is required for dental pain, consider alternative analgesics (NSAIDs) in patients taking narcotics for acute or chronic pain.
- Monitor and record vital signs.
- Avoid products that affect platelet function, such as aspirin and NSAIDs.
- Patient on chronic drug therapy may rarely present with symptoms of blood dyscrasias, which can include infection, bleeding, and poor healing. If dyscrasia is present, caution patient to prevent oral tissue trauma when using oral hygiene aids.
- Examine for oral manifestation of opportunistic infection.
- Palliative medication may be required for management of oral side effects.

Consultations:

- Medical consultation should include routine blood counts including platelet counts and bleeding time.
- Consult physician; prophylactic or therapeutic antiinfectives may be indicated if surgery or periodontal treatment is required.
- In a patient with symptoms of blood dyscrasias, request a medical consultation for blood studies and postpone treatment until normal values are reestablished.
- Medical consultation may be required to assess disease control and patient's ability to tolerate stress.

Teach Patient/Family:

- To use soft tooth brush to reduce risk of bleeding
- Importance of good oral hygiene to prevent soft tissue inflammation
- To prevent trauma when using oral hygiene aids
- To report oral lesions, soreness, or bleeding to dentist

S

scopolamine

skoe-pol′-a-meen
(Trans-Derm Scop, Transderm-V)

CATEGORY AND SCHEDULE

Pregnancy Risk Category: C

MECHANISM OF ACTION

An anticholinergic that reduces excitability of labyrinthine receptors, depressing conduction in the vestibular cerebellar pathway. ***Therapeutic Effect:*** Prevents motion-induced nausea and vomiting.

AVAILABILITY

Transdermal System: 1.5 mg.

INDICATIONS AND DOSAGES

▸ Prevention of Motion Sickness

TRANSDERMAL

Adults. 1 system q72h.

▸ Postoperative Nause or Vomiting

TRANSDERMAL

Adults, Elderly. 1 system no sooner than 1 h before surgery and removed 24 h after surgery.

CONTRAINDICATIONS

Angle-closure glaucoma, GI or GU obstruction, myasthenia gravis, paralytic ileus, tachycardia, thyrotoxicosis

INTERACTIONS

Drug

Antihistamines, tricyclic antidepressants: May increase the anticholinergic effects of scopolamine.
CNS depressants: May increase CNS depression.

Herbal

None known.

Food

None known.

Drug interactions of concern to dentistry

- Increased anticholinergic effects: propantheline and other anticholinergic drugs
- Increased risk of CNS depression: alcohol, all CNS depressants

DIAGNOSTIC TEST EFFECTS

May interfere with gastric secretion test.

SIDE EFFECTS

Frequent (> 15%)

Dry mouth, somnolence, blurred vision

Rare (5%–1%)

Dizziness, restlessness, hallucinations, confusion, difficulty urinating, rash

SERIOUS REACTIONS

! None known.

DENTAL CONSIDERATIONS

General:

- Avoid dental light in patient's eyes; offer dark glasses for patient comfort.
- Caution patients about driving or performing other tasks requiring mental alertness

Teach Patient/Family:

- To avoid mouth rinses with high alcohol content because of drying effects

secobarbital

see-koe-bar′-bi-tal

SCHEDULE II

(Seconal)

CATEGORY AND SCHEDULE

Pregnancy Risk Category: D
Controlled substance: Schedule II

MECHANISM OF ACTION

A barbiturate that depresses the central nervous system (CNS) activity by binding to barbiturate site at the GABA-receptor complex enhancing GABA activity and depressing reticular activity system. ***Therapeutic Effect:*** Produces hypnotic effect due to central nervous system (CNS) depression.

PHARMACOKINETICS

Well absorbed from the gastrointestinal (GI) tract. Protein binding: 52%–57%. Crosses blood-brain barrier. Widely distributed. Metabolized in liver by microsomal enzyme system to inactive and active metabolites. Primarily excreted in urine. Not removed by hemodialysis. ***Half-life:*** 15–40 hrs.

AVAILABILITY

Capsules: 50 mg (Seconal sodium).

INDICATIONS AND DOSAGES

▸ **Insomnia**

PO

Adults. 100 mg at bedtime.

▸ **Preoperative Sedation**

PO

Adults. 100–300 mg 1–2 hrs. before procedure.

Children. 2–6 mg/kg 1–2 hrs. before procedure. Maximum: 100 mg/dose.

▸ **Sedation, Daytime**

PO

Adults. 30–50 mg 3–4 times/day.

Children. 2 mg/kg 3 times/day.

OFF-LABEL USES

Chemotherapy-induced nausea and vomiting

CONTRAINDICATIONS

History of manifest or latent porphyria, marked liver dysfunction, marked respiratory disease in which dyspnea or obstruction is evident, and hypersensitivity to secobarbital or barbiturates

INTERACTIONS

Drug

Alcohol, CNS depressants: May increase the CNS depressant effects.
Anticoagulants: May decrease anticoagulant activity.
Corticosteroids: May increase metabolism of corticosteroids.
Doxycycline: May shorten the half-life of doxycycline.
Griseofulvin: May decrease levels of griseofulvin by interfering with its metabolism.
Estradiol, estrone, progesterone, other steroidal hormones: May decrease the effect of these hormones by increasing their metabolism.
MAOIs: May prolong the effects of secobarbital by inhibiting its metabolism.
Phenytoin, sodium valproate, valproic acid: May decreases the metabolism and increase the concentration and risk of toxicity with secobarbital.

Herbal

St. John's Wort, kava kava, gotu kola, valerian: May increase CNS depressant effects.

Food

None known.

Drug interactions of concern to dentistry

- Hepatotoxicity: halogenated hydrocarbon anesthetics
- Increased CNS depression: alcohol, all CNS depressants
- Increased metabolism of carbamazepine, tricyclic antidepressants, corticosteroids
- Decreased half-life of doxycycline

DIAGNOSTIC TEST EFFECTS

None known.

SIDE EFFECTS

Frequent

Somnolence

Occasional

Agitation, confusion, hyperkinesia, ataxia, CNS depression, nightmares, nervousness, psychiatric disturbance, hallucinations, insomnia, anxiety, dizziness, abnormality in thinking, hypoventilation, apnea, bradycardia, hypotension, syncope, nausea, vomiting, constipation, headache

Rare

Hypersensitivity reactions, fever, liver damage, megaloblastic anemia

SERIOUS REACTIONS

! Agranulocytosis, megaloblastic anemia, apnea, hypoventilation, bradycardia, hypotension, syncope, hepatic damage, and Stevens-Johnson syndrome rarely occur.
! Tolerance and physical dependence may occur with repeated use.

DENTAL CONSIDERATIONS

General:

- Determine why the patient is taking the drug.
- Monitor vital signs at every appointment because of CV side effects. Evaluate respiration characteristics and rate.
- Patients on chronic drug therapy may rarely have symptoms of blood dyscrasias, which can include infection, bleeding, and poor healing.
- *When used for sedation in dentistry:*
  - Assess vital signs before and q30min after use as sedative.
  - Observe respiratory dysfunction: respiratory depression, character, rate, rhythm; hold drug if respirations are <10/min or if pupils are dilated.
- After supine positioning, have patient sit upright for at least 2 min

before standing to avoid orthostatic hypotension.
• Have someone drive patient to and from dental office when drug used for conscious sedation.
• Barbiturates induce liver microsomal enzymes, which alter the metabolism of other drugs.
• Geriatric patients are more susceptible to drug effects; use a lower dose.

Consultations:
• In a patient with symptoms of blood dyscrasias, request a medical consultation for blood studies and postpone dental treatment until normal values are reestablished.

Teach Patient/Family:
• To avoid driving or other activities requiring mental alertness
• To avoid alcohol ingestion and CNS depressants; serious CNS depression may result
• Caution when using OTC preparations (antihistamines, cold remedies) that contain CNS depressants

selegiline hydrochloride

seh-leg′-ill-ene
(Apo-Selegiline[CAN], Eldepryl, Novo-Selegiline[CAN], Selgene[AUS])
Do not confuse selegiline with Stelazine, or Eldepryl with enalapril.

CATEGORY AND SCHEDULE
Pregnancy Risk Category: C

MECHANISM OF ACTION
An antiparkinson agent that irreversibly inhibits the activity of monoamine oxidase type B, the enzyme that breaks down dopamine, thereby increasing dopaminergic action. ***Therapeutic Effect:*** Relieves signs and symptoms of Parkinson's disease.

PHARMACOKINETICS
Rapidly absorbed from the GI tract. Crosses the blood-brain barrier. Metabolized in the liver to the active metabolites. Primarily excreted in urine. ***Half-life:*** 17 hr (amphetamine), 20 hr (methamphetamine).

AVAILABILITY
Capsules: 5 mg.
Tablets: 5 mg.

INDICATIONS AND DOSAGES
▸ Adjunctive Treatment for Parkinsonism
PO
Adults. 10 mg/day in divided doses, such as 5 mg at breakfast and lunch, given concomitantly with each dose of carbidopa and levodopa.
Elderly. Initially, 5 mg in the morning. May increase up to 10 mg/day.

CONTRAINDICATIONS
None known.

INTERACTIONS
Drug
Fluoxetine: May cause serotonin syndrome.
Meperidine: May cause a diaphoresis, excitation, hypertension or hypotension, coma, and even death.
Herbal
None known.
Food
Caffeine, tyramine-rich foods: Large amounts of these substances may produce a severe hypertensive reaction.

Drug interactions of concern to dentistry
• Fatal interaction: opioids (especially meperidine); do not administer together

- Risk of serotonin syndrome: serotonin uptake inhibitors (fluoxetine, sertraline, paroxetine)

DIAGNOSTIC TEST EFFECTS
None known.

SIDE EFFECTS
Frequent (10%–4%)
Nausea, dizziness, light-headedness, syncope, abdominal discomfort
Occasional (3%–2%)
Confusion, hallucinations, dry mouth, vivid dreams, dyskinesia
Rare (1%)
Headache, myalgia, anxiety, diarrhea, insomnia

SERIOUS REACTIONS
! Symptoms of overdose may vary from CNS depression, characterized by sedation, apnea, cardiovascular collapse, and death, to severe paradoxical reactions, such as hallucinations, tremor, and seizures.
! Other serious effects may include involuntary movements, impaired motor coordination, loss of balance, blepharospasm, facial grimaces, feeling of heaviness in the lower extremities, depression, nightmares, delusions, overstimulation, sleep disturbance, and anger.

DENTAL CONSIDERATIONS
General:
- Monitor vital signs at every appointment because of CV side effects.
- After supine positioning, have patient sit upright for at least 2 min before standing to avoid orthostatic hypotension.
- Assess for presence of extrapyramidal motor symptoms, such as tardive dyskinesia and akathisia. Extrapyramidal motor activity may complicate dental treatment.
- Assess salivary flow as a factor in caries, periodontal disease, and candidiasis.

Consultations:
- Medical consultation may be required to assess disease control and patient's ability to tolerate stress.
- If signs of tardive dyskinesia or akathisia are present, refer to physician.

Teach Patient/Family:
- To use electric toothbrush if patient has difficulty holding conventional devices
- *When chronic dry mouth occurs, advise patient:*
  - To avoid mouth rinses with high alcohol content because of drying effects
  - Of need for daily use of home fluoride products to prevent caries
  - To use sugarless gum, frequent sips of water, or saliva substitutes

sertaconazole
sir-tah-con′-ah-zole
(Ertaczo)

CATEGORY AND SCHEDULE
Pregnancy Risk Category: C

MECHANISM OF ACTION
An imidazole derivative that inhibits synthesis of ergosterol, a vital component of fungal cell formation. ***Therapeutic Effect:*** Damages the fungal cell membrane, altering its function.

AVAILABILITY
Cream: 2%.

INDICATIONS AND DOSAGES

▸ **Tinea Pedis**

TOPICAL

Adults, Elderly, Children 12 yr and older. Apply to affected area twice a day for 4 wk.

CONTRAINDICATIONS

None known.

INTERACTIONS

Drug

None known.

Herbal

None known.

Food

None known.

Drug interactions of concern to dentistry

- None reported

DIAGNOSTIC TEST EFFECTS

None known.

SIDE EFFECTS

Rare (2%)

Burning, tenderness, erythema, dryness, pruritus, hyperpigmentation, and contact dermatitis at application site

SERIOUS REACTIONS

! None known.

DENTAL CONSIDERATIONS

General:

- Determine why patient is taking this drug.

sertraline

sir′-trall-een

(Apo-Sertraline[CAN], Novo-Sertraline[CAN], PMS-Sertraline[CAN], Zoloft)

Do not confuse sertraline with Serentil.

CATEGORY AND SCHEDULE

Pregnancy Risk Category: B

MECHANISM OF ACTION

An antidepressant, anxiolytic, and obsessive-compulsive disorder adjunct that blocks the reuptake of the neurotransmitter serotonin at CNS neuronal presynaptic membranes, increasing its availability at postsynaptic receptor sites. ***Therapeutic Effect:*** Relieves depression, reduces obsessive-compulsive behavior, decreases anxiety.

PHARMACOKINETICS

Incompletely and slowly absorbed from the GI tract; food increases absorption. Protein binding: 98%. Widely distributed. Undergoes extensive first-pass metabolism in the liver to active compound. Excreted in urine and feces. Not removed by hemodialysis. ***Half-life:*** 26 hr.

AVAILABILITY

Oral Concentrate: 20 mg/ml.
Tablets: 25 mg, 50 mg, 100 mg.

INDICATIONS AND DOSAGES

▸ **Depression**

PO

Adults. Initially, 50 mg/day. May increase by 50 mg/day at 7-day intervals up to 200 mg/day.
Elderly. Initially, 25 mg/day. May increase by 25–50 mg/day at 7-day intervals up to 200 mg/day.

▸ **Obsessive-Compulsive Disorder**
PO
Adults, Children 13–17 yr. Initially, 50 mg/day with morning or evening meal. May increase by 50 mg/day at 7-day intervals.
Elderly, Children 6–12 yr. Initially, 25 mg/day. May increase by 25–50 mg/day at 7-day intervals. Maximum: 200 mg/day.
▸ **Panic Disorder, Posttraumatic Stress Disorder, Social Anxiety Disorder**
PO
Adults, Elderly. Initially, 25 mg/day. May increase by 50 mg/day at 7-day intervals. Range: 50–200 mg/day. Maximum: 200 mg/day.
▸ **Premenstrual Dysphoric Disorder**
PO
Adults. Initially, 50 mg/day. May increase up to 150 mg/day in 50-mg increments.

OFF-LABEL USES
Eating disorders, generalized anxiety disorder (GAD), impulse control disorders

CONTRAINDICATIONS
User within 14 days of MAOIs

INTERACTIONS
Drug
Highly protein-bound medications (e.g., digoxin and warfarin): May increase the blood concentration and risk of toxicity of these drugs.
MAOIs: May cause neuroleptic malignant syndrome, hypertensive crisis, hyperpyrexia, seizures, and serotonin syndrome (marked by diaphoresis, diarrhea, fever, mental changes, restlessness, and shivering).
Herbal
St. John's wort: May increase the risk of adverse effects.
Food
None known.

Drug interactions of concern to dentistry
- Increased CNS depression: alcohol, CNS depressants, St. John's wort (herb)
- Increased side effects: highly protein-bound drugs (aspirin), tricyclic antidepressants
- Increased half-life of diazepam
- Possible inhibition of sertraline metabolism: erythromycin, clarithromycin
- Potent inhibitor of CYP2D6 isoenzymes; use drugs metabolized by the enzyme only with caution
- Possible risk of serotonin syndrome with tramadol, oxycodone
- Decreased effects: carbamazepine
- First-time users of SSRIs also taking NSAIDs may have a higher risk of GI side effects; until more data are available, it may be advisable to avoid use of NSAIDs in these patients (*Br J Clin Pharmacol* 55:591–595, 2003)

DIAGNOSTIC TEST EFFECTS
May increase serum total cholesterol, triglyceride, AST, and ALT levels. May decrease serum uric acid level.

SIDE EFFECTS
Frequent (26%–12%)
Headache, nausea, diarrhea, insomnia, somnolence, dizziness, fatigue, rash, dry mouth
Occasional (6%–4%)
Anxiety, nervousness, agitation, tremor, dyspepsia, diaphoresis, vomiting, constipation, abnormal ejaculation, visual disturbances, altered taste
Rare (< 3%)
Flatulence, urinary frequency, paraesthesia, hot flashes, chills

SERIOUS REACTIONS
! None known.

S

DENTAL CONSIDERATIONS

General:

- Monitor vital signs at every appointment because of CV side effects.
- After supine positioning, have patient sit upright for at least 2 min before standing to avoid orthostatic hypotension.
- Assess salivary flow as a factor in caries, periodontal disease, and candidiasis.
- Avoid dental light in patient's eyes; offer dark glasses for patient comfort.
- Consider semisupine chair position for patient comfort if GI side effects occur.

Consultations:

- Medical consultation may be required to assess patient's ability to tolerate stress.
- Physician should be informed if significant xerostomic side effects occur (e.g., increased caries, sore tongue, problems eating or swallowing, difficulty wearing prosthesis) so that a medication change can be considered.

Teach Patient/Family:

- To use electric toothbrush if patient has difficulty holding conventional devices
- *When chronic dry mouth occurs, advise patient:*
  - To avoid mouth rinses with high alcohol content because of drying effects
  - Of need for daily use of home fluoride products to prevent caries
  - To use sugarless gum, frequent sips of water, or saliva substitutes

sevelamer hydrochloride

seh-vel′-a-mer

(Renagel)

Do not confuse Renagel with Reglan or Regonol.

CATEGORY AND SCHEDULE

Pregnancy Risk Category: C

MECHANISM OF ACTION

An antihyperphosphatemia agent that binds with dietary phosphorus in the GI tract, thus allowing phosphorus to be eliminated through the normal digestive process and decreasing the serum phosphorus level. ***Therapeutic Effect:*** Decreases incidence of hypercalcemic episodes in patients receiving calcium acetate treatment.

PHARMACOKINETICS

Not absorbed systemically. Unknown if removed by hemodialysis.

AVAILABILITY

Capsules: 403 mg.
Tablets: 400 mg, 800 mg.

INDICATIONS AND DOSAGES

▸ Hyperphosphatemia

PO

Adults, Elderly. 800–1,600 mg with each meal, depending on severity of hyperphosphatemia.

CONTRAINDICATIONS

Bowel obstruction, hypophosphatemia

INTERACTIONS

Drug

None known.

Herbal

None known.

Food

None known.

Drug interactions of concern to dentistry

- Possible decrease in bioavailability: orally administered, rapidly absorbed drugs; give at least 1 hr before or 3 hr after sevelamer doses

DIAGNOSTIC TEST EFFECTS

None known.

SIDE EFFECTS

Frequent (20%–11%)
Infection, pain, hypotension, diarrhea, dyspepsia, nausea, vomiting
Occasional (10%–1%)
Headache, constipation, hypertension, thrombosis, increased cough

SERIOUS REACTIONS

! None known.

DENTAL CONSIDERATIONS

General:

- Patients taking this drug may be undergoing renal dialysis; confirm the medical and drug history to plan appropriate management.
- If you prescribe medications for dental needs, have patient take medication 1 hr before or 3 hr after sevelamer doses.
- Monitor and record vital signs.
- Consider semisupine chair position for patient comfort if GI side effects occur.
- Patient may need assistance in getting into and out of dental chair. Adjust chair position for patient comfort.
- Consultation with physician may be necessary if sedation or general anesthesia is required.

Consultations:

- Medical consultation may be required to assess disease control and patient's ability to tolerate stress.

Teach Patient/Family:

- To report oral lesions, soreness, or bleeding to dentist
- Importance of good oral hygiene to prevent soft tissue inflammation
- To prevent trauma when using oral hygiene aids
    - Importance of updating health and medication history if physician makes any changes in evaluation or drug regimens; include OTC, herbal, and nonherbal remedies in the update

sibutramine

sih-byoo′-tra-meen
sih-byoo′-tra-meen
(Meridia)

CATEGORY AND SCHEDULE

Pregnancy Risk Category: C
Controlled substance: Schedule IV

MECHANISM OF ACTION

A central nervous system (CNS) stimulant inhibits reuptake of serotonin (enhancing satiety) and norepinephrine (raises metabolic rate) centrally.
Therapeutic Effect: Induces and maintains weight loss.

PHARMACOKINETICS

Rapidly absorbed from the gastrointestinal (GI) tract. Protein binding: 95%–97%. Metabolized in liver, undergoes first-pass metabolism. Primarily excreted in urine, minimal elimination in feces. ***Half-life:*** 1.1 hrs.

AVAILABILITY

Capsules: 5 mg, 10 mg, 15 mg (Meridia).

INDICATIONS AND DOSAGES

▸ Weight Loss

PO

Adults 16 years and older. Initially, 10 mg/day. May increase up to 15 mg/day. Maximum: 20 mg/day.

CONTRAINDICATIONS

Anorexia nervosa, concomitant MAOI use, concomitant use of centrally acting appetite suppressants, hypersensitivity to sibutramine or any component of the formulation

INTERACTIONS

Drug

CNS-acting appetite suppressants: May increase risk of hypertension and tachycardia.

Dextromethorphan, dihydroergotamine, ergotamine, fentanyl, lithium, meperidine, MAOIs, pentazocine, SSRIs, serotonin agonists, tryptophan: May increase risk of serotonin syndrome.

Herbal

St. John's Wort: May decrease sibutramine levels.

Yohimbine: May increase risk of adverse cardiovascular effects.

Food

None known.

Drug interactions of concern to dentistry

- Avoid use of meperidine: risk of serotonin syndrome

DIAGNOSTIC TEST EFFECTS

None known.

SIDE EFFECTS

Frequent

Headache, dry mouth, anorexia, constipation, insomnia, rhinitis, pharyngitis

Occasional

Back pain, flu syndrome, dizziness, nausea, asthenia (loss of strength, energy), arthralgia, nervousness, dyspepsia, sinusitis, abdominal pain, anxiety, dysmenorrheal

Rare

Depression, rash, cough, sweating, tachycardia, migraine, increased B/P, paresthesia, altered taste

SERIOUS REACTIONS

! Seizures, thrombocytopenia, and deaths have been reported.

! Serotonin syndrome can occur with concomitant use of drugs that increase serotonin.

! Large doses may produce extreme nervousness and tachycardia.

DENTAL CONSIDERATIONS

General:

- Monitor vital signs at every appointment because of CV side effects.
- Assess salivary flow as factor in caries, periodontal disease, and candidiasis.
- Information on any abuse liability is unknown.
- Determine why patient is taking the drug.

Teach Patient/Family:

- *When chronic dry mouth occurs, advise patient:*
  - To avoid mouth rinses with high alcohol content because of drying effects
  - Of need for daily use of home fluoride products to prevent caries
  - To use sugarless gum, frequent sips of water, or saliva substitutes

sildenafil citrate

sill-den′-a-fill
(Viagra)
Do not confuse Viagra with Vaniqa.

CATEGORY AND SCHEDULE

Pregnancy Risk Category: B

MECHANISM OF ACTION

An erectile dysfunction agent that inhibits phosphodiesterase type 5, the enzyme responsible for degrading cyclic guanosine monophosphate in the corpus cavernosum of the penis, resulting in smooth muscle relaxation and increased blood flow. ***Therapeutic Effect:*** Facilitates an erection.

AVAILABILITY

Tablets: 25 mg, 50 mg, 100 mg.

INDICATIONS AND DOSAGES

▸ Erectile Dysfunction

PO

Adults. 50 mg (30 min–4 hr before sexual activity). Range: 25–100 mg. Maximum dosing frequency is once daily.

Elderly older than 65 yr. Consider starting dose of 25 mg.

S

OFF-LABEL USES

Treatment of diabetic gastroparesis, sexual dysfunction associated with the use of selective serotonin reuptake inhibitors

CONTRAINDICATIONS

Concurrent use of sodium nitroprusside or nitrates in any form

INTERACTIONS

Drug

Cimetidine, erythromycin, itraconazole, ketoconazole: May increase sildenafil plasma concentration.

Nitrates: Potentiates the hypotensive effects of nitrates.

Herbal

None known.

Food

High-fat meals: Delay drug's maximum effectiveness by 1 hour.

Drug interactions of concern to dentistry

- Avoid use of nitroglycerin within 24 hr
- Increased plasma levels caused by interference with metabolism: cimetidine, erythromycin, ketoconazole, itraconazole
- Strong inhibitors of CYP3A4 or CYP2C9 isoenzymes: should be used with caution

DIAGNOSTIC TEST EFFECTS

None known.

SIDE EFFECTS

Frequent

Headache (16%), flushing (10%)

Occasional (7%–3%)

Dyspepsia, nasal congestion, UTI, abnormal vision, diarrhea

Rare (2%)

Dizziness, rash

SERIOUS REACTIONS

! Prolonged erections (lasting over 4 hours) and priapism (painful erections lasting over 6 hours) occur rarely.

DENTAL CONSIDERATIONS

General:

- This is an acute-use drug intended to be taken just before sexual activity, and the reported incidence of oral side effects does not differ from a placebo. However, the potential interacting drugs should be avoided.

silver sulfadiazine

sul-fa-dye′-a-zeen
(Flamazine[CAN], SSD, SSD AF, Silvadene)

CATEGORY AND SCHEDULE

Pregnancy Risk Category: B

MECHANISM OF ACTION

An anti-infective that acts upon cell wall and cell membraine. Releases silver slowly in concentrations selectively toxic to bacteria.
Therapeutic Effect: Produces bactericidal effect.

PHARMACOKINETICS

Variably absorbed. Significant systemic absorption may occur if applied to extensive burns. Absorbed medication excreted unchanged in urine. ***Half-life:*** 10 hrs (half-life increased with impaired renal function).

AVAILABILITY

Cream: 1% (Silvadene, SSD, SSD AF).

INDICATIONS AND DOSAGES

▸ **Burns**

TOPICAL

Adults, Elderly Children. Apply 1–2 times daily.

OFF-LABEL USES

Treatment of minor bacterial skin infection, dermal ulcer

CONTRAINDICATIONS

Hypersensitivity to silver sulfadiazine or any component of the formulation

INTERACTIONS

Drug

Collagenase, papain, sutilains: May be inactivated.

Herbal

None known.

Food

None known.

Drug interactions of concern to dentistry

- None reported

DIAGNOSTIC TEST EFFECTS

None known.

SIDE EFFECTS

Side effects characteristic of all sulfonamides may occur when systemically absorbed such as extensive burn areas, anorexia, nausea, vomiting, headache, diarrhea, dizziness, photosensitivity, joint pain

Frequent

Burning feeling at treatment site

Occasional

Brown-gray skin discoloration, rash, itching

Rare

Increased sensitivity or skin to sunlight

SERIOUS REACTIONS

! If significant systemic absorption occurs, less often but serious are hemolytic anemia, hypoglycemia, diuresis, peripheral neuropathy, Stevens-Johnson syndrome, agranulocytosis, disseminated lupus erythematosus, anaphylaxis, hepatitis, and toxic nephrosis.

! Fungal superinfections may occur.

! Interstitial nephritis occurs rarely.

DENTAL CONSIDERATIONS

General:

- Dental management depends on extent and severity of burns and patient's ability to cooperate; above all use aseptic techniques.
- Provide palliative dental care for dental emergencies only.

Consultations:
- Medical consultation may be required to assess disease control and patient's ability to tolerate stress.
- Consult patient's physician if an acute dental infection occurs and another antiinfective is required.

Teach Patient/Family:
- Importance of good oral hygiene to prevent soft tissue inflammation
- To prevent trauma when using oral hygiene aids

simethicone

si-meth′-i-kone
(Alka-Seltzer Gas Relief, Gas-X, Genasym, Infant Mylicon, Mylanta Gas, Ovol[CAN], Phazyme)

CATEGORY AND SCHEDULE
Pregnancy Risk Category: C
OTC

MECHANISM OF ACTION
An antiflatulent that changes surface tension of gas bubbles, allowing easier elimination of gas. ***Therapeutic Effect:*** Drug dispersal, prevents formation of gas pockets in the GI tract.

PHARMACOKINETICS
Does not appear to be absorbed from GI tract. Excreted unchanged in feces.

S

AVAILABILITY
Oral Drops (Infants Mylicon): 40 mg/0.6 ml .
Softgel (Alka-Seltzer Gas Relief, Gas-Z, Mylanta Gas): 125 mg.
Softgel (Phazyme): 180 mg.
Tablets (Chewable [Gas-X, Mylanta Gas]): 80 mg, 125 mg.

INDICATIONS AND DOSAGES
▸ **Antiflatulent**

PO
Adults, Elderly, Children 12 yr and older. 40–250 mg after meals and at bedtime. Maximum: 500 mg/day.
Children 2–11 yr. 40 mg 4 times a day.
Children younger than 2 yr. 20 mg 4 times a day.

OFF-LABEL USES
Adjunct to bowel radiography and gastroscopy

CONTRAINDICATIONS
None known.

INTERACTIONS
Drug
None known.
Herbal
None known.
Food
None known.
Drug interactions of concern to dentistry
- None reported

DIAGNOSTIC TEST EFFECTS
None known.

SIDE EFFECTS
None known.

SERIOUS REACTIONS
! None known.

DENTAL CONSIDERATIONS

General:
- Determine why patient is taking the drug.
- Consider semisupine chair position for patient comfort because of GI effects of disease.
- Question patient about tolerance of NSAIDS or aspirin related to GI disease.
- Patients with gastroesophageal reflux may present with oral symptoms. including burning mouth, secondary candidiasis, and signs of tooth erosion.

• Patients using this drug may have GI disease; review medical and drug history.

Teach Patient/Family:

• Importance of updating health and medication history if physician makes any changes in evaluation or drug regimens; include OTC, herbal, and nonherbal remedies in the update
• Importance of good oral hygiene to prevent soft tissue inflammation

simvastatin

sim′-va-sta-tin
(Apo-Simvastatin[CAN], Lipex[AUS], Zocor)
Do not confuse Zocor with Cozaar.

CATEGORY AND SCHEDULE

Pregnancy Risk Category: X

MECHANISM OF ACTION

A HMG-CoA reductase inhibitor that interferes with cholesterol biosynthesis by inhibiting the conversion of the enzyme HMG-CoA to mevalonate. ***Therapeutic Effect:*** Decreases serum LDL, cholesterol, VLDL, and plasma triglyceride levels; slightly increases serum HDL concentration.

PHARMACOKINETICS

Route	Onset	Peak	Duration
PO to reduce cholesterol	3 days	14 days	N/A

Well absorbed from the GI tract. Protein binding: 95%. Undergoes extensive first-pass metabolism. Hydrolyzed to active metabolite. Primarily eliminated in feces. Unknown if removed by hemodialysis.

AVAILABILITY

Tablets: 5 mg, 10 mg, 20 mg, 40 mg, 80 mg.

INDICATIONS AND DOSAGES

Adjunct to diet to decrease heterozygous familial hypercholesterolemia in adolescents 10–17 yrs of age (girls at least 1 year post-menarche).

▸ **Heterozygous Familial Hypercholesterolemia**

PO

Pediatric. 10 mg once daily in evening. Range: 10–40 mg/day. Maximum: 40 mg/day.

▸ **To Decrease Elevated Total and LDL Cholesterol in Hypercholesterolemia (types IIa and IIb), Lower Triglyceride Levels, and Increase HDL Levels; to Reduce Risk of Death and Prevent MI in Patients with Heart Disease and Elevated Cholesterol Level; to Reduce Risk of Revascularization Procedures; to Decrease Risk of Stroke or Transient Ischemic Attack; to Prevent Cardiovascular Events.**

PO

Adults. Initially, 10–40 mg/day in evening. Dosage adjusted at 4-wk intervals.

Elderly. Initially, 10 mg/day. May increase by 5–10 mg/day q4wk. Range: 5–80 mg/day. Maximum: 80 mg/day.

CONTRAINDICATIONS

Active hepatic disease or unexplained, persistent elevations of liver function test results, age younger than 18 years, pregnancy

INTERACTIONS

Drug

Cyclosporine, erythromycin, gemfibrozil, immunosuppressants, niacin: Increases the risk of acute renal failure and rhabdomyolysis.
Erythromycin, itraconazole, ketoconazole: May increase simvastatin blood concentration and cause muscle inflammation, myalgia, or weakness.

Herbal

None known.

Food

None known.

Drug interactions of concern to dentistry

- Increased myalgia, myositis: erythromycin, cyclosporin, itraconazole, ketoconazole
- Caution with use of drugs that are strong inhibitors of CYP3A4 isoenzymes

DIAGNOSTIC TEST EFFECTS

May increase serum CK and serum transaminase concentrations.

SIDE EFFECTS

Simvastatin is generally well tolerated. Side effects are usually mild and transient.

Occasional (3%–2%)
Headache, abdominal pain or cramps, constipation, upper respiratory tract infection

Rare (< 2%)
Diarrhea, flatulence, asthenia (loss of strength and energy), nausea or vomiting

SERIOUS REACTIONS

! Lens opacities may occur.
! Hypersensitivity reaction and hepatitis occur rarely.

DENTAL CONSIDERATIONS

General:

- Consider semisupine chair position for patient comfort because of GI side effects.

sirolimus

sir-oh-leem′-us
(Rapamune)

CATEGORY AND SCHEDULE

Pregnancy Risk Category: C

MECHANISM OF ACTION

An immunosuppressant that inhibits T-lymphocyte proliferation induced by stimulation of cell surface receptors, mitogens, alloantigens, and lymphokines. Prevents activation of the enzyme target of rapamycin, a key regulatory kinase in cell cycle progression. ***Therapeutic Effect:*** Inhibits proliferation of T and B cells, essential components of the immune response; prevents organ transplant rejection.

AVAILABILITY

Oral Solution: 1 mg/ml.
Tablets: 1 mg, 2 mg.

INDICATIONS AND DOSAGES

▸ Prevention of Organ Transplant Rejection

PO
Adults. Loading dose: 6 mg. Maintenance: 2 mg/day.
Children 13 yr and older weighing less than 40 kg. Loading dose: 3 mg/m^2. Maintenance: 1 mg/m^2/day.

CONTRAINDICATIONS

Hypersensitivity to sirolimus, malignancy

S

INTERACTIONS

Drug

Cyclosporine, diltiazem, ketoconazole: May increase the blood concentration and risk of toxicity of sirolimus.
Rifampin: May decrease the blood concentration and effects of sirolimus.

Herbal

None known.

Food

Grapefruit, grapefruit juice: May decrease the metabolism of sirolimus.

Drug interactions of concern to dentistry

• Increased blood levels: potent inhibitors of CYP3A4 isoenzymes (clarithromycin, clotrimazole, erythromycin, fluconazole, itraconazole, ritonavir, indinavir, grapefruit juice)
• Decreased blood levels: potent inducers of CYP3A4 isoenzymes (phenobarbital, carbamazepine, St. John's wort [herb])

DIAGNOSTIC TEST EFFECTS

May decrease blood Hgb level, Hct, and platelet count. May increase serum cholesterol, creatinine, and triglyceride levels.

SIDE EFFECTS

Occasional

Hypercholesterolemia, hyperlipidemia, hypertension, rash; with high doses (5 mg/day): anemia, arthralgia, diarrhea, hypokalemia, and thrombocytopenia

SERIOUS REACTIONS

! None known.

DENTAL CONSIDERATIONS

General:

• Caution: patients on immunosuppressive therapy may be at high risk for infection.
• Provide palliative dental care for dental emergencies only.
• Oral infections should be eliminated and/or treated aggressively.
• Patients may be at risk for bleeding; check oral signs.
• Examine for evidence of oral candidiasis Topically acting antifungals may be preferred: note potential drug interactions.
• Monitor and record vital signs.
• Avoid products that affect platelet function, such as aspirin and NSAIDs.
• Patient on chronic drug therapy may rarely present with symptoms of blood dyscrasias, which can include infection, bleeding, and poor healing. If dyscrasia is present, caution patient to prevent oral tissue trauma when using oral hygiene aids.
• Consider local hemostasis measures to prevent excessive bleeding.

Consultations:

• Medical consultation should include routine blood counts including platelet counts and bleeding time.
• Consult physician; prophylactic or therapeutic antiinfectives may be indicated if surgery or periodontal treatment is required.
• In a patient with symptoms of blood dyscrasias, request a medical consultation for blood studies and postpone treatment until normal values are reestablished.
• Medical consultation may be required to assess disease control and patient's ability to tolerate stress.

Teach Patient/Family:

• To use soft tooth brush to reduce risk of bleeding
• Importance of good oral hygiene to prevent soft tissue inflammation
• To prevent trauma when using oral hygiene aids

- To report oral lesions, soreness, or bleeding to dentist
- Use of electric toothbrush if patient has difficulty holding conventional devices

sotalol hydrochloride

soe′-ta-lole

(Apo-Sotalol[CAN], Betapace, Betapace AF, Cardol[AUS], Novo-Sotalol[CAN], PMS-Sotalol[CAN], Solavert[AUS], Sorine, Sotab[AUS], Sotacor[AUS], Sotahexal[AUS])

Do not confuse sotalol with Stadol.

CATEGORY AND SCHEDULE

Pregnancy Risk Category: B (D if used in second or third trimester)

MECHANISM OF ACTION

A beta-adrenergic blocking agent that prolongs action potential, effective refractory period, and QT interval. Decreases heart rate and AV node conduction; increases AV node refractoriness.
Therapeutic Effect: Produces antiarrhythmic activity.

PHARMACOKINETICS

Well absorbed from the GI tract. Protein binding: None. Widely distributed. Primarily excreted unchanged in urine. Removed by hemodialysis. ***Half-life:*** 12 hr (increased in the elderly and patients with impaired renal function).

S

AVAILABILITY

Tablets (Betapace): 80 mg, 120 mg, 160 mg, 240 mg.
Tablets (Betapace AF): 80 mg, 120 mg, 160 mg.
Tablets (Sorine): 80 mg, 120 mg, 160 mg, 240 mg.

INDICATIONS AND DOSAGES

▸ **Documented, Life-Threatening Arrhythmias**

PO

Adults, Elderly. Initially, 80 mg twice a day. May increase gradually at 2- to 3-day intervals. Range: 240–320 mg/day.

▸ **Dosage in Renal Impairment**

Dosage interval is modified on the basis of creatinine clearance.

Creatinine Clearance	Dosage Interval
31–60 ml/min	24 hr
10–30 ml/min	36–48 hr
less than 10 ml/min	Individualized

OFF-LABEL USES

Maintenance of normal heart rhythm in chronic or recurring atrial fibrillation or flutter; treatment of anxiety, chronic angina pectoris, hypertension, hypertrophic cardiomyopathy, MI, mitral valve prolapse syndrome, pheochromocytoma, thyrotoxicosis, tremors

CONTRAINDICATIONS

Bronchial asthma, cardiogenic shock, prolonged QT syndrome (unless functioning pacemaker is present), second- and third-degree heart block, sinus bradycardia, uncontrolled cardiac failure

INTERACTIONS

Drug

Antiarrhythmics, phenothiazine, tricyclic antidepressants: May prolong QT interval.
Calcium channel blockers: May increase effect on AV conduction and BP.
Clonidine: May potentiate rebound hypertension after clonidine is discontinued.
Digoxin: May increase risk of proarrhythmias.

Insulin, oral hypoglycemics: May mask signs of hypoglycemia and prolong the effects of insulin and oral hypoglycemics.
Sympathomimetics: May inhibit the effects of sympathomimetics.

Herbal
None known.

Food
None known.

Drug interactions of concern to dentistry
- Decreased hypotensive effect: NSAIDs, indomethacin
- Increased hypotension, myocardial depression: hydrocarbon inhalation anesthetics
- Hypertension, bradycardia: sympathomimetics
- Slow metabolism of lidocaine

DIAGNOSTIC TEST EFFECTS
May increase blood glucose, serum alkaline phosphatase, serum LDH, serum lipoprotein, AST (SGOT), ALT (SGPT), and serum triglyceride levels.

SIDE EFFECTS
Frequent
Diminished sexual function, drowsiness, insomnia, unusual fatigue or weakness
Occasional
Depression, cold hands or feet, diarrhea, constipation, anxiety, nasal congestion, nausea, vomiting
Rare
Altered taste, dry eyes, itching, numbness of fingers, toes, or scalp

SERIOUS REACTIONS
! Bradycardia, CHF, hypotension, bronchospasm, hypoglycemia, prolonged QT interval, torsades de pointes, ventricular tachycardia, and premature ventricular complexes may occur.

DENTAL CONSIDERATIONS
General:
- Monitor vital signs at every appointment because of CV side effects.
- After supine positioning, have patient sit upright for at least 2 min before standing to avoid orthostatic hypotension.
- Stress from dental procedures may compromise CV function; determine patient risk.
- Use vasoconstrictors with caution, in low doses, and with careful aspiration. Avoid use of gingival retraction cord with epinephrine.
- Short appointments and a stress reduction protocol may be required for anxious patients.

Consultations:
- Medical consultation should be made to assess disease control and patient's ability to tolerate stress.

sparfloxacin
spar-floks′-a-sin
(Zagam)

CATEGORY AND SCHEDULE
Pregnancy Risk Category: C

MECHANISM OF ACTION
A fluoroquinolone that interferes with DNA-gyrase in susceptible microorganisms. ***Therapeutic Effect:*** Inhibits DNA replication and repair. Bactericidal.

PHARMACOKINETICS
Well absorbed from the gastrointestinal (GI) tract after PO administration. Widely distributed. Metabolized in liver. Primarily excreted in urine with a lesser amount eliminated in the feces. ***Half-life:*** 16–30 hrs.

AVAILABILITY

Tablets: 200 mg (Zagam).

INDICATIONS AND DOSAGES

▸ Bronchitis, Pneumonia

PO

Adults 18 yrs and older, Elderly. Initially, two 200 mg tablets as a loading dose on first day. Then one 200 mg tablet q24h for a total of 10 days.

▸ Dosage in Renal Impairment (creatinine clearance <50 ml/min)

PO

Adults 18 yrs and older, Elderly. Initially, two 200 mg tablets as a loading dose on first day. Then one 200 mg tablet q48h for a total of 9 days.

CONTRAINDICATIONS

Hypersensitivity to fluoroquinolones, cinoxacin, nalidixic acid

INTERACTIONS

Drug

Antacids, sucralfate, iron preparations: May decrease sparfloxacin plasma concentration and half-life.

Phenothiazines, tricyclic antidepressants, erythromycin: Concurrent use of these drugs may increase the risk of QTc prolongation and life-threatening arrhythmias.

Cyclosporine: Increases the risk of nephrotoxicity.

Herbal

None known.

Food

None known.

Drug interactions of concern to dentistry

- Avoid concurrent use with erythromycin, pentamidine, tricyclic antidepressants, phenothiazines
- Concurrent administration with antacids greatly reduces oral absorption, can increase warfarin levels
- Increased risk of life-threatening arrhythmias: procainamide

DIAGNOSTIC TEST EFFECTS

May increase SGOT (AST), SGOT (ALT), alkaline phosphatase, WBC count.

SIDE EFFECTS

Occasional

Photosensitivity, diarrhea, nausea, headache

Rare

Dyspepsia, dizziness, insomnia, abdominal pain, change in taste

SERIOUS REACTIONS

! Superinfection (particularly enterococcal or fungal overgrowth of nonsusceptible organisms) due to altered bacterial balance may occur (genital-anal pruritus, ulceration or changes in oral mucosa, moderate to severe diarrhea, new or increased fever).

! Hypersensitivity reactions have occurred in those receiving fluoroquinolone therapy.

DENTAL CONSIDERATIONS

General:

- Contraindicated for patients whose lifestyle or employment will not permit compliance with photosensitivity precautions.
- Determine why patient is taking the drug.
- Assess salivary flow as factor in caries, periodontal disease, and candidiasis.
- Consider semisupine chair position for patient comfort if GI side effects occur.
- Avoid dental light in patient's eyes; offer dark glasses for patient comfort.

Consultations:

• Consult with patient's physician if an acute dental infection occurs and another antiinfective is required.

Teach Patient/Family:

• To avoid exposure to sunlight and wear sunscreen if sun exposure is planned during treatment and for 5 days after treatment is stopped

spironolactone

speer-on-oh-lak′-tone
(Aldactone, Novospiroton[CAN], Spiractin[AUS])
Do not confuse Aldactone with Aldactazide.

CATEGORY AND SCHEDULE

Pregnancy Risk Category: C (D if used in pregnancy-induced hypertension)

MECHANISM OF ACTION

An potassium-sparing diuretic that interferes with sodium reabsorption by competitively inhibiting the action of aldosterone in the distal tubule, thus promoting sodium and water excretion and increasing potassium retention. ***Therapeutic Effect:*** Produces diuresis; lowers BP; diagnostic aid for primary aldosteronism.

PHARMACOKINETICS

Route	Onset	Peak	Duration
PO	24–48 hr	48–72 hr	48–72 hr

Well absorbed from the GI tract (absorption increased with food). Protein binding: 91%–98%. Metabolized in the liver to active metabolite. Primarily excreted in urine. Unknown if removed by hemodialysis. ***Half-life:*** 0–24 hr (metabolite, 13–24 hr).

AVAILABILITY

Tablets: 25 mg, 50 mg, 100 mg.

INDICATIONS AND DOSAGES

▸ **Edema**

PO

Adults, Elderly. 25–200 mg/day as a single dose or in 2 divided doses.
Children. 1.5–3.3 mg/kg/day in divided doses.
Neonates. 1–3 mg/kg/day in 1–2 divided doses.

▸ **Hypertension**

PO

Adults, Elderly. 25–50 mg/day in 1–2 doses/day.
Children. 1.5–3.3 mg/kg/day in divided doses.

▸ **Hypokalemia**

PO

Adults, Elderly. 25–200 mg/day as a single dose or in 2 divided doses.

▸ **Male Hirsutism**

PO

Adults, Elderly. 50–200 mg/day as a single dose or in 2 divided doses.

▸ **Primary Aldosteronism**

PO

Adults, Elderly. 100–400 mg/day as a single dose or in 2 divided doses.
Children. 100–400 mg/m^2/day as a single dose or in 2 divided doses.

▸ **Dosage in Renal Impairment**

Dosage interval is modified on the basis of creatinine clearance.

Creatinine Clearance	Interval
10–50 ml/min	Usual dose q12–24h
less than 10 ml/min	Avoid use.

OFF-LABEL USES

Treatment of female hirsutism, polycystic ovary disease

CONTRAINDICATIONS

Acute renal insufficiency, anuria, BUN and serum creatinine levels

S

more than twice normal values, hyperkalemia

INTERACTIONS

Drug

ACE inhibitors (such as captopril), potassium-containing medications, potassium supplements: May increase the risk of hyperkalemia.
Anticoagulants, heparin: May decrease the effects of these drugs.
Digoxin: May increase the half-life of digoxin.
Lithium: May decrease the clearance and increase the risk of toxicity of lithium.
NSAIDs: May decrease the antihypertensive effect of spironolactone.

Herbal

None known.

Food

None known.

Drug interactions of concern to dentistry

- Nephrotoxicity: indomethacin and possibly other NSAIDs
- Decreased antihypertensive effect: indomethacin and possibly other NSAIDs

DIAGNOSTIC TEST EFFECTS

May increase urinary calcium excretion; BUN and blood glucose levels; serum creatinine, magnesium, potassium, and uric acid levels. May decrease serum sodium level.

S

SIDE EFFECTS

Frequent

Hyperkalemia (in patients with renal insufficiency and those taking potassium supplements), dehydration, hyponatremia, lethargy

Occasional

Nausea, vomiting, anorexia, abdominal cramps, diarrhea, headache, ataxia, somnolence, confusion, fever
Male: Gynecomastia, impotence, decreased libido
Female: Menstrual irregularities (including amenorrhea and postmenopausal bleeding), breast tenderness

Rare

Rash, urticaria, hirsutism

SERIOUS REACTIONS

! Severe hyperkalemia may produce arrhythmias, bradycardia, and ECG changes (tented T waves, widening QRS complex and ST segment depression). These may proceed to cardiac standstill or ventricular fibrillation.
! Cirrhosis patients are at risk for hepatic decompensation if dehydration or hyponatremia occurs.
! Patients with primary aldosteronism may experience rapid weight loss and severe fatigue during high-dose therapy.

DENTAL CONSIDERATIONS

General:

- Monitor vital signs at every appointment because of CV side effects.
- Assess salivary flow as a factor in caries, periodontal disease, and candidiasis.
- If dry mouth occurs, follow usual preventive and palliative measures, but consider hyponatremia as a contributing factor.
- Consider semisupine chair position for patient comfort if GI side effects occur.

Consultations:

- Medical consultation may be required to assess disease control and patient's ability to tolerate stress.

Teach Patient/Family:

- *When chronic dry mouth occurs, advise patient:*
  - To avoid mouth rinses with high alcohol content because of drying effects

• Of need for daily use of home fluoride products to prevent caries
• To use sugarless gum, frequent sips of water, or saliva substitutes

sucralfate

soo-kral′-fate
(Apo-Sucralate[CAN], Carafate, Novo-Sucralate[CAN], Ulcyte[AUS])
Do not confuse Carafate with Cafergot.

CATEGORY AND SCHEDULE

Pregnancy Risk Category: B

MECHANISM OF ACTION

An antiulcer agent that forms an ulcer-adherent complex with proteinaceous exudate, such as albumin, at ulcer site. Also forms a viscous, adhesive barrier on the surface of intact mucosa of the stomach or duodenum. ***Therapeutic Effect:*** Protects damaged mucosa from further destruction by absorbing gastric acid, pepsin, and bile salts.

PHARMACOKINETICS

Minimally absorbed from the GI tract. Eliminated in feces, with small amount excreted in urine. Not removed by hemodialysis.

AVAILABILITY

Oral Suspension: 500 mg/ 5 ml.
Tablets: 1 g.

INDICATIONS AND DOSAGES

▸ Active Duodenal Ulcers

PO

Adults, Elderly. 1 g 4 times a day (before meals and at bedtime) for up to 8 wk.

▸ Maintenance Therapy After Healing of Acute Duodenal Ulcers

PO

Adults, Elderly. 1 g twice a day.

OFF-LABEL USES

Prevention and treatment of stress-related mucosal damage, especially in acutely or critically ill patients; treatment of gastric ulcer and rheumatoid arthritis; relief of GI symptoms associated with NSAIDs; treatment of gastroesophageal reflux disease

CONTRAINDICATIONS

None known.

INTERACTIONS

Drug

Antacids: May interfere with binding of sucralfate.
Digoxin, phenytoin, quinolones, such as ciprofloxacin, theophylline: May decrease the absorption of these drugs.

Herbal

None known.

Food

None known.

Drug interactions of concern to dentistry

• Gastric irritation: chloral hydrate
• Decreased absorption of tetracyclines, fluoroquinolones
• Decreased effects of diclofenac, ketoconazole

DIAGNOSTIC TEST EFFECTS

None known.

SIDE EFFECTS

Frequent (2%)

Constipation

Occasional (< 2%)

Dry mouth, backache, diarrhea, dizziness, somnolence, nausea, indigestion, rash, hives, itching, abdominal discomfort

SERIOUS REACTIONS

! None known.

DENTAL CONSIDERATIONS

General:

- Prescribe acetaminophen for analgesia if needed. ASA and NSAIDs are contraindicated in active upper GI disease.
- Consider semisupine chair position for patient comfort because of GI effects of disease.
- Tetracycline doses should be given 2 hr before or after the sucralfate dose.

Teach Patient/Family:

- To avoid mouth rinses with high alcohol content because of drying effects

sulconazole nitrate

sul-**kon**-a-zole-**nye**-trate
(Exelderm)

CATEGORY AND SCHEDULE

Pregnancy Risk Category: C

MECHANISM OF ACTION

An imidazole derivative that inhibits synthesis of ergosterol (vital component of fungal cell formation), damaging cell membrane. ***Therapeutic Effect:*** Fungistatic.

PHARMACOKINETICS

Minimal systemic absorption following topical administration. Excreted in urine. ***Half-life:*** Unknown.

AVAILABILITY

Cream (Exelderm): 1%.
Topical Solution (Exelderm): 1%.

INDICATIONS AND DOSAGES

▸ Tinea Pedis

TOPICAL

Adults, Elderly, Children 12 yr and Older. Apply 2 times per day until signs and symptoms significantly improve.

▸ Tinea Corporis, Tinea Cruris, Tinea Versicolor

TOPICAL

Adults, Elderly, Children 12 yr Aand Older. Apply 1–2 times per day until signs and symptoms significantly improve.

CONTRAINDICATIONS

Hypersensitivity to sulconazole nitrate or any component of the formulation

INTERACTIONS

Drug

None known.

Herbal

None known.

Food

None known.

DIAGNOSTIC TEST EFFECTS

None known.

SIDE EFFECTS

Oral: Headache, nausea

Rare

Burning or stinging, pruritus, redness

SERIOUS REACTIONS

None known.

DENTAL CONSIDERATIONS

General:

- There are no significant dental considerations. One possible concern is the few patients with topical candidiasis, in whom broad-spectrum antiinfectives could potentially contribute to a superinfection.

S

sulfacetamide

sul-fa-see′-ta-mide
(AK-Sulf, Bleph-10, Isopto Cetamide, Diosulf[CAN], Ophthacet, Sodium Sulamyd, Sulfair)

CATEGORY AND SCHEDULE

Pregnancy Risk Category: C

MECHANISM OF ACTION

Interferes with synthesis of folic acid that bacteria require for growth.
Therapeutic Effect: Prevents further bacterial growth. Bacteriostatic.

PHARMACOKINETICS

Small amounts may be absorbed into the cornea. Excreted rapidly in urine.
Half-life: 7–13 hrs.

AVAILABILITY

Lotion: 10% (Carmol, Klaron, Ovace).
Ophthalmic ointment: 10% (AK-Sulf).
Ophthalmic solution: 10% (Bleph-10, Ocusulf, Sulf-10).

INDICATIONS AND DOSAGES

▸ **Treatment of Corneal Ulcers, Conjunctivitis and Other Superficial Infections of the Eye, Prophylaxis After Injuries to the Eye/Removal of Foreign Bodies, Adjunctive Therapy for Trachoma and Inclusion Conjunctivitis**

OPHTHALMIC

Adults, Elderly. Ointment: Apply small amount in lower conjunctival sac 1–4 times/day and at bedtime. Solution: 1–3 drops to lower conjunctival sac q2–3h. Seborrheic dermatitis, seborrheic sicca (dandruff), secondary bacterial skin infections

TOPICAL

Adults, Elderly. Apply 1–4 times/day.

OFF-LABEL USES

Treatment of bacterial blepharitis, blepharoconjunctivitis, bacterial keratitis, keratoconjunctivitis

CONTRAINDICATIONS

Hypersensitivity to sulfonamides or any component of preparation (some products contain sulfite), use in combination with silver-containing products

INTERACTIONS

Drug

Silver-containing preparations: These products are incompatible together.

Herbal

None known.

Food

None known.

Drug interactions of concern to dentistry

- None reported

DIAGNOSTIC TEST EFFECTS

None known.

SIDE EFFECTS

Frequent

Transient ophthalmic burning, stinging

Occasional

Headache

Rare

Hypersensitivity (erythema, rash, itching, swelling, photosensitivity)

SERIOUS REACTIONS

! Superinfection, drug-induced lupus erythematosus, Stevens-Johnson syndrome occur rarely; nephrotoxicity w/high dermatologic concentrations.

DENTAL CONSIDERATIONS

General:

- Protect patient's eye from accidental spatter during dental treatment.

- Avoid dental light in patient's eyes; offer dark glasses for patient comfort.

sulfasalazine

sul-fa-sal′-a-zeen
(Alti-Sulfasalazine[CAN], Azulfidine, Azulfidine EN-tabs, Pyralin EN[AUS], Salazopyrin[CAN], Salazopyrin EN[AUS], Salazopyrin EN-Tabs[CAN])

Do not confuse Azulfidine with azathioprine, or sulfasalazine with sulfadiazine or sulfisoxazole.

CATEGORY AND SCHEDULE

Pregnancy Risk Category: B (D if given near term)

MECHANISM OF ACTION

A sulfonamide that inhibits prostaglandin synthesis, acting locally in the colon. ***Therapeutic Effect:*** Decreases inflammatory response, interferes with GI secretion.

PHARMACOKINETICS

Poorly absorbed from the GI tract. Cleaved in colon by intestinal bacteria, forming sulfapyridine and mesalamine (5-ASA). Absorbed in colon. Widely distributed. Metabolized in the liver. Primarily excreted in urine. ***Half-life:*** sulfapyridine, 6–14 hr; 5-ASA, 0.6–1.4 hr.

S

AVAILABILITY

Tablets (Azulfidine): 500 mg.
Tablets (Delayed-Release [Azulfidine EN-Tabs]): 500 mg.

INDICATIONS AND DOSAGES

▸ **Ulcerative Colitis**

PO

Adults, Elderly. 1 g 3–4 times a day in divided doses q4–6h. Maintenance: 2 g/day in divided doses q6–12h. Maximum: 6 g/day.

Children. 40–75 mg/kg/day in divided doses q4–6h. Maintenance: 30–50 mg/kg/day in divided doses q4–8h. Maximum: 2 g/day. Maximum: 6 g/day.

▸ **Rheumatoid Arthritis**

PO

Adults, Elderly. Initially, 0.5–1 g/day for 1 wk. Increase by 0.5 g/wk, up to 3 g/day.

▸ **Juvenile Rheumatoid Arthritis**

PO

Children. Initially, 10 mg/kg/day. May increase by 10 mg/kg/day at weekly intervals. Range: 30–50 mg/kg/day. Maximum: 2 g/day.

OFF-LABEL USES

Treatment of ankylosing spondylitis

CONTRAINDICATIONS

Children younger than 2 years; hypersensitivity to carbonic anhydrase inhibitors, local anesthetics, salicylates, sulfonamides, sulfonylureas, sunscreens containing PABA, or thiazide or loop diuretics; intestinal or urinary tract obstruction; porphyria; pregnancy at term; severe hepatic or renal dysfunction

INTERACTIONS

Drug

Anticonvulsants, methotrexate, oral anticoagulants, oral antidiabetics: May increase the effects of these drugs.
Hemolytics: May increase the toxicity of sulfasalazine.
Hepatotoxic medications: May increase the risk of hepatotoxicity.

Herbal

None known.

Food

None known.

Drug interactions of concern to dentistry

- Increased photosensitizing effects: tetracycline
- Decreased absorption: folic acid

DIAGNOSTIC TEST EFFECTS

None known.

SIDE EFFECTS

Frequent (33%)

Anorexia, nausea, vomiting, headache, oligospermia (generally reversed by withdrawal of drug)

Occasional (3%)

Hypersensitivity reaction (rash, urticaria, pruritus, fever, anemia)

Rare (< 1%)

Tinnitus, hypoglycemia, diuresis, photosensitivity

SERIOUS REACTIONS

! Anaphylaxis, Stevens-Johnson syndrome, hematologic toxicity (leukopenia, agranulocytosis), hepatotoxicity, and nephrotoxicity occur rarely.

DENTAL CONSIDERATIONS

General:

- Patients on chronic drug therapy may rarely have symptoms of blood dyscrasias, which can include infection, bleeding, and poor healing.
- Question patient about response to antibiotics to avoid responses that might provoke pseudomembranous colitis.
- Palliative medication may be required for management of oral side effects.
- Consider semisupine chair position for patient comfort because of GI effects of disease.

Consultations:

- Medical consultation may be required to assess disease control and patient's ability to tolerate stress.
- In a patient with symptoms of blood dyscrasias, request a medical consultation for blood studies and postpone dental treatment until normal values are reestablished.

Teach Patient/Family:

- Caution to prevent injury when using oral hygiene aids

sulfinpyrazone

sul-fin-pyr′-a-zone
(Anturane, Apo-Sulfinpyrazone[CAN], Nu-Sufinpyrazone[CAN])
Do not confuse with Accutane.

CATEGORY AND SCHEDULE

Pregnancy Risk Category: C/D (near term)

MECHANISM OF ACTION

A uricosuric that increases urinary excretion of uric acid, thereby decreasing blood urate levels. ***Therapeutic Effect:*** Promotes uric acid excretion and reduces serum uric acid levels.

PHARMACOKINETICS

Rapidly and completely absorbed from gastrointestinal (GI) tract. Widely distributed. Metabolized in liver to two active metabolite, p-hydroxy-sulfinpyrazone and a sulfide analogue. Excreted primarily in urine. Not removed by hemodialysis. ***Half-life:*** 2.7–6 hrs.

AVAILABILITY

Tablets: 100 mg (Anturane).

INDICATIONS AND DOSAGES

▸ **Gout**

PO

Adults, Elderly. 100–200 mg 2 times/day. Maximum: 800 mg/day.

S

OFF-LABEL USES
Mitral valve replacement, myocardial infarction

CONTRAINDICATIONS
Active peptic ulcer, blood dyscrasias, GI inflammation, pregnancy (near term), hypersensitivity to sulfinpyrazone, phenylbutazone, other pyrazoles, or any of its components

INTERACTIONS
Drug
Acetaminophen: May increase risk of heptotoxicity and decrease effect of sulfinpyrazone.
Aspirin: May decrease uricosuric effect.
Oral anticoagulants: May increase anticoagulant effect.
Oral hypoglycemics: May increase hypoglycemic effect.
Salicylates, niacin: May decrease uricosuric activity.
Theophylline, verapamil: May decrease effects and levels of theophylline and verapamil.
Herbal
Arnica, astragalus, bilberry, black currant, cat's claw, chaparral, chondroitin, clove oil, evening primrose, feverfew, ginger, Ginkgo biloba, hawthorn, kava kava, skullcap, tan-shen: May increase risk of bleeding.
Dong quai, St. John's Wort: May increase risk of photosensitization.
Food
Rhubarb: May increase risk of bleeding.
Drug interactions of concern to dentistry
- Increased bleeding: NSAIDs, aspirin
- Decreased effects of salicylates

DIAGNOSTIC TEST EFFECTS
May alter serum uric acid levels.

SIDE EFFECTS
Frequent
Nausea, vomiting, stomach pain
Occasional
Flushed face, headache, dizziness, frequent urge to urinate, rash
Rare
Increased bleeding time, hepatic necrosis, nephrotic syndrome, uric acid stones

SERIOUS REACTIONS
! Hematological toxicity including anemia, leucopenia, agranulocytosis, thrombocytopenia, and aplastic anemia occur rarely.
! Overdose causes a drowsiness, dizziness, anorexia, abdominal pain, hemolytic anemia, acidosis, jaundice, fever, and agranulocytosis.

DENTAL CONSIDERATIONS
General:
- Consider local hemostasis measures to prevent excessive bleeding.
- Avoid prescribing aspirin-containing products.
- Patients on chronic drug therapy may rarely have symptoms of blood dyscrasias, which can include infection, bleeding, and poor healing.
- Consider semisupine chair position for patient comfort if GI side effects occur.
- Evaluate respiration characteristics and rate.

Consultations:
- In a patient with symptoms of blood dyscrasias, request a medical consultation for blood studies and postpone dental treatment until normal values are reestablished.

Teach Patient/Family:
- Caution to prevent injury when using oral hygiene aids

sulfisoxazole

sul-fi-sox′-a-zole

Gantrisin, Novo-Soxazole[CAN], Sulfizole[CAN], Truxazole

Do not confuse with sulfadiazine, sulfamethoxazole, sulfasalazine, Gastrosed

CATEGORY AND SCHEDULE

Pregnancy risk category: B/D (near term)

MECHANISM OF ACTION

An antibacterial sulphonamide that inhibits bacterial synthesis of dihydrofolic acid by preventing condensation of pteridine with aminobenzoic acid through competitive inhibition of the enzyme dihydropteroate synthetase. ***Therapeutic Effect:*** Bacteriostatic.

PHARMACOKINETICS

Rapidly and completely absorbed. Small intestine is major site of absorption, but some absorption occurs in the stomach. Exists in the blood as unbound, protein-bound and conjugated forms. Sulfisoxazole is metabolized primarily by acetylation and oxidation in the liver. The free form is considered to be the therapeutically active form. Protein binding: 85%. ***Half-life:*** 5–8 hrs.

AVAILABILITY

Tablet: *500 mg* *Powder:* 100%
Suspension: 500 mg/5 mL (Gantrisin)

INDICATIONS AND DOSAGES

▸ Acute, Recurrent or Chronic Urinary Tract Infections, Meningococcal Meningitis, Acute Otitis Media due to Haemophilus Influenzae

PO

Infants Older Than 2 Months of Age, Children: One-half of the 24-hr dose initially then 150 mg/kg daily or 4 g/M2 daily for maintanence divided q4–6h. Maximum dose: 6 g daily.
Adults: 2–4 g initially then 4–8 g daily divided q4–6h.

CONTRAINDICATIONS

Patients with a known hypersensitivity to sulfonamides, children younger than 2 months (except in the treatment of congenital toxoplasmosis as adjunctive therapy with pyrimethamine), pregnant women at term, and mothers nursing infants younger than 2 months of age.

INTERACTIONS

Drug

Warfarin: May prolong prothrombin time.
Thiopental: May increase effect of thiopental.
Methotrexate: May increase free Methotrexate concentrations.
Sulfonylureas: May increase hypoglycemic effect of sulfonylureas.

Herbal

Dong quai, St. John's Wort: May cause photosensitization.

Food

Folate: May decrease folate absorption.

Drug interactions of concern to dentistry

- Decreased effect: ester-type local anesthetics (procaine, tetracaine)
- Increased photosensitizing effect: tetracycline
- Decreased effect of penicillins, cephalosporins

DIAGNOSTIC TEST EFFECTS

May cause false-positive for protein in urine and urine glucose with Clinitest.

SIDE EFFECTS

Anaphylaxis, erythema multiforme (Stevens-Johnson syndrome), toxic epidermal necrolysis, exfoliative dermatitis, angioedema, arteritis and vasculitis, allergic myocarditis, serum sickness, rash, urticaria, pruritus, photosensitivity, conjunctival and scleral injection, generalized allergic reactions, generalized skin eruptions, tachycardia, palpitations, syncope, cyanosis, goiter, diuresis, hypoglycaemia, arthralgia, myalgia, headache, dizziness, peripheral neuritis, paresthesia, convulsions, tinnitus, vertigo, ataxia, intracranial hypertension, cough, shortness of breath, pulmonary infiltrates

SERIOUS REACTIONS

! Fatalities associated with the administration of sulfonamides including Stevens-Johnson Syndrome toxic epidermal necrolysis, fulminant hepatic necrosis, agranulocytosis, aplastic anemia, and other blood dyscrasias occur rarely.
! Clinical signs, such as rash, sore throat, fever, arthralgia, pallor, purpura or jaundice, may be early indications of serious reactions.

DENTAL CONSIDERATIONS

General:
- Patients on chronic drug therapy may rarely have symptoms of blood dyscrasias, which can include infection, bleeding, and poor healing.
- Determine why the patient is taking the drug.
- Palliative medication may be required for management of oral side effects.
- Consider semisupine chair position for patient comfort if GI side effects occur.

Consultations:
- Medical consultation may be required to assess disease control.
- In a patient with symptoms of blood dyscrasias, request a medical consultation for blood studies and postpone dental treatment until normal values are reestablished.

Teach Patient/Family:
- Importance of good oral hygiene to prevent soft tissue inflammation

sulindac

sul-in′-dak
(Aclin[AUS], Apo-Sulin[CAN], Clinoril, Novo Sundac[CAN])
Do not confuse Clinoril with Clozaril.

CATEGORY AND SCHEDULE

Pregnancy Risk Category: B (D if used in third trimester or near delivery)

MECHANISM OF ACTION

An NSAID that produces analgesic and anti-inflammatory effects by inhibiting prostaglandin synthesis.
Therapeutic Effect: Reduces inflammatory response and intensity of pain.

PHARMACOKINETICS

Route	Onset	Peak	Duration
PO (Antirheumatic)	7 days	2–3 wk	N/A

Well absorbed from the GI tract. Metabolized in liver to active metabolite. Primarily excreted in urine. Not removed by hemodialysis. ***Half-life:*** 7.8 hr; metabolite: 16.4 hr.

AVAILABILITY

Tablets: 150 mg, 200 mg.

INDICATIONS AND DOSAGES

▸ Rheumatoid Arthritis, Osteoarthritis, Ankylosing Spondylitis

PO

Adults, Elderly. Initially, 150 mg twice a day; may increase up to 400 mg/day.

▸ Acute Shoulder Pain, Gouty Arthritis, Bursitis, Tendinitis

PO

Adults, Elderly. 200 mg twice a day.

CONTRAINDICATIONS

Active peptic ulcer disease, chronic inflammation of GI tract, GI bleeding or ulceration, history of hypersensitivity to aspirin or NSAIDs

INTERACTIONS

Drug

Antacids: May decrease the sulindac blood concentration.

Antihypertensives, diuretics: May decrease the effects of these drugs.

Aspirin, other salicylates: May increase the risk of GI side effects, such as bleeding.

Bone marrow depressants: May increase the risk of hematologic reactions.

Heparin, oral anticoagulants, thrombolytics: May increase the effects of these drugs.

Lithium: May increase the blood concentration and risk of toxicity of lithium.

Methotrexate: May increase the risk of methotrexate toxicity.

Probenecid: May increase the sulindac blood concentration.

Herbal

Feverfew: May decrease the effects of feverfew.

Ginkgo biloba: May increase the risk of bleeding.

Food

None known.

Drug interactions of concern to dentistry

- Increased bleeding, GI effects: alcohol, aspirin, steroids, other NSAIDs
- Renal toxicity: acetaminophen (prolonged use)
- Possible risk of decreased renal function: cyclosporine
- Increased photosensitizing effect: tetracycline
- Increased toxicity of methotrexate, cyclosporine
- Decreased plasma levels: diflunisal
- First-time users of SSRIs also taking NSAIDs may have a higher risk of GI side effects; until more data are available, it may be advisable to avoid use of NSAIDs in these patients (*Br J Clin Pharmacol* 55:591–595, 2003)

DIAGNOSTIC TEST EFFECTS

May increase liver function test results and serum alkaline phosphatase level.

SIDE EFFECTS

Frequent (9%–4%)

Diarrhea or constipation, indigestion, nausea, maculopapular rash, dermatitis, dizziness, headache

Occasional (3%–1%)

Anorexia, abdominal cramps, flatulence

SERIOUS REACTIONS

! Rare reactions with long-term use include peptic ulcer disease, GI bleeding, gastritis, nephrotoxicity (glomerular nephritis, interstitial nephritis, nephrotic syndrome), severe hepatic reactions (cholestasis, jaundice), and severe hypersensitivity reactions (fever, chills, and joint pain).

DENTAL CONSIDERATIONS

General:

- Patients on chronic drug therapy may rarely have symptoms of blood dyscrasias, which can include infection, bleeding, and poor healing.

- Assess salivary flow as a factor in caries, periodontal disease, and candidiasis.
- Avoid prescribing in last trimester of pregnancy.
- Should oral inflammation or lesions occur, refer to physician and consider palliative treatment for the lesions.
- Consider semisupine chair position for patient comfort because of GI side effects.

Consultations:

- Medical consultation may be required to assess disease control.
- In a patient with symptoms of blood dyscrasias, request a medical consultation for blood studies and postpone dental treatment until normal values are reestablished.

Teach Patient/Family:

- To report oral lesions, soreness, or bleeding to dentist
- Caution to prevent injury in use of oral hygiene aids
- Importance of good oral hygiene to prevent soft tissue inflammation
- *When chronic dry mouth occurs, advise patient:*
  - To avoid mouth rinses with high alcohol content because of drying effects
  - Of need for daily use of home fluoride products to prevent caries
  - To use sugarless gum, frequent sips of water, or saliva substitutes

S

sumatriptan

soo-ma-trip′-tan
(Imigran[AUS], Imitrex, Suvalan[AUS])
Do not confuse sumatriptan with somatropin.

CATEGORY AND SCHEDULE

Pregnancy Risk Category: C

MECHANISM OF ACTION

A serotonin receptor agonist that binds selectively to vascular receptors, producing a vasoconstrictive effect on cranial blood vessels.
Therapeutic Effect: Relieves migraine headache.

PHARMACOKINETICS

Route	Onset	Peak	Duration
Nasal	15 min	N/A	24–48 h
PO	30 min	2 h	24–48 h
Subcutaneous	10 min	1 h	24–48 h

Rapidly absorbed after subcutaneous administration. Absorption after PO administration is incomplete, with significant amounts undergoing hepatic metabolism, resulting in low bioavailability (about 14%). Protein binding: 10%–21%. Widely distributed. Undergoes first-pass metabolism in the liver. Excreted in urine.
Half-life: 2 hr.

AVAILABILITY

Tablets: 25 mg, 50 mg, 100 mg.
Injection: 6 mg/0.5 ml.
Nasal Spray: 5 mg, 20 mg.

INDICATIONS AND DOSAGES

▸ Acute Migraine Attack

PO

Adults, Elderly. 25–50 mg. Dose may be repeated after at least 2 hr. Maximum: 100 mg/single dose; 200 mg/24 hr.

SUBCUTANEOUS

Adults, Elderly. 6 mg. Maximum: Two 6-mg injections/24 hr (separated by at least 1 hr).

INTRANASAL

Adults, Elderly. 5–20 mg; may repeat in 2 hr. Maximum: 40 mg/24 hr.

CONTRAINDICATIONS

CVA, ischemic heart disease (including angina pectoris, history of MI, silent ischemia, and Prinzmetal's angina), severe hepatic impairment, transient ischemic attack, uncontrolled hypertension, use within 14 days of MAOIs, use within 24 hr of ergotamine preparations

INTERACTIONS

Drug

Ergotamine-containing medications: May produce vasospastic reaction.
MAOIs: May increase sumatriptan blood concentration and half-life.

Herbal

None known.

Food

None known.

Drug interactions of concern to dentistry

- None reported; avoid ergot-containing medications

DIAGNOSTIC TEST EFFECTS

None known.

SIDE EFFECTS

Frequent

Oral (10%–5%): Tingling, nasal discomfort
Subcutaneous (> 10%): Injection site reactions, tingling, warm or hot sensation, dizziness, vertigo
Nasal (> 10%): Bad or unusual taste, nausea, vomiting

Occasional

Oral (5%–1%): Flushing, asthenia, visual disturbances
Subcutaneous (10%–2%): Burning sensation, numbness, chest discomfort, drowsiness, asthenia
Nasal (5%–1%): Nasopharyngeal discomfort, dizziness

Rare

Oral (< 1%): Agitation, eye irritation, dysuria
Subcutaneous (< 2%): Anxiety, fatigue, diaphoresis, muscle cramps, myalgia
Nasal (< 1%): Burning sensation

SERIOUS REACTIONS

! Excessive dosage may produce tremor, red extremities, reduced respirations, cyanosis, seizures, and paralysis.
! Serious arrhythmias occur rarely, especially in patients with hypertension, diabetes, or a strong family history of coronary artery disease; obese patients; and smokers.

DENTAL CONSIDERATIONS

- Be aware of the patient's disease, its severity, and its frequency, when known.
- Monitor vital signs at every appointment because of CV side effects.
- Avoid dental light in patient's eyes; offer dark glasses for patient comfort.

Consultations:

- If treating chronic orofacial pain, consult with physician of record.

Teach Patient/Family:

- That oral symptoms uncommonly occur and will disappear when drug is discontinued

S

suprofen

soo-proe′-fen
(Profenal)

CATEGORY AND SCHEDULE

Pregnancy Risk Category: C

MECHANISM OF ACTION

A nonsteroidal anti-inflammatory that inhibits prostaglandin synthesis and the intensity of pain stimulus

reaching sensory nerve endings. Constricts iris sphincter.
Therapeutic Effect: Produces analgesic and anti-inflammatory effect. Prevents miosis during cataract surgery.

PHARMACOKINETICS

No data available on systemic absorption.

AVAILABILITY

Ophthalmic Solution: 1% (Profenal).

INDICATIONS AND DOSAGES

▸ Miosis Inhibitor in Ophthalmic Surgery

OphthalmicAdults, Elderly. Apply 2 drops 3, 2, and 1 hour prior to surgery. If desired, 2 drops may be applied q4h while the patient is awake on the day prior to surgery.

CONTRAINDICATIONS

Rhinitis, urticaria, asthma, allergic reactions to aspirin or other anti-inflammatory agents, epithelial herpes keratitis, hypersensitivity to suprofen or any component of the formulation.

INTERACTIONS

Drug
None known.

Herbal
None known.

Food
None known.

Drug interactions of concern to dentistry
- None reported

DIAGNOSTIC TEST EFFECTS

None known.

SIDE EFFECTS

Frequent
Burning, stinging on instillation, ocular discomfort

Occasional
Itching, tearing

Rare
Headache, trouble sleeping, weakness

SERIOUS REACTIONS

! Nausea or vomiting, pain, sensitivity to light, trouble breathing, and shortness of breath occur rarely.

DENTAL CONSIDERATIONS

General:
- Protect patient's eyes from accidental spatter during dental treatment.
- Avoid dental light inpatient's eyes; offer dark glasses for patient comfort.

S

tacrine hydrochloride

tack′-rin
(Cognex)

CATEGORY AND SCHEDULE

Pregnancy Risk Category: C

MECHANISM OF ACTION

A cholinesterase inhibitor that inhibits the enzyme acetylcholinesterase, thus increasing the concentration of acetylcholine at cholinergic synapses and enhancing cholinergic function in the CNS. ***Therapeutic Effect:*** Slows the progression of Alzheimer's disease.

AVAILABILITY

Capsules: 10 mg, 20 mg, 30 mg, 40 mg.

INDICATIONS AND DOSAGES

▸ Alzheimer's Disease

PO

Adults, Elderly. Initially, 10 mg 4 times a day for 6 wk, followed by 20 mg 4 times a day for 6 wk, 30 mg 4 times a day for 12 wk, then 40 mg 4 times a day if needed.

▸ Dosage in Hepatic Impairment

For patients with ALT (SGPT) greater than 3–5 times normal, decrease the dose by 40 mg/day and resume the normal dose when ALT (SGPT) returns to normal. For patients with ALT (SGPT) greater than 5 times normal, stop treatment and resume it when ALT (SGPT) returns to normal.

CONTRAINDICATIONS

Known hypersensitivity to tacrine, patients previously treated with tacrine who developed jaundice

INTERACTIONS

Drug

Anticholinergics: May decrease the effects of tacrine oranticholinergics.
Cimetidine: May increase the tacrine blood concentration.
NSAIDs: May increase the adverse effects of NSAIDs.
Theophylline: May increase the theophylline blood concentration.

Herbal

None known.

Food

None known.

Drug interactions of concern to dentistry

- Potential increase in GI complaints: NSAIDs
- Action inhibited by anticholinergic drugs
- Increased effects with succinylcholine and other cholinergic agonists

DIAGNOSTIC TEST EFFECTS

Increases AST (SGOT) and ALT (SGPT) levels. Alters blood Hgb, Hct, and serum electrolyte levels.

SIDE EFFECTS

Frequent (28%–11%)
Headache, nausea, vomiting, diarrhea, dizziness

Occasional (9%–4%)
Fatigue, chest pain, dyspepsia, anorexia, abdominal pain, flatulence, constipation, confusion, agitation, rash, depression, ataxia, insomnia, rhinitis, myalgia

Rare (< 3%)
Weight loss, anxiety, cough, facial flushing, urinary frequency, back pain, tremor

SERIOUS REACTIONS

! Overdose can cause cholinergic crisis, marked by increased salivation, lacrimation, bradycardia, respiratory depression, hypotension, and increased muscle weakness. Treatment usually consists of supportive measures and an anticholinergic, such as atropine.

DENTAL CONSIDERATIONS

General:

- Patients on chronic drug therapy may rarely have symptoms of blood dyscrasias, which can include infection, bleeding, and poor healing.
- Monitor vital signs at every appointment because of CV and respiratory side effects.
- After supine positioning, have patient sit upright for at least 2 min before standing to avoid orthostatic hypotension.
- Assess salivary flow as a factor in caries, periodontal disease, and candidiasis.
- Take precautions if dental surgery is anticipated and anesthesia is required.
- Consider semisupine chair position for patient comfort because of GI effects of drug.
- Place on frequent recall because early attention to dental health is important for Alzheimer's patients.

Consultations:

- Medical consultation may be required to assess disease control.
- In a patient with symptoms of blood dyscrasias, request a medical consultation for blood studies and postpone dental treatment until normal values are reestablished.

Teach Patient/Family:

- Importance of good oral hygiene to prevent soft tissue inflammation
- To prevent injury when using oral hygiene aids
- Use of electric toothbrush if patient has difficulty holding conventional devices
- *When chronic dry mouth occurs, advise patient:*
  - To avoid mouth rinses with high alcohol content because of drying effects
  - Of need for daily home fluoride use to prevent caries
  - To use sugarless gum, frequent sips of water, or saliva substitutes

tacrolimus

tak-roe-leem′-us

(Prograf, Protopic)

Do not confuse Protopic with Protonix, Protopam, Protopin.

CATEGORY AND SCHEDULE

Pregnancy Risk Category: C

MECHANISM OF ACTION

An immunologic agent that inhibits T-lymphocyte activation by binding to intracellular proteins, forming a complex, and inhibiting phosphatase activity. ***Therapeutic Effect:*** Suppresses the immunologically mediated inflammatory response; prevents organ transplant rejection.

PHARMACOKINETICS

Variably absorbed after PO administration (food reduces absorption). Protein binding: 75%–97%. Extensively metabolized in the liver. Excreted in urine. Not removed by hemodialysis. ***Half-life:*** 11.7 hr.

AVAILABILITY

Capsules (Prograf): 0.5 mg, 1 mg, 5 mg.

T

Injection (Prograf): 5 mg/ml.
Ointment (Protopic): 0.03%, 0.1%.

INDICATIONS AND DOSAGES

▸ Prevention of Liver Transplant Rejection

PO

Adults, Elderly. 0.1–0.15 mg/kg/day in 2 divided doses 12 hr apart.
Children. 0.15–0.2 mg/kg/day in 2 divided doses 12 hr apart.

IV

Adults, Elderly, Children. 0.03–0.15 mg/kg/day as a continuous infusion.

▸ Prevention of Kidney Transplant Rejection

PO

Adults, Elderly. 0.2 mg/kg/day in 2 divided doses 12 hr apart

IV

Adults, Elderly. 0.03–0.15 mg/kg/day as continuous infusion.

▸ Atopic Dermatitis

TOPICAL

Adults, Elderly, Children 2 yr and older. Apply 0.03% ointment to affected area twice a day. 0.1% ointment may be used in adults and the elderly. Continue until 1 wk after symptoms have cleared.

OFF-LABEL USES

Prevention of organ rejection in patients receiving allogeneic bone marrow, heart, pancreas, pancreatic island cell, or small-bowel transplant, treatment of autoimmune disease, severe recalcitrant psoriasis

CONTRAINDICATIONS

Concurrent use with cyclosporine (increases the risk of nephrotoxicity), hypersensitivity to HCO-60 polyoxyl 60 hydrogenated castor oil (used in solution for injection), hypersensitivity to tacrolimus

INTERACTIONS

Drug

Aminoglycosides, amphotericin B, cisplatin: Increase the risk of renal dysfunction.
Antacids: Decrease the absorption of tacrolimus.
Antifungals, bromocriptine, calcium channel blockers, cimetidine, clarithromycin, cyclosporine, danazol, diltiazem, erythromycin, methylprednisolone, metoclopramide: Increase tacrolimus blood concentration.
Carbamazepine, phenobarbital, phenytoin, rifamycin: Decrease tacrolimus blood concentration.
Cyclosporine: Increases the risk of nephrotoxicity.
Live-virus vaccines: May potentiate virus replication, increase vaccine side effects, and decrease the patient's antibody response to the vaccine.
Other immunosuppressants: May increase the risk of infection or lymphomas.

Herbal

Echinacea: May decrease the effects of tacrolimus.

Food

Grapefruit, grapefruit juice: May alter the effects of the drug.

Drug interactions of concern to dentistry

tacrolimus (topical)

- No drug interactions are documented, but use with caution in patients taking CYP3A4 isoenzyme inhibitors: erythromycin, itraconazole, ketoconazole, fluconazole

tacrolimus (FK506)

- No confirmed studies to date: avoid drugs with potential for renal impairment
- Risk of increased blood levels with clotrimazole, fluconazole,

T

ketoconazole, clarithromycin, erythromycin, and methylprednisolone
• Risk of decreased blood levels with carbamazepine, phenobarbital, St. John's wort (herb)

DIAGNOSTIC TEST EFFECTS

May increase blood glucose, BUN, and serum creatinine levels, as well as WBC count. May decrease serum magnesium level and RBC and thrombocyte counts. May alter serum potassium level.

IV INCOMPATIBILITIES

No known drug incompatibilities. Do not mix tacrolimus with other medications if possible.

IV COMPATIBILITIES

Calcium gluconate, dexamethasone (Decadron), diphenhydramine (Benadryl), dobutamine (Dobutrex), dopamine (Intropin), furosemide (Lasix), heparin, hydromorphone (Dilaudid), insulin, leucovorin, lorazepam (Ativan), morphine, nitroglycerin, potassium chloride

SIDE EFFECTS

Frequent (> 30%)
Headache, tremor, insomnia, paresthesia, diarrhea, nausea, constipation, vomiting, abdominal pain, hypertension
Occasional (29%–10%)
Rash, pruritus, anorexia, asthenia, peripheral edema, photosensitivity

SERIOUS REACTIONS

! Nephrotoxicity (characterized by increased serum creatinine level and decreased urine output), neurotoxicity (including tremor, headache, and mental status changes), and pleural effusion are common adverse reactions.
! Thrombocytopenia, leukocytosis, anemia, atelectasis, sepsis, and infection occur occasionally.

DENTAL CONSIDERATIONS

TACROLIMUS (TOPICAL)

General:
• Advise patient if dental drugs prescribed have a potential for photosensitivity.

TACROLIMUS (FK506)

General:
• Patients on immunosuppressant therapy have increased susceptibility to infection.
• Patients on chronic drug therapy may rarely have symptoms of blood dyscrasias, which can include infection, bleeding, and poor healing.
• Monitor vital signs at every appointment because of CV side effects.
• Prophylactic antibiotics may be indicated to prevent infection if surgery or deep scaling is planned.
• Examine for evidence of oral candidiasis. Topically acting antifungals may be preferred.

Consultations:
• Medical consultation may be required to assess disease control.
• In a patient with symptoms of blood dyscrasias, request a medical consultation for blood studies and postpone dental treatment until normal values are reestablished.
• Consult with patient's physician for recommendations on possible antibiotic prophylaxis before dental treatment or when considering use of systemic antifungals.

Teach Patient/Family:

- Importance of good oral hygiene to prevent soft tissue inflammation
- Caution to prevent injury when using oral hygiene aids
- Use of electric toothbrush if patient has difficulty holding conventional devices
- That secondary oral infection may occur; must see dentist immediately if infection occurs
- To report oral lesions, soreness, or bleeding to dentist

tadalafil

tah-dal′-ah-fill
(Cialis)

CATEGORY AND SCHEDULE

Pregnancy Risk Category: B

MECHANISM OF ACTION

An erectile dysfunction agent that inhibits phosphodiesterase type 5, the enzyme responsible for degrading cyclic guanosine monophosphate in the corpus cavernosum of the penis, resulting in smooth muscle relaxation and increased blood flow. ***Therapeutic Effect:*** Facilitates an erection.

PHARMACOKINETICS

Route	Onset	Peak	Duration
PO	16 min	2 hr	36 hr

Rapidly absorbed after PO administration. Drug has no effect on penile blood flow without sexual stimulation. ***Half-life:*** 17.5 hour.

AVAILABILITY

Tablets: 5 mg, 10 mg, 20 mg.

INDICATIONS AND DOSAGES

▸ Erectile Dysfunction

PO

Adults, Elderly. 10 mg 30 min before sexual activity. Dose may be increased to 20 mg or decreased to 5 mg, based on patient tolerance. Maximum dosing frequency is once daily.

▸ Dosage in Renal Impairment

For patients with a creatinine clearance of 31–50 ml/min, the starting dose is 5 mg before sexual activity once a day and the maximum dose is 10 mg no more frequently than once q48h.
For patients with a creatinine clearance of less than 31 ml/min, the starting dose is 5 mg before sexual activity once a day.

▸ Dosage in Mild or Moderate Hepatic Impairment

Patients with Child-Pugh class A or B hepatic impairment should take no more than 10 mg once a day.

CONTRAINDICATIONS

Concurrent use of alpha-adrenergic blockers (other than the minimum dose tamsulosin), concurrent use of sodium nitroprusside or nitrates in any form, severe hepatic impairment

INTERACTIONS

Drug

Alcohol: Increases the risk of orthostatic hypotension.
Alpha-adrenergic blockers, nitrates: Potentiate the hypotensive effects of these drugs.
Doxazosin: May produce additive hypotensive effects.
Erythromycin, indinavir, itraconazole, ketoconazole, ritonavir: May increase tadalafil blood concentration.

Herbal

None known.

Food
None known.

Drug interactions of concern to dentistry

- Maximum dose in patients taking CYP3A4 isoenzyme inhibitors is 10 mg: includes ketoconazole, erythromycin, itraconazole, and other potent inhibitors of CYP3A4
- Avoid use of nitroglycerin within 24–36 hr

DIAGNOSTIC TEST EFFECTS
None known.

SIDE EFFECTS
Occasional
Headache, dyspepsia, back pain, myalgia, nasal congestion, flushing

SERIOUS REACTIONS
! Prolonged erections (lasting > 4 hours) and priapism (painful erections lasting > 6 hours) occur rarely.

DENTAL CONSIDERATIONS
General:

- This is an acute-use drug intended to be taken just before sexual activity. Be mindful of the drug interactions when prescribing potent inhibitors of CYP3A4 isoenzymes and warn patient.

T

tamoxifen citrate
ta-mox′-i-fen
(Apo-Tamox[CAN], Genox[AUS], Istubol, Nolvadex, Nolvadex-D[CAN], Novo-Tamoxifen[CAN], Tamofen[CAN], Tamosin[AUS])

CATEGORY AND SCHEDULE
Pregnancy Risk Category: D

MECHANISM OF ACTION
A nonsteroidal antiestrogen that competes with estradiol for estrogen-receptor binding sites in the breasts, uterus, and vagina. ***Therapeutic Effect:*** Inhibits DNA synthesis and estrogen response.

PHARMACOKINETICS
Well absorbed from the GI tract. Metabolized in the liver. Primarily eliminated in feces by biliary system. ***Half-life:*** 7 days.

AVAILABILITY
Tablets (Nolvadex): 10 mg, 20 mg.

INDICATIONS AND DOSAGES
▸ **Adjunctive Treatment of Breast Cancer**
PO
Adults, Elderly. 20–40 mg/day. Give doses greater than 20 mg/day in divided doses.

▸ **Prevention of Breast Cancer in High-Risk Women**
PO
Adults, Elderly. 20 mg/day.

OFF-LABEL USES
Induction of ovulation

CONTRAINDICATIONS
Concomitant coumarin-type therapy when used in the treatment of breast cancer in high-risk women,

history of deep vein thrombosis or pulmonary embolism in high-risk women, pregnancy

INTERACTIONS

Drug

Anticoagulants: May increase the risk of bleeding.
Estrogens: May decrease the effects of tamoxifen.

Herbal

Red clover, St. John's wort: May decrease tamoxifen's effectiveness.

Food

None known.

Drug interactions of concern to dentistry

- None reported

DIAGNOSTIC TEST EFFECTS

May increase serum cholesterol, calcium, and triglyceride levels.

SIDE EFFECTS

Frequent

Women (> 10%): Hot flashes, nausea, vomiting

Occasional

Women (9%–1%): Changes in menstruation, genital itching, vaginal discharge, endometrial hyperplasia or polyps
Men: Impotence, decreased libido
Men and women: Headache, nausea, vomiting, rash, bone pain, confusion, weakness, somnolence

SERIOUS REACTIONS

! Retinopathy, corneal opacity, and decreased visual acuity have been noted in patients receiving extremely high dosages (240–320 mg/day) for longer than 17 months.
! There have been an increased number of incidences of endometrial changes, thromboembolic events, and uterine malignancies while using tamoxifen.

DENTAL CONSIDERATIONS

General:

- Patients on chronic drug therapy may rarely have symptoms of blood dyscrasias, which can include infection, bleeding, and poor healing.
- Consider semisupine chair position for patient comfort if GI side effects occur.

Consultations:

- Medical consultation may be required to assess disease control.
- In a patient with symptoms of blood dyscrasias, request a medical consultation for blood studies and postpone dental treatment until normal values are reestablished.

Teach Patient/Family:

- Importance of good oral hygiene to prevent soft tissue inflammation

tamsulosin hydrochloride

tam-sool′-o-sin
(Flomax)
Do not confuse Flomax with Fosamax or Volmax.

CATEGORY AND SCHEDULE

Pregnancy Risk Category: B
(Not indicated for use in women.)

MECHANISM OF ACTION

An $alpha_1$ antagonist that targets receptors around bladder neck and prostate capsule. ***Therapeutic Effect:*** Relaxes smooth muscle and improves urinary flow and symptoms of prostatic hyperplasia.

PHARMACOKINETICS
Well absorbed and widely distributed. Protein binding: 94%–99%. Metabolized in the liver. Primarily excreted in urine. Unknown if removed by hemodialysis. ***Half-life:*** 9–13 hr.

AVAILABILITY
Capsules: 0.4 mg.

INDICATIONS AND DOSAGES
▸ Benign Prostatic Hyperplasia
PO
Adults. 0.4 mg once a day, approximately 30 min after same meal each day. May increase dosage to 0.8 mg if inadequate response in 2–4 wk.

CONTRAINDICATIONS
History of sensitivity to tamsulosin

INTERACTIONS
Drug
Other alpha-adrenergic blocking agents (such as cimetidine, doxazosin, prazosin, terazosin): May increase the alpha-blockade effects of both drugs.
Warfarin: May alter the effects of warfarin.
Herbal
None known.
Food
None known.
Drug interactions of concern to dentistry
- No interactions reported with usual dental drugs; it is possible but not known whether risk of orthostatic hypotension could be increased with conscious sedation techniques
- Opioids and anticholinergic drugs may enhance urinary retention; use alternative analgesics (NSAIDs)
- Caution in use or avoid concurrent use with other adrenergic antagonists

DIAGNOSTIC TEST EFFECTS
None known.

SIDE EFFECTS
Frequent (9%–7%)
Dizziness, somnolence
Occasional (5%–3%)
Headache, anxiety, insomnia, orthostatic hypotension
Rare (< 2%)
Nasal congestion, pharyngitis, rhinitis, nausea, vertigo, impotence

SERIOUS REACTIONS
! First-dose syncope (hypotension with sudden loss of consciousness) may occur within 30 to 90 minutes after administration of initial dose and may be preceded by tachycardia (pulse rate of 120–160 beats/minute).

DENTAL CONSIDERATIONS
General:
- Monitor vital signs at every appointment because of CV and respiratory side effects.
- Consider semisupine chair position for patient comfort when GI side effects occur.
- After supine positioning, have patient sit upright for at least 2 min before standing to avoid orthostatic hypotension.

tazarotene
ta-zare′-oh-teen
(Tazorac, Avage)

CATEGORY AND SCHEDULE
Pregnancy Risk Category: X

MECHANISM OF ACTION
Modulates differentiation and proliferation of epithelial tissue,

binds selectively to retinoic acid receptors. ***Therapeutic Effect:*** Restores normal differentiation of the epidermis and reduction in epidermal inflammation.

PHARMACOKINETICS

Minimal systemic absorption occurs through the skin. Binding to plasma proteins is greater than 99%. Metabolism is in the skin and liver. Elimination occurs through the fecal and renal pathways.
Half-life: 18 hours.

AVAILABILITY

Gel: 0.05%, 0.1% (Tazorac)
Cream: 0.05%, 0.1% (Tazorac)

INDICATIONS AND DOSAGES

▸ Psoriasis

TOPICAL

Adults, adolescents, children >12 years. Thin film applied once daily in the evening; only cover the lesions, and area should be dry before application

▸ Acne Vulgaris

TOPICAL

Adults, adolescents, children > 12 years. Thin film applied to affected areas once daily in the evening, after face is gently cleansed and dried.

▸ Fine Facial Wrinkles, Facial Mottled Hyperpigmentation (Liver Spots), Hypopigmentation Associated with Photoaging

TOPICAL

Adults. Thin film applied to affected areas once daily in the evening, after face is gently cleansed and dried.

CONTRAINDICATIONS

Should not be used in pregnant women, patients with hypersensitivity to tazarotene, benzyl alcohol, or any one of its components.

INTERACTIONS

Drug

Ethanol, benzoyl peroxide, resorcinol, salicylic acid, sulfur: Increases the drying effect.
Quinolones, phenothiazines, sulfonamides, sulfonylureas, tetracyclines, thiazide diuretics: Increase the risk of photosensitivity.

Herbal

None known.

Food

None known.

Drug interactions of concern to dentistry

- Increased risk of photosensitivity: tetracyclines, fluoroquinolones, phenothiazines
- Caution in use with systemic vitamin A

DIAGNOSTIC TEST EFFECTS

None known.

SIDE EFFECTS

Frequent

Desquamination, burning or stinging, dry skin, itching, erythema, worsening of psoriasis, irritation, skin pain, pruritis, xerosis, photosensitivity

Occasional

Irritation, skin pain, fissuring, localized edema, skin discoloration, rash, desquamation, contact dermatitis, skin inflammation, bleeding, dry skin, hypertriglyceridema, peripheral edema, acne vulgaris, cheilitis

DENTAL CONSIDERATIONS

General:

- Apply lubricant to dry lips for patient comfort before dental procedures.
- Advise patient if dental drugs prescribed have a potential for photosensitivity.

Teach Patient/Family:
- Should not be used if pregnant
- To avoid application to oral mucous membranes or lips

tegaserod

teh-gas′-er-od
(Zelnorm)

CATEGORY AND SCHEDULE
Pregnancy Risk Category: B

MECHANISM OF ACTION
An anti-irritable bowel syndrome (IBS) agent that binds to $5\text{-}HT_4$ receptors in the GI tract.
Therapeutic Effect: Triggers a peristaltic reflex in the gut, increasing bowel motility.

PHARMACOKINETICS
Rapidly absorbed. Widely distributed. Protein binding: 98%. Metabolized by hydrolysis in the stomach and by oxidation and conjugation of the primary metabolite. Primarily excreted in feces. ***Half-life:*** 11 hr.

AVAILABILITY
Tablets: 2 mg, 6 mg.

INDICATIONS AND DOSAGES
▸ **IBS**

PO

Adults, Elderly women. 6 mg twice a day for 4–6 wk.

▸ **Chronic Constipation**

PO

Adults. 6 mg twice a day.

CONTRAINDICATIONS
Abdominal adhesions, diarrhea, history of bowel obstruction, moderate to severe hepatic impairment, severe renal impairment, suspected sphincter of Oddi dysfunction, symptomatic gallbladder disease

INTERACTIONS
Drug
None known.
Herbal
None known.
Food
None known.
Drug interactions of concern to dentistry
- No dental drug interactions reported; does not induce CYP450 isoenzymes
- Avoid use of drugs (opioids, anticholinergics) that could lead to risk of constipation
- Use NSAIDs or acetaminophen for mild or moderate pain

DIAGNOSTIC TEST EFFECTS
None known.

SIDE EFFECTS
Frequency (> 5%)
Headache, abdominal pain, diarrhea, nausea, flatulence
Occasional (5%–2%)
Dizziness, migraine, back pain, extremity pain

SERIOUS REACTIONS
! None known.

DENTAL CONSIDERATIONS
General:
- Monitor vital signs at every appointment because of CV side effects.
- Consider semisupine chair position for patient comfort if GI side effects occur.

• Short appointments and a stress reduction protocol may be required for anxious patients.
• Avoid drugs with anticholinergic activity, such as antihistamines, opioids, benzodiazepines, propantheline, atropine, and scopolamine.
• Question patient about tolerance of NSAIDs or aspirin related to GI disease.

Consultations:

• Consult with physician before prescribing drugs that can cause constipation (opioids).
• Consultation with physician may be necessary if sedation or general anesthesia is required.
• Medical consultation may be required to assess disease control and patient's ability to tolerate stress.

Teach Patient/Family:

• Importance of updating health and drug history if physician makes any changes in evaluation or drug regimens

telmisartan

tel-meh-sar′-tan
(Micardis, Pritor[AUS])

CATEGORY AND SCHEDULE

Pregnancy Risk Category: C (D if used in second or third trimester)

MECHANISM OF ACTION

An angiotensin II receptor, type AT_1, antagonist that blocks vasoconstrictor and aldosterone-secreting effects of angiotensin II, inhibiting the binding of angiotensin II to the AT_1 receptors. ***Therapeutic Effect:*** Causes vasodilation, decreases peripheral resistance, and decreases BP.

PHARMACOKINETICS

Rapidly and completely absorbed after PO administration. Protein binding: greater than 99%. Undergoes metabolism in the liver to inactive metabolite. Excreted in feces. Unknown if removed by hemodialysis. ***Half-life:*** 24 hr.

AVAILABILITY

Tablets: 20 mg, 40 mg, 80 mg.

INDICATIONS AND DOSAGES

▸ **Hypertension**

PO

Adults, Elderly. 40 mg once a day. Range: 20–80 mg/day.

OFF-LABEL USES

Treatment of CHF

CONTRAINDICATIONS

None known.

INTERACTIONS

Drug

Digoxin: Increases digoxin plasma concentration.

Warfarin: Slightly decreases warfarin plasma concentration.

Herbal

None known.

Food

None known.

Drug interactions of concern to dentistry

• None reported; CYP450 isoenzymes are not involved with metabolism of this drug

DIAGNOSTIC TEST EFFECTS

May increase serum creatinine level. May decrease blood Hgb and Hct levels.

SIDE EFFECTS

Occasional (7%–3%)
Upper respiratory tract infection, sinusitis, back or leg pain, diarrhea
Rare (1%)
Dizziness, headache, fatigue, nausea, heartburn, myalgia, cough, peripheral edema

SERIOUS REACTIONS

! Overdosage may manifest as hypotension and tachycardia. Bradycardia occurs less often.

DENTAL CONSIDERATIONS

General:

- Monitor vital signs at every appointment because of CV side effects.
- Stress from dental procedures may compromise CV function; determine patient risk.
- Use precaution if sedation or general anesthesia is required; risk of hypotensive episode.
- Short appointments and a stress reduction protocol may be required for anxious patients.
- Limit use of sodium-containing products, such as saline IV fluids, for patients with a dietary salt restriction.

Consultations:

- Medical consultation may be required to assess disease control and patient's ability to tolerate stress.

temazepam

te-maz′-e-pam
Schedule IV
(Apo-Temazepam[CAN], Novo-Temazepam[CAN], PMS-Temazepam[CAN], Restoril)
Do not confuse Restoril with Vistaril or Zestril.

CATEGORY AND SCHEDULE

Pregnancy Risk Category: X
Controlled Substance: Schedule IV

MECHANISM OF ACTION

A benzodiazepine that enhances the action of the inhibitory neurotransmitter gamma-aminobutyric acid, resulting in CNS depression.
Therapeutic Effect: Induces sleep.

PHARMACOKINETICS

Well absorbed from the GI tract. Protein binding: 96%. Widely distributed. Crosses the blood-brain barrier. Metabolized in the liver. Primarily excreted in urine.
Not removed by hemodialysis.
Half-life: 4–18 hr.

AVAILABILITY

Capsules: 7.5 mg, 15 mg, 22.5 mg, 30 mg.

INDICATIONS AND DOSAGES

▸ Insomnia

PO
Adults, Children 18 yr and older. 15–30 mg at bedtime.
Elderly, Debilitated. 7.5–15 mg at bedtime.

CONTRAINDICATIONS

Angle-closure glaucoma; CNS depression; pregnancy or breast-feeding; severe, uncontrolled pain; sleep apnea

INTERACTIONS

Drug

Alcohol, other CNS depressants: May increase CNS depression.

Herbal

Kava kava, valerian: May increase CNS depression.

Food

None known.

Drug interactions of concern to dentistry

• Increased action of both drugs: alcohol, all CNS depressants
• Increased bioavailability: macrolide antibiotics

DIAGNOSTIC TEST EFFECTS

None known.

SIDE EFFECTS

Frequent

Somnolence, sedation, rebound insomnia (may occur for 1–2 nights after drug is discontinued), dizziness, confusion, euphoria

Occasional

Asthenia, anorexia, diarrhea

Rare

Paradoxical CNS excitement or restlessness (particularly in elderly or debilitated patients)

SERIOUS REACTIONS

! Abrupt or too-rapid withdrawal may result in pronounced restlessness, irritability, insomnia, hand tremor, abdominal or muscle cramps, vomiting, diaphoresis, and seizures.
! Overdose results in somnolence, confusion, diminished reflexes, respiratory depression, and coma.

DENTAL CONSIDERATIONS

General:

• Psychologic and physical dependence may occur with chronic administration.
• Geriatric patients are more susceptible to drug effects; use lower dose.

Teach Patient/Family:

• Importance of good oral hygiene to prevent soft tissue inflammation

temozolomide

teh-moe-zoll′-oh-mide
(Temodal[AUS], Temodar)

CATEGORY AND SCHEDULE

Pregnancy Risk Category: D

MECHANISM OF ACTION

An imidazotetrazine derivative that acts as a prodrug and is converted to a highly active cytotoxic metabolite. Its cytotoxic effect is associated with methylation of DNA. ***Therapeutic Effect:*** Inhibits DNA replication, causing cell death.

PHARMACOKINETICS

Rapidly and completely absorbed after PO administration. Protein binding: 15%. Peak plasma concentration occurs in 1 hr. Penetrates the blood-brain barrier. Eliminated primarily in urine and, to a much lesser extent, in feces. ***Half-life:*** 1.6–1.8 hr.

AVAILABILITY

Capsules: 5 mg, 20 mg, 100 mg, 250 mg.

INDICATIONS AND DOSAGES

▸ **Anaplastic Astrocytoma**

PO

Adults, Elderly. Initially, 150 mg/m^2/day for 5 consecutive days of a 28-day treatment cycle. Subsequent doses based on platelet

T

count and ANC during previous cycle. ANC greater than 1500 per microliter and platelet: more than 100,000 per microliter. Maintenance: 200 mg/m^2/day for 5 days q4wks. Continue until disease progression. Minimum: 100 mg/m^2/day for 5 days q4wks.

CONTRAINDICATIONS

Hypersensitivity to dacarbazine, pregnancy

INTERACTIONS

Drug

Live-virus vaccines: May potentiate virus replication, increase vaccine side effects, and decrease the patient's antibody response to the vaccine.
Valproic acid: Decreases the clearance of temozolomide.

Herbal

None known.

Food

All foods: Decrease the rate of drug absorption.

Drug interactions of concern to dentistry

- None reported

DIAGNOSTIC TEST EFFECTS

May decrease blood Hgb levels and neutrophil, platelet, and WBC counts.

SIDE EFFECTS

Frequent (53%–33%)
Nausea, vomiting, headache, fatigue, constipation
Occasional (16%–10%)
Diarrhea, asthenia, fever, dizziness, peripheral edema, incoordination, insomnia
Rare (9%–5%)
Paraesthesia, drowsiness, anorexia, urinary incontinence, anxiety, pharyngitis, cough

SERIOUS REACTIONS

! Elderly patients and women are at increased risk for developing severe myelosuppression, characterized by neutropenia and thrombocytopenia and usually occurring within the first few cycles. Neutrophil and platelet counts reach their nadirs approximately 26–28 days after administration and recover within 14 days of the nadir.

DENTAL CONSIDERATIONS

General:

- Caution: patients may be at high risk for infection.
- Provide palliative dental care for dental emergencies only.
- Oral infections should be eliminated and/or treated aggressively.
- Patients may be at risk for bleeding; check oral signs.
- Caution: potential drug interactions with drugs used in dentistry.
- Monitor and record vital signs.
- If additional analgesia is required for dental pain, consider alternative analgesics (NSAIDs) in patients taking narcotics for acute or chronic pain.
- Avoid products that affect platelet function, such as aspirin and NSAIDs.
- Patient on chronic drug therapy may rarely present with symptoms of blood dyscrasias, which can include infection, bleeding, and poor healing. If dyscrasia is present, caution patient to prevent oral tissue trauma when using oral hygiene aids.
- Consider local hemostasis measures to prevent excessive bleeding.
- Consider semisupine chair position for patient comfort if GI side effects occur.

Consultations:

- Medical consultation should include routine blood counts including platelet counts and bleeding time.

• Consult physician; prophylactic or therapeutic antiinfectives may be indicated if surgery or periodontal treatment is required.
• In a patient with symptoms of blood dyscrasias, request a medical consultation for blood studies and postpone treatment until normal values are re-established.
• Medical consultation may be required to assess disease control and patient's ability to tolerate stress.

Teach Patient/Family:
• To use soft tooth brush to reduce risk of bleeding
• Importance of good oral hygiene to prevent soft tissue inflammation
• To prevent trauma when using oral hygiene aids
• To report oral lesions, soreness, or bleeding to dentist
• Use of electric toothbrush if patient has difficulty holding conventional devices

tenecteplase

ten-eck′-teh-place
(Metalyse[AUS], TNKase)

CATEGORY AND SCHEDULE

Pregnancy Risk Category: C

MECHANISM OF ACTION

A tissue plasminogen activator produced by recombinant DNA that binds to fibrin and converts plasminogen to plasmin. Initiates fibrinolysis by degrading fibrin clots, fibrinogen, other plasma proteins. ***Therapeutic Effect:*** Exerts thrombolytic action.

PHARMACOKINETICS

Extensively distributed to tissues. Completely eliminated by hepatic metabolism. ***Half-life:*** 11–20 min.

AVAILABILITY

Powder for Injection: 50 mg.

INDICATIONS AND DOSAGES

▸ **Acute MI**

IV

Adults. Dosage is based on patient's weight. Treatment should be initiated as soon as possible after onset of symptoms.

Weight (kg)	(mg)	(ml)
90 or more	50	10
80 to less than 90	45	9
70 to less than 80	40	8
60 to less than 70	35	7
less than 60	30	6

CONTRAINDICATIONS

Active internal bleeding, aneurysm, AV malformation, bleeding diathesis, history of cerebrovascular accident, intracranial or intraspinal surgery or trauma within past 2 months, intracranial neoplasm, severe uncontrolled hypertension

INTERACTIONS

Drug

Anticoagulants (such as heparin, warfarin), aspirin, dipyridamole, glycoprotein IIb/IIIa inhibitors: Increase the risk of bleeding.

Herbal

Ginkgo biloba: May increase the risk of bleeding.

Food

None known.

Drug interactions of concern to dentistry

• Increased risk of bleeding: drugs that interfere with coagulation or platelet function, such as NSAIDs and aspirin, ginkgo biloba (herb)

DIAGNOSTIC TEST EFFECTS

Decreases plasminogen and fibrinogen levels during infusion, decreasing clotting time and confirming presence of lysis. Decreases Hct and Hgb.

IV INCOMPATIBILITIES

Do not mix with other medications.

SIDE EFFECTS

Frequent

Bleeding (major, 4.7%; minor, 21.8%)

SERIOUS REACTIONS

! Bleeding at internal sites may occur, including intracranial, retroperitoneal, GI, GU, and respiratory sites.
! Lysis or coronary thrombi may produce atrial or ventricular arrhythmias and stroke.

DENTAL CONSIDERATIONS

General:

- An acute use drug for use in hospitals or emergency departments.
- Patients are at risk for bleeding; check for oral signs.
- Avoid products that affect platelet function, such as aspirin and NSAIDs.
- Monitor and record vital signs.
- Review medical and drug history.

Consultations:

- Medical consultation should include routine blood counts including platelet counts and bleeding time.
- In a patient with symptoms of blood dyscrasias, request a medical consultation for blood studies and postpone treatment until normal values are re-established.
- Medical consultation may be required to assess disease control and patient's ability to tolerate stress.

Teach Patient/Family:

- To use soft tooth brush to reduce risk of bleeding
- Importance of good oral hygiene to prevent soft tissue inflammation
- To report oral lesions, soreness, or bleeding to dentist
- To prevent trauma when using oral hygiene aids
- Importance of updating health and medication history if physician makes any changes in evaluation or drug regimens; include OTC, herbal, and nonherbal remedies in the update

teniposide

ten-ih′-poe-side
(Vumon)

CATEGORY AND SCHEDULE

Pregnancy Risk Category: D

MECHANISM OF ACTION

An epipodophyllotoxin that induces single- and double-strand breaks in DNA, inhibiting or altering DNA synthesis. Acts in the late S and early G_2 phases of cell cycle. ***Therapeutic Effect:*** Prevents cells from entering mitosis.

AVAILABILITY

Injection: 50 mg.

INDICATIONS AND DOSAGES

▸ **Induction Therapy in Patients with Refractory Childhood Acute Lymphoblastic Leukemia (in Combination with Other Antineoplastic Agents)**

Children. Dosage is individualized on the basis of the patient's clinical response and tolerance of the drug's adverse effects. When used in combination therapy, consult specific protocols for optimum dosage or sequence of drug administration.

CONTRAINDICATIONS

Absolute neutrophil count less than 500/mm^3; hypersensitivity to Cremophor EL (polyoxyethylated castor oil), etoposide, or teniposide; platelet count less than 50,000/mm^3

INTERACTIONS

Drug

Bone marrow depressants: May increase myelosuppression.
Live-virus vaccines: May potentiate virus replication, increase vaccine side effects, and decrease the patient's antibody response to the vaccine.
Methotrexate: May increase intracellular accumulation of this drug.
Vincristine: May increase the severity of peripheral neuropathy.

Herbal

None known.

Food

None known.

Drug interactions of concern to dentistry

- None reported

DIAGNOSTIC TEST EFFECTS

None significant.

SIDE EFFECTS

Frequent (> 30%)

Mucositis, nausea, vomiting, diarrhea, anemia

Occasional (5%–3%)

Alopecia, rash

Rare (< 3%)

Hepatic dysfunction, fever, renal dysfunction, peripheral neurotoxicity

SERIOUS REACTIONS

! Myelosuppression manifested as hematologic toxicity (principally leukopenia, neutropenia, and thrombocytopenia) may be severe and may increase the risk of infection or bleeding.
! Hypersensitivity reaction may include anaphylaxis (marked by chills, fever, tachycardia, bronchospasm, dyspnea, and facial flushing).

DENTAL CONSIDERATIONS

General:

- If additional analgesia is required for dental pain, consider alternative analgesics (NSAIDs) in patients taking narcotics for acute or chronic pain.
- Examine for oral manifestation of opportunistic infection.
- Avoid products that affect platelet function, such as aspirin and NSAIDs.
- This drug may be used in the hospital or on an outpatient basis. Confirm the patient's disease and treatment status.
- Chlorhexidine mouth rinse prior to and during chemotherapy may reduce severity of mucositis.
- Patient on chronic drug therapy may rarely present with symptoms of blood dyscrasias, which can include infection, bleeding, and poor healing. If dyscrasia is present, caution patient to prevent oral tissue trauma when using oral hygiene aids.
- Palliative medication may be required for management of oral side effects.
- Short appointments and a stress reduction protocol may be required for anxious patients.
- Consider semisupine chair position for patient comfort if GI side effects occur.
- Caution: patients may be at high risk for infection.
- Patients may be at risk for bleeding; check oral signs.

- Oral infections should be eliminated and/or treated aggressively.

Consultations:

- Medical consultation should include routine blood counts including platelet counts and bleeding time.
- Consult physician; prophylactic or therapeutic antiinfectives may be indicated if surgery or periodontal treatment is required.
- Medical consultation may be required to assess immunologic status during cancer chemotherapy and determine safety risk, if any, posed by the required dental treatment.
- Medical consultation may be required to assess disease control and patient's ability to tolerate stress.
- In a patient with symptoms of blood dyscrasias, request a medical consultation for blood studies and postpone treatment until normal values are re-established.

Teach Patient/Family:

- Secondary oral infection may occur; need to see dentist immediately if infection occurs.
- To be aware of oral side effects
- Importance of good oral hygiene to prevent soft tissue inflammation
- To report oral lesions, soreness, or bleeding to dentist
- To prevent trauma when using oral hygiene aids
- Importance of updating health and medication history if physician makes any changes in evaluation or drug regimens; include OTC, herbal, and nonherbal remedies in the update

tenofovir

ten-oh′-foh-veer
(Viread)

CATEGORY AND SCHEDULE

Pregnancy Risk Category: B

MECHANISM OF ACTION

A nucleotide analogue that inhibits HIV reverse transcriptase by being incorporated into viral DNA, resulting in DNA chain termination.
Therapeutic Effect: Slows HIV replication and reduces HIV RNA levels (viral load).

AVAILABILITY

Tablets: 300 mg.

INDICATIONS AND DOSAGES

▸ HIV Infection (in Combination with Other Antiretrovirals)

PO

Adults, Elderly, Children 18 yr and older. 300 mg once a day.

CONTRAINDICATIONS

None known.

INTERACTIONS

Drug

Didanosine: May increase didanosine blood concentration.
Indinavir, lamivudine, lopinavir, ritonavir: May decrease the blood concentrations of these drugs.

Herbal

None known.

Food

High-fat food: Increases tenofovir bioavailability.

Drug interactions of concern to dentistry

- Potential for competition for renal clearance: acyclovir, valacyclovir

DIAGNOSTIC TEST EFFECTS

May elevate liver function test results. May alter serum CK, GGT, uric acid, AST (SGOT), ALT (SGPT), and triglyceride levels, as well as creatinine clearance.

SIDE EFFECTS

Occasional

GI disturbances (diarrhea, flatulence, nausea, vomiting)

SERIOUS REACTIONS

! Lactic acidosis and hepatomegaly with steatosis occur rarely, but may be severe.

DENTAL CONSIDERATIONS

General:

• Examine for oral manifestation of opportunistic infection.

Consultations:

• Medical consultation may be required to assess disease control and patient's ability to tolerate stress.

Teach Patient/Family:

• Importance of good oral hygiene to prevent soft tissue inflammation/ infection

terazosin hydrochloride

ter-a′-zoe-sin

(Apo-Terazosin[CAN], Hytrin, Novo-Terazosin[CAN])

CATEGORY AND SCHEDULE

Pregnancy Risk Category: C

MECHANISM OF ACTION

An antihypertensive and benign prostatic hyperplasia agent that blocks alpha-adrenergic receptors. Produces vasodilation, decreases peripheral resistance, and targets receptors around bladder neck and prostate. ***Therapeutic Effect:*** In hypertension, decreases BP. In benign prostatic hyperplasia, relaxes smooth muscle and improves urine flow.

PHARMACOKINETICS

Route	Onset	Peak	Duration
PO	15 min	1–2 hr	12–24 hr

Rapidly, completely absorbed from the GI tract. Protein binding: 90%–94%. Metabolized in the liver to active metabolite. Primarily eliminated in feces via biliary system; excreted in urine. Not removed by hemodialysis. ***Half-life:*** 12 hr.

AVAILABILITY

Capsules: 1 mg, 2 mg, 5 mg, 10 mg.
Tablets: 1 mg, 2 mg, 5 mg, 10 mg.

INDICATIONS AND DOSAGES

▸ **Mild to Moderate Hypertension**

PO

Adults, Elderly. Initially, 1 mg at bedtime. Slowly increase dosage to desired levels. Range: 1–5 mg/day as single or 2 divided doses. Maximum: 20 mg.

▸ **Benign Prostatic Hyperplasia**

PO

Adults, Elderly. Initially, 1 mg at bedtime. May increase up to 10 mg/day. Maximum: 20 mg/day.

T

CONTRAINDICATIONS

None known.

INTERACTIONS

Drug

Estrogen, NSAIDs, other sympathomimetics: May decrease the effects of terazosin.

Hypotension-producing medications, such as antihypertensives and diuretics: May increase the effects of terazosin.

Herbal

Dong quai, ginseng, garlic, yohimbe: May decrease the effects of terazosin.

Food

None known.

Drug interactions of concern to dentistry

- Decreased antihypertensive effects: NSAIDs, indomethacin

DIAGNOSTIC TEST EFFECTS

May decrease blood Hgb and Hct levels, serum albumin level, total serum protein level, and WBC count.

SIDE EFFECTS

Frequent (9%–5%)

Dizziness, headache, unusual tiredness

Rare (< 2%)

Peripheral edema, orthostatic hypotension, myalgia, arthralgia, blurred vision, nausea, vomiting, nasal congestion, somnolence

SERIOUS REACTIONS

! First-dose syncope (hypotension with sudden loss of consciousness) may occur 30 to 90 minutes after initial dose of 2 mg or more, a too rapid increase in dosage, or addition of another antihypertensive agent to therapy. First-dose syncope may be preceded by tachycardia (pulse rate of 120–160 beats/minute).

T

DENTAL CONSIDERATIONS

General:

- Monitor vital signs at every appointment because of CV side effects.
- After supine positioning, have patient sit upright for at least 2 min before standing to avoid orthostatic hypotension.
- Assess salivary flow as a factor in caries, periodontal disease, and candidiasis.
- Limit use of sodium-containing products, such as saline IV fluids, for patients with a dietary salt restriction.
- Consider semisupine chair position for patient comfort if GI side effects occur.

Teach Patient/Family:

- *When chronic dry mouth occurs, advise patient:*
  - To avoid mouth rinses with high alcohol content because of drying effects
  - Of need for daily home fluoride use to prevent caries
  - To use sugarless gum, frequent sips of water, or saliva substitutes

terbinafine hydrochloride

ter-been′-a-feen

(Apo-Terbinafine[CAN], Lamisil, Lamisil AT, Novo-Terbinafine [CAN])

Do not confuse terbinafine with terbutaline or Lamisil with Lamictal.

CATEGORY AND SCHEDULE

Pregnancy Risk Category: B

MECHANISM OF ACTION

A fungicidal antifungal that inhibits the enzyme squalene epoxidase, thereby interfering with fungal biosynthesis. ***Therapeutic Effect:*** Results in death of fungal cells.

AVAILABILITY

Tablets (Lamisil): 250 mg.
Cream (Lamisil AT): 1%.

Topical Solution (Lamisil, Lamisil AT): 1% .

INDICATIONS AND DOSAGES

▸ **Tinea Pedis**

TOPICAL

Adults, Elderly, Children 12 yr and older. Apply twice a day until signs and symptoms significantly improve.

▸ **Tinea Cruris, Tinea Corporis**

TOPICAL

Adults, Elderly, Children 12 yr and older. Apply 1–2 times a day until signs and symptoms significantly improve.

▸ **Onychomycosis**

PO

Adults, Elderly, Children 12 yr and older. 250 mg/day for 6 wk (fingernails) or 12 wk (toenails).

▸ **Tinea Versicolor**

TOPICAL SOLUTION

Adults, Elderly. Apply to the affected area twice a day for 7 days.

▸ **Systemic Mycosis**

PO

Adults, Elderly. 250–500 mg/day for up to 16 mo.

CONTRAINDICATIONS

Oral: Children younger than 12 years, preexisting hepatic or renal impairment (creatinine clearance of ≤ 50 ml/min)

INTERACTIONS

Drug

Alcohol, other hepatotoxic medications: May increase the risk of hepatotoxicity.

Hepatic enzyme inducers, including rifampin: May increase terbinafine clearance.

Hepatic enzyme inhibitors, including cimetidine: May decrease terbinafine clearance.

Herbal

None known.

Food

None known.

Drug interactions of concern to dentistry

- None reported

Drug interactions of concern to dentistry terbinafine HCL (topical)

- None reported

DIAGNOSTIC TEST EFFECTS

May increase AST(SGOT) and ALT(SGPT) levels.

SIDE EFFECTS

Frequent (13%)

Oral: Headache

Rare

Occasional (6%–3%)

Oral: Diarrhea, rash, dyspepsia, pruritus, taste disturbance, nausea

Oral: Abdominal pain, flatulence, urticaria, visual disturbance

Topical: Irritation, burning, pruritus, dryness

SERIOUS REACTIONS

! Hepatobiliary dysfunction (including cholestatic hepatitis), serious skin reactions, and severe neutropenia occur rarely.

! Ocular lens and retinal changes have been noted.

DENTAL CONSIDERATIONS

General:

- Determine why patient is taking the drug.
- Consider semisupine chair position for patient comfort if GI side effects occur.
- Patients on chronic drug therapy may rarely have symptoms of blood dyscrasias, which can include infection, bleeding, and poor healing.

Consultations:

- In a patient with symptoms of blood dyscrasias, request a

medical consultation for blood studies and postpone treatment until normal values are reestablished.

Teach Patient/Family:

- Importance of good oral hygiene to prevent soft tissue inflammation
- To prevent trauma when using oral hygiene aids

terconazole

ter-kon′-a-zole
(Terazol[CAN], Terazol 3, Terazol 7)

CATEGORY AND SCHEDULE

Pregnancy Risk Category: C

MECHANISM OF ACTION

An antifungal that disrupts fungal cell membrane permeability. ***Therapeutic Effect:*** Produces antifungal activity.

PHARMACOKINETICS

Extent of systemic absorption after vaginal administration may be dependent on presence of a uterus, 5%–8% in women who had a hysterectomy versus 12%–16% in nonhysterectomy women.

T

AVAILABILITY

Suppository: 80 mg (Terazol 3).
Cream: 0.4 % (Terazol 7), 0.8% (Terazol 3).

INDICATIONS AND DOSAGES

▸ Vulvovaginal Candidiasis

INTRAVAGINAL

Adults, Elderly. 1 suppository vaginally at bedtime for 3 days.

Adults, Elderly. 1 applicatorful at bedtime for 7 days (0.4% cream) or for 3 days (0.8% cream).

CONTRAINDICATIONS

Hypersensitivity to terconazole or any component of the formulation

INTERACTIONS

Drug

None known.

Herbal

None known.

Food

None known.

DIAGNOSTIC TEST EFFECTS

None known.

SIDE EFFECTS

Frequent

Headache, vulvovaginal burning

Occasional

Dysmenorrhea, pain in femail fenitalia, abdominal pain, fever, itching

Rare

Chills

SERIOUS REACTIONS

! Flulike syndrome has been reported.

DENTAL CONSIDERATIONS

General:

- Broad-spectrum antibiotics can exacerbate vaginal candidiasis.

teriparatide

ter-i-par′-a-tide
(Forteo)

CATEGORY AND SCHEDULE

Pregnancy Risk Category: C

MECHANISM OF ACTION

A synthetic polypeptide hormone that acts on bone to mobilize calcium; also acts on kidney to reduce calcium clearance, increase phosphate excretion. ***Therapeutic effect:*** Promotes an increased rate of release of calcium from bone into blood, stimulates new bone formation.

AVAILABILITY

Injection: 3 ml pre-filled pen containing 750 mcg teriparatide (Forteo).

INDICATIONS AND DOSAGES

▸ Osteoporosis

SC

Adults, Elderly. 20 mcg once daily into the thigh or abdominal wall.

CONTRAINDICATIONS

Serum calcium above normal level, those at increased risk for osteosarcoma (Paget's disease, unexplained elevations of alkaline phosphatase, open epiphyses, prior radiation therapy that include the skeleton), hypercalcemic disorder (e.g., hyperparathyroidism), hypersensitivity to teriparatide or any of the components of the formulation

INTERACTIONS

Drug

Digoxin: May increase serum digoxin concentration.

Herbal

None known.

Food

None known.

Drug interactions of concern to dentistry

- None reported

DIAGNOSTIC TEST EFFECTS

May increase serum calcium.

IV INCOMPATIBILITIES

Do not mix with other medications.

SIDE EFFECTS

Occasional

Leg cramps, nausea, dizziness, headache, orthostatic hypotension, increased heart rate

SERIOUS REACTIONS

! None known.

DENTAL CONSIDERATIONS

General:

- Patients with osteoporosis and risk of fracture should be asked if they use this drug; otherwise some patients may not report its use.
- Patients may need special assistance in the dental office to avoid risk of falling.

Teach Patient/Family:

- Importance of updating health and drug history, reporting changes in health status, drug regimen, or disease/treatment status
- To contact physician if symptoms of hypercalcemia appear (nausea, vomiting, constipation, lethargy, muscle weakness)

testosterone

tess-toss′-ter-one
Schedule III
(Andriol[CAN], Androderm, AndroGel, Andropository[CAN], Delatestryl, Depotest[CAN], Depo-Testosterone, Everone[CAN], Striant, Testim, Testoderm, Testoprel, Virilon IM[CAN])
Do not confuse testosterone with testolactone.

CATEGORY AND SCHEDULE

Pregnancy Risk Category: X

MECHANISM OF ACTION

A primary endogenous androgen that promotes growth and development of male sex organs and maintains secondary sex characteristics in androgen-deficient males.
Therapeutic Effect: Helps relieve androgen deficiency.

PHARMACOKINETICS

Well absorbed after IM administration. Protein binding: 98%. Undergoes first-pass metabolism in the liver. Primarily excreted in urine. Unknown if removed by hemodialysis. ***Half-life:*** 10–20 min.

AVAILABILITY

Cypionate Injection (Depo-Testosterone): 100 mg/ml, 200 mg/ml.
Ethanate Injection (Delatestryl): 200 mg/ml.
Subcutaneous Pellets (Testopel): 75 mg .
Topical Gel (AndroGel): 25 mg/2.5 g, 50 mg/5 g.
Topical Gel (Testim): 50 mg/5 g.
Transdermal Patch (Androderm): 2.5 mg/day, 5 mg/day.
Transdermal Patch (Testoderm): 4 mg/day, 6 mg/day.
Buccal (Striant): 30 mg.

T

INDICATIONS AND DOSAGES

▸ Male Hypogonadism

IM
Adults. 50–400 mg q2–4wk.
Adolescents. Initially 40–50 mg/m^2/dose monthly until growth rate falls to prepubertal levels. 100 mg/m^2/dose until growth ceases. Maintenance virilizing dose: 100 mg/m^2/dose twice a month.
SUBCUTANEOUS (Pellets)
Adults, adolescents. 150–450 mg q3–6mo.
TRANSDERMAL (Patch [Testoderm])
Adults, Elderly. Start therapy with 6 mg/day patch. Apply patch to scrotal skin.
TRANSDERMAL (Patch [Testoderm TTS])
Adults, Elderly. Apply TTS patch to arm, back, or upper buttocks.
TRANSDERMAL (Patch [Androderm])
Adults, Elderly. Start therapy with 5 mg/day patch applied at night. Apply patch to abdomen, back, thighs, or upper arms.
TRANSDERMAL (Gel [AndroGel])
Adults, Elderly. Initial dose of 5 mg delivers 50 mg testosterone and is applied once daily to the abdomen, shoulders, or upper arms. May increase to 7.5 g, then to 10 g, if necessary.
TRANSDERMAL (Gel [Testim])
Adults, Elderly. Initial dose of 5 g delivers 50 mg testosterone and is applied once a day to the shoulders or upper arms. May increase to 10 g.
BUCCAL SYSTEM (Striant)
Adults, Elderly: 30 mg q12h.

▸ Delayed Puberty

IM
Adults. 50–200 mg q2–4wk.
Adolescents. 40–50 mg/m^2/dose every month for 6 mo.
SUBCUTANEOUS (Pellets)
Adults, Adolescents. 150–450 mg q3–6mo.

▸ **Breast Carcinoma**
IM (testosterone aqueous)
Adults. 50–100 mg 3 times a week.
IM (testosterone cypionate or testosterone ethanate)
Adults. 200–400 mg q2–4wk.
IM (testosterone propionate)
Adults. 50–100 mg 3 times a week.

CONTRAINDICATIONS
Cardiac impairment, hypercalcemia, pregnancy, prostate or breast cancer in males, severe hepatic or renal disease

INTERACTIONS
Drug
Hepatotoxic medications: May increase the risk of hepatotoxicity.
Oral anticoagulants: May increase the effects of oral anticoagulants.
Herbal
None known.
Food
None known.
Drug interactions of concern to dentistry
- Edema: ACTH, adrenal steroids

DIAGNOSTIC TEST EFFECTS
May increase blood Hgb level and Hct, as well as serum LDL, alkaline phosphatase, bilirubin, calcium, potassium, sodium, and AST (SGOT) levels. May decrease serum HDL level.

SIDE EFFECTS
Frequent
Gynecomastia, acne
Females: Hirsutism, amenorrhea or other menstrual irregularities, deepening of voice, clitoral enlargement that may not be reversible when drug is discontinued
Occasional
Edema, nausea, insomnia, oligospermia, priapism, male-pattern baldness, bladder irritability, hypercalcemia (in immobilized patients or those with breast cancer), hypercholesterolemia, inflammation and pain at IM injection site
Transdermal: Pruritus, erythema, skin irritation
Rare
Polycythemia (with high dosage), hypersensitivity

SERIOUS REACTIONS
! Peliosis hepatitis (presence of blood-filled cysts in parenchyma of liver), hepatic neoplasms, and hepatocellular carcinoma have been associated with prolonged high-dose therapy.
! Anaphylactic reactions occur rarely.

DENTAL CONSIDERATIONS
General:
- Determine why the patient is taking the drug.
- Consider local hemostasis measures to prevent excessive bleeding.
- Short appointments and a stress reduction protocol may be required for anxious patients.
- Prophylactic antibiotics may be indicated to prevent infection if surgery or deep scaling is planned.

Consultations:
- Physician consultation may be required if signs of anemia are observed in oral tissues.
- Medical consultation may be required to assess disease control and patient's ability to tolerate stress.

• Medical consultation should include partial prothrombin time or prothrombin time.

Teach Patient/Family:

• Importance of good oral hygiene to prevent soft tissue inflammation
• To be aware of the possibility of secondary oral infection and the need to see dentist immediately if infection occurs

tetracaine

tet′-ra-cane
(AK-T Caine, Cepacol, Viractin, Pontocaine, Opticaine)
Do not confuse with procaine, lidocaine.

CATEGORY AND SCHEDULE

Pregnancy Risk Category: C

MECHANISM OF ACTION

Tetracaine causes a reversible blockade of nerve conduction by decreasing nerve membrance permeability to sodium. ***Therapeutic Effect:*** Local anesthetic.

PHARMACOKINETICS

Systemic absorption of tetracaine is variable. Metabolized by plasma pseudocholinesterasis. Excreted in the urine.

T

AVAILABILITY

Solution for injection: 0.2%, 0.3%, 1%, 2% (Pontocaine)
Cream: 1%
Ointment: 0.5%

INDICATIONS AND DOSAGES

▸ **Anesthetize Lower Abdomen**
SPINAL
Adults. 3–4 ml (9–12 mg) of a 0.3% solution

▸ **Anesthetize Perineum**
SPINAL
Adults. 1–2 ml (3–6 mg) of a 0.3% solution

▸ **Anesthetize Upper Abdomen**
SPINAL
Adults. 5 ml (15 mg) of a 0.3% solution

▸ **Obstetric Anesthesia, Low Spinal (Saddle Block) Anesthesia**
SPINAL
Adults. 1–2 ml (2–14 mg) of a 0.2% solution

▸ **Anesthesia of the Perineum**
INTRATHECAL
Adults. 0.5 ml (5 mg) as a 1% solution, diluted with equal amount of CSF or 10% dextrose injection.

▸ **Anesthesia of the Perineum and Lower Extremeties**
INTRATHECAL
Adults. 1 ml (10 mg) as a 1% solution, diluted with equal amount of CSF or 10% dextrose injection.

▸ **Anesthesia up to the Costal Margin**
INTRATHECAL
Adults. 1.5–2 ml (15–20 mg) as a 1% solution, diluted with equal amount of CSF.

▸ **Topical Anesthesia**
TOPICAL
Adults. Apply to the affected areas as needed. Maximum dosage is 28 g per 24 hours.
Children. Apply to the affected areas as needed. Maximum dosage is 7 g in a 24 hour period.

▸ **Topical Anesthesia of Nose and Throat, Abolish Laryngeal and Esophageal Reflexes Prior to Diagnostic Procedure**
TOPICAL
Adults. Direct application of a 0.25% or 0.5% topical solution or by oral inhalation of a nebulized 0.5% solution. Total dose should not exceed 20 mg.

▸ **Mild Pain, Burning and/or Pruritis Associated with Herpes Labialis (Cold Sores or Fever Blisters)**
TOPICAL
Adults and children 2 years and older. Apply to the affected area no more than 3–4 times a day.
▸ **Ophthalmic Anesthesia**
TOPICAL
Adults. 1–2 drops of a 0.5% solution.

CONTRAINDICATIONS
Hypersensitivity to esther local anesthetics, sulfites, PABA; infection or inflammation at the injection site, bactermia, platelet abnormalities, thrombocytopenia, increased bleeding time, uncontrolled coagulopathy, or anticoagulant therapy, sulfonamide therapy.

INTERACTIONS
Drug
Local anesthetics: The toxic effects are additive.
Cholinesterase inhibitors: Local anesthetics can antagonize the effects of these medications.
Neuromuscular blockers: Local anesthetics prolong and enhance the effects of these medications.
Anihypertensives, nitrates, vasodilators: Additive hypotensive effects.
Opiate agonists: May lead to increased depression of the CNS
Class IA and III antiarrhythmics, macrolide and ketolide antibiotics, quinolone antibiotics, alfuzosin, arsenic trioxide, astemizole, beta agonists, amoxapine, bepridil, cisapride, chloroquine, clozapine, cyclobenzaprine, dolasetron, droperidol, flecainide, halofantrine, haloperidol, halogenated anesthetics, levomethadyl, maprotiline, methadone, octreotide, palonosetron, pentamidine, chlorpromazine, fluphenazine, mesoridazine, pimozide, probucol, propafenone, risperidone, sertindole, tacrolimus, terfenadine,vardenafil, ziprasidone: May increase the risk of cardiotoxicity, including QT prolongation.
MAOIs: Increased risk of hypotension.
Herbal
None known.
Food
None known.
Drug interactions of concern to dentistry
• Specific drug interactions are not listed; it would be wise to use with caution in patients taking tocainide, mexiletine; significant systemic absorption could lead to synergistic and potentially toxic effects

DIAGNOSTIC TEST EFFECTS
None known.
IV COMPATIBILITIES
Water, physiologic saline solution, dextrose solution, CSF

SIDE EFFECTS
Frequent
Burning stinging, or tenderness, skin rash, itching, redness, or inflammation, numbness or tingling of the face or mouth, pain at the injection site, sensitivity to light, swelling of the eye or eyelid, watering of the eyes, acute ocular pain and ocular irritation (burning, stinging, or redness)
Occasional
Paresthesias, weakness and paralysis of lower extremity, hypotension, high or total spinal block, urinary retention or incontinence, fecal incontinence, headache, back pain, septic meningitis, meningismus, arachnoiditis, shivering cranial nerve

palsies due to traction on nerves from loss of CSF, and loss of perineal sensation and sexual function

Rare

Anxiety, restlessness, difficulty breathing, shortness of breath, dizziness, drowsiness, lightheadedness, nausea, vomiting, seizures (convulsions), slow, irregular heartbeat (palpitations), swelling of the face or mouth, skin rash, itching (hives), tremors, visual impairment.

SERIOUS REACTIONS

! Tetracaine-induced CNS toxicity usually presents with symptoms of a CNS stimulation, such as anxiety, apprehension, restlessness, nervousness, disorientation, confusion, dizziness, tinnitus, blurred vision, tremor, and/or seizures. Subsequently, depressive symptoms may occur including drowsiness, respiratory arrest, or coma.

! Depression or cardiac excitability and contractility may cause AV block, ventricular arrhythmias, or cardiac arrest. Symptoms of local anesthetic CNS toxicity, such as dizziness, tongue numbness, visual impairment or disturbances, and muscular twitching appear to occur before cardiotoxic effects. Cardiotoxic effects include angina, QT prolongation, PR prolongation, atrial fibrillation, sinus bradycardia, hypotension, palpitations, and cardiovascular collapse. Maternal seizures and cardiovascular collapse may occur following paracervical block in early pregnancy due to rapid systemic absorption.

Alert

! Tetracaine is more likely than any other topical anesthetic to cause contact reactions including, skin rash (unspecified), mucous membrane irritation, erythema, pruritis, urticaria, burning, stinging, edema, or tenderness.

Alert

! During labor and obstetric delivery, local anesthetics can cause varying degrees of maternal, fetal, and neonatal toxicities. Fetal heart rate should be monitored continuously because fetal bradycardia may occur in patients receiving tetracaine anesthesia and may be associated with fetal acidosis. Maternal hypotension can result from regional anesthesia; patient position can alleviate this problem. Spinal tetracaine may cause decreased uterine contractility or maternal expulsion efforts and alter the forces of parturition.

DENTAL CONSIDERATIONS

General:

- Apply smallest effective dose; apply to small area because significant absorption can occur, especially from denuded areas.
- Absorption of excessive amounts of drug may lead to signs of local anesthetic toxicity; with correct use, toxicity is a rare event.
- Use for topical anesthesia or temporary relief of symptoms; reevaluate if symptoms persist.
- Toxic amounts can be absorbed from denuded mucosa or skin.
- Apply with cotton-tipped applicator by pressing, not rubbing, paste on lesion.

Teach Patient/Family:

- How to apply
- Not to chew gum or eat while numbness is present after dental treatment
- Symptoms of systemic toxicity, which can include nervousness,

T

nausea, excitement followed by drowsiness, convulsions, and cardiac and respiratory depression
- That symptoms may vary because they depend on the amount of drug actually absorbed

tetracycline hydrochloride

tet-ra-sye′-kleen
(Apo-Tetra[CAN], Latycin[AUS], Mysteclin[AUS], Novotetra[CAN], Nu-Tetra[CAN], Sumycin, Tetrex[AUS])

CATEGORY AND SCHEDULE

Pregnancy Risk Category: D (B with topical form)

MECHANISM OF ACTION

A tetracycline antibiotic that inhibits bacterial protein synthesis by binding to ribosomes. ***Therapeutic Effect:*** Bacteriostatic.

PHARMACOKINETICS

Readily absorbed from the GI tract. Protein binding: 30%–60%. Widely distributed. Excreted in urine; eliminated in feces through biliary system. Not removed by hemodialysis. ***Half-life:*** 6–11 hr (increased in impaired renal function).

AVAILABILITY

Capsules: 250 mg, 500 mg.
Oral Suspension: 125 mg/5 ml.
Tablets: 250 mg, 500 mg.
Topical Solution. 2.2 mg/ml.
Topical Ointment: 3%.

INDICATIONS AND DOSAGES

▸ Inflammatory Acne Vulgaris, Lyme Disease, Mycoplasmal Disease, *Legionella* Infections, Rocky Mountain Spotted Fever, Chlamydial Infections in Patients with Gonorrhea

PO

Adults, Elderly. 250–500 mg q6–12h.

Children 8 yr and older. 25–50 mg/kg/day in 4 divided doses. Maximum: 3 g/day.

▸ *Helicobacter pylori* Infections

PO

Adults, Elderly. 500 mg 2–4 times a day (in combination).

▸ Topical

Adults, Elderly. Apply twice a day (once in the morning, once in the evening).

▸ Dosage in Renal Impairment

Dosage interval is modified on the basis of creatinine clearance.

Creatinine Clearance	Dosage Interval
50–80 ml/min	Usual dose q8–12h
10–50 ml/min	Usual dose q12–24h
less than 10 ml/min	Usual dose q24h

CONTRAINDICATIONS

Children 8 years and younger, hypersensitivity to tetracyclines or sulfites

INTERACTIONS

Drug

Carbamazepine, phenytoin: May decrease tetracycline blood concentration.
Cholestyramine, colestipol: May decrease tetracycline absorption.
Oral contraceptives: May decrease the effects of oral contraceptives.

Herbal

St. John's wort: May increase the risk of photosensitivity.

Food

Dairy products: Inhibit tetracycline absorption.

Drug interactions of concern to dentistry

- Decreased absorption: $NaHCO_3$, other antacids
- Decreased effect of penicillins, cephalosporins
- Possible increase in serum levels of methotrexate
- Suspected increase in effects of warfarin, theophylline

DIAGNOSTIC TEST EFFECTS

May increase BUN and serum alkaline phosphatase, amylase, bilirubin, AST (SGOT), and ALT (SGPT) levels.

SIDE EFFECTS

Frequent

Dizziness, light-headedness, diarrhea, nausea, vomiting, abdominal cramps, possibly severe photosensitivity
Topical: Dry, scaly skin; stinging or burning sensation

Occasional

Pigmentation of skin or mucous membranes, rectal or genital pruritus, stomatitis
Topical: Pain, redness, swelling, or other skin irritation.

T

SERIOUS REACTIONS

! Superinfection (especially fungal), anaphylaxis, and benign intracranial hypertension may occur.
! Bulging fontanelles occur rarely in infants.

DENTAL CONSIDERATIONS

General:

- Determine why the patient is taking tetracycline.
- Broad-spectrum antibiotics may be a factor in oral or vaginal *Candida* infections.
- Advise patient if dental drugs prescribed have a potential for photosensitivity.

Consultations:

- Medical consultation may be required to assess disease control.

Teach Patient/Family:

- Importance of good oral hygiene to prevent soft tissue inflammation
- Caution to prevent injury when using oral hygiene aids
- To avoid milk products; to take with a full glass of water
- To take tetracycline doses 1 hr before or 2 hr after air polishing device (Prophy-Jet), if used
- *When used for dental infection, advise patient:*
  - If taking birth control pill to use additional method of contraception for duration of cycle
  - To report sore throat, oral burning sensation, fever, fatigue, any of which could indicate superinfection
  - To take at prescribed intervals and complete dosage regimen
  - To immediately notify the dentist if signs or symptoms of infection increase

thalidomide

thah-lid′-owe-mide
(Thalomid)

CATEGORY AND SCHEDULE

Pregnancy Risk Category: X

MECHANISM OF ACTION

An immunomodulator whose exact mechanism is unknown. Has sedative, anti-inflammatory, and immunosuppressive activity, which may be due to selective inhibition of the production of tumor necrosis factor-alpha. ***Therapeutic Effect:*** Improves muscle wasting in HIV patients; reduces local and systemic effects of leprosy.

AVAILABILITY

Capsules: 50 mg.

INDICATIONS AND DOSAGES

▸ AIDS-Related Muscle Wasting

PO

Adults. 100–300 mg a day.

▸ Leprosy

PO

Adults, Elderly. Initially, 100–300 mg/day as single bedtime dose, at least 1 hr after the evening meal. Continue until active reaction subsides, then reduce dose q2–4 wk in 50 mg increments.

OFF-LABEL USES

Treatment of Crohn's disease, recurrent aphthous ulcers in HIV patients, wasting syndrome associated with HIV or cancer

CONTRAINDICATIONS

Neutropenia, peripheral neuropathy; pregnancy, sensitivity to thalidomide

INTERACTIONS

Drug

Alcohol, other CNS depressants: May increase sedative effects.
Medications associated with peripheral neuropathy (such as isoniazid, lithium, metronidazole, phenytoin): May increase peripheral neuropathy.
Medications that decrease effectiveness of hormonal contraceptives (such as carbamazepine, protease inhibitors, rifampin): May decrease the effectiveness of the contraceptive; patient must use two other methods of contraception.

Herbal

None known.

Food

None known.

Drug interactions of concern to dentistry

- Increased sedative effects of: alcohol, barbiturates, phenothiazines
- Increased risk of peripheral neuropathy: metronidazole
- May interfere with hormonal contraceptives: patient must use two alternative methods of contraception

DIAGNOSTIC TEST EFFECTS

None known.

SIDE EFFECTS

Frequent

Somnolence, dizziness, mood changes, constipation, dry mouth, peripheral neuropathy

Occasional

Increased appetite, weight gain, headache, loss of libido, edema of face and limbs, nausea, alopecia, dry skin, rash, hypothyroidism

SERIOUS REACTIONS

! Neutropenia, peripheral neuropathy, and thromboembolism occur rarely.

DENTAL CONSIDERATIONS

General:

- Determine why patient is taking the drug.
- Consider semisupine chair position for patient comfort if GI side effects occur.
- Assess salivary flow as a factor in caries, periodontal disease, and candidiasis.
- Examine for oral manifestation of opportunistic infection.
- Patient on chronic drug therapy may rarely present with symptoms of blood dyscrasias, which can include infection, bleeding, and poor healing. If dyscrasia is present, caution patient to prevent oral tissue trauma when using oral hygiene aids.
- After supine positioning, have patient sit upright for at least 2 min before standing to avoid orthostatic hypotension.
- Can be prescribed only by S.T.E.P.S. (System for Thalidomide Education and Prescribing Safety) registered prescribers.
- Absolutely contraindicated in pregnancy.

Consultations:

- Refer patients to attending physician if symptoms of peripheral neuropathy is present (numbness, tingling or pain in hands or feet).
- Consultation with physician may be necessary if sedation or general anesthesia is required.
- Medical consultation may be required to assess disease control and patient's ability to tolerate stress.
- In a patient with symptoms of blood dyscrasias, request a medical consultation for blood studies and postpone treatment until normal values are reestablished.
- Precaution if dental surgery is anticipated or general anesthesia required.

Teach Patient/Family:

- Caution patients about driving or performing other tasks requiring mental alertness.
- *When chronic dry mouth occurs, advise patient:*
  - To avoid mouth rinses with high alcohol content due to drying effects
  - To use daily home fluoride products for anticaries effect
  - To use sugarless gum, frequent sips of water or saliva substitutes
- Importance of good oral hygiene to prevent soft tissue inflammation
- To prevent trauma when using oral hygiene aids
- To report oral lesions, soreness, or bleeding to dentist
- Importance of updating health and medication history if physician makes any changes in evaluation or drug regimens; include OTC, herbal, and nonherbal remedies in the update

T

theophylline

thee-off′-i-lin

Aerobin[Germany]; Aerodyne Retard[Austria]; Afonilum Forte[Germany]; Afonilum Mite [Germany]; Afonilum Retard [Germany]; Almarion[Thailand]; Armophylline[France]; Asmasalon [Philippines]; Asperal-T[Belgium]; Austyn[Korea]; Bronchoretard [Germany]; Bronsolvan [Indonesia]; Cronasma[Germany]; Deo-Q Syrup[Korea]; Ditenaten [Germany]; Elixofilina[Mexico, Peru]; Elixophyllin; Euphylong [Israel, Hong Kong]; Euphylong Retardkaps[Germany]; Euphylong SR[Philippines]; Godafilin[Spain]; Lasma[Israel, England]; Nefoben[Argentina]; Neobiphyllin[China]; Neulin SA[South Africa]; Neulin-SR [Taiwan]; Nuelin[Puerto Rico, Costa Rica, Denmark, Dominican Republic, El Salvador, Finland, Honduras, Malaysia, Norway, Panama, Philippines]; Nuelin SA [South Africa, Israel, Costa Rica, Dominican Republic, El Salvador, Guatemala, Honduras, Panama]; Nuelin SR[Israel, Australia, Hong Kong, Malaysia, Thailand]; Pharphylline[Netherlands]; Phylobid[South Africa, India]; Protheo[China]; Pulmidur [Austria, Germany]; Slo-Bid Gyrocaps; Quibron-T; Quibron T SR[US, Canada, Indonesia]; Slo-Theo [Hong Kong]; Solosin[Germany]; Somofillina[Italy]; Teobid[Colombia]; Teoclear[Korea]; Teoclear LA [Argentina]; Teofilina Retard [Colombia]; Teolixir[Spain]; Teolong[Mexico]; Teosona [Argentina]; Theo-2 [Belgium]; Theo-24; Theo-Bros[Greece]; Theochron; Theo-Dur; Theolair; Theolair SR; Theolair S[Peru]; Theolan[Korea, Taiwan]; Theolin[Singapore]; Theolin SR[Singapore]; Theolong [Japan]; Theomax[Spain]; Theon [Switzerland]; Theo PA[India]; Theoplus[Bulgaria, Singapore, Spain]; Theoplus Retard[Austria, Greece]; Theospirex Retard [Austria, Switzerland]; Theostat LP[France]; Theotard[Israel]; Theo-Time; Theotrim[Israel]; Theovent LA[Hong Kong]; Theo von CT[Germany]; Tiodilax [Argentina]; T-Phyl; Truxophyllin; Tyrex[Peru]; Unicontin-400 Continus[India]; Uni-Dur; Unifyl Retard[Switzerland]; Uniphyl; Uniphyl CR[Korea]; Uniphyllin[Taiwan]; UniphyllinContinus[South Africa]; Xanthium[Singapore]; Xantivent[Switzerland]

CATEGORY AND SCHEDULE

Pregnancy risk category: C

MECHANISM OF ACTION

An antiasthmatic medication with two distinct actions in the airways of patients with reversible obstruction; smooth muscle relaxation and suppression of the response of airways to stimuli. Mechanisms of action are not known with certainty. It is known that theophylline increases force of contraction of diaphragmatic muscles by enhancing calcium uptake through adenosine-mediated channels. ***Therapeutic Effect:*** Causes bronchodilation and decreased airway reactivity.

PHARMACOKINETICS

The pharmacokinetics of theophylline vary widely among

similar patients and cannot be predicted by age, sex, body weight or other demographic characteristics. Rapidly and completely absorbed after oral administration in solution or immediate-release solid oral dosage form. Distributed freely into fat-free tissues. Extensively metabolized in liver. ***Half-life:*** 4–8 hrs.

AVAILABILITY

Capsule, extended release: 100 mg (Slo-Bid Gyrocaps); 125 mg; 200 mg (Slo-Bid Gyrocaps); 300 mg (Slo-Bid Gyrocaps)
Elixir: 80 mg/15 mL (Elixophyllin)
Solution, intravenous: 40 mg/100 mL, 80 mg/100 mL, 160 mg/100 mL, 200 mg/100 mL, 200 mg/50 mL, 320 mg/100 mL, 400 mg/100 mL
Solution, oral: 80 mg/15 mL (Truxophyllin)
Tablet: 100 mg
Tablet, extended release: 100 mg (Theo-Dur, Theochron, Theo-Time); 200 mg (Theo-Dur, Theochron, Theo-Time); 300 mg (Theo-Dur, Theochron, Theo-Time); 400 mg (Uni-Dur); 450 mg (Theochron)

INDICATIONS AND DOSAGES

▸ Chronic Asthma/Lung Diseases

PO
Adults. Acute symptoms: 5 mg/kg as a loading dose, maintenance 3 mg/kg every 8 hours (nonsmokers), 3 mg/kg every 6 hours (smokers), 2 mg/kg every 8 hours (older patients), 1–2 mg/kg every 12 hours (CHF); IV 5 mg/kg load over 20 minutes, maintenance 0.2 mg/kg/hour (CHF, elderly), 0.43 mg/kg/hour (nonsmokers), 0.7 mg/kg/hour (young adult smokers).
Slow titration. initial dose 16 mg/kg/day or 400mg daily, whichever is less, doses divided every 6–8 hours
Dosage adjustment after serum theophylline measurement. Serum level 5–10 mcg/ml, maintain dose by 25%, recheck level in 3 days. Serum level 10–20 mcg/ml, maintain dosage if tolerated, recheck level every 6–12 months. Serum level 20–25 mcg/ml, decrease dose by 10%, recheck level in 3 days. Serum level 25–30 mcg/ml, skip next dose, decrease dose by 25%, recheck level in 3 days. Serum level > 30 mcg/ml, skip next 2 doses, decrease dose by 50%, recheck level in 3 days.
Children 9–16 years. 5 mg/kg as a loading dose, maintenance 3 mg/kg every 6 hours; IV 5 mg/kg load over 20 minutes, maintenance 0.7 mg/kg/hour.
Children 1–9 years. 5 mg/kg as a loading dose, maintenance 4 mg/kg every 6 hours; IV 5 mg/kg load over 20 minutes, maintenance 0.8 mg/kg/hour.
Infants. [(0.2 × age in weeks) +5] × kg = 24 hour dose in mg; divide into every 8 hour dosing (6 weeks to 6 months), every 6 hour dosing (6–12 months); IV 5 mg/kg load over 20 minutes, maintenance dose in mg/kg/hour [(0.0008 × age in weeks) + 0.21]

OFF-LABEL USES

Apnea, bradycardia of prematurity

CONTRAINDICATIONS

Hypersensitivity to theophylline or any component of the formulation, active peptic ulcer disease, underlying seizure disorders unless receiving appropriate anti-convulsant medication.

INTERACTIONS

Drug

Adenosine, diazepam, flurazepam, lorazepam, midazolam: May decrease therapeutic effect at adenosine receptors.

T

Alcohol, allopurinol, cimetidine, ciprofloxacin, clarithromycin, disulfiram, erythromycin, enoxacin, estrogen, fluvoxamine, interferon alpha-A, methotrexate, mexiletine, pentoxifylline, propafenone, propranolol, thiabendazole, ticlopidine, troleandomycin, verapamil: May decrease theophylline clearance.
Aminoglutethimide, carbamazepine, isoprotereno, moricizinel, phenobarbital, phenytoin, rifampin, sulfinpyrazone: May increase theophylline clearance.
Ephedrine: May cause synergistic CNS effects.
Halothane: May cause ventricular arrhythmia.
Ketamine: May decrease seizure threshold.
Lithium: May increase lithium clearance.

Herbal

Capsicum: May increase absorption and effect.
Ipriflavone, St. John's Wort: May decrease metabolism of theophylline.

Food

High-fat content meals: May decrease theophylline absorption.
Charbroiled foods: May increase elimination of theophylline.
Caffeine, dietary protein and carbohydrates: May increase the activity and side effects caused by theophylline. Large amounts should be avoided. Low-carbohydrate, high-protein diets, charbroiled beef, and large amounts of cruciferous vegetables (broccoli, Brussels sprouts, cabbage, and cauliflower) can reduce theophylline activity.

Drug interactions of concern to dentistry

- Increased action: erythromycin, ciprofloxacin, glucocorticoids
- Increased risk of cardiac dysrhythmia: halothane inhalation anesthesia, CNS stimulants
- Decreased effect: barbiturates, carbamazepine, ketoconazole
- May decrease sedative effects of benzodiazepines

DIAGNOSTIC TEST EFFECTS

None known.

SIDE EFFECTS

Anxiety, dizziness, headache, insomnia, lightheadedness, muscle twitching, restlessness, seizures, dysrhythmias, fluid retention with tachycardia, hypotension, palpitations, pounding heartbeat, sinus tachycardia, anorexia, bitter taste, diarrhea, dyspepsia, gastroesophageal reflux, nausea, vomiting, urinary frequency, increased respiratory rate, flushing, urticaria

SERIOUS REACTIONS

! Severe toxicity from theophylline overdose is a relatively rare event.

DENTAL CONSIDERATIONS

General:

- Consider semisupine chair position for patients with respiratory disease.
- Monitor vital signs at every appointment because of CV side effects.
- Assess salivary flow as a factor in caries, periodontal disease, and candidiasis.
- Be aware that aspirin or sulfite preservatives in vasoconstrictor-containing products can exacerbate asthma.
- Acute asthmatic episodes may be precipitated in the dental office. Sympathomimetic inhalants should be available for emergency use.
- Midday appointments and a stress reduction protocol may be required for anxious patients.

Consultations:
- Medical consultation may be required to assess disease control.

Teach Patient/Family:
- *When chronic dry mouth occurs, advise patient:*
  - To avoid mouth rinses with high alcohol content because of drying effects
  - Of need for daily home fluoride use to prevent caries
  - To use sugarless gum, frequent sips of water, or saliva substitutes

thiabendazole

thye-a-ben′-da-zole
(Mintezol)

CATEGORY AND SCHEDULE

Pregnancy Risk Category: C

MECHANISM OF ACTION

An anthelmintic agent that inhibits helminth-specific mitochondrial fumarate reductase. ***Therapeutic Effect:*** Suppresses parasite production.

PHARMACOKINETICS

Rapidly and well absorbed from the gastrointestinal (GI) tract. Rapidly metabolized in liver. Primarily excreted in urine; partially eliminated in feces. Removed ***Half-life:*** 1.2 hrs.

AVAILABILITY

Suspension: 500 mg/5 ml (Mintezol).
Tablets: 500 mg (Mintezol).

INDICATIONS AND DOSAGES

Dose is based on patient's body weight

▸ **Cutaneous Lava Migrans (Creeping Eruption)**
PO
Adults, Elderly, Children.
50 mg/kg/day q12h for 2 days. Maximum: 3 g/day.

▸ **Intestinal Roundworms**
PO
Adults, Elderly, Children.
50 mg/kg/day q12h for 2 days. Maximum: 3 g/day.

▸ **Strongloidiasis (Thread Worms)**
PO
Adults, Elderly, Children.
50 mg/kg/day q12h for 2 days. Maximum: 3 g/day.

▸ **Trichinosis**
PO
Adults, Elderly, Children.
50 mg/kg/day q12h for 2–4 days. Maximum: 3 g/day.

▸ **Visceral Larva Migrans**
PO
Adults, Elderly, Children.
50 mg/kg/day q12h for 7 days. Maximum: 3 g/day.

OFF-LABEL USES

Angiostrongyliasis, capillaria infestations, dracunculus infestations, pediculosis capitis, tinea infections

CONTRAINDICATIONS

Prophylactic treatment of pinworm infestation, hypersensitivity to thiabendazole or its components

INTERACTIONS

Drug

Theophylline, other xanthines: May increase levels of theophylline or other xanthinges.

Herbal

None known.

Food

None known.

T

Drug interactions of concern to dentistry

- Suspected interference with xanthine metabolism

DIAGNOSTIC TEST EFFECTS

None known.

SIDE EFFECTS

Occasional

Dizziness, drowsiness, nausea, vomiting, diarrhea

Rare

Erythema multiform, liver damage

SERIOUS REACTIONS

! Overdose includes symptoms of altered mental status and visual problems.

! Erythema multiform, liver damage, and Stevens-Johnsons syndrome occur rarely.

DENTAL CONSIDERATIONS

General:

- Determine why patient is taking the drug.
- Patient on chronic drug therapy may rarely present with symptoms of blood dyscrasias, which can include infection, bleeding, and poor healing. If dyscrasia is present, caution patient to prevent oral tissue trauma when using oral hygiene aids.
- Assess salivary flow as a factor in caries, periodontal disease, and candidiasis.
- Pinworm infections are easily spread to persons in close contact.
- Question patients about other drugs they may be using.

Consultations:

- In a patient with symptoms of blood dyscrasias, request a medical consultation for blood studies and postpone treatment until normal values are reestablished.
- Medical consultation may be required to assess disease control in the patient.

Teach Patient/Family:

- *When chronic dry mouth occurs, advise patient:*
  - To avoid mouth rinses with high alcohol content due to drying effects
  - To use daily home fluoride products for anticaries effect
  - To use sugarless gum, frequent sips of water or saliva substitutes

thiamine hydrochloride (vitamin B_1)

thy′-a-min

(Beta-Sol[AUS], Betaxin[CAN], Thiamilate)

CATEGORY AND SCHEDULE

Pregnancy Risk Category: A (C if used in doses above recommended daily allowance)

OTC (tablets)

MECHANISM OF ACTION

A water-soluble vitamin that combines with adenosine triphosphate in the liver, kidneys, and leukocytes to form thiamine diphosphate, a coenzyme that is necessary for carbohydrate metabolism. ***Therapeutic Effect:*** Prevents and reverses thiamine deficiency.

PHARMACOKINETICS

Readily absorbed from the GI tract, primarily in duodenum, after IM administration. Widely distributed. Metabolized in the liver. Primarily excreted in urine.

T

AVAILABILITY
Tablets: 50 mg, 100 mg, 250 mg, 500 mg.
Injection: 100 mg/ml.

INDICATIONS AND DOSAGES
▸ Dietary Supplement
PO
Adults, Elderly. 1–2 mg/day.
Children. 0.5–1 mg/day.
Infants. 0.3–0.5 mg/day.
▸ Thiamine Deficiency
PO
Adults, Elderly. 5–30 mg/day, as a single dose or in 3 divided doses, for 1 mo.
Children. 10–50 mg/day in 3 divided doses.
▸ Thiamine Deficiency in Patients Who Are Critically Ill or Have Malabsorption Syndrome
IV, IM
Adults, Elderly. 5–100 mg, 3 times a day.
Children. 10–25 mg/day.
▸ Metabolic Disorders
PO
Adults, Elderly, Children. 10–20 mg/day; increased up to 4 g/day in divided doses.

CONTRAINDICATIONS
None known.

INTERACTIONS
Drug
None known.
Herbal
None known.
Food
None known.

DIAGNOSTIC TEST EFFECTS
None known.

IV INCOMPATIBILITIES
sodium bicarbonate

IV COMPATIBILITIES
Famotidine (Pepcid), multivitamins

SIDE EFFECTS
Frequent
Pain, induration, and tenderness at IM injection site

SERIOUS REACTIONS
! IV administration may result in a rare, severe hypersensitivity reaction marked by a feeling of warmth, pruritus, urticaria, weakness, diaphoresis, nausea, restlessness, tightness in throat, angioedema, cyanosis, pulmonary edema, GI tract bleeding, and cardiovascular collapse.

DENTAL CONSIDERATIONS
General:
- Determine why the patient is taking this vitamin.

Teach Patient/Family:
- Food sources to be included in diet: yeast, whole grain, beef, liver, legumes

thiethylperazine
thye-eth-il-per′-azeen
(Torecan)
Do not confuse with thioridazine.

CATEGORY AND SCHEDULE
Pregnancy Risk Category: X

MECHANISM OF ACTION
A piperazine phenothiazine that acts centrally to block dopamine receptors in chemoreceptor trigger zone (CTZ) in central nervous system (CNS). ***Therapeutic Effect:*** Relieves nausea and vomiting.

AVAILABILITY
Injection: 5 mg/ml (Torecan).
Tablets: 10 mg (Torecan).

T

INDICATIONS AND DOSAGES

▸ **Nausea or Vomiting**

PO/RECTAL/IM

Adults, Elderly. 10 mg 1–3 times/day.

CONTRAINDICATIONS

Comatose states, severe CNS depression, pregnancy, hypersensitivity to phenothiazines

INTERACTIONS

Drug

Alcohol, CNS depressants: May increase respiratory depression and the hypotensive effects of thiethylperazine.

Epinephrine: May block alpha-adrenergic effects of epinephrine causing hypotension and tachycardia.

Extrapyramidal symptom-producing medications: Increased risk of extrapyramidal symptoms (EPS).

Levodopa: May decrease the effects of levodopa.

Quinidine: May increase cardiac effects.

Herbal

None known.

Food

None known.

Drug interactions of concern to dentistry

- Increased anticholinergic action: anticholinergics
- Increased CNS depression, hypotension: alcohol, CNS depressants

DIAGNOSTIC TEST EFFECTS

None known.

SIDE EFFECTS

Frequent

Drowsiness, dizziness

Occasional

Blurred vision, decreased color/night vision, fever, headache, orthostatic hypotension, rash, ringing in ears, constipation, dry mouth, decreased sweating.

SERIOUS REACTIONS

! Extrapyramidal symptoms manifested as torticollis (neck muscle spasm), oculogyric crisis (rolling back of eyes), and akathisia (motor restlessness, anxiety) occur rarely.

DENTAL CONSIDERATIONS

General:

- Postpone elective dental treatment when symptoms are present.

Consultations:

- Medical consultation may be required to assess disease control.

thioridazine

thye-or-rid′-a-zeen

(Aldazine[AUS], Apo-Thioridazine[CAN], Mellaril, Melleril[AUS], Thioridazine Intensol)

Do not confuse thioridazine with thiothixene or Thorazine, or Mellaril with Mebaral.

CATEGORY AND SCHEDULE

Pregnancy Risk Category: C

MECHANISM OF ACTION

A phenothiazine that blocks dopamine at postsynaptic receptor sites. Possesses strong anticholinergic and sedative effects.

Therapeutic Effect: Suppresses behavioral response in psychosis; reduces locomotor activity and aggressiveness.

AVAILABILITY

Oral Solution (Concentrate [Thioridazine Intensol]): 30 mg/ml.
Tablets (Melleril): 10 mg, 15 mg, 25 mg, 50 mg, 100 mg, 150 mg, 200 mg.

INDICATIONS AND DOSAGES

▸ Psychosis

PO
Adults, Elderly, Children 12 yr and older. Initially, 25–100 mg 3 times a day; dosage increased gradually. Maximum: 800 mg/day.
Children 2–11 yr. Initially, 0.5 mg/kg/day in 2–3 divided doses. Maximum: 3 mg/kg/day.

OFF-LABEL USES

Treatment of behavioral problems in children, dementia, depressive neurosis

CONTRAINDICATIONS

Angle-closure glaucoma, blood dyscrasias, cardiac arrhythmias, cardiac or hepatic impairment, concurrent use of drugs that prolong QT interval, severe CNS depression

INTERACTIONS

Drug

Alcohol, other CNS depressants: May increase respiratory depression and the hypotensive effects of thioridazine.
Antithyroid agents: May increase the risk of agranulocytosis.
Extrapyramidal symptom-producing medications: May increase the risk of extrapyramidal symptoms.
Hypotension-producing agents: May increase hypotension.
Levodopa: May decrease the effects of levodopa.
Lithium: May decrease the absorption of thioridazine and produce adverse neurologic effects.
MAOIs, tricyclic antidepressants: May increase the anticholinergic and sedative effects of thioridazine.

Herbal

None known.

Food

None known.

Drug interactions of concern to dentistry

- Increased sedation: other CNS depressants, alcohol, barbiturate anesthetics, opioid analgesics
- Hypotension, tachycardia: epinephrine (systemic)
- Increased extrapyramidal effects: phenothiazines and related drugs (haloperidol, droperidol), metoclopramide
- Additive photosensitization: tetracyclines
- Increased anticholinergic effects: anticholinergics

DIAGNOSTIC TEST EFFECTS

May cause ECG changes. Therapeutic serum level is 0.2–2.6 mcg/ml; toxic serum level is not established.

SIDE EFFECTS

Occasional

Drowsiness during early therapy, dry mouth, blurred vision, lethargy, constipation or diarrhea, nasal congestion, peripheral edema, urine retention

Rare

Ocular changes, altered skin pigmentation (in those taking high doses for prolonged periods), photosensitivity, darkening of urine

SERIOUS REACTIONS

! Prolonged QT interval may produce torsades de pointes, a form of ventricular tachycardia, and sudden death.

T

DENTAL CONSIDERATIONS

General:

- Monitor vital signs at every appointment because of CV side effects.
- Patients on chronic drug therapy may rarely have symptoms of blood dyscrasias, which can include infection, bleeding, and poor healing.
- After supine positioning, have patient sit upright for at least 2 min before standing to avoid orthostatic hypotension.
- Assess salivary flow as a factor in caries, periodontal disease, and candidiasis.
- Avoid dental light in patient's eyes; offer dark glasses for patient comfort.
- Assess for presence of extrapyramidal motor symptoms, such as tardive dyskinesia and akathisia. Extrapyramidal motor activity may complicate dental treatment.
- Geriatric patients are more susceptible to drug effects; use lower dose.
- Use vasoconstrictors with caution, in low doses, and with careful aspiration.

Consultations:

- In a patient with symptoms of blood dyscrasias, request a medical consultation for blood studies and postpone dental treatment until normal values are reestablished.
- Take precautions if dental surgery is anticipated and anesthesia is required.
- Refer to physician if signs of tardive dyskinesia or akathisia are present.
- Physician should be informed if significant xerostomic side effects occur (e.g., increased caries, sore tongue, problems eating or swallowing, difficulty wearing prosthesis) so that a medication change can be considered.

Teach Patient/Family:

- Importance of good oral hygiene to prevent soft tissue inflammation
- Caution to prevent injury when using oral hygiene aids
- To use electric toothbrush if patient has difficulty holding conventional devices
- *When chronic dry mouth occurs, advise patient:*
  - To avoid mouth rinses with high alcohol content because of drying effects
  - Of need for daily home fluoride use to prevent caries
  - To use sugarless gum, frequent sips of water, or saliva substitutes

thiotepa

thigh-oh-teh′-pah
(Thioplex)

CATEGORY AND SCHEDULE

Pregnancy Risk Category: D

MECHANISM OF ACTION

An alkylating agent that inhibits DNA and RNA protein synthesis by cross-linking with DNA and RNA strands, preventing cell growth. Cell cycle-phase nonspecific.

Therapeutic Effect: Interferes with DNA and RNA function.

AVAILABILITY

Powder for Injection: 15 mg.

INDICATIONS AND DOSAGES

▸ **Adenocarcinoma of Breast and Ovary, Hodgkin's Disease, Lymphosarcoma, Superficial**

T

Papillary Carcinoma of Urinary Bladder
IV
Adults, Elderly. Initially, 0.3–0.4 mg/kg every 1–4 wk. Maintenance dose adjusted weekly on the basis of blood counts.
Children. 25–65 mg/m^2 as a single dose every 3–4 wk.

▸ **Control of Pericardial, Peritoneal, or Pleural Effusions Due to Metastatic Tumors**
INTRACAVITARY INJECTION
Adults, Elderly. 0.6–0.8 mg/kg every 1–4wk.

OFF-LABEL USES
Treatment of lung carcinoma

CONTRAINDICATIONS
Pregnancy, severe myelosuppression (leukocyte count < 3000/mm^3 or platelet count less than 150,000/mm^3)

INTERACTIONS
Drug
Antigout medications: May decrease the effects of these drugs.
Bone marrow depressants: May increase myelosuppression.
Live-virus vaccines: May potentiate virus replication, increase vaccine side effects, and decrease the patient's antibody response to the vaccine.

T

Herbal
None known.
Food
None known.
Drug interactions of concern to dentistry
- Suspected decrease in effects: probenecid
- Prolonged neuromuscular blockade: pancuronium

DIAGNOSTIC TEST EFFECTS
May increase serum uric acid levels.

IV INCOMPATIBILITIES
Cisplatin (Platinol-AQ), filgrastim (Neupogen)

IV COMPATIBILITIES
Allopurinol (Aloprim), bumetanide (Bumex), calcium gluconate, carboplatin (Paraplatin), cyclophosphamide (Cytoxan), dexamethasone (Decadron), diphenhydramine (Benadryl), doxorubicin (Adriamycin), etoposide (VePesid), fluorouracil, gemcitabine (Gemzar), granisetron (Kytril), heparin, hydromorphone (Dilaudid), leucovorin, lorazepam (Ativan), magnesium sulfate, morphine, ondansetron (Zofran), paclitaxel (Taxol), potassium chloride, vincristine (Oncovin), vinorelbine (Navelbine)

SIDE EFFECTS
Occasional
Pain at injection site, headache, dizziness, urticaria, rash, nausea, vomiting, anorexia, stomatitis
Rare
Alopecia, cystitis, hematuria (after intravesical dose)

SERIOUS REACTIONS
! Hematologic toxicity, manifested as leukopenia, anemia, thrombocytopenia, and pancytopenia, may occur from bone marrow depression.
! Although the WBC count falls to its lowest point 10–14 days after initial therapy, the initial effects on bone marrow may not evident for 30 days.
! Stomatitis and ulceration of intestinal mucosa may occur.

DENTAL CONSIDERATIONS
General:
- If additional analgesia is required for dental pain, consider alternative

analgesics (NSAIDs) in patients taking narcotics for acute or chronic pain.
• Examine for oral manifestation of opportunistic infection.
• Avoid products that affect platelet function, such as aspirin and NSAIDs.
• This drug may be used in the hospital or on an outpatient basis. Confirm the patient's disease and treatment status.
• Patient on chronic drug therapy may rarely present with symptoms of blood dyscrasias, which can include infection, bleeding, and poor healing. If dyscrasia is present, caution patient to prevent oral tissue trauma when using oral hygiene aids.
• Palliative medication may be required for management of oral side effects.
• Patient may need assistance in getting into and out of dental chair. Adjust chair position for patient comfort.
• Consider semisupine chair position for patient comfort if GI side effects occur.
• Caution: patients may be at high risk for infection.
• Patients may be at risk for bleeding; check oral signs.
• Oral infections should be eliminated and/or treated aggressively.

Consultations:
• Medical consultation should include routine blood counts including platelet counts and bleeding time.
• In a patient with symptoms of blood dyscrasias, request a medical consultation for blood studies and postpone treatment until normal values are reestablished.
• Consult physician; prophylactic or therapeutic antiinfectives may be indicated if surgery or periodontal treatment is required.
• Medical consultation may be required to assess immunologic status during cancer chemotherapy and determine safety risk, if any, posed by the required dental treatment.
• Medical consultation may be required to assess disease control and patient's ability to tolerate stress.

Teach Patient/Family:
• Importance of good oral hygiene to prevent soft tissue inflammation
• To report oral lesions, soreness, or bleeding to dentist
• To prevent trauma when using oral hygiene aids
• Importance of updating health and medication history if physician makes any changes in evaluation or drug regimens; include OTC, herbal, and nonherbal remedies in the update

thiothixene

thye-oh-thix′-een
(Navane)
Do not confuse thiothixene with thioridazine.

CATEGORY AND SCHEDULE

Pregnancy Risk Category: C

T

MECHANISM OF ACTION

An antipsychotic that blocks postsynaptic dopamine receptor sites in brain. Has alpha-adrenergic blocking effects, and depresses the release of hypothalamic and hypophyseal hormones. ***Therapeutic Effect:*** Suppresses psychotic behavior.

PHARMACOKINETICS
Well absorbed from the GI tract after IM administration. Widely distributed. Metabolized in the liver. Primarily excreted in urine. Unknown if removed by hemodialysis. ***Half-life:*** 34 hr.

AVAILABILITY
Capsules: 1 mg, 2 mg, 5 mg, 10 mg, 20 mg.
Oral Concentrate: 5 mg/ml.
Injection: 5 mg of thiothixene and 59.6 mg of mannitol per ml when reconstituted with 2.2 ml of sterile water for injection.

INDICATIONS AND DOSAGES
▸ Psychosis
PO
Adults, Elderly, Children older than 12 yr. Initially, 2 mg 3 times a day. Maximum: 60 mg/day.
IM
Adults, Elderly, Children older than 12 yr. Initially, 4 mg 2–4 times a day. Maximum: 30 mg/day.

CONTRAINDICATIONS
Blood dyscrasias, circulatory collapse, CNS depression, coma, history of seizures

INTERACTIONS
Drug
Alcohol, other CNS depressants: May increase CNS and respiratory depression and the hypotensive effects of thiothixene.
Extrapyramidal symptom-producing medications: May increase the risk of extrapyramidal symptoms.
Levodopa: May inhibit the effects of levodopa.
Quinidine: May increase cardiac effects.
Herbal
Kava kava, St. John's wort, valerian: May increase CNS depression.
Food
None known.
Drug interactions of concern to dentistry
- Increased sedation: other CNS depressants, alcohol, barbiturate anesthetics, opioid analgesics
- Hypotension, tachycardia: epinephrine (systemic)
- Increased extrapyramidal effects: phenothiazines and related drugs (haloperidol, droperidol), metoclopramide
- Additive photosensitization: tetracyclines
- Increased anticholinergic effects: anticholinergics

DIAGNOSTIC TEST EFFECTS
May decrease serum uric acid level.

SIDE EFFECTS
Expected
Hypotension, dizziness, syncope (occur frequently after first injection, occasionally after subsequent injections, and rarely with oral form)
Frequent
Transient drowsiness, dry mouth, constipation, blurred vision, nasal congestion
Occasional
Diarrhea, peripheral edema, urine retention, nausea
Rare
Ocular changes, altered skin pigmentation (in those taking high doses for prolonged periods), photosensitivity

SERIOUS REACTIONS
! The most common extrapyramidal reaction is akathisia, characterized by motor restlessness and anxiety. Akinesia, marked by rigidity, tremor, increased salivation, masklike facial expression, and reduced voluntary movements, occurs less frequently. Dystonias, including torticollis,

opisthotonos, and oculogyric crisis, occur rarely.

! Tardive dyskinesia, characterized by tongue protrusion, puffing of the cheeks, and chewing or puckering of the mouth, occurs rarely but may be irreversible. Elderly female patients have a greater risk of developing this reaction.

! Grand mal seizures may occur in epileptic patients, especially those receiving the drug by IM administration.

! Neuroleptic malignant syndrome occurs rarely.

DENTAL CONSIDERATIONS

General:

- Monitor vital signs at every appointment because of CV side effects.
- Patients on chronic drug therapy may rarely have symptoms of blood dyscrasias, which can include infection, bleeding, and poor healing.
- After supine positioning, have patient sit upright for at least 2 min before standing to avoid orthostatic hypotension.
- Assess salivary flow as a factor in caries, periodontal disease, and candidiasis.
- Assess for presence of extrapyramidal motor symptoms, such as tardive dyskinesia and akathisia. Extrapyramidal motor activity may complicate dental treatment.
- Use vasoconstrictors with caution, in low doses, and with careful aspiration.
- Avoid dental light in patient's eyes; offer dark glasses for patient comfort.
- Geriatric patients are more susceptible to drug effects; use lower dose.

Consultations:

- In a patient with symptoms of blood dyscrasias, request a medical consultation for blood studies and postpone dental treatment until normal values are reestablished.
- Take precautions if dental surgery is anticipated and anesthesia is required.
- If signs of tardive dyskinesia or akathisia are present, refer to physician.

Teach Patient/Family:

- Importance of good oral hygiene to prevent soft tissue inflammation
- Caution to prevent injury when using oral hygiene aids
- To use electric toothbrush if patient has difficulty holding conventional devices
- *When chronic dry mouth occurs, advise patient:*
  - To avoid mouth rinses with high alcohol content because of drying effects
  - Of need for daily home fluoride use to prevent caries
  - To use sugarless gum, frequent sips of water, or saliva substitutes

thrombin, topical (thrombinar, thrombin-JMI, thrombostat, etc.)

throm-**bin**

CATEGORY AND SCHEDULE

Pregnancy Risk Category: C

MECHANISM OF ACTION

A protein substance produced through a conversion reaction in which prothrombin of bovine origin is activated by tissue thromboplastin in the presence of calcium chloride. It directly clots fibrinogen in the blood. ***Therapeutic Effect:*** Controls bleeding.

PHARMACOKINETICS

The speed with which thrombin clots blood is dependent upon the concentration of both thrombin and fibrinogen.

AVAILABILITY

Topical Kit: 10,000 units (Thrombogen), 20,000 units (Thrombin-JMI, Thrombogen).
Topical Powder for Reconstitution: 1000 units (Thrombin-JMI), 5000 units (Thrombinar, Thrombogen), 10,000 units (Thrombin-JMI, Thrombogen).

INDICATIONS AND DOSAGES

▸ **Hemorrhage, Mild**
TOPICAL
Adults. Apply 100 units/ml as needed

▸ **Hemorrhage, Severe**
TOPICAL
Adults. Apply 1000 units/ml as needed.

CONTRAINDICATIONS

Sensitivity to thrombin, any of its components and/or to material of bovine origin

INTERACTIONS

Drug
None known.
Herbal
None known.
Food
None known.
Drug interactions of concern to dentistry
- None reported

DIAGNOSTIC TEST EFFECTS

None known.

SIDE EFFECTS

Occasional
Allergic reaction

SERIOUS REACTIONS

! Because of its action in the clotting mechanism, thrombin must not be injected or otherwise allowed to enter large blood vessels. Extensive intravascular clotting and even death may result.

DENTAL CONSIDERATIONS

General:
- Solutions (~ 100 U/ml) are prepared with sterile normal saline or sterile distilled water.
- Can be used with absorbable gelatin sponge but not microfibrillar collagen.

Teach Patient/Family:
- To report oral lesions, soreness, or bleeding to dentist

thyroid

thye′-roid
(Armour Thyroid, Nature-Throid NT, Westhroid)

CATEGORY AND SCHEDULE

Pregnancy Risk Category: A

MECHANISM OF ACTION

A natural hormone derived from animal sources, usually beef or pork, that is involved in normal metabolism, growth, and development, especially the central nervous system (CNS) of infants. Possesses catabolic and anabolic effects. Provides both levothyroxine and liothyronine hormones. ***Therapeutic Effect:*** Increases basal metabolic rate,

T

enhances gluconeogenesis, stimulates protein synthesis.

PHARMACOKINETICS

Partially absorbed from the gastrointestinal (GI) tract. Protein binding: 99%. Widely distributed. Metabolized in liver to active, liothyronine (T_3), and inactive, reverse triiodothyronine (rT_3), metabolites. Eliminated by biliary excretion. ***Half-life:*** 2–7 days.

AVAILABILITY

Capsules: 15 mg, 30 mg, 60 mg, 90 mg, 120 mg, 180 mg, 240 mg.
Tablets: 30 mg, 32.5 mg, 60 mg, 65 mg, 120 mg, 130 mg, 180 mg.
15 mg, 30 mg, 60 mg, 90 mg, 120 mg, 180 mg, 240 mg, 300 mg (Armour Thyroid).
32.4 mg, 64.8 mg, 129.6 mg, 194.4 mg (Nature-Throid NT, Westhroid).

INDICATIONS AND DOSAGES

▸ Hypothyroidism

PO

Adults, Elderly. Initially, 15–30 mg. May increase by 15 mg increments q2–4wks. Maintenance: 60–120 mcg/day. Use 15 mg in patients with cardiovascular disease or myxedema.
Children 12 yrs and older. 90 mg/day.
Children 6–12 yrs. 60–90 mg/day.
Children older than 1–5 yrs. 45–60 mg/day.
Children older than 6–12 mos. 30–45 mg/day.
Children 3 mos and younger. 15–30 mg/day.

CONTRAINDICATIONS

Uncontrolled adrenal cortical insufficiency, untreated thyrotoxicosis, treatment of obesity, uncontrolled angina, uncontrolled hypertension, uncontrolled myocardial infarction, and hypersensitivity to any component of the formulations

INTERACTIONS

Drug

Cholestyramine, colestipol: May decrease absorption of thyroid hormones.
Estrogens, oral contraceptives: May decrease effects of thyroid hormones.
Insulin, oral hypoglycemics: May decrease effects of insulin and oral hypoglycemics.
Oral anticoagulants: May increase hypoprothrombinemic effects of oral anticoagulants
Tricyclic antidepressants: May increase risk of toxicity of both drugs.

Herbal

Bugleweed: May decrease effects of thyroid hormones.

Food

None known.

Drug interactions of concern to dentistry

- Increased effects of sympathomimetics when thyroid doses are not carefully monitored or with coronary artery disease

SIDE EFFECTS

Rare

Dry skin, GI intolerance, skin rash, hives, severe headache

SERIOUS REACTIONS

! Excessive dosage produces signs and symptoms of hyperthyroidism including weight loss, palpitations, increased appetite, tremors, nervousness, tachycardia, hypertension, headache, insomnia, and menstrual irregularities.
! Cardiac arrhythmias occur rarely.

DENTAL CONSIDERATIONS

General:

- Increased nervousness, excitability, sweating, or tachycardia may indicate uncontrolled hyperthyroidism or a dose of medication that is too high. Uncontrolled patients should be referred for medical treatment.

Consultations:

- Medical consultation may be required to assess disease control.

tiagabine

ti-ah-ga′-bean

(Gabitril)

CATEGORY AND SCHEDULE

Pregnancy Risk Category: C

MECHANISM OF ACTION

An anticonvulsant that enhances the activity of gamma-aminobutyric acid, the major inhibitory neurotransmitter in the CNS. ***Therapeutic Effect:*** Inhibits seizures.

AVAILABILITY

Tablets: 2 mg, 4 mg, 12 mg, 16 mg.

INDICATIONS AND DOSAGES

▸ **Adjunctive Treatment of Partial Seizures**

PO

Adults, Elderly. Initially, 4 mg once a day. May increase by 4–8 mg/day at weekly intervals. Maximum: 56 mg/day.

Children 12–18 yr. Initially, 4 mg once a day. May increase by 4 mg at week 2 and by 4–8 mg at weekly intervals thereafter. Maximum: 32 mg/day.

CONTRAINDICATIONS

None known.

INTERACTIONS

Drug

Carbamazepine, phenobarbital, phenytoin: May increase tiagabine clearance.

Valproic acid: May alter the effects of valproic acid.

Herbal

None known.

Food

None known.

Drug interactions of concern to dentistry

- Increased tiagabine clearance: carbamazepine, phenobarbital
- Use CNS depressants with caution because of possible additional effects

DIAGNOSTIC TEST EFFECTS

None known.

SIDE EFFECTS

Frequent (34%–20%)

Dizziness, asthenia, somnolence, nervousness, confusion, headache, infection, tremor

Occasional

Nausea, diarrhea, abdominal pain, impaired concentration

SERIOUS REACTIONS

! Overdose is characterized by agitation, confusion, hostility, and weakness. Full recovery occurs within 24 hours.

DENTAL CONSIDERATIONS

General:

- Monitor vital signs at every appointment because of CV and respiratory side effects.
- Consider semisupine chair position for patient comfort when GI side effects occur.

• Short appointments and a stress reduction protocol may be required for anxious patients.
• Determine type of epilepsy, seizure frequency, and quality of seizure control.
• Assess salivary flow as factor in caries, periodontal disease, and candidiasis.
• Place on frequent recall if oral side effects occur.

Consultations:
• Consultation with physician may be necessary if sedation or general anesthesia is required.

Teach Patient/Family:
• Caution to prevent trauma when using oral hygiene aids
• Use of electric toothbrush if patient has difficulty holding conventional devices
• Importance of good oral hygiene to prevent soft tissue inflammation
• Importance of updating health and drug history if physician makes any changes in evaluation or drug regimens
• To be aware of oral side effects and potential sequelae
• *When chronic dry mouth occurs, advise patient:*
  • To avoid mouth rinses with high alcohol content because of drying effects
  • To use daily home fluoride products for anticaries effect
  • To use sugarless gum, frequent sips of water, or saliva substitutes

ticarcillin
(Ticar)

CATEGORY AND SCHEDULE
Pregnancy Risk Category: B

MECHANISM OF ACTION
Binds to bacterial cell wall, inhibiting bacterial cell wall synthesis. ***Therapeutic Effect:*** Causes cell lysis, death. Bactericidal.

PHARMACOKINETICS
Well absorbed. Widely distributed. Protein binding: 45%–60%. Minimal metabolism in liver. Primarily excreted unchanged in urine. Moderately dialyzable. ***Half-life:*** 1.2 hrs (half-life is increased in those with impaired renal function).

AVAILABILITY
Powder for reconstitution: 1g, 3 g, 20 g (Ticar).

INDICATIONS AND DOSAGES
▸ Septicemia; Skin and Skin-Structure, Bone, Joint, and Lower Respiratory Tract Infections; and Endometriosis
IV
Adults, Elderly, Children over 40 kg. 200–300 mg/kg/day q4–6h or 3 g q4h or 4 g q6h. Maximum: 18 g/day.
Children and infants under 40 kg. 200–300 mg/kg/day q4–6h. Maximum: 18 g/day.
Neonates over 2000 g. 75 mg/kg IV q8h under 7 days old; 100 mg/kg IV q8h over 7 old.
Neonates under 2000 g. 75 mg/kg IV q12h under 7 days old; 75 mg/kg q8h over 7 days old.
▸ Urinary Tract Infection (UTI), Complicated
IV
Adults, Elderly, Children over 40 kg. 150–200 mg/kg/day divided q4–6h or 3 g q6h.
Children under 40 kg. 150–200 mg/kg/day in divided doses q6–8h.

T

Urinary Tract Infection (UTI), Uncomplicated
IV/IM
Adults, Elderly, Children over 40 kg. 1 g q6h.
Children under 40 kg.
50–100 mg/kg/day in divided doses q6–8h.

Dosage in Renal Impairment

Creatinine Clearance	Dosage Interval
30–60 ml/min	2 g q4h
10–30 ml/min	2 g q8h
less than 10 ml/min	2 g q12h

CONTRAINDICATIONS
Hypersensitivity to any penicillin

INTERACTIONS
Drug
Anticoagulants, heparin, NSAIDs, thrombolytics: May increase the risk of hemorrhage with high dosages of ticarcillin.
Probenecid: May increase ticarcillin blood concentration and risk of toxicity.
Herbal
None known.
Food
None known.
Drug interactions of concern to dentistry
- Possible increase in bleeding: anticoagulants, thrombolytic drugs, diflunisal (high doses), platelet aggregation inhibitors
- Decreased antimicrobial effectiveness: erythromycins, sulfonamides tetracyclines
- Oral contraceptives: advise patient of a potential risk for decreased contraceptive action, to maintain compliance with oral contraceptive while using antibiotics, and to consider the use of additional nonhormonal contraception
- Possible increase in methotrexate toxicity
- Increased or prolonged plasma levels: probenecid

DIAGNOSTIC TEST EFFECTS
May cause positive Coombs' test. May increase bleeding time, serum alkaline phosphatase, serum bilirubin, serum creatinine, serum LDH, SGOT (AST), and SGPT (ALT) levels. May decrease serum potassium, sodium, and uric acid levels.

IV INCOMPATIBILITIES
Amphotericin B complex (Abelcet, AmBisome, Amphotec), vancomycin (Vancocin)
IV COMPATIBILITIES
Diltiazem (Cardizem), heparin, insulin, morphine, propofol (Diprivan)

SIDE EFFECTS
Frequent
Phlebitis, thrombophlebitis with IV dose, rash, urticaria, pruritus, smell or taste disturbances
Occasional
Nausea, diarrhea, vomiting
Rare
Headache, fatigue, hallucinations, bleeding or bruising

SERIOUS REACTIONS
! Overdosage may produce seizures and neurologic reactions.
! Superinfections including potentially fatal antibiotic-associated colitis, may result from bacterial imbalance.
! Severe hypersensitivity reactions, including anaphylaxis, occur rarely.

DENTAL CONSIDERATIONS
General:
- For selected infections in the hospital setting; provide emergency dental treatment only.
- Caution regarding allergy to medication.

- Examine for oral manifestation of opportunistic infection.
- Determine why patient is taking the drug.

Consultations:

- Medical consultation may be required to assess disease control.
- CONIF

Teach Patient/Family:

- Importance of good oral hygiene to prevent soft tissue inflammation
- To report oral lesions, soreness, or bleeding to dentist
- To prevent trauma when using oral hygiene aids

ticarcillin disodium/ clavulanate potassium

tie-car-sill′-in/klah-view-lan′-ate (Timentin)

CATEGORY AND SCHEDULE

Pregnancy Risk Category: B

MECHANISM OF ACTION

Ticarcillin binds to bacterial cell walls, inhibiting cell wall synthesis. Clavulanate inhibits the action of bacterial beta-lactamase. ***Therapeutic Effect:*** Ticarcillin is bactericidal in susceptible organisms. Clavulanate protects ticarcillin from enzymatic degradation.

PHARMACOKINETICS

Widely distributed. Protein binding: ticarcillin 45%–60%, clavulanate 9%–30%. Minimally metabolized in the liver. Primarily excreted unchanged in urine. Removed by hemodialysis. ***Half-life:*** 1–1.2 hr (increased in impaired renal function).

AVAILABILITY

Powder for Injection: 3.1 g.
Premixed Solution for Infusion: 3.1 g/100 ml.

INDICATIONS AND DOSAGES

▸ Skin and Skin-Structure, Bone, Joint, and Lower Respiratory Tract Infections; Septicemia; Endometriosis

IV

Adults, Elderly. 3.1 g (3 g ticarcillin) q4–6h. Maximum: 18–24 g/day.
Children 3 mo and older. 200–300 mg (as ticarcillin) q4–6h.

▸ UTIs

IV

Adults, Elderly. 3.1 g q6–8h.

▸ Dosage in Renal Impairment

Dosage interval is modified on the basis of creatinine clearance.

Creatinine Clearance	Dosage Interval
10–30 ml/min	Usual dose q8h
less than 10 ml/min	Usual dose q12h

CONTRAINDICATIONS

Hypersensitivity to any penicillin

INTERACTIONS

Drug

Anticoagulants, heparin, NSAIDs, thrombolytics: May increase the risk of hemorrhage with high dosages of ticarcillin.
Probenecid: May increase ticarcillin blood concentration and risk of toxicity.

Herbal

None known.

Food

None known.

Drug interactions of concern to dentistry

- Possible increase in bleeding: anticoagulants, thrombolytic drugs,

T

diflunisal (high doses), platelet aggregation inhibitors
- Decreased antimicrobial effectiveness: erythromycins, sulfonamides, tetracyclines
- Oral contraceptives: advise patient of a potential risk for decreased contraceptive action, to maintain compliance with oral contraceptive while using antibiotics, and to consider the use of additional nonhormonal contraception
- Possible increase in methotrexate toxicity
- Increased or prolonged plasma levels: probenecid

DIAGNOSTIC TEST EFFECTS

May increase bleeding time and serum alkaline phosphatase, bilirubin, creatinine, LDH, AST (SGOT), and ALT (SGPT) levels. May decrease serum potassium, sodium, and uric acid levels. May cause a positive Coombs' test.

IV INCOMPATIBILITIES

Amphotericin B complex (Abelcet, AmBisome, Amphotec), vancomycin (Vancocin)

IV COMPATIBILITIES

Diltiazem (Cardizem), heparin, insulin, morphine, propofol (Diprivan)

SIDE EFFECTS

Frequent
Phlebitis or thrombophlebitis (with IV dose), rash, urticaria, pruritus, altered smell or taste
Occasional
Nausea, diarrhea, vomiting
Rare
Headache, fatigue, hallucinations, bleeding, or ecchymosis

SERIOUS REACTIONS

! Overdosage may produce seizures and other neurologic reactions.
! Antibiotic-associated colitis and other superinfections may result from bacterial imbalance.
! Severe hypersensitivity reactions including anaphylaxis occur rarely.

DENTAL CONSIDERATIONS

General:
- For selected infections in the hospital setting; provide emergency dental treatment only.
- Caution regarding allergy to medication.
- Examine for oral manifestation of opportunistic infection.
- Determine why patient is taking the drug.

Consultations:
- Medical consultation may be required to assess disease control.
- CONIF

Teach Patient/Family:
- Importance of good oral hygiene to prevent soft tissue inflammation
- To report oral lesions, soreness, or bleeding to dentist
- To prevent trauma when using oral hygiene aids

ticlopidine hydrochloride

tye-klo′-pa-deen
(Apo-Ticlopidine[CAN], Ticlid, Tilodene[AUS])

CATEGORY AND SCHEDULE

Pregnancy Risk Category: B

MECHANISM OF ACTION

An aggregation inhibitor that inhibits the release of adenosine diphosphate from activated platelets, which prevents fibrinogen from binding to glycoprotein IIb/IIIa receptors on the surface of activated platelets. ***Therapeutic Effect:*** Inhibits platelet aggregation and thrombus formation.

AVAILABILITY

Tablets: 250 mg.

INDICATIONS AND DOSAGES

▸ **Prevention of Stroke**

PO

Adults, Elderly. 250 mg twice a day.

OFF-LABEL USES

Treatment of intermittent claudication, sickle cell disease, subarachnoid hemorrhage

CONTRAINDICATIONS

Active pathologic bleeding, such as bleeding peptic ulcer and intracranial bleeding, hematopoietic disorders including neutropenia and thrombocytopenia; presence of hemostatic disorder; severe hepatic impairment

INTERACTIONS

Drug

Aspirin, heparin, oral anticoagulants, thrombolytics: May increase the risk of bleeding with these drugs.

Herbal

None known.

Food

None known.

Drug interactions of concern to dentistry

• Increased bleeding tendencies: aspirin, NSAIDs

DIAGNOSTIC TEST EFFECTS

May increase serum cholesterol, serum alkaline phosphatase, bilirubin, triglyceride, AST(SGOT), and ALT(SGPT) levels. May prolong bleeding time. May decrease neutrophil and platelet counts.

SIDE EFFECTS

Frequent (13%–5%)

Diarrhea, nausea, dyspepsia including heartburn, indigestion GI discomfort, and bloating

Rare (2%–1%)

Vomiting, flatulence, pruritus, dizziness

SERIOUS REACTIONS

! Neutropenia occurs in approximately 2% of patients.

! Thrombotic thrombocytopenia purpura, agranulocytosis, hepatitis, cholestatic jaundice, and tinnitus occur rarely.

DENTAL CONSIDERATIONS

General:

• Patients on chronic drug therapy may rarely have symptoms of blood dyscrasias, which can include infection, bleeding, and poor healing.

• Consider local hemostatic measures to prevent excessive bleeding.

Consultations:

• Medical consultation may be required to assess disease control and patient's ability to tolerate stress. Consultation should include data on hematologic profile.

Teach Patient/Family:

• Caution to prevent injury when using oral hygiene aids

tiludronate
ti-loo′-dro-nate
(Skelid)

CATEGORY AND SCHEDULE
Pregnancy Risk Category: C

MECHANISM OF ACTION
A calcium regulator that inhibits functioning osteoclasts through disruption of cytoskeletal ring structure and inhibition of osteoclastic proton pump. ***Therapeutic Effect:*** Inhibits bone resorption.

AVAILABILITY
Tablets: 200 mg.

INDICATIONS AND DOSAGES
▸ **Paget's Disease**

PO

Adults, Elderly. 400 mg once a day for 3 mo. Must take with 6–8 ounces plain water. Do not give within 2 hr of food intake. Avoid giving aspirin, calcium supplements, mineral supplements, or antacids within 2 hr of tiludronate administration.

CONTRAINDICATIONS
GI disease, such as dysphagia and gastric ulcer, impaired renal function.

INTERACTIONS
Drug

Antacids containing aluminum or magnesium, calcium, salicylates: May interfere with the absorption of tiludronate.

Herbal

None known.

Food

None known.

Drug interactions of concern to dentistry

- Bioavailability decreased by calcium, food, aluminum or magnesium antacids
- Do not take indomethacin, aspirin, or calcium supplements 2 hr before or after tiludronate

DIAGNOSTIC TEST EFFECTS
None known.

SIDE EFFECTS
Frequent (9%–6%)

Nausea, diarrhea, generalized body pain, back pain, headache

Occasional

Rash, dyspepsia, vomiting, rhinitis, sinusitis, dizziness

DENTAL CONSIDERATIONS
General:

- Be aware of oral manifestations of Paget's disease (macrognathia, alveolar pain).
- Consider semisupine chair position for patient comfort when GI side effects occur.
- Consider short appointments for patient comfort.
- Assess salivary flow as a factor in caries, periodontal disease, and candidiasis.

Consultations:

- Medical consultation may be required to assess disease control.

Teach Patient/Family:

- Caution to prevent trauma when using oral hygiene aids
- Importance of good oral hygiene to prevent soft tissue inflammation
- Importance of updating health and drug history if physician makes any changes in evaluation or drug regimens
- *When chronic dry mouth occurs, advise patient:*
  - To avoid mouth rinses with high alcohol content because of drying effects

• To use daily home fluoride products for anticaries effect
• To use sugarless gum, frequent sips of water, or saliva substitutes

timolol maleate

tim′-oh-lole
(Apo-Timol[CAN], Apo-Timop[CAN], Betimol, Blocadren, Gen-Timolol[CAN], Istadol, Optimol[AUS], PMS-Timolol [CAN], Tenopt[AUS], Timoptic, Timoptic OccuDose, Timoptic XE, Timoptol[AUS], Timoptol XE [AUS])

Do not confuse timolol with atenolol, or Timoptic with Viroptic.

CATEGORY AND SCHEDULE

Pregnancy Risk Category: C (D if used in second or third trimester)

MECHANISM OF ACTION

An antihypertensive, antimigraine, and antiglaucoma agent that blocks $beta_1$- and $beta_2$-adrenergic receptors. ***Therapeutic Effect:*** Reduces intraocular pressure (IOP) by reducing aqueous humor production, lowers BP, slows the heart rate, and decreases myocardial contractility.

PHARMACOKINETICS

Route	Onset	Peak	Duration
PO	15–45 min	0.5–2.5 hr	4 hr
Ophthalmic	30 min	1–2 hr	12–24 hr

Well absorbed from the GI tract. Protein binding: 60%. Minimal absorption after ophthalmic administration. Metabolized in the liver. Primarily excreted in urine. Not removed by hemodialysis. ***Half-life:*** 4 hr. Systemic absorption may occur with ophthalmic administration.

AVAILABILITY

Tablets (Blocadren): 5 mg, 10 mg, 20 mg.
Ophthalmic Gel (Timoptic-XE): 0.25%, 0.5%.
Ophthalmic Solution (Betimol, Timoptic, Timoptic OccuDose): 0.25%, 0.5%.

INDICATIONS AND DOSAGES

▸ **Mild to Moderate Hypertension**

PO

Adults, Elderly. Initially, 10 mg twice a day, alone or in combination with other therapy. Gradually increase at intervals of not less than 1 wk. Maintenance: 20–60 mg/day in 2 divided doses.

▸ **Reduction of Cardiovascular Mortality in Definite or Suspected Acute MI**

PO

Adults, Elderly. 10 mg twice a day, beginning 1–4 wk after infarction.

▸ **Migraine Prevention**

PO

Adults, Elderly. Initially, 10 mg twice a day. Range: 10–30 mg/day.

▸ **Reduction of IOP in Open-Angle Glaucoma, Aphakic Glaucoma, Ocular Hypertension, and Secondary Glaucoma**

OPHTHALMIC

Adults, Elderly, Children. 1 drop of 0.25% solution in affected eye(s) twice a day. May be increased to 1 drop of 0.5% solution in affected eye(s) twice a day. When IOP is controlled, dosage may be reduced to 1 drop once a day. If patient is switched to timolol from another antiglaucoma agent, administer

concurrently for 1 day. Discontinue other agent on following day.
Ophthalmic (Timoptic XE)
Adults, Elderly. 1 drop/day
Ophthalmic (Istalol)
Adults, Elderly. Apply once daily.

OFF-LABEL USES

Systemic: Treatment of anxiety, cardiac arrhythmias, chronic angina pectoris, hypertrophic cardiomyopathy, migraine, pheochromocytoma, thyrotoxicosis, tremors
Ophthalmic: To decrease IOP in acute or chronic angle-closure glaucoma, treatment of angle-closure glaucoma during and after iridectomy, malignant glaucoma, secondary glaucoma

CONTRAINDICATIONS

Bronchial asthma, cardiogenic shock, CHF unless secondary to tachyarrhythmias, COPD, patients receiving MAOI therapy, second- or third-degree heart block, sinus bradycardia, uncontrolled cardiac failure

INTERACTIONS

Drug

Diuretics, other antihypertensives: May increase hypotensive effect.
Insulin, oral hypoglycemics: May mask symptoms of hypoglycemia and prolong hypoglycemic effects of these drugs.
NSAIDs: May decrease antihypertensive effect.
Sympathomimetics, xanthines: May mutually inhibit effects.

Herbal

None known.

Food

None known.

Drug interactions of concern to dentistry

- Increased hypotension, bradycardia: anticholinergics, sympathomimetics (epinephrine)
- Decreased antihypertensive effects: indomethacin and other NSAIDs
- Suspected increase in plasma levels: diphenhydramine
- May slow metabolism of lidocaine

Drug interactions of concern to dentistry timolol maleate (optic)

- Avoid use of anticholinergic drugs, atropine-like drugs, propantheline, and diazepam (benzodiazepines)

DIAGNOSTIC TEST EFFECTS

May increase antinuclear antibody titer and BUN, serum LDH, serum lipoprotein, serum alkaline phosphatase, serum bilirubin, serum creatinine, serum potassium, serum uric acid, AST (SGOT), ALT (SGPT), and serum triglyceride levels.

SIDE EFFECTS

Frequent

Diminished sexual function, drowsiness, difficulty sleeping, unusual tiredness or weakness
Ophthalmic: Eye irritation, visual disturbances

Occasional

Depression, cold hands or feet, diarrhea, constipation, anxiety, nasal congestion, nausea, vomiting

Rare

Altered taste, dry eyes, itching, numbness of fingers, toes, or scalp

SERIOUS REACTIONS

! Overdose may produce profound bradycardia, hypotension, and bronchospasm.
! Abrupt withdrawal may result in diaphoresis, palpitations, headache, and tremors.
! Timolol administration may precipitate CHF and MI in patients with cardiac disease; thyroid storm in those with thyrotoxicosis; and peripheral ischemia in those

with existing peripheral vascular disease.

! Hypoglycemia may occur in patients with previously controlled diabetes.

! Ophthalmic overdose may produce bradycardia, hypotension, bronchospasm, and acute cardiac failure.

DENTAL CONSIDERATIONS

General:

- Monitor vital signs at every appointment because of CV side effects.
- Patients on chronic drug therapy may rarely have symptoms of blood dyscrasias, which can include infection, bleeding, and poor healing.
- Assess salivary flow as a factor in caries, periodontal disease, and candidiasis.
- Limit use of sodium-containing products, such as saline IV fluids, for patients with a dietary salt restriction.
- After supine positioning, have patient sit upright for at least 2 min before standing to avoid orthostatic hypotension.
- Stress from dental procedures may compromise CV function; determine patient risk.
- Short appointments and a stress reduction protocol may be required for anxious patients.
- Consider semisupine chair position for patients with nausea or respiratory distress.

Consultations:

- In a patient with symptoms of blood dyscrasias, request a medical consultation for blood studies and postpone dental treatment until normal values are reestablished.
- Medical consultation may be required to assess disease control and patient's ability to tolerate stress.

Teach Patient/Family:

- Importance of good oral hygiene to prevent soft tissue inflammation
- Caution to prevent injury when using oral hygiene aids
- *When chronic dry mouth occurs, advise patient:*
  - To avoid mouth rinses with high alcohol content because of drying effects
  - Of need for daily home fluoride use to prevent caries
  - To use sugarless gum, frequent sips of water, or saliva substitutes

TIMOLOL MALEATE (OPTIC)

General:

- Check compliance of patient with prescribed drug regimen for glaucoma.
- Avoid dental light in patient's eyes; offer dark glasses for patient comfort.

Consultations:

- Consultation with physician may be necessary if sedation or anesthesia is required.

tinzaparin sodium

tin-za-pair′-in
(Innohep)

CATEGORY AND SCHEDULE

Pregnancy Risk Category: B

MECHANISM OF ACTION

A low-molecular-weight heparin that inhibits factor Xa. Causes less inactivation of thrombin, inhibition of platelets, and bleeding than standard heparin. Does not significantly influence bleeding time, PT, aPTT. ***Therapeutic Effect:*** Produces anticoagulation.

PHARMACOKINETICS

Well absorbed after subcutaneous administration. Primarily eliminated in urine. ***Half-life:*** 3–4 hr.

AVAILABILITY

Injection: 20,000 anti-Xa international units/ml.

INDICATIONS AND DOSAGES

▸ Deep Vein Thrombosis

SUBCUTANEOUS

Adults, Elderly. 175 anti-Xa international units/kg once a day. Continue for at least 6 days and until patient is sufficiently anticoagulated with warfarin (International Normalizing Ratio [INR] of 2 or more for 2 consecutive days).

CONTRAINDICATIONS

Active major bleeding, concurrent heparin therapy, hypersensitivity to heparin or pork products, thrombocytopenia associated with positive in vitro test for antiplatelet antibody

INTERACTIONS

Drug

Anticoagulants, platelet inhibitors: May increase the risk of bleeding.

Herbal

Ginkgo biloba: May increase the risk of bleeding.

Food

None known.

Drug interactions of concern to dentistry

- Increased risk of bleeding: drugs that interfere with coagulation or platelet function, such as NSAIDs and aspirin

DIAGNOSTIC TEST EFFECTS

Increases (reversible) LDH, serum alkaline phosphatase, AST(SGOT), and ALT(SGPT) levels.

SIDE EFFECTS

Frequent (16%)

Injection site reaction, such as inflammation, oozing, nodules, and skin necrosis

Rare (< 2%)

Nausea, asthenia, constipation, epistaxis

SERIOUS REACTIONS

! Overdose may lead to bleeding complications ranging from local ecchymoses to major hemorrhage. Antidote: Dose of protamine sulfate (1% solution) should be equal to dose of tinzaparin injected. One mg protamine sulfate neutralizes 100 units of tinzaparin. A second dose of 0.5 mg tinzaparin per 1 mg protamine sulfate may be given if aPTT tested 2–4 hours after the initial infusion remains prolonged.

DENTAL CONSIDERATIONS

General:

- Determine why patient is taking the drug.
- Consider local hemostasis measures to prevent excessive bleeding.
- Avoid products that affect platelet function, such as aspirin and NSAIDs.
- Antibiotic prophylaxis prior to dental treatment may be required for joint prosthesis (see 1997 ADA guidelines).
- Patient may need assistance in getting into and out of dental chair. Adjust chair position for patient comfort.
- Product may be used in outpatient therapy. Delay elective dental

treatment until patient completes tinzaparin therapy.

Consultations:

- Medical consultation should include routine blood counts including platelet counts and bleeding time.

Teach Patient/Family:

- To prevent trauma when using oral hygiene aids
- To report oral lesions, soreness, or bleeding to dentist
- Importance of good oral hygiene to prevent soft tissue inflammation

tioconazole

tyo-con′-a-zole
(Gynecure[CAN], Monistat-1, Trosyd[CAN], Vagistat)

CATEGORY AND SCHEDULE

Pregnancy Risk Category: C

MECHANISM OF ACTION

An imidazole derivative that inhibits synthesis of ergosterol (vital component of fungal cell formation). ***Therapeutic Effect:*** Damaging fungal cell membrane. Fungistatic.

PHARMACOKINETICS

Negligible absorption from vaginal application.

AVAILABILITY

Vaginal Ointment: 6.5% (Monistat-1, Vagistat).

INDICATIONS AND DOSAGES

▸ **Vulvovaginal Candidiasis**

INTRAVAGINAL

Adults, Elderly. 1 applicatorful just before bedtime as a single dose.

CONTRAINDICATIONS

Hypersensitivity to tioconazole or other imidazole antifungal agents

INTERACTIONS

Drug

None known.

Herbal

None known.

Food

None known.

Drug interactions of concern to dentistry

- None reported

DIAGNOSTIC TEST EFFECTS

None known.

SIDE EFFECTS

Frequent (25%)

Headache

Occasional (6%–1%)

Burning, itching

Rare (< 1%)

Irritation, vaginal pain, dysuria, dryness of vaginal secretions, vulvar edema/swelling

SERIOUS REACTIONS

! None reported.

DENTAL CONSIDERATIONS

General:

- Be aware that broad-spectrum antibiotics can exacerbate vaginal candidiasis.

T

tiotropium bromide

tee-oh-trow′-pea-um
(Spiriva)

CATEGORY AND SCHEDULE

Pregnancy Risk Category: C

MECHANISM OF ACTION

An anticholinergic that binds to recombinant human muscarinic receptors at the smooth muscle, resulting in long-acting bronchial smooth-muscle relaxation. ***Therapeutic Effect:*** Relieves bronchospasm.

PHARMACOKINETICS

Route	Onset	Peak	Duration
Inhalation	N/A	N/A	24–36 hr

Binds extensively to tissue. Protein binding: 72%. Metabolized by oxidation. Excreted in urine. ***Half-life:*** 5–6 days.

AVAILABILITY

Powder for Inhalation:
18 mcg/capsule (in blister packs containing 6 capsules with inhaler).

INDICATIONS AND DOSAGES

▸ COPD

INHALATION

Adults, Elderly. 18 mcg (1 capsule)/day via *HandiHaler* inhalation device.

CONTRAINDICATIONS

History of hypersensitivity to atropine or its derivatives, including ipratropium

INTERACTIONS

Drug

Ipratropium: Concurrent administration with this drug is not recommended.

Herbal

None known.

Food

None known.

Drug interactions of concern to dentistry

- Dental drug interactions have not been studied

DIAGNOSTIC TEST EFFECTS

None known.

SIDE EFFECTS

Frequent (16%–6%)
Dry mouth, sinusitis, pharyngitis, dyspepsia, UTI, rhinitis
Occasional (5%–4%)
Abdominal pain, peripheral edema, constipation, epistaxis, vomiting, myalgia, rash, oral candidiasis

SERIOUS REACTIONS

! Angina pectoris, depression, and flulike symptoms occur rarely.

DENTAL CONSIDERATIONS

General:

- Monitor vital signs, especially respiration.
- Ask patient about exercise and activity tolerance.
- Caution: Not for acute episodes or emergency use.
- Assess salivary flow as a factor in caries, periodontal disease, and candidiasis.
- Place on frequent recall due to oral side effects.
- Acute asthmatic episodes may be precipitated in the dental office. A rapid-acting sympathomimetic inhalant (rescue inhaler) should be available for emergency use. Many patients may already have a prescribed rescue inhaler they normally use for acute asthmatic events.
- Consider semisupine chair position for patients with respiratory disease.

Consultations:

- Medical consultation may be required to assess disease control and patient's ability to tolerate stress.

T

Teach Patient/Family:

- *When chronic dry mouth occurs, advise patient:*
  - To avoid mouth rinses with high alcohol content due to drying effects
  - To use daily home fluoride products for anticaries effect
  - To use sugarless gum, frequent sips of water or saliva substitutes
- Importance of gargling, rinsing mouth with water and expectorating after each aerosol dose

tirofiban

tye-roe-fye′-ban
(Aggrastat)
Do not confuse Aggrastat with Aggrenox.

CATEGORY AND SCHEDULE

Pregnancy Risk Category: B

MECHANISM OF ACTION

An antiplatelet and antithrombotic agent that binds to platelet receptor glycoprotein IIb/IIIa, preventing binding of fibrinogen. ***Therapeutic Effect:*** Inhibits platelet aggregation and thrombus formation.

PHARMACOKINETICS

Poorly bound to plasma proteins; unbound fraction in plasma: 35%. Limited metabolism. Primarily eliminated in the urine (65%) and, to a lesser amount, in the feces. Removed by hemodialysis. ***Half-life:*** 2 hr. Clearance is significantly decreased in severe renal impairment (creatinine clearance < 30 ml/min).

AVAILABILITY

Injection Premix: 12.5 mg/250 ml, 25 mg/500 ml (50 mcg/ml).
Vial: 250 mcg/ml.

INDICATIONS AND DOSAGES

▸ **Inhibition of Platelet Aggregation**

IV

Adults, Elderly. Initially, 0.4 mcg/kg/min for 30 min; then continue at 0.1 mcg/kg/min through procedure and for 12–24 hrs after procedure.

▸ **Severe Renal Insufficiency (Creatinine Clearance < 30 ml/min)**

Adults, Elderly. Half the usual rate of infusion.

CONTRAINDICATIONS

Active internal bleeding or a history of bleeding diathesis within previous 30 days, arteriovenous malformation or aneurysm, history of intracranial hemorrhage, history of thrombocytopenia after prior exposure to tirofiban, intracranial neoplasm, major surgical procedure within previous 30 days, severe hypertension, stroke

INTERACTIONS

Drug

Drugs that affect hemostasis (such as aspirin, heparin, NSAIDs, and warfarin): May increase the risk of bleeding

Herbal

None known.

Food

None known.

Drug interactions of concern to dentistry

- Increased risk of bleeding: drugs that interfere with coagulation or platelet function, such as NSAIDs and aspirin

DIAGNOSTIC TEST EFFECTS
Decreases Hct, Hgb and platelet count.

IV INCOMPATIBILITIES
Do not mix with other medications.

SIDE EFFECTS
Occasional (6%–3%)
Pelvis pain, bradycardia, dizziness, leg pain
Rare (2%–1%)
Edema and swelling, vasovagal reaction, diaphoresis, nausea, fever, headache

SERIOUS REACTIONS
! Signs and symptoms of overdose include generally minor mucocutaneous bleeding and bleeding at the femoral artery access site.
! Thrombocytopenia occurs rarely.

DENTAL CONSIDERATIONS
General:
- An acute-use drug for use in hospitals or emergency departments. If a patient should report this drug in his/her medical history, question about cardiovascular disease and drugs he/she may be taking.
- Patients are at risk for bleeding while receiving this drug; provide palliative dental care for dental emergencies only.
- Avoid products that affect platelet function, such as aspirin and NSAIDs.

Consultations:
- Medical consultation should include routine blood counts including platelet counts and bleeding time.
- Medical consultation may be required to assess disease control and patient's ability to tolerate stress.

Teach Patient/Family:
- To inform dentist of unusual bleeding episodes following dental treatment

T

tobramycin
toe-bra-mye′-sin
(Nebcin, Nebcin Pediatric, Tobi)

CATEGORY AND SCHEDULE
Pregnancy Risk Category: C

MECHANISM OF ACTION
An aminoglycoside antibiotic that irreversibly binds to protein on bacterial ribosomes. ***Therapeutic Effect:*** Interferes in protein synthesis of susceptible microorganisms.

PHARMACOKINETICS
Rapid, complete absorption after IM administration. Protein binding: less than 30%. Widely distributed but does not cross the blood-brain barrier and is in low concentrations in cerebrospinal fluid (CSF). Excreted unchanged in urine. Removed by hemodialysis. ***Half-life:*** 2 hrs. Half-life is increased with impaired renal function and in neonates. Half-life is decreased in cystic fibrosis, febrile, or burn patients.

AVAILABILITY
Inhalation solution: 60 mg/ml (Tobi).
Injection: 10 mg/ml, 40 mg/ml (Nebcin).
Powder for Injection: 1.2 g (Nebcin).

INDICATIONS AND DOSAGES
▸ **Skin/skin Structure, Bone, Joint, Respiratory Tract Infections, Postoperative, Burn, Intra-Abdominal Infections, Complicated Urinary Tract Infections, Septicemia, Meningitis**
IM/IV
Adults, Elderly. 3mg/kg/day in 3 divided doses. May use up to 5 mg/kgday in 3 to 4 equal doses.

▸ **Cystic Fibrosis**
INHALATION
Adult, Elderly, Children 6 yrs and older. 1 ampule (300 mg) via nebulizer twice daily (28 days on, 28 days off). Consider starting elderly patients at 3 mg/kg IV q8h.

▸ **Dosage in Renal Impairment**
Dosage and frequency are modified on the basis of degree of renal impairment and the serum concentration of the drug. After a loading dose of 1–2 mg/kg, the maintenance dose and frequency are based on serum creatinine levels and creatinine clearance. Dosage should be reduced to 3 mg/kg/day as soon as clinically indicated. Dosage should not exceed 5 mg/kg/day.

CONTRAINDICATIONS
Hypersensitivity to aminoglycosides (cross-sensitivity)

INTERACTIONS
Drug
Other aminoglycosides, nephrotoxic and ototoxic-producing medications: May increase the risk of tobramycin toxicity.
Neuromuscular blocking agents: May increase the effects of neuromuscular blocking agents.
Herbal
None known.
Food
None known.
Drug interactions of concern to dentistry
- Increased risk of nephrotoxicity: cephalosporins, enflurane, vancomycin
- Increased neuromuscular blocking effects: neuromuscular blockers

DIAGNOSTIC TEST EFFECTS
May increase serum bilirubin, BUN, serum creatinine, serum LDH concentrations, SGOT (AST), and SGPT (ALT) levels. May decrease serum calcium, magnesium, potassium, and sodium concentrations. Therapeutic blood level: Peak is 5–20 mcg/ml; trough is 0.5–2 mcg/ml. Toxic blood level: Peak is greater than 20 mcg/ml; trough is greater than 2 mcg/ml.

IV INCOMPATIBILITIES
Amphotericin B complex (Abelcet, AmBisome, Amphotec), heparin, hetastarch (Hespan), indomethacin (Indocin), propofol (Diprivan), sargramostim (Leukine, Prokine)

IV COMPATIBILITIES
Amiodarone (Cordarone), calcium gluconate, diltiazem (Cardizem), furosemide (Lasix), hydromorphone (Dilaudid), insulin, magnesium sulfate, midazolam (Versed), morphine, theophylline

SIDE EFFECTS
Occasional
IM: Pain, induration at IM injection site
IV: Phlebitis, thrombophlebitis
Rare
Hypotension, nausea, vomiting

SERIOUS REACTIONS
! Nephrotoxicity, as evidenced by increased BUN and serum creatinine and decreased creatinine clearance, may be reversible if the drug is stopped at the first sign of nephrotoxic symptoms.
! Irreversible ototoxicity, manifested as tinnitus, dizziness, ringing or roaring in ears, impaired hearing and neurotoxicity, as evidenced by headache, dizziness, lethargy, tremors, and visual disturbances, occur occasionally. The risk of irreversible neurotoxicity and ototoxicity is greater with higher dosages, prolonged therapy, or if the solution is applied directly to the mucosa.

! Superinfections, particularly with fungi, may result from bacterial imbalance with any route of administration.
! Anaphylaxis may occur.

DENTAL CONSIDERATIONS

General:

- For selected infections in the hospital setting; provide emergency dental treatment only.
- Caution regarding allergy to medication.
- Examine for oral manifestation of opportunistic infection.
- Determine why patient is taking the drug.

Consultations:

- Medical consultation may be required to assess disease control in the patient.
- CONIF

Teach Patient/Family:

- Importance of good oral hygiene to prevent soft tissue inflammation
- To report oral lesions, soreness, or bleeding to dentist
- To prevent trauma when using oral hygiene aids

tobramycin sulfate

tow-bra-my′-sin
(AK-Tob, Apo-Tobramycin[CAN], Nebcin, PMS-Tobramycin, TOBI, Tobrex)

CATEGORY AND SCHEDULE

Pregnancy Risk Category: C (B, ophthalmic form)

MECHANISM OF ACTION

An aminoglycoside antibiotic that irreversibly binds to protein on bacterial ribosomes. ***Therapeutic Effect:*** Interferes with protein synthesis of susceptible microorganisms.

PHARMACOKINETICS

Rapid, complete absorption after IM administration. Protein binding: less than 30%. Widely distributed (doesn't cross the blood-brain barrier; low concentrations in CSF. Excreted unchanged in urine. Removed by hemodialysis. ***Half-life:*** 2–4 hr (increased in impaired renal function and neonates; decreased in cystic fibrosis and febrile or burn patients).

AVAILABILITY

Injection Solution (Nebcin): 10 mg/ml, 40 mg/ml.
Injection Powder for Reconstitution (Nebcin): 1.2 g.
Ophthalmic Ointment (Tobrex): 0.3%.
Ophthalmic Solution (AKTob, Tobrex): 0.3%.
Nebulization Solution (TOBI): 60 mg/ml.

INDICATIONS AND DOSAGES

▸ **Skin and Skin-Structure, Bone, Joint, Respiratory Tract, Postoperative, Intra-Abdominal, and Burn Wound Infections; Complicated UTIs; Septicemia; Meningitis**

IV, IM
Adults, Elderly. 3–6 mg/kg/day in 3 divided doses or 4–6.6 mg/kg once a day.

▸ **Superficial Eye Infections Including Blepharitis, Conjunctivitis, Keratitis, and Corneal Ulcers**

OPHTHALMIC OINTMENT
Adults, Elderly. Usual dosage, apply a thin strip to conjunctiva q8–12h (q3–4h for severe infections).

OPHTHALMIC SOLUTION
Adults, Elderly. Usual dosage, 1–2 drops in affected eye q4h (2 drops/hr for severe infections).

▸ Bronchopulmonary Infections in Patients with Cystic Fibrosis
INHALATION SOLUTION
Adults. Usual dosage, 60–80 mg twice a day for 28 days, then off for 28 days.
Children. 40–80 mg 2–3 times/day.

▸ Dosage in Renal Impairment
Dosage and frequency are modified on the basis of the degree of renal impairment and the serum drug concentration. After a loading dose of 1–2 mg/kg, the maintenance dose and frequency are based on serum creatinine levels and creatinine clearance.

CONTRAINDICATIONS

Hypersensitivity to tobramycin, other aminoglycosides (cross-sensitivity), and their components

INTERACTIONS

Drug

Nephrotoxic medications, other aminoglycosides, ototoxic medications: May increase the risk of nephrotoxicity and ototoxicity.
Neuromuscular blockers: May increase neuromuscular blockade.

Herbal

None known.

Food

None known.

DIAGNOSTIC TEST EFFECTS

May increase serum bilirubin, BUN, serum creatinine, serum LDH, AST(SGOT), and ALT(SGPT) levels. May decrease serum calcium, magnesium, potassium, and sodium concentrations. Therapeutic peak serum level is 5–20 mcg/ml; therapeutic trough serum level is 0.5–2 mcg/ml. Toxic peak serum level is greater than 20 mcg/ml; toxic trough serum level is greater than 2 mcg/ml.

IV INCOMPATIBILITIES

Amphotericin B complex (Abelcet, AmBisome, Amphotec), heparin, hetastarch (Hespan), indomethacin (Indocin), propofol (Diprivan), sargramostim (Leukine, Prokine)

IV COMPATIBILITIES

Amiodarone (Cordarone), calcium gluconate, diltiazem (Cardizem), furosemide (Lasix), hydromorphone (Dilaudid), insulin, magnesium sulfate, midazolam (Versed), morphine, theophylline

SIDE EFFECTS

Occasional

IM: Pain, induration
IV: Phlebitis, thrombophlebitis
Topical: Hypersensitivity reaction (fever, pruritus, rash, urticaria)
Ophthalmic: Tearing, itching, redness, eyelid swelling

Rare

Hypotension, nausea, vomiting

SERIOUS REACTIONS

! Nephrotoxicity (as evidenced by increased BUN and serum creatinine levels and decreased creatinine clearance) may be reversible if the drug is stopped at the first sign of nephrotoxic symptoms.

! Irreversible ototoxicity (manifested as tinnitus, dizziness, ringing or roaring in ears, and hearing loss) and neurotoxicity (manifested as headache, dizziness, lethargy, tremor, and visual disturbances) occur occasionally. The risk of these reactions increases with higher dosages or prolonged therapy and when the solution is applied directly to the mucosa.

! Superinfections, particularly fungal infections, may result from bacterial imbalance with any administration route.
! Anaphylaxis may occur.

DENTAL CONSIDERATIONS

General:

- Avoid directing dental light into patient's eyes; provide dark glasses during treatment to avoid irritation.
- Protect patient's eyes from accidental spatter during dental treatment.

tocainide hydrochloride

toe-kay′-nide
(Tonocard)

CATEGORY AND SCHEDULE

Pregnancy Risk Category: C

MECHANISM OF ACTION

An amide-type local anesthetic that shortens the action potential duration and decreases the effective refractory period and automaticity in the His-Purkinje system of the myocardium by blocking sodium transport across myocardial cell membranes. ***Therapeutic Effect:*** Suppresses ventricular arrhythmias.

T

AVAILABILITY

Tablets: 400 mg, 600 mg.

INDICATIONS AND DOSAGES

▸ Suppression and Prevention of Ventricular Arrhythmias

PO

Adults, Elderly. Initially, 400 mg q8h. Maintenance: 1.2–1.8 g/day in divided doses q8h.
Maximum: 2400 mg/day.

CONTRAINDICATIONS

Hypersensitivity to local anesthetics, second- or third-degree AV block

INTERACTIONS

Drug

Beta-adrenergic blockers: May increase pulmonary wedge pressure and decrease cardiac index.
Other antiarrhythmics: May increase risk of adverse cardiac effects.

Herbal

None known.

Food

None known.

Drug interactions of concern to dentistry

- No specific interactions are reported with dental drugs; however, any drug that could affect the cardiac action of tocainide (local anesthetics, vasoconstrictors, and anticholinergics) should be used in the least effective dose

DIAGNOSTIC TEST EFFECTS

None known.

SIDE EFFECTS

Tocainide is generally well tolerated.

Frequent (10%–3%)

Minor, transient light-headedness, dizziness, nausea, paraesthesia, rash, tremor

Occasional (3%–1%)

Clammy skin, night sweats, myalgia

Rare (< 1%)

Restlessness, nervousness, disorientation, mood changes, ataxia (muscular incoordination), visual disturbances

SERIOUS REACTIONS

! High dosage may produce bradycardia or tachycardia, hypotension, palpitations, increased ventricular arrhythmias, premature ventricular contractions (PVCs), chest pain, and exacerbation of CHF.

DENTAL CONSIDERATIONS

General:

- Monitor vital signs at every appointment because of CV and respiratory side effects.
- After supine positioning, have patient sit upright for at least 2 min before standing to avoid orthostatic hypotension.
- Patients on chronic drug therapy may rarely have symptoms of blood dyscrasias, which can include infection, bleeding, and poor healing.
- Assess salivary flow as a factor in caries, periodontal disease, and candidiasis.
- Stress from dental procedures may compromise CV function; determine patient risk.

Consultations:

- In a patient with symptoms of blood dyscrasias, request a medical consultation for blood studies and postpone dental treatment until normal values are reestablished.
- Medical consultation may be required to assess disease control and patient's ability to tolerate stress.

Teach Patient/Family:

- Importance of good oral hygiene to prevent soft tissue inflammation
- Caution to prevent injury when using oral hygiene aids
- *When chronic dry mouth occurs, advise patient:*
  - To avoid mouth rinses with high alcohol content because of drying effects
  - Of need for daily home fluoride use to prevent caries
  - To use sugarless gum, frequent sips of water, or saliva substitutes

tolazamide

tole-az′-a-mide

(Tolinase)

Do not confuse with tolubutamide, tocainide, or tolazine.

CATEGORY AND SCHEDULE

Pregnancy Risk Category: D

MECHANISM OF ACTION

A first-generation sulfonylurea that promotes release of insulin from beta cells of pancreas. ***Therapeutic Effect:*** Lowers blood glucose concentration.

PHARMACOKINETICS

Well absorbed from the gastrointestinal (GI) tract. Extensively metabolized in liver to five metabolites, three of which are active. Primarily excreted in urine. Unknown if removed by hemodialysis. ***Half-life:*** 7 hrs.

AVAILABILITY

Tablets: 100 mg, 250 mg, 500 mg; 100 mg, 250 mg (Tolinase).

INDICATIONS AND DOSAGES

▸ Diabetes Mellitus

PO

Adults, Elderly. Initially, 100–250 mg once a day, with breakfast or first main meal. Maintenance: 100–1000 mg once a day. May increase by increments of 100–250 mg weekly on the basis of blood glucose response. May increase by 100–250 mg/day at weekly intervals. Maximum: 1000 mg/day. Doses more than 500 mg/day should be given in 2 divided doses with meals.

OFF-LABEL USES
None known.

CONTRAINDICATIONS
Diabetic complications, such as ketosis, acidosis, and diabetic coma, sole therapy for type 1 diabetes mellitus, hypersensitivity to tolazamide or its components

INTERACTIONS
Drug
Beta-blockers: May increase hypoglycemic effect and mask signs of hypoglycemia.
Cimetidine, fluoroquinolones, fluconazole, MAOIs, quinidine, ranitidine, large doses of salicylates: May increase effects of tolazamide.
Corticosteroids, lithium, thiazide diuretics: May decrease effects of tolazamide.
Oral anticoagulants: May increase effects of oral anticoagulants.
Herbal
Bitter melon, fenugreek, ginseng, glucomannan, glucosamine, gymnema extracts, licorice, psyllium, St. John's Wort: May increase risk of hypoglycemia.
Food
None known.
Drug interactions of concern to dentistry
• Increased hypoglycemic reaction: NSAIDs, salicylates, ketoconazole, miconazole
• Decreased action of tolazamide: corticosteroids, sympathomimetics (epinephrine)

DIAGNOSTIC TEST EFFECTS
May increase BUN, LDH concentrations, serum alkaline phosphatase, creatinine, and SGOT (AST) levels.

IV INCOMPATIBILITIES
None known.

IV COMPATIBILITIES
None known.

SIDE EFFECTS
Frequent
Altered taste sensation, dizziness, drowsiness, weight gain, constipation, diarrhea, heartburn, nausea, vomiting, stomach fullness, headache
Occasional
Increased sensitivity of skin to sunlight, peeling of skin, itching, rash

SERIOUS REACTIONS
! Severe hypoglycemia may occur due to overdosage and insufficient food intake, especially with increased glucose demands.
! GI hemorrhage, cholestatic hepatic jaundice, leukopenia, thrombocytopenia, pancytopenia, agranulocytosis, and aplastic or hemolytic anemia occur rarely.

DENTAL CONSIDERATIONS
General:
• Patients on chronic drug therapy may rarely have symptoms of blood dyscrasias, which can include infection, bleeding, and poor healing.
• Place on frequent recall to evaluate healing response.
• Short appointments and a stress reduction protocol may be required for anxious patients.
• Diabetics may be more susceptible to infection and have delayed wound healing.
• Ensure that patient is following prescribed diet and regularly takes medication.
• Question patient about self-monitoring of drug's antidiabetic effect.

• Avoid prescribing aspirin-containing products.

Consultations:

• In a patient with symptoms of blood dyscrasias, request a medical consultation for blood studies and postpone dental treatment until normal values are reestablished.

• Medical consultation may be required to assess disease control.

Teach Patient/Family:

• Importance of good oral hygiene to prevent soft tissue inflammation

• To avoid mouth rinses with high alcohol content because of drying effects

tolbutamide

tole-byoo′-ta-mide

(Apo-Tolbutamide[CAN], Orinase, Orinase Diagnositic, Rastinon[AUS], Tol-Tab)

Do not confuse with tolazamide, tocainide, or tolazine.

CATEGORY AND SCHEDULE

Pregnancy Risk Category: C

MECHANISM OF ACTION

A first-generation sulfonylurea that promotes the release of insulin from beta cells of pancreas. ***Therapeutic Effect:*** Lowers blood glucose concentration.

PHARMACOKINETICS

Route	Onset	Peak	Duration
PO	1 hr	5–8 hrs	12–24 hrs
IV	N/A	30–45 min	90–181 min

Well absorbed from the gastrointestinal (GI) tract. Protein binding: 80%–99%. Extensively metabolized in liver to 2 inactive metabolites, primarily via oxidation. Excreted in urine. Removed by hemodialysis. ***Half-life:*** 4.5–6.5 hrs.

AVAILABILITY

Tablets: 500 mg (Orinase, Tol-Tab).
Injection, powder for reconstitution: 1 g (Orinase Diagnostic).

INDICATIONS AND DOSAGES

▸ Diabetes Mellitus

PO

Adults. Initially, 1 g daily, with breakfast or first main meal, or in divided doses. Maintenance: 0.25–3 g once a day. After dose of 2 g is reached, dosage should be increased in increments of up to 2 mg q1–2wks, based on blood glucose response. Maximum: 3 g/day.

▸ Endocrine Tumor Diagnosis

IV

Adults. 1 g infused over 2–3 minutes.

CONTRAINDICATIONS

Diabetic ketoacidosis with or without coma, sole therapy for type 1 diabetes mellitus, use in children, hypersensitivity to tolbutamide or any component of its formulation

INTERACTIONS

Drug

Beta-blockers: May increase the hypoglycemic effect and mask signs of hypoglycemia.

Cimetidine, fluoroquinolones, fluconazole, MAOIs, quinidine, ranitidine, large doses of salicylates: May increase the effects of tolbutamide.

T

Corticosteroids, lithium, thiazide diuretics: May decrease the effects of tolbutamide.
Oral anticoagulants: May increase the effects of oral anticoagulants.
Fosphenytoin, phenytoin: May increase the risk of phenytoin toxicity.
Rifampin: May decrease effectiveness of tolbutamide.
Sertraline: May decrease the clearance of tolbutamide.

Herbal

Bitter melon, fenugreek, ginseng, glucomannan, glucosamine, gymnema extracts, licorice, psyllium, St. John's Wort: May increase the risk of hypoglycemia.

Food

None known.

Drug interactions of concern to dentistry

- Increased hypoglycemic reactions: NSAIDs, salicylates, ketoconazole, miconazole
- Decreased effects: corticosteroids, sympathomimetics

DIAGNOSTIC TEST EFFECTS

May increase BUN, LDH concentrations, serum alkaline phosphatase, creatinine, and SGOT (AST) levels.

SIDE EFFECTS

Frequent

Increased sensitivity of skin to sunlight, peeling of skin, itching, rash, dizziness, drowsiness, weight gain, constipation, diarrhea, heartburn, nausea, headache, pain at injection site, oral lichenoid reaction

Occasional

Altered taste sensation, constipation, vomiting, stomach fullness

SERIOUS REACTIONS

! Severe hypoglycemia may occur because of overdosage or insufficient food intake, especially with increased glucose demands.

! Cardiovascular mortality has been reported higher in patients treated with tolbutamide.

! GI hemorrhage, cholestatic hepatic jaundice, leukopenia, thrombocytopenia, pancytopenia, agranulocytosis and aplastic or hemolytic anemia occurs rarely.

DENTAL CONSIDERATIONS

General:

- Patients on chronic drug therapy may rarely have symptoms of blood dyscrasias, which can include infection, bleeding, and poor healing.
- Ensure that patient is following prescribed diet and regularly takes medication.
- Question patient about self-monitoring of drug's antidiabetic effect including blood glucose values or finger-stick records.
- Place on frequent recall to evaluate healing response.
- Short appointments and a stress reduction protocol may be required for anxious patients.
- Diabetics may be more susceptible to infection and have delayed wound healing.
- Avoid prescribing aspirin-containing products.

Consultations:

- In a patient with symptoms of blood dyscrasias, request a medical consultation for blood studies and postpone dental treatment until normal values are reestablished.
- Medical consultation may be required to assess disease control.
- Medical consultation may include data from patient's blood glucose monitoring including glycosylated hemoglobin or HbA_{1c} testing.

T

Teach Patient/Family:
• Importance of good oral hygiene to prevent soft tissue inflammation
• To avoid mouth rinses with high alcohol content because of drying effects

tolcapone

toll′-ka-pone
(Tasmar)

CATEGORY AND SCHEDULE

Pregnancy Risk Category: C

MECHANISM OF ACTION

An antiparkinson agent that inhibits the enzyme catechol-*O*-methyltransferase (COMT), potentiating dopamine activity and increasing the duration of action of levodopa. ***Therapeutic Effect:*** Relieves signs and symptoms of Parkinson's disease.

PHARMACOKINETICS

Rapidly absorbed after PO administration. Protein binding: 99%. Metabolized in the liver. Eliminated primarily in urine (60%) and, to a lesser extent, in feces (40%). Unknown if removed by hemodialysis. ***Half-life:*** 2–3 hr.

AVAILABILITY

Tablets: 100 mg, 200 mg.

INDICATIONS AND DOSAGES

▸ Adjunctive Treatment of Parkinson's Disease

PO

Adults, Elderly. Initially, 100–200 mg 3 times a day concomitantly with each dose of carbidopa and levodopa. Maximum: 600 mg/day.

▸ Dosage in Hepatic Impairment

Patients with moderate to severe cirrhosis should not receive more than 200 mg tolcapone 3 times a day.

CONTRAINDICATIONS

None known.

INTERACTIONS

Drug

Levodopa: Increases the duration of action of this drug.

Herbal

None known.

Food

All foods: Decrease tolcapone bioavailability by 10%–20% if given within 1 hour before or 2 hour after drug administration.

Drug interactions of concern to dentistry

• Increased sedation: alcohol and all CNS depressants
• No other data for dental drugs reported

DIAGNOSTIC TEST EFFECTS

May increase AST (SGOT) and ALT (SGPT) levels.

SIDE EFFECTS

Alert

Frequency of side effects increases with dosage. The following effects are based on a 200-mg dose.

Frequent (35%–16%)

Nausea, insomnia, somnolence, anorexia, diarrhea, muscle cramps, orthostatic hypotension, excessive dreaming, dry mouth

Occasional (11%–4%)

Headache, vomiting, confusion, hallucinations, constipation, diaphoresis, bright yellow urine, dry eyes, abdominal pain, dizziness, flatulence

Rare (3%–2%)

Dyspepsia, neck pain, hypotension, fatigue, chest discomfort

SERIOUS REACTIONS

! Upper respiratory tract infection and UTI occur in 7%–5% of patients.
! Too-rapid withdrawal from therapy may produce withdrawal-emergent hyperpyrexia, characterized by fever, muscular rigidity, and altered LOC.
! Dyskinesia and dystonia occur frequently.

DENTAL CONSIDERATIONS

General:

- Notify physician immediately if symptoms of liver failure are observed (bleeding, jaundice, etc.).
- Assess salivary flow as a factor in caries, periodontal disease, and candidiasis.
- After supine positioning, have patient sit upright for at least 2 min before standing to avoid orthostatic hypotension.
- Consider semisupine chair position for patient comfort because of GI side effects of drug.

Consultations:

- Medical consultation may be required to assess disease control.
- Take precaution if dental surgery is anticipated and general anesthesia is required.

Teach Patient/Family:

- Use of electric toothbrush if patient has difficulty holding conventional devices
- *When chronic dry mouth occurs, advise patient:*
  - To avoid mouth rinses with high alcohol content because of drying effects
  - To use daily home fluoride products for anticaries effect
  - To use sugarless gum, frequent sips of water, or saliva substitutes

T

tolmetin

tole′-met-in
(Novo-Tolmetin[CAN], Tolectin, Tolectin DS)

CATEGORY AND SCHEDULE

Pregnancy Risk Category: C, D if used in third trimester or near delivery

MECHANISM OF ACTION

A nonsteroidal anti-inflammatory that produces analgesic and anti-inflammatory effect by inhibiting prostaglandin synthesis. ***Therapeutic Effect:*** Reduces inflammatory response and intensity of pain stimulus reaching sensory nerve endings.

PHARMACOKINETICS

Rapdily absorbed from the gastrointestinal (GI) tract. Metabolized in liver. Excreted in urine. Minimally removed by hemodialysis. ***Half-life:*** 5 hrs.

AVAILABILITY

Tablets: 200 mg, 600 mg (Tolectin).
Capsules: 400 mg (Tolectin DS).

INDICATIONS AND DOSAGES

▸ **Rheumatoid Arthritis, Osteoarthritis**

PO

Adults, Elderly. Initially, 400 mg 3 times/day (including 1 dose upon arising, 1 dose at bedtime). Adjust dose at 1–2 wk intervals.
Maintenance: 600–1,800 mg/day in 3–4 divided doses.

▸ **Juvenile Rheumatoid Arthritis**

PO

Children more than 2 yrs. Initially, 20 mg/kg/day in 3–4 divided doses.
Maintenance: 15–30 mg/kg/day in 3–4 divided doses.

OFF-LABEL USES
Treatment of ankylosing spondylitis, psoriatic arthritis

CONTRAINDICATIONS
Severely incapacitated, bedridden, wheelchair bound, hypersensitivity to aspirin or other NSAIDs

INTERACTIONS
Drug
Antacids: May decrease concentrations of tolmetin.
Antihypertensives, diuretics: May decrease the effects of antihypertensives and diuretics.
Aspirin, salicylates: May increase the risk of GI bleeding and side effects.
Bone marrow depressants: May increase the risk of hematologic reactions.
Heparin, oral anticoagulants, thrombolytics: May increase the effects of heparin, oral anticoagulants and thrombolytics.
Lithium: May increase the blood concentration and risk of toxicity of lithium.
Methotrexate: May increase the risk of toxicity of methotrexate.
Probenecid: May increase tolmetin blood concentration.
Herbal
Ginkgo biloba: May increase the risk of bleeding.
Feverfew: May decrease the effects of feverfew.
Food
None known.
Drug interactions of concern to dentistry
- Increased risk of GI side effects: ASA, NSAIDs, ethanol (alcohol)
- Nephrotoxicity: acetaminophen (prolonged use and high doses)
- Possible risk of decreased renal function: cyclosporine
- Decreased antihypertensive effect of diuretics, β-adrenergic blockers, and ACE inhibitors
- First-time users of SSRIs also taking NSAIDs may have a higher risk of GI side effects; until more data are available, it may be advisable to avoid use of NSAIDs in these patients (*Br J Clin Pharmacol* 55:591–595, 2003)

DIAGNOSTIC TEST EFFECTS
May increase BUN, potassium, liver function tests. May decrease Hgb, Hct. May prolong bleeding time.

SIDE EFFECTS
Occasional
Nausea, vomiting, diarrhea, abdominal cramping, dyspepsia (heartburn, indigestion, epigastric pain), flatulence, dizziness, headache, weight decrease or increase
Rare
Constipation, anorexia, rash, pruritus

SERIOUS REACTIONS
! Peptic ulcer, GI bleeding, gastritis, and severe hepatic reaction (cholestasis, jaundice) occur rarely.
! Nephrotoxicity (dysuria, hematuria, proteinuria, nephrotic syndrome) and severe hypersensitivity reaction (fever, chills, bronchospasm) occur rarely.

DENTAL CONSIDERATIONS
General:
- Patients on chronic drug therapy may rarely have symptoms of blood dyscrasias, which can include infection, bleeding, and poor healing.
- Monitor vital signs at every appointment because of CV side effects.
- Assess salivary flow as a factor in caries, periodontal disease, and candidiasis.
- Avoid prescribing for dental use in last trimester of pregnancy.

- Possibility of cross-allergenicity when patient is allergic to aspirin.

Consultations:

- Medical consultation may be required to assess disease control.
- In a patient with symptoms of blood dyscrasias, request a medical consultation for blood studies and postpone dental treatment until normal values are reestablished.

Teach Patient/Family:

- Importance of good oral hygiene to prevent soft tissue inflammation
- Caution to prevent injury when using oral hygiene aids
- *When chronic dry mouth occurs, advise patient:*
  - To avoid mouth rinses with high alcohol content because of drying effects
  - Of need for daily home fluoride use to prevent caries
  - To use sugarless gum, frequent sips of water, or saliva substitutes

tolterodine tartrate

tol-tare′-oh-deen
(Detrol, Detrol LA)

CATEGORY AND SCHEDULE

Pregnancy Risk Category: C

MECHANISM OF ACTION

An antispasmodic that exhibits potent antimuscarinic activity by interceding via cholinergic muscarinic receptors, thereby inhibiting urinary bladder contraction. ***Therapeutic Effect:*** Decreases urinary frequency, urgency.

PHARMACOKINETICS

Rapidly and well absorbed after PO administration. Protein binding: 96%. Extensively metabolized in the liver to active metabolite. Primarily excreted in urine. Unknown if removed by hemodialysis. ***Half-life:*** 1.9–3.7 hr.

AVAILABILITY

Tablets (Detrol): 1 mg, 2 mg.
Capsules (Extended-Release [Detrol LA]): 2 mg, 4 mg.

INDICATIONS AND DOSAGES

▸ Overactive Bladder

PO

Adults, Elderly. 1–2 mg twice a day.

▸ Dosage in Severe Renal or Hepatic Impairment

PO

Adults, Elderly. 1 mg twice a day.

PO (Extended-Release)

Adults, Elderly. 2–4 mg once a day.

CONTRAINDICATIONS

Uncontrolled angle-closure glaucoma, urine retention

INTERACTIONS

Drug

Clarithromycin, erythromycin, itraconazole, ketoconazole, miconazole: May increase tolterodine blood concentration.
Fluoxetine: May inhibit tolterodine metabolism.

Herbal

None known.

Food

None known.

Drug interactions of concern to dentistry

- Studies not available; however, drugs that inhibit cytochrome P-450 3A4 enzymes, such as erythromycin, clarithromycin, ketoconazole, itraconazole, and fluoxetine, require a dose reduction to 1 mg bid
- Increased anticholinergic effects: possibly with other anticholinergic drugs

DIAGNOSTIC TEST EFFECTS
None known.

SIDE EFFECTS
Frequent (40%)
Dry mouth
Occasional (11%–4%)
Headache, dizziness, fatigue, constipation, dyspepsia (heartburn, indigestion, epigastric discomfort), upper respiratory tract infection, UTI, dry eyes, abnormal vision (accommodation problems), nausea, diarrhea
Rare (3%)
Somnolence, chest or back pain, arthralgia, rash, weight gain, dry skin

SERIOUS REACTIONS
! Overdose can result in severe anticholinergic effects including abdominal cramps, facial warmth, excessive salivation or lacrimation, diaphoresis, pallor, urinary urgency, blurred vision, and prolonged QT interval.

DENTAL CONSIDERATIONS
General:
- Assess salivary flow as a factor in caries, periodontal disease, and candidiasis.
- Consider semisupine chair position for patient comfort because of GI side effects of drug.
- Avoid dental light in patient's eyes; offer dark glasses for patient comfort.
- Avoid drugs with anticholinergic activity, such as antihistamines, opioids, benzodiazepines, propantheline, atropine, and scopolamine.

Consultations:
- Physician should be informed if significant xerostomic side effects occur (e.g., increased caries, sore tongue, problems eating or swallowing, difficulty wearing prosthesis) so that a medication change can be considered.

Teach Patient/Family:
- Importance of good oral hygiene to prevent soft tissue inflammation
- *When chronic dry mouth occurs, advise patient:*
  - To avoid mouth rinses with high alcohol content because of drying effects
  - To use daily home fluoride products for anticaries effect
  - To use sugarless gum, frequent sips of water, or saliva substitutes

topiramate
toe-peer′-a-mate
(Topamax)
Do not confuse topiramate or Topamax with Toprol XL.

CATEGORY AND SCHEDULE
Pregnancy Risk Category: C

MECHANISM OF ACTION
An anticonvulsant that blocks repetitive, sustained firing of neurons by enhancing the ability of gamma-aminobutyric acid to induce an influx of chloride ions into the neurons; may also block sodium channels. **Therapeutic Effect:** Decreases seizure activity.

PHARMACOKINETICS
Rapidly absorbed after PO administration. Protein binding: 13%–17%. Not extensively metabolized. Primarily excreted unchanged in urine. Removed by hemodialysis. ***Half-life:*** 21 hr.

AVAILABILITY

Capsules (Sprinkle): 15 mg, 25 mg.
Tablets: 25 mg, 50 mg, 100 mg, 200 mg.

INDICATIONS AND DOSAGES

▸ Adjunctive Treatment of Partial Seizures, Lennox-Gastant Syndrome

PO

Adults, Elderly, Children older than 17 yr. Initially, 25–50 mg for 1 wk. May increase by 25–50 mg/day at weekly intervals. Maximum: 1,600 mg/day.
Children 2–16 yr. Initially, 1–3 mg/kg/day to maximum of 25 mg. May increase by 1–3 mg/kg/day at weekly intervals. Maintenance: 5–9 mg/kg/day in 2 divided doses.

▸ Tonic-Clonic Seizures

PO

Adults, Elderly, Children. Dosage is individualized and titrated.

▸ Migraine Prevention

PO

Adults, Elderly. 100 mg/day in 2 divided doses.

▸ Dosage in Renal Impairment

Expect to reduce drug dosage by 50% in patients with tonic-clonic seizures who have a creatinine clearance of less than 70 ml/min.

OFF-LABEL USES

Prevention of migraine headaches, treatment of alcohol dependence

CONTRAINDICATIONS

None known.

INTERACTIONS

Drug

Alcohol, other CNS depressants: May increase CNS depression.
Carbamazepine, phenytoin, valproic acid: May decrease topiramate blood concentration.
Carbonic anhydrase inhibitors: May increase the risk of renal calculi.
Oral contraceptives: May decrease the effectiveness of oral contraceptives.

Herbal

None known.

Food

None known.

Drug interactions of concern to dentistry

- Increased CNS depression: opioids, sedatives, ethanol, and other CNS depressants
- Decreased serum levels: carbamazepine

DIAGNOSTIC TEST EFFECTS

None known.

SIDE EFFECTS

Frequent (30%–10%)
Somnolence, dizziness, ataxia, nervousness, nystagmus, diplopia, paresthesia, nausea, tremor
Occasional (9%–3%)
Confusion, breast pain, dysmenorrhea, dyspepsia, depression, asthenia, pharyngitis, weight loss, anorexia, rash, musculoskeletal pain, abdominal pain, difficulty with coordination, sinusitis, agitation, flulike symptoms
Rare (3%–2%)
Mood disturbances, such as irritability and depression; dry mouth; aggressive behavior

SERIOUS REACTIONS

! Psychomotor slowing, impaired concentration, language problems (such as word-finding difficulties), and memory disturbances occur occasionally. These reactions are generally mild to moderate but may be severe enough to require discontinuation of drug therapy.

DENTAL CONSIDERATIONS

General:

- Patients on chronic drug therapy may rarely have symptoms of blood dyscrasias, which can include infection, bleeding, and poor healing.
- Short appointments and a stress reduction protocol may be required for anxious patients.
- Assess salivary flow as factor in caries, periodontal disease, and candidiasis.
- Avoid dental light in patient's eyes; offer dark glasses for patient comfort.
- Determine type of epilepsy, seizure frequency, and quality of seizure control. A stress reduction protocol may be required.

Consultations:

- In a patient with symptoms of blood dyscrasias, request a medical consultation for blood studies and postpone dental treatment until normal values are reestablished.
- Medical consultation may be required to assess disease control.

Teach Patient/Family:

- Importance of good oral hygiene to prevent soft tissue inflammation
- Caution to prevent trauma when using oral hygiene aids
- Use of electric toothbrush if patient has difficulty holding conventional devices
- Importance of updating health and drug history if physician makes any changes in evaluation or drug regimens
- *When chronic dry mouth occurs, advise patient:*
  - To avoid mouth rinses with high alcohol content because of drying effects
  - To use daily home fluoride products for anticaries effect
  - To use sugarless gum, frequent sips of water, or saliva substitutes

topotecan

toe-poh'-teh-can
(Hycamtin)

CATEGORY AND SCHEDULE

Pregnancy Risk Category: D

MECHANISM OF ACTION

A DNA topoisomerase inhibitor that interacts with topoisomerase I, an enzyme that allows DNA replication by producing reversible single-strand breaks in DNA that relieve torsional strain. Topotecan prevents religation of the DNA strand, resulting in damage to double-strand DNA and cell death. ***Therapeutic Effect:*** Kills cancer cells.

PHARMACOKINETICS

Hydrolyzed to active form after IV administration. Protein binding: 35%. Excreted in urine. ***Half-life:*** 2–3 hr (increased in impaired renal function).

AVAILABILITY

Powder for Injection: 4 mg (single-dose vial).

INDICATIONS AND DOSAGES

▸ Ovarian Carcinoma, Small-Cell Lung Cancer

IV

Adults, Elderly. 1.5 $mg/m^2/day$ over 30 min for 5 consecutive days, beginning on day 1 of a 21-day course. Minimum of four courses recommended. If severe neutropenia (neutrophil count < $1500/mm^2$) occurs during treatment, reduce dose for subsequent courses by 0.25 mg/m^2 or administer filgrastim (G-CSF) no sooner than 24 hr after the last dose of topotecan.

▸ Dosage in Renal Impairment

No dosage adjustment is necessary in patients with mild renal impairment

T

(creatinine clearance of 40–60 ml/min). For moderate renal impairment (creatinine clearance of 20–39 ml/min), give 0.75 mg/m^2.

OFF-LABEL USES

Treatment of solid tumors including osteosarcoma, neuroblastoma, pediatric leukemia, rhabdomyosarcoma

CONTRAINDICATIONS

Baseline neutrophil count less than 1500 cells/mm^3, breast-feeding, pregnancy, severe myelosuppression

INTERACTIONS

Drug

Cisplatin: May increase the severity of myelosuppression.
Live-virus vaccines: May potentiate virus replication, increase vaccine side effects, and decrease the patient's antibody response to the vaccine.
Other bone marrow depressants: May increase the risk of myelosuppression.

Herbal

None known.

Food

None known.

Drug interactions of concern to dentistry

- None reported

DIAGNOSTIC TEST EFFECTS

T

May increase serum bilirubin, AST (SGOT), and ALT (SGPT) levels. May decrease RBC, leukocyte, neutrophil, and platelet counts.

IV INCOMPATIBILITIES

Dexamethasone (Decadron), 5-fluorouracil, mitomycin (Mutamycin)

IV COMPATIBILITIES

Carboplatin (Paraplatin), cisplatin (Platinol AQ), cyclophosphamide (Cytoxan), doxorubicin (Adriamycin), etoposide (VePesid), gemcitabine (Gemzar), granisetron (Kytril), ondansetron (Zofran), paclitaxel (Taxol), vincristine (Oncovin)

SIDE EFFECTS

Frequent

Nausea (77%); vomiting (58%); diarrhea, total alopecia (42%); headache (21%); dyspnea (21%)

Occasional

Paraesthesia (9%); constipation, abdominal pain (3%)

Rare

Anorexia, malaise, arthralgia, asthenia, myalgia

SERIOUS REACTIONS

! Severe neutropenia (neutrophil count < 500 cells/mm^3) occurs in 60% of patients, usually during the first course of therapy. The neutrophil nadir usually occurs at a median of 11 days after starting therapy.
! Thrombocytopenia (platelet count < 25,000/mm^3) occurs in 26% of patients, and severe anemia (RBC count < 8 g/dl) occurs in 40% of patients. The platelet and RBC nadirs usually occur at a median of 15 days after starting the first course of therapy.

DENTAL CONSIDERATIONS

General:

- If additional analgesia is required for dental pain, consider alternative analgesics (NSAIDs) in patients taking narcotics for acute or chronic pain.
- Examine for oral manifestation of opportunistic infection.
- This drug may be used in the hospital or on an outpatient basis. Confirm the patient's disease and treatment status.

- Chlorhexidine mouth rinse prior to and during chemotherapy may reduce severity of mucositis.
- Patient on chronic drug therapy may rarely present with symptoms of blood dyscrasias, which can include infection, bleeding, and poor healing. If dyscrasia is present, caution patient to prevent oral tissue trauma when using oral hygiene aids.
- Palliative medication may be required for management of oral side effects.
- Short appointments and a stress reduction protocol may be required for anxious patients.
- Consider semisupine chair position for patient comfort if GI side effects occur.
- Caution: patients may be at high risk for infection.
- Patients may have received other chemotherapy or radiation; confirm medical and drug history.
- Oral infections should be eliminated and/or treated aggressively.

Consultations:

- Medical consultation should include routine blood counts including platelet counts and bleeding time.
- Consult physician; prophylactic or therapeutic antiinfectives may be indicated if surgery or periodontal treatment is required.
- Medical consultation may be required to assess immunologic status during cancer chemotherapy and determine safety risk, if any, posed by the required dental treatment.
- Medical consultation may be required to assess disease control and patient's ability to tolerate stress.
- In a patient with symptoms of blood dyscrasias, request a medical consultation for blood studies and postpone treatment until normal values are reestablished.

Teach Patient/Family:

- Secondary oral infection may occur; need to see dentist immediately if infection occurs.
- To be aware of oral side effects.
- Importance of good oral hygiene to prevent soft tissue inflammation.
- To report oral lesions, soreness, or bleeding to dentist.
- To prevent trauma when using oral hygiene aids.
- Importance of updating health and medication history if physician makes any changes in evaluation or drug regimens; include OTC, herbal, and nonherbal remedies in the update.
- To use soft tooth brush to reduce risk of bleeding.

toremifene citrate

tore′-mih-feen
(Fareston)

CATEGORY AND SCHEDULE

Pregnancy Risk Category: D

MECHANISM OF ACTION

A nonsteroidal antiestrogen and antineoplastic agent that binds to estrogen receptors on tumors, producing a complex that decreases DNA synthesis and inhibits estrogen effects. ***Therapeutic Effect:*** Blocks growth-stimulating effects of estrogen in breast cancer.

PHARMACOKINETICS

Well absorbed after PO administration. Metabolized in the liver. Eliminated in feces. ***Half-life:*** Approximately 5 days.

AVAILABILITY

Tablets: 60 mg.

INDICATIONS AND DOSAGES

Breast Cancer

PO

Adults. 60 mg/day until disease progression is observed.

OFF-LABEL USES

Treatment of desmoid tumors, endometrial carcinoma

CONTRAINDICATIONS

History of thromboembolic disease

INTERACTIONS

Drug

Carbamazepine, phenobarbital, phenytoin: May decrease toremifene blood concentration.

Warfarin: May increase PT.

Herbal

None known.

Food

None known.

Drug interactions of concern to dentistry

- None reported

DIAGNOSTIC TEST EFFECTS

May increase serum alkaline phosphatase, bilirubin, calcium, and AST (SGOT) levels.

SIDE EFFECTS

Frequent

Hot flashes (35%); diaphoresis (20%); nausea (14%); vaginal discharge (13%); dizziness, dry eyes (9%)

Occasional (5%–2%)

Edema, vomiting, vaginal bleeding

Rare

Fatigue, depression, lethargy, anorexia

SERIOUS REACTIONS

! Ocular toxicity (cataracts, glaucoma, decreased visual acuity) and hypercalcemia may occur.

DENTAL CONSIDERATIONS

General:

- Patients on chronic drug therapy may rarely have symptoms of blood dyscrasias, which can include infection, bleeding, and poor healing.
- Consider semisupine chair position for patient comfort because of GI side effects of drug.

Consultations:

- Medical consultation may be required to assess disease control.

Teach Patient/Family:

- Importance of good oral hygiene to prevent soft tissue inflammation

torsemide

tor′-se-mide

(Demadex)

Do not confuse torsemide with furosemide.

CATEGORY AND SCHEDULE

Pregnancy Risk Category: B

MECHANISM OF ACTION

A loop diuretic that enhances excretion of sodium, chloride, potassium, and water at the ascending limb of the loop of Henle; also reduces plasma and extracellular fluid volume.

Therapeutic Effect: Produces diuresis; lowers BP.

PHARMACOKINETICS

Route	Onset	Peak	Duration
PO	1 hr	1–2 hr	6–8 hr
IV	10 min	1 hr	6–8 hr

T

Rapidly and well absorbed from the GI tract. Protein binding: 97%–99%. Metabolized in the liver. Primarily excreted in urine. Not removed by hemodialysis. ***Half-life:*** 3.3 hr.

AVAILABILITY

Tablets: 5 mg, 10 mg, 20 mg, 100 mg.
Injection: 10 mg/ml.

INDICATIONS AND DOSAGES

▸ Hypertension

PO

Adults, Elderly. Initially, 5 mg/day. May increase to 10 mg/day if no response in 4–6 wk. If no response, additional antihypertensive added.

▸ CHF

PO, IV

Adults, Elderly. Initially, 10–20 mg/day. May increase by approximately doubling dose until desired therapeutic effect is attained. Doses greater than 200 mg have not been adequately studied.

▸ Chronic Renal Failure

PO, IV

Adults, Elderly. Initially, 20 mg/day. May increase by approximately doubling dose until desired therapeutic effect is attained. Doses greater than 200 mg have not been adequately studied.

▸ Hepatic Cirrhosis

PO, IV

Adults, Elderly. Initially, 5 mg/day given with aldosterone antagonist or potassium-sparing diuretic. May increase by approximately doubling dose until desired therapeutic effect is attained. Doses greater than 40 mg have not been adequately studied.

CONTRAINDICATIONS

Anuria, hepatic coma, severe electrolyte depletion

INTERACTIONS

Drug

Amphotericin B, nephrotoxic medications, ototoxic medications: May increase the risk of nephrotoxicity and ototoxicity.
Anticoagulants, heparin, thrombolytics: May decrease the effects of these drugs.
Digoxin: May increase the risk of digoxin toxicity associated with torsemide-induced hypokalemia.
Lithium: May increase the risk of lithium toxicity.
NSAIDs, probenecid: May decrease the diuretic effect of torsemide.
Other antihypertensives: May increase the risk of hypotension.
Other hypokalemia-causing medications: May increase the risk of hypokalemia.

Herbal

None known.

Food

None known.

Drug interactions of concern to dentistry

• Increased electrolyte imbalance: systemic corticosteroids
• Masked ototoxicity: phenothiazines
• Decreased antihypertensive effects: NSAIDs, especially indomethacin
• Increased sweating, hot flashes, weakness, CV symptoms: chloral hydrate (rare)

DIAGNOSTIC TEST EFFECTS

May increase BUN, serum creatinine, and serum uric acid levels. May decrease serum calcium, chloride, magnesium, potassium, and sodium levels.

IV INCOMPATIBILITIES

Don't mix torsemide with any other medications except for milrinone (Primacor).

IV COMPATIBILITIES
Milrinone (Primacor)

SIDE EFFECTS
Frequent (10%–4%)
Headache, dizziness, rhinitis
Occasional (3%–1%)
Asthenia, insomnia, nervousness, diarrhea, constipation, nausea, dyspepsia, edema, ECG changes, pharyngitis, cough, arthralgia, myalgia
Rare (< 1%)
Syncope, hypotension, arrhythmias

SERIOUS REACTIONS
! Ototoxicity may occur with high doses or a too-rapid IV administration.
! Overdose produces acute, profound water loss; volume and electrolyte depletion; dehydration; decreased blood volume; and circulatory collapse.

DENTAL CONSIDERATIONS
General:
- Monitor vital signs at every appointment because of CV side effects.
- After supine positioning, have patient sit upright for at least 2 min before standing to avoid orthostatic hypotension.
- Patients on high-potency loop diuretics should be questioned about serum potassium levels or potassium supplement use.
- Short appointments and a stress reduction protocol may be required for anxious patients.
- Consider semisupine chair position for patient comfort if GI side effects occur.

Consultations:
- Medical consultation may be required to assess disease control and patient's ability to tolerate stress.

Teach Patient/Family:
- Importance of updating health history/drug record if physician makes any changes in evaluation or drug regimens

T

tramadol hydrochloride
tray′-mah-doal
(Tramal[AUS], Tramal SR[AUS], Ultram, Zydol[AUS])
Do not confuse tramadol with Toradol, or Ultram with Ultane.

CATEGORY AND SCHEDULE
Pregnancy Risk Category: C

MECHANISM OF ACTION
An analgesic that binds to mu-opioid receptors and inhibits reuptake of norepinephrine and serotonin. Reduces the intensity of pain stimuli reaching sensory nerve endings.
Therapeutic Effect: Alters the perception of and emotional response to pain.

PHARMACOKINETICS

Route	Onset	Peak	Duration
PO	less than 1 hr	2–3 hr	4–6 hr

Rapidly and almost completely absorbed after PO administration. Protein binding: 20%. Extensively metabolized in the liver to active metabolite (reduced in patients with advanced cirrhosis). Primarily excreted in urine. Minimally removed by hemodialysis.
Half-life: 6–7 hr.

AVAILABILITY
Tablets: 50 mg.

INDICATIONS AND DOSAGES
▸ **Moderate to Moderately Severe Pain**
PO
Adults, Elderly. 50–100 mg q4–6h. Maximum: 400 mg/day for patients 75 yr and younger; 300 mg/day for patients older than 75 yr.
▸ **Dosage in Renal Impairment**
For patients with creatinine clearance of less than 30 ml/min, increase dosing interval to q12h. Maximum: 200 mg/day.
▸ **Dosage in Hepatic Impairment**
Dosage is decreased to 50 mg q12h.

CONTRAINDICATIONS
Acute alcohol intoxication; concurrent use of centrally acting analgesics, hypnotics, opioids, or psychotropic drugs

INTERACTIONS
Drug
Alcohol, other CNS depressants: May increase CNS or respiratory depression and hypotension.
Carbamazepine: Decreases tramadol blood concentration.
MAOIs: Increase tramadol blood concentration.
Herbal
None known.
Food
None known.
Drug interactions of concern to dentistry
- Increased risk of respiratory depression: anesthetics, alcohol
- Significant increase in metabolism: carbamazepine
- Increased serum concentrations: quinidine
- Increased risk of seizures: MAOIs, tricyclic antidepressants, selective serotonin reuptake inhibitors
- Increased risk of sedation: other CNS depressant drugs, alcohol

DIAGNOSTIC TEST EFFECTS
May increase serum creatinine, AST (SGOT), and ALT (SGPT)hepatic levels. May decrease blood Hgb level. May cause proteinuria.

SIDE EFFECTS
Frequent (25%–15%)
Dizziness or vertigo, nausea, constipation, headache, somnolence
Occasional (10%–5%)
Vomiting, pruritus, CNS stimulation (such as nervousness, anxiety, agitation, tremor, euphoria, mood swings, and hallucinations), asthenia, diaphoresis, dyspepsia, dry mouth, diarrhea
Rare (< 5%)
Malaise, vasodilation, anorexia, flatulence, rash, blurred vision, urine retention or urinary frequency, menopausal symptoms

SERIOUS REACTIONS
! Overdose results in respiratory depression and seizures.
! Tramadol may have a prolonged duration of action and cumulative effect in patients with hepatic or renal impairment.

DENTAL CONSIDERATIONS
General:
- Determine why the patient is taking the drug.
- Patients taking opioids for acute or chronic pain should be given alternative analgesics for dental pain.
- Geriatric patients are more susceptible to drug effects; use lower dose.
- Assess salivary flow as a factor in caries, periodontal disease, and candidiasis.

- Take precautions if dental surgery is anticipated and general anesthesia is required.
- Risk of cross-hypersensitivity to other opioid analgesics.

Teach Patient/Family:

- Caution to prevent trauma when using oral hygiene aids
- That opioid drugs may alter reaction time; caution patient about driving or operating complex equipment
- *When chronic dry mouth occurs, advise patient:*
  - To avoid mouth rinses with high alcohol content because of drying effects
  - To use daily home fluoride products for anticaries effect
  - To use sugarless gum, frequent sips of water, or saliva substitutes

trandolapril

tran-doe′-la-pril

(Gopten[AUS], Mavik, Odrik[AUS])

Do not confuse trandolapril with tramadol.

CATEGORY AND SCHEDULE

Pregnancy Risk Category: C (D if used in second or third trimester)

T

MECHANISM OF ACTION

An ACE inhibitor that suppresses the renin-angiotensin-aldosterone system and prevents the conversion of angiotensin I to angiotensin II, a potent vasoconstrictor; may also inhibit angiotensin II at local vascular and renal sites. Decreases plasma angiotensin II, increases plasma renin activity, and decreases aldosterone secretion. ***Therapeutic Effect:*** Reduces peripheral arterial resistance and pulmonary capillary wedge pressure; improves cardiac output and exercise tolerance.

PHARMACOKINETICS

Slowly absorbed from the GI tract. Protein binding: 80%. Metabolized in the liver and GI mucosa to active metabolite. Primarily excreted in urine. Removed by hemodialysis. ***Half-life:*** 24 hr.

AVAILABILITY

Tablets: 1 mg, 2 mg, 4 mg.

INDICATIONS AND DOSAGES

▸ Hypertension (without Diuretic)

PO

Adults, Elderly. Initially, 1 mg once a day in nonblack patients, 2 mg once a day in black patients. Adjust dosage at least at 7-day intervals. Maintenance: 2–4 mg/day. Maximum: 8 mg/day.

▸ CHF

PO

Adults, Elderly. Initially, 0.5–1 mg, titrated to target dose of 4 mg/day.

CONTRAINDICATIONS

History of angioedema from previous treatment with ACE inhibitors

INTERACTIONS

Drug

Alcohol, antihypertensives, diuretics: May increase the effects of trandolapril.

Lithium: May increase lithium blood concentration and risk of lithium toxicity.

NSAIDs: May decrease the effects of trandolapril.

Potassium-sparing diuretics, potassium supplements: May cause hyperkalemia.

Herbal

None known.

Food
None known.

Drug interactions of concern to dentistry
• Decreased absorption of tetracycline
• Drugs that lower blood pressure could possibly exaggerate hypotensive effects

DIAGNOSTIC TEST EFFECTS

May increase BUN, serum alkaline phosphatase, serum bilirubin, serum creatinine, serum potassium, AST (SGOT), and ALT (SGPT) levels. May decrease serum sodium levels. May cause positive antinuclear antibody titer.

SIDE EFFECTS

Frequent (35%–23%)
Dizziness, cough

Occasional (11%–3%)
Hypotension, dyspepsia (heartburn, epigastric pain, indigestion), syncope, asthenia (loss of strength), tinnitus

Rare (< 1%)
Palpitations, insomnia, drowsiness, nausea, vomiting, constipation, flushed skin

SERIOUS REACTIONS

! Excessive hypotension ("first-dose syncope") may occur in patients with CHF and in those who are severely salt or volume depleted.
! Angioedema and hyperkalemia occur rarely.
! Agranulocytosis and neutropenia may be noted in those with collagen vascular disease including scleroderma and systemic lupus erythematosus and impaired renal function.
! Nephrotic syndrome may be noted in those with history of renal disease.

DENTAL CONSIDERATIONS

General:
• Monitor vital signs at every appointment because of CV disease.
• Limit use of sodium-containing products, such as saline IV fluids, for patients with a dietary salt restriction.
• Stress from dental procedures may compromise CV function; determine patient risk.
• Short appointments and a stress reduction protocol may be required for anxious patients.
• Use precaution if sedation or general anesthesia is required; risk of hypotensive episode.
• After supine positioning, have patient sit upright for at least 2 min before standing to avoid orthostatic hypotension.
• Consider semisupine chair position for patient comfort because of respiratory side effects of drug.
• Patients on chronic drug therapy may rarely have symptoms of blood dyscrasias, which can include infection, bleeding, and poor healing.

Consultations:
• Medical consultation may be required to assess disease control and patient's ability to tolerate stress.

Teach Patient/Family:
• Importance of good oral hygiene to prevent soft tissue inflammation
• Caution to prevent trauma when using oral hygiene aids
• Importance of updating health and drug history if physician makes any changes in evaluation or drug regimens

tranexamic acid

tran-ex-**am**-ik
(Cyklokapron)

CATEGORY AND SCHEDULE

Pregnancy Risk Category: B

MECHANISM OF ACTION

A competitive inhibitor of plasminogen activation and, at much higher concentrations, a noncompetitive inhibitor of plasmin (i.e., actions similar to aminocaproic acid), which exerts its antifibrinolytic effects primarily by forming a reversible complex with a modified plasminogen. ***Therapeutic Effect:*** Prevents fibrin clots from forming.

PHARMACOKINETICS

Absorption after PO administration represents 30%–50% of the ingested dose, and bioavailability is not affected by food intake. Protein binding: 3%. Site of metabolism is not established. Excreted in urine. ***Half-life:*** Unknown.

AVAILABILITY

Tablets (Cyklokapron): 500 mg.
Injection (Cyklokapron): 100 mg/ml.

INDICATIONS AND DOSAGES

▸ Hemorrhage Prophylaxis, Tooth Extraction

IV/PO

Adults, Children. 10 mg/kg body weight immediately before dental extraction. Following surgery, a dose of 25 mg/kg body weight can be given orally 3 or 4 times daily for 2–8 days. Alternatively, tranexamic acid can be administered entirely orally, 25 mg/kg body weight 3–4 times per day beginning 1 day before surgery.

T

▸ Dosage in Renal Impairment

Serum Creatinine	IV Dosage	Tablets
120–250 μmol/L (1.36–2.83 mg/dl)	10 mg/kg bid	15 mg/kg bid
250–500 μmol/L (2.83–5.66 mg/dl)	10 mg/kg daily	15 mg/kg daily
>500 μmol/L (>5.66 mg/dl)	10 mg/kg q48h or 5 mg/kg q24h	15 mg/kg q48h or 7.5 mg/kg q24h

UNLABELED USES

Hereditary angioedema, hemorrhage

CONTRAINDICATIONS

Acquired defective color vision, subarachnoid hemorrhage, active intravascular clotting process, hypersensitivity to tranexamic acid or any component of the formulation

INTERACTIONS

Drug

None known.

Herbal

None known.

Food

None known.

Drug interactions of concern to dentistry

- Increased risk of bleeding: drugs that affect coagulation
- Factor IX complex: increased risk of thrombotic complications when used concurrently

DIAGNOSTIC TEST EFFECTS

None known.

IV INCOMPATIBILITIES

Blood, solutions containing penicillin

IV COMPATIBILITIES

Can be mixed with most solutions for infusion, such as electrolyte solutions, carbohydrate solutions, amino acid solutions, and Dextran solutions. Heparin can be added to tranexamic acid injection.

SIDE EFFECTS

Occasional

Hypotension, diarrhea, nausea, vomiting, dizziness

SERIOUS REACTIONS

! Thromboembolic events (e.g., deep vein thrombosis, pulmonary embolism, cerebral thrombosis, acute renal cortical necrosis, central retinal artery and vein obstruction) have been reported.

DENTAL CONSIDERATIONS

General:

• Has been used as an antifibrinolytic mouthwash following oral surgery to prevent hemorrhage in patients taking oral anticoagulants.

Consultations:

• Hematologist consultation is strongly recommended.

Teach Patient/Family:

• Importance of updating health and drug history if physician makes any changes in evaluation or drug regimens

• To report hemorrhage or bleeding not responding to postsurgical hemostasis

• Caution to prevent trauma when using oral hygiene aids

tranylcypromine sulfate

tran-ill-sip′-roe-meen
(Parnate)

CATEGORY AND SCHEDULE

Pregnancy Risk Category: C

MECHANISM OF ACTION

An MAOI that inhibits the activity of the enzyme monoamine oxidase at CNS storage sites, leading to increased levels of the neurotransmitters epinephrine, norepinephrine, serotonin, and dopamine at neuronal receptor sites. ***Therapeutic Effect:*** Relieves depression.

PHARMACOKINETICS

Well absorbed from GI tract. Metabolized in the liver. Primarily excreted in urine. Removed by hemodialysis. ***Half-life:*** 1.5–3.5 hr.

AVAILABILITY

Tablets: 10 mg.

INDICATIONS AND DOSAGES

▸ Depression Refractory to or Intolerant of Other Therapy

PO

Adults, Elderly. Initially, 10 mg twice a day. May increase by 10 mg/day at 1- to 3-wk intervals up to 60 mg/day in divided doses.

OFF-LABEL USES

Post-traumatic stress disorder

CONTRAINDICATIONS

CHF, children younger than 16 years, pheochromocytoma, severe hepatic or renal impairment, uncontrolled hypertension

INTERACTIONS

Drug

Alcohol, other CNS depressants: May increase CNS depressant effects.
Buspirone: May increase BP.
Caffeine-containing medications: May increase the risk of cardiac arrhythmias and hypertension.
Carbamazepine, cyclobenzaprine, maprotiline, other MAOIs: May precipitate hypertensive crisis.

Dopamine, tryptophan: May cause sudden, severe hypertension.
Fluoxetine, trazodone, tricyclic antidepressants: May cause serotonin syndrome and neuroleptic malignant syndrome.
Insulin, oral antidiabetics: May increase the effects of these drugs.
Meperidine, other opioid analgesics: May produce diaphoresis, immediate excitation, rigidity, and severe hypertension or hypotension, sometimes leading to severe respiratory distress, vascular collapse, seizures, coma, and death.

Herbal
None known.

Food
Caffeine, chocolate, tyramine-containing foods (such as aged cheese): May cause sudden, severe hypertension.

Drug interactions of concern to dentistry
- Increased pressor effects: indirect-acting sympathomimetics (ephedrine)
- Hyperpyretic crisis, convulsions, hypertensive episode, and death: carbamazepine, meperidine, and possibly other opioids
- Increased anticholinergic effects: anticholinergics and antihistamines
- Increased effects of alcohol, barbiturates, benzodiazepines, CNS depressants, fluoxetine, tricyclic antidepressants

T

DIAGNOSTIC TEST EFFECTS
None known.

SIDE EFFECTS
Frequent
Orthostatic hypotension, restlessness, GI upset, insomnia, dizziness, lethargy, weakness, dry mouth, peripheral edema

Occasional
Flushing, diaphoresis, rash, urinary frequency, increased appetite, transient impotence

Rare
Visual disturbances

SERIOUS REACTIONS
! Hypertensive crisis occurs rarely and is marked by severe hypertension, occipital headache radiating frontally, neck stiffness or soreness, nausea, vomiting, diaphoresis, fever or chills, clammy skin, dilated pupils, palpitations, tachycardia or bradycardia, and constricting chest pain.
! Intracranial bleeding has been reported in association with severe hypertension.

DENTAL CONSIDERATIONS
General:
- After supine positioning, have patient sit upright for at least 2 min before standing to avoid orthostatic hypotension.
- Monitor vital signs at every appointment because of CV side effects.
- Assess salivary flow as a factor in caries, periodontal disease, and candidiasis.
- Hypertensive episodes are possible even though there are no specific contraindications to vasoconstrictor use in local anesthetics.

Consultations:
- Medical consultation may be required to assess patient's ability to tolerate stress.

Teach Patient/Family:
- To use electric toothbrush if patient has difficulty holding conventional devices
- *When chronic dry mouth occurs, advise patient:*
  - To avoid mouth rinses with high alcohol content because of drying effects

- Of need for daily home fluoride use to prevent caries
- To use sugarless gum, frequent sips of water, or saliva substitutes

trastuzumab

traz-two′-zoo-mab
(Herceptin)

CATEGORY AND SCHEDULE

Pregnancy Risk Category: B

MECHANISM OF ACTION

Binds to the HER-2 protein, which is overexpressed in 25%–30% of primary breast cancers, thereby inhibiting proliferation of tumor cells. ***Therapeutic Effect:*** Inhibits the growth of tumor cells and mediates antibody-dependent cellular cytotoxicity.

PHARMACOKINETICS

Half-life: 5.8 days (range: 1–32 days).

AVAILABILITY

Injection, Powder for Reconstitution: 440 mg.

INDICATIONS AND DOSAGES

▸ Breast Cancer

IV

Adults, Elderly. Initially, 4 mg/kg as a 30–90-min infusion, then 2 mg/kg weekly as a 30-min infusion.

CONTRAINDICATIONS

Preexisting cardiac disease

INTERACTIONS

Drug

Cyclophosphamide, doxorubicin, epirubicin: May increase the risk of cardiac dysfunction.

Herbal

None known.

Food

None known.

Drug interactions of concern to dentistry

- Dental drug interactions have not been studied

DIAGNOSTIC TEST EFFECTS

None known.

IV INCOMPATIBILITIES

Don't mix trastuzumab with any other medications or with D_5W.

SIDE EFFECTS

Frequent (> 20%)

Pain, asthenia, fever, chills, headache, abdominal pain, back pain, infection, nausea, diarrhea, vomiting, cough, dyspnea

Occasional (15%–5%)

Tachycardia, CHF, flulike symptoms, anorexia, edema, bone pain, arthralgia, insomnia, dizziness, paresthesia, depression, rhinitis, pharyngitis, sinusitis

Rare (< 5%)

Allergic reaction, anemia, leukopenia, neuropathy, herpes simplex

SERIOUS REACTIONS

! Cardiomyopathy, ventricular dysfunction, and CHF occur rarely.

! Pancytopenia may occur.

DENTAL CONSIDERATIONS

General:

- If additional analgesia is required for dental pain, consider alternative analgesics (NSAIDs) in patients taking narcotics for acute or chronic pain.
- Monitor and record vital signs.
- Avoid products that affect platelet function, such as aspirin and NSAIDs.

- This drug may be used in the hospital or on an outpatient basis. Confirm the patient's disease and treatment status.
- Patient on chronic drug therapy may rarely present with symptoms of blood dyscrasias, which can include infection, bleeding, and poor healing. If dyscrasia is present, caution patient to prevent oral tissue trauma when using oral hygiene aids.
- Consider semisupine chair position for patient comfort if GI side effects occur.
- Caution: patients may be at high risk for infection.
- Patients may be at risk for bleeding; check oral signs.
- Oral infections should be eliminated and/or treated aggressively.

Consultations:

- Medical consultation should include routine blood counts including platelet counts and bleeding time.
- In a patient with symptoms of blood dyscrasias, request a medical consultation for blood studies and postpone treatment until normal values are reestablished.
- Consult physician; prophylactic or therapeutic antiinfectives may be indicated if surgery or periodontal treatment is required.
- Medical consultation may be required to assess immunologic status during cancer chemotherapy and determine safety risk, if any, posed by the required dental treatment.
- Medical consultation may be required to assess disease control and patient's ability to tolerate stress.

Teach Patient/Family:

- To inform dentist of unusual bleeding episodes following dental treatment
- Secondary oral infection may occur; need to see dentist immediately if infection occurs.
- Importance of good oral hygiene to prevent soft tissue inflammation
- To report oral lesions, soreness, or bleeding to dentist
- To prevent trauma when using oral hygiene aids
- Importance of updating health and medication history if physician makes any changes in evaluation or drug regimens; include OTC, herbal, and nonherbal remedies in the update

travoprost

tra′-voe-prost
(Apo-Timop[CAN], Gen-Timolol[CAN], Optimol[AUS], Tenopt[AUS], Travatan)

CATEGORY AND SCHEDULE

Pregnancy Risk Category: C

MECHANISM OF ACTION

An ophthalmic agent that is a prostanoid selective FP receptor agonist. ***Therapeutic Effect:*** Reduces intraocular pressure (IOP) by reducing aqueous humor production.

PHARMACOKINETICS

Absorbed through the cornea and hydrolyzed to the active free acid form. Metabolized in cornea and liver. Metabolites are inactive. Excreted in urine. ***Half-life:*** 17–86 min.

T

AVAILABILITY

Ophthalmic Solution: 0.004% (Travatan).

INDICATIONS AND DOSAGES

▸ **Open-Angle Glaucoma, Ocular Hypertension**

OPHTHALMIC

Adults, Elderly. 1 drop in affected eye(s) once daily, in the evening.

CONTRAINDICATIONS

Hypersensitivity to travoprost or benzalkonium chloride, or any other component of the formulation

INTERACTIONS

Drug

None known.

Herbal

None known.

Food

None known.

Drug interactions of concern to dentistry

- None reported

DIAGNOSTIC TEST EFFECTS

None known.

SIDE EFFECTS

Frequent

Ocular hyperemia

Occasional

Ocular pain, pruritus, eye discomfort, decreased visual acuity, foreign body sensation

Rare

Abnormal vision, cataract, conjunctivitis, dry eye, eye disorder, flare, iris discoloration, keratitis, lid margin crusting, photophobia, subconjunctival hemorrhage, and tearing

SERIOUS REACTIONS

! Ocular adverse events including accidental injury, angina pectoris, anxiety, arthritis, back pain, bradycardia, bronchitis, chest pain, cold syndrome, depression, dyspepsia, gastrointestinal disorder, headache, hypercholesterolemia, hypertension, hypotension, infection, pain, prostate disorder, sinusitis, urinary incontinence, and urinary tract infection, occur rarely.

DENTAL CONSIDERATIONS

General:

- Monitor vital signs at every appointment because of CV and respiratory side effects and question patient about occurrence of CV side effects.
- Avoid drugs with anticholinergic activity, such as antihistamines, opioids, benzodiazepines, propantheline, atropine, and scopolamine.
- Protect patient's eyes from accidental spatter during dental treatment.
- Avoid dental light in patient's eyes; offer dark glasses for patient comfort.

Consultations:

- Medical consultation may be required to assess disease control.

Teach Patient/Family:

- Importance of updating health and drug history if physician makes any changes in evaluation or drug regimens

trazodone hydrochloride

tray′-zoe-done
(Apo-Trazodone[CAN], Desyrel, Novo-Trazodone[CAN], PMS-Trazodone[CAN])
Do not confuse Desyrel with Delsym or Zestril.

CATEGORY AND SCHEDULE

Pregnancy Risk Category: C

MECHANISM OF ACTION

An antidepressant that blocks the reuptake of serotonin at neuronal presynaptic membranes, increasing its availability at postsynaptic receptor sites. ***Therapeutic Effect:*** Relieves depression.

PHARMACOKINETICS

Well absorbed from the GI tract. Protein binding: 85%–95%. Metabolized in the liver. Primarily excreted in urine. Unknown if removed by hemodialysis.
Half-life: 5–9 hr.

AVAILABILITY

Tablets: 50 mg, 100 mg, 150 mg, 300 mg.

INDICATIONS AND DOSAGES

▸ Depression

PO

Adults. Initially, 150 mg/day in equally divided doses. Increase by 50 mg/day at 3-to 4–day intervals until therapeutic response is achieved. Maximum: 600 mg/day.
Elderly. Initially, 25–50 mg at bedtime. May increase by 25–50 mg every 3–7 days. Range: 75–150 mg/day.
Children 6–18 yr. Initially, 1.5–2 mg/kg/day in divided doses. May increase gradually to 6 mg/kg/day in 3 divided doses.

OFF-LABEL USES

Treatment of neurogenic pain

CONTRAINDICATIONS

None known.

INTERACTIONS

Drug

Alcohol, CNS depression-producing medications: May increase CNS depression.
Antihypertensives: May increase the effects of antihypertensives.
Digoxin, phenytoin: May increase the blood concentration of these drugs.
Indinavir, ketoconazole, ritonavir: May increase the blood concentration and toxicity of trazodone.

Herbal

St. John's wort: May increase the adverse effects of trazodone.

Food

None known.

Drug interactions of concern to dentistry

- Increased anticholinergic effects: anticholinergic drugs
- Increased CNS depression: alcohol, all other CNS depressants

DIAGNOSTIC TEST EFFECTS

May decrease serum WBC and neutrophil counts.

SIDE EFFECTS

Frequent (9%–3%)

Somnolence, dry mouth, light-headedness, dizziness, headache, blurred vision, nausea, vomiting

Occasional (3%–1%)

Nervousness, fatigue, constipation, generalized aches and pains, mild hypotension

Rare
Photosensitivity reaction

SERIOUS REACTIONS

! Priapism, diminished or improved libido, retrograde ejaculation, and impotence occur rarely.
! Trazodone appears to be less cardiotoxic than other antidepressants, although arrhythmias may occur in patients with preexisting cardiac disease.

DENTAL CONSIDERATIONS

General:
- Monitor vital signs at every appointment because of CV side effects.
- Patients on chronic drug therapy may rarely have symptoms of blood dyscrasias, which can include infection, bleeding, and poor healing.
- Assess salivary flow as a factor in caries, periodontal disease, and candidiasis.
- After supine positioning, have patient sit upright for at least 2 min before standing to avoid orthostatic hypotension.

Consultations:
- In a patient with symptoms of blood dyscrasias, request a medical consultation for blood studies and postpone dental treatment until normal values are reestablished.
- Medical consultation may be required to assess disease control.
- Physician should be informed if significant xerostomic side effects occur (e.g., increased caries, sore tongue, problems eating or swallowing, difficulty wearing prosthesis) so that a medication change can be considered.

Teach Patient/Family:
- To report oral lesions, soreness, or bleeding to dentist
- *When chronic dry mouth occurs, advise patient:*
  - To avoid mouth rinses with high alcohol content because of drying effects
  - Of need for daily home fluoride use to prevent caries
  - To use sugarless gum, frequent sips of water, or saliva substitutes

treprostinil sodium

treh-prost′-in-ill
(Remodulin)

CATEGORY AND SCHEDULE

Pregnancy Risk Category: B

MECHANISM OF ACTION

An antiplatelet that directly dilates pulmonary and systemic arterial vascular beds, inhibiting platelet aggregation. ***Therapeutic Effect:*** Reduces symptoms of pulmonary arterial hypertension associated with exercise.

PHARMACOKINETICS

Rapidly, completely absorbed after subcutaneous infusion; 91% bound to plasma protein. Metabolized by the liver. Excreted mainly in the urine with a lesser amount eliminated in the feces. ***Half-life:*** 2–4 hr.

AVAILABILITY

Injection: 1 mg/ml, 2.5 mg/ml, 5 mg/ml, 10 mg/ml.

INDICATIONS AND DOSAGES

▸ Pulmonary Arterial Hypertension
Continuous subcutaneous infusion
Adults, Elderly. Initially, 1.25 ng/kg/min. Reduce infusion

rate to 0.625 ng/kg/min if initial dose cannot be tolerated. Increase infusion rate in increments of no more than 1.25 ng/kg/min per week for the first 4 wk and then no more than 2.5 ng/kg/min per week for the duration of infusion.

▸ **Hepatic Impairment (Mild to Moderate)**

Adults, Elderly. Decrease the initial dose to 0.625 ng/kg/min on the basis of ideal body weight and increase cautiously.

CONTRAINDICATIONS

None known.

INTERACTIONS

Drug

Anticoagulants, aspirin, heparin, thrombolytics: May increase the risk of bleeding.

Drugs that alter BP, including antihypertensive agents, diuretics, vasodilators: Reduced BP caused by treprostinil may be exacerbated by these drugs.

Herbal

None known.

Food

None known.

Drug interactions of concern to dentistry

• Increased risk of bleeding: drugs that interfere with coagulation or platelet function, such as NSAIDs and aspirin

T

DIAGNOSTIC TEST EFFECTS

None known.

SIDE EFFECTS

Frequent

Infusion site pain, erythema, induration, rash

Occasional

Headache, diarrhea, jaw pain, vasodilation, nausea

Rare

Dizziness, hypotension, pruritus, edema

SERIOUS REACTIONS

! Abrupt withdrawal or sudden large reductions in dosage may result in worsening of pulmonary arterial hypertension symptoms.

DENTAL CONSIDERATIONS

General:

• An acute use drug for use in hospitals or emergency departments.

• If a patient reports this drug in his/her medical history, question about cardiovascular disease and drugs he/she may be taking.

• Patients are at risk for bleeding while receiving this drug; provide palliative dental care for dental emergencies only.

• Avoid products that affect platelet function, such as aspirin and NSAIDs.

Consultations:

• Medical consultation should include routine blood counts including platelet counts and bleeding time.

• Medical consultation may be required to assess disease control and patient's ability to tolerate stress.

Teach Patient/Family:

• To inform dentist of unusual bleeding episodes following dental treatment

tretinoin

tret′-i-noyn

(Altinac, Avita, Renova, Retin-A, Retin-A Micro, Vesanoid)

CATEGORY AND SCHEDULE

Pregnancy Risk Category: D (oral), C (topical)

MECHANISM OF ACTION

A retinoid that decreases cohesiveness of follicular epithelial cells. Increases turnover of follicular epithelial cells. Bacterial skincounts are not altered. Transdermal: Exerts its effects on growth and differentiation of epithelial cells. Antineoplastic: Induces maturation, decreases proliferation of acute promyelocytic leukemia (APL) cells ***Therapeutic Effect:*** Causes expulsion of blackheads; alleviates fine wrinkles, hyperpigmentation; causes repopulation of bone marrow and blood by normal hematopoietic cells.

PHARMACOKINETICS

Topical: Minimally absorbed. Oral: Well absorbed following oral administration. Protein binding: 95%. Metabolized in liver. Primarily excreted in urine, minimal excretion in feces. ***Half-life:*** 0.5–2 hrs.

AVAILABILITY

Capsules: 10 mg (Vesanoid).
Cream: 0.025% (Altinac, Avita, Retin-A), 0.02% (Renova), 0.05% (Altinac, Renova, Retin-A), 0.1 % (Altinac, Retin-A).
Gel: 0.01% (Retin-A), 0.025% (Avita, Retin-A), 0.04% (Retin-A Micro), 0.1% (Retin-A Micro).
Topical Liquid: 0.05% (Retin-A).

INDICATIONS AND DOSAGES

▸ Acne

TOPICAL
Adults. Apply once daily at bedtime.

▸ Transdermal

TRANSDERMAL
Adults. Apply to face once daily at bedtime.

▸ Acute Promyelocytic Leukemia

PO
Adults. 45 mg/m2/day given as two evenly divided doses until complete remission is documented. Discontinue therapy 30 days after complete remission or after 90 days of treatment, whichever comes first.

OFF-LABEL USES

Treatment of disorders of keratinization, including photo-aged skin, liver spots

CONTRAINDICATIONS

Sensitivity to parabens (used as preservative in gelatin capsule)

INTERACTIONS

Drug

Topical
Keratolytic agents (e.g., sulfur, benzoyl peroxide, salicylic acid), medicated soaps, shampoos, astringents, spice or lime cologne, permanent wave solutions, hair depilatories: May increase skin irritation.
Photosensitive medication (thiazides, tetracyclines, fluoroquinolones, phenothiazines, sulfonamides): May augment phototoxicity.
PO
Ketoconazole: May increase tretinoin concentration.

Herbal

Vitamin A: May increase risk of vitamin A toxicity.

Food

None known.

Drug interactions of concern to dentistry

- Increased peeling: medication-containing agents, such as alcohol or astringents
- Avoid concurrent use with photosensitizing drugs: tetracycline, fluoroquinolones, sulfonamides

DIAGNOSTIC TEST EFFECTS

PO: Leukocytosis occurs commonly (40%). May elevate liver function tests, cholesterol, triglycerides.

SIDE EFFECTS

Expected

Topical

Temporary change in pigmentation, photosensitivity. Local inflammatory reactions (peeling, dry skin, stinging, erythema, pruritus) are to be expected and are reversible with discontinuation of tretinoin

Frequent

PO

Headache, fever, dry skin/oral mucosa, bone pain, nausea, vomiting, rash

Occasional

PO

Mucositis, earache or feeling of fullness in ears, flushing, pruritus, increased sweating, visual disturbances, hypo/hypertension, dizziness, anxiety, insomnia, alopecia, skin changes

Rare

PO

Change in visual acuity, temporary hearing loss

SERIOUS REACTIONS

PO

! Retinoic acid syndrome (fever, dyspnea, weight gain, abnormal chest auscultatory findings, episodic hypotension) occurs commonly, as does leukocytosis.

! Syndrome generally occurs during first month of therapy (sometimes occurs following first dose).

! Pseudo tumor cerebri may be noted, especially in children (headache, nausea, vomiting, visual disturbances).

! Possible tumorigenic potential when combined with ultraviolet radiation.

Topical

! Possible tumorigenic potential when combined with ultraviolet radiation.

DENTAL CONSIDERATIONS

General:

- May cause dry, peeling skin if used around lips; provide lip lubricant for patient comfort during dental treatment.
- Advise patient if dental drugs prescribed have a potential for photosensitivity.

Teach Patient/Family:

- To avoid application on normal skin or getting cream in eyes, mouth, or other mucous membranes

T

triamcinolone/ triamcinolone acetonide/ triamcinolone diacetate/triamcinol one hexacetonide

trye-am-sin′-oh-lone

(triamcinolone) Aristocort(triamcinolone acetonide) Aristocort, Azmacort, Kenacort A[AUS], Kenalog, Kenalog in Orabase[AUS], Nasacort AQ, Triaderm[CAN] (triamcinolone diacetate) Amcort, Aristocort Intralesional (triamcinolone hexacetonide) Aristospan

Do not confuse triamcinolone with Triaminicin or Triaminicol.

CATEGORY AND SCHEDULE

Pregnancy Risk Category: C (D if used in first trimester)

MECHANISM OF ACTION

An adrenocortical steroid that inhibits accumulation of inflammatory cells at inflammation sites, phagocytosis, lysosomal enzyme release and synthesis, and release of mediators of inflammation. ***Therapeutic Effect:*** Prevents or suppresses cell-mediated immune reactions. Decreases or prevents tissue response to inflammatory process.

AVAILABILITY

Oral (Topical Paste [Kenalog in Orabase]): 0.1% or 5 g.
Tablets (Aristocort): 4 mg.
Inhalation (Oral [Azmacort]): 100 mcg/actuation.
Nasal spray (Tri-Nasal): 50 mcg/inhalation.
Nasal Spray (Vasacort AQ): 55 mcg/inhalation.
Cream (Aristocort A): 0.025%, 0.05%, 0.1%.
Cream (Kenalog, Triderm): 0.1%.
Oinment (Aristocort A, Kenalog): 0.025%, 0.1%.
Injection (acetonide, Kenalog): 10 mg/ml, 40 mg/ml.
Injection (diacetate, Aristocort): 25 mg/ml), 40 mg/ml.
Injection (hexacetonide, Aristospan): 5 mg/ml, 20 mg/ml.

INDICATIONS AND DOSAGES

▸ Immunosuppression, Relief of Acute Inflammation

PO
Adults, Elderly. 4–60 mg/day.
IM (triamcinolone acetonide)
Adults, Elderly. Initially, 2.5–60 mg/day.
IM (triamcinolone diacetate)
Adults, Elderly. 40 mg/wk.
IM (triamcinolone hexacetonide)
Adults, Elderly. Initially, 2.5–40 mg up to 100 mg; 2–20 mg.
Intra-articular, Intralesional
Adults, Elderly. 5–40 mg.

▸ Control of Bronchial Asthma

INHALATION
Adults, Elderly. 2 inhalations 3–4 times a day.
Children 6–12 yr. 1–2 inhalations 3–4 times a day.
Maximum: 12 inhalations/day.

▸ Rhinitis

INTRANASAL
Adults, Children 6 yr and older. 2 sprays each nostril each day.

▸ Relief of Inflammation or Pruritus Associated with Corticoid-Responsive Dermatoses

TOPICAL
Adults, Elderly. 2–4 times a day. May give 1–2 times a day or as intermittent therapy.

CONTRAINDICATIONS

Administration of live virus vaccines, especially smallpox vaccine; hypersensitivity to corticosteroids or tartrazine; IM injection or oral inhalation in children younger than 6 years; peptic ulcer disease (except life-threatening situations); systemic fungal infection
Topical: Marked circulation impairment

INTERACTIONS

Drug

Amphotericin: May increase hypokalemia.
Digoxin: May increase the risk of digoxin toxicity caused by hypokalemia.
Diuretics, insulin, oral hypoglycemics, potassium supplements: May decrease the effects of these drugs.
Hepatic enzyme inducers: May decrease the effects of triamcinolone.
Live-virus vaccines: May decrease the patient's antibody response to vaccine, increase vaccine side effects, and potentiate virus replication.

Herbal

None known.

T

Food
None known.
Drug interactions of concern to dentistry
(Inhaler only)
- None reported

Drug interactions of concern to dentistry trimcinolone/triamcinolone acetonide/triamcinolone hexacetonide
- Decreased action: barbiturates, rifampin, rifabutin
- Increased GI side effects: alcohol, salicylates, NSAIDs
- Increased action: ketoconazole, macrolide antibiotics

DIAGNOSTIC TEST EFFECTS

May increase blood glucose and serum lipid, amylase, and sodium levels. May decrease serum calcium, potassium, and thyroxine levels.

SIDE EFFECTS

Frequent
Insomnia, dry mouth, heartburn, nervousness, abdominal distention, diaphoresis, acne, mood swings, increased appetite, facial flushing, delayed wound healing, increased susceptibility to infection, diarrhea or constipation
Occasional
Headache, edema, change in skin color, frequent urination
Rare
Tachycardia, allergic reaction (including rash and hives), mental changes, hallucinations, depression
Topical: Allergic contact dermatitis

SERIOUS REACTIONS

! Long-term therapy may cause muscle wasting in the arms or legs, osteoporosis, spontaneous fractures, amenorrhea, cataracts, glaucoma, peptic ulcer disease, and CHF.
! Abruptly withdrawing the drug following long-term therapy may cause anorexia, nausea, fever, headache, arthralgia, rebound inflammation, fatigue, weakness, lethargy, dizziness, and orthostatic hypotension.
! Anaphylaxis occurs rarely with parenteral administration.
! Suddenly discontinuing triamcinolone may be fatal.
! Blindness has occurred rarely after intralesional injection around face and head.

DENTAL CONSIDERATIONS

General:
- Place on frequent recall because of oral side effects.
- Evaluate respiration characteristics and rate.
- Midday appointments and a stress reduction protocol may be required for anxious patients.
- Acute asthmatic episodes may be precipitated in the dental office. Rapid-acting sympathomimetic inhalants should be available for emergency use. Triamcinolone is not a rapid-acting drug and is not intended for use in acute asthmatic attacks.
- Be aware that aspirin or sulfite preservatives in vasoconstrictor-containing products can exacerbate asthma.
- Examine for oral manifestation of opportunistic infection.

Consultations:
- Medical consultation may be required to assess disease control.

Teach Patient/Family:
- Importance of good oral hygiene to prevent soft tissue inflammation
- Importance of gargling, rinsing mouth with water, and expectorating after each aerosol dose

T

DENTAL CONSIDERATIONS

TRIAMCINOLONE/TRIAMCINOLONE ACETONIDE/TRIAMCINOLONE DIACETATE/TRIAMCINOLONE HEXACETONIDE

General:

• Symptoms of oral infections may be masked.
• Examine for oral manifestation of opportunistic infections.
• Oral side effects may be more common with inhalation products; significant steroid side effects are more likely to occur with chronic systemic doses.
• Acute asthmatic episodes may be precipitated in the dental office. Rapid-acting sympathomimetic inhalants should be available for emergency use. A stress reduction protocol may be required.
• Monitor vital signs at every appointment because of CV side effects.
• Assess salivary flow as a factor in caries, periodontal disease, and candidiasis.
• Prophylactic antibiotics may be indicated to prevent infection.
• Place on frequent recall to monitor healing response.
• Determine dose and duration of steroid therapy for each patient to assess risk for stress tolerance and immunosuppression.
• Be aware that aspirin or sulfite preservatives in vasoconstrictor-containing products can exacerbate asthma.
• Patients who have been or are currently on chronic steroid therapy (>2 wk) may require supplemental steroids for dental treatment.

Consultations:

• Medical consultation may be required to assess disease control.
• Consultation may be required to confirm steroid dose and duration of use.

Teach Patient/Family:

• Importance of good oral hygiene to prevent soft tissue inflammation
• To report oral lesions, soreness, or bleeding to dentist
• *When chronic dry mouth occurs, advise patient:*
  • To avoid mouth rinses with high alcohol content because of drying effects
  • To use daily home fluoride products for anticaries effect
  • To use sugarless gum, frequent sips of water, or saliva substitutes

TRIAMCINOLONE ACETONIDE (TOPICAL)

General:

• Apply approximately 0.25 inch; measure with cotton-tipped applicator; press on lesion, do not rub. Use after brushing and eating and at bedtime for optimal effect.
• When used for oral lesions, return for oral evaluation if response of oral tissues has not occurred in 7–14 days.

Teach Patient/Family:

• To avoid sunlight on affected area; burns may occur
• Not to use on herpetic lesions

triamterene

try-am′-ter-een
(Dyrenium)
Do not confuse triamterene with trimipramine.

CATEGORY AND SCHEDULE

Pregnancy Risk Category: C
(D if used in pregnancy-induced hypertension)

MECHANISM OF ACTION

A potassium-sparing diuretic that inhibits sodium, potassium, ATPase. Interferes with sodium and potassium exchange in distal tubule, cortical collecting tubule, and collecting duct. Increases sodium and decreases potassium excretion. Also increases magnesium, decreases calcium loss. ***Therapeutic Effect:*** Produces diuresis and lowers BP.

PHARMACOKINETICS

Route	Onset	Peak	Duration
PO	2–4 hr	N/A	7–9 hr

Incompletely absorbed from the GI tract. Widely distributed. Metabolized in the liver. Primarily eliminated in feces via biliary route. ***Half-life:*** 1.5–2.5 hr (increased in renal impairment).

T

AVAILABILITY

Capsules: 50 mg, 100 mg.

INDICATIONS AND DOSAGES

▸ Edema, Hypertension

PO

Adults, Elderly. 25–100 mg/day as a single dose or in 2 divided doses. Maximum: 300 mg/day.

Children. 2–4 mg/kg/day as a single dose or in 2 divided doses. Maximum: 6 mg/kg/day or 300 mg/day.

OFF-LABEL USES

Treatment adjunct for hypertension, prevention and treatment of hypokalemia

CONTRAINDICATIONS

Drug-induced or preexisting hyperkalemia, progressive or severe renal disease, severe hepatic disease

INTERACTIONS

Drug

ACE inhibitors (such as captopril), potassium-containing medications, potassium supplements: May increase the risk of hyperkalemia.
Anticoagulants, heparin: May decrease the effects of these drugs.
Lithium: May decrease the clearance and increase the risk of toxicity of lithium.
NSAIDs: May decrease the antihypertensive effect of triamterene.

Herbal

None known.

Food

None known.

Drug interactions of concern to dentistry

- Nephrotoxicity: possible risk with indomethacin, NSAIDs
- Decreased antihypertensive effect: possible risk with NSAIDs, indomethacin
- Decreased effect of folic acid

DIAGNOSTIC TEST EFFECTS

May increase urinary calcium excretion; BUN and blood glucose levels; and serum calcium, creatinine, potassium, magnesium, and uric acid levels. May decrease serum sodium levels.

SIDE EFFECTS

Occasional

Fatigue, nausea, diarrhea, abdominal pain, leg cramps, headache

Rare

Anorexia, asthenia, rash, dizziness

SERIOUS REACTIONS

! Triamterene use may result in hyponatremia (somnolence, dry mouth, increased thirst, lack of energy) or severe hyperkalemia (irritability, anxiety, heaviness of legs, paresthesia, hypotension, bradycardia, ECG changes [tented T waves, widening QRS complex, ST segment depression]).

! Agranulocytosis, nephrolithiasis, and thrombocytopenia occur rarely.

DENTAL CONSIDERATIONS

General:

- Limit use of sodium-containing products, such as saline IV fluids, for patients with a dietary salt restriction.
- Assess salivary flow as a factor in caries, periodontal disease, and candidiasis.
- Monitor vital signs at every appointment because of CV effects and possible hyperkalemia.
- Patients on chronic drug therapy may rarely have symptoms of blood dyscrasias, which can include infection, bleeding, and poor healing.

Consultations:

- In a patient with symptoms of blood dyscrasias, request a medical consultation for blood studies and postpone dental treatment until normal values are reestablished.
- Medical consultation may be required to assess disease control.

Teach Patient/Family:

- Importance of good oral hygiene to prevent soft tissue inflammation
- Caution to prevent injury when using oral hygiene aids
- To report oral lesions, soreness, or bleeding to dentist
- *When chronic dry mouth occurs, advise patient:*
  - To avoid mouth rinses with high alcohol content because of drying effects
  - Of need for daily home fluoride use to prevent caries
  - To use sugarless gum, frequent sips of water, or saliva substitutes

triazolam

trye-ay′-zoe-lam

Schedule IV

(Apo-Triazo[CAN], Halcion)

Do not confuse Halcion with Haldol or Healon.

CATEGORY AND SCHEDULE

Pregnancy Risk Category: X

Controlled Substance: Schedule IV

MECHANISM OF ACTION

A benzodiazepine that enhances the action of the inhibitory neurotransmitter gamma-aminobutyric acid, resulting in CNS depression. ***Therapeutic Effect:*** Induces sleep.

AVAILABILITY

Tablets: 0.125 mg, 0.25 mg.

INDICATIONS AND DOSAGES

▸ Insomnia

PO

Adults, Children 18 yr and older. 0.125–0.5 mg at bedtime.

Elderly. 0.0625–0.125 mg at bedtime.

CONTRAINDICATIONS

Angle-closure glaucoma; CNS depression; pregnancy or breast-feeding; severe, uncontrolled pain; sleep apnea

INTERACTIONS

Drug

Alcohol, other CNS depressants: May increase CNS depression.

Herbal

Kava kava, valerian: May increase CNS depression.

Food

Grapefruit, grapefruit juice: May alter the absorption of triazolam.

Drug interactions of concern to dentistry

- Increased effects: erythromycin, clarithromycin
- Increased sedation: alcohol, CNS depressants, opioid analgesics, diltiazem, anesthetics
- Avoid use with ketoconazole, itraconazole, ritonavir, indinavir, nelfinavir
- Caution if used with fluvoxamine, reduce dose by 50%
- Caution when used with drugs that are strong inhibitors of CYP3A4 isoenzymes

DIAGNOSTIC TEST EFFECTS

None known.

SIDE EFFECTS

Frequent

Somnolence, sedation, dry mouth, headache, dizziness, nervousness, light-headedness, incoordination, nausea, rebound insomnia (may occur for 1–2 nights after drug is discontinued)

Occasional

Euphoria, tachycardia, abdominal cramps, visual disturbances

Rare

Paradoxical CNS excitement or restlessness (particularly in elderly or debilitated patients)

SERIOUS REACTIONS

! Abrupt or too-rapid withdrawal may result in pronounced restlessness, irritability, insomnia, hand tremors, abdominal or muscle cramps, vomiting, diaphoresis, and seizures.

! Overdose results in somnolence, confusion, diminished reflexes, respiratory depression, and coma.

DENTAL CONSIDERATIONS

General:

- Assess salivary flow as a factor in caries, periodontal disease, and candidiasis.
- If dizziness occurs, provide assistance when escorting patient to and from dental chair.
- When used for conscious sedation, have someone drive patient to and from dental office.
- Avoid the use of this drug in a patient with a history of drug abuse or alcoholism.
- Geriatric patients are more susceptible to drug effects; use a lower dose.
- Psychologic and physical dependence may occur with chronic administration.
- Determine why the patient is taking the drug.
- Patients on chronic drug therapy may rarely have symptoms of blood dyscrasias, which can include infection, bleeding, and poor healing.

Teach Patient/Family:

- *When chronic dry mouth occurs, advise patient:*
  - To avoid mouth rinses with high alcohol content because of drying effects
  - Of need for daily home fluoride use to prevent caries
  - To use sugarless gum, frequent sips of water, or saliva substitutes

trifluoperazine hydrochloride

trye-floo-oh-per′-a-zeen
(Apo-Trifluoperazine[CAN], Nono-Trifluzine[CAN], PMS-Trifluoperazine[CAN], Stelazine)
Do not confuse trifluoperazine with triflupromazine, or Stelazine with selegiline.

CATEGORY AND SCHEDULE
Pregnancy Risk Category: C

MECHANISM OF ACTION
A phenothiazine derivative that blocks dopamine at postsynaptic receptor sites. Possesses strong extrapyramidal and antiemetic effects and weak anticholinergic and sedative effects. ***Therapeutic Effect:*** Suppresses behavioral response in psychosis; reduces locomotor activity and aggressiveness.

AVAILABILITY
Tablets: 1 mg, 2 mg, 5 mg, 10 mg.
Injection: 2 mg/ml.

INDICATIONS AND DOSAGES
▸ Psychotic Disorders
PO
Adults, Elderly, Children 12 yr and older. Initially, 2–5 mg once or twice a day. Range: 15–20 mg/day. Maximum: 40 mg/day.
Children 6–11 yr. Initially, 1 mg once or twice a day. Maintenance: Up to 15 mg/day.
IM
Adults. 1–2 mg q4–6h. Maximum: 10 mg/24h.
Elderly. 1 mg q4–6h. Maximum: 6 mg/24h.
Children. 1 mg 2 times/day.

CONTRAINDICATIONS
Angle-closure glaucoma, circulatory collapse, myelosuppression, severe cardiac or hepatic disease, severe hypertension or hypotension

INTERACTIONS
Drug
Alcohol, other CNS depressants: May increase CNS and respiratory depression and the hypotensive effects of trifluoperazine.
Antacids: May inhibit absorption of trifluoperzine if given within 1 hour of drug.
Antithyroid agents: May increase the risk of agranulocytosis.
Extrapyramidal symptom-producing medications: May increase extrapyramidal symptoms.
Hypotension-producing agents: May increase hypotension.
Levodopa: May decrease the effects of levodopa.
Lithium: May decrease the absorption of trifluoperazine and produce adverse neurologic effects.
MAOIs, tricyclic antidepressants: May increase the anticholinergic and sedative effects of trifluoperazine.
Herbal
None known.
Food
None known.
Drug interactions of concern to dentistry
- Increased sedation: other CNS depressants, alcohol, barbiturate anesthetics, opioid analgesics
- Hypotension, tachycardia: epinephrine
- Increased extrapyramidal effects: phenothiazines and related drugs (haloperidol, droperidol), metoclopramide
- Additive photosensitization: tetracyclines
- Increased anticholinergic effects: anticholinergics

T

DIAGNOSTIC TEST EFFECTS

May cause ECG changes.

SIDE EFFECTS

Frequent

Hypotension, dizziness, and syncope (occur frequently after first injection, occasionally after subsequent injections, and rarely with oral form)

Occasional

Drowsiness during early therapy, dry mouth, blurred vision, lethargy, constipation or diarrhea, nasal congestion, peripheral edema, urine retention

Rare

Ocular changes, altered skin pigmentation (in those taking high doses for prolonged periods), photosensitivity

SERIOUS REACTIONS

! Extrapyramidal symptoms appear to be dose related (particularly high doses) and are divided into 3 categories: akathisia (inability to sit still, tapping of feet), parkinsonian symptoms (such as masklike face, tremors, shuffling gait, and hypersalivation), and acute dystonias (such as torticollis, opisthotonos, and oculogyric crisis). Dystonic reactions may also produce diaphoresis and pallor.

! Tardive dyskinesia, marked by tongue protrusion, puffing of the cheeks, and chewing or puckering of the mouth, occurs rarely but may be irreversible.

! Abrupt withdrawal after long-term therapy may precipitate nausea, vomiting, gastritis, dizziness, and tremors.

! Blood dyscrasias, particularly agranulocytosis, and mild leukopenia may occur.

! Trifluoperazine may lower the seizure threshold.

DENTAL CONSIDERATIONS

General:

- Monitor vital signs at every appointment because of CV side effects.
- Patients on chronic drug therapy may rarely have symptoms of blood dyscrasias, which can include infection, bleeding, and poor healing.
- After supine positioning, have patient sit upright for at least 2 min before standing to avoid orthostatic hypotension.
- Assess salivary flow as a factor in caries, periodontal disease, and candidiasis.
- Avoid dental light in patient's eyes; offer dark glasses for patient comfort.
- Assess for presence of extrapyramidal motor symptoms, such as tardive dyskinesia and akathisia. Extrapyramidal motor activity may complicate dental treatment.
- Geriatric patients are more susceptible to drug effects; use lower dose.
- Use vasoconstrictors with caution, in low doses, and with careful aspiration.

Consultations:

- In a patient with symptoms of blood dyscrasias, request a medical consultation for blood studies and postpone dental treatment until normal values are reestablished.
- Take precautions if dental surgery is anticipated and anesthesia is required.
- Physician should be informed if significant xerostomic side effects occur (e.g., increased caries, sore tongue, problems eating or swallowing, difficulty wearing prosthesis) so that a medication change can be considered.

- If signs of tardive dyskinesia or akathisia are present, refer to physician.

Teach Patient/Family:

- Importance of good oral hygiene to prevent soft tissue inflammation
- Caution to prevent injury when using oral hygiene aids
- To use electric toothbrush if patient has difficulty holding conventional devices
- *When chronic dry mouth occurs, advise patient:*
  - To use daily home fluoride products for anticaries effect
  - To avoid mouth rinses with high alcohol content because of drying effects
  - To use sugarless gum, frequent sips of water, or saliva substitutes

trifluridine

trye-flure′-i-deen

(Viroptic)

Do not confuse with Zostrix.

CATEGORY AND SCHEDULE

Pregnancy Risk Category: C

MECHANISM OF ACTION

An antiviral agent that incorporates into DNS causing increased rate of mutation and errors in protein formation. ***Therapeutic Effect:*** Prevents viral replication.

PHARMACOKINETICS

Intraocular solution is undetectable in serum. ***Half-life:*** 12 min.

AVAILABILITY

Ophthalmic solution: 1% (Viroptic).

INDICATIONS AND DOSAGES

▸ Herpes Simplex Virus Ocular Infections

OPHTHALMIC

Adults, Elderly, Children older than 6 yrs. 1 drop onto cornea q2h while awake. Maximum: 9 drops/day. Continue until corneal ulcer has completely reepithelialized; then, 1 drop q4h while awake (minimum: 5 drops/day) for an additional 7 days.

CONTRAINDICATIONS

Hypersensitivity to trifluridine or any component of the formulation

INTERACTIONS

Drug

None known.

Herbal

None known.

Food

None known.

Drug interactions of concern to dentistry

- None reported

DIAGNOSTIC TEST EFFECTS

None known.

SIDE EFFECTS

Frequent

Transient stinging or burning with instillation

Occasional

Edema of eyelid

Rare

Hypersensitivity reaction

SERIOUS REACTIONS

! Ocular toxicity may occur if used longer than 21 days.

DENTAL CONSIDERATIONS

General:

- Protect patient's eyes from accidental spatter during dental treatment.

T

- Avoid dental light in patient's eyes; offer dark glasses for patient comfort.
- Evaluate:
  - Therapeutic response: absence of redness, inflammation, tearing
  - Allergy: itching, lacrimation, redness, swelling

trihexyphenidyl

trye-hex-ee-fen′-i-dill
(Artane, Apo-Trihex[CAN])

CATEGORY AND SCHEDULE

Pregnancy Risk Category: C

MECHANISM OF ACTION

An anticholinergic agent that blocks central cholinergic receptors (aids in balancing cholinergic and dopaminergic activity). ***Therapeutic Effect:*** Decreases salivation, relaxes smooth muscle.

PHARMACOKINETICS

Well absorbed from gastrointestinal (GI) tract. Primarily excreted in urine. ***Half-life:*** 3.3–4.1 hrs.

AVAILABILITY

Elixer: 2 mg/5ml (Artane).
Tablets: 2 mg, 5 mg (Artane).

T

INDICATIONS AND DOSAGES

▸ **Parkinsonism**

PO

Adults, Elderly. Initially, 1 mg on first day. May increase by 2 mg/day at 3–5 day intervals up to 6–10 mg/day (12–15 mg/day in patients with postencephalitic parkinsonism).

▸ **Drug-Induced Extrapyramidal Symptoms**

PO

Adults, Elderly. Initially, 1 mg/day. Range: 5–15 mg/day.

CONTRAINDICATIONS

Angle closure glaucoma, GI obstruction, paralytic ileus, intestinal atony, severe ulcerative colitis, prostatic hypertrophy, myasthenia gravis, megacolon, hypersensitivity to trihexyphenidyl or any component of the formulation

INTERACTIONS

Drug

Alcohol, CNS depressants: May increase sedative effect.
Amantadine, anticholinergics, MAOIs: May increase anticholinergic effects.
Antacids, antidiarrheals: May decrease absorption and effects of trihexyphenidyl.

Herbal

None known.

Food

None known.

Drug interactions of concern to dentistry

- Increased anticholinergic effects: scopolamine, atropine, phenothiazines, antihistamines, and other anticholinergics
- Increased CNS depression: alcohol, CNS depressants
- Decreased effects of phenothiazines

DIAGNOSTIC TEST EFFECTS

None known.

SIDE EFFECTS

Elderly (older than 60 yrs) tend to develop mental confusion, disorientation, agitation, psychotic-like symptoms

Frequent
Drowsiness, dry mouth
Occasional
Blurred vision, urinary retention, constipation, dizziness, headache, muscle cramps
Rare
Seizures, depression, rash

SERIOUS REACTIONS

! Hypersensitivity reaction (eczema, pruritus, rash, cardiac disturbances, photosensitivity) may occur.
! Overdosage may vary from CNS depression (sedation, apnea, cardiovascular collapse, death) to severe paradoxical reaction (hallucinations, tremor, seizures).

DENTAL CONSIDERATIONS

General:
- Assess salivary flow as a factor in caries, periodontal disease, and candidiasis.
- Place on frequent recall because of oral side effects.
- After supine positioning, have patient sit upright for at least 2 min before standing to avoid orthostatic hypotension.
- Avoid dental light in patient's eyes; offer dark glasses for patient comfort.

Teach Patient/Family:
- Importance of good oral hygiene to prevent soft tissue inflammation
- To use electric toothbrush if patient has difficulty holding conventional devices
- *When chronic dry mouth occurs, advise patient:*
  - To avoid mouth rinses with high alcohol content because of drying effects
  - Of need for daily home fluoride use to prevent caries
  - To use sugarless gum, frequent sips of water, or saliva substitutes

trimethobenzamide hydrochloride

trye-meth-oh-ben′-za-mide
(Tigan)

CATEGORY AND SCHEDULE

Pregnancy Risk Category: C

MECHANISM OF ACTION

An anticholinergic that acts at the chemoreceptor trigger zone in the medulla oblongata. ***Therapeutic Effect:*** Relieves nausea and vomiting.

PHARMACOKINETICS

Route	Onset	Peak	Duration
PO	10–40 min	N/A	3–4 hr
IM	15–30 min	N/A	2–3 hr

Partially absorbed from the GI tract. Distributed primarily to the liver. Metabolic fate unknown. Excreted in urine. ***Half-life:*** 7–9 hr.

AVAILABILITY

Capsules: 100 mg, 300 mg.
Injection: 100 mg/ml.
Suppositories: 100 mg, 200 mg.

INDICATIONS AND DOSAGES

▸ **Nausea and Vomiting**

PO

Adults, Elderly. 300 mg 3–4 times a day.
Children weighing 30–100 lb. 100–200 mg 3–4 times a day.

IM

Adults, Elderly. 200 mg 3–4 times a day.

RECTAL

Adults, Elderly. 200 mg 3–4 times a day.
Children weighing 30–100 lb. 100–200 mg 3–4 times a day.

T

Children weighing less than 30 lb. 100 mg 3–4 times a day.

CONTRAINDICATIONS
Hypersensitivity to benzocaine or similar local anesthetics; use of parenteral form in children or suppositories in premature infants or neonates

INTERACTIONS
Drug
CNS depressants: May increase CNS depression.
Herbal
None known.
Food
None known.
Drug interactions of concern to dentistry
- Increased effect: CNS depressants
- May mask ototoxic symptoms associated with antibiotics or large doses of salicylates

DIAGNOSTIC TEST EFFECTS
None known.

SIDE EFFECTS
Frequent
Somnolence
Occasional
Blurred vision, diarrhea, dizziness, headache, muscle cramps
Rare
Rash, seizures, depression, opisthotonos, parkinsonian syndrome, Reye's syndrome (marked by vomiting, seizures)

SERIOUS REACTIONS
! A hypersensitivity reaction, manifested as extrapyramidal symptoms such as muscle rigidity and allergic skin reactions, occurs rarely.
! Children may experience paradoxical reactions, marked by restlessness, insomnia, euphoria, nervousness, and tremor.
! Overdose may produce CNS depression (manifested as sedation, apnea, cardiovascular collapse, and death) or severe paradoxical reactions (such as hallucinations, tremor, and seizures).

DENTAL CONSIDERATIONS
General:
- Nausea and vomiting may be accompanied by dehydration and electrolyte imbalance and should be corrected as part of treatment.
- Postpone elective dental treatment when symptoms are present.

trimetrexate
try-meh-trex-ate
(Neutrexin)
Do not confuse with Amicar.

CATEGORY AND SCHEDULE
Pregnancy Risk Category: D

MECHANISM OF ACTION
A folate antagonist that inhibits the enzyme dihydrofolate reductase (DHFR). ***Therapeutic Effect:*** Disrupts purine, DNA, RNA, protein synthesis, with consequent cell death.

PHARMACOKINETICS
Following IV administration, distributed readily into ascitic fluid. Metabolized in liver. Eliminated in urine. ***Half-life:*** 11–20 hrs.

AVAILABILITY
Powder for Injection: 25 mg (Neutrexin).

INDICATIONS AND DOSAGES

▸ Pneumocystis Carinii Pneumonia (PCP)

IV INFUSION

Adults. Trimetrexate: 45 mg/m^2 once daily over 60–90 min. Leucovorin: 20 mg/m^2 over 5–10 min q6h for total daily dose of 80 mg/m^2, or orally as 4 doses of 20 mg/m^2 spaced equally throughout the day. Round up the oral dose to the next higher 25 mg increment. Recommended course of therapy: 21 days trimetrexate, 24 days leucovorin.

OFF-LABEL USES

Treatment of non–small cell lung, prostate, and colorectal cancer

CONTRAINDICATIONS

Clinically significant hypersensitivity to trimetrexate, leucovorin, or methotrexate

INTERACTIONS

Drug

Erythromycin, rifampin, rifabutin, ketoconazole, fluconazole, acetaminophen: May alter timetrexate plasma concentration.
Cimetidine: May reduce trimetrexate metabolism.
Clotrimazole, ketoconazole, miconazole: May inhibit trimetrexate metabolism.

Herbal

None known.

Food

None known.

Drug interactions of concern to dentistry

- Alteration of plasma levels: concurrent use with erythromycin, ketoconazole, and fluconazole
- Alteration in trimetrexate metabolites: acetaminophen
- Caution with use of drugs that are strong inhibitors of CYP3A4 isoenzymes

DIAGNOSTIC TEST EFFECTS

May increase SGOT (AST), SGPT (ALT), alkaline phosphatase, bilirubin, BUN, serum creatinine. May decrease Hgb, Hct, leukocytes, platelet counts.

IV INCOMPATIBILITIES

Foscarnet (Foscavir), indomethacin (Indocin)

SIDE EFFECTS

Occasional

Fever, rash, pruritus, nausea, vomiting, confusion

Rare

Fatigue

SERIOUS REACTIONS

! Trimetrexate given without concurrent leucovorin may result in serious or fatal hematologic, hepatic, and/or renal complications, including bone marrow suppression, oral and GI mucosal ulceration, and renal and hepatic dysfunction.

! In event of overdose, stop trimetrexate and give leucovorin 40 mg/m^2 q6h for 3 days.

! Anaphylaxis occurs rarely.

DENTAL CONSIDERATIONS

General:

- Examine for evidence of oral manifestations of blood dyscrasia (infection, bleeding, poor healing).
- Place on frequent recall because of oral side effects.
- Determine why the patient is taking the drug.
- Examine for oral manifestations of opportunistic infections.
- Consider local hemostasis measures to prevent excessive bleeding.
- Palliative treatment may be required for stomatitis.
- Refer to physician if oral ulcerative lesions occur.

• Consider semisupine chair position for patient comfort because of GI effects of disease.

Consultations:

• Obtain a medical consultation for blood studies (CBC) because leukopenic or thrombocytopenic side effects may result in infection, delayed healing, and excessive bleeding. Postpone elective dental treatment until normal values are maintained.
• Medical consultation may be required to assess disease control.

Teach Patient/Family:

• Importance of good oral hygiene to prevent soft tissue inflammation
• Caution to prevent injury when using oral hygiene aids
• That secondary oral infection may occur; must see dentist immediately if infection occurs

trimipramine

trye-mih-prah-meen
(Apo-Trimip[CAN], Novo-Tripramine[CAN], Nu-Trimipramine[CAN], Rhotrimine[CAN], Surmontil)
Do not confuse with desipramine.

CATEGORY AND SCHEDULE

Pregnancy Risk Category: C

MECHANISM OF ACTION

A tricyclic antibulimic, anticataplectic, antidepressant, antinarcoleptic, antineuralgic, antineuritic, and antipanic agent that blocks the reuptake of neurotransmitters, such as norepinephrine and serotonin, at presynaptic membranes, increasing their concentration at postsynaptic receptor sites. May demonstrate less autonomic toxicity than other tricyclic antidepressants.
Therapeutic Effect: Results in antidepressant effect. Anticholinergic effect controls nocturnal enuresis.

PHARMACOKINETICS

Rapidly, completely absorbed after PO administration, and not affected by food. Protein binding: 95%. Metabolized in liver (significant first-pass effect). Primarily excreted in urine. Not removed by hemodialysis. ***Half-life:*** 16–40 hrs.

AVAILABILITY

Capsules: 25 mg, 50 mg, 100 mg (Surmontil).

INDICATIONS AND DOSAGES

▸ Depression

PO

Adults. 50–150 mg/day at bedtime. Maximum: 200 mg/day for outpatients, 300 mg/day for inpatients.
Elderly. Initially, 25 mg/day at bedtime. May increase by 25 mg q3–7days. Maximum: 100 mg/day.

CONTRAINDICATIONS

Acute recovery period after myocardial infarction (MI), within 14 days of MAOI ingestion, hypersensitivity to trimipramine or any component of the formulation

INTERACTIONS

Drug

Alcohol, central nervous system (CNS) depressants: May increase CNS and respiratory depression and the hypotensive effects of trimipramine.
Anticoagulants: May increase risk of bleeding.

T

Antipsychotics (amisulpride, haloperidol, risperidone, sertindole, quetiapine, sultopride, zotepine): May increase the cardiac effects (QT prolongation, torsades de pointes, cardia arrest).
Antithyroid agents: May increase the risk of agranulocytosis.
Amprenavir, atazanavir: May increase serum concentrations and risk of toxicity of trimipramine.
Atomoxetine: May increase plasma concentrations of atomoxetine.
Barbituates: May decrease trimipramine serum concentrations and possible additive adverse effects.
Baclofen: May increase the risk of memory loss and/or muscle tone.
Cimetidine: May increase trimipramine blood concentration and risk of toxicity.
Cisapride: May increase the cardiac effects.
Class 1, 1A and III antiarrhythmic agents: May increase the cardiac effects.
Clonidine, guanadrel: May decrease the effects of clonidine and guanadrel.
Cotrimoxazole, fluconazole: May increase the cardiac effects.
Duloxetine, fluoxetine, paroxetine, sertraline: May increase serum concentrations and risk of toxicity.
Estrogens: May increase the antidepressant effectiveness and risk of tricyclic toxicity.
Gatifloxacin, gemifloxacin, grepafloxacin, sparfloxacin, telithromycin: May increase the cardiac effects.
Halofantrine, halothane: May increase the cardiac effects.
MAOIs: May increase the risk of hyperpyrexia, hypertensive crisis, and seizures.
Phenothiazines: May increase anticholinergic and sedative effects of trimipramine.
Phenytoin: May decrease trimipramine blood concentration.
Quinidine: May increase the risk of trimipramine toxicity.
Sympathomimetics: May increase the cardiac effects.
Vasopressin: May increase the cardiac effects.
Zolmitriptan: May increase the cardiac effects.

Herbal

Ginkgo biloba: May decrease seizure threshold.
St. John's wort: May have additive effect.

Drug interactions of concern to dentistry

- Increased anticholinergic effects: muscarinic blockers, antihistamines, phenothiazines
- Increased effects of direct-acting sympathomimetics (epinephrine, levonordefrin)
- Possible risk of increased CNS depression: alcohol, barbiturates, benzodiazepines, and other CNS depressants
- Decreased antihypertensive effects: clonidine, guanadrel, guanethidine

DIAGNOSTIC TEST EFFECTS

May alter blood glucose levels and ECG readings.

SIDE EFFECTS

Frequent

Drowsiness, fatigue, dry mouth, blurred vision, constipation, delayed micturition, postural hypotension, diaphoresis, disturbed concentration, increased appetite, urinary retention, photosensitivity.

Occasional

Gastrointestinal (GI) disturbances, such as nausea, and a metallic taste sensation.

Rare

Paradoxical reaction, marked by agitation, and restlessness, nightmares, insomnia, and extrapyramidal symptoms, particularly fine hand tremors.

SERIOUS REACTIONS

! High dosage may produce cardiovascular effects, such as severe postural hypotension, dizziness, tachycardia, palpitations, arrhythmias and seizures. High dosage may also result in altered temperature regulation, including hyperpyrexia or hypothermia.

! Abrupt withdrawal from prolonged therapy may produce headache, malaise, nausea, vomiting, and vivid dreams.

DENTAL CONSIDERATIONS

General:

- Monitor vital signs at every appointment because of CV side effects.
- Assess salivary flow as a factor in caries, periodontal disease, and candidiasis.
- Patients on chronic drug therapy may rarely have symptoms of blood dyscrasias, which can include infection, bleeding, and poor healing.
- After supine positioning, have patient sit upright for at least 2 min before standing to avoid orthostatic hypotension.
- Use vasoconstrictors with caution, in low doses, and with careful aspiration. Avoid use of gingival retraction cord with epinephrine.
- Place on frequent recall because of oral side effects.

Consultations:

- In a patient with symptoms of blood dyscrasias, request a medical consultation for blood studies and postpone dental treatment until normal values are reestablished.
- Medical consultation may be required to assess disease control.
- Physician should be informed if significant xerostomic side effects occur (e.g., increased caries, sore tongue, problems eating or swallowing, difficulty wearing prosthesis) so that a medication change can be considered.

Teach Patient/Family:

- Importance of good oral hygiene to prevent soft tissue inflammation
- Caution to prevent injury when using oral hygiene aids
- *When chronic dry mouth occurs, advise patient:*
  - To avoid mouth rinses with high alcohol content because of drying effects
  - Of need for daily home fluoride use to prevent caries
  - To use sugarless gum, frequent sips of water, or saliva substitutes

triptorelin pamoate

trip-toe-ree′-linn

(Trelstar Depot, Trelstar LA)

CATEGORY AND SCHEDULE

Pregnancy Risk Category: X

MECHANISM OF ACTION

A gonadotropin-releasing hormone (GnRH) analogue and antineoplastic agent that inhibits gonadotropin hormone secretion through a negative feedback mechanism. Circulating levels of luteinizing hormone, follicle-stimulating hormone, testosterone, and estradiol rise initially, then subside with continued therapy. ***Therapeutic Effect:*** Suppresses growth of abnormal prostate tissue.

AVAILABILITY

Powder for Injection (Trelstar Depot): 3.75 mg.
Powder for Injection (Trelstar LA): 11.25 mg.

INDICATIONS AND DOSAGES

▸ Prostate Cancer

IM (Trelstar Depot)
Adults, Elderly. 3.75 mg once q28days.
IM (Trelstar LA)
Adults, Elderly. 11.25 mg q84days.

CONTRAINDICATIONS

Hypersensitivity to luteinizing hormone-releasing hormone (LHRH) or LHRH agonists

INTERACTIONS

Drug

Hyperprolactinemic drugs: Reduce the number of pituitary gonadrotropin-releasing hormone (GnRH) receptors.

Herbal

None known.

Food

None known.

Drug interactions of concern to dentistry

• Dental drug interactions have not been studied

DIAGNOSTIC TEST EFFECTS

May alter serum pituitary-gonadal function test results. May cause transient increase in serum testosterone levels, usually during first week of treatment.

SIDE EFFECTS

Frequent (> 5%)

Hot flashes, skeletal pain, headache, impotence

Occasional (5%–2%)

Insomnia, vomiting, leg pain, fatigue

Rare (< 2%)

Dizziness, emotional lability, diarrhea, urine retention, UTIs, anemia, pruritus

SERIOUS REACTIONS

! Bladder outlet obstruction, skeletal pain, hematuria, and spinal cord compression (with weakness or paralysis of the lower extremities) may occur.

DENTAL CONSIDERATIONS

General:

• If additional analgesia is required for dental pain, consider alternative analgesics (NSAIDs) in patients taking narcotics for acute or chronic pain.
• This drug may be used in the hospital or on an outpatient basis. Confirm the patient's disease and treatment status.
• Patients may have received other chemotherapy or radiation; confirm medical and drug history.
• When urinary retention is a problem, use anticholinergic drugs with care.

Consultations:

• Consult patient's physician if an acute dental infection occurs and another antiinfective is required.
• Medical consultation may be required to assess disease control and patient's ability to tolerate stress.

Teach Patient/Family:

• Importance of good oral hygiene to prevent soft tissue inflammation
• To prevent trauma when using oral hygiene aids
• Importance of updating health and medication history if physician makes any changes in evaluation or drug regimens; include OTC, herbal, and nonherbal remedies in the update

T

tropicamide

troe-pik′-a-mide
(Diotrope[CAN], Mydriacyl, Opticyl, Tropicacyl)

CATEGORY AND SCHEDULE

Pregnancy Risk Category: C

MECHANISM OF ACTION

An antimuscarininc agent that produces competitive antagonism of the actions of acetylcholine.
Therapeutic Effect: Produces dilation of pupil (mydriasis); produces paralysis of accommodation (cycloplegia).

PHARMACOKINETICS

Onset of action occurs within 20 to 40 minutes. The duration is about 6 hours.

AVAILABILITY

Ophthalmic Solution: 0.5% (Mydriacyl, Opticyl, Tropicacyl), 1% (Mydriacyl).

INDICATIONS AND DOSAGES

▸ **Ocular Diagnostic Procedure, Examination of Fundus**

OPHTHALMIC

Adults, Elderly, Children. 1–2 drops in the eye(s) 15–20 min prior to exam

▸ **Ocular Diagnostic Procedure, Refractive Procedures**

OPHTHALMIC

Adults, Elderly, Children. 1–2 drops in the eye(s). May be repeated in 5 min.

CONTRAINDICATIONS

Primary glaucoma or tendency toward glaucoma, hypersensitivity to tropicamide or any component of the formulation

INTERACTIONS

Drug

Cisapride: May decrease the efficacy of cisapride.

Herbal

None known.

Food

None known.

Drug interactions of concern to dentistry

- None reported

DIAGNOSTIC TEST EFFECTS

None known.

SIDE EFFECTS

Occasional

Blurred vision, ocular irritation, headache

Rare

Photophobia, increased intraocular pressure

SERIOUS REACTIONS

! Cardiorespiratory collapse has been reported.

! Systemic absorption, including behavioral disturbances, confusion, dry mouth, fast heartbeat, and psychotic reactions, occurs rarely.

DENTAL CONSIDERATIONS

General:

- An acute use drug for diagnostic purposes.
- Protect patient's eyes from accidental spatter during dental treatment.
- Avoid dental light in patient's eyes; offer dark glasses for patient comfort.

unoprostone isopropyl

yoo-noh-prost′-ohn eye-se-pro′-pel
(Rescula)

CATEGORY AND SCHEDULE

Pregnancy Risk Category: C

MECHANISM OF ACTION

An ophthalmic agent that increases the outflow of aqueous humor.
Therapeutic Effect: Decreases intraocular pressure.

PHARMACOKINETICS

Peak response occurs in 4 to 8 weeks. The duration of a single dose is about 10 hours. Hydrolyzed to unoprostone free acid form in the cornea. Rapidly eliminated from plasma. Excreted as metabolites in urine. ***Half-life:*** 14 min.

AVAILABILITY

Ophthalmic solution: 0.15% (Rescula).

INDICATIONS AND DOSAGES

▸ **Glaucoma, Ocular Hypertension**
OPHTHALMIC
Adults, Elderly. Instill 1 drop in affected eye(s) 2 times/day.

CONTRAINDICATIONS

Hypersensitivity to unoprostone isopropyl, benzalkonium chloride or any other component of the formulation

INTERACTIONS

Drug
None known.
Herbal
None known.
Food
None known.

Drug interactions of concern to dentistry
• None reported; avoid use of anticholinergic drugs: atropine-like drugs, propantheline, diazepam, other benzodiazepines

DIAGNOSTIC TEST EFFECTS

None known.

SIDE EFFECTS

Frequent (25%–10%)
Burning, stinging, dry eyes, itching, increased eyelash length and redness.
Occasional (< 10%)
Abnormal vision, eyelid disorder, foreign body sensation.

SERIOUS REACTIONS

! Elevated intraocular pressure occurs rarely.

DENTAL CONSIDERATIONS

General:
• Check compliance of patient with prescribed drug regimen for glaucoma.
• Protect patient's eyes from accidental spatter during dental treatment.
• Avoid dental light in patient's eyes; offer dark glasses for patient comfort.
Consultations:
• Medical consultation may be required to assess disease control.

U

ursodiol

your-soo′-dee-ol
(Actigall, Urso)

CATEGORY AND SCHEDULE

Pregnancy Risk Category: B

MECHANISM OF ACTION

A gallstone solubilizing agent that suppresses hepatic synthesis and secretion of cholesterol; inhibits intestinal absorption of cholesterol. ***Therapeutic Effect:*** Changes the bile of patients with gallstones from precipitating (capable of forming crystals) to cholesterol solubilizing (capable of being dissolved).

AVAILABILITY

Capsules: 300 mg.
Tablets: 250 mg.

INDICATIONS AND DOSAGES

▸ Dissolution of Radiolucent, Noncalcified Gallstones When Cholecystectomy Is not Recommended; Treatment of Biliary Cirrhosis

PO

Adults, Elderly. 8–10 mg/kg/day in 2–3 divided doses. Treatment may require months. Obtain ultrasound image of gallbladder at 6-mo intervals for first year. If gallstones have dissolved, continue therapy and repeat ultrasound within 1–3 mo.

▸ Prevention of Gallstones

PO

Adults, Elderly. 300 mg twice a day.

OFF-LABEL USES

Treatment of alcoholic cirrhosis, biliary atresia, chronic hepatitis, gallstone formation, sclerosing cholangitis, prophylaxis of liver transplant rejection

U

CONTRAINDICATIONS

Allergy to bile acids, calcified cholesterol stones, chronic hepatic disease, radiolucent bile pigment stones, radiopaque stones

INTERACTIONS

Drug

Aluminum-containing antacids, cholestyramine: May decrease the absorption and effects of ursodiol.
Estrogens, oral contraceptives: May decrease the effects of ursodiol.

Herbal

None known.

Food

None known.

Drug interactions of concern to dentistry

- Reduced action: aluminum-based antacids

DIAGNOSTIC TEST EFFECTS

May alter liver functions test results.

SIDE EFFECTS

Occasional

Diarrhea

SERIOUS REACTIONS

! None significant.

DENTAL CONSIDERATIONS

General:

- Consider semisupine chair position for patient comfort because of GI effects of disease.
- Some opioids can cause spasm of bile duct leading to epigastric distress. Use caution in use for sedation or pain control. NSAIDs may be better choice.
- Consider drug as a factor in the diagnosis of altered taste.

valacyclovir

val-a-sye′-kloe-ver
(Valtrex)

CATEGORY AND SCHEDULE

Pregnancy Risk Category: B

MECHANISM OF ACTION

A virustatic antiviral that is converted to acyclovir triphosphate, becoming part of the viral DNA chain. ***Therapeutic Effect:*** Interferes with DNA synthesis and replication of herpes simplex virus and varicella-zoster virus.

PHARMACOKINETICS

Rapidly absorbed after PO administration. Protein binding: 13%–18%. Rapidly converted by hydrolysis to the active compound acyclovir. Widely distributed to tissues and body fluids (including CSF). Primarily eliminated in urine. Removed by hemodialysis. ***Half-life:*** 2.5–3.3 hr (increased in impaired renal function).

AVAILABILITY

Caplets: 500 mg, 1000 mg.

INDICATIONS AND DOSAGES

▸ **Herpes Zoster (Shingles)**

PO

Adults, Elderly. 1 g 3 times a day for 7 days.

▸ **Herpes Simplex (Cold Sores)**

PO

Adults, Elderly. 2 g twice a day for 1 day.

▸ **Initial Episode of Genital Herpes**

PO

Adults, Elderly. 1 g twice a day for 10 days.

▸ **Recurrent Episodes of Genital Herpes**

PO

Adults, Elderly. 500 mg twice a day for 3 days.

▸ **Prevention of Genital Herpes**

PO

Adults, Elderly. 500–1000 mg/day.

▸ **Dosage in Renal Impairment**

Dosage and frequency are modified on the basis of creatinine clearance.

Creatinine Clearance	Herpes Zoster	Genital Herpes
50 ml/min or higher	1 g q8h	500 mg q12h
30–49 ml/min	1 g q12h	500 mg q12h
10–29 ml/min	1 g q24h	500 mg q24h
less than 10 ml/min	500 mg q24h	500 mg q24h

OFF-LABEL USES

To reduce the risk of heterosexual transmission of genital herpes

CONTRAINDICATIONS

Hypersensitivity to or intolerance of acyclovir, valacyclovir, or their components

INTERACTIONS

Drug

Cimetidine, probenecid: May increase acyclovir blood concentration.

Herbal

None known.

Food

None known.

Drug interactions of concern to dentistry

• None reported in otherwise uncompromised patients

DIAGNOSTIC TEST EFFECTS

None known.

V

SIDE EFFECTS

Frequent

Herpes zoster (17%–10%): Nausea, headache

Genital herpes (17%): Headache

Occasional

Herpes zoster (7%–3%): Vomiting, diarrhea, constipation (50 yr or older), asthenia, dizziness (50 yr and older)

Genital herpes (8%–3%): Nausea, diarrhea, dizziness

Rare

Herpes zoster (3%–1%): Abdominal pain, anorexia

Genital herpes (3%–1%): Asthenia, abdominal pain

SERIOUS REACTIONS

! None known.

DENTAL CONSIDERATIONS

General:

- Determine why the patient is taking the drug.
- Be aware of general discomfort associated with shingles; acute symptoms may preclude patient's routine dental visit or mandate short appointments.
- Patients on chronic drug therapy may rarely have symptoms of blood dyscrasias, which can include infection, bleeding, and poor healing.

Consultations:

- Medical consultation may be required to assess disease control.
- In a patient with symptoms of blood dyscrasias, request a medical consultation for blood studies and postpone dental treatment until normal values are reestablished.

Teach Patient/Family:

- Importance of good oral hygiene to prevent soft tissue inflammation
- Caution to prevent trauma when using oral hygiene aids

valdecoxib

val-de-cocks′-ib

(Bextra)

ALERT

Valdecoxib has been withdrawn from the market.

CATEGORY AND SCHEDULE

Pregnancy Risk Category: C

MECHANISM OF ACTION

An NSAID that inhibits cyclooxygenase-2, the enzyme responsible for producing prostaglandins, which cause pain and inflammation.

Therapeutic Effect: Reduces inflammatory response and intensity of pain.

PHARMACOKINETICS

Rapidly and almost completely absorbed from the GI tract. Widely distributed. Extensively metabolized in the liver. Primarily eliminated in urine. ***Half-life:*** 8–11 hr.

AVAILABILITY

Tablets: 10 mg, 20 mg.

INDICATIONS AND DOSAGES

▸ Osteoarthritis, Rheumatoid Arthritis

PO

Adults, Elderly. 10 mg once a day.

▸ Primary Dysmenorrhea

PO

Adults, Elderly. 20 mg twice a day.

CONTRAINDICATIONS

Hypersensitivity to aspirin or NSAIDs, severe hepatic or renal impairment

INTERACTIONS

Drug

Anticoagulants: May increase the effects of anticoagulants.

Aspirin, other salicylates: May increase the risk of GI side effects, such as bleeding.
Dextromethorphan: May increase the plasma level of dextromethorphan.
Fluconazole, ketoconazole: May increase the plasma concentration of valdecoxib.

Herbal

None known.

Food

None known.

Drug interactions of concern to dentistry

- Increased plasma levels: fluconazole, ketoconazole, probenecid
- Increased risk of GI side effects: aspirin, methotrexate
- Decreased antihypertensive effects: diuretics, calcium channel blockers, ACE inhibitors, β-blockers
- Decreased renal clearance of lithium
- Monitor PT time: anticoagulants
- Increased renal toxicity: cyclosporine
- First-time users of SSRIs also taking NSAIDs may have a higher risk of GI side effects; until more data are available, it may be advisable to avoid use of NSAIDs in these patients (*Br J Clin Pharmacol* 55:591–595, 2003)

DIAGNOSTIC TEST EFFECTS

May increase BUN and serum creatinine levels and liver function test results.

SIDE EFFECTS

Frequent (8%–4%)
Headache
Occasional (3%–2%)
Dizziness
Rare (< 2%)
Dyspepsia, nausea, diarrhea, sinusitis, peripheral edema

SERIOUS REACTIONS

! None known.

DENTAL CONSIDERATIONS

General:

- Patients on chronic drug therapy may rarely have symptoms of blood dyscrasias, which can include infection, bleeding, and poor healing.
- Use aspirin or NSAIDs with caution.
- Consider altering chair position for comfort of arthritic patients.
- Assess salivary flow as a factor in caries, periodontal disease, and candidiasis.
- Monitor vital signs at every appointment because of CV side effects.

Consultations:

- In a patient with symptoms of blood dyscrasias, request a medical consultation for blood studies and postpone treatment until normal values are reestablished.

Teach Patient/Family:

- Importance of good oral hygiene to prevent soft tissue inflammation
- Importance of updating health and drug history if physician makes any changes in evaluation or drug regimens
- *When chronic dry mouth occurs, advise patient:*
  - To avoid mouth rinses with high alcohol content because of drying effects
  - To use fluoride products for anticaries effects
  - To use sugarless gum, frequent sips of water, or saliva substitutes

valganciclovir hydrochloride

val-gan-sye′-kloh-veer
(Valcyte)

CATEGORY AND SCHEDULE

Pregnancy Risk Category: C

MECHANISM OF ACTION

A synthetic nucleoside that competes with viral DNA esterases and is incorporated directly into growing viral DNA chains. ***Therapeutic Effect:*** Interferes with DNA synthesis and viral replication.

PHARMACOKINETICS

Well absorbed and rapidly converted to ganciclovir by intestinal and hepatic enzymes. Widely distributed. Slowly metabolized intracellularly. Primarily excreted unchanged in urine. Removed by hemodialysis. ***Half-life:*** 18 hr (increased in impaired renal function).

AVAILABILITY

Tablets: 450 mg.

INDICATIONS AND DOSAGES

▸ Cytomegalovirus (CMV) Retinitis in Patients with Normal Renal Function

PO

Adults. Initially, 900 mg (two 450-mg tablets) twice a day for 21 days. Maintenance: 900 mg once a day.

▸ Prevention of CMV After Transplant

PO

Adults, Elderly. 900 mg once a day beginning within 10 days of transplant and continuing until 100 days post-transplant.

▸ Dosage in Renal Impairment

Dosage and frequency are modified on the basis of creatinine clearance.

Creatinine Clearance	Induction Dosage	Maintenance Dosage
60 ml/min or more	900 mg twice/day	900 mg once/day
40–59 ml/min	450 mg twice/day	450 mg once/day
25–39 ml/min	450 mg once/day	450 mg q2 days
10–24 ml/min	450 mg q2 days	450 mg twice/week

CONTRAINDICATIONS

Hypersensitivity to acyclovir or ganciclovir

INTERACTIONS

Drug

Amphotericin B, cyclosporine: May increase the risk of nephrotoxicity.
Bone marrow depressants: May increase bone marrow depression.
Imipenem and cilastatin: May increase the risk of seizures.
Probenecid: Decreases renal clearance of valganciclovir.
Zidovudine (AZT): May increase the risk of hematologic toxicity.

Herbal

None known.

Food

All foods: Maximize drug bioavailability.

Drug interactions of concern to dentistry

- Increased risk of blood dyscrasias: dapsone, carbamazepine, phenothiazines
- Increased risk of seizures: imipenem/cilastatin (Primaxin)
- Low platelet counts may prevent the use of aspirin, NSAIDs

DIAGNOSTIC TEST EFFECTS

May decrease blood Hct and Hgb levels, serum creatinine level, platelet count, and WBC count

SIDE EFFECTS

Frequent (16%–9%)
Diarrhea, neutropenia, headache
Occasional (8%–3%)
Nausea, anemia, thrombocytopenia
Rare (< 3%)
Insomnia, paraesthesia, vomiting, abdominal pain, fever

SERIOUS REACTIONS

! Hematologic toxicity including severe neutropenia (most common), anemia, and thrombocytopenia may occur.
! Retinal detachment occurs rarely.
! An overdose may result in renal toxicity.
! Valganciclovir may decrease sperm production and fertility.

DENTAL CONSIDERATIONS

General:

- Patients on chronic drug therapy may rarely have symptoms of blood dyscrasias, which can include infection, bleeding, and poor healing.
- Examine for oral manifestation of opportunistic infection.
- Place on frequent recall to evaluate healing response.
- Consider local hemostasis measures to control excessive bleeding.

Consultations:

- Medical consultation for blood studies (CBC); leukopenic or thrombocytopenic side effects may result in infection, delayed healing, and excessive bleeding. Postpone elective dental treatment until normal values are maintained.
- Medical consultation may be required to assess disease control.

Teach Patient/Family:

- To prevent trauma when using oral hygiene aids
- About the possibility of secondary oral infection and the need to see dentist immediately if signs of infection occur
- Importance of good oral hygiene to prevent soft tissue inflammation

valproic acid/ valproate sodium/ divalproex sodium

val-pro′-ick
(valproic acid)
Depakene(valproate sodium)
Depakene syrup, Epilim[AUS], Valpro[AUS](divalproex sodium)
Depacon, Depakote, Depakote ER, Depakote Sprinkle

CATEGORY AND SCHEDULE

Pregnancy Risk Category: D

MECHANISM OF ACTION

An anticonvulsant, antimanic, and antimigraine agent that directly increases concentration of the inhibitory neurotransmitter gamma-aminobutyric acid. ***Therapeutic Effect:*** Reduces seizure activity.

PHARMACOKINETICS

Well absorbed from the GI tract. Protein binding: 80%–90%. Metabolized in the liver. Primarily excreted in urine. Not removed by hemodialysis. ***Half-life:*** 6–16 hr (may be increased in hepatic impairment, the elderly, and children younger than 18 mo).

AVAILABILITY

Capsules (Depakene): 250 mg.
Syrup (Depakene): 250 mg/5 ml.
Tablets (Delayed-Release [Depakote]): 125 mg, 250 mg, 500 mg.

Tablets (Extended-Release [Depakote ER]): 500 mg.
Capsules Sprinkles (Depakote Sprinkle): 125 mg.
Injection (Depacon): 100 mg/ml.

INDICATIONS AND DOSAGES

Seizures

PO

Adults, Elderly, Children 10 yr and older. Initially, 10–15 mg/kg/day in 1–3 divided doses. May increase by 5–10 mg/kg/day at weekly intervals up to 30–60 mg/kg/day. Usual adult dosage: 1000–2500 mg/day.

IV

Adults, Elderly, Children. Same as oral dose but given q6h.

Manic Episodes

PO

Adults, Elderly. Initially, 750 mg/day in divided doses. Maximum: 60 mg/kg/day.

Prevention of Migraine Headaches

PO (Extended-Release)

Adults, Elderly. Initially, 500 mg/day for 7 days. May increase up to 1000 mg/day.

PO (Delayed-Release)

Adults, Elderly. Initially, 250 mg twice a day. May increase up to 1000 mg/day.

OFF-LABEL USES

Treatment of myoclonic, simple partial, and tonic-clonic seizures

CONTRAINDICATIONS

Active hepatic disease

INTERACTIONS

Drug

Alcohol, other CNS depressants: May increase CNS depressant effects.
Amitriptyline, primidone: May increase the blood concentration of these drugs.
Anticoagulants, heparin, platelet aggregation inhibitors, thrombolytics: May increase the risk of bleeding.
Carbamazepine: May decrease valproic acid blood concentration.
Hepatotoxic medications: May increase the risk of hepatotoxicity.
Phenytoin: May increase the risk of phenytoin toxicity and decrease the effects of valproic acid.

Herbal

None known.

Food

None known.

Drug interactions of concern to dentistry

- Increased effects: CNS depressants; carbamazepine, phenobarbital levels may be increased; phenothiazines can lower the seizure threshold
- Increased bleeding and toxicity: salicylates, NSAIDs
- Increased blood levels: erythromycin
- Increased serum levels of amitriptyline, nortriptyline (start with low dose and monitor)
- Decreased effects of diazepam

DIAGNOSTIC TEST EFFECTS

May increase serum LDH, bilirubin, AST (SGOT), and ALT (SGPT) levels. Therapeutic serum level is 50–100 mcg/ml; toxic serum level is greater than 100 mcg/ml.

IV INCOMPATIBILITIES

Do not mix valproic acid with any other medications.

SIDE EFFECTS

Frequent

Epilepsy: Abdominal pain, irregular menses, diarrhea, transient alopecia, indigestion, nausea, vomiting, tremors, weight gain or loss
Mania (22%–19%): Nausea, somnolence

Occasional
Epilepsy: Constipation, dizziness, drowsiness, headache, skin rash, unusual excitement, restlessness
Mania (12%–6%): Asthenia, abdominal pain, dyspepsia (heartburn, indigestion, epigastric distress), rash
Rare
Epilepsy: Mood changes, diplopia, nystagmus, spots before eyes, unusual bleeding or ecchymosis

SERIOUS REACTIONS

! Hepatotoxicity may occur, particularly in the first 6 months of valproic acid therapy. It may be preceded by loss of seizure control, malaise, weakness, lethargy, anorexia, and vomiting rather than abnormal serum liver function test results.
! Blood dyscrasias may occur.

DENTAL CONSIDERATIONS

General:
- Patients on chronic drug therapy may rarely have symptoms of blood dyscrasias, which can include infection, bleeding, and poor healing.
- Evaluate for clotting ability during gingival instrumentation because inhibition of platelet aggregation may occur.
- Consider semisupine chair position for patient comfort if GI side effects occur.
- Place on frequent recall if gingival overgrowth occurs.
- Ask about type of epilepsy, seizure frequency, and quality of seizure control.

Consultations:
- In a patient with symptoms of blood dyscrasias, request a medical consultation for blood studies and postpone dental treatment until normal values are reestablished.
- Medical consultation may be required to assess disease control.

Teach Patient/Family:
- Importance of good oral hygiene to prevent soft tissue inflammation and minimize gingival overgrowth
- Caution to prevent injury when using oral hygiene aids
- To use electric toothbrush if patient has difficulty holding conventional devices
- Need for frequent oral prophylaxis if gingival overgrowth occurs
- To report oral lesions, soreness, or bleeding to dentist

valrubicin

val-rue′-bih-sin
(VaHaxan[CAN], Valstar)
Do not confuse valrubicin with valsartan.

CATEGORY AND SCHEDULE

Pregnancy Risk Category: C

MECHANISM OF ACTION

An anthracycline antibiotic that inhibits incorporation of nucleosides into nucleic acids after penetrating cells. ***Therapeutic Effect:*** Causes chromosomal damage, arresting cells in the G_2 phase of cell division, and interferes with DNA synthesis.

AVAILABILITY

Solution for Intravesical Instillation: 40 mg/ml.

INDICATIONS AND DOSAGES

▸ **Bladder Cancer**
INTRAVESICAL
Adults, Elderly. 800 mg once weekly for 6 wk.

CONTRAINDICATIONS
Perforated bladder, sensitivity to valrubicin, severe irritated bladder, small bladder capacity, UTI

INTERACTIONS
Drug interactions of concern to dentistry
- None reported

SIDE EFFECTS
Frequent
Local intravesical reaction (10%): Local bladder symptoms, urinary frequency or urgency, dysuria, hematuria, bladder pain, cystitis, bladder spasms
Systemic (15%–5%): Abdominal pain, nausea, UTI
Occasional
Local intravesical reaction (less than 10%): Nocturia, local burning, urethral pain, pelvic pain, gross hematuria
Systemic (5%–2%): Diarrhea, vomiting, urine retention, microscopic hematuria, asthenia, headache, malaise, back pain, chest pain, dizziness, rash, anemia, fever, vasodilation
Rare
Systemic (1%): Flatus, peripheral edema, hyperglycemia, pneumonia, myalgia

DENTAL CONSIDERATIONS
General:
- If additional analgesia is required for dental pain, consider alternative analgesics (NSAIDs) in patients taking narcotics for acute or chronic pain.
- This drug may be used in the hospital or on an outpatient basis. Confirm the patient's disease and treatment status.
- Offer patient frequent breaks if urinary frequency is a concern.
- Avoid prescribing drugs that could cause urinary retention, such as drugs with anticholinergic activity.

Consultations:
- Medical consultation may be required to assess disease control and patient's ability to tolerate stress.

Teach Patient/Family:
- Importance of good oral hygiene to prevent soft tissue inflammation
- Importance of updating health and medication history if physician makes any changes in evaluation or drug regimens; include OTC, herbal, and nonherbal remedies in the update

valsartan
val-sar′-tan
(Diovan)
Do not confuse valsartan with Valstan.

CATEGORY AND SCHEDULE
Pregnancy Risk Category: C (D if used in second or third trimester)

MECHANISM OF ACTION
An angiotensin II receptor, type AT_1, antagonist that blocks vasoconstrictor and aldosterone-secreting effects of angiotensin II, inhibiting the binding of angiotensin II to the AT_1 receptors. ***Therapeutic Effect:*** Causes vasodilation, decreases peripheral resistance, and decreases BP.

PHARMACOKINETICS
Poorly absorbed after PO administration. Food decreases peak plasma concentration. Protein binding: 95%.

Metabolized in the liver. Recovered primarily in feces and, to a lesser extent, in urine. Unknown if removed by hemodialysis.
Half-life: 6 hr.

AVAILABILITY
Tablets: 40 mg, 80 mg, 160 mg, 320 mg.

INDICATIONS AND DOSAGES
▸ Hypertension
PO
Adults, Elderly. Initially, 80–160 mg/day in patients who are not volume depleted. May increase up to a maximum: 320 mg/day.
▸ CHF
PO
Adults, Elderly. Initially, 40 mg twice a day. May increase up to 160 mg twice a day. Maximum: 320 mg/day.

CONTRAINDICATIONS
Bilateral renal artery stenosis, biliary cirrhosis or obstruction, hypoaldosteronism, severe hepatic impairment

INTERACTIONS
Drug
Diuretics: Produces additive hypotensive effects.
Herbal
None known.
Food
All foods: Decreases peak plasma concentration of valsartan.
Drug interactions of concern to dentistry
- Possible reduction in effect: ketoconazole

DIAGNOSTIC TEST EFFECTS
May increase AST (SGOT), ALT (SGPT), and serum bilirubin, creatinine, and potassium levels. May decrease blood Hgb and Hct levels.

SIDE EFFECTS
Rare (2%–1%)
Insomnia, fatigue, heartburn, abdominal pain, dizziness, headache, diarrhea, nausea, vomiting, arthralgia, edema

SERIOUS REACTIONS
! Overdosage may manifest as hypotension and tachycardia. Bradycardia occurs less often.
! Viral infection and upper respiratory tract infection (cough, pharyngitis, sinusitis, rhinitis) occur rarely.

DENTAL CONSIDERATIONS
General:
- Monitor vital signs at every appointment because of CV side effects.
- Limit use of sodium-containing products, such as saline IV fluids, for patients with a dietary salt restriction.
- Stress from dental procedures may compromise CV function; determine patient risk.
- Short appointments and a stress reduction protocol may be required for anxious patients.
- Use precaution if sedation or general anesthesia is required; risk of hypotensive episode.

Consultations:
- Medical consultation may be required to assess disease control and patient's ability to tolerate stress.

vancomycin hydrochloride

van-koe-mye′-sin
(Vancocin, Vancocin CP[AUS], Vancocin HCl Pulvules[AUS])

CATEGORY AND SCHEDULE

Pregnancy Risk Category: B

MECHANISM OF ACTION

A tricyclic glycopeptide antibiotic that binds to bacterial cell walls, altering cell membrane permeability and inhibiting RNA synthesis. ***Therapeutic Effect:*** Bactericidal.

PHARMACOKINETICS

PO: Poorly absorbed from the GI tract. Primarily eliminated in feces. Parenteral: Widely distributed. Protein binding: 55%. Primarily excreted unchanged in urine. Not removed by hemodialysis. ***Half-life:*** 4–11 hr (increased in impaired renal function).

AVAILABILITY

Capsules: 125 mg, 250 mg.
Powder for Oral Suspension (Vancocin): 1 g (provides 250 mg/5 ml after mixing).
Powder for Injection: 500 mg, 1 g.
Infusion (Premix): 500 mg/100 ml, 1 g/200 ml.

INDICATIONS AND DOSAGES

▸ **Treatment of Bone, Respiratory Tract, Skin and Soft Tissue Infections, Endocarditis, Peritonitis, and Septicemia; Prevention of Bacterial Endocarditis in Those at Risk (if Penicillin Is Contraindicated) When Undergoing Biliary, Dental, GI, GU, or Respiratory Surgery or Invasive Procedures**

IV

Adults, Elderly. 500 mg q6h or 1 g q12h.
Children older than 1 mo. 40 mg/kg/day in divided doses q6–8h. Maximum: 3–4 g/day.
Neonates. Initially, 15 mg/kg, then 10 mg/kg q8–12h.

▸ **Staphylococcal Enterocolitis, Antibiotic-Associated Pseudomembranous Colitis Caused by *Clostridium Difficile***

PO

Adults, Elderly. 0.5–2 g/day in 3–4 divided doses for 7–10 days.
Children. 40 mg/kg/day in 3–4 divided doses for 7–10 days. Maximum: 2 g/day.

▸ **Dosage in Renal Impairment**

After a loading dose, subsequent dosages and frequency are modified on the basis of creatinine clearance, the severity of the infection, and the serum concentration of the drug.

OFF-LABEL USES

Treatment of brain abscess, perioperative infections, staphylococcal or streptococcal meningitis

CONTRAINDICATIONS

None known.

INTERACTIONS

Drug

Aminoglycosides, amphotericin B, aspirin, bumetanide, carmustine, cisplatin, cyclosporine, ethacrynic acid, furosemide, streptozocin: May increase the risk of ototoxicity and nephrotoxicity of parenteral vancomycin.
Cholestyramine, colestipol: May decrease the effects of oral vancomycin.

Herbal

None known.

Food

None known.

V

Drug interactions of concern to dentistry

• Ototoxicity or nephrotoxicity: aminoglycosides and high-dose salicylates
• Increased effects of nondepolarizing muscle relaxants

DIAGNOSTIC TEST EFFECTS

May increase BUN level. Therapeutic peak serum level is 20–40 mcg/ml; therapeutic trough serum level is 5–15 mcg/ml. Toxic peak serum level is greater than 40 mcg/ml; toxic trough serum level is greater than 15 mcg/ml.

IV INCOMPATIBILITIES

Albumin, amphotericin B complex (Abelcet, AmBisome, Amphotec), aztreonam (Azactam), cefazolin (Ancef), cefepime (Maxipime), cefotaxime (Claforan), cefotetan (Cefotan), cefoxitin (Mefoxin), ceftazidime (Fortaz), ceftriaxone (Rocephin), cefuroxime (Zinacef), foscarnet (Foscavir), heparin, idarubicin (Idamycin), nafcillin (Nafcil), piperacillin and tazobactam (Zosyn), ticarcillin and clavulanate (Timentin)

IV COMPATIBILITIES

Amiodarone (Cordarone), calcium gluconate, diltiazem (Cardizem), hydromorphone (Dilaudid), insulin, lorazepam (Ativan), magnesium sulfate, midazolam (Versed), morphine, potassium chloride, propofol (Diprivan)

SIDE EFFECTS

Frequent

PO: Bitter or unpleasant taste, nausea, vomiting, mouth irritation (with oral solution)

Rare

Parenteral: Phlebitis, thrombophlebitis, or pain at peripheral IV site; dizziness; vertigo; tinnitus; chills; fever; rash; necrosis with extravasation
PO: Rash.

SERIOUS REACTIONS

! Nephrotoxicity and ototoxicity may occur.
! "Red-neck" syndrome (redness on face, neck, arms, and back; chills; fever; tachycardia; nausea or vomiting; pruritus; rash; unpleasant taste) may result from too-rapid injection.

DENTAL CONSIDERATIONS

General:

• Monitor vital signs at every appointment because of CV side effects.
• Administer IV slowly over 1 hr; administration that is too rapid can lead to a fall in blood pressure (monitor) and a red rash on the face, neck, and chest caused by local histamine release. No specific treatment is required for this reaction; evaluate recovery progress.
• Determine why the patient is taking the drug.

Consultations:

• Medical consultation may be required to assess disease control.

vardenafil

var-den′-ah-fill
(Levitra)
Do not confuse Levitra with Lexiva.

CATEGORY AND SCHEDULE

Pregnancy Risk Category: B

MECHANISM OF ACTION

An erectile dysfunction agent that inhibits phosphodiesterase type 5, the enzyme responsible for degrading cyclic guanosine monophosphate in the corpus cavernosum of the penis, resulting in smooth muscle relaxation and increased blood flow. ***Therapeutic Effect:*** Facilitates an erection.

PHARMACOKINETICS

Rapidly absorbed after PO administration. Extensive tissue distribution. Protein binding: 95%. Metabolized in the liver. Excreted primarily in feces; a lesser amount eliminated in urine. Drug has no effect on penile blood flow without sexual stimulation. ***Half-life:*** 4–5 hr.

AVAILABILITY

Tablets: 2.5 mg, 5 mg, 10 mg, 20 mg.

INDICATIONS AND DOSAGES

▸ Erectile Dysfunction

PO

Adults. 10 mg approximately 1 hr before sexual activity. Dose may be increased to 20 mg or decreased to 5 mg, based on patient tolerance. Maximum dosing frequency is once daily.

Elderly, older than 65 yr. 5 mg.

▸ Dosage in Moderate Hepatic Impairment

PO

For patients with Child-Pugh class B hepatic impairment, dosage is 5 mg 60 min before sexual activity.

▸ Dosage with Concurrent Ritonavir

PO

Adults. 2.5 mg in a 72-hr period.

▸ Dosage with Concurrent Ketoconazole or Itraconazole (at 400 mg/day), or Indinavir

PO

Adults. 2.5 mg in a 24-hr period.

▸ Dosage with Concurrent ketoconazole or Itraconazole (at 200 mg/day), or Erythromycin

PO

Adults. 5 mg in a 24-hr period.

CONTRAINDICATIONS

Concurrent use of alpha-adrenergic blockers, sodium nitroprusside, or nitrates in any form

INTERACTIONS

Drug

Alpha-adrenergic blockers, nitrates: Potentiates the hypotensive effects of these drugs.

Erythromycin, indinavir, itraconazole, ketoconazole, ritonavir: May increase vardenafil blood concentration.

Herbal

None known.

Food

High-fat meals: Delay drug's maximum effectiveness.

Drug interactions of concern to dentistry

- Dose adjustments caused by potential drug interactions—do not exceed the maximum single dose of 2.5 mg in a 72-hr period: ritonavir
- Do not exceed 2.5 mg in a 24-hr period: indinavir, ketoconazole (400 mg), itraconazole (400 mg)
- Do not exceed 5 mg in a 24-hr period: ketoconazole (200 mg), itraconazole (200 mg), erythromycin
- Increased plasma levels: drugs that are potent inhibitors of CYP3A4 isoenzymes (erythromycin, ketoconazole)
- Avoid nitroglycerin within a 24-hr period

DIAGNOSTIC TEST EFFECTS

None known.

SIDE EFFECTS

Occasional
Headache, flushing, rhinitis, indigestion
Rare (< 2%)
Dizziness, changes in color vision, blurred vision

SERIOUS REACTIONS

! Prolonged erections (lasting over 4 hours) and priapism (painful erections lasting > 6 hours) occur rarely.

DENTAL CONSIDERATIONS

General:

• This is an acute-use drug intended to be taken just before sexual activity. Be sure to include drug use in medical history and avoid use of potentially interacting drugs or warn patient of the interaction when CYP3A4 isoenzyme inhibitors are required.
• If signs of angina pectoris occur during dental treatment, do not use sublingual nitroglycerin.

vasopressin

vay-soe-press′-in
(Pitressin, Pressyn[CAN])
Do not confuse Pitressin with Pitocin.

CATEGORY AND SCHEDULE

Pregnancy Risk Category: B

MECHANISM OF ACTION

A posterior pituitary hormone that increases reabsorption of water by the renal tubules. Increases water permeability at the distal tubule and collecting duct. Directly stimulates smooth muscle in the GI tract.
Therapeutic Effect: Causes peristalsis and vasoconstriction.

PHARMACOKINETICS

Route	Onset	Peak	Duration
IV	N/A	N/A	0.5–1 hr
IM, Subcutaneous	1–2 hr	N/A	2–8 hr

Distributed throughout extracellular fluid. Metabolized in the liver and kidney. Primarily excreted in urine.
Half-life: 10–20 min.

AVAILABILITY

Injection: 20 units/ml.

INDICATIONS AND DOSAGES

▸ **Cardiac Arrest**

IV
Adults, Elderly. 40 units as a one-time bolus.

▸ **Diabetes Insipidus**

IV INFUSION
Adults, Children. 0.5 mUnits/kg/hr. May double dose q30min. Maximum: 10 mUnits/kg/hr.
IM, SUBCUTANEOUS
Adults, Elderly. 5–10 units 2–4 times a day. Range: 5–60 unit/day.
Children. 2.5–10 units, 2–4 times a day.

▸ **Abdominal Distention, Intestinal Paresis**

IM
Adults, Elderly. Initially, 5 units. Subsequent doses, 10 units q3–4h.

▸ **GI Hemorrhage**

IV INFUSION
Adults, Elderly. Initially, 0.2–0.4 unit/min progressively increased to 0.9 unit/min.
Children. 0.002–0.005 unit/kg/min. Titrate as needed. Maximum: 0.01 unit/kg/min.

Vasodilatory Shock

IV

Adults, Elderly. Initially, 0.04–0.1 unit/min. Titrate to desired effect.

OFF-LABEL USES

Adjunct in treatment of acute, massive hemorrhage

CONTRAINDICATIONS

None known.

INTERACTIONS

Drug

Alcohol, demeclocycline, lithium, norepinephrine: May decrease the effects of vasopressin.

Carbamazepine, chlorpropamide, clofibrate: May increase the effects of vasopressin.

Herbal

None known.

Food

None known.

Drug interactions of concern to dentistry

- Decreased effects: demeclocycline, alcohol
- Increased effects: carbamazepine

DIAGNOSTIC TEST EFFECTS

None known.

IV INCOMPATIBILITIES

Amphotericin B complex (Abelcet, AmBisome, Amphotec), diazepam (Valium), etomidate (Amidate), furosemide (Lasix), thiopentothal

IV COMPATIBILITIES

Dobutamine (Dobutrex), dopamine (Intropin), heparin, lorazepam (Ativan), midazolam (Versed), milrinone (Primacor), verapamil (Calan, Isoptin)

SIDE EFFECTS

Frequent

Pain at injection site (with vasopressin tannate)

Occasional

Abdominal cramps, nausea, vomiting, diarrhea, dizziness, diaphoresis, pale skin, circumoral pallor, tremors, headache, eructation, flatulence

Rare

Chest pain; confusion; allergic reaction, including rash or hives, pruritus, wheezing or difficulty breathing, facial and peripheral edema; sterile abscess (with vasopressin tannate)

SERIOUS REACTIONS

! Anaphylaxis, MI, and water intoxication have occurred.

! The elderly and very young are at higher risk for water intoxication.

DENTAL CONSIDERATIONS

General:

- Normally for acute use in the hospital or emergency department setting.
- Determine why patient is taking the drug.

Consultations:

- Medical consultation may be required to assess disease control and patient's ability to tolerate stress.

venlafaxine

ven-la-fax′-een

(Effexor, Effexor XR)

CATEGORY AND SCHEDULE

Pregnancy Risk Category: C

MECHANISM OF ACTION

A phenethylamine derivative that potentiates CNS neurotransmitter

activity by inhibiting the reuptake of serotonin, norepinephrine and, to a lesser degree, dopamine.
Therapeutic Effect: Relieves depression.

PHARMACOKINETICS

Well absorbed from the GI tract. Protein binding: 25%–30%. Metabolized in the liver to active metabolite. Primarily excreted in urine. Not removed by hemodialysis. ***Half-life:*** 3–7 hr; metabolite, 9–13 hr (increased in hepatic or renal impairment.

AVAILABILITY

Capsules (Extended-Release [Effexor XL]): 37.5 mg, 75 mg, 150 mg.
Tablets (Effexor): 25 mg, 37.5 mg, 50 mg, 75 mg, 100 mg.

INDICATIONS AND DOSAGES

▸ Depression

PO

Adults, Elderly. Initially, 75 mg/day in 2–3 divided doses with food. May increase by 75 mg/day at intervals of 4 days or longer. Maximum: 375 mg/day in 3 divided doses.

PO (Extended-Release)

Adults, Elderly. 75 mg/day as a single dose with food. May increase by 75 mg/day at intervals of 4 days or longer. Maximum: 225 mg/day.

▸ Anxiety Disorder

PO (Extended-Release)

Adults. 37.5–225 mg/day.

▸ Dosage in Renal and Hepatic Impairment

Expect to decrease venlafaxine dosage by 50% in patients with moderate hepatic impairment, 25% in patients with mild to moderate renal impairment, and 50% in patients on dialysis (withhold dose until completion of dialysis).

OFF-LABEL USES

Prevention of relapses of depression; treatment of attention-deficit hyperactivity disorder, autism, chronic fatigue syndrome, obsessive-compulsive disorder

CONTRAINDICATIONS

Use within 14 days of MAOIs

INTERACTIONS

Drug

MAOIs: May cause neuroleptic malignant syndrome, autonomic instability (including rapid fluctuations of vital signs), extreme agitation, hyperthermia, mental status changes, myoclonus, rigidity, and coma.

Herbal

St. John's wort: May increase the sedative-hypnotic effect of venlafaxine.

Food

None known.

Drug interactions of concern to dentistry

- None reported; however, because this drug is similar in action to other antidepressants, it would be wise to avoid excessive amounts of vasoconstrictors, especially in gingival retraction cords
- Increased CNS depression: all CNS depressants
- Risk of serotonin syndrome: St. John's wort (herb)

DIAGNOSTIC TEST EFFECTS

May increase BUN level and serum alkaline phosphatase, bilirubin, cholesterol, uric acid, AST (SGOT), and ALT (SGPT) levels. May decrease serum phosphate and sodium levels. May alter blood glucose and serum potassium levels.

SIDE EFFECTS

Frequent (> 20%)
Nausea, somnolence, headache, dry mouth
Occasional (20%–10%)
Dizziness, insomnia, constipation, diaphoresis, nervousness, asthenia, ejaculatory disturbance, anorexia
Rare (< 10%)
Anxiety, blurred vision, diarrhea, vomiting, tremor, abnormal dreams, impotence

SERIOUS REACTIONS

! A sustained increase in diastolic BP of 10–15 mm Hg occurs occasionally.

DENTAL CONSIDERATIONS

General:
- Monitor vital signs at every appointment because of CV side effects.
- After supine positioning, have patient sit upright for at least 2 min before standing to avoid orthostatic hypotension.
- Assess salivary flow as a factor in caries, periodontal disease, and candidiasis.
- Examine for evidence of oral manifestations of blood dyscrasias (infection, bleeding, poor healing).
- Place on frequent recall to evaluate healing response.
- Consider semisupine chair position for patient comfort because of GI effects of disease.

Consultations:
- Medical consultation may be required to assess disease control.
- Physician should be informed if significant xerostomic side effects occur (e.g., increased caries, sore tongue, problems eating or swallowing, difficulty wearing prosthesis) so that a medication change can be considered.
- Obtain a medical consultation for blood studies (CBC) because leukopenic or thrombocytopenic side effects may result in infection, delayed healing, and excessive bleeding. Postpone elective dental treatment until normal values are maintained.

Teach Patient/Family:
- Importance of good oral hygiene to prevent soft tissue inflammation
- Caution to prevent injury when using oral hygiene aids
- *When chronic dry mouth occurs, advise patient:*
  - To avoid mouth rinses with high alcohol content because of drying effects
  - Of need for daily use of home fluoride products to prevent caries
  - To use sugarless gum, frequent sips of water, or saliva substitutes

verapamil hydrochloride

ver-ap′-a-mill
(Anpec[AUS], Apo-Verap[CAN], Calan, Calan SR, Chronovera [CAN], Cordilox SR[AUS], Covera-HS, Isoptin[AUS], Isoptin SR, Novo-Veramil[CAN], Novo-Veramil SR[CAN], Veracaps SR[AUS], Verahexal [AUS], Verelan, Verelan PM)
Do not confuse Isoptin with Intropin, or Verelan with Virilon, Vivarin, or Voltaren.

CATEGORY AND SCHEDULE

Pregnancy Risk Category: C

MECHANISM OF ACTION

A calcium channel blocker and antianginal, antiarrhythmic, and antihypertensive agent that inhibits calcium ion entry across cardiac and vascular smooth-muscle cell membranes. This action causes the dilation of coronary arteries, peripheral arteries, and arterioles. ***Therapeutic Effect:*** Decreases heart rate and myocardial contractility and slows SA and AV conduction. Decreases total peripheral vascular resistance by vasodilation.

PHARMACOKINETICS

Route	Onset	Peak	Duration
PO	30 min	1–2 hr	6–8 hr
PO (Extended-release)	30 min	N/A	N/A
IV	1–2 min	3–5 min	10–60 min

Well absorbed from the GI tract. Protein binding: 90% (60% in neonates.) Undergoes first-pass metabolism in the liver to active metabolite. Primarily excreted in urine. Not removed by hemodialysis. ***Half-life:*** 2–8 hr.

AVAILABILITY

Caplet (Calan SR): 120 mg, 180 mg, 240 mg.
Capsules (Extended-Release [Verelan PM]): 100 mg, 200 mg, 300 mg.
Capsules (Sustained-Release [Verelan]): 120 mg, 180 mg, 240 mg, 360 mg.
Tablets (Calan): 40 mg, 80 mg, 120 mg.
Tablets (Extended-Release [Covera HS]). 180 mg, 240 mg.
Tablets (Sustained-Release [Isoptin SR]): 120 mg, 180 mg, 240 mg.
Injection: 2.5 mg/ml.

INDICATIONS AND DOSAGES

▸ **Supraventricular Tachyarrhythmias, Temporary Control of Rapid Ventricular Rate with Atrial Fibrillation or Flutter**

IV

Adults, Elderly. Initially, 5–10 mg; repeat in 30 min with 10-mg dose.
Children 1 to 15 yr. 0.1 mg/kg. May repeat in 30 min up to a maximum second dose of 10 mg. Not recommended in children younger than 1 yr.

▸ **Arrhythmias, Including Prevention of Recurrent Paroxysmal Supraventricular Tachycardia and Control of Ventricular Resting Rate in Chronic Atrial Fibrillation or Flutter (with Digoxin)**

PO

Adults, Elderly. 240–480 mg/day in 3–4 divided doses.

▸ **Vasospastic Angina (Prinzmetal's Variant), Unstable (Crescendo or Preinfarction) Angina, Chronic Stable (Effort-Associated) Angina**

PO

Adults. Initially, 80–120 mg 3 times a day. For elderly patients and those with hepatic dysfunction, 40 mg 3 times a day. Titrate to optimal dose. Maintenance: 240–480 mg/day in 3–4 divided doses.

PO (Covera-HS)

Adults, Elderly. 180–480 mg/day at bedtime.

▸ **Hypertension**

PO

Adults, Elderly. Initially, 40–80 mg 3 times a day. Maintenance: 480 mg or less a day.

PO (Covera-HS)

Adults, Elderly. 180–480 mg/day at bedtime.

PO (Extended-Release)

Adults, Elderly. 120–240 mg/day. May give 480 mg or less a day in 2 divided doses.
PO (Verelan PM)
Adults, Elderly. 100–300 mg/day.

OFF-LABEL USES

Treatment of hypertrophic cardiomyopathy, vascular headaches

CONTRAINDICATIONS

Atrial fibrillation or flutter and an accessory bypass tract, cardiogenic shock, heart block, sinus bradycardia, ventricular tachycardia

INTERACTIONS

Drug

Beta blockers: May have additive effect.
Carbamazepine, quinidine, theophylline: May increase verapamil blood concentration and risk of toxicity.
Digoxin: May increase digoxin blood concentration.
Disopyramide: May increase negative inotropic effect.
Procainamide, quinidine: May increase risk of QT-interval prolongation.

Herbal

None known.

Food

Grapefruit, grapefruit juice: May increase verapamil blood concentration.

Drug interactions of concern to dentistry

- Decreased effect: indomethacin, possibly other NSAIDs, phenobarbital
- Increased effect: parenteral and inhalation general anesthetics or other drugs with hypotensive actions, benzodiazepines
- Increased effects of nondepolarizing muscle relaxants
- Increased effects of carbamazepine
- Caution in use of strong inhibitors of CYP3A4 isoenzymes, itraconazole

DIAGNOSTIC TEST EFFECTS

ECG waveform may show increased PR interval. Therapeutic serum level is 0.08–0.3 mcg/ml.

IV INCOMPATIBILITIES

Amphotericin B complex (Abelcet, AmBisome, Amphotec), nafcillin (Nafcil), propofol (Diprivan), sodium bicarbonate

IV COMPATIBILITIES

Amiodarone (Cordarone), calcium chloride, calcium gluconate, dexamethasone (Decadron), digoxin (Lanoxin), dobutamine (Dobutrex), dopamine (Intropin), furosemide (Lasix), heparin, hydromorphone (Dilaudid), lidocaine, magnesium sulfate, metoclopramide (Reglan), milrinone (Primacor), morphine, multivitamins, nitroglycerin, norepinephrine (Levophed), potassium chloride, potassium phosphate, procainamide (Pronestyl), propranolol (Inderal)

SIDE EFFECTS

Frequent (7%)
Constipation
Occasional (4%–2%)
Dizziness, light-headedness, headache, asthenia (loss of strength, energy), nausea, peripheral edema, hypotension
Rare (< 1%)
Bradycardia, dermatitis or rash

SERIOUS REACTIONS

! Rapid ventricular rate in atrial flutter or fibrillation, marked hypotension, extreme bradycardia, CHF, asystole, and second- and third-degree AV block occur rarely.

DENTAL CONSIDERATIONS

General:

• Monitor cardiac status; take vital signs at every appointment because of CV side effects. Consider a stress reduction protocol to prevent stress-induced angina during the dental appointment.
• After supine positioning, have patient sit upright for at least 2 min before standing to avoid orthostatic hypotension.
• Place on frequent recall to monitor gingival condition.
• Limit use of sodium-containing products, such as saline IV fluids, for patients with a dietary salt restriction.
• Assess salivary flow as a factor in caries, periodontal disease, and candidiasis.
• Use vasoconstrictors with caution, in low doses, and with careful aspiration. Avoid use of gingival retraction cord with epinephrine.

Consultations:

• In a patient with symptoms of blood dyscrasias, request a medical consultation for blood studies and postpone dental treatment until normal values are reestablished.
• Medical consultation may be required to assess disease control and patient's ability to tolerate stress.

Teach Patient/Family:

• Importance of good oral hygiene to prevent soft tissue inflammation and minimize gingival overgrowth
• Need for frequent oral prophylaxis if gingival overgrowth occurs
• *When chronic dry mouth occurs, advise patient:*
  • To avoid mouth rinses with high alcohol content because of drying effects
  • Of need for daily use of home fluoride products to prevent caries
  • To use sugarless gum, frequent sips of water, or saliva substitutes

vidarabine

vye-dare′-a-been
(Ara-A, Vira-A)
Do not confuse with Zostrix.

CATEGORY AND SCHEDULE

Pregnancy Risk Category: C

MECHANISM OF ACTION

An antiviral agent that appears to interfere with viral DNS synthesis. ***Therapeutic Effect:*** Regenerates corneal epithelium.

PHARMACOKINETICS

None reported.

AVAILABILITY

Ophthalmic ointment: 3% (Vira-A).

INDICATIONS AND DOSAGES

▸ Treatment of Keratitis, Keratoconjunctivitis Caused by Herpes Simplex virus, Types 1 and 2

OPHTHALMIC

Adults, Elderly. Apply 0.5 inch into lower conjunctival sac 5 times/day at 3 hr intervals. After re-epithelialization, treat for additional 7 days at dosage of 2 times/day.

CONTRAINDICATIONS

Hypersensitivity to vidarabine or any component of the formulation

INTERACTIONS

Drug

None known.

Herbal

None known.

Food

None known.

Drug interactions of concern to dentistry

• None reported

V

DIAGNOSTIC TEST EFFECTS
None known.

SIDE EFFECTS
Frequent
Burning, itching, irritation
Occasional
Foreign body sensation, tearing, sensitivity to light, pain, photophobia

SERIOUS REACTIONS
! None significant.

DENTAL CONSIDERATIONS
General:
- Protect patient's eyes from spatter during dental procedures.
- Avoid dental light in patient's eyes; offer dark glasses for patient comfort.

DENTAL CONSIDERATIONS
VIDARABINE (VIRA-A)
General:
- Protect patient's eyes from accidental spatter during dental treatment.
- Avoid dental light in patient's eyes; offer dark glasses for patient comfort.

Teach Patient/Family:
- To seek evaluation if healing has not occurred in 7 to 10 days.

vinblastine sulfate
vin-blass′-teen
(Oncovin[AUS], Velban, Velbe[AUS])
Do not confuse vinblastine with vincristine or vinorelbine.

V

CATEGORY AND SCHEDULE
Pregnancy Risk Category: D

MECHANISM OF ACTION
A vinca alkaloid that binds to microtubular protein of mitotic spindle, causing metaphase arrest. ***Therapeutic Effect:*** Inhibits cell division.

PHARMACOKINETICS
Does not cross the blood-brain barrier. Protein binding: 75%. Metabolized in the liver to active metabolite. Primarily eliminated in feces by biliary system. ***Half-life:*** 24.8 hr.

AVAILABILITY
Injection: 1 mg/ml.
Powder for Injection: 10 mg.

INDICATIONS AND DOSAGES
▸ **Remission Induction in Advanced Testicular Carcinoma, Advanced Mycosis Fungoides, Breast Carcinoma, Choriocarcinoma, Disseminated Hodgkin's Disease, Non-Hodgkin's Lymphoma, Kaposi's Sarcoma, or Letterer-Siwe Disease**
IV
Adults, Elderly. Initially, 3.7 mg/m^2 as a single dose. Increase dose by about 1.8 mg/m^2 at weekly intervals until desired therapeutic response is attained, WBC count falls below 3,000/mm^3, or maximum weekly dose of 18.5 mg/m^2 is reached.
Children. Initially, 2.5 mg/m^2 as a single dose. Increase dose by about 1.25 mg/m^2 at weekly intervals until desired therapeutic response is attained, WBC count falls below 3,000/mm^3, or maximum weekly dose of 7.5–12.5 mg/m^2 is reached.
▸ **Maintenance Dose for Treatment of Advanced Testicular Carcinoma, Advanced Mycosis Fungoides, Breast Carcinoma, Choriocarcinoma, Disseminated Hodgkin's Disease, Non-Hodgkin's**

Lymphoma, Kaposi's Sarcoma, or Letterer-Siwe Disease

IV

Adults, Elderly, Children.
Administer one increment less than dose required to produce WBC count of 3000/mm^3. Each subsequent dose given when WBC count returns to 4000/mm^3 and at least 7 days have elapsed since previous dose.

OFF-LABEL USES

Treatment of bladder, head and neck, kidney, or lung carcinoma; chronic myelocytic leukemia; germ cell ovarian tumors; neuroblastoma

CONTRAINDICATIONS

Bacterial infection, severe leukopenia, significant granulocytopenia (unless it stems from disease being treated)

INTERACTIONS

Drug

Antigout medications: May decrease the effects of these drugs.
Bone marrow depressants: May increase myelosuppression.
Live-virus vaccines: May potentiate virus replication, increase vaccine side effects, and decrease the patient's antibody response to the vaccine.

Herbal

None known.

Food

None known.

Drug interactions of concern to dentistry

• Suspected increase in metabolism: strong inhibitors of CYP3A4 isoenzymes (erythromycin, clarithromycin, fluconazole, itraconazole, ketoconazole, metronidazole)

DIAGNOSTIC TEST EFFECTS

May increase serum uric acid levels.

IV INCOMPATIBILITIES

Cefepime (Maxipime), furosemide (Lasix)

IV COMPATIBILITIES

Allopurinol (Aloprim), cisplatin (Platinol AQ), cyclophosphamide (Cytoxan), doxorubicin (Adriamycin), etoposide (VePesid), 5-fluorouracil, gemcitabine (Gemzar), granisetron (Kytril), heparin, leucovorin, methotrexate, ondansetron (Zofran), paclitaxel (Taxol), vinorelbine (Navelbine)

SIDE EFFECTS

Frequent

Nausea, vomiting, alopecia

Occasional

Constipation or diarrhea, rectal bleeding, headache, paraesthesia (occur 4–6 hr after administration and persist for 2–10 hr); malaise; asthenia; dizziness; pain at tumor site; jaw or face pain; depression; dry mouth

Rare

Dermatitis, stomatitis, phototoxicity, hyperuricemia

SERIOUS REACTIONS

! Hematologic toxicity is manifested as leukopenia and, less commonly, anemia. The WBC count reaches its nadir 4 to 10 days after initial therapy and recovers within 7 to 14 days (21 days with high vinblastine dosages).
! Thrombocytopenia is usually mild and transient, with recovery occurring in few days.
! Hepatic insufficiency may increase the risk of toxic drug effects.
! Acute shortness of breath or bronchospasm may occur, particularly when vinblastine is administered concurrently with mitomycin.

DENTAL CONSIDERATIONS

General:

- If additional analgesia is required for dental pain, consider alternative analgesics (NSAIDs) in patients taking narcotics for acute or chronic pain.
- This drug may be used in the hospital or on an outpatient basis. Confirm the patient's disease and treatment status.
- Short appointments and a stress reduction protocol may be required for anxious patients.
- Patient on chronic drug therapy may rarely present with symptoms of blood dyscrasias, which can include infection, bleeding, and poor healing. If dyscrasia is present, caution patient to prevent oral tissue trauma when using oral hygiene aids.
- Examine for oral manifestation of opportunistic infection.
- Palliative medication may be required for management of oral side effects.
- Chlorhexidine mouth rinse prior to and during chemotherapy may reduce severity of mucositis.
- Advise patient if dental drugs prescribed have a potential for photosensitivity.
- Assess salivary flow as a factor in caries, periodontal disease, and candidiasis.
- Patients may have received other chemotherapy and radiation; confirm medical and drug history.
- Patients presenting with Kaposi's sarcoma also may be HIV positive.
- Patients may be at risk for infection.

Consultations:

- Medical consultation may be required to assess immunologic status during cancer chemotherapy and determine safety risk, if any, posed by the required dental treatment.
- Medical consultation may be required to assess disease control and patient's ability to tolerate stress.
- In a patient with symptoms of blood dyscrasias, request a medical consultation for blood studies and postpone treatment until normal values are reestablished.

Teach Patient/Family:

- To maintain fastidious oral hygiene
- Importance of good oral hygiene to prevent soft tissue inflammation
- To report oral lesions, soreness, or bleeding to dentist
- To prevent trauma when using oral hygiene aids
- *When chronic dry mouth occurs, advise patient:*
  - To avoid mouth rinses with high alcohol content due to drying effects
  - To use daily home fluoride products for anticaries effect
  - To use sugarless gum, frequent sips of water or saliva substitutes
- Importance of updating health and medication history if physician makes any changes in evaluation or drug regimens; include OTC, herbal, and nonherbal remedies in the update

vincristine sulfate

vin-cris′-teen

(Oncovin, Vincasar PFS)

Do not confuse vincristine with vinblastine, or Oncovin with Ancobon.

CATEGORY AND SCHEDULE

Pregnancy Risk Category: D

MECHANISM OF ACTION
A vinca alkaloid that binds to microtubular protein of mitotic spindle, causing metaphase arrest. ***Therapeutic Effect:*** Inhibits cell division.

PHARMACOKINETICS
Does not cross the blood-brain barrier. Protein binding: 75%. Metabolized in the liver. Primarily eliminated in feces by biliary system. ***Half-life:*** 10–37 hr.

AVAILABILITY
Injection: 1 mg/ml.

INDICATIONS AND DOSAGES
▸ Acute Leukemia, Advanced Non-Hodgkin's Lymphoma, Disseminated Hodgkin's Disease, Neuroblastoma, Rhabdomyosarcoma, Wilms' Tumor
IV
Adults, Elderly. 0.4–1.4 mg/m^2 once a week.
Children. 1–2 mg/m^2 once a week.
Children weighing less than 10 kg or with a body surface area less than 1 m^2. 0.05 mg/kg. Maximum: 2 mg.
▸ Dosage in Hepatic Impairment
Reduce dosage by 50% in patients with a direct serum bilirubin concentration more than 3 mg/dl.

OFF-LABEL USES
Treatment of breast, cervical, colorectal, lung, and ovarian carcinomas; chronic lymphocytic and chronic myelocytic leukemias; germ cell ovarian tumors; idiopathic thrombocytopenic purpura; malignant melanoma; multiple myeloma; mycosis fungoides

CONTRAINDICATIONS
Patients receiving radiation therapy through ports that include the liver

INTERACTIONS
Drug
Asparaginase, neurotoxic medications: May increase the risk of neurotoxicity.
Antigout medications: May decrease the effects of these drugs.
Doxorubicin: May increase the risk of myelosuppression.
Live-virus vaccines: May potentiate virus replication, increase vaccine side effects, and decrease the patient's antibody response to the vaccine.
Herbal
None known.
Food
None known.
Drug interactions of concern to dentistry
- None reported

DIAGNOSTIC TEST EFFECTS
May increase serum uric acid levels.

IV INCOMPATIBILITIES
Cefepime (Maxipime), furosemide (Lasix), idarubicin (Idamycin)
IV COMPATIBILITIES
Allopurinol (Aloprim), cisplatin (Platinol AQ), cyclophosphamide (Cytoxan), cytarabine (Ara-C, Cytosar), doxorubicin (Adriamycin), etoposide (VePesid), 5-fluorouracil, gemcitabine (Gemzar), granisetron (Kytril), leucovorin, methotrexate, ondansetron (Zofran), paclitaxel (Taxol), vinorelbine (Navelbine)

SIDE EFFECTS
Expected
Peripheral neuropathy (occurs in nearly every patient; first clinical sign is depression of Achilles tendon reflex)
Frequent
Peripheral paraesthesia, alopecia, constipation or obstipation (upper

colon impaction with empty rectum), abdominal cramps, headache, jaw pain, hoarseness, diplopia, ptosis or drooping of eyelid, urinary tract disturbances

Occasional

Nausea, vomiting, diarrhea, abdominal distention, stomatitis, fever

Rare

Mild leukopenia, mild anemia, thrombocytopenia

SERIOUS REACTIONS

! Acute shortness of breath and bronchospasm may occur, especially when vincristine is administered concurrently with mitomycin.

! Prolonged or high-dose therapy may produce foot or wrist drop, difficulty walking, slapping gait, ataxia, and muscle wasting.

! Acute uric acid nephropathy may occur.

DENTAL CONSIDERATIONS

General:

- If additional analgesia is required for dental pain, consider alternative analgesics (NSAIDs) in patients taking narcotics for acute or chronic pain.
- This drug may be used in the hospital or on an outpatient basis. Confirm the patient's disease and treatment status.
- Short appointments and a stress reduction protocol may be required for anxious patients.
- Patient on chronic drug therapy may rarely present with symptoms of blood dyscrasias, which can include infection, bleeding, and poor healing. If dyscrasia is present, caution patient to prevent oral tissue trauma when using oral hygiene aids.
- Examine for oral manifestation of opportunistic infection.
- Assess salivary flow as a factor in caries, periodontal disease, and candidiasis.
- Palliative medication may be required for management of oral side effects.
- Chlorhexidine mouth rinse prior to and during chemotherapy may reduce severity of mucositis.
- Patients may have received other chemotherapy or radiation; confirm medical and drug history.
- Patients may be at risk for infection.

Consultations:

- Medical consultation may be required to assess immunologic status during cancer chemotherapy and determine safety risk, if any, posed by the required dental treatment.
- Medical consultation may be required to assess disease control and patient's ability to tolerate stress.
- In a patient with symptoms of blood dyscrasias, request a medical consultation for blood studies and postpone treatment until normal values are reestablished.
- Refer patients to attending physician if symptoms of peripheral neuropathy are present (numbness, tingling or pain in hands or feet).

Teach Patient/Family:

- To maintain fastidious oral hygiene
- Importance of good oral hygiene to prevent soft tissue inflammation
- To report oral lesions, soreness, or bleeding to dentist
- To prevent trauma when using oral hygiene aids
- *When chronic dry mouth occurs, advise patient:*
  - To avoid mouth rinses with high alcohol content due to drying effects
  - To use daily home fluoride products for anticaries effect

- To use sugarless gum, frequent sips of water, or saliva substitutes
- Importance of updating health and medication history if physician makes any changes in evaluation or drug regimens; include OTC, herbal, and nonherbal remedies in the update

vinorelbine

vin-oh-rell′-bean
(Navelbine)
Do not confuse vinorelbine with vinblastine.

CATEGORY AND SCHEDULE

Pregnancy Risk Category: D

MECHANISM OF ACTION

A semisynthetic vinca alkaloid that interferes with mitotic microtubule assembly. ***Therapeutic Effect:*** Prevents cell division.

PHARMACOKINETICS

Widely distributed after IV administration. Protein binding: 80%–90%. Metabolized in the liver. Primarily eliminated in feces by biliary system. ***Half-life:*** 28–43 hr.

AVAILABILITY

Injection: 10 mg/ml (1-ml, 5-ml vials).

INDICATIONS AND DOSAGES

▸ Unresectable, Advanced Non–Small-Cell Lung Cancer (as Monotherapy or in Combination with Cisplatin)

IV

Adults, Elderly. 30 mg/m² administered weekly over 6–10 min.

▸ Dosage Adjustment Guidelines

Dosage adjustments should be based on granulocyte count obtained on the day of treatment, as follows:

Granulocyte count (cells/mm³) on Day of Treatment	Dose
1500 or higher	30 mg/m²
1000–1499	15 mg/m²
less than 1000	Do not administer

▸ Combination Therapy (with Cisplatin)

IV INJECTION

Adults, Elderly. 25 mg/m² every week or 30 mg/m² on days 1 and 29, then q6wk.

OFF-LABEL USES

Treatment of breast cancer, cisplatin-resistant ovarian carcinoma, Hodgkin's disease

CONTRAINDICATIONS

Granulocyte count before treatment of fewer than 1000 cells/mm³

INTERACTIONS

Drug

Bone marrow depressants: May increase the risk of myelosuppression.
Cisplatin: Significantly increases the risk of granulocytopenia.
Live-virus vaccines: May potentiate virus replication, increase vaccine side effects, and decrease the patient's antibody response to the vaccine.
Mitomycin: May produce an acute pulmonary reaction.

Herbal

None known.

Food

None known.

Drug interactions of concern to dentistry
- None reported

DIAGNOSTIC TEST EFFECTS
May increase total serum bilirubin and AST (SGOT) levels and liver function test results. Decreases granulocyte, leukocyte, thrombocyte, and RBC counts.

IV INCOMPATIBILITIES
Acyclovir (Zovirax), allopurinol (Aloprim), amphotericin B (Fungizone), amphotericin B complex (Abelcet, AmBisome, Amphotec), ampicillin (Omnipen), cefazolin (Ancef), cefoperazone (Cefobid), cefotetan (Cefotan), ceftriaxone (Rocephin), cefuroxime (Zinacef), 5-fluorouracil, furosemide (Lasix), ganciclovir (Cytovene), methylprednisolone (Solu-Medrol), sodium bicarbonate

IV COMPATIBILITIES
Calcium gluconate, carboplatin (Paraplatin), cisplatin (Platinol AQ), cyclophosphamide (Cytoxan), cytarabine (ARA-C, Cytosar), dacarbazine (DTIC-Dome), daunorubicin (Cerubidine), dexamethasone (Decadron), diphenhydramine (Benadryl), doxorubicin (Adriamycin), etoposide (VePesid), gemcitabine (Gemzar), granisetron (Kytril), hydromorphone (Dilaudid), idarubicin (Idamycin), methotrexate, morphine, ondansetron (Zofran), teniposide (Vumon), vinblastine (Velban), vincristine (Oncovin)

V

SIDE EFFECTS
Frequent
Asthenia (35%); mild or moderate nausea (34%); constipation (29%); erythema, pain, or vein discoloration at injection site (28%); fatigue (27%); peripheral neuropathy manifested as paresthesia and hyperesthesia (25%); diarrhea (17%); alopecia (12%)
Occasional
Phlebitis (10%), dyspnea (7%), loss of deep tendon reflexes (5%)
Rare
Chest pain, jaw pain, myalgia, arthralgia, rash

SERIOUS REACTIONS
! Bone marrow depression is manifested mainly as granulocytopenia, which may be severe. Other hematologic toxicities, including neutropenia, thrombocytopenia, leukopenia, and anemia, increase the risk of infection and bleeding.
! Acute shortness of breath and severe bronchospasm occur infrequently, particularly in patients with preexisting pulmonary dysfunction and in those receiving mitomycin concurrently.

DENTAL CONSIDERATIONS
General:
- If additional analgesia is required for dental pain, consider alternative analgesics (NSAIDs) in patients taking narcotics for acute or chronic pain.
- Avoid products that affect platelet function, such as aspirin and NSAIDs.
- This drug may be used in the hospital or on an outpatient basis. Confirm the patient's disease and treatment status.
- Patient on chronic drug therapy may rarely present with symptoms of blood dyscrasias, which can include infection, bleeding, and poor healing. If dyscrasia is present, caution patient to prevent oral tissue trauma when using oral hygiene aids.
- Consider semisupine chair position for patients with respiratory disease.

• Caution: patients may be at high risk for infection.
• Patient may have received other chemotherapy or radiation; confirm medical and drug history.
• Oral infections should be eliminated and/or treated aggressively.

Consultations:
• Medical consultation should include routine blood counts including platelet counts and bleeding time.
• In a patient with symptoms of blood dyscrasias, request a medical consultation for blood studies and postpone treatment until normal values are reestablished.
• Consult physician; prophylactic or therapeutic antiinfectives may be indicated if surgery or periodontal treatment is required.
• Medical consultation may be required to assess immunologic status during cancer chemotherapy and determine safety risk, if any, posed by the required dental treatment.
• Medical consultation may be required to assess disease control and patient's ability to tolerate stress.

Teach Patient/Family:
• Secondary oral infection may occur; need to see dentist immediately if infection occurs
• Importance of good oral hygiene to prevent soft tissue inflammation
• To report oral lesions, soreness, or bleeding to dentist
• To prevent trauma when using oral hygiene aids
• Importance of updating health and medication history if physician makes any changes in evaluation or drug regimens; include OTC, herbal, and nonherbal remedies in the update

vitamin A

vight′-ah-myn A
(Aquasol A, Palmitate A)
Do not confuse Aquasol A with Anusol.

CATEGORY AND SCHEDULE

Pregnancy Risk Category: A (X if used in doses above recommended daily allowance)

MECHANISM OF ACTION

A fat-soluble vitamin that may act as a cofactor in biochemical reactions. ***Therapeutic Effect:*** Is essential for normal function of retina, visual adaptation to darkness, bone growth, testicular and ovarian function, and embryonic development; preserves integrity of epithelial cells.

PHARMACOKINETICS

Rapidly absorbed from the GI tract if bile salts, pancreatic lipase, protein, and dietary fat are present. Transported in blood to the liver, where it's metabolized; stored in parenchymal hepatic cells, then transported in plasma as retinol, as needed. Excreted primarily in bile and, to a lesser extent, in urine.

AVAILABILITY

Capsules: 10,000 units, 25,000 units.
Injection (Aquasol A): 50,000 units/ml .
Tablets (Palmitate A): 5,000 units, 15,000 units.

INDICATIONS AND DOSAGES

▸ Severe Vitamin A Deficiency

PO

Adults, Elderly, Children 8 yr and older. 500,000 units/day for 3 days; then 50,000 units/day for 14 days, then 10,000–20,000 units/day for 2 mo.

Children 1–7 yr. 5000 units/kg/day for 5 days, then 5000–10000 units/day for 2 mo.
Children younger than 1 yr. 5000–10000 units/day for 2 mo.
IM
Adults, Elderly, Children 8 yr and older. 100,000 units/day for 3 days; then 50,000 units/day for 14 days.
Children 1–7 yr. 17,500–35,000 units/day for 10 days.
Children younger than 1 yr. 7500–15,000 units/day.

▸ **Malabsorption Syndrome**
PO
Adults, Elderly, Children 8 yr and older. 10,000–50,000 units/day.

▸ **Dietary Supplement**
PO
Adults, Elderly. 4000–5000 units/day.
Children 7–10 yr. 3300–3500 units/day.
Children 4–6 yr. 2500 units/day.
Children 6 mo–3 yr. 1500–2000 units/day.
Neonates younger than 5 mos. 1500 units/day.

CONTRAINDICATIONS
Hypervitaminosis A

INTERACTIONS
Drug
Cholestyramine, colestipol, mineral oil: May decrease the absorption of vitamin A.
Isotretinoin: May increase the risk of toxicity.
Herbal
None known.
Food
None known.

DIAGNOSTIC TEST EFFECTS
May increase BUN and serum cholesterol, calcium, and triglyceride levels. May decrease blood erythrocyte and leukocyte counts.

SIDE EFFECTS
None known.

SERIOUS REACTIONS
! Chronic overdose produces malaise, nausea, vomiting, drying or cracking of skin or lips, inflammation of tongue or gums, irritability, alopecia, and night sweats.
! Bulging fontanelles have occurred in infants.

DENTAL CONSIDERATIONS
General:
- Oral manifestation of side effects could indicate hypervitaminosis.
- May cause dry/peeling skin around lips; provide lip lubricant for patient comfort during dental treatment.

vitamin D
vight′-ah-myn D
(Calciferol, Drisdol, Ostoforet[CAN])

CATEGORY AND SCHEDULE
Pregnancy Risk Category: A (D if used in doses above recommended daily allowance)

MECHANISM OF ACTION
A fat-soluble vitamin that stimulates calcium and phosphate absorption from small intestine, promotes secretion of calcium from bone to blood, and promotes resorption of phosphate in renal tubules; also acts on bone cells to stimulate skeletal growth and on parathyroid gland to suppress hormone synthesis and secretion. ***Therapeutic Effect:*** Essential for absorption and utilization of calcium and phosphate and normal bone calcification. Reduces parathyroid hormone level.

Improves phosphorus and calcium homeostasis in chronic renal failure.

PHARMACOKINETICS

Readily absorbed from small intestine. Concentrated primarily in liver and fat deposits. Activated in the liver and kidneys. Eliminated by biliary system; excreted in urine. ***Half-life:*** 19–48 hr for ergocalciferol.

AVAILABILITY

Capsules (Drisdol): 50,000 units (1.25 mg).
Injection (Calciferol): 500,000 units/ml (12.5 mg).
Oral Liquid Drops (Calciferol, Drisdol): 8000 units/ml.

INDICATIONS AND DOSAGES

AlertOral dosing is preferred. Administer the drug IM only in patients with GI, hepatic, or biliary disease associated with malabsorption of vitamin D

▸ **Dietary Supplement**
PO
Adults, Elderly, Children. 10 mcg (400 units)/day.
Neonates. 10–20 mcg (400–800 units)/day.

▸ **Renal Failure**
PO
Adults, Elderly. 0.5 mg/day.
Children. 0.1–1 mg/day.

▸ **Hypoparathyroidism**
PO
Adults, Elderly. 625 mcg–5 mg/day (with calcium supplements).
Children. 1.25–5 mg/day (with calcium supplements).

▸ **Nutritional Rickets, Osteomalacia**
PO
Adults, Elderly, Children. 25–125 mcg/day for 8–12 wk.
Adults, Elderly (with malabsorption syndrome). 250–7,500 mcg/day.
Children (with malabsorption syndrome). 250–625 mcg/day.

▸ **Vitamin D–Dependent Rickets**
PO
Adults, Elderly. 250 mcg–1.5 mg/day.
Children. 75–125 mcg/day.
Maximum: 1500 mcg/day.

▸ **Vitamin D-Resistant Rickets**
PO
Adults, Elderly. 250–1500 mcg/day (with phosphate supplements).
Children. Initially 1000–2000 mcg/day (with phosphate supplements). May increase in 250- to 600-mcg increments q3–4mo.

CONTRAINDICATIONS

Hypercalcemia, malabsorption syndrome, vitamin D toxicity

INTERACTIONS

Drug

Aluminum-containing antacids (long-term use): May increase aluminum blood concentration and risk of aluminum bone toxicity.
Calcium-containing preparations, thiazide diuretics: May increase the risk of hypercalcemia.
Magnesium-containing antacids: May increase magnesium blood concentration.
Mineral oil: Excessive use of mineral oil decreases vitamin D absorption.

Herbal

None known.

Food

None known.

Drug interactions of concern to dentistry

- Reduction in calcitriol levels: ketoconazole

DIAGNOSTIC TEST EFFECTS

May increase serum cholesterol, calcium, magnesium, and phosphate levels. May decrease serum alkaline phosphatase level.

SIDE EFFECTS

None known.

SERIOUS REACTIONS

! Early signs and symptoms of overdose are weakness, headache, somnolence, nausea, vomiting, dry mouth, constipation, muscle and bone pain, and metallic taste.

! Later signs and symptoms of overdose include polyuria, polydipsia, anorexia, weight loss, nocturia, photophobia, rhinorrhea, pruritus, disorientation, hallucinations, hyperthermia, hypertension, and cardiac arrhythmias.

DENTAL CONSIDERATIONS

General:

- Sensitivity of eyes to dental light may indicate late toxicity.

Teach Patient/Family:

- That oral side effects are associated with early symptoms of overdose

vitamin E

vight′-ah-myn E
(Aqua Gem E, Aquasol E, E-Gems, Key-E, Key-E Kaps)
Do not confuse Aquasol E with Anusol.

CATEGORY AND SCHEDULE

Pregnancy Risk Category: A (C if used in doses above recommended daily allowance)
OTC

V

MECHANISM OF ACTION

An antioxidant that prevents oxidation of vitamins A and C, protects fatty acids from attack by free radicals, and protects RBCs from hemolysis by oxidizing agents. ***Therapeutic Effect:*** Prevents and treats vitamin E deficiency.

PHARMACOKINETICS

Variably absorbed from the GI tract (requires bile salts, dietary fat, and normal pancreatic function). Primarily concentrated in adipose tissue. Metabolized in the liver. Primarily eliminated by biliary system.

AVAILABILITY

Capsules (E-Gems): 100 units, 600 units, 800 units, 1,000 units, 1200 units.
Capsules (Aqua-Gem E, Key-E Kaps): 200 units, 400 units.
Tablets (Key-E): 100 units, 200 units, 400 units, 800 units.

INDICATIONS AND DOSAGES

▸ **Vitamin E Deficiency**

PO

Adults, Elderly. 60–75 units/day.
Children. 1 unit/kg/day.

OFF-LABEL USES

To decrease severity of tardive dyskinesia

CONTRAINDICATIONS

None known.

INTERACTIONS

Drug

Cholestyramine, colestipol, mineral oil: May decrease the absorption of vitamin E.
Iron (large doses): May increase vitamin E requirements.

Herbal

None known.

Food

None known.

Drug interactions of concern to dentistry

- With doses >400 IU: increased action of oral anticoagulants

DIAGNOSTIC TEST EFFECTS

None known.

SIDE EFFECTS

None known.

SERIOUS REACTIONS

! Chronic overdose may produce fatigue, weakness, nausea, headache, blurred vision, flatulence, and diarrhea.

DENTAL CONSIDERATIONS

General:

- Determine why the patient is taking the drug.

warfarin sodium

war′-far-in

(Apo-Warfarin[CAN], Coumadin, Gen-Warfarin[CAN], Jantoven, Marevan[AUS], Tar-Warfarin[CAN])

Do not confuse Coumadin with Kemadrin.

CATEGORY AND SCHEDULE

Pregnancy Risk Category: D

MECHANISM OF ACTION

A coumarin derivative that interferes with hepatic synthesis of vitamin K-dependent clotting factors, resulting in depletion of coagulation factors II, VII, IX, and X. ***Therapeutic Effect:*** Prevents further extension of formed existing clot; prevents new clot formation or secondary thromboembolic complications.

PHARMACOKINETICS

Route	Onset	Peak	Duration
PO	1.5–3 days	5–7 days	N/A

Well absorbed from the GI tract. Metabolized in the liver. Primarily excreted in urine. Not removed by hemodialysis. ***Half-life:*** 1.5–2.5 days.

AVAILABILITY

Tablets (Coumadin, Jantoven): 1 mg, 2 mg, 2.5 mg, 3 mg, 4 mg, 5 mg, 6 mg, 7.5 mg, 10 mg.

INDICATIONS AND DOSAGES

▸ **Anticoagulant**

PO

Adults, Elderly. Initially, 5–15 mg/day for 2–5 days; then adjust based on International Normalized Ratio (INR). Maintenance: 2–10 mg/day.

Children. Initially, 0.1–0.2 mg/kg (maximum 10 mg). Maintenance: 0.05–0.34 mg/kg/day.

▸ **Usual Elderly Dosage (Maintenance)**

PO, IV

Elderly. 2–5 mg/day.

OFF-LABEL USES

Prevention of recurrent cerebral embolism, myocardial reinfarction; treatment adjunct in transient ischemic attacks

CONTRAINDICATIONS

Neurosurgical procedures, open wounds, pregnancy, severe hypertension, severe hepatic or renal damage, uncontrolled bleeding, ulcers

INTERACTIONS

Drug

Acetaminophen, allopurinol, amiodarone, anabolic steroids, androgens, aspirin, cefamandole, cefoperazone, chloral hydrate, chloramphenicol, cimetidine, clofibrate, danazol, dextrothyroxine, diflunisal, disulfiram, erythromycin, fenoprofen, gemfibrozil, indomethacin, methimazole, metronidazole, oral hypoglycemics, phenytoin, plicamycin, propylthiouracil, quinidine, salicylates, sulfinpyrazone, sulfonamides, sulindac: Warfarin increases the effects of these drugs.

Alcohol: May enhance warfarin's anticoagulant effect.

Barbiturates, carbamazepine, cholestyramine, colestipol, estramustine, estrogens, griseofulvin, primidone, rifampin, vitamin K: Warfarin decreases the effects of these drugs.

Herbal

American ginseng, St. John's wort: May decrease the effectiveness of warfarin.

Feverfew, garlic, ginkgo biloba, ginseng, glucosamine-chondroitin: May increase the risk of bleeding.

Food

None known.

Drug interactions of concern to dentistry

- Increased action: diflunisal, salicylates, propoxyphene, metronidazole, erythromycin, clarithromycin, ketoconazole, itraconazole, fluconazole, NSAIDs, indomethacin, chloral hydrate, tetracyclines, fluoroquinolones, acetaminophen, ciprofloxacin, levofloxacin
- If NSAIDs must be used, monitor patient
- Decreased action: barbiturates, carbamazepine
- Possible increase in anticoagulant effects with celecoxib, rofecoxib, acetaminophen (monitor INR levels)
- Herbal products with some anticoagulant activity: feverfew, garlic, ginger, ginkgo, ginseng

DIAGNOSTIC TEST EFFECTS

None known.

SIDE EFFECTS

Occasional

GI distress, such as nausea, anorexia, abdominal cramps, diarrhea

Rare

Hypersensitivity reaction including dermatitis and urticaria, especially in those sensitive to aspirin

SERIOUS REACTIONS

! Bleeding complications ranging from local ecchymoses to major hemorrhage may occur. Drug should be discontinued immediately and vitamin K or phytonadione administered. Mild hemorrhage: 2.5–10 mg PO, IM, or IV. Severe hemorrhage: 10–15 mg IV and repeated q4h, as necessary.

! Hepatotoxicity, blood dyscrasias, necrosis, vasculitis, and local thrombosis occur rarely.

DENTAL CONSIDERATIONS

General:

- Reports on concomitant use of acetaminophen and warfarin seem to suggest a possible increase in anticoagulant effects, especially in patients with other diseases or contributing factors (diarrhea, age, debilitation, etc.). Patients taking warfarin should be questioned about recent use of acetaminophen and current INR values. Acetaminophen has been shown to increase the INR, depending on the amount of acetaminophen taken and duration of use. A new PT or INR value may be required if surgical procedures are planned. Data from one study indicated that use of four regular-strength acetaminophen tablets (325 mg) qd for 1 wk can increase INR values. Use of acetaminophen over a long duration and in higher doses suggests that it is important to closely monitor INR values (*JAMA* 279:657–662, 1998).
- Patients on chronic drug therapy may rarely have symptoms of blood dyscrasias, which can include infection, bleeding, and poor healing.
- Consider local hemostasis measures to prevent excessive bleeding.
- Increased bleeding may occur with IM injections.

Consultations:

- Medical consultation should include partial prothrombin time, prothrombin time, or INR.
- For dental surgical procedures that may result in excessive bleeding, consider requesting dose reduction

before dental treatment so that PT is no more than twice normal.

- In a patient with symptoms of blood dyscrasias, request a medical consultation for blood studies and postpone dental treatment until normal values are reestablished.

Teach Patient/Family:

- Importance of good oral hygiene to prevent soft tissue inflammation
- Caution to prevent injury when using oral hygiene aids
- To report oral lesions, soreness, or bleeding to dentist

zafirlukast

za-feer′-loo-kast
(Accolate)
Do not confuse Accolate with Accupril or Aclovate.

CATEGORY AND SCHEDULE

Pregnancy Risk Category: B

MECHANISM OF ACTION

An antiasthmic that binds to leukotriene receptors, inhibiting bronchoconstriction due to sulfur dioxide, cold air, and specific antigens, such as grass, cat dander, and ragweed. ***Therapeutic Effect:*** Reduces airway edema and smooth muscle constriction; alters cellular activity associated with the inflammatory process.

PHARMACOKINETICS

Rapidly absorbed after PO administration (food reduces absorption). Protein binding: 99%. Extensively metabolized in the liver. Primarily excreted in feces. Unknown if removed by hemodialysis. ***Half-life:*** 10 hr.

AVAILABILITY

Tablets: 10 mg, 20 mg.

INDICATIONS AND DOSAGES

▸ Bronchial Asthma

PO

Adults, Elderly, Children 12 yr and older. 20 mg twice a day.
Children 5–11 yr. 10 mg twice a day.

CONTRAINDICATIONS

None known.

INTERACTIONS

Drug

Aspirin: Increases zafirlukast blood concentration.
Erythromycin, theophylline: Decreases zafirlukast blood concentration.
Warfarin: Increases PT.

Herbal

None known.

Food

None known.

Drug interactions of concern to dentistry

- Increased PT with concurrent use of warfarin
- Reduced plasma levels: erythromycin, terfenadine, theophylline
- Increased plasma levels with aspirin
- Inhibits CYP2C9 and CYP3A4 isoenzymes: use with caution when drugs metabolized by these enzymes are used

DIAGNOSTIC TEST EFFECTS

May increase ALT(SGPT) level.

SIDE EFFECTS

Frequent (13%)
Headache
Occasional (3%)
Nausea, diarrhea
Rare (< 3%)
Generalized pain, asthenia, myalgia, fever, dyspepsia, vomiting, dizziness

SERIOUS REACTIONS

! Concurrent administration of inhaled corticosteroids increases the risk of upper respiratory tract infection.

DENTAL CONSIDERATIONS

General:

- Midday appointments and a stress reduction protocol may be required for anxious patients.
- Avoid prescribing aspirin-containing products.
- Acute asthmatic episodes may be precipitated in the dental office.

Sympathomimetic inhalants should be available for emergency use. A stress reduction protocol may be required.
• Be aware that aspirin or sulfite preservatives in vasoconstrictor-containing products can exacerbate asthma.
• Consider semisupine chair position for patients with respiratory disease or if GI side effects occur.

Consultations:
• Medical consultation may be required to assess disease control.

Teach Patient/Family:
• Use of electric toothbrush if patient has difficulty holding conventional devices
• Importance of updating health and drug history if physician makes any changes in evaluation or drug regimens

zalcitabine
zal-site′-a-been
(Hivid)

CATEGORY AND SCHEDULE
Pregnancy Risk Category: C

MECHANISM OF ACTION
A nucleoside reverse transcriptase inhibitor that inhibits viral DNA synthesis. ***Therapeutic Effect:*** Prevents replication of HIV-1.

PHARMACOKINETICS
Readily absorbed from the GI tract (absorption decreased by food). Protein binding: less than 4%. Undergoes phosphorylation intracellularly to the active metabolite. Primarily excreted in urine. Removed by hemodialysis. ***Half-life:*** 1–3 hr; metabolite, 2.6–10 hr (increased in impaired renal function).

AVAILABILITY
Tablets: 0.375 mg, 0.75 mg.

INDICATIONS AND DOSAGES
▸ HIV Infection (in Combination with Other Antiretrovirals)
PO
Adults, Children 13 yr and older. 0.75 mg q8h.
Children younger than 13 yr. 0.01 mg/kg q8h. Range: 0.005–0.01 mg/kg q8h.

▸ Dosage in Renal Impairment
Dosage and frequency are modified on the basis of creatinine clearance.

Creatinine Clearance	Dose
10–40 ml/min	0.75 mg q12h
less than 10 ml/min	0.75 mg q24h

CONTRAINDICATIONS
Moderate or severe peripheral neuropathy

INTERACTIONS
Drug
Medications associated with peripheral neuropathy (including cisplatin, disulfiram, phenytoin, vincristine): May increase the risk of neuropathy.
Medications causing pancreatitis (including IV pentamidine): May increase the risk of pancreatitis.
Herbal
None known.
Food
None known.
Drug interactions of concern to dentistry
• Increased peripheral neuropathy: metronidazole, dapsone, or other

drugs associated with peripheral neuropathy

DIAGNOSTIC TEST EFFECTS

May increase serum alkaline phosphatase, amylase, bilirubin, lipase, AST (SGOT), ALT (SGPT), and triglyceride levels. May decrease serum calcium, magnesium, and phosphate levels. May alter blood glucose and sodium levels.

SIDE EFFECTS

Frequent (28%–11%)
Peripheral neuropathy, fever, fatigue, headache, rash
Occasional (10%–5%)
Diarrhea, abdominal pain, oral ulcers, cough, pruritus, myalgia, weight loss, nausea, vomiting
Rare (4%–1%)
Nasal discharge, dysphagia, depression, night sweats, confusion

SERIOUS REACTIONS

! Peripheral neuropathy (characterized by numbness, tingling, burning, and pain in the lower extremities) occurs in 17% to 31% of patients. These symptoms may be followed by sharp, shooting pain and progress to a severe, continuous, burning pain that may be irreversible if the drug is not discontinued in time.
! Pancreatitis, leukopenia, neutropenia, eosinophilia, and thrombocytopenia occur rarely.

DENTAL CONSIDERATIONS

General:
- Examine oral cavity for side effects if on long-term drug therapy.
- Monitor vital signs at every appointment because of CV side effects.
- Palliative medication may be required for management of oral side effects.
- Assess salivary flow as a factor in caries, periodontal disease, and candidiasis.
- Prophylactic antibiotics may be indicated to prevent infection if surgery or deep scaling is planned.
- Patients may be more susceptible to infection and have delayed wound healing.

Consultations:
- Medical consultation may be required to assess disease control and patient's ability to tolerate stress.

Teach Patient/Family:
- Importance of good oral hygiene to prevent soft tissue inflammation
- Caution to prevent injury when using oral hygiene aids
- That secondary oral infection may occur; must see dentist immediately if infection occurs
- *When chronic dry mouth occurs, advise patient:*
  - To avoid mouth rinses with high alcohol content because of drying effects
  - Of need for daily use of home fluoride products to prevent caries
  - To use sugarless gum, frequent sips of water, or saliva substitutes

zaleplon

zal'-e-plon
(Sonata, Stamoc[CAN])

CATEGORY AND SCHEDULE

Pregnancy Risk Category: C

MECHANISM OF ACTION

A nonbenzodiazepine that enhances the action of the inhibitory neurotransmitter gamma-aminobutyric acid. *Therapeutic Effect:* Induces sleep.

AVAILABILITY

Capsules: 5 mg, 10 mg.

INDICATIONS AND DOSAGES

▸ Insomnia

PO

Adults. 10 mg at bedtime.
Range: 5–20 mg.
Elderly. 5 mg at bedtime.

CONTRAINDICATIONS

Severe hepatic impairment

INTERACTIONS

Drug

Alcohol, other CNS depressants: May increase CNS depression.
Cimetidine: May increase the effect of zaleplon.
Rifampin: Decreases the zaleplon blood concentration.

Herbal

None known.

Food

High-fat, heavy meals: May delay onset of sleep by approximately 2 hours.

Drug interactions of concern to dentistry

- Caution when using dental drugs that inhibit or induce cytochrome P-450 enzymes; this drug is a minor substrate for CYP3A4; however, use caution (see Appendix I)
- CNS depression: all CNS depressant drugs

DIAGNOSTIC TEST EFFECTS

None known.

SIDE EFFECTS

Expected

Somnolence, sedation, mild rebound insomnia (on first night after drug is discontinued)

Frequent (28%–7%)

Nausea, headache, myalgia, dizziness

Occasional (5%–3%)

Abdominal pain, asthenia, dyspepsia, eye pain, paresthesia

Rare (2%)

Tremors, amnesia, hyperacusis (acute sense of hearing), fever, dysmenorrhea

SERIOUS REACTIONS

! Zaleplon may produce altered concentration, behavior changes, and impaired memory.
! Taking the drug while up and about may result in adverse CNS effects, such as hallucinations, impaired coordination, dizziness, and light-headedness.
! Overdose results in somnolence, confusion, diminished reflexes, and coma.

DENTAL CONSIDERATIONS

General:

- Assess salivary flow as a factor in caries, periodontal disease, and candidiasis.
- Determine why patient is taking the drug.
- Consider semisupine chair position for patient comfort if GI side effects occur.

Consultations:

- Medical consultation may be required to assess disease control and patient's ability to tolerate stress.

Teach Patient/Family:

- *When chronic dry mouth occurs, advise patient:*
  - To avoid mouth rinses with high alcohol content because of drying effects
  - To use daily home fluoride products for anticaries effect
  - To use sugarless gum, frequent sips of water, or saliva substitutes

zanamivir

za-na′-mi-veer
(Relenza)

CATEGORY AND SCHEDULE

Pregnancy Risk Category: B

MECHANISM OF ACTION

An antiviral that appears to inhibit the influenza virus enzyme neuraminidase, which is essential for viral replication. ***Therapeutic Effect:*** Prevents viral release from infected cells.

AVAILABILITY

Powder for Inhalation: 5 mg/blister.

INDICATIONS AND DOSAGES

▸ **Influenza Virus**

INHALATION

Adults, Elderly, Children 7 yr and older. 2 inhalations (one 5-mg blister per inhalation for a total dose of 10 mg) twice a day (~ 12 hr apart) for 5 days.

▸ **Prevention of Influenza Virus**

INHALATION

Adults, Elderly. 2 inhalations once a day for the duration of the exposure period.

CONTRAINDICATIONS

None known.

INTERACTIONS

Drug

None known.

Herbal

None known.

Food

None known.

Drug interactions of concern to dentistry

- None reported

DIAGNOSTIC TEST EFFECTS

May increase serum CK level and liver function test results.

SIDE EFFECTS

Occasional (3%–2%)

Diarrhea, sinusitis, nausea, bronchitis, cough, dizziness, headache

Rare (< 1.5%)

Malaise, fatigue, fever, abdominal pain, myalgia, arthralgia, urticaria

SERIOUS REACTIONS

! Neutropenia may occur.

! Bronchospasm may occur in those with a history of COPD or bronchial asthma.

DENTAL CONSIDERATIONS

General:

- Acute influenza patients are unlikely to be seen in the dental office except for dental emergencies.

ziconotide

zi-koe′-no-tide
(Prialt)

CATEGORY AND SCHEDULE

Pregnancy Risk Category: C

MECHANISM OF ACTION

A synthetic peptide that selectively binds to N-type voltage-sensitive calcium channels located on afferent nerves in the spinal cord. This binding is thought to block N-type calcium channels. ***Therapeutic Effect:*** Blocks excitatory neurotransmitter release, reducing sensitivity to painful stimuli.

AVAILABILITY
Solution: 25-mcg/ml (20-ml), 100-mcg/ml (1-ml, 2-ml, 5-ml) vials.

INDICATIONS AND DOSAGES
▸ Pain control
INTRATHECAL
Adults, Elderly. Initially, 2.4 mcg/day (0.1 mcg/hour). May titrate to maximum of 19.2 mcg/day (0.8 mcg/hr).

CONTRAINDICATIONS
History of psychosis, presence of infection at the injection site, uncontrolled bleeding, or spinal canal obstruction that impairs CSF circulation, IV administration

INTERACTIONS
Drug
Other CNS depressants: May enhance the adverse and toxic effects of these drugs.
Herbal
None known.
Food
None known.
Drug interactions of concern to dentistry
- Enhanced CNS depression: all CNS depressants

DIAGNOSTIC TEST EFFECTS
May increase serum kinase levels.

SIDE EFFECTS
Frequent (47%–11%)
Dizziness, nausea, somnolence, weakness, diarrhea, confusion, ataxia, headache, vomiting, gait disturbance, memory impairment, hypertonia
Occasional (10%–7%)
Anorexia, visual disturbances, anxiety, urinary retention, speech disorder, aphasia, nystagmus, paresthesia, fever, hallucinations, nervousness, vertigo
Rare
Insomnia, dry skin, constipation, arthralgia, myalgia, tremor

SERIOUS REACTIONS
! Atrial fibrillation, cerebral vascular accident, seizures, kidney failure (acute), myoclonus, and psychosis occurs rarely.

DENTAL CONSIDERATIONS
General:
- Determine why patient is taking the drug.
- For use in the hospital setting.

Consultations:
- Medical consultation may be required to assess disease control and patient's ability to tolerate stress.

Teach Patient/Family:
- Importance of good oral hygiene to prevent soft tissue inflammation
- Importance of updating health and medication history if physician makes any changes in evaluation or drug regimens; include OTC, herbal, and nonherbal remedies in the update

zidovudine
zyde-o′-vue-deen
(Apo-Zidovudine[CAN], AZT, Novo-AZT[CAN], Retrovir)
Do not confuse Retrovir with ritonavir.

CATEGORY AND SCHEDULE
Pregnancy Risk Category: C

MECHANISM OF ACTION
A nucleoside reverse transcriptase inhibitor that interferes with viral RNA-dependent DNA polymerase,

an enzyme necessary for viral HIV replication. ***Therapeutic Effect:*** Interferes with HIV replication, slowing the progression of HIV infection.

PHARMACOKINETICS

Rapidly and completely absorbed from the GI tract. Protein binding: 25%–38%. Undergoes first-pass metabolism in the liver. Crosses the blood-brain barrier and is widely distributed, including to CSF. Primarily excreted in urine. Minimal removal by hemodialysis. ***Half-life:*** 0.8–1.2 hr (increased in impaired renal function).

AVAILABILITY

Capsules: 100 mg.
Syrup: 50 mg/5 ml.
Tablets: 300 mg.
Injection: 10 mg/ml.

INDICATIONS AND DOSAGES

▸ HIV Infection

PO

Adults, Elderly, Children older than 12 yr. 200 mg q8h or 300 mg q12h.
Children 12 yr and younger. 160 mg/m^2/dose q8h. Range: 90–180 mg/m^2/dose q6–8h.
Neonates. 2 mg/kg/dose q6h.

IV

Adults, Elderly, Children older than 12 yr. 1–2 mg/kg/dose q4h.
Children 12 yr and younger. 120 mg/m^2/dose q6h.
Neonates. 1.5 mg/kg/dose q6h.

OFF-LABEL USES

Prophylaxis in health care workers at risk of acquiring HIV after occupational exposure

CONTRAINDICATIONS

Life-threatening allergic reactions to zidovudine or its components

INTERACTIONS

Drug

Bone marrow depressants, ganciclovir: May increase myelosuppression.
Clarithromycin: May decrease zidovudine blood concentration.
Probenecid: May increase zidovudine blood concentrations and the risk of zidovudine toxicity.

Herbal

None known.

Food

None known.

Drug interactions of concern to dentistry

- Decreased blood levels: acetaminophen, clarithromycin
- Increased serum levels: fluconazole

DIAGNOSTIC TEST EFFECTS

May increase mean corpuscular volume.

IV INCOMPATIBILITIES

None known.

IV COMPATIBILITIES

Dexamethasone (Decadron), dobutamine (Dobutrex), dopamine (Intropin), heparin, lorazepam (Ativan), morphine, potassium chloride

SIDE EFFECTS

Expected (46%–42%)
Nausea, headache
Frequent (20%–16%)
Abdominal pain, asthenia, rash, fever, acne
Occasional (12%–8%)
Diarrhea, anorexia, malaise, myalgia, somnolence
Rare (6%–5%)
Dizziness, paresthesia, vomiting, insomnia, dyspnea, altered taste

SERIOUS REACTIONS

! Serious reactions include anemia, which occurs most commonly after 4–6 weeks of therapy, and granulocytopenia; both effects are more likely to occur in patients who have a low Hgb level or granulocyte count before beginning therapy.

! Neurotoxicity (as evidenced by ataxia, fatigue, lethargy, nystagmus, and seizures) may occur.

DENTAL CONSIDERATIONS

General:

- Examine for oral manifestations of opportunistic infections.
- Patients on chronic drug therapy may rarely have symptoms of blood dyscrasias, which can include infection, bleeding, and poor healing.
- Avoid dental light in patient's eyes; offer dark glasses for patient comfort.
- Place on frequent recall because of oral side effects.

Consultations:

- In a patient with symptoms of blood dyscrasias, request a medical consultation for blood studies and postpone dental treatment until normal values are reestablished.
- Medical consultation may be required to assess disease control.

Teach Patient/Family:

- Importance of good oral hygiene to prevent soft tissue inflammation
- Caution to prevent injury when using oral hygiene aids
- That secondary oral infection may occur; must see dentist immediately if infection occurs

zileuton

zye-lew-ton

(Zyflo)

Do not confuse Zyban.

CATEGORY AND SCHEDULE

Pregnancy Risk Category: C

MECHANISM OF ACTION

A leukotriene inhibitor that inhibits the enzyme responsible for producing inflammatory response. Prevents formation of leukotrienes (leukotrienes induce bronchoconstricton response, enhances vascular permeability, stimulates mucus secretion).

Therapeutic Effect: Prevents airway edema, smooth muscle contraction, and the inflammatory process, relieving signs and symptoms of bronchial asthma.

PHARMACOKINETICS

Rapidly absorbed from gastrointestinal (GI) tract. Protein binding: 93%. Metabolized in liver. Primarily excreted in urine. Unknown if removed by hemodialysis.

Half-life: 2.1–2.5 hrs.

AVAILABILITY

Tablets: 600 mg (Zyflo).

INDICATIONS AND DOSAGES

▸ **Bronchial Asthma**

PO

Adults, Elderly, Children 12 yrs and older. 600 mg 4 times/day. Total daily dosage: 2400 mg.

CONTRAINDICATIONS

Active liver disease, impaired liver function, hypersensitivity to zileuton or any component of the formulation

INTERACTIONS

Drug

Beta blockers: May increase effects of beta blockers.
Cyclosporine, calcium channel blockers, theophylline: May increase concentration/toxicity of these drugs.
Warfarin: May increase PT in those receiving warfarin.

Drug interactions of concern to dentistry

- Increased plasma levels of theophylline, propranolol
- Significant increase in PT when taking warfarin
- Use caution when prescribing dental drugs that are strong inhibitors of CYP1A2 isoenzymes

DIAGNOSTIC TEST EFFECTS

May increase liver transaminase, SGOT (ALT).

SIDE EFFECTS

Frequent

Headache

Occasional

Dyspepsia, nausea, abdominal pain, asthenia (loss of strength), myalgia

Rare

Conjunctivitis, constipation, dizziness, flatulence, insomnia

SERIOUS REACTIONS

! Liver dysfunction occurs rarely and may be manifested as right upper quadrant pain, nausea, fatigue, lethargy, pruritus, jaundice or flulike symptoms.

DENTAL CONSIDERATIONS

General:

- Consider semisupine chair position for patient comfort because of GI side effects of disease.
- Acute asthmatic episodes may be precipitated in the dental office. Sympathomimetic inhalants should be available for emergency use.
- Midday appointments and a stress reduction protocol may be required for anxious patients.
- Be aware that aspirin or sulfite preservatives in vasoconstrictor-containing products can exacerbate asthma.

Consultations:

- Medical consultation may be required to assess disease control.

Teach Patient/Family:

- Importance of updating health and drug history if physician makes any changes in evaluation or drug regimens

zinc oxide/zinc sulfate

zink′- ox′-eyed/zink′- sul′-fate
(zinc oxide) Balmex, Desitin (zinc sulfate) Orazinc, Zincaps[AUS]

CATEGORY AND SCHEDULE

Pregnancy Risk Category: C

MECHANISM OF ACTION

A mineral that acts as a cofactor for enzymes that are important for protein and carbohydrate metabolism. ***Therapeutic Effect:*** Zinc oxide acts as a mild astringent and skin protectant. Zinc sulfate helps maintain normal growth and tissue repair, as well as skin hydration.

AVAILABILITY

Zinc Oxide
Ointment: 10%, 20%, 40%.

Zinc Sulfate
Capsules: 110 mg, 220 mg.
Tablets: 110 mg.
Injection: 1 mg/ml.

INDICATIONS AND DOSAGES

▸ Mild Skin Irritations and Abrasions (Such as Chapped Skin, Diaper Rash)
TOPICAL (zinc oxide)
Adults, Elderly, Children. Apply as needed.

▸ Treatment and Prevention of Zinc Deficiency, Wound Healing.
PO (zinc sulfate)
Adults, Elderly. 220 mg 3 times a day.

CONTRAINDICATIONS

None known.

INTERACTIONS

Drug

H_2 blockers (such as famotidine): May decrease zinc absorption.
Quinolones (such as ciprofloxacin, tetracycline): May decrease the absorption of these drugs.

Herbals

None known.

Food

Coffee, dairy products: May decrease zinc sulfate (capsules, tablets) absorption.

Drug interactions of concern to dentistry

- Decreased absorption: tetracyclines, fluoroquinolones

DIAGNOSTIC TEST EFFECTS

None known.

SIDE EFFECTS

None known.

SERIOUS REACTIONS

! None known.

DENTAL CONSIDERATIONS

General:

- Determine why patient is taking the drug.

ziprasidone

zye-pray′-za-done
(Geodon)

CATEGORY AND SCHEDULE

Pregnancy Risk Category: C

MECHANISM OF ACTION

A piperazine derivative that antagonizes alpha-adrenergic, dopamine, histamine, and serotonin receptors; also inhibits reuptake of serotonin and norepinephrine.
Therapeutic Effect: Diminishes symptoms of schizophrenia and depression.

PHARMACOKINETICS

Well absorbed after PO administration. Food increases bioavailability. Protein binding: 99%. Extensively metabolized in the liver. Not removed by hemodialysis. ***Half-life:*** 7 hr.

AVAILABILITY

Capsules: 20 mg, 40 mg, 60 mg, 80 mg.
Injection: 20 mg/ml.

INDICATIONS AND DOSAGES

▸ Schizophrenia
PO
Adults, Elderly. Initially, 20 mg twice a day with food. Titrate at intervals of no less than 2 days. Maximum: 80 mg twice a day.

IM
Adults, Elderly. 10 mg q2h or 20 mg q4h. Maximum: 40 mg/day.

▸ Bipolar Mania
PO
Adults, Elderly. 40 mg 2 times/day.

CONTRAINDICATIONS
Conditions that prolong the QT interval, such as congenital long QT syndrome

INTERACTIONS
Drug
Alcohol, other CNS depressants: May increase CNS depression.
Carbamazepine: May decrease ziprasidone blood concentration.
Ketoconazole: May increase ziprasidone blood concentration.
Herbal
None known.
Food
All foods: Enhance the bioavailability of ziprasidone.
Drug interactions of concern to dentistry
- Avoid use of any drug that prolongs the QT interval
- Caution in use of other CNS depressants: increased risk of CNS depressant effects
- Reduced plasma levels: carbamazepine
- Increased plasma levels: ketoconazole and other strong inhibitors of CYP3A4 isoenzymes (see Appendix I)
- Drugs that lower blood pressure (BP): increased risk of hypotension
- Increased extrapyramidal effects: phenothiazines and related drugs (haloperidol, droperidol), metoclopramide

DIAGNOSTIC TEST EFFECTS
May prolong the QT interval.

SIDE EFFECTS
Frequent (30%–16%)
Headache, somnolence, dizziness
Occasional
Rash, orthostatic hypotension, weight gain, restlessness, constipation, dyspepsia

SERIOUS REACTIONS
! Prolongation of QT interval may produce torsades de pointes, a form of ventricular tachycardia. Patients with bradycardia, hypokalemia, or hypomagnesemia are at increased risk.

DENTAL CONSIDERATIONS
General:
- Monitor vital signs at every appointment because of CV side effects.
- After supine positioning, have patient sit upright for at least 2 min before standing to avoid orthostatic hypotension.
- Assess salivary flow as a factor in caries, periodontal disease, and candidiasis.
- Consider semisupine chair position for patient comfort if GI side effects occur.
- Assess for presence of extrapyramidal motor symptoms, such as tardive dyskinesia and akathisia. Extrapyramidal motor activity may complicate dental treatment.
- Use vasoconstrictors with caution, in low doses, and with careful aspiration; avoid use of epinephrine-impregnated gingival retraction cord.

Consultations:
- Consultation with physician may be necessary if sedation or general anesthesia is required.
- Physician should be informed if significant xerostomic side effects occur (e.g., increased caries, sore tongue, problems eating or

swallowing, difficulty wearing prosthesis) so that a medication change can be considered.
- Medical consultation may be required to assess disease control and patient's ability to tolerate stress.

Teach Patient/Family:
- Importance of good oral hygiene to prevent soft tissue inflammation
- To prevent trauma when using oral hygiene aids
- Use of electric toothbrush if patient has difficulty holding conventional devices
- *When chronic dry mouth occurs, advise patient:*
  - To avoid mouth rinses with high alcohol content because of drying effects
  - To use daily home fluoride products for anticaries effect
  - To use sugarless gum, frequent sips of water, or saliva substitutes

zoledronic acid

zole-eh-drone′-ick
(Zometa)

CATEGORY AND SCHEDULE

Pregnancy Risk Category: C

MECHANISM OF ACTION

A bisphosphonate that inhibits the resorption of mineralized bone and cartilage; inhibits increased osteoclastic activity and skeletal calcium release induced by stimulatory factors produced by tumors. ***Therapeutic Effect:*** Increases urinary calcium and phosphorus excretion; decreases serum calcium and phosphorus levels.

AVAILABILITY

Injection Powder for Reconstitution: 4 mg.
Injection Solution: 4 mg/5 ml.

INDICATIONS AND DOSAGES

▸ Hypercalcemia

IV INFUSION
Adults, Elderly. 4 mg IV infusion given over no less than 15 min. Retreatment may be considered, but at least 7 days should elapse to allow for full response to initial dose.

▸ Multiple Myeloma

IV
Adults, Elderly. 4 mg q3–4wk.

CONTRAINDICATIONS

Hypersensitivity to other bisphosphonates, including alendronate, etidronate, pamidronate, risedronate, and tiludronate. Dental implants are contraindicated for patients taking this drug.

INTERACTIONS

Drug

Calcium-containing medications, vitamin D: May antagonize the effects of zoledronic acid in treatment of hypercalcemia.

Herbal

None known.

Food

None known.

Drug interactions of concern to dentistry
- None reported

DIAGNOSTIC TEST EFFECTS

May decrease serum magnesium, calcium, and phosphate levels.

IV INCOMPATIBILITIES

Do not mix with other medications.

SIDE EFFECTS

Frequent (44%–26%)

Fever, nausea, vomiting, constipation

Occasional (15%–10%)
Hypotension, anxiety, insomnia, flulike symptoms (fever, chills, bone pain, myalgia, and arthralgia)
Rare
Conjunctivitis

SERIOUS REACTIONS

! Renal toxicity may occur if IV infusion is administered in less than 15 minutes.

DENTAL CONSIDERATIONS

General:

- This drug is used only in oncology units or hospitals.
- Examine for oral manifestation of opportunistic infection.
- Consider semisupine chair position for patient comfort if GI side effects occur.
- Short appointments may be required.
- If oral candidiasis occurs, treat with suitable antifungal drug.

Consultations:

- Medical consultation may be required to assess disease control.

zolmitriptan

zohl-mih-trip′-tan
(Zomig, Zomig Rapimelt[CAN], Zomig-ZMT)

CATEGORY AND SCHEDULE

Pregnancy Risk Category: C

MECHANISM OF ACTION

A serotonin receptor agonist that binds selectively to vascular receptors, producing a vasoconstrictive effect on cranial blood vessels. ***Therapeutic Effect:*** Relieves migraine headache.

PHARMACOKINETICS

Rapidly but incompletely absorbed after PO administration. Protein binding: 15%. Undergoes first-pass metabolism in the liver to active metabolite. Eliminated primarily in urine (60%) and, to a lesser extent, in feces (30%). ***Half-life:*** 3 hr.

AVAILABILITY

Tablets (Zomig): 2.5 mg, 5 mg.
Tablets (Orally Disintegrating [Zomig-ZMT]): 2.5 mg, 5 mg.
Nasal Spray (Zomig): 5 mg/0.1 ml.

INDICATIONS AND DOSAGES

▸ Acute Migraine Attack

PO
Adults, Elderly, Children older than 18 yr. Initially, 2.5 mg or less. If headache returns, may repeat dose in 2 hr. Maximum: 10 mg/24 hr.
INTRANASAL
Adults, Elderly. 5 mg. May repeat in 2 hr. Maximum: 10 mg/24hr.

CONTRAINDICATIONS

Arrhythmias associated with conduction disorders, basilar or hemiplegic migraine, coronary artery disease, ischemic heart disease (including angina pectoris, history of MI, silent ischemia, and Prinzmetal's angina), uncontrolled hypertension, use within 24 hr of ergotamine-containing preparations or another serotonin receptor agonist, use within 14 days of MAOIs, Wolff-Parkinson-White syndrome

INTERACTIONS

Drug

Ergotamine-containing medications: May produce a vasospastic reaction.
Fluoxetine, fluvoxamine, paroxetine, sertraline: May produce hyperreflexia, incoordination, and weakness.

MAOIs: May dramatically increase plasma concentration of zolmitriptan.
Oral contraceptives: Decrease zolmitriptan clearance and volume of distribution.

Herbal

None known.

Food

None known.

Drug interactions of concern to dentistry

- Potential serotonin crises: selective serotonin reuptake inhibitors, ergot-containing drugs (avoid use within 24 hr of taking this drug)
- Decreased plasma levels: cimetidine

DIAGNOSTIC TEST EFFECTS

None known.

SIDE EFFECTS

Frequent (8%–6%)

Oral: Dizziness; tingling; neck, throat, or jaw pressure; somnolence
Nasal: Altered taste, paraesthesia

Occasional (5%–3%)

Oral: Warm or hot sensation, asthenia, chest pressure
Nasal: Nausea, somnolence, nasal discomfort, dizziness, asthenia, dry mouth

Rare (2%–1%)

Diaphoresis, myalgia, paresthesia

SERIOUS REACTIONS

! Cardiac reactions (including ischemia, coronary artery vasospasm, and MI) and noncardiac vasospasm-related reactions (such as hemorrhage and CVA) occur rarely, particularly in patients with hyper-tension, diabetes, or a strong family history of coronary artery disease; obese patients; smokers; males older than 40 years; and postmenopausal women.

DENTAL CONSIDERATIONS

General:

- This is an acute-use drug; thus it is doubtful that patients will come to the office if acute migraine is present.
- Be aware of patient's disease, its severity, and its frequency, when known.
- Advise patient if dental drugs prescribed have potential for photosensitivity.

Consultations:

- If treating chronic orofacial pain, consult with physician of record.
- Medical consultation may be required to assess disease control and patient's ability to tolerate stress.

Teach Patient/Family:

- That dryness of the mouth may occur when taking this drug
- To avoid mouth rinses with high alcohol content because of drying effects
- Importance of updating health and drug history if physician makes any changes in evaluation or drug regimens

zolpidem tartrate

zole-pi′-dem
Schedule IV
(Ambien, Stilnox[AUS])
Do not confuse Ambien with Amen.

CATEGORY AND SCHEDULE

Pregnancy Risk Category: B
Controlled Substance: Schedule IV

MECHANISM OF ACTION

A nonbenzodiazepine that enhances the action of the inhibitory neurotransmitter gamma-aminobutyric acid. ***Therapeutic Effect:*** Induces sleep and improves sleep quality.

PHARMACOKINETICS

Route	Onset	Peak	Duration
PO	30 min	N/A	6–8hr

Rapidly absorbed from the GI tract. Protein binding: 92%. Metabolized in the liver; excreted in urine. Not removed by hemodialysis. ***Half-life:*** 1.4–4.5 hr (increased in hepatic impairment).

AVAILABILITY

Tablets: 5 mg, 10 mg.

INDICATIONS AND DOSAGES

▸ Insomnia

PO

Adults. 10 mg at bedtime.

Elderly, Debilitated. 5 mg at bedtime.

CONTRAINDICATIONS

None known.

INTERACTIONS

Drug

Alcohol, other CNS depressants: May increase CNS depression.

Herbal

None known.

Food

None known.

Drug interactions of concern to dentistry

- Increased CNS depression: alcohol, all CNS depressants, fluconazole, ketoconazole, itraconazole

DIAGNOSTIC TEST EFFECTS

None known.

SIDE EFFECTS

Occasional (7%)

Headache

Rare (< 2%)

Dizziness, nausea, diarrhea, muscle pain

SERIOUS REACTIONS

! Overdose may produce severe ataxia, bradycardia, altered vision (such as diplopia), severe drowsiness, nausea and vomiting, difficulty breathing, and unconsciousness.

! Abrupt withdrawal of the drug after long-term use may produce asthenia, facial flushing, diaphoresis, vomiting, and tremor.

! Drug tolerance or dependence may occur with prolonged, high-dose therapy.

DENTAL CONSIDERATIONS

General:

- Assess salivary flow as a factor in caries, periodontal disease, and candidiasis.
- Monitor vital signs at every appointment because of CV side effects.

Consultations:

- Medical consultation may be required to assess disease control.

Teach Patient/Family:

- *When chronic dry mouth occurs, advise patient:*
  - To avoid mouth rinses with high alcohol content because of drying effects
  - Of need for daily use of home fluoride products to prevent caries
  - To use sugarless gum, frequent sips of water, or saliva substitutes

zonisamide

zoh-nis′-a-mide
(Zonegran)

CATEGORY AND SCHEDULE

Pregnancy Risk Category: C

MECHANISM OF ACTION

A succinimide that may stabilize neuronal membranes and suppress neuronal hypersynchronization by blocking sodium and calcium channels. ***Therapeutic Effect:*** Reduces seizure activity.

PHARMACOKINETICS

Well absorbed after PO administration. Extensively bound to RBCs. Protein binding: 40%. Primarily excreted in urine. ***Half-life:*** 63 hr (plasma), 105 hr (RBCs).

AVAILABILITY

Capsules: 25 mg, 50 mg, 100 mg.

INDICATIONS AND DOSAGES

▸ Partial Seizures

PO

Adults, Elderly, Children older than 16 yr. Initially, 100 mg/day for 2 wk. May increase by 100 mg/day at intervals of 2 wk or longer. Range: 100–600 mg/day.

OFF-LABEL USES

Treatment of obesity, weight loss

CONTRAINDICATIONS

Allergy to sulfonamides

INTERACTIONS

Drug

Alcohol, other CNS depressants: May increase zonisamide's sedative effect.

Carbamazepine, phenobarbital, phenytoin, valproic acid: May increase the metabolism and decrease the effect of zonisamide.

Herbal

None known.

Food

None known.

Drug interactions of concern to dentistry

- No dental drug interactions reported; it has been proposed that drugs which either induce or inhibit CYP3A4 enzymes may not significantly alter serum levels
- Carbamazepine increases renal clearance

DIAGNOSTIC TEST EFFECTS

May increase BUN and serum creatinine levels.

SIDE EFFECTS

Frequent (17%–9%)

Somnolence, dizziness, anorexia, headache, agitation, irritability, nausea

Occasional (8%–5%)

Fatigue, ataxia, confusion, depression, impaired memory or concentration, insomnia, abdominal pain, diplopia, diarrhea, speech difficulty

Rare (4%–3%)

Paresthesia, nystagmus, anxiety, rash, dyspepsia, weight loss

SERIOUS REACTIONS

! Overdose is characterized by bradycardia, hypotension, respiratory depression, and coma.

! Leukopenia, anemia, and thrombocytopenia occur rarely.

DENTAL CONSIDERATIONS

General:

- Determine type of epilepsy, seizure frequency, and quality of seizure control.

• Patients on chronic drug therapy may rarely have symptoms of blood dyscrasias, which can include infection, bleeding, and poor healing.
• Short appointments and a stress reduction protocol may be required for anxious patients.
• Place on frequent recall to evaluate gingival condition and self-care.
• Consider semisupine chair position for patient comfort if GI side effects occur.
• Warn patient of increased CNS side effects when sedation is used. Advise not to drive a car to and from dental appointment.

Consultations:

• Consultation with physician may be necessary if sedation or general anesthesia is required.
• In a patient with symptoms of blood dyscrasias, request a medical consultation for blood studies and postpone treatment until normal values are reestablished.
• Medical consultation may be required to assess disease control and patient's ability to tolerate stress.

Teach Patient/Family:

• Importance of good oral hygiene to prevent soft tissue inflammation
• To prevent trauma when using oral hygiene aids
• Importance of updating health and drug history if physician makes any changes in evaluation or drug regimens
• To see physician immediately if rash develops because of drug

Based on Material from AAOM *Clinician's Guide to Treatment of Common Oral Conditions* and Appendix B from *Dental Management of the Medically Compromised Patient*

This is a quick reference to the etiologic factors, clinical description, currently accepted therapeutic management, and patient education of the more common oral conditions. Some of the recommended treatments have been investigated more thoroughly than others, but all have been reported to be of clinical value.

Many oral conditions described here have no cure, but treatment modalities are available that can relieve discomfort, shorten the clinical duration and frequency, and minimize recurrences.

Clinicians are reminded that an accurate diagnosis is imperative for clinical success. Every effort should be made to determine the diagnosis before initiating treatment. Infection and malignancy must be ruled out. Where signs, symptoms, and microscopic and other laboratory evidence do not support a definitive diagnosis, empirical treatment may be initiated and evaluated as a therapeutic trial basis.

Patient management should be governed by the natural history of the oral condition and whether a palliative, supportive, or curative treatment exists. Referral of patients should be made when the patient's problems are beyond the scope of the clinician trial. Further treatment can be determined by the patient's response. However, when healing of a lesion or an expected response to treatment is not achieved within an expected period of time, a biopsy is recommended.

All drugs require a prescription unless identified as over-the-counter (OTC) drugs. Please note that in recent years, the Food and Drug Administration (FDA) has been active in allowing OTC status for drugs formerly available by prescription only. Be sure to check the dosages of the newly released OTC drugs because they usually are of a different strength than those available by prescription.

SUPPORTIVE CARE

Management of oral mucosal conditions may require topical and systemic interventions. Therapy should address patient nutrition and hydration, oral discomfort, oral hygiene, management of secondary infection, and local control of the disease process. Depending on the extent, severity, and location of oral lesions, consideration should be given to obtaining a consultation from a dentist who specializes in oral medicine, oral pathology, or oral surgery. When a question arises involving a medical condition, a physician should be consulted.

Symptomatic relief of painful conditions can be provided with topical preparations, such as 2% viscous lidocaine hydrochloride or 0.5% dyclonine hydrochloride. Topical anesthetics can be used as a rinse in adults but should be applied with a cotton swab in a child so that the child does not swallow the medication. Swallowing these anesthetics is contraindicated, in part, because they may interfere with the patient's gag reflex. Symptomatic relief also can be obtained by mixing equal parts of diphenhydramine hydrochloride elixir and magnesium hydroxide/aluminum hydroxide. Children's formula diphenhydramine hydrochloride elixir does not contain alcohol. Sucralfate suspension also can be used before meals. The diphenhydramine mixture and the sucralfate coat the ulcerated lesions and may allow the patient to eat more comfortably.

Meticulous oral hygiene is absolutely mandatory for these patients. Mucosal lesions contacting bacterial plaque present on the dentition are more likely to become secondarily infected. Patients should be seen by the dentist or hygienist for scaling and root planing, under local anesthesia when necessary, in all cases in which oral hygiene is suboptimal. Patients must be encouraged to brush and floss their teeth after meals in a gentle yet efficient manner. This may be enhanced by placing a soft toothbrush under hot water to further soften the bristles. Tartar control toothpastes containing calcium pyrophosphate should be avoided because of their caustic nature and reported involvement in circumoral dermatitis.

HERPES SIMPLEX

Infection with the herpes simplex virus produces a disease that has a primary, or acute, phase and a secondary, or recurrent, phase.

Primary Herpetic Gingivostomatitis

Etiology: A transmissible infection with herpes simplex virus, usually type I or, less commonly, type II.

Clinical description: Clear, then yellowish, vesicles develop intraorally and extraorally. These vesicles rupture within hours and form shallow, painful ulcers. The gingivae often are red, enlarged, and painful. The patient may have systemic signs and symptoms including regional lymphadenitis, fever, and malaise. Usually it is self-limiting, with healing in 7 to 10 days.

Rationale for treatment: Relieve symptoms, prevent secondary infection, and support general health. Supportive therapy includes forced fluids, protein, vitamin and mineral food supplements, and rest. Systemic acyclovir is effective in treating herpes in immunocompromised patients. Topical steroids should be avoided because they tend to permit spread of the viral infection on mucous membranes, particularly ocular. Patients should be cautioned to avoid touching the herpetic lesions and then touching the eyes, genital, or other body areas because of the possibility of self-inoculation.

Topical Anesthetics and Coating Agents

Rx

Diphenhydramine (Benadryl) elixir 12.5 mg/5 ml (Note: Elixir is Rx and syrup [Benylin] is OTC) 4 oz mixed with Kaopectate OTC 4 oz (to make a 50% mixture by volume).

Disp: 8 oz

Sig: Rinse with 1 teaspoonful every 2 hours and spit out.

Maalox OTC can be used in place of Kaopectate.

Rx

Diphenhydramine (Benadryl) elixir 12.5 mg/5 ml

Disp: 4-oz bottle

Sig: Rinse with 1 teaspoonful for 2 minutes every 2 hours and before each meal and spit out.

Systemic Antiviral Therapy

Acyclovir oral capsules may relieve and decrease the duration of symptoms.

Rx

Acyclovir (Zovirax) capsules 200 mg

Disp: 50 (or 60) capsules

Sig: Take 1 capsule 5 times per day for 10 days (or 2 capsules 3 times per day for 10 days).

(Current FDA recommendation is that systemic acyclovir be used to treat oral herpes only for immunocompromised patients.)

Systemic Antibiotics

(For secondary bacterial infection in susceptible individuals. Do not use routinely.)

Rx

Penicillin V tablets 500 mg

Disp: 40 tablets

Sig: Take 1 tablet qid.

For patients allergic to penicillin:

Rx

Erythromycin tablets 250 mg

Disp: 40 tablets

Sig: Take 1 tablet qid.

If nausea or stomach cramps occur, prescribe enteric-coated preparations (e.g., E-Mycin, ERYC, PCE, etc.) or a second-generation erythromycin (e.g., clarithromycin [Biaxin]).

Nutritional Supplements

Rx

Meritene (protein-vitamin-mineral food supplement) OTC

Disp: 1-lb can (plain vanilla, chocolate, and eggnog flavors)

Sig: Take 3 servings per day. Prepare as indicated on the label. Serve cold.

Rx

Ensure Plus (protein-vitamin-mineral food supplement) OTC

Disp: 20 cans

Sig: Drink 3 to 5 cans in divided doses throughout the day as tolerated. Serve cold.

Analgesic

Rx

Acetaminophen tablets 325 mg OTC

Sig: Take 2 tablets q4h PRN for pain and fever. Limit 4 g per 24 hours.

For Moderate to Severe Pain

Acetaminophen 300 mg with codeine 30 mg (Tylenol no. 3)

Sig: Take 1 or 2 tablets q4h for pain (requires Drug Enforcement Agency [DEA] number).

Recurrent (Orofacial) Herpes Simplex

Etiology: Reactivation of the latent virus that resides in the sensory ganglion of the trigeminal nerve. Precipitating factors include fever, stress, exposure to sunlight, trauma, and hormonal alterations.

Clinical description: *Intraoral*–single or small clusters of vesicles that quickly rupture, forming painful ulcers.
The lesions usually occur on the keratinized tissue of the hard palate and gingiva.

Labialis–clusters of vesicles on the lips that rupture within hours and then crust.

Rationale for treatment: Should be initiated as early as possible in the prodromal stage, with the objective of reducing the duration and symptoms of the lesion.
Oral acyclovir, prophylactically and therapeutically, can be considered when frequent recurrent herpetic episodes interfere with daily function and nutrition.
(Current FDA recommendation is that systemic acyclovir be used to treat oral herpes only for immunocompromised patients.)

Prevention

Rx

PreSun 15-sunscreen lotion (OTC)

Disp: 4 fl oz
Sig: Apply to susceptible area 1 hour before sun exposure and every hour thereafter.
Rx
PreSun 15-lip gel (OTC)
Disp: 15 oz
Sig: Apply to lips 1 hour before sun exposure and every hour thereafter.

If a recurrence on the lips usually is precipitated by exposure to sunlight, the lesion may be prevented by applying a sunscreen with a high skin protection factor (SPF ≥15) to the area.

Topical Antiviral Agents

Antiviral creams and ointments are of minimal efficacy for recurrent herpes simplex. Their value may be attributable to coating of the lesion by the petrolatum vehicle, which reduces the possibility of self-inoculation. Constant or intermittent application of ice to the area for 90 minutes during the prodromal phase may result in aborting the lesion. Cocoa butter ointment, lanolin-based lip preparations, or petrolatum (Vaseline) as an emollient may be palliative.
Rx
Penciclovir (Denavir) topical ointment 5%
Disp: 15-g tube
Sig: Apply to area q2h during waking hours, beginning when symptoms first occur.
Rx
Docosanol (Abreva) cream (OTC)
Disp: 2-g tube
Sig: Dab on lesion 5 times per day during waking hours for 4 days, beginning when symptoms first occur.

VARICELLA ZOSTER (SHINGLES)

Etiology: Reactivation of latent herpes varicella virus present since an original varicella infection through chickenpox.
Precipitating factors include thermal, inflammatory, radiologic, or mechanical trauma.
Clinical description: Usually painful segmental eruption of small vesicles that later rupture to form punctate or confluent ulcers. Acute zoster follows a portion of the trigeminal nerve distribution in approximately 20% of cases. It is rare in the young, more common in the elderly.
Rationale for treatment: Promptly initiate antiviral therapy to reduce duration and symptoms of the lesions. Patients older than 60 years are particularly prone to postherpetic neuralgia. In the absence of specific contraindications, consideration should be given to prescribing short-term, high-dose corticosteroid prophylaxis for postherpetic neuralgia, in conjunction with oral acyclovir.
Rx
Acyclovir (Zovirax) capsules 200 mg
Disp: 200 capsules
Sig: Take 4 capsules 5 times per day for 10 days.
Rx
Valacyclovir (Valtrex) HCl caplets 500 mg
Disp: 42 capsules
Sig: Take 2 capsules 3 times per day for 7 days.
Use with caution in immunocompromised patients.

RECURRENT APHTHOUS STOMATITIS

Etiology: An altered local immune response is the predisposing factor. Patients with frequent recurrences should be screened for diseases, such as anemia, diabetes mellitus, vitamin deficiency, inflammatory bowel disease, and immunosuppression.

Precipitating factors include stress, trauma, allergies, endocrine alterations, dietary components, such as acidic foods and juices, and foods that contain gluten. Inspect the oral cavity closely for sources of trauma.

Clinical description: Minor aphthae (canker sore), less than 0.6 cm, small, shallow, painful ulceration covered by a gray membrane and surrounded by a narrow erythematous halo. They usually occur on nonkeratinized (moveable) oral mucosa.

Major aphthae, greater than 0.6 cm, large painful ulcers. A more severe form of aphthae that may last weeks or months. They may mimic other diseases, such as granulomatous or malignant lesions.

Herpetiform ulcers, crops of small, shallow, painful ulcers. They may occur anywhere on nonkeratinized oral mucosa and resemble recurrent intraoral herpes simplex clinically but are of unknown etiology.

Rationale for treatment: Effective treatment involves barriers, amlexanox, topical or systemic corticosteroids, and immunosuppressants or combination therapy, when indicated. Treatment should be initiated as early as possible in the course of lesions. Identification and elimination of precipitating factors may minimize recurrent episodes. Medications such as mycophenolate mofetil, pentoxifylline, and thalidomide are used to treat patients with severe, persistent, recurrent aphthous ulcers but should not be routinely used.

Nonsteroidal

Rx

Amlexanox oral paste 5%
Disp: 5-g tube
Sig: Dab on affected area qid until healed.

Rx

Orabase Soothe-N-Seal Protective Barrier (OTC)
Disp: 1 package
Sig: Apply as per the package directions every 6 hours when necessary.

Therapies with steroids and immunomodulating drugs are presented to inform the clinician that such modalities are available. Because of the potential for side effects, close collaboration with the patient's physician is recommended if these medications are prescribed. These modalities may be beyond the scope of clinical experience of general dentists, and referral to a specialist in oral medicine or to an appropriate physician may be necessary.

Topical Steroids

Prolonged use of topical steroids (>2 weeks of continuous use) may result in mucosal atrophy or secondary candidiasis and may increase the potential for systemic absorption. It may be necessary to prescribe antifungal therapy with steroids.

Rx

Triamcinolone acetonide (Kenalog) in Orabase 0.1%
Disp: 5-g tube
Sig: Coat the lesion with a thin film after each meal and at bedtime.

Other topical steroid preparations (cream, gel rinse, ointment) include:

Ultra-Potent:

Clobetasol propionate (Temovate) 0.05%

Halobetasol propionate (Ultravate) 0.05%

Potent:

Dexamethasone (Decadron) 0.5 mg/5 ml

Intermediate:

Betamethasone valerate (Valisone) 0.1%

Triamcinolone acetonide (Kenalog) 0.1%

Low:

Hydrocortisone 1%

(Mixing ointments with equal parts of Orabase B paste promotes adhesion.)

Rx

Dexamethasone (Decadron) elixir 0.5 mg/5 ml

Disp: 100 ml

Sig: Rinse with 1 teaspoon for 2 minutes qid and expectorate. Discontinue when lesions become asymptomatic.

Oral candidiasis may result from topical steroid therapy. The oral cavity should be monitored for emergence of fungal infection in patients who are placed on therapy. Prophylactic antifungal therapy should be initiated in patients with a history of fungal infections with previous steroid administration (see Candidiasis/Candidosis).

System Steroids and Immunosuppressants

For Severe Cases

Rx

Dexamethasone (Decadron) elixir 0.5 mg/5 ml

Disp: 320 ml

Sig:

1. For 3 days, rinse with 1 tablespoon (15 ml) qid and swallow. Then
2. For 3 days, rinse with 1 teaspoonful (5 ml) qid and swallow. Then
3. For 3 days, rinse with 1 teaspoonful (5 ml) qid and swallow every other time. Then
4. Rinse with 1 teaspoonful (5 ml) qid and spit out. Discontinue medication when mouth becomes comfortable.

If mouth discomfort recurs, restart treatment at step 3. Rinsing should be done after meals and at bedtime. Refill one time.

Rx

Prednisone tablets 5 mg

Disp: 40 tablets

Sig: Take 5 tablets in the morning for 5 days, then 5 tablets in the morning every other day until gone.

For Very Severe Cases

Rx

Prednisone tablets 10 mg

Disp: 26 tablets

Sig: Take 4 tablets in the morning for 5 days, then decrease by 1 tablet on each successive day.

Therapy with medications, such as systemic steroids, immunosuppressants, and immunomodulators are presented to inform the clinician that such modalities have been reported effective for patients suffering from severe, persistent, recurrent aphthous stomatitis. Medications such as azathioprine, pentoxifylline, levamisole, colchicine, dapsone, and thalidomide are used to treat patients with severe, persistent recurrent aphthous stomatitis but should not be routinely used because of the potential for side effects. Close collaboration with the patient's physician is recommended when these medications are prescribed.

CANDIDIASIS

Etiology: *Candida albicans*, a yeastlike fungus. *Candida* is an opportunistic organism that tends to proliferate with the use of broad-spectrum antibiotics, corticosteroids, medicines that reduce salivary output, and cytotoxic agents. Conditions that contribute to candidiasis include xerostomia, diabetes mellitus, poor oral hygiene, prosthetic appliances, and suppression of the immune system (i.e., AIDS or the side effects of some medications). It is important to determine the predisposing factors.

Clinical description: The disease is characterized by soft, white, slightly elevated plaques that usually can be wiped away, leaving an erythematous area (pseudomembranous type). Candidiasis also may appear as generalized erythematous, sensitive areas (atrophic or erythematous type) or as confluent white areas (hypertrophic form). When the clinical diagnosis is questionable, it is advisable to culture for *C. albicans* concurrent with starting medication.

Rationale for treatment: To reestablish a normal balance of oral flora and improve oral hygiene. Medication should be continued for 48 hours after disappearance of clinical signs to prevent immediate recurrence.

Topical Antifungal Agents

Rx
Nystatin (Mycostatin, Nilstat) oral suspension 100,000 units/ml
Disp: 60 ml
Sig: Take 2–5 ml qid. Rinse for 2 minutes and swallow. Nystatin suspension has a high sugar content; therefore good oral hygiene should be reinforced. A few drops of nystatin oral suspension can be added to the water used for soaking acrylic prostheses.

Rx
Nystatin ointment
Disp: 15-g tube
Sig: Apply a thin coat to inner surface of denture and to the affected area after each meal.

Rx
Nystatin topical powder
Disp: 15 g
Sig: Apply a thin layer under the prosthesis after each meal.

Rx (Mycostatin)
Nystatin pastilles 200,000 units
Disp: 50 pastilles
Sig: Let 1 pastille dissolve in mouth 5 times per day.

Rx
Nystatin vaginal suppositories 100,000 units
Sig: Let suppository dissolve in mouth qid. Do not rinse for 30 minutes.

Rx
Clotrimazole (Mycelex) troches 10 mg
Disp: 70 troches
Sig: Let 1 troche dissolve in mouth 5 times per day. If concern exists about sugar content of the nystatin and clotrimazole troches, vaginal tablets can be substituted.

Rx
Ketoconazole (Nizoral) cream 2%
Disp: 15-g tube
Sig: Apply thin coat to inner surface of denture and affected areas after meal.

Rx
Clotrimazole (Gyne-Lotrimin, Mycelex-G) Vaginal Cream 1% (OTC)
Disp: 1 tube
Sig: Apply small dab to tissue side of denture or to the infected oral mucosa 4 times per day.

Rx
Miconazole (Monistat 7) Vaginal Cream 2% (OTC)
Disp: 1 tube
Sig: Apply small dab to tissue side of denture or to the infected oral mucosa 4 times per day.

Systemic Antifungal Agents

Note: In many cases, combinations of these antifungal preparations (liquids, troches, and ointments) can be used depending upon clinical considerations and response to therapy.

When topical therapy is not practical or is ineffective, ketoconazole (Nizoral) and fluconazole (Diflucan) are effective, well-tolerated, systemic drugs for mucocutaneous candidiasis. They should be used with caution in patients with impaired liver function (i.e., with history of alcoholism or hepatitis). Liver function tests should be performed initially and conducted monthly when ketoconazole is prescribed for an extended period. Several drug interactions have been reported with ketoconazole.

Rx
Ketoconazole (Nizoral) tablets 200 mg
Disp: 20 tablets
Sig: Take 1 tablet per day with a meal or orange juice.

Rx
Fluconazole (Diflucan) tablets 100 mg
Disp: 20 tablets
Sig: Take 2 tablets stat, then 1 tablet per day.

Rx
Itraconazole (Sporanox) tablets 100 mg
Disp: 28 tablets
Sig: Take 1 tablet bid or 2 tablets per day with meal or orange juice.

Rx
Amphotericin B (Fungizone) oral suspension 100 mg/ml
Disp: 48 ml
Sig: 1 ml qid. Swish in mouth 3–4 minutes then swallow.

CHEILITIS AND CHEILOSIS

Angular Cheilitis and Cheilosis

Etiology: Fissured lesions in the corners of the mouth are caused by a mixed infection of the microorganisms *C. albicans*, *Staphylococcus*, and *Streptococcus*. Predisposing factors include local habits, drooling, a decrease in intermaxillary space, anemia, immunosuppression, and an extension of oral infections.

Clinical description: The commissures may appear wrinkled, red, fissured, cracked, or crusted.

Rationale for treatment: Identification and correction of predisposing factors and elimination of the secondary infection and inflammation.

Rx
Nystatin plus triamcinolone acetonide (Mycolog II) ointment
Disp: 15-g tube
Sig: Apply to affected area after each meal and at bedtime. Concomitant intraoral antifungal treatment may be indicated.

Rx
Ketoconazole (Nizoral) cream 2%
Disp: 15-g tube
Sig: Apply a small dab to corners of mouth daily at bedtime.

Rx
Clotrimazole (Gyne-Lotrimin, Mycelex-G) vaginal cream 1% (OTC)
Disp: 1 tube
Sig: Apply small dab to corner of mouth qid.

Rx
Miconazole (Monistat 7) nitrate vaginal cream 2% (OTC)
Disp: 1 tube
Sig: Apply small dab to corner of mouth qid.

Actinic Cheilitis and Solar Cheilosis

Etiology: Prolonged exposure to sunlight results in irreversible degenerative changes in the vermilion of the lips, especially the everted lower lip.

Clinical description: The normal red translucent vermilion with regular vertical fissuring of a smooth surface is replaced by a white flat surface that may exhibit periodic ulceration.

Rationale for treatment: If exposure to the ultraviolet light in the sun's rays is allowed to continue, the degenerative changes may progress to a malignancy. Sunscreens with a high skin protection factor (SPF >15) should be used constantly.

Rx
Several OTC sunscreen preparations are available (e.g., PreSun 15 lotion and lip gel). For those patients allergic to paraaminobenzoic acid, non–paraaminobenzoic acid sunscreens should be prescribed.

GEOGRAPHIC TONGUE (BENIGN MIGRATORY GLOSSITIS; ERYTHEMA MIGRANS)

Etiology: The etiology is unknown. Because its histologic appearance is similar to psoriasis, some have associated it with psoriasis. This may be purely coincidental. Oral lesions should not be associated with psoriasis if no cutaneous signs exist of this disorder. It has been associated with Reiter's syndrome and atopy.
Clinical description: A benign inflammatory condition caused by desquamation of superficial keratin and filiform papillae. It is characterized by both red, denuded, irregularly shaped patches of the tongue dorsum and lateral borders surrounded by a raised white-yellow border.
Rationale for treatment: Generally no treatment is necessary as most patients are asymptomatic. When symptoms are present, they may be associated with secondary infection with *C. albicans* (see Supportive Care). Topical steroids, especially in combination with topical antifungal agents, are the treatment modality of choice. Patients must be told that this condition does not suggest a more serious disease and is not contagious. In most cases, biopsy is not indicated because of the pathognomonic clinical appearance.
Rx
Nystatin-triamcinolone acetonide (Mycolog II, Mytrex) ointment
Disp: 15-g tube
Sig: Apply to affected areas after meals and at bedtime.
Rx
Clotrimazole-betamethasone dipropionate (Lotrisone) cream
Disp: 15-g tube
Sig: Apply to affected area after each meal and at bedtime.
Rx
Betamethasone Valerate ointment, 0.1%
Disp: 15-g tube
Sig: Apply to affected areas after meals and at bedtime.
Rx
Nystatin ointment
Disp: 15-g tube
Sig: Apply to affected areas after meals and at bedtime.

XEROSTOMIA

Etiology: Acute or chronic reduced salivary flow may result from drug therapy, mechanical blockage, dehydration, emotional stress, infection of the salivary glands, local surgery, avitaminosis, diabetes, anemia, connective tissue diseases, Sjögren's syndrome, radiation therapy, and congenital factors (e.g., ectodermal dysplasia) (see Box 21-9).
Clinical description: The tissues may be dry, pale, or red and atrophic. The tongue may be devoid of papillae, atrophic, fissured, and inflamed. Multiple carious lesions may be present, especially at the gingival margin and on exposed root surfaces.
Rationale for treatment: Salivary stimulation or replacement therapy to keep mouth moist, prevention of caries and candidal infection, and palliative relief.

Saliva Substitutes

Rx
Sodium carboxymethyl cellulose 0.5% aqueous solution (OTC)

Disp: 8 fl oz
Sig: Use as a rinse as frequently as needed.
Saliva substitutes (OTC): Optimoist, MouthKote, Sage Moist Plus, Xero-Lube, Salivart, Moi-Stir, Orex
Commercial oral moisturizing gels (OTC): Sage Mouth Moisturizer, Oral Balance
Relief from oral dryness and accompanying discomfort can be achieved conservatively by sipping water frequently all day long, letting ice melt in the mouth, restricting caffeine intake, not using mouth rinses that contain alcohol, humidifying sleeping area, and coating lips with Blistex or Vaseline

Saliva Stimulants

Chewing sugarless gum and sucking sugarless mints are conservative methods to temporarily stimulate salivary flow in patients with medication xerostomia or with salivary gland dysfunction. Patients should be cautioned against using products that contain sugar.

Rx
Pilocarpine HCl solution 1 mg/ml
Disp: 100 ml
Sig: Take 1 teaspoonful qid.
(The dosage should be adjusted to increase saliva while minimizing the adverse side effects [sweating, stomach upset].)

Rx
Pilocarpine HCl (Salagen) tablets 5 mg
Disp: 100 tablets
Sig: Take 1 tablet tid. *An extra tablet* (10 mg) may be taken at bedtime.

Rx
Cevimeline HCl (Evoxac) tablets 30 mg
Disp: 100 tablets
Sig: Take 1 tablet PO tid or qid

Rx
Bethanechol (Urecholine) 25 mg
Disp: 21 tablets
Sig: Take 1 tablet tid.

Caries Prevention

Rx
Stannous fluoride gel 0.4%
Disp: 4.3 oz
Sig: Apply to teeth daily for 5 minutes; 5–10 drops in a custom tray. Do not swallow the gel.
SnF_2 gels available include IDP Gel-Oh, Stan-Gard, Perfect Choice, Flo-Gel, True Gel, Nova Gel, Omni-Gel, Control, Gel-Pro, Perfect Choice, Basic Gel, Gel-Tin, IDP Gel-Oh, Gel-Kam, Stan-Gard, Easy-Gel, Thera-Flur
When the taste of acidulated SnF_2 gels is poorly tolerated or where there is etching of ceramic restorations, neutral pH sodium fluoride gel 1% (Thera-Flur-N) should be considered.

Rx
Neutral NaF gel (Thera-Flur-N) 1.0% or PreviDent (Colgate) 1.1% neutral NaF
Disp: 24 ml
Sig: Place 1 drop per tooth in custom tray; apply for 5 minutes daily. Avoid rinsing or eating for 30 minutes following treatment.

FDA regulations have limited the size of bottles of fluoride because of toxicity if ingested by infants. Because most preparations do not come in childproof bottles, the sizes of topical fluoride preparations vary; 24 ml is an approximately 2-week supply for application to a full dentition in custom carriers.
Xerostomia provides an excellent environment for overgrowth of *C. albicans*. The patient is likely to require treatment for candidiasis along with treatment for dry mouth. In a dry oral environment, plaque control becomes more difficult. Scrupulous oral hygiene is essential.

LICHEN PLANUS

Etiology: Postulated to be a chronic mucocutaneous autoimmune disorder with a genetic predisposition that is initiated by a variety of factors, including emotional stress, hypersensitivity to drugs, dental products, or foods.

Clinical description: Lichen planus varies in clinical appearance. Oral forms of this disorder include lacy white lines representing Wickham's striae (reticular), an erythematous form (atrophic), and an ulcerating form that often is accompanied by striae peripheral to the ulceration (ulcerative).

The lesions are commonly found on the buccal mucosa, gingiva, and tongue, but they can be found on the lips and palate. Lichen planus lesions are chronic and also may affect the skin.

Any refractory lesion should be considered for biopsy to establish a diagnosis and to rule out a malignancy.

Rationale for treatment: To provide oral comfort if the lesions are symptomatic. No known cure exists. Systemic and local relief with antiinflammatory and immunosuppressant agents is indicated. Identification of any dietary component, dental product, or medication (lichenoid drug reaction) should be undertaken to ensure against a hypersensitivity reaction. Treatment or prevention of a secondary fungal infection with a systemic antifungal agent also should be considered.

Therapies with steroids and immunomodulating drugs are presented to inform the clinician that such modalities are available. Because of the potential for side effects, close collaboration with the patient's physician is recommended when these medications are prescribed. These modalities may be beyond the scope of clinical experience of general dentists, and referral to a specialist in oral medicine or to an appropriate physician may be necessary.

Topical steroids

Prolonged use of topical steroids (for a period >2 weeks of continuous use) may result in mucosal atrophy and secondary candidiasis and may increase the potential for systemic absorption. The prescribing of antifungal therapy with steroids may be necessary. Therapy with topical steroids, once the lichen planus is under control, should be tapered to alternate day therapy or less depending on control of the disease and the tendency for recurrence.

Rx

Fluocinonide (Lidex) gel 0.05%

Disp: 30-g tube

Sig: Coat the lesion with a thin film after each meal and at bedtime.

Rx

Dexamethasone (Decadron) elixir 0.5 mg/5 ml

Disp: 100 ml

Sig: Rinse with 1 teaspoonful for 2 minutes qid and spit out. Discontinue when lesions become asymptomatic.

Other topical steroid preparations (cream, gel ointment) include:

Ultra-Potent:

Clobetasol propionate (Temovate) 0.05%

Halobetasol propionate (Ultravate) 0.05%

Potent:

Dexamethasone (Decadron) 0.5 mg/5 ml

Fluocinonide (Lidex) 0.05%

Intermediate:

Betamethasone valerate (Valisone) 0.1%

Triamcinolone acetonide (Kenalog) 0.1%

Low:

Hydrocortisone 1%

Oral candidiasis may result from topical steroid therapy. The oral cavity should be monitored for emergence of fungal infection in patients who are placed on therapy. Prophylactic antifungal therapy should be initiated in patients with a history of fungal infection with prior steroid administration (see Candidiasis/Candidosis).

Systemic Steroids and Immunosuppressants

For Severe Cases

Rx
Dexamethasone (Decadron) elixir 0.5 mg/5 ml
Disp: 320 ml
Sig:
1. For 3 days, rinse with 1 tablespoonful (15 ml) qid and swallow. Then
2. For 3 days rinse with 1 teaspoonful (5 ml) qid and swallow. Then
3. For 3 days, rinse with 1 teaspoonful (5 ml) qid and swallow every other time. Then
4. Rinse with 1 teaspoonful (5 ml) qid and expectorate.

Rx
Prednisone tablets 10 mg
Disp: 26 tablets
Sig: Take 4 tablets in the morning for 5 days, then decrease by 1 tablet on each successive day.

Rx
Prednisone tablets 5 mg
Disp: 40 tablets
Sig: Take 5 tablets in the morning for 5 days, then 5 tablets in the morning every other day until gone. If oral discomfort recurs, the patient should return to the clinician for reevaluation.

Many studies suggest that oral lichen planus has an intrinsic property predisposing to malignant transformation. However, the etiology is complex, with interaction among genetic, infectious agents, environmental, and lifestyle factors. Prospective studies have demonstrated that lichen planus patients have a slightly increased risk to develop oral squamous cell carcinoma. All patients exhibiting lichen planus intraorally, particularly those who have had the ulcerative form, should receive periodic follow-up.

Therapy with medications such as systemic steroids, immunosuppressants, and immunomodulators is presented to inform the clinician that such modalities have been reported effective for patients suffering from ulcerative lichen planus. Medications such as azathioprine, mycophenolate mofetil, tacrolimus hydroxychloroquine sulfate, acitretin, and cyclosporin A are used to treat patients with severe persistent ulcerative lichen planus but should not be routinely used because of the potential for side effects. Close collaboration with the patient's physician is recommended when these medications are prescribed.

Pemphigus and Mucous Membrane Pemphigoid

Pemphigus and mucous membrane pemphigoid are relatively uncommon lesions. They should be suspected when chronic, multiple oral ulcerations and a history of oral and skin blisters exist. Often they may occur only in the mouth. Diagnosis is based on history and on histologic and immunofluorescent characteristics of a biopsy specimen of the primary lesion.

Etiology: Both are autoimmune diseases with autoantibodies against antigens appearing in different portions of the epithelium (mucosa). In pemphigus the antigens are within the epithelium (desmosomes), whereas in pemphigoid the antigens are located at the base of the epithelium in the hemidesmosomes.

Clinical description: In pemphigus the lesion may stay in one location for a long period of time with small placid bullae. The bullae may rupture, leaving an ulcer. Approximately 80% to 90% of patients have oral lesions. The oral manifestations are the first signs of the disease in approximately two thirds of patients. All parts of the mouth may be involved. The bullae rupture almost immediately in the mouth but may stay intact for some time on the skin. One of the classic signs, the Nikolsky's sign (blister formation induced with gentle rubbing of an affected mucosal site), is positive in pemphigus but is not pathognomic because it also has been found positive in other disorders. Because the vesicle or bullae are intraepithelial, they often are filled with clear fluid. Histologically, a cleavage (Tzanck cells, acantholytic cells) exist within the spinous layer of the epithelium.

In pemphigoid the cleavage or split is beneath the epithelium, resulting in bullae that usually are blood filled. Mucous membrane pemphigoid often is limited to the oral cavity, but some patients have ocular lesions (symblepharon, ankyloblepharon) that must be evaluated by an ophthalmologist. Gingiva is the most common oral site involved. Pemphigoid may appear clinically as a red, nonulcerated gingival lesion.

Rationale for treatment: Because both pemphigus and pemphigoid are autoimmune disorders, the primary treatment is topical or systemic steroids or other immunomodulating drugs. Custom trays can be used to localize topical steroid medications on the gingival tissues (occlusive therapy).

Because they can resemble other ulcerative bullous diseases, a biopsy is necessary for a definitive diagnosis. Specimens should be submitted for light microscopic, immunofluorescent, and immunologic testing. Because of the potential serious nature, referral to a specialist in oral medicine, dermatology, and ophthalmology must be considered. When eye lesions are present, an ophthalmologist must be consulted immediately to prevent blindness.

Therapy with medications such as systemic steroids, immunosuppressants, and immunomodulators are presented to inform the clinician that such modalities have been reported effective for patients suffering from vesiculobullous disorders such as pemphigus vulgaris and mucous membrane pemphigoid. Therapies such as dapsone, methotrexate, mycophenolate mofetil, cyclosporine A, niacinamide with tetracycline, and plasmapheresis are used to treat patients with vesiculobullous disorders such as pemphigus vulgaris and mucous membrane pemphigoid but should not be routinely used because of the potential for side effects. Close collaboration with the patient's physician is recommended when these medications are prescribed.

Injectable Steroids

Dexamethasone phosphate injectable, 1 ampule (4 mg/ml), can be used in the following manner. After anesthetizing the area with lidocaine, inject 0.5 to 1 ml around margins of ulcer with a 25-gauge needle twice per week until ulcer heals. Therapy with systemic or injectable steroids should be coordinated with the patient's physician because of side effects and potential systemic complications.

ORAL ERYTHEMA MULTIFORME

Etiology: Oral erythema multiforme is believed to be an autoimmune condition. It can occur at any age. Drug reactions to medications such as penicillin and sulfonamides may play a role in some cases. In a few patients who developed oral erythema multiforme, a herpetic infection occurred immediately before the onset of clinical signs.

Clinical description: Signs of oral erythema multiforme include "blood-crusted" lips, "targetoid" or "bull's-eye" skin lesions, and a nonspecific mucosal slough. The name *multiforme* is used because its appearance may take multiple different forms.

A severe form of erythema multiforme is called *Stevens-Johnson syndrome*, or erythema multiforme major. Erythema multiforme as a skin disease occurs most frequently because of an allergic reaction.

Rationale for treatment: Treatment is primarily anti-inflammatory in nature. Steroids are initiated then tapered. Because of the possible relationship or oral erythema multiforme with herpes simplex virus, suppressive antiviral therapy may be necessary before initiation of steroid therapy. Patients should be questioned carefully about a previous history of recurrent herpetic infections and prodromal symptoms that might have preceded the onset of erythema multiforme.

Dosing must be titrated to specific situations.

Steroid Therapy

Rx
Prednisone tablets 10 mg
Disp: 100 tablets
Sig: Take 6 tablets in the morning until lesions recede, then decrease by 1 tablet on each successive day.

Suppressive Antiviral Therapy

Renew as needed to following:

Rx
Acyclovir (Zovirax) capsules 400 mg
Disp: 90 capsules
Sig: Take 1 tablet 3 times per day.

Rx
Valacyclovir (Valtrex) capsules 500 mg
Disp: 30 capsules
Sig: Take 1 tablet per day.

DENTURE SORE MOUTH

Etiology: Discomfort under oral prosthetic appliances may result from combinations of candidal infections, poor denture hygiene, an occlusive syndrome, overextension, or excessive movement of the appliance. This condition may be erroneously attributed to an allergy to denture material, which is a rare occurrence. The retention and fit of the denture should be idealized, and mechanical irritation should be ruled out.

Clinical description: The tissue covered by the appliance, especially one made of acrylic, is erythematous and smooth or granular, and it may be asymptomatic or associated with burning.

Rationale for treatment: Therapy is directed toward controlling all possible etiologies and improving oral comfort. If therapy is ineffective, consider underlying systemic conditions such as diabetes mellitus and poor nutrition.

Treatment:

1. Institute appropriate antifungal medication (see Candidiasis/Candidosis).
2. Improve oral and appliance hygiene. The patient may have to leave the appliance out for extended periods of time and should be instructed to leave the denture out overnight.

The appliance should be soaked in a commercially available denture cleanser or soaked in a 1% sodium hypochlorite solution (1 teaspoon of sodium hypochlorite in a denture cup of water) for 15 minutes and thoroughly rinsed for at least 2 minutes under running water.

3. Reline, rebase, or construct a new appliance.
4. Apply an artificial saliva or oral lubricant gel, such as Laclede Oral Balance or Sage gel, to the tissue contact surface of the denture to reduce frictional trauma.

If all the above actions fail to control symptoms, a biopsy or short trial of topical steroid therapy can be used to rule out contact mucositis (an allergic reaction to denture materials). If a therapeutic trial fails to resolve the condition, a biopsy should be performed to establish the diagnosis.

BURNING MOUTH SYNDROME

Etiology: Multiple conditions have been implicated in the causation of burning mouth syndrome. Current literature favors neurogenic, vascular, and psychogenic etiologies. However, other conditions such as xerostomia, candidiasis, referred pain from the tongue musculature, chronic infections, reflux of gastric acid, medications, blood dyscrasias, nutritional deficiencies, hormonal imbalances, and allergic and inflammatory disorders must be considered.

Clinical description: Burning mouth syndrome is characterized by the absence of clinical signs.

Rationale for treatment: To reduce discomfort by addressing possible etiologic factors.

Treatment: On the basis of the history, physical evaluation, and specific laboratory studies, rule out all possible organic etiologies. Minimal blood studies should include CBC and differential, fasting glucose, iron, ferritin, folic acid, and B_{12} levels, and thyroid profile (TSH, T_3, T_4).

Rx

Diphenhydramine (Children's Benadryl) elixir 12.5 mg/5 ml (OTC)
Disp: 1 bottle
Sig: Rinse with 1 teaspoon for 2 minutes before each meal and swallow.

Children's Benadryl is alcohol free.

When the burning mouth is considered psychogenic or idiopathic, a tricyclic or benzodiazepine in low doses exhibits the properties of analgesia and sedation and frequently is successful in reducing or eliminating the symptoms after several weeks or months. The dosage is adjusted according to patient reaction and clinical symptomatology.

Rx

Clonazepam (Klonopin) tablets 0.5 mg
Disp: 100 tablets
Sig: Take 1 tablet tid, then adjust dose after 3-day intervals.

This therapy probably is best managed by an appropriate specialist or the patient's physician at this time.

Rx

Amitriptyline (Elavil) tablets 25 mg
Disp: 50 tablets
Sig: Take 1 tablet at bedtime for 1 week, then 2 tablets HS. Increase to 3 tablets HS after 2 weeks and maintain at that dosage or titrate as appropriate.

Rx

Chlordiazepoxide (Librium) tablets 5 mg
Disp: 50 tablets
Sig: Take 1 or 2 tablets tid.

Rx

Alprazolam (Xanax) tablets 0.25 mg
Disp: 50 tablets
Sig: Take 1 tablet tid.

Rx
Diazepam (Valium) tablets 2 mg
Disp: 50 tablets
Sig: Take 1 or 2 tablets.

The dosage should be adjusted according to the patient's response. Anticipated side effects are dry mouth and morning drowsiness. The rationale for use of tricyclic antidepressants and other psychotropic drugs should be thoroughly explained to the patient, and the patient's physician should be made aware of the therapy. Those medications have a potential for addiction and dependence.

Rx
Tabasco sauce (Capsaicin) (OTC)
Disp: 1 bottle
Sig: Place 1 part Tabasco sauce in 2–4 parts of water. Rinse for 1 minute qid and expectorate.

Rx
Capsaicin (Zostrix) cream 0.025% (OTC)
Disp: 1 tube
Sig: Apply sparingly to affected site(s) qid.
Wash hands after each application and do not use near the eyes. Topical capsaicin may improve the burning sensation in some individuals. As with topical capsaicin, an increase in discomfort for a 2- to 3-week period should be anticipated.

CHAPPED OR CRACKED LIPS

Etiology: Alternate wetting and drying, resulting in inflammation and possible secondary infection.
Clinical description: The surface of the vermilion is rough and peeling and may be ulcerated with crusting. The normal vertical fissuring may be lost.
Rationale for treatment: An interrupted and chronically inflamed surface invites secondary infection. An antiinflammatory agent in a petrolatum or adhesive base will interrupt the irritating factors and allow healing.

Rx
Betamethasone valerate (Valisone) ointment 0.1%
Disp: 15-g tube
Sig: Apply to lips after each meal and at bedtime.

Prolonged use of corticosteroids can result in thinning of the tissue. Their use should be closely monitored.

For maintenance, the frequent application of lip care products (e.g., Blistex, Chapstick, Vaseline, or cocoa butter) should be suggested.

If the lesions do not resolve with treatment, consider biopsy to rule out dysplasia or malignancy.

GINGIVAL ENLARGEMENT

Etiology: Phenytoin sodium (Dilantin), calcium channel-blocking agents (nifedipine and others), and cyclosporine therapy are drugs known to predispose some patients to gingival enlargement. Blood dyscrasias and hereditary fibromatosis should be ruled out by history and indicated laboratory tests.
Clinical description: The gingival tissues, especially in the anterior region, are dense, resilient, insensitive, and enlarged but essentially of normal color.
Rationale for treatment: Local factors, such as plaque and calculus accumulation, contribute to secondary inflammation and the hyperplastic process. This further interferes with plaque control. Specific drugs tend to deplete serum folic acid levels, which result in compromised tissue integrity. Folic acid and drug serum levels should be determined every 6 months. This should be coordinated with the patient's physician.

Treatment: Consists of (1) meticulous plaque control, (2) gingivoplasty when indicated, and (3) folic acid oral rinse.

Rx

Folic acid oral rinse 1 mg/ml
Disp: 16 oz
Sig: Rinse with 1 teaspoonful for 2 minutes bid and spit out.

Rx

Chlorhexidine gluconate (Peridex) 0.12%
Disp: 16 oz
Sig: Rinse with 1/2 oz bid for 30 seconds and spit out.

TASTE DISORDERS

Etiology: Taste acuity may be affected by neurologic and physiologic changes and by drugs. Diagnostic procedures should first rule out a neurologic deficiency, olfactory deficit, and systemic influences such as malnutrition, metabolic disturbances, drugs, chemical and physical trauma, and radiation sequelae. Blood tests for trace elements should be conducted to identify any deficiencies.

Rationale for treatment: A reduction in salivary flow may concentrate the electrolytes in the saliva, resulting in a salty or metallic taste (see treatment for xerostomia.) A deficiency of zinc has been associated with a loss of taste (and smell) sensation.

For Zinc Replacement (In Patients with Proven Zinc Deficiency)

Rx

Orazinc capsules 220 mg (OTC)
Disp: 100 capsules
Sig: Take 1 capsule with milk 3 times per day for at least 1 month.

Rx

Z-Bec tablets (OTC)
Disp: 60 tablets
Sig: Take 1 tablet per day with food or after meals.

MANAGEMENT OF PATIENTS RECEIVING ANTINEOPLASTIC AGENTS AND RADIATION THERAPY

Etiology: Cancer chemotherapy and radiation to the head and neck tend to reduce the volume and alter the character of the saliva. The balance of the oral flora is disrupted, allowing overgrowth of opportunistic organisms (e.g., *C. albicans*). Anticancer therapy damages fast-growing tissues, especially the oral mucosa.

Clinical description: The oral mucosa becomes red and inflamed. The saliva is viscous or absent.

Rationale for treatment: The treatment of these patients is symptomatic and supportive. Patient education, frequent monitoring, and close cooperation with the patient's physician are important. The oral discomfort may be relieved with topical anesthetics, such as diphenhydramine elixir (Benadryl) and dyclonine (Dyclone). Artificial salivas (i.e., Sage Moist Plus, Moi-Stir, Salivart, Xero-Lube) will reduce oral dryness. Mouth moisturizing gels (i.e., Sage Mouth Moisturizer or Oral Balance gel) may be helpful. Nystatin and clotrimazole preparations will control fungal overgrowth. Chlorhexidine rinses help control plaque and candidiasis. Fluorides are applied for caries control. The patient information sheet that follows this topic can be reproduced and given to the patient.

Mouth Rinses

Rx

Alkaline saline (salt/bicarbonate) mouth rinse. (Mix 1/2 teaspoonful each of salt and baking soda in a glass of water)
Sig: Rinse with copious amounts qid.

Commercially available as Sage Salt and Soda Rinse.

Gingivitis Control

Rx

Chlorhexidine gluconate mouthwash (Peridex) 0.12%

Disp: 32 oz

Sig: Rinse with 1/2 oz bid for 30 seconds and spit out. Avoid rinsing or eating for 30 minutes following treatment. (Rinse after breakfast and at bedtime.)

In xerostomic patients, chlorhexidine (Peridex) should be used concurrently with artificial saliva to provide the needed protein-binding agent for efficacy and substantivity.

Caries Control

(See Xerostomia)

Rx

Neutral NaF gel (Thera-Flur-N) 1.0%

Disp: 24 ml

Sig: Place 1 drop per tooth in the custom tray; apply for 5 minutes daily. Avoid rinsing or eating for 30 minutes after treatment.

Topical Anesthetics

Rx

Diphenhydramine (Benadryl) elixir 12.5 mg/5 ml. 4 oz, mixed with Kaopectate (OTC) 4 oz (to make a 50% mixture by volume).

Disp: 8 oz

Sig: Rinse with 1 teaspoonful every 2 hours and spit out.

Maalox (OTC) can be used in place of Kaopectate. Dyclonine (Dyclone) HCl 0.5% 1 oz can be added to the above for greater anesthetic efficacy.

Rx

Diphenhydramine (Benadryl) elixir 12.5 mg/5 ml.

(*Note:* Elixir is Rx and syrup [Benylin] is OTC.)

Disp: 4-oz bottle

Sig: Rinse with 1 teaspoonful for 2 minutes before each meal and spit out.

Rx

Clotrimazole (Mycelex) troches 10 mg

Disp: 70 troches

Sig: Let 1 troche dissolve in the mouth 5 times per day.

Rx

Nystatin pastilles 200,000 units

Disp: 50 pastilles

Sig: Let 1 pastille dissolve in the mouth 5 times per day.

(See Candidiasis for additional antifungal therapy.)

KEY POINTS TO REMEMBER

- When topical anesthetics are used, patients should be warned about a reduced gag reflex and the need for caution while eating and drinking to avoid possible airway compromise. Allergies are rare but may occur.
- In immunocompromised patients, herpes simplex virus lesions can occur on any mucosal surface and may have atypical appearances. They can resemble major aphthae and allergic responses.
- Mixing ointments with equal parts of Orabase promotes adhesion.
- Therapy with systemic steroids and immunosuppressants is presented to inform the clinician that such modalities are available. Because of the potential for side effects, close collaboration with the patient's physician is recommended when these medications are prescribed.
- Although some consultants disagree with the use of vaginal creams intraorally, the efficacy of the creams has been observed clinically in selected cases in which other topical antifungal agents have failed.
- Generic carboxymethyl cellulose solutions may be prepared by a pharmacist. These cholinergics should be prescribed in consultation with a physician because of significant side effects.

• The rationale for use of tricyclic antidepressants and other psychotropic drugs should be thoroughly explained to patients, and their physician also should be made aware of the therapy. These medications have a potential for addiction and dependency.

• When testing for serum folate level, it is judicious to also check for the vitamin B_{12} level because a B_{12} deficiency can be masked by the patient's use of folic acid supplement. The phenytoin level also should be assessed for future reference.

Patient Information Sheet

The oral regimen for patients receiving chemotherapy and radiotherapy is outlined earlier in this chapter. The following are general guidelines to be individualized by your doctor. Follow your doctor's advice or discuss any questions with your doctor if these guidelines differ from what you have been told or have heard.

A. RINSES

1. Rinse with warm, dilute solution of sodium bicarbonate (baking soda) or salt and bicarbonate every 2 hours to bathe the tissues and control oral acidity. Take 2 teaspoonfuls of bicarbonate (or 1 teaspoonful of table salt plus 1 teaspoonful of bicarbonate) per quart of water.
2. If you are experiencing pain, rinse with 1 teaspoonful of elixir of Benadryl before each meal. Be careful when eating while your mouth is numb to avoid choking.
3. If your mouth is dry, sip cool water frequently (every 10 minutes) all day long. Allowing ice chips to melt in the mouth is comforting. Artificial salivas (e.g., Moi-Stir, Salivart, Xero-Lube, Orex) can be used as frequently as needed to make the mouth moist and "slick." Keep the lips lubricated with petrolatum or a lanolin-containing lip preparation. Commercial mouth rinses containing alcohol or coffee, tea, and colas should be avoided because they tend to dry the mouth.
4. If an oral yeast infection develops, antifungal medications can be prescribed.
   a. Nystatin pastille,* let one dissolve in mouth 5 times per day or
   b. Let a 10-mg clotrimazole (Mycelex)* troche dissolve in the mouth 5 times per day.

B. CARE OF TEETH AND GUMS

1. Floss your teeth after each meal. Be careful not to cut the gums.
2. Brush your teeth after each meal. Use a soft even-bristle brush and a bland toothpaste containing fluoride (e.g., Aim, Crest, Colgate). Brushing with a sodium bicarbonate–water paste is also helpful. Arm & Hammer Dental Care toothpaste and tooth powder are bicarbonate based. If a toothbrush is too irritating, cotton-tip swabs (Q-Tips) or foam sticks (Toothettes) can provide some mechanical cleaning.

*Drugs that must be prescribed by your dentist or physician.

Continued

3. A pulsating water device (e.g., Water-Pik) will remove loose debris. Use warm water with a half teaspoonful of salt and baking soda and low pressure to prevent damage to tissue.
4. Have custom, flexible vinyl trays made by your dentist to self-apply fluoride gel to the teeth for 5 minutes once per day after brushing.
5. Rinse with an antiplaque solution (Peridex) (if prescribed by your dentist) 2 or 3 times per day when you cannot follow other oral hygiene procedures.
6. Follow any alternative oral hygiene instructions prescribed by your dentist.

C. NUTRITION

Adequate nutrition and fluid intake are very important for oral and general health. Use diet supplements (e.g., Carnation Instant Breakfast, Meritene, Ensure). If your mouth is sore, a blender can be used to soften food.

D. MAINTENANCE

Have your oral health status reevaluated at regularly scheduled intervals by your dentist.

E. SUPPORTIVE

A humidifier in the sleeping area will alleviate or reduce nighttime oral dryness.

The above regimen is also applicable to patients with AIDS.

Suggested Readings

1. Boger J, Araujo O, Flowers F: Sunscreens: efficacy, use and misuse, *South Med J* 77:1421-1427, 1984.
2. Brooke RI, Sapp JP: Herpetiform ulceration, *Oral Surg Oral Med Oral Pathol* 42:182-188, 1976.
3. Brown RS, Bottomley WK: Combination immunosuppressant and topical steroid therapy for treatment of recurrent major aphthae, *Oral Surg Oral Med Oral Pathol* 69:42-44, 1990.
4. Browning S, et al: The association between burning mouth syndrome and psychosocial disorders, *Oral Surg Oral Med Oral Pathol* 64:171-174, 1987.
5. Burns RA, Davis WJ: Recurrent aphthous stomatitis, *Am Fam Physician* 32:99-104, 1988.
6. Bystryn JC: Adjuvant therapy of pemphigus, *Arch Dermatol* 120: 941-951, 1984.
7. Dilley D, Blozis G: Common oral lesions and oral manifestations of systemic illnesses and therapies, *Pediatr Clin North Am* 29:585-611, 1982.
8. Drew H, et al: Effect of folate on phenytoin hyperplasia, *J Clin Periodontol* 14:350-356, 1987.
9. Duxbury AJ, et al: Clinical trial of a mucin-containing artificial saliva, *IRCS Med Sci* 13:1197-1198, 1985.
10. Fardal O, Turnbull RS: A review of the literature on use of chlorhexidine in dentistry, J Am Dent Assoc 112:863-869, 1986.
11. Feinmann C: Pain relief by antidepressants: possible modes of action, *Pain* 23:1-8, 1985.
12. Fenske NA, Greenberg SS: Solar-induced skin changes, *Am Fam Physician* 25:109-117, 1982.

13. Fharav V, et al: The analgesic effect of amitriptyline on chronic facial pain, *Pain* 31:199-207, 1987.
14. Fox PC, et al: Systemic therapy of salivary gland hypofunction, *J Dent Res* 66:689-692, 1987 (special issue).
15. Gabriel SA, et al: Lichen planus: possible mechanisms of pathogenesis, *J Oral Med* 40:56-59, 1985.
16. Gorsku M, Silverman S, Chinn H: Clinical characteristics and management outcome in the burning mouth syndrome, *Oral Surg Oral Med Oral Pathol* 72:192-195, 1991.
17. Gorsline J, Bradlow HL, Sherman MR: Triamcinolone acetonide 21-oic acid methyl ester: a potent local anti-inflammatory steroid without detectable systemic effects, *Endocrinology* 116:263-273, 1985.
18. Greenberg MS: Oral herpes simplex infections in immunosuppressed patients, *Compendium* 9(suppl): 289-291, 1988.
19. Grushka M: Clinical features of burning mouth syndrome, *Oral Surg Oral Med Oral Pathol* 63:30-36, 1987.
20. Hay KD, Reade PC: The use of an elimination diet in the treatment of recurrent aphthous ulceration of the oral cavity, *Oral Surg Oral Med Oral Pathol* 57:504-507, 1984.
21. Holst E: Natamycin and nystatin for treatment of oral candidiasis during and after radiotherapy, *J Prosthet Dent* 51:226-231, 1984.
22. Huff JC et al: Therapy of herpes zoster with oral acyclovir, *Am J Med* 85:85-89, 1988.
23. Hughes WT, et al: Ketoconazole and candidiasis: a controlled study, *J Infect Dis* 147:1060-1063, 1983.
24. Katz S: The use of fluoride and chlorhexidine for the prevention of radiation caries, *J Am Dent Assoc* 104:164-169, 1982.
25. Lamey PJ, et al: Vitamin status of patients with burning mouth syndrome and the response to replacement therapy, *Br Dent J* 160:81-84, 1986.
26. Lang NP, Brecx MC: Chlorhexidine digluconate–an agent for chemical plaque control and prevention of gingival inflammation, *J Periodont Res* 43(suppl):74-89, 1986.
27. Lever WF, Schaumburg-Lever G: Treatment of pemphigus vulgaris: results obtained in 84 patients between 1961 and 1982, *Arch Dermatol* 120:44-47, 1984.
28. Lozada F, Silverman S Jr, Migliorati C: Adverse side effects associated with prednisone in the treatment of patients with oral inflammatory ulcerative diseases, *J Am Dent Assoc* 109:269-270, 1984.
29. Lucatorto FM, et al: Treatment of refractory oral candidiasis with fluconazole: A case report, *Oral Surg Oral Med Oral Pathol* 71:42-44, 1991.
30. Lundeen RC, Langlais RP, Terezhalmy GT: Sunscreen protection for lip mucosa: a review and update, *J Am Dent Assoc* 111:617-621, 1985.
31. O'Neil T, Figures K: The effects of chlorhexidine and mechanical methods of plaque control on the recurrence of gingival hyperplasia in young patients taking phenytoin, *Br Dent J* 152:130-133, 1982.
32. Owens NJ, et al: Prophylaxis of oral candidiasis with clotrimazole troches, *Arch Intern Med* 144:290-293, 1984.
33. Poland JM: The spectrum of HSV-1 infections in nonimmunosuppressed patients, *Compendium* 9(suppl): 310-312, 1988.
34. Porter SR, Sculy C, Flint S: Hematologic status in recurrent aphthous stomatitis compared with other oral disease, *Oral Surg Oral Med Oral Pathol* 66:41-44, 1988.
35. Raborn GW, et al: Oral acyclovir and herpes labialis: a randomized, double-blind, placebo-controlled study, *J Am Dent Assoc* 11:38-42, 1987.
36. Rhodus NL, et al: Candia albicans levels in patients with Sjögren's syndrome before and after long-term use of pilocarpine hydrochloride, *Quintessence Int* 29:705-710, 1998.
37. Rhodus, NL, Schuh, MJ: The effects of pilocarpine on salivary flow in patients with Sjögren's syndrome, *Oral Surg Oral Med Oral Pathol* 72:545-549.36, 1991

38. Rowe NJ: Diagnosis and treatment of herpes simplex virus disease, *Compendium* 9(suppl):292-295, 1988.
39. Schiffman SS: Taste and smell in disease (pts a and b), *N Engl J Med* 308:1275-1279, 1337-1343, 1983.
40. Scully C, Mason DK: Therapeutic measures in oral medicine. In Jones JH, Mason DK, editors: *Oral manifestations of systemic disease*, London, 1980, WB Saunders.
41. Silverman S Jr, et al: Oral mucous membrane pemphigoid, *Oral Surg Oral Med Oral Pathol* 61:233-237, 1986.
42. Silverman S, et al: A prospective of findings and management in 214 patients with oral lichen planus, *Oral Surg Oral Med Oral Pathol* 72:665-670, 1991.
43. Sonis ST, Sonis AL, Lieberman A: Oral complications in patients receiving treatment for malignancies other than of the head and neck, *JAMA* 97:468-471, 1978.
44. Straus SE, moderator: Herpes simplex virus infection: biology, treatment, and prevention, *Ann Intern Med* 103:404-419, 1985.
45. Thompson PJ, et al: Assessment of oral candidiasis in patients with respiratory disease and efficacy of a new nystatin formulation, *Br Med J* 292:699-700, 1986.
46. Vincent SD, et al: Oral lichen planus: the clinical, historical and therapeutic features of 100 cases, *Oral Surg Oral Med Oral Pathol* 70:165-171, 1990.
47. Wood MJ, et al: Efficacy of oral acyclovir treatment of acute herpes zoster, *Am J Med* 85:79-83, 1988.
48. Wright WE, et al: An oral disease prevention program for patients receiving radiation and chemotherapy, *J Am Dent Assoc* 110:43-47, 1985.

ENDOCARDITIS AND ENDARTERITIS PREVENTION

The American Heart Association (AHA) recommends that patients with prosthetic heart valves, history of endocarditis, single-ventricle states, tetralogy of Fallot, acquired heart valve dysfunction, hypertrophic cardiomyopathy, or mitral valve prolapse with regurgitation receive antibiotic prophylaxis prior to certain dental procedures to prevent bacterial endocarditis. The dental procedures recommended for prophylaxis include extractions; periodontal surgery, scaling, root planning, probing, and recall maintenance; placement of dental implants; reimplantation of avulsed teeth; endodontic instrumentation or surgery only beyond the apex; subgingival placement of antibiotic fibers/strips; initial placement of orthodontic bands but not brackets; intraligamentary local anesthetic injections; and prophylactic cleaning of teeth or implants when bleeding is anticipated.

The most current set of guidelines were published in 1997.

The AHA is expected to publish new guidelines sometime in 2006.

Standard regimen:
- Amoxicillin 2 g orally, 1 hour before procedure

Patients unable to take oral medications:
- Ampicillin 2 g IV, 30 minutes before procedure

Patients allergic to penicillin:
- Clindamycin 600 mg orally, 1 hour before procedure

Patients allergic to penicillin and unable to take oral medicines:
- Clindamycin 600 mg/kg IV, 30 minutes before procedure

NONVALVULAR CARDIOVASCULAR DEVICE–RELATED INFECTIONS

In 2003, the AHA published guidelines regarding the use of antibiotic prophylaxis for patients with nonvalvular cardiovascular devices undergoing dental, respiratory, gastrointestinal, or genitourinary procedures. The devices considered included pacemakers, defibrillators, total artificial hearts, ventriculoatrial shunts, patent ductus arteriosus occlusion devices (plugs, umbrellas, buttons, discs, embolization coils), atrial septal defect and ventricular septal defect closure devices (Bard clamshell occluders, discs, buttons, double umbrellas), conduits, patches, peripheral vascular stents, vascular grafts (including hemodialysis), coronary artery stents, and vena caval filters.

Antibiotic prophylaxis is not routinely recommended after device placement for patients undergoing dental procedures. It is recommended for dental patients having these devices if they undergo incision and drainage of oral abscesses. Antibiotic prophylaxis also is recommended for patients with residual leak after device placement for attempted closure of the leak associated with patent ductus arteriosus, atrial septal defect, or ventricular septal defect. In these patients, prophylaxis is indicated for the dental procedures listed in the Endocarditis section. Also, the antibiotic regimens listed in that section can be used as indicated by presence or absence of penicillin allergy.

ORTHOPEDIC DEVICES: SCREWS, PLATES, PINS, AND PROSTHETIC JOINTS

In 1997 and 2002, the American Dental Association (ADA) and the

American Academy of Orthopedic Surgeons (AAOS) jointly published an advisory on antibiotic prophylaxis for dental patients with total joint replacements. Antibiotic prophylaxis was not indicated for patients with pins, plates, or pins. Antibiotic prophylaxis was not suggested for most patients with total joint replacements. However, they do suggest that prophylaxis **be considered** for patients who may be at "high risk" for hematogenous infection, including patients with inflammatory arthropathies, immunosuppression, type 1 diabetes mellitus, joint replacement within 2 years, previous prosthetic joint infection (PJI), malnourishment, or hemophilia. (Of note, there is no evidence that even these "higher-risk" patients are at increased risk from dentally induced bacteremias. In fact, the microbiology of PJI in these "higher-risk" patients is the same as for other patients with PJI. A more appropriate interpretation is that these patients are at increased risk for PJI from the usual sources, such as wound contamination and acute infection from distant sites.)

The advisory statement also makes clear that the final decision as to whether or not to provide antibiotic prophylaxis lies with the dentist, who must weigh perceived potential benefits against the risks. The advisory statement provides suggested antibiotic regimens should the practitioner elect to provide antibiotic prophylaxis. If prophylaxis is selected, it should be used only for the dental procedures listed in the Endocarditis section.

Nonallergic (penicillin) patients:
- Amoxicillin 2 g orally, 1 hour before dental procedure
- Cephalexin 2 g orally, 1 hour before dental procedure

Patients allergic to penicillin:
- Clindamycin 600 mg orally, 1 hour before dental procedure

ADRENAL INSUFFICIENCY (PRIMARY AND SECONDARY): PREVENTION OF ADRENAL CRISIS

Patients with primary (Addison's disease) or secondary (exogenous corticosteroid induced) adrenal insufficiency may be at risk for adrenal crisis during or following surgical procedures performed in dentistry. Adrenal crisis is a medical emergency that requires prompt intervention to save the patient's life. In order to prevent adrenal crisis, supplemental steroids in rather large doses have been recommended since the mid 1950s for patients with adrenal insufficiency. Adrenal crisis is a rare event in dentistry, especially in patients with secondary adrenal insufficiency. Four factors appear to be associated with the risk for adrenal crisis: (1) magnitude of surgery, (2) general anesthesia, (3) health status and stability of the patient, and (4) degree of pain control.

The most significant acute adverse outcome of adrenal insufficiency is adrenal crisis. This event can occur when a patient with adrenal insufficiency, most commonly Addison's disease, is challenged by stress (e.g., illness, infection, or surgery) and in response is unable to synthesize adequate amounts of cortisol and aldosterone. This potentially life-threatening emergency usually evolves slowly over a few hours and then is manifested by severe exacerbation of the condition, including profuse sweating, hypotension, weak pulse, cyanosis, nausea, vomiting, weakness, headache, dehydration, fever, sunken eyes, dyspnea, myalgias, arthralgia, hyponatremia, and eosinophilia.

If not treated rapidly, the patient may develop hypothermia, severe hypotension, hypoglycemia, confusion, and circulatory collapse that can culminate in death.

Four factors appear to contribute to the risk of "adrenal crisis" during the perioperative period of oral surgery: (1) magnitude of surgery, (2) general anesthesia, (3) overall health of the patient (e.g., stable vs. ongoing infection) and (4) degree of pain control.

Negligible Risk: Nonsurgical Dental Procedures

The vast majority of patients with adrenal insufficiency can undergo routine, nonsurgical dental treatment without the need for supplemental glucocorticoids. This is supported by the fact that routine, nonsurgical dental procedures do not stimulate cortisol production at levels comparable to oral surgery, and local anesthesia blocks neural stress pathways required for adrenocorticotropic hormone (ACTH) secretion. This guideline does not advocate dental treatment on patients whose adrenal insufficiency is uncontrolled or undiagnosed. However, stable patients with adrenal insufficiency and those with a history of steroid use in whom glucocorticoid medication was discontinued prior to surgery have withstood general surgical procedures without developing adrenal crisis.

Mild-Risk Regimen

For minor oral and periodontal surgery (e.g., few simple extractions, soft tissue surgery), evidence suggests that adrenal insufficiency is prevented when **circulating levels of glucocorticoids are** approximately **25 mg hydrocortisone equivalent per day. This is equivalent to a dose of approximately 5 mg prednisone.** The clinician should confirm that the patient has taken the recommended amount of steroid within 2 hours of the surgical procedure and schedule the surgery in the morning when normal cortisol levels are highest. Stress reduction measures should be implemented. Benefits can be gained from use of (1) oral, inhalation, or intravenous sedation, which provides stress reduction; (2) intravenous fluids (i.e., 5% dextrose), which can prevent hypovolemia and hypoglycemia; (3) long-acting local anesthetics; and (4) adequate postoperative analgesics.

Moderate-Risk to Major-Risk Regimen

Adrenally insufficient patients undergoing major oral surgery are at increased risk for adrenal crisis when compared with minor surgery. Major surgical procedures are more stressful than minor surgical procedures. They increase the demand for cortisol because of postoperative pain. Blood loss is greater, thus increasing the risk for hypovolemia and hypotension.

For major oral surgical stress (multiple extractions, quadrant periodontal surgery, extraction of bony impactions, osseous surgery, osteomy, bone resections, cancer surgery), surgical procedures involving use of general anesthesia, procedures lasting more than 1 hour, or procedures associated with significant blood loss, **the glucocorticoid target is approximately 50 to 100 mg/day hydrocortisone equivalent for the day of surgery and at least 1 postoperative day.** Higher doses may be necessary if excessive bleeding or complications are encountered. Patients should take their normal steroid dose prior to the procedure and be provided supplemental intravenous hydrocortisone intraoperatively to achieve a total of 100 mg. Hospitalization should be considered for these patients because blood pressure can be more closely monitored postoperatively in this setting. Hydrocortisone 25 mg usually is prescribed every 8 hours following surgery for 24 to 48 hours, depending on the procedure and anticipated level of postoperative pain.

Following the recommendations listed will further minimize the risk of adrenal crisis associated with surgical stress in adrenally insufficient individuals:

- Define the risk for adrenal insufficiency with a thorough medical history and clinical examination. Patients with a past or present history of tuberculosis or human immunodeficiency virus infection are at increased risk for adrenal insufficiency because opportunistic infectious agents can attack the adrenal glands.
- Ensure that adrenally insufficient patients take their glucocorticoid prior to a stressful surgery.
- Schedule surgery in the morning when cortisol levels normally are highest.
- Provide proper stress reduction because anxiety can increase cortisol demand.
- Minor surgeries require minimal steroid coverage. The patient's customary daily dose usually is sufficient.
- Major surgeries and those procedures lasting more than 1 hour or requiring use of general anesthesia should be performed in a hospital with steroid supplementation.
- Use of nitrous oxide-oxygen or intravenous or oral benzodiazepine sedation is helpful, as plasma cortisol levels are not reduced by these agents.
- Avoid outpatient general anesthesia, as general anesthesia increases glucocorticoid demand. Also, avoid use of barbiturates, which increase the metabolism of cortisol and reduce blood levels of cortisol.

SUMMARY OF NEED FOR SUPPLEMENTATION

Negligible-Risk Category

Nonsurgical dental procedures

Regimen: No supplementation required.

Mild-Risk Category

Minor oral surgery
- Few simple extractions, biopsy

Minor periodontal surgery

Regimen: Target 25 mg hydrocortisone equivalent (5 mg prednisone), day of surgery

Moderate-Risk to Major-Risk Category

Major oral surgery
- Multiple extractions
- Quadrant periodontal surgery
- Extraction of bony impactions
- Osseous surgery
- Osteomy
- Bone resections
- Cancer surgery
- Surgical procedures involving use of general anesthesia
- Procedures lasting more than 1 hour
- Procedures associated with significant blood loss

Regimen: Target glucocorticoid target is approximately 50 to 100 mg/day hydrocortisone equivalent, day of surgery and at least 1 postoperative day.

CONTROL OF BLEEDING IN PATIENTS ON ANTICOAGULANT THERAPY

If the history establishes that a patient is receiving one of the coumarin drugs, the dentist should consult the patient's physician regarding the patient's reason for taking the drug and the level of anticoagulation reported as the international normalized ratio (INR). Most patients are held at an INR of approximately 2 to 3, whereas patients with mechanical prosthetic heart valves are held at an INR of 2.5 to 3.5. The AMA and the ADA suggest that an INR value 2 and 3 before a surgical procedure is attempted. Local measures can be used to control bleeding if it occurs.

In patients with INR >3, the dentist should consult with the patient's physician regarding possible reduction of the anticoagulant dosage before surgery. Minor surgery usually can be performed safely in patients with an INR up to 3.5. In general, treating these patients without reducing the anticoagulant dose is safer than stopping the anticoagulant. Current information does not support stopping the drug, which increases the risk for thrombotic events. If the physician desires a reduced dosage, he or she will direct the patient to reduce the anticoagulant dosage. At least 3 to 4 days must pass before the effect of the reduced dosage will be reflected in a decreased INR. The INR value should be checked on the scheduled day of surgery to be certain that the desired reduction of anticoagulation effect has occurred.

If acute infection is present, surgery should be delayed until the infection has been treated. When the patient is free of acute infection and the INR is ≤3.5, surgery can be performed. The procedure should be done with as little trauma as possible. If excessive postoperative bleeding (slow blood flow and oozing) occurs, one or more of the following measures can be used to control it:

Use a splint constructed before surgery (in cases with multiple extractions)

Pressure using gauze pack

Absorbable gelatin sponge (Gelfoam)

Dental packing blocks: 20 × 20 × 7 mm, can be cut to fit and applied to bleeding site.

Powder: Apply to bleeding site.

Gelfoam with thrombin

Thrombogen: Powder with isotonic saline diluent (5,000-unit container with isotonic saline). For bleeding from skin or mucosa, use solution of 100 units/ml. Do not use with Oxycel, Surgicel, or microfibrillar collagen because they inactivate the thrombin.

Oxidized cellulose (Oxycel)

Pad: 3 3 inch; pledget: 2 × 1 × 1 inch; strip: 18 × 2, 5 × ½, 36 × ½ inch. Cut to appropriate size and apply dry.

Tranexamic acid (Cyklokapron)

Solution: 100 mg/ml in 10-ml vials; tablets: 500 mg, after surgery 25 mg/kg orally tid.

Oxidized regenerated cellulose (Surgicel absorbable hemostat)

Surgicel sheets: 2 × 14, 4 × 8, 2 × 3, ½ × 2 inch; Surgicel Nu-Knit sheets: 1 × 1, 3 × 4, 6 × 9 inch. Pick appropriate size and lay over extraction site to control bleeding.

Microfibrillar collagen hemostat (Avitene, CollaTape, Instat MCH)

Avitene sheets: 35 × 35, 70 × 35, 70 × 70 mm; CollaTape: 1 × 3, ¾ × 1½, ⅜ × ¾ inch.

Instat MCH: Coherent fibers packaged in 0.5- and 1.0-g containers. Apply topically, and it adheres firmly to bleeding surfaces.

Collagen hemostat
Pads: 1 × 2, 3 × 4 inch. Apply directly to bleeding surface with pressure. It is more effective when applied dry.

MANAGEMENT OF ANXIETY IN THE DENTAL PATIENT

Anxiety

The dentist may detect anxiety in a patient on the basis of his or her physical appearance, speech, dress, and presence of certain signs and symptoms. The anxious person looks overalert, displayed in ways such as sitting forward in a chair; moving fingers, arms, or legs; getting up and moving; pacing around the room; checking certain parts of clothing; and straightening ties or scarves. On the other hand, sloppy dress habits and other signs, just the opposite of a concern with perfection, may be seen. An anxious person may show signs of being watchful of possessions, always trying to keep them in sight.

The anxious person may speak mechanically and rapidly and at times may seem to block out or not connect thoughts together. The anxious person may respond to questions quickly, often not allowing the dentist to finish a question.

Signs of sweating, tension in muscles, increased breathing, and rapid heart rate may be seen. The patient may complain of an inability to sleep, may wake at an early hour, and may not be able to go back to sleep. Attacks of diarrhea and increased frequency of urination may occur. In general, anxious persons are overalert and tense, feel apprehensive, and have a sense of impending disaster that has no apparent cause. Insomnia, tension, and apprehension lead to fatigue, which makes it even more difficult for the individual to deal with anxiety.

The dentist should talk with the patient and show personal interest. Verbal and nonverbal communication must be consistent. The dentist should confront the patient with the observation that the patient appears anxious, then ask if the individual would like to talk about feelings, which may include the person's attitude toward the dentist. During these discussions, tension-free pauses should be allowed to develop between ideas, as a temporary state of regression will help the patient return to a more anxiety-free state. Some patients may respond well to this approach without ever indicating why they were anxious.

If the patient remains anxious in the dental situation, the dentist can plan to use hypnosis, oral or parenteral sedation agents or nitrous oxide, and oxygen to better manage the dental treatment.

Anxiety or a history of panic attacks may be associated with mitral valve prolapse. Patients with mitral valve prolapse and regurgitation require antibiotic prophylaxis for dental procedures resulting in significant bleeding. If no regurgitation is associated with the mitral valve prolapse, antibiotic prophylaxis is not indicated on the basis of the 1997 AHA guidelines. If the patient is unaware of his or her status regarding the presence of absence of valvular regurgitation, a medical referral is indicated.

Patients with uncontrolled hyperthyroidism may have associated anxiety. Epinephrine must not be used in these patients, including even the small amounts that are used in local anesthetics. Patients with signs and symptoms of hyperthyroidism should be referred for medical evaluation and treatment.

Dental Management of the Anxious Patient

1. Preoperative

A. Behavioral
- Establish effective communication with the patient
- Be open and honest; let the patient see who you are
- Consistent verbal and nonverbal communication
- Explain procedures and answer any questions
- Explain possible discomfort associated with a procedure
- Explain what you will do to make procedures "pain free"
- Possibly confront patient who appears anxious:
  - "You seem tense today."
  - "Would you like to talk about it?"

B. Pharmacologic
- Oral sedation: benzodiazepines
- Night before appointment: aid patient in getting a good night's sleep
- Day of appointment: reduce anxiety prior to appointment
- Select a fast-acting drug, at the lowest dosage that will be effective

2. Operative

A. Behavioral
- Allow patient to ask questions about what is happening
- Let patient know if any discomfort is about to be felt
- Reassure patient that procedure is going well

B. Pharmacologic
- Effective local anesthesia
- Oral sedation: benzodiazepines
- Inhalation sedation: nitrous oxide
- Intramuscular sedation: midazolam, promethazine, meperidine
- Intravenous sedation: diazepam, midazolam, fentanyl

3. Postoperative

A. Behavioral
- Explain what usually occurs after the procedure
- Explain what the patient needs to do
- Explain what the patient needs to avoid
- Describe complications that can occur:
  - Pain
  - Bleeding
  - Infection
  - Allergic reaction to medication
- Tell patient to inform you if any complications develop

B. Pharmacologic
- Effective postoperative pain control is essential
- Select the most appropriate medication for pain control
- Analgesics: nonsteroidal antiinflammatory drugs (NSAIDs), salicylates, acetaminophen, codeine, oxycodone, fentanyl, morphine, others
- Adjunctive medications: antidepressants, muscle relaxants, steroids, anticonvulsants, antibiotics

Specific Drugs and Dosage for Anxiety Control (Dosage for Older Adults and Children Must Be Reduced):

- Nitrous oxide, inhalation, 20%–50%
- Diazepam (Valium), oral (2-, 5-, or 10-mg tablets), bid or tid
- Triazolam (Halcion), oral (0.125- or 0.25-mg tablets), first dose 1–2 hours before procedure
- Lorazepam (Ativan), oral (1- or 3-mg tablets), bid or tid
- Meperidine (Demerol), intramuscular (25, 50, 75, or 100 mg/ml) 50 to 100 mg, 30 to 90 minutes before procedure

Midazolam (Versed), intramuscular (0.07–0.08 mg/kg)
30–60 minutes before procedure
Midazolam (Versed), intravenous (1.5 mg/ml), ≤2.5 mg given over 2 minutes just before procedure
Fentanyl (Sublimaze), intravenous (50 mg/ml), 0.07–2.0 μg/kg given minutes before the procedure

DEPRESSION IN DENTAL PATIENTS

Signs of low-grade chronic depression include fatigue (even after getting enough sleep); difficulty getting up in the morning; restlessness; loss of interest in family, work, and sex; inability to make decisions; anger and resentment; chronic complaining; self-criticism; feelings of inferiority; and excessive daydreaming. Signs of more severe depression include excessive crying, change in sleeping habits, thoughts of food making one sick, weight loss without dieting, strong feelings of guilt, nightmares, thoughts about suicide, feeling unreal or in a "fog," and an inability to concentrate.

Patients with major depression are depressed most of the day, show a marked decrease in interest or pleasure in most activities, have a marked gain or loss in weight, and manifest insomnia or hypersomnia. These symptoms must be present for at least 2 weeks before major depression can be diagnosed.

Dental Management

Significant impairment of all personal hygiene may occur during the depth of a depressive episode, including a total lack of oral hygiene. Salivary flow may be reduced, and patients may complain of xerostomia (dry mouth), an increased rate of dental caries, and periodontal disease. The xerostomia may be compounded by the side effects of the medications used to treat depression. Complaints of glossodynia and various facial pain syndromes are common.

The dentist should provide an aggressive preventive dental education program for depressed patients, including the use of artificial salivary products, antiseptic mouthwash, and daily fluoride mouth rinses. Table 6 lists the various methods used to manage xerostomia. Xerostomia provides an excellent environment for overgrowth of *Candida albicans*; as a result, patients are likely to require treatment for candidiasis along with treatment for dry mouth.

Small amounts of epinephrine (1:100,000) can be used in patients taking tricyclic or heterocyclic antidepressants, provided the dentist aspirates before injecting and injects the anesthetic slowly. In general, no more than two cartridges should be injected at any appointment. Excessive amounts of epinephrine can result in hypertension. Levonordefrin is contraindicated in patients taking tricyclics or heterocyclics because of the possibility of an exaggerated hypertensive response. A lower dosage of sedative medications may be necessary to avoid excessive CNS depression.

Patients taking tricyclic or heterocyclic antidepressant drugs may be prone to orthostatic hypotension. Dentists should avoid rapid changes in chair position for these patients and provide support when patients first get out of the dental chair. Atropine should be used with care because increased intraocular pressure can result. Acetaminophen should be used with care because it can decrease the metabolic rate of the heterocyclics, which could lead to toxic levels of the tricyclic antidepressant.

Phenobarbital increases the metabolism of tricyclic antidepressants, which can attenuate their antidepressant effects.

No medical contraindication exists for dental treatment during a depressive episode; however, most depressed patients may be best managed by dealing with their immediate dental needs only during the depression. More complex dental procedures can be performed once the patient has responded to medical treatment.

The dentist can use two simple screening questions to identify patients who are believed to be depressed. According to a 2003 report from the National Institute of Mental Health, these questions will detect more than 50% of depressed individuals.

Patients with signs and symptoms of severe depression must be referred for medical evaluation and treatment. If the patient is not responsive to this recommendation, the problem should be shared with a family member and every attempt made to get the individual to medical attention. During severe depression, suicide is always a possibility; however, medical treatment currently is able to reduce this possibility.

Suicidal Patients

Studies have shown that questions about suicide do not prompt these patients to act. The dentist should ask the very depressed patient if he or she has had any thoughts about suicide. Patients who state they have had these thoughts must be referred for immediate medical care; members of the family need to be involved if possible.

Drug Interactions of Significance to Dentistry

Dental Drug	Interacting Drug	Medical Condition/Situation	Effect
Antibiotics Antibiotics	Oral contraceptives (birth control pills)	Contraception	Decreased effectiveness of oral contraceptives has been suggested for several antibiotic classes because of elimination of gut bacteria responsible for second round cleavage and activation of contraceptive. However, most well-designed studies do not show any reduction in estrogen serum levels in patients taking antibiotics (except rifampin). **RECOMMENDATION: Okay to use dental antibiotics.**
β-Lactams (penicillins, cephalosporins)	Allopurinol (Lopurin, Zyloprim)	Gout	Incidence of minor allergic reactions to ampicillin is increased. Other penicillins have not been implicated. **RECOMMENDATION: Avoid ampicillin.**
	β-blockers (Tenormin, Lopressor, Inderal, Corgard)	Hypertension	Serum levels of atenolol are reduced after prolonged use of ampicillin. Anaphylactic reactions to penicillins or other drugs may be more severe in patients taking β-blockers because of increased mediator release from mast cells. **RECOMMENDATION: Use ampicillin cautiously, advise patient of potential reaction.**
	Tetracyclines and other bacteriostatic antibiotics	Infection, acne, periodontal disease	Effectiveness of penicillins and cephalosporins may be reduced by bacteriostatic agents. **RECOMMENDATION: Avoid interaction.**

Tetracyclines	Antacids	Dyspepsia, gastroesophageal reflux, peptic ulcer	Antacids, dairy products, and other agents containing divalent and trivalent cations will chelate tetracyclines and limit their absorption in the gut. Doxycycline is least influenced by this interaction. **RECOMMENDATION: Avoid interaction.**
	Insulin	Diabetes mellitus	Doxycycline and oxytetracycline have been documented as enhancing the hypoglycemic effects of exogenously administered insulin. **RECOMMENDATION: Select different antibiotic or increase carbohydrate intake.**
Metronidazole	Ethanol	Alcohol use or abuse	Severe disulfiramlike reactions are well documented. **RECOMMENDATION: Avoid interaction.**
	Lithium	Manic depression	Inhibits renal excretion of lithium, leading to elevated/toxic levels of lithium. Lithium toxicity produces confusion, ataxia, and kidney damage. **RECOMMENDATION: Avoid interaction.**
	Benzodiazepines	Anxiety	Delayed metabolism of benzodiazepine, increasing the pharmacologic effects can result in excessive sedation and irrational behavior. **RECOMMENDATION: Reduce dose of benzodiazepine.**
	Carbamazepine (Tegretol)	Seizure disorder	Increased blood levels of carbamazepine leading to toxicity (symptoms include drowsiness, dizziness, nausea, headache, and blurred vision). Hospitalization has been required. **RECOMMENDATION: Avoid interaction.**
	Cyclosporine	Organ transplant	Enhanced immunosuppression and nephrotoxicity. **RECOMMENDATION: Avoid interaction, monitor patient.**

Continued

Drug Interactions of Significance to Dentistry—cont'd

Dental Drug	Interacting Drug	Medical Condition/Situation	Effect
	H_1 histamine blocker astemizole (Hismanal)	Allergy	Blocks metabolism of parent molecule, resulting in accumulation of antihistamine and ventricular arrhythmia (torsade de pointes), potentially life threatening. **RECOMMENDATION: Avoid interaction.**
	Lovastatin, pravastatin, simvastatin, other statins	Hyperlipidemia	Muscle (eosinophilia) myalgia and rhabdomyolysis. **RECOMMENDATION: Avoid interaction.**
	Prednisone, methylprednisol one	Autoimmune disorders, organ transplant	Increased risk of Gushing's syndrome and immunosuppression. **RECOMMENDATION: Monitor patient, shorten duration of antibiotic administration if possible.**
	Theophylline (Theo-Dur)	Asthma	Erythromycins inhibit metabolism of theophylline, leading to toxic serum levels (symptoms of toxicity: headache, nausea, vomiting, confusion, thirst, cardiac arrhythmias, convulsions). Conversely, theophylline reduces serum levels of erythromycin. **RECOMMENDATION: Avoid prescribing erythromycin.**
Antibiotics (especially erythromycin and tetracycline)	Digoxin (Lanoxin)	Congestive heart failure	Alters gastrointestinal flora and retards metabolism of digoxin in approximately 10% of patients, resulting in dangerously high digoxin serum levels that may persist for several weeks after discontinuation of antibiotic. Strongest documentation for erythromycin and tetracycline. Patients should be cautioned to report any signs of digitalis toxicity (salivation, visual disturbances, arrhythmias) during antibiotic therapy. **RECOMMENDATION: Safe in 90%, should monitor digoxin levels during antimicrobial therapy.**

Antibiotics (cephalosporins, erythromycin, clarithromycin, metronidazole)	Warfarin (Coumadin)	Atrial fibrillation, myocardial infarction, post major surgery, stroke prevention	Anticoagulant effect of warfarin may be increased by several antibiotic classes. Reduced synthesis of vitamin K by gut flora is a putative mechanism, but several antibiotics have antiplatelet and anticoagulant activity. Most convincing documentation for cephalosporins, macrolide antibiotics, and metronidazole. **RECOMMENDATION:** Penicillins, tetracyclines, and clindamycin are preferred choices but must be used cautiously.
Analgesics			
Acetaminophen	Alcohol	Alcohol use and abuse	Increased risk of liver toxicity, especially during fasting state or ≥4 g/day acetaminophen. **RECOMMENDATION: Use lower dose, encourage discontinuation of alcohol use.**
Aspirin	Oral hypoglycemics (sulfonylureas: glyburide, chlorpropamide, acetohexamide)	Diabetes type 2	Increased hypoglycemic effects. **RECOMMENDATION: Avoid interaction.**
Aspirin NSAIDs	Anticoagulants (coumarins)	Atrial fibrillation, myocardial infarction, postsurgery	Increased risk of gastrointestinal bleeding. **RECOMMENDATION: Avoid interaction.**
Aspirin NSAIDs	Alcohol	Alcohol use and abuse	Increases risk of gastrointestinal bleeding. **RECOMMENDATION: Lower dose, encourage discontinuation of alcohol use.**
NSAIDs	β-Blocker angiotensin-converting enzyme inhibitor	Hypertension, postmyocardial infarction	Decreased antihypertensive effect. **RECOMMENDATION: Limit duration of NSAID dosage to approximately 4 days.**

Continued

Drug Interactions of Significance to Dentistry—cont'd

Dental Drug	Interacting Drug	Medical Condition/Situation	Effect
NSAIDs	Lithium	Manic depression	Produces symptoms of lithium toxicity, including nausea, vomiting, slurred speech, and mental confusion. **RECOMMENDATION: NSAIDs should not be prescribed to patients with manic depression who take lithium. It can result in toxic levels of lithium.**
NSAIDs	Methotrexate (MTX)	Connective tissue disease, cancer therapy	Toxic levels of methotrexate may accumulate. **RECOMMENDATION: Avoid interaction if patient on high-dose MTX for cancer therapy. Low-dose MTX for arthritis is not a concern.**
Anesthetics			
Lidocaine	Bupivacaine		Additive effect of these two local anesthetics increases risk. **RECOMMENDATION: Limit dose of each.**
Mepivacaine	Meperidine (Demerol)		Sedation with opioids may increase risk of local anesthetic toxicity, especially in children. **RECOMMENDATION: Reduce anesthetic dose.**
Sedatives			
Barbiturates	Digoxin, theophylline, corticosteroids, oral anticoagulants	Congestive heart failure, asthma, autoimmune disease, atrial fibrillation	Barbiturates bind cytochrome P450 system in liver, enhance metabolism of many drugs. **RECOMMENDATION: Limit dose, observe for adverse effects.**
	Benzodiazepines, alcohol, antihistamines	Anxiety, alcohol use and abuse, seasonal allergies	Additive effects for sedation and respiratory depression. **RECOMMENDATION: Reduce dose, administer combination of sedatives with extreme caution.**

Benzodiazepines (BZDP; e.g., alprazolam, chlordiazepoxide, diazepam)	Cimetidine, oral contraceptives, fluoxetine, isoniazid (INH), alcohol	Peptic ulcer disease, depression, tuberculosis, alcohol use and abuse	Delayed metabolism of BZDP, increasing pharmacologic effects can result in excessive sedation and irrational behavior. **RECOMMENDATION: Reduce dose of benzodiazepine.** Delayed metabolism of BZDP, increasing pharmacologic effects can result in excessive sedation and irrational behavior. **RECOMMENDATION: Reduce dose of benzodiazepine.**
	Digoxin (Lanoxin), phenytoin, theophylline (Theo-Dur)	Congestive heart failure, epilepsy, asthma	Serum concentrations of digoxin, phenytoin may be increased, resulting in toxicity. Antagonize sedative effects of benzodiazepine. **RECOMMENDATION: Avoid interaction.**
	Protease inhibitors (Indinavir, Nelfinavir)	HIV, AIDS	Increased bioavailability and effects of benzodiazepines, especially triazolam and oral midazolam. **RECOMMENDATION: Avoid interaction.**
Vasoconstrictor			
Epinephrine and levonordephrine (Neo-Cobefrin)	Nonselective β-blockers: propranolol (Inderal), nadolol (Corgard), penbutolol (Levatol), pindolol (Visken), sotalol (Betapace), timolol (Blocadren)	Angina pectoris, hypertension, glaucoma, migraine, headache, hyperthyroidism, panic syndromes	Unopposed effects: increased blood pressure with secondary bradycardia. **RECOMMENDATION: Initial dose is 1/2 cartridge containing 1:100,000 epinephrine, aspirate to avoid intravascular injection, inject slowly. Monitor vital signs; if no adverse cardiovascular change, up to two cartridges containing a vasoconstrictor can be administered at 5-minute intervals with continual monitoring. Avoid epinephrine-containing retraction cord and higher concentrations of epinephrine in the dental anesthetic.**

Continued

Drug Interactions of Significance to Dentistry—cont'd

Dental Drug	Interacting Drug	Medical Condition/Situation	Effect
	Cocaine	Illicit use, topical anesthetic for mucous membrane procedures	Blocks reuptake of norepinephrine and intensifies postsynaptic response to epinephrine-like drugs. This potentiates the adrenergic effects on the heart, with potential for a heart attack. **RECOMMENDATION: Recognize signs and symptoms of cocaine abuse. Avoid use of vasoconstrictors in these patients until cocaine has been withheld for at least 24 hours.**
	Halothane	General anesthetic for surgical procedures	Stimulation of 1 and receptors resulting in arrhythmia at doses >2 g/kg. **RECOMMENDATION: Limit dose to remain <2 g/kg threshold, aspirate to avoid intravascular injection. Monitor vital signs. Avoid epinephrine-containing retraction cord and concentrations of epinephrine >1:100,000.**
	Tricyclic antidepressants (amitriptyline [Elavil], doxepin [Sinequan], imipramine [Tofranil])	Depression, severe anxiety, neuropathic pain, attention deficit disorder	Blocks reuptake of norepinephrine resulting in unopposed effects (increased blood pressure, increased heart rate), potential cardiac arrhythmias; effect is greater with levonordefrin. **RECOMMENDATION: Avoid levonordephrin. Limit dose to 2 cartridges containing 1:100,000 epinephrine (36 g), aspirate to avoid intravascular injection. Monitor vital signs. Avoid epinephrine-containing retraction cord and higher concentrations of epinephrine in the dental anesthetic.**

	Peripheral adrenergic antagonists (reserpine [Serpasil], guanethidine [Ismelin], guanadrel [Hylorel])	Hypertension	Potential for increased sensitivity of adrenergic receptors to epinephrine and levonordefrin. **RECOMMENDATION: Administer cautiously. Monitor vital signs during and following administration of first cartridge. Limit dose to 2 cartridges containing 1:100,000 epinephrine (36 g) or less depending on vital signs and patient response. Aspirate to avoid intravascular injection. Avoid epinephrine-containing retraction cord and higher concentrations of epinephrine in the dental anesthetic.**
	Catechol-*O*-methyltransferase inhibitors (tolcapone [Tasmar], entacapone [Comtan])	Parkinson's disease	Potential for increased sensitivity of adrenergic receptors to epinephrine and levonordefrin, resulting in increased heart rate and blood pressure and arrhythmias. **RECOMMENDATION: Administer cautiously. Monitor vital signs during and after administration of first cartridge. Limit dose to 2 cartridges containing 1:100,000 epinephrine (36 g) or less depending on vital signs and patient response. Aspirate to avoid intravascular injection. Avoid epinephrine-containing retraction cord and higher concentrations of epinephrine in the dental anesthetic.**

AIDS, Acquired immunodeficiency virus; *HIV,* human immunodeficiency virus.

COMPLEMENTARY MEDICINES AND DENTISTRY

The term *alternative medicine* is used to describe practices that are used instead of mainstream medical practice. *Complementary medicine* refers to practices that are used as adjuncts to conventional medicine. These systems are divided into five major categories: alternative medical systems (traditional Chinese medicine, Ayurveda medicine of India, and Native-American healing approaches), biologically based therapies (natural products), manipulative and body-based methods (chiropractic and osteopathic manipulation), mind–body interventions (hypnosis, cognitive therapies and biofeedback), and energy therapies (use of magnets and acupuncture). Both of these systems use treatments that often have no established efficacy. An estimated 42% of Americans use alternative and complementary medicine therapies.

Complementary medicines are defined as herbal medicines, homeopathic remedies, and essential oils. The basic principle of homeopathy is selection of a remedy, which, if given to a healthy individual, will produce a range of symptoms similar to those observed in the ill patient (like cures like). Only minute amounts are given to avoid toxicity. Only one remedy is used at any one time. Dilute tinctures are used rather than concentrated ones. In homeopathic practice, medication in tablet form is commonly used.

The standard tinctures used in Western tradition herbal medicine are very different from those used in homoeopathy. Alcohol is used to dissolve the plant, and the final product is not diluted. Thus these remedies are concentrated, highly potent preparations and usually are taken as the unmodified liquid tincture. Other preparations used in herbal remedies include lotions and creams for topical application. Tablet form of medication is not used very often (<5%)

Efficacy of Herbal Medicines

Many herbal remedies have been used for hundreds of years. However, traditional use is not a good indication of efficacy. The gold standard for testing efficacy is the randomized clinical trial (RCT). This standard should apply as much to herbal medicines as for conventional medicines. A number of RCTs of herbal medical products have been conducted. However, many of these studies differ with regard to how they were conducted and in their findings. Ernst suggests that the best way to evaluate a number of RCTs on the efficacy of a specific herbal medicine is to do a systematic review or meta-analysis of all RCTs for that product.

Herbal medicines with proven efficacy

Several herbal remedies have been repeatedly tested in placebo-controlled RCTs. Systematic reviews of these studies have shown that some herbal medicines are effective for certain conditions. For example, ginkgo biloba has been shown to be effective for symptomatic treatment of dementia and intermittent claudication. Table 1 lists the more commonly used herbal medicines that have proved to be effective for the condition(s) listed.

TABLE 1
Claims for Herbal Actions Supported by Clinical Trials

Herb	Claimed Action	Effectiveness Supported by Clinical Trials
Kava	Used to treat anxiety.	Clinical trials have shown it reduces anxiety significantly more than placebo.
Artichoke	Used to lower the lipid levels in blood.	Only one randomized clinical study shows it moderately lowers elevated total cholesterol levels when given orally for several weeks.
Feverfew	Used for women's ailments and inflammatory diseases. Recently has been suggested for headache and migraine.	Three studies showed greater effect than placebo in alleviating symptoms of headache or migraine.
Garlic	Used to reduce blood pressure and lower blood lipid levels.	Data show a small but statistically significant reduction in systolic and diastolic blood pressures. No data support claims for lipid-lowering properties of garlic.
Ginger	Used to treat nausea and vomiting.	Several studies support the antiemetic use for ginger. Used to treat or prevent nausea or vomiting.
Ginkgo biloba	Used to treat cerebral insufficiency, prevent loss of cognitive function, and tinnitus.	Studies have shown it is effective in the treatment of cerebral insufficiency when given for 4–6 weeks. Data show that regular oral intake of ginkgo biloba slows the loss of cognitive function in patients with dementia.
Hawthorn	Used to treat heart failure.	Various studies show it is effective for the early signs of congestive heart failure.
Horse chestnut	Used to treat venous congestion.	Studies have shown it is effective in reducing signs and symptoms of chronic venous insufficiency.
Saw palmetto	Used in Europe to treat prostate enlargement.	Clinical trials support its use for symptoms of benign prostatic hypertrophy.
St. John's wort	Used to treat depression.	Studies show that it is effective for treating mild to moderate depression. The question of its effectiveness for severe depression remains to be answered.

Herbal medicines with doubtful or no efficacy
Asian ginseng, one of the most popular herbal medicines in the United States, showed no convincing evidence for efficacy as a general tonic or in enhancing mental and physical performance. A review of studies regarding the use of valerian as a hypnotic agent was inconclusive because of flaws in the study designs. A systematic review of RCTs found no evidence that evening primrose was effective for treatment of premenstrual syndrome in women. Garlic was not found to be effective as a cholesterol-lowering drug.
Table 2 lists some of the more common herbal medicines that were found not to be effective for the conditions listed.

TABLE 2
Claims for Herbal Actions Unsupported by Clinical Trials

Herb	Claimed Action	Effectiveness Supported by Clinical Trials
Aloe vera	Used as an adjunct oral treatment for diabetes and skin conditions such as herpes and psoriasis.	Currently, compelling data support none of the claims made for aloe vera.
Echinacea	Used to prevent and treat the common cold.	Overall there is insufficient evidence that echinacea extracts are effective for treatment or prevention of the common cold.
Evening primrose	Used for treatment of premenstrual syndrome.	Current evidence suggests uncertain value when it is used to treat premenstrual syndrome.
Ginseng	Used to treat type 2 diabetes and herpes simplex infections. Also has been used to increase physical and psychomotor performance and enhance cognitive function.	None of the 16 double-blinded, randomized clinical trials support any effective action on physical performance, psychomotor performance, and cognitive function, type 2 diabetes, and herpes simplex infections.
Guar Gum	Used to treat obesity and overweight.	Clinical trials have not supported this use.
Mistletoe	Has been suggested for treatment of cancer.	Current studies do not support these claims.
Peppermint	Used to treat to irritable bowel syndrome.	Studies show that it alleviates the symptoms of irritable bowel syndrome. However, many of the trials had flaws.
Valerian	Used to promote sleep.	Randomized clinical trials are necessary to demonstrate effectiveness. Studies to date have been flawed.

Side Effects and Adverse Reactions

Recent increased use of herbal remedies seems to come from the public's view that natural products are harmless or at least have fewer side effects than regular drugs. The assumption that phytomedicines (herbal medicines) have only beneficial effects has proved be incorrect.

Toxicity can be associated with use of herbal remedies. These reactions can be caused by accidental or deliberate contamination of the product. For example, lead, mercury, cadmium, pesticides, microorganisms, and fumigants have been found to contaminate some herbal products. Substitution of animal substances such as enzymes, hormones, or organ extracts and synthetic drugs has accounted for some of the toxic reactions to herbal products. Adulteration by accidental or deliberate substitution of the original plant material by other plant species has been reported to be a source of toxic reactions to herbal products.

Other sources of adverse reactions to herbal products are intrinsic or plant associated. In some cases, the manufacturer ignored the known toxicity of a plant or constituent in the herbal product. In other cases, the product contains plants for which no or insufficient data regarding safety are available. If a highly concentrated or specifically processed extract is used, toxic reactions may occur. If a plant contains constituents known to affect the bioavailability and/or pharmacokinetics of other drugs, serious drug interactions can occur.

Long-term users, consumers of large amounts of phytomedicines, or people who use many different medicinal products may be prone to side effects. Pregnant or nursing women, babies, and the elderly, sick, and undernourished are at higher risk for side effects. Some of the more common side effects associated with herbal remedies include bleeding with ginkgo biloba; upset stomach, fatigue, dizziness, confusion, dry mouth, and photosensitivity with St. John's wort; high blood pressure, arrhythmias, nervousness, headaches, heart attack, or stroke with ephedra; and sleepiness, rash, and motor dysfunction of skeletal muscles with kava. Table 3 lists some of the serious adverse reactions that can occur with use of natural products.

TABLE 3
Selected Herbal Medicines with Potentially Serious Adverse Effects

Product	Effect
Aristolochia	Nephrotoxicity Carcinogenicity
Chaparral	Cholestatic hepatitis
Comfrey	Acute and chronic hepatitis
Digitalis leaf	Arrhythmias
Ephedra	Hypertension Stroke Myocardial infarction
Germander	Acute and chronic hepatitis
Kava	Hepatitis
Khat	Tachycardia Psychosis
Kombucha	Hepatotoxicity Lactic acidosis
Mistletoe	Anaphylaxis
Skullcap	Seizures Acute and chronic hepatitis
St. John's wort	Photosensitivity Possible hypertension with tyramine-containing foods

Medical Problems

Certain medical problems can make consumption of herbal medicines unsafe. Individuals with high blood pressure, thyroid disease, psychiatric disorders, Parkinson's disease, enlarged prostate gland, diabetes mellitus, heart disease, epilepsy, glaucoma, blood clotting problems, and a history of stroke should check with their physician before taking any herbal remedies. Patients with a history of aspirin allergy can be at risk if they take an herb containing willow bark.

Drug Interactions

Important drug interactions can occur between certain herbal products and conventional medications (Table 4). The most common drug involved with drug–herb interactions is warfarin. The most common herb involved with these interactions is St. John's wort. In a study evaluating the potential of St. John's wort to alter the cytochrome P450 enzymes, Markowitz found that a 14-day course of the herbal product significantly induced the activity of CYP3A4 as measured by changes in alprazolam pharmacokinetics. Markowitz concluded that long-term administration of St. John's wort may result in diminished clinical effectiveness or increased dosage requirements for all CYP3A4 substrates, which represent approximately 50% of all marketed medications. In contrast, in another study Markowitz found little evidence that garlic extracts alter the disposition of coadministered medications metabolized by the CYP3A4 pathway.

Patients taking aspirin, warfarin, ticlopidine, clopidogrel, or dipyridamole should not take ginkgo biloba because bleeding may occur. Patients taking an antidepressant should not take St. John's wort. Patients taking a decongestant, a stimulant drug, or who drink caffeinated beverages should not take ephedra. Individuals taking a benzodiazepine, a barbiturate, an antipsychotic medication, or any medicine used to treat Parkinson's disease should not take kava products. It is important that patients notify their general practitioner if they are taking phytomedicines concurrently with conventional drugs, especially those with cardiac, diuretic, sedative, hypotensive or other properties. Individuals taking a prescription medicine should check with their physician before taking any herbal health product.

TABLE 4
Selected Natural Medicines That Potentiate or Interfere with Approved Drugs

Natural Medicine	Approved Drug
Ephedra	Theophylline (P) Antihypertensives (I) Corticosteroids (I)
Evening primrose	Anticoagulants (P) Antiplatelet agents (P) Low-molecular-weight heparins (P) Anticonvulsants (I)
Garlic	Aspirin (P) Clopidogrel (P) Ticlopidine (P)
Ginkgo leaf extract	Anticoagulants (P) Antiplatelet (P) Anticonvulsants (I)
Glucosamine	Antidiabetic drugs (I)
Panax ginseng	Anticoagulants (P) Diabetic agents (possible P) Nifedipine (P)
Saw palmetto	Hormone replacement therapies (P)
Soy	Estrogenic drugs (P)
St. John's wort	Antidepressants (P) HIV protease inhibitors (I) Cyclosporine (I)
Valerian	Sedatives (P)
Yohimbe	Antihypertensives (I)

HIV = Human immunodeficiency virus; *I* = interferes; *P* = potentiates.

Dental Implications

A limited number of papers describe the use of complementary and alternative medical systems for dental problems. Two of these papers describe the use of herbal products for treatment of periodontal disease. In a series of five papers, Goldstein suggests that unconventional or alternative dentistry is analogous to and conceptually inseparable from unconventional or alternative medicine. He suggests that dentists should learn about these procedures in terms of the evidence for effectiveness and safety. Dentists should accept and encompass science-based advances and reject unproved or disproved methods. Selected unconventional treatments can be incorporated into conventional dentistry in certain patients for specific purposes that will be beneficial to the patient.

Information for Dentists

Herbal remedies have the potential to affect on the safety of invasive or prolonged dental procedures. Excessive bleeding can occur with some of these medications. Other herbal medicines may affect the cardiovascular system and render the patient more susceptible to cardiac arrhythmias and other cardiovascular complications. Ginseng may cause hypoglycemia. Chinese cancer patients undergoing chemotherapy who were users of Chinese herbal medicine were found to have higher scores of mucositis. It is important for the dentist to include a section in the patient's medical history on the consumption of herbal medications and over-the-counter drugs. Because most U.S. dental schools teach very little on the use, side effects, toxicity, and drug interactions associated with herbal remedies, the dentist must find a way to become informed regarding these issues.

Important references for dentists are the Physicians Desk Reference for Herbal Medicines, Third Edition, 2004 and the Physicians Desk Reference for Nonprescription Drugs, Dietary Supplements and Herbs, 2006, both published by Thomson. Dentists should use only treatment procedures that have been established to be effective and with minimal risks involved. As clinical trials demonstrate certain alternative and complementary treatments to be effective and safe, they can be incorporated into conventional medicine and dentistry. The dentist may find a medically compromised patient is taking an herbal remedy that is potentially harmful. This should be discussed with the patient and the patient referred to his or her physician for evaluation and management.

Sources for Major Topics Covered Parts I and II

ADA and AAOS: Advisory statement for dental patients with total joint replacements, *JADA* 128:1004, 1997.

American Dental Association: *ADA guide to dental therapeutics,* ed 3, Chicago, 2003, ADA Publishing Division.

Baddour LM, Bettmann MA, Bolger AF, Epstein AE, Ferrieri P: AHA scientific statement: nonvalvular cardiovascular device-related infections, *Circulation* 108:2015, 2003.

Dajani AS, Taubert KA, Wilson W, Bolger AF, Bayer A, Ferrieri P, et al: Prevention of bacterial endocarditis. Recommendations by the American Heart Association, *JAMA* 277:1794, 1997.

Miller CS: Drug interactions of significance to dentistry. In Little JW, Falace DA, Miller CS, Rhodus NL, editors: *Dental management of the medically compromised patient,* ed 6, St. Louis, 2002, Mosby.

Miller CS, Little JW, Falace DA: Need of supplemental corticosteroids for dental patients with adrenal insufficiency: reconsideration of the problem, *JADA* 132:1570, 2001.

Little JW, Miller CS, Henry RG, McIntosh BA: Antithrombotic agents: implications in dentistry, *Oral Surg Oral Med Oral Path Oral Radiol Endod* 93:544, 2002.

Little JW: Behavioral and psychiatric disorders. In Little JW, Falace DA, Miller CS, Rhodus NL. editors: *Dental management of the medically compromised patient*, ed 6, St. Louis, 2002, Mosby.

Little, JW: Anxiety disorders: dental implications, *J Gen Dent* 51:562-570, 2003.

Little JW: Dental implication of mood disorders, *J Gen Dent* 52:442, 2004.

Little JW: Complementary and alternative medicine: impact on dentistry, *Oral Surg Oral Med Oral Path Oral Radiol Endod* 98:137, 2004.

Little JW: Drugs, drugs, and more drugs: their impact on dentistry, *J Northwest Dent* July-August:23, 2005.

Rhodus NL: Therapeutic management of common oral lesions. In Little JW, Falace DA, Miller CS, Rhodus NL, editors: *Dental management of the medically compromised patient,* ed 6, St. Louis, 2002, Mosby.

Siegel MA, Silverman S, Sollecato TP, editors: *American Academy of Oral Medicine: clinician's guide to treatment of common oral conditions*, ed 5, Baltimore, 2001.

Many drugs are available in fixed combinations of two or more medications. Some of the most common trade names for combination drugs in the United States are listed, along with their generic components and classifications. The list is alphabetical by the brand name of the combination product. Brand names for identical drug combinations are listed together. When the patient's drug history includes one of these combination products, it can be easily accessed through the index.

Combination Product Name	Generic Components
AC Gel	Cocaine (an anesthetic)/epinephrine (a vasopressor)
Accuretic	Quinapril (an ACE inhibitor)/hydrochlorothiazide (a diuretic)
Activella	Estradiol (an estrogen)/norethindrone (a hormone)
Advair	Fluticasone (a corticosteroid)/salmeterol (a bronchodilator)
Advil Cold	Pseudoephedrine (a sympathomimetic)/ibuprofen (an NSAID)
Aggrenox	Aspirin (an antiplatelet and nonnarcotic analgesic)/ dipyridamole (an antiplatelet)
Aldactazide	Spironolactone (a potassium-sparing diuretic)/ hydrochlorothiazide (a diuretic)
Aldoril	Methyldopa (an antihypertensive)/hydrochlorothiazide (a diuretic)
Allegra-D	Fexofenadine (an antihistamine)/pseudoephedrine (a nasal decongestant)
Allegra-D 24 Hour	Fexofenadine (an antihistamine)/pseudoephedrine (a sympathomimetic)
Anexsia	Hydrocodone (a narcotic analgesic)/acetaminophen (a nonnarcotic analgesic)
Apresazide	Hydralazine (a vasodilator)/hydrochlorothiazide (a diuretic)
Arthrotec	Diclofenac (an NSAID)/misoprostol (an antisecretory gastric protectant)
Atacand HCT	Candesartan (an angiotensin II receptor antagonist)/ hydrochlorothiazide (a diuretic)
Avalide	Irbesartan (an angiotensin II receptor antagonist)/ hydrochlorothiazide (a diuretic)
Avandamet	Rosiglitazone (an antidiabetic)/metformin (an antidiabetic)
Bactrim	Sulfamethoxazole (a sulfonamide)/trimethoprim (an antiinfective)
Bellergal-S	Ergotamine (an antimigraine)/belladonna (an anticholinergic)/ phenobarbital (an anticonvulsant)
Benicar HCT	Olmesartan (an angiotensin II receptor antagonist)/ hydrochlorothiazide (a diuretic)

Combination Product Name	Generic Components
Bicillin CR	Penicillin G benzathine (a penicillin)/penicillin procaine (a penicillin)
Blephamide	Sulfacetamide (an antiinfective)/prednisolone (an adrenocortical steroid)
Caduet	Amlodipine (a calcium channel blocker)/atorvastatin (an antihyperlipidemic)
Caladryl	Calamine (an astringent)/diphenhydramine (an antihistamine)/ camphor (a counterirritant)
Capital with Codeine	Acetaminophen (a nonnarcotic analgesic)/codeine (a narcotic analgesic)
Capozide	Captopril (an ACE inhibitor)/hydrochlorothiazide (a diuretic)
Children's Advil Cold	Ibuprofen (an NSAID)/pseudoephedrine (a nasal decongestant)
Ciprodex Otic	Ciprofloxacin (an antiinfective)/dexamethasone (an adrenocortical steroid)
Cipro HC Otic	Ciprofloxacin (an antiinfective)/hydrocortisone (an adrenocortical steroid)
Claritin-D	Loratadine (an antihistamine)/pseudoephedrine (a nasal decongestant)
CombiPatch	Estradiol (an estrogen)/norethindrone (a hormone)
Combipres	Clonidine (an antihypertensive)/chlorthalidone (a diuretic)
Combivent	Ipratropium (a bronchodilator)/albuterol (a bronchodilator)
Combivir	Lamivudine (an antiretroviral)/zidovudine (an antiretroviral)
Combunox	Ibuprofen (an NSAID)/oxycodone (a narcotic analgesic)
Cortisporin	Neomycin (an antiinfective)/polymyxin B (an antiinfective)/ hydrocortisone (an adrenocortical steroid)
Corzide	Nadolol (a β-blocker)/bendroflumethiazide (a diuretic)
Cosopt	Dorzolamide (a carbonic anhydrase inhibitor)/timolol (a β-blocker)
Darvocet A500	Propoxyphene (a narcotic analgesic)/acetaminophen (a nonnarcotic analgesic)
Darvocet-N	Propoxyphene (a narcotic analgesic)/acetaminophen (a nonnarcotic analgesic)
Dexacidin	Neomycin (an antiinfective)/polymyxin (an antiinfective)/dexamethasone (an adrenocortical steroid)
Dilantin with PB	Phenobarbital (an anticonvulsant)/phenytoin (an anticonvulsant)
Diovan HCT	Valsartan (an angiotensin II receptor antagonist)/ hydrochlorothiazide (a diuretic)
Donnatal	Atropine (an anticholinergic)/hyoscyamine (an anticholinergic)/ phenobarbital (a sedative)/scopolamine (an anticholinergic)
Duocet	Acetaminophen (a nonnarcotic analgesic)/hydrocodone (a narcotic analgesic)

Combination Product Name	Generic Components
DuoNeb	Ipratropium (a bronchodilator)/albuterol base (a bronchodilator)
Dyazide	Triamterene (a potassium-sparing diuretic)/hydrochlorothiazide (a diuretic)
EMLA	Lidocaine (a local anesthetic)/prilocaine (an anesthetic)
Epzicom	Abacavir (an antiretroviral)/lamivudine (an antiretroviral)
Eryzole	Erythromycin (a macrolide)/sulfisoxazole (a sulfonamide)
Etrafon	Perphenazine (an antipsychotic)/amitriptyline (an antidepressant)
Extra Strength Maalox	Magnesium hydroxide (an antacid)/simethicone (an antiflatulent)
Femhrt	Norethindrone (a hormone)/estradiol (an estrogen)
Ferro-Sequels	Ferrous fumarate (a hematinic)/docusate (a laxative)
Fioricet	Butabarbital (a sedative-hypnotic)/acetaminophen (a nonnarcotic analgesic)/caffeine (a CNS stimulant)
Fiorinal	Butabarbital (a sedative-hypnotic)/aspirin (a nonnarcotic analgesic)/caffeine (a CNS stimulant)
Gaviscon (oral suspension)	Aluminum hydroxide (an antacid)/magnesium carbonate (an antacid)
Gaviscon (tablets)	Aluminum hydroxide (an antacid)/magnesium trisilicate (an antacid)
Gelusil	Aluminum hydroxide (an antacid)/magnesium hydroxide (a laxative)/simethicone (an antiflatulent)
Gentlax-S	Senna (a laxative)/docusate (a laxative)
Glucovance	Glyburide (an antidiabetic)/metformin (an antidiabetic)
Haley's M-O	Magnesium (a laxative)/mineral oil (a lubricant laxative)
Helidac	Bismuth (an antidiarrheal)/metronidazole (an antiinfective)/tetracycline (an antiinfective)
Humalog Mix 75/25	Insulin: lispro suspension 75% and lispro solution 25%
Humulin 50/50	Insulin: NPH 50% and regular 50%
Humulin 70/30	Insulin: NPH 70% and rapid-acting regular 30%
Hyzaar	Losartan (an angiotensin II receptor antagonist)/hydrochlorothiazide (a diuretic)
Imodium Advanced	Loperamide (an antidiarrheal)/simethicone (an antiflatulent)
Inderide	Propranolol (a β-blocker)/hydrochlorothiazide (a diuretic)
Inderide LA	Propranolol (a β-blocker)/hydrochlorothiazide (a diuretic)
Lexxel	Enalapril (an ACE inhibitor)/felodipine (a calcium channel blocker)
Librax	Chlordiazepoxide (an antianxiety agent)/clidinium (an anticholinergic)

Combination Product Name	Generic Components
Lidocaine with epinephrine	Lidocaine (a local anesthetic)/epinephrine (a vasoconstrictor)
LidoSite	Epinephrine (a sympathomimetic)/lidocaine (an anesthetic)
Limbitrol	Chlordiazepoxide (an antianxiety agent)/amitriptyline (an antidepressant)
Lomotil	Diphenoxylate (an antidiarrheal)/atropine (an anticholinergic/antispasmodic)
Lopressor HCT	Metoprolol (a β-blocker)/hydrochlorothiazide (a diuretic)
Lorcet	Acetaminophen (a nonnarcotic analgesic)/hydrocodone (a narcotic analgesic)
Lortab	Hydrocodone (a narcotic analgesic)/acetaminophen (a nonnarcotic analgesic)
Lortab Elixir	Hydrocodone (a narcotic analgesic)/acetaminophen (a nonnarcotic analgesic)
Lortab/ASA	Hydrocodone (a narcotic analgesic)/aspirin (a nonnarcotic analgesic)
Lotensin HCT	Benazepril (an ACE inhibitor)/hydrochlorothiazide (a diuretic)
Lotrel	Amlodipine (a calcium channel blocker)/benazepril (an ACE inhibitor)
Lotrisone	Clotrimazole (an antifungal)/betamethasone (an adrenocortical steroid)
Lunelle	Medroxyprogesterone (a progestin)/estradiol (an estrogen)
Maalox	Aluminum hydroxide (an antacid)/magnesium hydroxide (an antacid)
Maalox Plus	Aluminum hydroxide (an antacid)/magnesium hydroxide (an antacid)/simethicone (an antiflatulent)
Maxitrol	Neomycin (an antiinfective)/polymyxin (an antiinfective)/dexamethasone (an adrenocortical steroid)
Maxzide	Triamterene (a potassium-sparing diuretic)/hydrochlorothiazide (a diuretic)
Metaglip	Glipizide (an antidiabetic)/metformin (an antidiabetic)
Micardis HCT	Telmisartan (an angiotensin II receptor antagonist)/hydrochlorothiazide (a diuretic)
Minizide	Prazosin (an antihypertensive)/polythiazide (a diuretic)
Moduretic	Amiloride (a potassium-sparing diuretic)/hydrochlorothiazide (a diuretic)
Motrin Cold	Pseudoephedrine (a sympathomimetic)/ibuprofen (an NSAID)
Mucinex D	Guaifenesin (an expectorant)/pseudoephedrine (a sympathomimetic)
Mucinex DM	Guaifenesin (an expectorant)/dextromethorphan (an expectorant)
Mycitracin	Neomycin (an aminoglycoside)/polymyxin B (an antiinfective)/bacitracin (an antiinfective)
Myco II	Nystatin (an antifungal)/triamcinolone (an adrenocortical steroid)

Combination Product Name	Generic Components
Mycolog II	Nystatin (an antifungal)/triamcinolone (an adrenocortical steroid)
Myco-Triacet	Nystatin (an antifungal)/triamcinolone (an adrenocortical steroid)
Mylanta (oral suspension)	Aluminum hydroxide (an antacid)/magnesium hydroxide (an antacid)/simethicone (an antiflatulent)
Mylanta (tablets)	Calcium carbonate/magnesium hydroxide
Naphcon-A	Naphazoline (a nasal decongestant/pheniramine (an antihistamine)
Neosporin GU Irrigant	Neomycin (an aminoglycoside)/polymyxin B (an antiinfective)
Neosporin Ointment, Triple Antibiotic	Neomycin (an aminoglycoside)/polymyxin B (an antiinfective)/ bacitracin (an antiinfective)
Norco	Hydrocodone (a narcotic analgesic)/acetaminophen (a nonnarcotic analgesic)
Normozide	Labetalol (a β-blocker)/hydrochlorothiazide (a diuretic)
Novolin 70/30	Insulin: NPH 70% and rapid-acting regular 30%
NovoLog 70/30	Insulin: aspart suspension 70% and aspart solution 30%
Pediazole	Erythromycin (a macrolide)/sulfisoxazole (a sulfonamide)
Pepcid Complete	Famotidine (an H_2 antagonist)/calcium chloride (an antacid)/ magnesium hydroxide (an antacid)
Percocet	Oxycodone (a narcotic analgesic)/acetaminophen (a nonnarcotic analgesic)
Percodan	Oxycodone (a narcotic analgesic)/aspirin (a nonnarcotic analgesic)
Phenergan with Codeine	Promethazine (an antihistamine)/codeine (a cough suppressant)
Phenergan VC	Promethazine (an antihistamine)/phenylephrine (a vasopressor)
Phenergan VC with Codeine	Promethazine (an antihistamine)/phenylephrine (a vasopressor)/codeine (a cough suppressant)
Polysporin	Polymyxin B (an antiinfective)/bacitracin (an antiinfective)
Pravigard	Aspirin (an antiplatelet)/pravastatin (an antihyperlipidemic)
Premphase	Conjugated estrogens (an estrogen)/medroxyprogesterone (an androgen)
Prempro	Conjugated estrogens (an estrogen)/medroxyprogesterone (an androgen)
Prevacid NapraPAC	Lansoprazole (a proton pump inhibitor)/naproxen (an NSAID)
Prinzide	Lisinopril (an ACE inhibitor)/hydrochlorothiazide (a diuretic)
Rebetron	Ribavirin (an antiviral)/interferon alfa 2b (an immunologic agent)
Reprexain CIII	Ibuprofen (an NSAID)/hydrocodone (a narcotic analgesic)
Rifamate	Rifampin (an antitubercular)/isoniazid (an antitubercular)
Rifater	Rifampin (an antitubercular)/isoniazid (an antitubercular)/ pyrazinamide (an antitubercular)
Robitussin AC	Guaifenesin (an antitussive)/codeine (a narcotic analgesic)

Combination Product Name	Generic Components
Robitussin DM	Dextromethorphan (a cough suppressant)/guaifenesin (an antitussive)
Roxicet	Oxycodone (a narcotic analgesic)/acetaminophen (a nonnarcotic analgesic)
Senokot-S	Senna (a laxative)/docusate (a laxative)
Septra	Sulfamethoxazole (a sulfonamide)/trimethoprim (an antiinfective)
Silain-Gel	Magnesium hydroxide (an antacid)/aluminum hydroxide (an antacid)/simethicone (an antiflatulent)
Stalevo	Carbidopa-levodopa (an antiparkinson agent)/entacapone (an antiparkinson agent)
Suboxone	Buprenorphine (a nonnarcotic analgesic)/naloxone (a narcotic antagonist)
Symbyax	Fluoxetine (an antidepressant)/olanzapine (an antipsychotic)
TAC	Tetracaine (an anesthetic)/epinephrine (a vasoconstrictor)/cocaine (an anesthetic)
Tarka	Trandolapril (an ACE inhibitor)/verapamil (a calcium channel blocker)
Teczem	Enalapril (an ACE inhibitor)/diltiazem (a calcium channel blocker)
Tenoretic	Atenolol (a β-blocker)/chlorthalidone (a diuretic)
Teveten HCT	Eprosartan (an angiotensin II receptor antagonist)/hydrochlorothiazide (a diuretic)
Thyrolar	Liothyronine (a thyroid agent)/levothyroxine (a thyroid agent)
Timolide	Timolol (a β-blocker)/hydrochlorothiazide (a diuretic)
TobraDex	Tobramycin (an aminoglycoside)/dexamethasone (an adrenocortical steroid)
Triavil	Perphenazine (an antipsychotic)/amitriptyline (an antidepressant)
Trizivir	Abacavir (an antiretroviral)lamivudine (an antiretroviral)/zidovudine (an antiretroviral)
Truvada	Emtricitabine (an antiretroviral)/tenofovir (an antiretroviral)
Tylenol with Codeine	Acetaminophen (a nonnarcotic analgesic)/codeine (a narcotic analgesic)
Tylox	Acetaminophen (a nonnarcotic analgesic)/oxycodone (a narcotic analgesic)
Ultracet	Tramadol (a nonnarcotic analgesic)/acetaminophen (a nonnarcotic analgesic)
Uniretic	Moexipril (an ACE inhibitor)/hydrochlorothiazide (a diuretic)
Vaseretic	Enalapril (an ACE inhibitor)/hydrochlorothiazide (a diuretic)
Vasocidin	Sulfacetamide (an antiinfective)/prednisolone (an adrenocortical steroid)

Combination Product Name	Generic Components
Vicodin	Hydrocodone (a narcotic analgesic)/acetaminophen (a nonnarcotic analgesic)
Vicodin ES	Hydrocodone (a narcotic analgesic)/acetaminophen (a nonnarcotic analgesic)
Vicodin HP	Hydrocodone (a narcotic analgesic)/acetaminophen (a nonnarcotic analgesic)
Vicoprofen	Hydrocodone (a narcotic analgesic)/ibuprofen (an NSAID)
Vytorin	Ezetimibe (an antihyperlipidemic)/simvastatin (an antihyperlipidemic)
Zestoretic	Lisinopril (an ACE inhibitor)/hydrochlorothiazide (a diuretic)
Ziac	Bisoprolol (a β-blocker)/hydrochlorothiazide (a diuretic)
Zotrim	Trimethoprim (an antiinfective)/sulfamethoxazole (a sulfonamide)/phenazopyridine (a spasmolytic)
Zydone	Hydrocodone (a narcotic analgesic)/acetaminophen (a nonnarcotic analgesic)
Zyrtec D 12 hour tablets	Cetirizine (an antihistamine)/pseudoephedrine (a nasal decongestant)

From *Mosby's 2006 drug consult for nurses,* St. Louis, 2006, Mosby.
ACE, Angiotensin-converting enzyme inhibitor, *CNS,* central nervous system; *NSAID,* nonsteroidal antiinflammatory drug.

aloe vera

(Aloe vera, Aloe barbadensis)

OTHER NAMES:
Burn plant, curaçao aloes

CLASS:
Herbal remedy

MAJOR INGREDIENTS

The term *aloe vera* conventionally refers to the gel within the aloe leaf. (The glands in the leaf surface contain a different and unsafe substance called *drug aloe*, which is not present, except in trace amounts, in aloe gel products.) The major active ingredients of aloe vera gel are thought to be its polysaccharides, especially one called *acemannan*. Other potentially important constituents include sitosterols and lignins.

CLAIMED ACTIONS

Aloe vera juice is widely credited with the ability to enhance skin regeneration after burns or wounds, but randomized controlled trials (RCTs) of aloe for speeding resolution of sunburn, skin damage caused by radiation therapy, and wounds have generally failed to find benefit. On the basis of the same putative tissue healing effect, aloe has been recommended for treatment of stomach ulcers and other gastrointestinal (GI) tract diseases, but no meaningful evidence supports these uses. Other claimed effects that lack supporting evidence from properly designed RCTs include immune stimulation and suppression of human immunodeficiency (HIV) infection (however, acemannan is approved by the U.S. Food and Drug Administration for treatment of fibrosarcoma in cats and dogs.) Two RCTs indicate that oral aloe gel might have a hypoglycemic effect in patients with type 2 diabetes, but it has been suggested that these benefits were due to trace contamination of the aloe gel with parts of the leaf glands, supplying some drug aloe.

USES

Preliminary RCTs of moderate to low quality suggest that aloe vera cream offers benefit for treatment of seborrhea, psoriasis, and genital herpes, reducing symptoms and speeding resolution. Other uses based on the claimed actions noted previously lack RCT support.

ADMINISTRATION

In most of the studies that produced positive results for seborrhea, psoriasis, and genital herpes, aloe was applied as a cream containing 0.5% of aloe extract administered three times daily. One study used a cream containing 30% aloe gel. Whole aloe gel (rather than cream) applied topically has generally shown less benefit. A typical oral dose of aloe vera juice is 1 tablespoon twice daily. Maximum safe doses in pregnant or nursing women, young children, and individuals with severe hepatic or renal disease are not established.

SIDE EFFECTS

Use of aloe gel, either internally or externally, has not been associated with any significant side effects other than nonspecific GI distress or allergic reactions. Drug aloe (made from the leaf glands and not generally available in the United States) is a strong laxative and should not be used.

DENTAL CONSIDERATIONS

Some people may swish or gargle with aloe preparation in hopes of treating periodontal disease. There is no evidence for or against this use.

DRUG INTERACTIONS

If aloe vera products can, in fact, reduce blood sugar in type 2 diabetes, potentiation interactions with oral hypoglycemics are a possibility. However, no such interactions have yet been reported.

bilberry fruit

(Vaccinium myrtillus)

OTHER NAMES:
Blueberry, huckleberry, hurtleberry, Myrtilli fructus

CLASS:
Herbal remedy

MAJOR INGREDIENTS

The *fruit* is the medicinal part under discussion. (Bilberry *leaf* is an entirely different and much less common product, with different uses, often proposed for glucose control.) The proposed active ingredients of bilberry fruit are its anthocyanosides. Other constituents include flavone glycosides, iridoids, tannins, caffeic acid derivatives, and fruit acids.

CLAIMED ACTIONS

The anthocyanosides in bilberry have antioxidant properties. In vitro and other highly preliminary evidence suggests that they influence collagen metabolism by increasing cross-linkage of collagen fibers, inhibiting collagen degradation, promoting collagen biosynthesis, reducing inflammatory activity, and scavenging free radicals. The net effect may be decreased capillary permeability and hence reduced capillary leakage in venous insufficiency and ischemia reperfusion. Other in vitro studies hint that anthocyanosides have an affinity for the retina, where they speed recovery of rhodopsin and alter enzymatic reactions in retinal tissues. At very high doses, anthocyanosides inhibit platelet aggregation.

USES

Bilberry fruit is widely used in the belief that it enhances night vision, but the basis for this use rests largely on anecdotes and a few poorly controlled studies performed in the 1960s. More recent and better-designed RCTs have failed to find any benefit. However, weak evidence from small, poor-quality clinical trials hints at benefits in diabetic or hypertensive retinopathy, as well as venous insufficiency.

ADMINISTRATION

Typical dose of bilberry fruit is 160 mg twice per day of an extract standardized to contain 25% bilberry anthocyanosides. Maximum safe doses in pregnant or nursing women, young children, and individuals with severe hepatic or renal disease are not established, but pregnant women have been given bilberry at the aforementioned dose in clinical trials.

SIDE EFFECTS

Animal and human trials indicate that bilberry fruit has a low level of toxicity. Reported side effects are limited to rare allergic reactions and nonspecific GI effects.

DENTAL CONSIDERATIONS

Ask why the product is being used.

DRUG INTERACTIONS

If taken in high doses, bilberry conceivably could potentiate anticoagulant or antiplatelet agents, but no such interactions have been reported.

bistort

(Polygonum bistorta)

OTHER NAMES:

Adder wort, dragonwort, Easter mangiant, English serpentary, oderwort, osterick, passions, patience dock, snakeweed, sweet dock, twice writhen

CLASS:

Herbal remedy

MAJOR INGREDIENTS

Tannins.

CLAIMED ACTIONS

Astringent, antidote for selected poisons or venoms, antidiarrheal, and antiinflammatory.

USES

Uses have included all forms of diarrhea and cholera. It has been used in a mouth rinse for gum disease, canker sores, and stomatitis. External uses include sores, wounds, and hemorrhage. It was used traditionally to treat insect bites, snake bites, gonorrhea, smallpox, measles, and intestinal worms.

ADMINISTRATION

The leaves, roots, and rhizomes can be used to form a powder; also used as a tea, tincture, infusion, or ointment.

SIDE EFFECTS

Increase in mucous production, irritation of the GI tract, and possible hepatic damage.

DENTAL CONSIDERATIONS

Awareness of patient use of product for sore throat or mouth rinse.

DRUG INTERACTIONS

Tinctures contain alcohol and should not be used with disulfiram.

black cohosh

(Cimicifuga racemosa, Cimicifuga racemosa rhizoma)

OTHER NAMES:

Black snakeroot, baneberry

CLASS:

Herbal remedy

MAJOR INGREDIENTS

The active chemicals are described as triterpene glycosides (acetin, 27-deoxyacetin, cimigoside, cimicifugoside, and racemoside), along with phytosterin and flavone derivatives. Other constituents include ferulic acids, isoflavones, fatty acids, and a volatile oil. The fresh and dried rhizomes are the portions of the plant used.

CLAIMED ACTIONS

Black cohosh is not a typical phytoestrogen (plant-based substance with estrogenic actions) because none of its constituents bind to estrogen receptors. It has been hypothesized, though, that some unknown constituent(s) of black cohosh undergo metabolic activation and acquire selective estrogen receptor modifier activity. Effects have been noted on estrogen receptors in bone (possibly reducing bone breakdown), brain/hypothalamus (altering luteinizing hormone release and reducing vasomotor symptoms), and vaginal cell wall (partially reversing atrophy). Uterus and breast estrogen receptors appear to be relatively unaffected.

USES
Black cohosh is primarily used to treat menopausal syndrome. Limited evidence from placebo-controlled RCTs suggests that it can reduce hot flashes and vaginal dryness, without causing uterine hypertrophy. Black cohosh is sometimes recommended for treatment of premenstrual syndrome (PMS) and dysmenorrhea disorders, but no meaningful evidence supports these uses.

ADMINISTRATION
The typical dosage of black cohosh is one or two tablets twice daily of a standardized extract manufactured to contain 1 mg of 27-deoxyaceteine per tablet. It has been suggested that black cohosh should not be used for more than 6 months except under the supervision of a physician.

CONTRAINDICATIONS
Not recommended for use by pregnant or nursing women.

SIDE EFFECTS
Use of black cohosh in clinical trials has not been associated with any significant side effects other than occasional allergic reactions or nonspecific GI distress. However, there is one case report of autoimmune hepatitis apparently induced by the use of black cohosh. Overdosage may cause vomiting, headache, hypotension, and other symptoms.

DENTAL CONSIDERATIONS
Ask why the product is being used.

DRUG INTERACTIONS
Weak evidence hints that black cohosh can potentiate antihypertensive drugs.

boswellia
(Boswellia serrata)

OTHER NAMES:
Frankincense, salai guggul

CLASS:
Herbal remedy

MAJOR INGREDIENTS
Boswellia is the dried oleores made from the sap of the *Boswellia serrata* tree. Its major ingredients include boswellic acids and volatile oils.

CLAIMED ACTIONS
Whole boswellia, as well as isolated boswellic acids, have shown antiinflammatory effects in in vitro, animal, and preliminary human trials.

USES
Preliminary RCTs suggest that boswellia might reduce symptoms of asthma, osteoarthritis, and inflammatory bowel disease,

presumably through antiinflammatory effects. RCTs on boswellia for rheumatoid arthritis were of low quality and produced inconsistent results. Boswellic acids are undergoing study for palliative treatment of malignant glioma, in which they may reduce cerebral edema and possibly slow tumor growth.

ADMINISTRATION

In most clinical trials, boswellia was taken at a dose of 300 to 400 mg three times per day, in the form of an extract standardized to contain 37.5% boswellic acids. Higher doses have been tried. Safety in pregnant or nursing women, young children, and individuals with severe hepatic or renal disease is not established.

SIDE EFFECTS

Use of boswellia in clinical trials has not been associated with any significant side effects other than rare allergic reactions and nonspecific GI distress. However, these trials generally used a pharmaceutical-grade extract of the herb boswellia or simply purified boswellic acids. Preparations made from the whole herb or use under less careful supervision might present additional risks.

DENTAL CONSIDERATIONS

Ask why the product is being used.

DRUG INTERACTIONS

No dental drug interactions are reported.

butterbur

(Petasites hybridus, P. albus, P. vulgaris)

OTHER NAMES:
Petasin, blatterdock, butterfly dock, capdockin, flapperdock, umbrella leaves

CLASS:
Herbal remedy

MAJOR INGREDIENTS

The entire plant is used medically. The major active ingredients are thought to be the sesquiterpene alcohol esters petasin and isopetasin. Hepatotoxic pyrrolizidine alkaloids are present in the crude herb but are removed during the manufacturing process for standardized products.

CLAIMED ACTIONS

Preliminary evidence suggests that butterbur, presumably through its petasin and isopetasin content, has antiinflammatory, antispasmodic, and antihistaminic properties. Its proposed antiinflammatory effect appears to be mediated through peptido-leukotrienes rather than prostaglandins.

USES

Standardized butterbur extract is widely used for prophylaxis of migraine headaches, but only one RCT supports this use. A double-blind comparative study without a placebo group found weak evidence that butterbur extract might have utility in allergic rhinitis. Another RCT failed to find butterbur to be effective for allergic skin disease. Other proposed uses based on the apparent actions of butterbur but lacking meaningful supporting evidence include asthma, bladder spasms, gallbladder pain, irritable bowel syndrome, musculoskeletal pain, and tension headaches.

ADMINISTRATION

The typical dosage of butterbur is 50 mg twice daily of an extract standardized to contain 7.5 mg of petasin and isopetasin. Only products that are certified free from pyrrolizidine alkaloids should be used.

CONTRAINDICATIONS

Until further safety studies are performed, butterbur extract is not recommended for use by pregnant or nursing women, young children, or those with liver disease.

SIDE EFFECTS

Use of pharmaceutical-grade standardized butterbur extract in clinical trials has not been associated with any significant side effects other than occasional allergic reactions and nonspecific GI distress. However, there is one case report of cholestatic hepatitis apparently linked to use of butterbur extract. Unprocessed butterbur contains toxic pyrrolizidine alkaloids and should not be used at all.

DENTAL CONSIDERATIONS

Ask why the product is being used.

DRUG INTERACTIONS

No dental drug interactions are reported.

chamomile

(Matricaria chamomilla, Matricaria recutita, Anthemis nobilis, Matricaria flos)

OTHER NAMES:

Roman chamomile, common chamomile, German chamomile

CLASS:

Herbal remedy

MAJOR INGREDIENTS

Volatile oil containing α-bisabolol and other bisabolol derivatives (chamazulene, apigenin), various flavonoids, umbelliferone (coumarin-like ingredient), and many other components. The portion of the plant used is the dried flower.

CLAIMED ACTIONS

Antiinflammatory, antispasmodic, antibacterial, carminative, and to promote wound healing.

USES

Chamomile cream is widely used to treat eczema and minor wounds, but only scant preliminary evidence supports this use. One RCT failed to find chamomile cream helpful for treatment of radiation therapy-induced skin damage; another failed to find benefit for aphthous ulcers caused by 5-fluorouracil chemotherapy. One RCT did find evidence that inhalation of chamomile essential oil can reduce common cold symptoms. Oral chamomile has been used to treat inflammation and spasm in the GI tract, but this indication has no reliable supporting evidence.

ADMINISTRATION

Available in a variety of dose forms including teas, infusions (external use), mouth rinse, and oral dose forms.

SIDE EFFECTS

Slight risk of contact dermatitis; possible cross allergies with ragweed.

DENTAL CONSIDERATIONS

Ask why the product is being used. Inquire about bleeding history in patients taking warfarin or other oral anticoagulant. Inquire about unusual bleeding episodes following dental treatment.

DRUG INTERACTIONS

Evidence is lacking, but theoretically patients taking oral anticoagulants could show increased bleeding times. Possible risk of increased sedation with central nervous system (CNS) depressants. Black cohosh may inhibit CYP3A4 activity, potentially changing serum levels of numerous drugs, but case reports are lacking.

chaste tree, chasteberry

(Vitex agnus-castus, Agni casti fructus)

OTHER NAMES:
Chaste tree fruit, monk's pepper, chaste tree

CLASS:
Herbal remedy

MAJOR INGREDIENTS

Iridoid glycosides (agnuide and aucubin), flavonoids, progestins, testosterone, and multiple essential oils. The portion of the plant used is the dried, ripe fruit.

CLAIMED ACTIONS

Chasteberry is thought to inhibit the release of prolactin through action on dopamine receptors, although the evidence for this effect remains incomplete. It does not have a direct estrogenlike or progesteronelike effect.

USES

Chasteberry is primarily used for treatment of cyclic breast pain, a use supported by several RCTs. It may produce benefits in PMS, although the evidence for this indication is largely limited to one well-designed RCT. Other proposed uses, all based on its prolactin-related actions and lacking significant clinical trial support, include amenorrhea, luteal phase defect, and infertility. No evidence or rationale indicates that chasteberry is helpful for menopausal syndrome, but it is sometimes recommended for that purpose.

ADMINISTRATION

The typical dosage of chasteberry extract is 20 to 40 mg daily, usually in one morning dose.

CONTRAINDICATIONS

Because of its effect on prolactin, chasteberry should not be used by pregnant or nursing women. Possible risk of increased ovulation and pregnancy in some women.

SIDE EFFECTS

Chasteberry was well tolerated in clinical trials, producing no more than nonspecific reactions. There is one case report of ovarian hyperstimulation apparently caused by chasteberry.

DENTAL CONSIDERATIONS

Ask why the product is being used.

DRUG INTERACTIONS
Based on its presumed mechanism of action, chasteberry might potentiate the action of bromocriptine. Dopamine receptor antagonists theory could block some herbal effects.

chondroitin sulfate

OTHER NAMES:
Chondroitin

CLASS:
Nonherbal remedy

MAJOR INGREDIENT
Chondroitin sulfate is a mucopolysaccharide, that is, a glycosaminoglycan (GAG). It is found in mammalian cartilaginous tissue and is believed to play a role in flexibility. It is highly viscous and related chemically to sodium hyaluronate.

CLAIMED ACTIONS
It has useful viscoelastic properties suitable for use in selected types of ocular surgery, usually in combination with sodium hyaluronate. Orally administered GAGs are believed to concentrate in cartilage. Chondrocytes use GAGs to form a new cartilage matrix. It may inhibit leukocyte elastase when high concentrations are associated with rheumatoid arthritis. Other properties may include bringing synovial fluid into the joint. All of these may contribute to reduced inflammatory activity in joints. Serum lipid-lowering and antithrombogenic effects have been suggested.

USES
The primary use of chondroitin as a dietary supplement is for treatment of osteoarthritis, often in combination with glucosamine. The results of several RCTs of varying quality indicate that chondroitin can reduce symptoms to approximately the same extent as nonsteroidal antiinflammatory drugs (NSAIDs). Weaker evidence supports a possible disease-modifying effect (slowing progressive joint damage). Chondroitin in an ophthalmic solution has been used to treat dry eyes. In combination with sodium hyaluronate it is used to support ocular surgery during cataract removal and lens implantation surgery. Its use in cardiovascular diseases remains in doubt.

ADMINISTRATION
A variety of oral dose forms are available, many in combination with glucosamine. Professionally used ophthalmic preparations are available.

SIDE EFFECTS
Long-term side effects are unknown. GI complaints are reported occasionally.

DENTAL CONSIDERATIONS
Ask why the product is being used. Arthritic patients may also be taking aspirin, NSAIDs, or arthritic disease-modifying drugs in addition to chondroitin. Question the patient about other antiarthritic drugs used including over-the-counter (OTC) drugs.

DRUG INTERACTIONS
None reported with dental drugs.

conjugated linoleic acids

OTHER NAMES:
CLAs

CLASS:
Nonherbal remedy

MAJOR INGREDIENTS

Conjugated linoleic acids are mixed isomers of the essential ω-6 fatty acid linoleic acid.

CLAIMED ACTIONS

The essential fatty acids in CLAs are hypothesized to affect fat metabolism. Limited and inconsistent evidence suggests that CLA supplements increase fat metabolism while retaining lean muscle mass. CLA has functional similarities to thiazolidinedione, which led to investigation of potential hypoglycemic effects; however, the limited evidence available suggests a possible hyperglycemic effect instead. Chemopreventive and hypolipidemic effects have also been hypothesized.

USES

The most common use of CLA is as an aid to enhancing body composition, said to "burn fat" while helping to increase muscle mass. However, the clinical evidence for this effect is limited to small RCTs with inconsistent results. CLA does not appear to aid weight loss per se.

ADMINISTRATION

Typical dose is 3 to 5 g daily.

CONTRAINDICATIONS

At this time, CLA should not be used by nursing mothers because one clinical trial found that CLA supplements reduced the fat content of breast milk.

SIDE EFFECTS

CLA generally causes no side effects other than nonspecific GI distress. Safety in pregnant women, young children, and individuals with liver disease is not established.

DENTAL CONSIDERATIONS

Ask why the product is being used.

DRUG INTERACTIONS

One study found potential hyperglycemic effects with CLA, suggesting antagonistic interactions with hypoglycemic agents. However, no such interactions have been reported.

coenzyme Q10

OTHER NAMES:
CoQ10, ubiquinone

CLASS:
Nonherbal remedy

MAJOR INGREDIENTS

Coenzyme Q10 is a cofactor found in all animal and plant cells. No dietary intake is necessary because the body manufactures it from other, widely available precursors.

CLAIMED ACTIONS

CoQ10 is an essential cofactor in the Krebs cycle, playing a role in the aerobic production of adenosine triphosphate (ATP). Because heart muscle depends entirely on aerobic energy production, CoQ10 supplementation has been suggested as a way to enhance myocardial function. Further support for this treatment approach comes from evidence of reduced myocardial CoQ10 in people with congestive heart failure. In addition, certain medications often taken by individuals with heart disease, most notably statins, are thought to either suppress the endogenous production of CoQ10 or interfere with its function. This suggests a need for repletion; however, little evidence as yet indicates that exogenous CoQ10 provides any objective or subjective benefit for people using such medications (other than restoring normal CoQ10 levels). Other proposed uses of CoQ10 are based on its antioxidant properties or other unknown mechanisms.

USES

Incomplete and somewhat inconsistent evidence from double-blind trials suggests that CoQ10 may offer benefit as adjuvant therapy for congestive heart failure, enhancing cardiac performance. Weaker and again inconsistent evidence suggests possible benefits in cardiomyopathy, hypertension, cardiac reperfusion injury, and diabetes. Weak evidence hints that CoQ10 might reduce doxorubicin cardiotoxicity, improve renal function in chronic renal failure, enhance antibody response to hepatitis B vaccine, aid recovery from periodontal disease, reduce symptoms of muscular dystrophy and neurogenic atrophy, and slow the progression of Parkinson's disease. CoQ10 does not appear to be helpful as a sports supplement. See Drug Interactions for a list of the medications for which CoQ10 has been recommended as a repletion agent.

ADMINISTRATION

Typical dosage of CoQ10 is 30 to 150 mg taken two or three times daily. Maximum safe doses in pregnant or nursing women, young children, and individuals with severe hepatic or renal disease are not established.

SIDE EFFECTS

CoQ10 appears to offer little to no toxic risk. Use of CoQ10 in human trials continuing for up to 6 years has shown no serious side effects. Mild nonspecific GI distress may occur. There have been a few questionable case reports of a CoQ10 withdrawal syndrome in individuals using the supplement for congestive heart failure.

DENTAL CONSIDERATIONS

Patients who believe that CoQ10 offers benefit for periodontal disease may be advised that the evidence for benefit with this expensive supplement is exceedingly weak.

DRUG INTERACTIONS

CoQ10 has a molecular similarity to vitamin K, which has led to concerns that CoQ10 use might antagonize the effects of warfarin. However, one study designed to evaluate this possibility found that use of CoQ10 caused no change in international normalized ratio or warfarin dosage. Drugs thought to interfere with the production or action of CoQ10, and therefore to potentially benefit from repletion, include the following: β-blocking agents (alprenolol, metoprolol, and propranolol to a greater extent than timolol), clonidine, hydrochlorothiazide, methyldopa, oral hypoglycemics acetohexamide [Dymelor], glyburide, phenformin, and tolazamide to a greater extent than chlorpropamide, glipizide, and tolbutamide), phenothiazines, statins, and tricyclic antidepressants. The best evidence for tangible benefit with exogenous CoQ10 supplementation exists for statins and tricyclics, but the evidence is not strong.

cranberry

(Vaccinium macrocarpon)

CLASS:

Herbal remedy

MAJOR INGREDIENTS

The berries are the medicinal part used. Cranberries contain a variety of proanthocyanidins, which are its presumed active ingredients. Other constituents include fructose and various plant acids, such as citric acid and malic acid.

CLAIMED ACTIONS

Proanthocyanidin complexes in cranberry are thought to reduce bacterial adhesion to uroepithelial cells by impairing the action of bacterial adhesins, thus interfering with the early stages of infection. This proposed mechanism does not tend to suggest benefits for infections that already are under way.

USES

Limited evidence from RCTs indicates that regular use of cranberry juice concentrate can reduce the incidence of acute urinary tract infections in women. There is no evidence of benefit once an acute infection has begun. Effectiveness for treatment of chronic bacteriuria/pyuria is unclear. One small study suggests that cranberry juice might increase insulin secretion in individuals with type 2 diabetes, but the clinical significance of this finding is unclear.

ADMINISTRATION

Dry cranberry juice extract often is taken at a dose of 500 to 2000 mg, three times daily, depending on the product's concentration. Cranberry juice itself is very bad tasting, and palatable cranberry beverages contain little cranberry. Maximum safe doses in pregnant or nursing women, young children, and individuals with severe hepatic or renal disease are not established.

SIDE EFFECTS

Use of cranberry concentrate is not associated with side effects other than occasional allergic reactions and nonspecific, mild GI distress. Some concerns have been expressed about possible lithogenic actions of cranberry, but it appears that balance intake is more likely to reduce risk of urolithiasis than to increase it.

DENTAL CONSIDERATIONS

Weak evidence hints that the proanthocyanidins in cranberry might offer dental benefits by impairing aggregation of the bacteria involved in plaque formation. However, because the taste of pure cranberry is difficult to tolerate unless sweetener is added, this finding will not have practical use unless an artificial sweetener can be used.

DRUG INTERACTIONS

On the basis of case reports, it appears that high intake of cranberry can increase the action of warfarin, leading to excess anticoagulation. In addition, because cranberries reduce urinary pH, excretion of various drugs might be increased, including opiates, antidepressants, antipsychotics, and some antibiotics. However, there are no actual case reports of such interactions.

creatine

OTHER NAMES:
Creatine monohydrate

CLASS:
Nonherbal remedy

MAJOR INGREDIENT
Creatine is manufactured in the body from arginine, glycine, and methionine. There is no dietary requirement for creatine.

CLAIMED ACTIONS
Exogenous creatine is thought to increase muscle supplies of phosphocreatine, enabling more rapid restoration of ATP levels after a short, high-intensity burst of exertion. Increased creatine levels may also enhance nerve function. These two effects combined are the basis for use of creatine in neuromuscular disorders. In mitochondrial disorders, exogenous creatine is thought to stabilize mitochondrial creatine kinase, decreasing demand on the damaged mitochondria. Creatine may also reduce lipid levels through an as-yet unidentified mechanism.

USES
Numerous small RCTs indicate that creatine may slightly increase performance in high-intensity repetitive burst exercise. However, the evidence is not entirely consistent, and rather specific parameters of duration and rest appear to be necessary for benefit. Creatine is not helpful in endurance exercise, and it may or may not enhance resistance exercise capacity. Other small RCTs suggest possible benefit in congestive heart failure (increasing exercise tolerance) and hyperlipidemia. Results of studies on creatine as an aid to recovery of muscle strength after limb immobilization or as treatment for a variety of neuromuscular and mitochondrial disorders have been mixed.

ADMINISTRATION
Typical daily dose of creatine is 2 to 5 g daily. Athletes typically begin with a loading dose of 15 to 30 g daily for several days, but there is no evidence that this offers additional value.

SIDE EFFECTS
Creatine has a low level of toxicity, but long-term safety studies have not been performed. Common side effects of creatine supplementation include weight gain, mostly from water retention, as well as mild GI distress and possibly muscle cramping and dehydration.
Contrary to some reports, there is no evidence that creatine diminishes the body's ability to tolerate increased environmental temperatures.
Maximum safe doses in pregnant or nursing women, young children, and individuals with severe hepatic or renal disease are not established.

DENTAL CONSIDERATIONS
Ask why the product is being used.

DRUG INTERACTIONS
No dental drug interactions are reported.

dong quai
(Angelica sinensis)

OTHER NAMES:
Chinese angelica, dang-gui

CLASS:
Herbal remedy

MAJOR INGREDIENTS
Active constituents of dong quai may include butylidene phthalide, ferulic acid, β-sitosterol, a variety of coumarins (oxypeucedanin, osthol, and others), an essential oil, polysaccharides, lactones, and vitamins E and B_{12}. The portion of the plant used is the root.

CLAIMED ACTIONS
Vasodilation, antispasmodic in blood vessels, CNS stimulation, and immunosuppressant and antiinflammatory properties. The mechanism of action of these effects is unclear. Contrary to some reports, dong quai does not appear to have phytoestrogen constituents.

USES
It is used in Chinese herbal medicine in combination with other herbs. Uses include dysmenorrhea, other menstrual problems, and menopausal symptoms. Other uses include arthritis, hypertension, and ulcers. However, significant clinical studies are lacking. One RCT failed to find dong quai helpful for menopausal symptoms. The remedy does not appear in the German Commission E monographs.

ADMINISTRATION
Administered orally as an infusion, a tincture, or a chewable root.

CONTRAINDICATIONS
Women who have had breast cancer should not use dong quai. Despite a lack of estrogenic action, dong quai may stimulate breast cancer cell growth (in vitro evidence only).

SIDE EFFECTS
In clinical trials, dong quai has been generally well tolerated. Photosensitization is possible on theoretic grounds. Safety for pregnant or nursing women, young children, and individuals with severe liver or kidney disease is not established.

DENTAL CONSIDERATIONS
Ask why the product is being used. Inquire about bleeding history in patients taking warfarin or other oral anticoagulant. Inquire about unusual bleeding episodes following dental treatment. Caution suggested for combination treatment with photosensitizing drugs.

DRUG INTERACTIONS
Dong quai may interact adversely with anticoagulants or antiplatelet agents.

echinacea
(Echinacea angustifolia, Echinacea purpurea, Echinacea pallida)

OTHER NAMES:
American cone flower, Kansas snakeroot, purple cone flower

CLASS:
Herbal remedy

MAJOR INGREDIENTS
Caffeic acid glycoside (echinacoside), alkylamides (echinacein and others), essential oils (humulene and others), variety of flavonoids, and many other components. As with any plant, the contents vary with the species, the parts of the plant used, and whether the plant is dried or fresh. The portions of the plant used are the flower, other aboveground parts, and even the roots. Most studies finding benefit for the common cold involved preparations made from the aboveground portion of the *E. purpurea* species.

CLAIMED ACTIONS
Stimulation of the immune system (some laboratory data suggest an increase in macrophage phagocytic activity and numbers of neutrophils); possible antibacterial, antiviral, and antiinflammatory activity lack strong support.

USES
Considerable (but not entirely consistent) evidence from RCTs indicates that acute use of echinacea may reduce the symptoms and duration of the common cold and influenza. Chronic use of echinacea does not appear to offer prophylactic benefits against colds. Other uses proposed but lacking meaningful supporting evidence include wound healing, *Candida* infections, supportive therapy for lower urinary tract infections, rheumatoid arthritis, and supportive use in colon cancer.

ADMINISTRATION
Available in a variety of preparations for internal (oral administration) and external use.

CONTRAINDICATIONS
On theoretical grounds, echinacea should not be used in patients with autoimmune diseases or progressive infectious diseases, including tuberculosis, multiple sclerosis, leukocytosis, and collagen diseases, or individuals taking immunosuppressive medications.

SIDE EFFECTS
Generally limited to parenteral doses only. Fatigue, headache, and dizziness were reported with oral doses. Possible risk of cross-allergic reaction with chamomile or ragweed.

DENTAL CONSIDERATIONS
Ask why it is being used. Avoid use during immunosuppression. Use with caution in asthma, atopy, or allergic rhinitis because of potential for allergic reactions.

DRUG INTERACTIONS
May decrease effectiveness of immunosuppressants. Discontinue before use of general anesthetics.

eleutherococcus
(Eleutherococcus senticosus, Acanthopanax senticosus)

OTHER NAMES:
Siberian ginseng, Russian ginseng, eleutheroginseng

CLASS:
Herbal remedy

MAJOR INGREDIENTS
Major constituents include a variety of unrelated lignans, setoids,

phenylacrylic acid derivatives, polysaccharides, steroid glycosides, and triterpene saponins, all somewhat misleadingly named eleutherosides (eleutheroside A, B, etc.). The root and rhizome are the parts used medicinally. Note that despite the common name "Russian ginseng," *Eleutherococcus* has no botanic or biochemical similarity to true ginseng, *Panax ginseng*.

CLAIMED ACTIONS

Eleutherococcus is said to act as an "adaptogen," a substance that enhances an organism's general ability to adapt to stress of all kinds. However, the supporting evidence that eleutherococcus (or any other substance) has adaptogenic properties is limited to human and animal trials of substandard methodology. Some evidence indicates that eleutherococcus may increase maximal oxygen intake during intense exercise. Immunomodulatory effects have been seen in some studies, specifically increases in helper/inducer T lymphocytes.

USES

One RCT found evidence that regular use of eleutherococcus by individuals with chronic recurrent genital herpes reduced the rate of flareups. One RCT failed to find eleutherococcus helpful for chronic fatigue syndrome. The majority of RCTs evaluating eleutherococcus for possible sports performance enhancement effects have failed to find benefit.

ADMINISTRATION

Typical dose of eleutherococcus is 2 to 3 g daily of the whole herb or 300 to 400 mg of a standardized extract. Maximum safe doses in pregnant or nursing women, young children, and individuals with severe hepatic or renal disease are not established.

SIDE EFFECTS

Eleutherococcus is thought to have a low level of toxicity; however, most safety studies were performed in the former Soviet Union, and whether the results can be fully relied upon is not clear. Use of eleutherococcus in clinical trials has not been associated with any significant side effects.

DENTAL CONSIDERATIONS

Ask why the product is being used.

DRUG INTERACTIONS

There is one case report in which use of eleutherococcus appears to have interfered with a laboratory test for serum digoxin levels, causing the test to falsely report an elevation that did not exist. On the basis of its possible immunomodulatory actions, eleutherococcus conceivably could interfere with the action of immunosuppressive drugs, but no such interactions have been reported.

evening primrose oil

(Oenothera biennis)

OTHER NAMES:
Evening primrose

CLASS:
Herbal remedy

MAJOR INGREDIENTS

The oil is a mixture of fatty acids, including linoleic acid (50%–80%), γ-linolenic acid (GLA, 6%–11%), and smaller amounts of other fatty acids, including palmitic acid, oleic acid, and stearic acid. Other ingredients include tannins, sitosterol, and trace minerals. The portion of the plant used is the seed.

CLAIMED ACTIONS

Antiatherosclerotic, relief of premenstrual tension, relief of mastalgia, and antiinflammatory actions for arthritis and dermatologic conditions. The fatty acids contained in the oil may function like essential oils and act as precursors of prostaglandins that help regulate metabolic functions.

USES

Evening primrose is primarily used as a source of GLA. Some RCT evidence suggests that evening primrose or GLA can reduce symptoms of diabetic neuropathy after many months of use. Weak RCT evidence hints that GLA from borage oil may help adult periodontitis. Other potential indications of GLA or evening primrose oil, with weak supporting evidence at best, include hyperlipidemia, PMS, rheumatoid arthritis, and weight loss. Claims are also made that GLA is effective in controlling symptoms of atopic dermatitis, but the most recent and best-designed RCTs failed to find benefit. The same can be said of GLA for treatment of cyclic mastitis. One RCT failed to find evening primrose oil effective for attention deficit/hyperactivity disorder. This herb is not listed in the German Commission E monographs.

ADMINISTRATION

Available as capsules for oral administration.

SIDE EFFECTS

Side effects are few and occur only occasionally. They generally include digestive complaints such as GI distress and nausea.

DENTAL CONSIDERATIONS

Ask why the product is being used. As noted previously, has shown some promise for periodontitis.

DRUG INTERACTIONS

No dental drug interactions are reported.

feverfew

(Tanacetum parthenium, Chrysanthemum parthenium)

OTHER NAMES:

Featherfew, feverfew leaf, bachelor's button

CLASS:

Herbal remedy

MAJOR INGREDIENTS

Sesquiterpene lactones, especially parthenolide 85%, once were considered the active ingredients in feverfew. However, studies using parthenolide-rich extracts found no benefit, and attention now is focused elsewhere. One bioactive candidate is tanetin, a lipophilic avonol (6-hydroxykaempferol 3,7,4′-trimethyl ether) that inhibits proinflammatory eicosanoids. Other constituents include volatile oils (camphor, *trans*-chrysanthylacetate), flavonoids (luteolin, apigenin), and many other constituents. The portion of the plant used is the leaf.

CLAIMED ACTIONS

Inhibition of proinflammatory eicosanoids resulting in antiinflammatory actions.
May decrease platelet aggregation and serotonin release (laboratory studies). It is not listed in the German Commission E monographs.

USES

A few small RCTs have found that regular use of feverfew leaf can reduce the severity, duration, or incidence of migraines. Studies using feverfew extracts standardized to parthenolide content, however, have failed to find benefits.
Other proposed uses, including osteoarthritis, rheumatoid arthritis, and stimulation of menstruation, lack RCT support.

ADMINISTRATION

Available in many oral dose forms or used to make an infusion. Safety in nursing women or individuals with severe hepatic or renal disease is not established.

CONTRAINDICATIONS

Because of its history of use as an abortifacient, feverfew should not be used by pregnant women.

SIDE EFFECTS

Oral products produce few complaints; chewing the leaves may lead to oral ulcerations and swelling of circumoral tissues. Potential risk for increased bleeding time.

DENTAL CONSIDERATIONS

Ask why the product is being used. Inquire about bleeding history in patients taking warfarin or other oral anticoagulant. Inquire about unusual bleeding episodes following dental treatment.

DRUG INTERACTIONS

On a theoretic basis, feverfew might potentiate the effects of antiplatelet agents and increase gastric side effects of NSAIDs. However, no such interactions have been reported. Advise patients not to take this herb for 2 to 3 weeks before surgery.

garlic

(Allium sativum)

OTHER NAMES:

Allium, poor man's treacle

CLASS:

Herbal remedy

MAJOR INGREDIENTS

A volatile oil containing several sulfur compounds, a sulfur-containing amino acid identified as alliin. With grinding, alliin is converted to allicin, which is responsible for the typical odor of garlic, as well as much of its bioactivity. Ajoene and *S*-allylcysteine are other active compounds. The portions of the plant used are whole (fresh or dried) garlic clove and oil of garlic.

CLAIMED ACTIONS

With oral use, actions claimed for garlic include hypolipidemic, antiplatelet aggregation, antihypertensive, antioxidant, antiatherosclerotic, and immune stimulant activity. In vitro studies have found topical antibiotic, antifungal, and antiviral actions. Antithrombotic effects have been documented in vitro and in vivo.

USES
Despite widespread use for hyperlipidemia, current evidence from well-designed RCTs suggests that garlic does not improve lipid levels to more than a minimal extent. Some evidence from preliminary RCTs indicates that regular use of standardized garlic extracts may reduce the incidence of the common cold in adults and children. Weak RCT evidence indicates possible antihypertensive and antiatherosclerotic actions. One RCT suggests that oral use of garlic can decrease insect (tick) bites. Topically, garlic has been used to treat a wide array of bacterial, fungal, and viral infections, but there are no rigorous supporting data. Oral antibiotic effectiveness is unlikely. Use in GI fungal infections remains in doubt. Long-term effects are unknown.

ADMINISTRATION
Available in a variety of oral dose forms. The best-studied form of garlic is garlic powder specially stabilized to provide alliin, which can be converted to allicin. Raw garlic also provides alliin/allicin, but other forms of garlic, such as cooked garlic, garlic oil, and aged garlic products, do not provide alliin. (Nonetheless, some pharmacologic effects have been seen with these other forms, presumably from other constituents.)

SIDE EFFECTS
The taste and odor of garlic are by far the most common complaints. Rarely GI symptoms occur with larger doses. Halitosis and burning of the mouth have been reported. There is one case report of spontaneous spinal epidural hematoma attributed to use of garlic products. Note that standardized garlic is more similar to raw garlic than to cooked garlic; therefore the common food use of cooked garlic cannot be taken as evidence of safety.

DENTAL CONSIDERATIONS
Ask why the product is being used. Inquire about unusual bleeding episodes following dental treatment.

DRUG INTERACTIONS
Garlic might potentiate antiplatelet or anticoagulant agents. Because of increased risk of bleeding, advise patients not to take this herb for 2 to 3 weeks before surgery. Garlic has been found to reduce plasma concentrations of saquinavir and possibly increase the GI toxicity of ritonavir (drugs used for HIV).

ginger
(Zingiber officinale, Zingiberis rhizoma)

OTHER NAMES:
Ginger root

CLASS:
Herbal remedy

MAJOR INGREDIENTS
The root contains a volatile oil and other chemicals termed *pungent principals.* These latter compounds are collectively known as gingerols, shogaols, and gingerdiols. The portion of the plant used is the root.

CLAIMED ACTIONS
Motion sickness prevention, promotion of salivary and gastric

secretions, positive inotropic action, and antiplatelet and antiinflammatory effects have all been claimed for this herb. Gluonolactone, an active ingredient, has been reported to have serotonin (5-HT) antagonist activity, and gingerols may have a positive inotropic effect.

USES

Incomplete and somewhat inconsistent evidence from multiple RCTs of varying quality suggests that ginger can reduce motion sickness symptoms. Other RCTs suggest benefits for nausea and vomiting of pregnancy (morning sickness). Results on benefits for postsurgical anesthesia are contradictory. Ginger has been used for nausea of chemotherapy, but supporting evidence is weak. RCTs have shown equivocal results regarding efficacy in osteoarthritis.

ADMINISTRATION

Only the rhizome (rootlike stalk) of the plant is used. The German Commission E monographs list the dose at 2 to 4 g daily. Despite ginger's medical use in nausea and vomiting of pregnancy, safety during pregnancy and lactation is not established.

SIDE EFFECTS

Generally not reported except for toxic doses that could include CNS depression and arrhythmia.

DENTAL CONSIDERATIONS

Ask why the product is being used.

DRUG INTERACTIONS

Although ginger has shown antiplatelet rather than anticoagulant effects, there is one case report in which use of ginger apparently potentiated phenprocoumon. Interactions with other anticoagulants or antiplatelet agents are possible.

ginkgo

(Ginkgo biloba, Ginkgo folium)

OTHER NAMES:

Maidenhair tree, ginkyo

CLASS:

Herbal remedy

MAJOR INGREDIENTS

Common ingredients with claimed pharmacologic activity include multiple flavonoids (biobetin, ginkgetin), flavone glycosides (quercetin), bioflavones, terpenoids (ginkgolides A, B, and C), and bilobalide. The only portion of the plant used is the leaf, made in a specific 50:1 extract. Thus the commonly tested treatment is more properly called *ginkgo biloba extract* (GBE) rather than ginkgo. The seeds are toxic.

CLAIMED ACTIONS

Improvement in blood flow in the microcirculation, inhibition of development of trauma-induced or toxin-induced cerebral edema, improved hypoxic tolerance in cerebral tissues, reduction in retinal edema, increased memory performance, inhibition of age-related reduction in muscarinic receptors, and antagonism of platelet-activating factor (PAF). It may have monoamine oxidase (MAO) inhibition properties.

USES
Significant, but not entirely consistent, evidence from multiple RCTs supports use in Alzheimer's dementia and other forms of dementia. Significant evidence also exists for benefit in intermittent claudication. Weaker evidence from RCTs supports use in normal age-related memory impairment, PMS, Raynaud's phenomenon, and vertiginous syndromes. Other potential uses with limited support include idiopathic sudden hearing loss, glaucoma, macular degeneration, and diabetic microvascular disease. Contrary to earlier reports, ginkgo does not appear to be effective for sexual dysfunction (in men or women), tinnitus, or mountain sickness.

ADMINISTRATION
Capsules and tablets of leaf extracts are available for use. Doses range from 120 to 240 mg of 50:1 dry extract for 8 weeks for chronic diseases. Use for longer than 3 months requires reevaluation of benefits.

CONTRAINDICATIONS
Not recommended for use by pregnant or nursing women. Individuals with seizure disorders should not use ginkgo.

SIDE EFFECTS
In clinical trials, ginkgo has been well tolerated, producing no more than occasional mild allergies and nonspecific GI distress. There are several reports of internal bleeding attributable to use of ginkgo, including bleeding episodes during surgery. Seizures have been reported. One report of oral ulcerations is noted.

DENTAL CONSIDERATIONS
Ask why the product is being used. Inquire about unusual bleeding episodes following dental treatment.

DRUG INTERACTIONS
There is considerable evidence for anticoagulant and antiplatelet activity with ginkgo; do not combine with other anticoagulant or antiplatelet agents except under close supervision. Discontinue ginkgo use 2 weeks before surgery and general anesthesia. Ginkgo might decrease effectiveness of calcium channel blockers and increase ototoxicity of aminoglycosides. Possible interaction between ginkgo and trazodone (Desyrel) may cause excess stimulation of γ-aminobutyric acid (GABA) receptors leading to CNS depression and possible coma.

ginseng
(Panax quinquefolius, American; Panax ginseng, Korean)

CLASS:
Herbal remedy

MAJOR INGREDIENTS
Constituents vary with the species of ginseng used. Contains steroidlike compounds called *ginsenosides* or *panaxosides.* Other ingredients include a volatile oil and flavonoids, along with smaller quantities of other substances.

CLAIMED ACTIONS
Panax ginseng is said to act as an "adaptogen," a substance that

enhances an organism's general ability to adapt to stress of all kinds. However, the supporting evidence that ginseng (or any other substance) has adaptogenic properties is limited to animal studies and a few human trials of substandard methodology. Despite earlier reports, ginseng itself does not appear to have estrogenic effects.

USES

Preliminary RCTs suggest that American ginseng but not Panax ginseng may improve glucose control in type 2 diabetes. Other uses with limited and in some cases inconsistent RCT support include increasing immune response to influenza vaccine, enhancing mental function, improving blood sugar control in diabetes, correcting erectile dysfunction, and enhancing sports performance.

ADMINISTRATION

The root is used for teas and various other oral preparations.

CONTRAINDICATIONS

Worrisome data from animal studies suggest possible teratogenic effects. Not recommended for use by pregnant women.

SIDE EFFECTS

Ginseng appears to have a low level of toxicity. Use of ginseng in clinical trials was associated with few side effects other than occasional allergic reactions and nonspecific GI distress. However, adulterants included with ginseng products may increase risk for other side effects.

DENTAL CONSIDERATIONS

Ask why the product is being used.

DRUG INTERACTIONS

No specific dental drug interactions are reported, but ginseng may interact with monoamine oxidase inhibitors (MAOIs). Interactions with warfarin are unclear. Discontinue 7 days before general anesthesia and general surgical procedures.

glucosamine sulfate

OTHER NAMES:

Chitosamine, glucosamine

CLASS:

Nonherbal remedy

MAJOR INGREDIENT

Glucosamine sulfate, an aminomonosaccharide (2-amino-2-deoxyglucose), is a component of mucopolysaccharides and mucoproteins. Other salt forms may also be used.

CLAIMED ACTIONS

Glucosamine is used in the synthesis of glycoproteins and GAGs. It is formed in the body from glucose through intermediary metabolic steps to be incorporated into GAGs, which are essential for cartilage function in joints. Exogenous glucosamine is thought to enhance joint proteoglycan content, thereby improving function of the failing joint.

USES

Most but not all published RCTs indicate that glucosamine is superior to placebo and equally effective (though slower acting) than standard NSAIDs for treatment of osteoarthritis. Incomplete RCT evidence also points toward a possible disease-modifying effect (retarding progressive joint damage). Other proposed uses include prevention and treatment of tendon and other soft tissue injuries, but no meaningful evidence supports these indications.

ADMINISTRATION
Usual dose is 500 mg three times daily.

SIDE EFFECTS
Side effects are uncommon but can include GI effects such as nausea, heartburn, diarrhea, and epigastric pain. CNS side effects are rarely observed and may include headache, insomnia, and drowsiness. Contrary to earlier reports, glucosamine does not appear to be harmful for patients with diabetes. However, arthritic patients may be taking aspirin, NSAIDs, or disease-modifying osteoarthritis drugs in addition to glucosamine and chondroitin. Question the patient about other antiarthritic drugs used, including OTC drugs.

DENTAL CONSIDERATIONS
Ask why the product is being used.

DRUG INTERACTIONS
No dental drug interactions are reported.

goldenseal
(Hydrastis canadensis)

OTHER NAMES:
Eye root, yellow root, turmeric root

CLASS:
Herbal remedy

MAJOR INGREDIENTS
Contains the isoquinoline alkaloids hydrastine and berberine, other related alkaloids, and a volatile oil.

CLAIMED ACTIONS
Astringent and antiseptic. May stimulate bile and may have laxative action. Hydrastine has been shown to cause vasoconstriction in peripheral vessels. Berberine may have some antibacterial actions. This herb is not included in the German Commission E monographs.

USES
No proposed uses of goldenseal are supported by RCTs. Goldenseal is frequently added to preparations designed to treat the common cold, but no evidence (or traditional history) suggests that it is effective for this purpose. Goldenseal is widely used topically for minor skin wounds and mucous membrane irritation, again without supporting evidence. Its constituent, berberine, may have some action against intestinal infections, but unrealistically high doses of goldenseal would be required to match the dose of berberine used in studies. Berberine (not goldenseal) has been used for treatment of eye infections. Numerous other proposed uses of goldenseal that lack evidence of efficacy include "masking"

a positive drug screen, treating minor cardiac arrhythmias, and reducing crampy intestinal pain and dyspepsia.

ADMINISTRATION

Typical dosages for oral use are 500 mg three times daily, often in combination with other herbs. Topical goldenseal preparations vary in concentration.

CONTRAINDICATIONS

Not recommended for use by pregnant or nursing women or by individuals with hepatic disease.

SIDE EFFECTS

Safe in usual doses. Adverse effects are more often observed with toxic doses (may include hypertension, convulsions, and breathing difficulties). Photosensitivity is a theoretical possibility.

DENTAL CONSIDERATIONS

Ask why the product is being used.

DRUG INTERACTIONS

No dental drug interactions are reported.

gotu kola

(Centella asiatica)

OTHER NAMES:

TECA (titrated extract of Centella asiatica), TTFCA (total triterpenic fraction of Centella asiatica), hydrocotyle, Indian pennywort

CLASS:

Herbal remedy

MAJOR INGREDIENTS

The aboveground parts of the plant are used medicinally. The major constituents are the triterpene acids and esters known as asiaticosides, asiatic acid, madecassic acid, and madecassoside. *(Note:* Gotu kola, unlike the unrelated kola nut, does not contain caffeine.)

CLAIMED ACTIONS

Gotu kola, or its triterpenic extract, is said to enhance the structure and function of connective tissues, an effect possibly mediated by actions on collagen cross-linking and fibronectin production. This is the basis for most of its proposed uses. However, the supporting evidence for such an effect is generally weak. Gotu kola extracts may weaken the protective outer coating of *Mycobacterium leprae* and on that basis has been used for treatment of leprosy.

USES

Several small RCTs found that gotu kola can decrease pain, edema, and leg fatigue in chronic venous insufficiency of the lower extremity. There is no evidence that it can alter the appearance of visible varicosities. Other small RCTs suggest benefit in the treatment of keloids and leprosy and in reducing the startle reflex to sudden loud noises. Oral and topical gotu kola have been recommended for virtually all diseases of the skin or diseases that have skin manifestations, but no RCT evidence supports these uses.

ADMINISTRATION

The studied dose of gotu kola is 20 to 40 mg three times daily of a triterpenic extract standardized to contain 40% asiaticoside,

29% to 30% asiatic acid, 29% to 30% madecassic acid, and 1% to 2% madecassoside. Safety in pregnant women is not established, but pregnant women have been in enrolled in clinical trials, with no harmful effects seen.

SIDE EFFECTS

Gotu kola appears to have a low level of toxicity. In clinical trials, use of gotu kola has not been associated with any significant side effects other than occasional allergic reactions and mild nonspecific GI distress. However, on the basis of a study in mice, there are some concerns that topical gotu kola might have cancer-promoting actions.

DENTAL CONSIDERATIONS

Ask why the product is being used.

DRUG INTERACTIONS

No dental drug interactions are reported.

grape seed extract

(Vitis vinifera, Vitis coignetiae)

OTHER NAMES:

Grape seed extract, grape seed oil, muskat, de pepins de raisin

CLASS:

Herbal remedy

MAJOR INGREDIENTS

The oil of the grape seed is one of the two major sources of oligomeric proanthocyanidin complexes (OPCs), less commonly called *procyanidolic oligomers* (PCOs). (The other is the bark of maritime pine.) Other constituents include essential fatty acids and tocopherols (vitamin E). Pycnogenol, a trademarked and patented herbal product and dietary supplement, contains similar but not identical OPCs from the bark of the maritime pine *(Pinus maritime*, sometimes called *Pinus nigra var. maritime)*. *Vitis coignetiae* also contains epsilon-viniferin, oligos-tilbenes and amyelopsins, and 51-nucleotidase inhibitors. Resveratrol (3,5, 41-trihydroxystilbene) is present when herbal preparations are mixed with grape skin extract. The seed and sometimes the skin of the grape are used medicinally.

CLAIMED ACTIONS

OPCs have significant free-radical scavenging actions and may protect connective tissue by inhibiting hyaluronidase, elastase, and collagenase and increasing collagen cross-linking. These and other effects may lead to decreased capillary permeability. OPCs inhibit platelet aggregation and alter prostaglandin metabolism.

USES

The best-documented use of OPCs is treatment of chronic venous insufficiency. Several RCTs suggest that OPC treatment can reduce lower extremity pain, edema, and fatigue. Effects on visible varicosities have not been documented. Weaker RCT evidence suggests possible benefit in reducing edema caused by surgery or minor injury. Other indications for OPCs from grape seed that have some support from small RCTs include reducing capillary fragility in liver cirrhosis and alleviating symptoms of allergic rhinitis. Related OPCs from pine bark have shown some potential benefit for periodontal disease, when used in the form of chewing gum. Grape seed OPCs have failed to prove effective for reducing lipid levels. Supposed benefits for cardiovascular disease are entirely theoretical, on the basis of antioxidant and antiplatelet properties.

ADMINISTRATION
Administered orally in tablets or capsules. Doses range from 40 to 300 mg/day, with maintenance doses at 40 to 80 mg daily.

CONTRAINDICATIONS
OPCs are thought to have antiplatelet activity, and on this basis they should not be taken by individuals using anticoagulant or antiplatelet agents.

SIDE EFFECTS
Grape seed OPCs have undergone extensive safety testing and appear to have a low level of toxicity.

DENTAL CONSIDERATIONS
Determine why the patient is taking botanic products. Patients should discontinue use 2 weeks before surgery. As noted previously, OPCs from pine bark have shown some promise for periodontitis.

DRUG INTERACTIONS
There are theoretical concerns that OPCs could potentiate antiplatelet or anticoagulant agents, but no well-documented case reports support this concern.

green tea
(Camellia sinensis)

OTHER NAMES:
EGCG, Camellia thea, Camellia theifera, epigallocatechin gallate, green tea polyphenols, thea bohea, thea sinensis, thea viridis

CLASS:
Herbal remedy

MAJOR INGREDIENTS
The major constituents of green tea include catechin polyphenols (especially epigallocatechin gallate), as well as triterpene saponins, caffeine, theobromine, theophylline, flavonoids, caffeic acid derivatives, and volatile oil. The product is made by steaming the fresh-cut leaf of the plant.

CLAIMED ACTIONS
Observational studies have inconsistently suggested that green tea might reduce cancer and heart disease risk. The polyphenols in green tea have antioxidant properties. Other reported actions of green tea with weak supporting evidence include enhanced thermogenesis, hypolipidemic effects, anti-inflammatory actions in periodontal disease, hepatoprotection, and protection of skin from sun damage.

USES
Green tea or extracts made from green tea are widely used with the expectation that they will reduce the risk of heart disease and cancer. However, at present the supporting evidence for benefit is weak, and no meaningful RCTs indicate benefit. One small double-blind, placebo-controlled trial did provide evidence

that sugarless green tea candy chews have a favorable effect on periodontal disease, as shown by relative improvements in approximal plaque index and sulcus bleeding index. More recently, green tea has become a common ingredient in weight loss products, based only on scant preliminary evidence. The one RCT on this proposed use failed to find benefit for preventing weight regain after weight loss. Neither topical nor oral green teas have proved to provide the same level of protection from the sun as standard sunblocks, although they may provide some protection.

ADMINISTRATION

Three cups of green tea daily, or 100 to 150 mg three times daily of a green tea extract standardized to contain 80% total polyphenols and 50% epigallocatechin gallate.

SIDE EFFECTS

Green tea contains less caffeine and related stimulants than does black tea, but caffeine-related side effects, such as agitation and insomnia, may occur.

DENTAL CONSIDERATIONS

Ask why the product is being used. Individuals who chew green tea candy for putative antiperiodontal disease actions should be cautioned not to consider it a substitute for standard care.

DRUG INTERACTIONS

Green tea contains high levels of vitamin K and therefore would be expected to decrease the effectiveness of warfarin (Coumadin) and related drugs. The caffeine in green tea could interact with MAOIs.

guggul

(Commiphora mukul)

OTHER NAMES:
False myrrh, gum guggul, gugulipid, mukul myrrh tree

CLASS:
Herbal remedy

MAJOR INGREDIENTS

Guggul is the oleo gum resin obtained by drying the sap of the *Commiphora mukul* tree. Its active ingredients are thought to be ketonic steroids known as *guggulsterones*.

CLAIMED ACTIONS

Guggulsterones are strong antagonists of two nuclear hormone receptors involved in cholesterol metabolism, which provides a plausible basis for the use of guggul in the treatment of hyperlipidemia, its major proposed use. It is widely claimed that guggul increases thyroid activity and thereby aids weight loss, but there is no meaningful supporting evidence for either part of this claim.

USES

Although earlier RCTs performed by researchers in India did report hypolipidemic actions, a more recent, larger, and better-designed RCT performed in the United States failed to find benefits; in fact, guggul appeared to increase levels of low-density lipoprotein cholesterol. One RCT found guggul ineffective as a weight loss aid. Other proposed uses of guggul that lack reliable supporting evidence include improving glucose control in diabetes, aiding weight loss, and treating acne.

ADMINISTRATION
Guggul typically is used in a standardized extract form to provide 100 mg of guggulsterones daily (especially E- and Z-guggulsterone). Safety in pregnant or nursing women and in individuals with severe hepatic or renal disease is not established.

SIDE EFFECTS
Guggul appears to have a low level of toxicity. Use of standardized guggul extract in clinical trials has not been associated with any significant side effects other than occasional allergic reactions (especially skin rash) and nonspecific GI distress.

DENTAL CONSIDERATIONS
Ask why the product is being used.

DRUG INTERACTIONS
No dental drug interactions are reported.

hawthorn
(Crataegus oxyacantha, Crataegus folium cum flore, C. monogyna, C. laevigata)

OTHER NAMES:
English hawthorn, maybush

CLASS:
Herbal remedy

MAJOR INGREDIENTS
Flavonoids (hyperoside, vitexin-rhamnose, rutin, proanthocyanidins) with vasodilating properties, as well as inhibition of vasoconstriction. Proanthocyanidins reportedly block angiotensin-converting enzyme (ACE). It also contains tyramine, a biogenic amine. The flowers, leaves, fruits, and mixtures of other plant parts are used medicinally.

CLAIMED ACTIONS
Hawthorn appears to have inotropic actions. In addition, some evidence suggests that hawthorn has antiarrhythmic actions by blocking repolarizing potassium currents in ventricular myocardium, a mechanism similar to that of class III antiarrhythmics. Other reported effects include inhibition of ACE and of cyclic adenosine monophosphate phosphodiesterase.

USES
Moderately strong evidence from multiple RCTs indicates that hawthorn improves signs and symptoms of class I or II congestive heart failure. However, there is no evidence that hawthorn reduces risk of morbidity and mortality (a benefit shown with ACE inhibitors). Weaker RCT support indicates benefits in angina. Other proposed indications that lack substantive support include atherosclerosis, hypertension, benign cardiac arrhythmias, and prevention of postischemic arrhythmias.

ADMINISTRATION
Available in oral dose forms as an extract and plant parts for brewing teas.

SIDE EFFECTS
No contraindications or side effects are reported.

DENTAL CONSIDERATIONS
Ask why the product is being used. Monitor vital signs in patients with cardiovascular disease.

DRUG INTERACTIONS
There are theoretical concerns of possible adverse interactions if the herb is used with other drugs that may affect cardiac function.

horse chestnut extract
(Aesculus hippocastanum)

OTHER NAMES:
HCE; raw form—buckeye, conkers

CLASS:
Herbal remedy

MAJOR INGREDIENTS
The major constituents of horse chestnut are triterpene saponins, especially escin (also spelled "aescin"). Other constituents include flavonoids, polysaccharides, and oligomeric proanthocyanidins. Whole horse chestnut contains the toxic coumarin glycoside esculin (also spelled "aesculin"), but the esculin has been removed from the standard horse chestnut extract product. Horse chestnut seed and leaf both are used medicinally.

CLAIMED ACTIONS
Horse chestnut extract (HCE) is thought to reduce capillary permeability. Proposed mechanisms include venotonic, antiinflammatory, antihydrolase, and antineutrophil adherence properties.

USES
Several moderate-size RCTs of varying quality have found evidence that HCE can reduce symptoms of venous insufficiency in the lower extremities including edema, pain, and fatigue. Benefits (prevention or treatment) regarding visible varicosities have not been documented. One RCT suggests benefits for hemorrhoids. Weaker evidence suggests potential benefits for aiding resolution of phlebitis and reducing edema after surgery or injury. Topical horse chestnut for bruising has similarly weak supporting evidence.

ADMINISTRATION
HCE is taken at a dose of 300 mg twice daily, in a form standardized to contain 50 mg escin per dose. Enteric-coated capsules are used to prevent otherwise predictable stomach discomfort. Safety in pregnant women is not established, but animal data are reassuring, and pregnant women have been enrolled in RCTs of horse chestnut.

SIDE EFFECTS
Whole horse chestnut, as opposed to HCE, is a toxic herb and should not be used. HCE predictably causes gastric irritation if it is not delivered in an enteric-coated capsule. Enteric-coated HCE is not associated with any significant side effects other than occasional allergic reactions.

DENTAL CONSIDERATIONS
Ask why the product is being used.

DRUG INTERACTIONS
Because of its saponin content, horse chestnut might potentiate the effects of antiplatelet or anticoagulant agents.

hydroxymethyl butyrate (HMB)

OTHER NAMES:
Beta-hydroxy beta-methylbutyric acid

CLASS:
Nonherbal remedy

MAJOR INGREDIENTS
Hydroxymethyl butyrate is a naturally occurring degradation product of the amino acid leucine.

CLAIMED ACTIONS
During intense exercise, muscle tissue degradation occurs, which leads to leakage of leucine and its subsequent transformation to HMB. It has been hypothesized that increased HMB levels from exogenous sources provides a downstream feedback signal that slows muscle protein degradation.

USES
Several small RCTs, some published only in abstract form, indicate that use of HMB may enhance response to weight training, resulting in increased muscle mass. On this basis, HMB has become a popular supplement for bodybuilders. However, the supporting evidence must be regarded as weak, and the benefits, if any, are modest. Even weaker evidence hints that HMB might have an antihypertensive or hypolipidemic effect.

ADMINISTRATION
Typical dosage of HMB is 1 g three times daily. Maximum safe doses in young children, pregnant or nursing women, and individuals with severe hepatic or renal disease are not established.

SIDE EFFECTS
HMB appears to have a low level of toxicity. Use of HMB in clinical trials has not been associated with any significant side effects other than occasional nonspecific GI distress. However, long-term safety studies have not been performed.

DENTAL CONSIDERATIONS
Ask why the product is being used.

DRUG INTERACTIONS
No dental drug interactions are reported.

kava

(Piper methysticum, Piperis methystici rhizoma)

OTHER NAMES:
Kava-kava, kew, tonga

CLASS:
Herbal remedy

MAJOR INGREDIENTS
Kava lactones (kava α-pyrones), including methysticin, kawain, and others. The dried rhizomes are the parts used medicinally.

CLAIMED ACTIONS
These lactones have demonstrable pharmacologic activity on the CNS. Reported actions include sedation, muscle relaxation, and anticonvulsive and antispasmodic effects. Suggested mechanisms of action range from GABA receptor modification to dopamine antagonist activity. A local anesthetic action is also claimed.

USES

Meaningful evidence from multiple RCTs demonstrates significant improvement of symptoms in various anxiety disorders. Other proposed uses lack support including relief of general tension, stress, and insomnia. An intoxicating effect has been reported with use of very high doses.

ADMINISTRATION

Standardized products for oral administration are available; in some areas the kava-kava is chewed. Use should be limited to no more than 3 months.

Warning: Kava has been taken off the market in numerous countries because of reports of severe liver injury, in some cases requiring transplantation. This appears to be a rare idiosyncratic or allergic reaction rather than ordinary liver toxicity, but it has been seen even with traditionally prepared kava, as well as with pharmaceutical-grade standardized products. Until further is known, kava should be considered an unsafe herb.

CONTRAINDICATIONS

Reports of dystonic reactions suggest that kava should not be used by patients taking antipsychotic medications. Apparent anti-dopaminergic actions contraindicate use in Parkinson's disease. CNS effects and possible potentiation of alcohol toxicity contraindicate use in alcoholism. Should not be used in patients with endogenous depression. Not recommended for use by pregnant or nursing women. Whether or not the risk of liver damage (see *Warning)* is increased in patients with preexisting liver disease is unknown.

SIDE EFFECTS

Kava in normal doses is generally well tolerated. GI complaints occasionally accompany use. Chewing kava-kava can result in circumoral numbness. Patients using kava-kava may have reduced mental alertness, and very high intake can cause inebriation. See *Warning* concerning liver damage.

DENTAL CONSIDERATIONS

Caution against use of kava in all patients, especially those with existing liver disease.

DRUG INTERACTIONS

May potentiate CNS sedation if used in combination with other CNS depressants. May increase risk of dystonic reactions if given in combination with antipsychotics. Discontinue 24 hours before general anesthesia and surgical procedures.

lemon balm

(Melissa officinalis)

OTHER NAMES:
Honey plant, Melissa, sweet Mary, balm mint

CLASS:
Herbal remedy

MAJOR INGREDIENTS

Volatile oil extract by distillation from leaves or whole plant contains geranial, neral, citronellal, linalool, and other compounds. Other constituents include glycosides, caffeic acids, flavonoids, and titerpene acids.

CLAIMED ACTIONS

Some evidence indicates that topical lemon balm extract blocks herpes virus receptors on host cells. It also may inhibit viral-related protein synthesis by action on elongation factor eEF-2. Taken internally, lemon balm may cause sedation through CNS nicotinic and muscarinic receptor-binding properties, although this mechanism is not well established.

USES

Several RCTs of moderate to low quality found evidence that use of topical lemon balm preparations can reduce the severity of acute genital or oral herpes recurrences if applied at the beginning of symptoms. There are no meaningful data on possible prophylactic effect. For oral use, lemon balm alone or combined with valerian has shown some potential value for insomnia, but not all data are consistent. One RCT found that lemon balm extract reduced agitation in individuals with Alzheimer's disease. Other proposed uses of lemon balm lack supporting evidence. These include anxiety disorders, dry skin, headache, influenza, menstrual problems, and muscle spasms.

ADMINISTRATION

Topical lemon balm for herpes is used in the form of a 70:1 extract cream, applied twice daily, and standardized using bioassay for inhibition of viral cellular lysis. Typical oral doses are 1.5 to 4.5 g/day of dried herb daily, or the equivalent in a standardized extract form. Maximum safe dosages of oral lemon balm for young children, pregnant or nursing women, and individuals with severe hepatic or renal disease are not established.

SIDE EFFECTS

Use of topical lemon balm has not been associated with any significant side effects other than occasional allergic reactions. Oral lemon balm is generally regarded as safe. However, on the basis of weak evidence indicating a possible sedative effect, people taking oral lemon balm might be at increased risk if they drive or operate heavy machinery or engage in activities that require a high level of mental alertness.

DENTAL CONSIDERATIONS

Ask why the product is being used. Pregnant women should be cautioned not to regard topical lemon balm as effective prevention against transmission of herpes to the newborn. See Drug Interactions.

DRUG INTERACTIONS

In animal studies, lemon balm extracts have produced dose-dependent potentiation of pentobarbital.

licorice

(Glycyrrhiza glabra)

OTHER NAMES:

Licorice root, liquorice, licorice, deglycyrrhizinated licorice, DGL, sweet wood, Yasti Madhu, sweet wort, Reglisse, Subholz

CLASS:

Herbal remedy

MAJOR INGREDIENTS

Whole licorice contains as its principal presumed active ingredient a terpenoid called *glycyrrhizin glycoside* (glycyrrhizinic acid). Deglycyrrhizinated licorice (DGL) is a popular form of licorice from which this constituent has been removed. Other constituents include asparagine, biotin, choline, fat, gum, inositol, lecithin, glycosides, volatile oil, coumarins, estrogenic substances, sterols, saponins, manganese, para-aminobenzoic acid, pantothenic acid, various pentacyclic triterpenes, phosphorous, B vitamins (1, 2, 3, 6, and 9), vitamin E, and a yellow dye.

CLAIMED ACTIONS

Glycyrrhizin has mineralocorticoid effects when used in high doses or with prolonged use. Possibly because of its glycyrrhizin content, licorice is thought to potentiate topical or oral corticosteroids and exert an estrogenlike effect. Other claimed actions with less substantiation include demulcent, diuretic, expectorant, antitussive, laxative, emetic, emollient, antiinflammatory, tissue healing, and antiarthritic effects.

USES

There are no well-documented uses of licorice or DGL. DGL has shown some promise for peptic ulcer disease, but published studies involved combination products with other active ingredients such as antacids. Various additional claims of effectiveness have been made for whole licorice including hypoglycemia, bronchitis, colitis, cystitis, stress, colds, high cholesterol levels, fever, nausea, inflammation, coughs, laryngitis, chronic fatigue syndrome, and general debility. Externally, licorice preparations have been used for eczema, psoriasis, burns, boils, sores, ulcers, and redness of the skin. DGL lozenges have been recommended for mouth ulcers. However, there is no reliable substantiation for any of these uses.

SIDE EFFECTS

Glycyrrhizin has direct mineralocorticoid effects and increases corticosteroid activity by inhibiting metabolic inactivation of cortisol. Signs of pseudohyperaldosteronism have been seen within a few weeks of usage including headache, muscle weakness, muscle cramps, hypertension, heart failure, arrhythmias, water retention, sodium retention, and potassium loss. The DGL form has not been associated with any significant side effects other than occasional allergic reactions or nonspecific GI distress.

ADMINISTRATION

Given as powder, liquid, or capsules. Topically a 2% licorice juice has been used as an antibacterial ointment. A mouthwash with 200 mg deglycyrrhizinated licorice in 200 ml warm water has been used. Snuff often contains a great deal of licorice.

CONTRAINDICATIONS

Not recommended for use by pregnant women (may cause reduced gestational age at birth), by women with a history of breast cancer (potential estrogenic effects), or by men with a history of infertility or decreased libido (may reduce testosterone levels). Because of its mineralocorticoid effects, licorice should not be used by patients taking thiazide or loop diuretics, digitalis, or potassium-sparing diuretics. However, DGL products should not interact with these medications.

DENTAL CONSIDERATIONS

Limit use of whole licorice to no more than 6 weeks. DGL lozenges have been proposed for aphthous ulcers, but no evidence supports this use.

DRUG INTERACTIONS
Tobacco may alter metabolism leading to toxicity. May potentiate corticosteroid drugs, so use in combination only with caution. May potentiate or antagonize diuretics, and increased potassium loss caused by licorice presents increased risks for individuals using digoxin or antiarrhythmic drugs.

myrrh
(Commiphora myrrha)

OTHER NAMES:
Bola, gum myrrh tree, mu-yao

CLASS:
Herbal remedy

MAJOR INGREDIENTS
Volatile oil (primarily sesquiterpenes), triterpenes, and gum resin

CLAIMED ACTIONS
Analgesic, antifungal, antiseptic, astringent, carminative, emmenagogue, expectorant, antispasmodic, disinfectant, immune stimulant, circulatory stimulant, stomachic, tonic, and vulnerary.

USES
Has been used as a disinfectant, as an astringent, and to treat disorders of the female reproductive system. It has long been used for treatment of oral ulcers, gingivitis, halitosis, denture-irritated mouth, and sore teeth and gums. Other uses include nonspecified chest problems and diphtheria. Used in Chinese medicine for rheumatism, arthritis, and circulatory problems.

ADMINISTRATION
Infusion, mouthwash, tincture, incense, capsules, and dental powder.

CONTRAINDICATIONS
Not recommended for use by pregnant women because of claimed uterine stimulant effects or by individuals with diabetes because of enhancement of oral hypoglycemic agents.

SIDE EFFECTS
Because of resin content and difficult clearance from the body, myrrh may cause minor renal damage if used over an extended period of time. Avoid high dose for chronic use.

DENTAL CONSIDERATIONS
Myrrh has been approved by Commission E (Germany) for treatment of inflammation of the mouth and pharynx, but topical uses are not substantiated.
A tea, prepared by placing 1 to 2 teaspoonfuls in one cup of boiling water and steeping for 10 to 15 minutes, has been used for oral administration three times daily.

DRUG INTERACTIONS
Enhancement of oral hypoglycemic agents.

nettle root

(Urtica dioica radix)

OTHER NAMES:
Stinging nettle

CLASS:
Herbal remedy

MAJOR INGREDIENTS

The presumed active constituents of nettle root are β-sitosterol and other related sitosterols. Other possibly active constituents include lectins, lignans, polysaccharides, and hydroxycoumarins. Note that nettle leaf is an entirely different herbal product from the nettle root discussed here.

CLAIMED ACTIONS

The sitosterols in nettle root, especially β-sitosterol, have multiple actions of possible relevance to prostate disease, including reducing inflammation in the prostate and alteration of sex hormone binding properties.

USES

Several small RCTs indicate that nettle root can improve symptoms of benign prostatic hyperplasia (BPH).

ADMINISTRATION

When taken for BPH, the typical dose is 120 mg of the dry extract twice daily, or 4 to 6 g daily of the whole root. Nettle root often is sold in combination with other herbs thought to be effective for BPH including saw palmetto and pygeum, and there is some evidence of a potentiating effect with the latter. Maximum safe dosages in young children, nursing women, and individuals with severe hepatic or renal disease are not established.

CONTRAINDICATIONS

On the basis of animal studies showing uterotonic action and on its traditional use as an abortifacient, nettle is not recommended for use by pregnant women.

SIDE EFFECTS

Although extensive safety studies have not been reported, nettle root appears to have a low level of toxicity. In drug monitoring studies, side effects were rare and nonspecific.

DENTAL CONSIDERATIONS

Ask why the product is being used.

DRUG INTERACTIONS

None known, but there are weak theoretic concerns regarding interactions with antihypertensive, hypoglycemic, and sedative pharmaceuticals.

passionflower

(Passiflora incarnate)

OTHER NAMES:
Passion vine

CLASS:
Herbal remedy

MAJOR INGREDIENTS

Passionflower contains harman and harmaline, alkaloids with possible MAOI activity. Other constituents include cyanogenic glycosides, flavonoids, and maltol. The aerial parts of the plant are used medicinally.

CLAIMED ACTIONS
Sedative and antispasmodic uses are claimed, based primarily on animal studies.

USES
Scant preliminary evidence from small RCTs found suggestive evidence that passionflower might be helpful for treatment of anxiety, as well as for withdrawal from opiate dependency. Its common use for "nervous stomach" has not been formally investigated.

ADMINISTRATION
Typical dosage of crude passionflower is 1 g three times daily. Concentrated extracts and tinctures are available. Maximum safe doses in nursing women, young children, and individuals with severe hepatic or renal disease are not established.

CONTRAINDICATIONS
Because of the uterotropic actions of harman and harmaline, passionflower is not recommended for use by pregnant women.

SIDE EFFECTS
Passionflower is generally well tolerated when taken in usual doses.

DENTAL CONSIDERATIONS
Ask why the product is being used.

DRUG INTERACTIONS
Passionflower might potentiate the action of sedative drugs, including those used for dental anesthesia. Interactions with MAOI drugs are possible.

peppermint
(Mentha piperita)

OTHER NAMES:
Peppermint oil, essential oil of peppermint, mint, brandy mint, menthol

CLASS:
Herbal remedy

MAJOR INGREDIENTS
The primary active constituent in peppermint is assumed to be menthol. Other constituents of the essential oil include menthone, menthofurane, menthyl acetate, neomenthol, and isomenthone. The whole leaf additionally contains caffeic acids and flavonoids. The leaf and flowers are the parts used medicinally. Most tested uses of peppermint involved preparations of the essential oil rather than whole leaf.

CLAIMED ACTIONS
Some evidence indicates that menthol relaxes GI smooth muscle. Peppermint oil has a cooling effect on the skin. It may have cholagogue properties.

USES
Several preliminary RCTs inconsistently suggest that peppermint oil can alleviate symptoms of irritable bowel syndrome. Other RCTs suggest that peppermint oil can decrease intestinal spasm during a barium enema. Other uses of peppermint oil with only minimal supporting evidence include functional dyspepsia and dissolution of gallstones. Inhaled peppermint oil has shown some promise for upper

respiratory infections. Peppermint oil applied to the temples may produce a subjective decrease in headache sensation. There are no well-documented uses of peppermint leaf.

ADMINISTRATION

In clinical trials, peppermint oil was given in enteric-coated form at a dose of 0.2 to 0.4 ml three times per day. Whole peppermint leaf is taken in tea form.

CONTRAINDICATIONS

Because of the potential toxicity of excessive peppermint oil, peppermint is not recommended for use by pregnant or nursing women or by individuals with severe hepatic or renal disease.

SIDE EFFECTS

Peppermint leaf has a low level of toxicity and is generally regarded as safe. At normal doses, peppermint oil generally causes few side effects. However, even at normal doses, peppermint oil can cause esophageal reflux, which is the reason for usage of enteric-coated capsules. Excessive intake of peppermint oil can cause CNS and renal damage. Inhalation occasionally causes hypersensitivity reactions.

DENTAL CONSIDERATIONS

Ask why the product is being used.

DRUG INTERACTIONS

Animal studies suggest that oral peppermint oil can increase cyclosporine bioavailability. This could cause cyclosporine levels to rise to toxic levels; conversely, if cyclosporine levels are adjusted while an individual is taking peppermint oil, discontinuation could cause a fall to subtherapeutic levels.

probiotics

OTHER NAMES:
Friendly bacteria, acidophilus

CLASS:
Nonherbal remedy

MAJOR INGREDIENTS

Probiotics in common use include *Lactobacillus acidophilus*, *Lactobacillus GG*, and other lactobacilli; *Bifidobacterium bifidum; Saccharomyces boulardii* (a yeast); *Streptococcus thermophilus;* and *Streptococcus salivarius*.

CLAIMED ACTIONS

Probiotics are microorganisms (usually bacteria, but also yeasts) that colonize the digestive tract and other tissues and exist in healthy symbiosis with the body. They compete with and potentially inhibit pathogenic organisms, and they may aid digestion and assist in the formation of vitamin K. Altered bowel flora may cause immunomodulatory effects.

USES

Numerous RCTs have evaluated the use of probiotics for preventing or treating various forms of diarrhea, including acute viral diarrhea, traveler's diarrhea, antibiotic-associated diarrhea, and chemotherapy- or radiation-induced diarrhea. In general, the results have been supportive. Probiotics may help prevent caries. One large RCT found that use of *Lactobacillus GG* in milk given to children ages 1 to 6 years reduced incidence of caries as compared with unfortified milk. Other RCTs suggest benefits for inflammatory bowel disease, irritable bowel syndrome, and eczema. Weaker or mixed evidence has been presented regarding usefulness for urinary tract infection prophylaxis, hyperlipidemia, and prevention of upper respiratory tract infections.

ADMINISTRATION
Typical dose of bacterial probiotics supplies approximately five billion live organisms daily. *S. boulardii* yeast is taken at a dose of 500 mg twice daily. Surveys of products on the market have shown wide variations in quality.

SIDE EFFECTS
Use of probiotics by healthy people has not been associated with any significant side effects other than a short-term increase in intestinal gas production. However, immunocompromised individuals may be at risk for invasive infection by the probiotic.

DENTAL CONSIDERATIONS
Ask why the product is being used. As noted previously, some evidence indicates potential benefit for caries prophylaxis in children.

DRUG INTERACTIONS
No dental drug interactions are reported. Use of probiotics during and for a short while after antibiotic usage may prevent antibiotic-associated diarrhea and restore normal bowel flora.

proteolytic enzymes

OTHER NAMES:
Pancreatic enzymes, digestive enzymes

CLASS:
Nonherbal remedy

MAJOR INGREDIENTS
Commercial products generally include one or more of the following proteolytic enzymes: bromelain, chymotrypsin, pancreatin, papain, or trypsin.

CLAIMED ACTIONS
Although the primary physiologic use of proteolytic enzymes is protein digestion, some portion of exogenously delivered proteolytic enzymes appears to enter systemic circulation and exerts an antiinflammatory effect.

USES
Results of numerous reported RCTs on the use of proteolytic enzyme mixtures for reducing pain and edema following surgery have been mixed. Other RCTs suggest possible benefits for sports injuries and other minor injuries, again reducing pain and edema. Proteolytic enzymes have shown some promise for osteoarthritis and herpes zoster. Other claimed uses that lack RCT support include treatment of food allergies and rheumatoid arthritis.

ADMINISTRATION
Proteolytic enzymes are delivered orally in a variety of enteric-coated or non–enteric-coated forms. Dosage depends on the particular product. Maximum safe doses for pregnant or

nursing women, young children, and individuals with severe hepatic or renal disease are not established.

SIDE EFFECTS

Use of proteolytic enzymes in clinical trials has not been associated with any significant side effects other than occasional allergic reactions or nonspecific GI distress.

DENTAL CONSIDERATIONS

Ask why the product is being used.

DRUG INTERACTIONS

Papain might potentiate anticoagulant and antiplatelet agents. Pancreatin could interfere with absorption of folic acid supplements.

pyruvate

OTHER NAMES:
Dihydroxyacetone pyruvate, DHAP

CLASS:
Nonherbal remedy

MAJOR INGREDIENTS

Pyruvate is a product of aerobic glycolysis. It enters the mitochondria to form acetyl-coenzyme A (CoA) by oxidative decarboxylation. There is little pyruvate in the diet; it is synthesized endogenously.

CLAIMED ACTIONS

Some evidence suggests that exogenous pyruvate has a feedback-inhibition effect on lipid synthesis. Weaker evidence hints that increased supply of pyruvate might enable a higher rate of ATP synthesis during exercise.

USES

Limited evidence from small RCTs indicates that pyruvate supplements may aid weight loss or body composition (fat/muscle proportion). In general, evidence from clinical trials does not support use of pyruvate as a sports performance-enhancing agent.

ADMINISTRATION

Typical dose is 30 g daily, taken in divided doses. It often is sold in combination with dihydroxyacetone, under the name DHAP (dihydroxy-acetone pyruvate). Maximum safe doses for pregnant or nursing women, young children, and individuals with severe hepatic or renal disease are not established.

SIDE EFFECTS

Use of pyruvate in clinical trials has not been associated with any significant side effects other than occasional allergic reactions and nonspecific GI distress.

DENTAL CONSIDERATIONS

Ask why the product is being used.

DRUG INTERACTIONS

No dental drug interactions are reported.

quercetin

OTHER NAMES:
Quercetin chalcone

CLASS:
Nonherbal remedy

MAJOR INGREDIENTS

Quercetin is a bioflavonoid found in many foods, particularly apples, black tea, grapefruit, onions, and red wine.

CLAIMED ACTIONS

Some evidence suggests that exogenous quercetin has antiinflammatory effects and inhibits nitric oxide and tyrosine kinase. Quercetin, like many bioflavonoids, has antioxidant and chemopreventive properties in vitro. It is said to have the cromolynlike effect of stabilizing mast cells, but the supporting evidence for this claim is weak, and no RCTs show actual clinical effect on allergies.

USES

One small RCT found limited evidence that quercetin may be effective for treatment of chronic prostatitis. Another small RCT hints at benefits for interstitial cystitis. Other proposed uses that lack RCT substantiation include allergies (eczema, asthma, allergic rhinitis), viral infections, and prevention of cataracts, cancer, and heart disease.

ADMINISTRATION

Quercetin usually is taken orally at a dose of 500 mg two times daily. Quercetin chalcone is marketed as having better oral absorption than quercetin, but this claim has not been reliably substantiated. Maximum safe doses in young children and in individuals with severe hepatic or renal disease are not established.

CONTRAINDICATIONS

Weak evidence hints that use of quercetin by pregnant or nursing women might increase the risk of infant leukemia.

SIDE EFFECTS

Use of quercetin in clinical trials has not been associated with any significant side effects other than occasional allergic reactions and nonspecific GI distress. However, despite in vitro evidence of chemoprevention, there are some indications that quercetin could have a carcinogenic effect under certain circumstances that are not yet well defined.

DENTAL CONSIDERATIONS

Ask why the product is being used.

DRUG INTERACTIONS

No dental drug interactions are reported.

sage

(Salvia officinalis)

OTHER NAMES:

Broad-leaf sage, common sage, Dalmatian sage, garden sage, true sage

CLASS:

Herbal remedy

MAJOR INGREDIENTS

Volatile oils, phenolic acids, tannins, diterpene bitter principles, triterpenes, steroids, flavones, and flavonoid glycosides

CLAIMED ACTIONS

Antibacterial, fungistatic, virustatic, astringent, carminative, secretion promotion, and perspiration inhibition.

USES
From the earliest of times, uses have included treatment of open sores and wounds, sore throat, and fertility problems. Sage is also used to treat gum disease, canker sores, and halitosis. Other uses include antioxidant effects, menstrual pain, menopausal symptoms, and muscle spasms. Orally ingested sage reportedly reduces perspiration and encourages appetite. Other uses include stomatitis, gingivitis, pharyngitis, and hyperhidrosis. It has been used topically to treat itching associated with insect bites, along with herpes lesions, shingles, and psoriasis.

ADMINISTRATION
Dried leaves, extract, tincture, and essential oil.

CONTRAINDICATIONS
Not recommended for use by pregnant women.

SIDE EFFECTS
Reported side effects include vertigo; tachycardia; and, for patients prone to seizures, a risk of seizures.

DENTAL CONSIDERATIONS
Efficacy for use of sage gargle for gum disease is not established.

DRUG INTERACTIONS
Interactions with insulin, oral hypoglycemics, and seizure medications. Some sage products may contain alcohol (tincture) and should not be used with disulfiram.

SAMe

OTHER NAMES:
Ademethionine, adenosylmethionine, *S*-adenosyl-methionine, *S*-adenosyl-L-methionine

CLASS:
Nonherbal remedy

MAJOR INGREDIENTS
S-adenosyl-methionine.

CLAIMED ACTIONS
A naturally occurring molecule found in most body tissues, SAMe (pronounced “Sammy”) is an active methyl carrier playing an essential role in transmethylation. It is involved in the synthesis, metabolism, and activation of hormones, neurotransmitters, phospholipids, proteins, nucleic acids, and some natural medications. SAMe is intimately linked to vitamin B_{12} and folic acid metabolism. When these vitamins are absent, reduced levels of SAMe can result, such that SAMe affects serotonin and many body tissues, including cartilage and membranes. It functions as an antidepressant via an unknown mechanism but is associated with increased levels of serotonin, dopamine, and norepinephrine.

USES
Moderate evidence from placebo-controlled and comparative RCTs indicates that oral SAMe can reduce symptoms of osteoarthritis, to approximately the same extent as low doses of NSAIDs. Weaker RCT evidence supports efficacy in

depression, fibromyalgia, and cholestasis. In highly preliminary studies, SAMe has shown promise for treatment of Gilbert's disease and other liver disorders.

ADMINISTRATION
Oral dose forms have variable bioavailability; doses used in clinical trials were generally 1200 to 1600 mg daily, taken in divided doses.

CONTRAINDICATIONS
None reported; however, there is a possible risk of hypomania in patients with bipolar disorder.

SIDE EFFECTS
GI complaints such as diarrhea, nausea, and vomiting, and CNS effects such as hypomania in bipolar disorder and anxiety.

DENTAL CONSIDERATIONS
Determine why the patient is taking the drug.

DRUG INTERACTIONS
SAMe might interfere with the effectiveness of L-dopa, which is used for Parkinson's disease. Based on a case report of a toxic interaction with clomipramine, combination of SAMe with standard antidepressants should be used only with caution.

saw palmetto
(Serenoa repens, Sabal fructus)

OTHER NAMES:
Sabal, cabbage palm, saw palmetto berry

CLASS:
Herbal remedy

MAJOR INGREDIENTS
Contains various sitosterols (phytosterols) such as β-sitosterol and other sitosterol compounds, flavonoids, polysaccharides, and free fatty acids. The ripe, dried fruit of the plant is used medicinally.

CLAIMED ACTIONS
Reported to be antiandrogenic and antiinflammatory. May have some low-level estrogenic activity. The antiandrogenic activity is suggested to occur by inhibition of the enzyme testosterone-5-α-reductase. This action prevents the conversion of testosterone to dihydrotestosterone, the active androgenic hormone. Some data support blockade of dihydrotestosterone to receptors in the cell nucleus. Limited data seem to support the estrogenic effects. The antiinflammatory effects remain doubtful. Use of saw palmetto does not affect prostate-specific antigen levels.

USES
This herbal product has been used for treatment of symptoms associated with BPH, particularly urinary difficulties. Clinical trials show better results than placebo and apparent comparative results to finasteride (Proscar) and other pharmaceuticals for BPH.

Saw palmetto appears to cause some reduction in prostate gland size, although not to the same extent as finasteride. *(Note:* Several effective pharmaceuticals for BPH cause no change in prostate gland size.) Use in prostatitis and baldness remains speculative.

ADMINISTRATION
Saw palmetto is taken at a dose of 160 mg twice per day of an extract standardized to contain 85% to 95% fatty acids and sterols.

CONTRAINDICATIONS
Not recommended for use by pregnant women or by women of childbearing age because of unclear influence of saw palmetto on other androgens and possible estrogenic effects.

SIDE EFFECTS
Use of saw palmetto in clinical trials was associated with a few, nonspecific side effects. There is one case report of saw palmetto apparently causing increased bleeding during surgery; for this reason, use of saw palmetto should be discontinued 2 weeks before surgery.

DENTAL CONSIDERATIONS
Ask why the product is being used.

DRUG INTERACTIONS
No dental drug interactions are reported.

St. John's wort
(Hypericum perforatum, Hyperici herba)

OTHER NAMES:
Hypericum, kaimath weed, John's wort

CLASS:
Herbal remedy

MAJOR INGREDIENTS
Contains quinoids (hypericin, pseudohypericin), anthraquinones, flavonoids (hyperoside, quercitin, rutin), bioflavonoids, and a volatile oil. One of the pharmacologically active components is hyperforin; another, hypericin, has photosensitizing properties. Flavonoids including amentaflavone may contribute to the pharmacologic action of the herb. The aboveground parts of the plant harvested during the flowering season are used medicinally.

CLAIMED ACTIONS
The primary actions are antidepressant, antiinflammatory, and antimicrobial. The constituent hyperforin appears to inhibit uptake of serotonin, dopamine, and norepinephrine.

USES
Used for treatment of mild to moderate major depression. According to most but not all of the many RCTs performed, it is more effective than placebo and, except in severe major depression, as effective as tricyclics or selective serotonin reuptake inhibitors. The volatile oil seems to increase the healing of burns. Hypericin has shown in vitro activity against the HIV virus, but

human trials indicate that hypericin must be taken in toxic doses in order to produce any clinical effect. One RCT failed to find St. John's wort helpful for polyneuropathy. Topical St. John's wort has shown some promise for treatment of eczema.

ADMINISTRATION

A variety of oral preparations are available, standardized to either hypericin or hyperforin.

SIDE EFFECTS

In the extensive clinical trial experience with St. John's wort, side effects have been limited and generally nonspecific. Photosensitization may occur at higher doses or with topical use. Like all antidepressants, St. John's wort can cause episodes of mania in people with bipolar disorder. There are some reports that use of St. John's wort by individuals with Alzheimer's disease may increase agitation. Safety during pregnancy and lactation is not established.

DENTAL CONSIDERATIONS

Ask why the product is being used.

DRUG INTERACTIONS

St. John's wort affects a variety of cytochromes, as well as the transport protein P-glycoprotein, and can reduce levels and thereby activity of numerous medications to a clinically significant extent. Interacting drugs include oral contraceptives (leading to unwanted pregnancy), protease inhibitors and nonnucleoside reverse transcriptase inhibitors (leading to reduced anti-HIV effectiveness), cyclosporine (leading to organ rejection), clozapine, digoxin, losartan, metronidazole, olanzapine, omeprazole, statins, warfarin, and various chemotherapy drugs. Note that if blood levels of a drug are stabilized while a patient is taking St. John's wort, discontinuation of the herb may cause a dangerous rise in levels. In addition, St. John's wort should be used only with caution, if at all, in patients taking other antidepressive medications, including MAOIs, tricyclic antidepressants, and selective serotonin reuptake inhibitors, because case reports suggest a risk of serotonin syndrome. Combined use with tramadol might present a similar risk. Although St. John's wort does not appear to have MAOI actions at normal doses, there is one case report of an MAO-like interaction between St. John's wort and tyramine-containing foods. Discontinue use 2 weeks before general anesthesia. Avoid dental (or other) drugs with a potential for photosensitivity.

stevia

(Stevia rebaudiana)

OTHER NAMES:

Caa'inhem, Paraguayan sweet herb, sweet herb, sweet leaf of Paraguay, sweetleaf

CLASS:

Herbal remedy

MAJOR INGREDIENTS

Major active constituents include diterpene steviosides and rebaudioside. Flavonoids and volatile oil are present as well. The leaves of the plant are used medicinally.

CLAIMED ACTIONS
Steviosides are sweeter than sucrose by weight, producing a taste said to be preferable to saccharine, though not entirely without aftertaste. Steviosides have shown an antihypertensive effect, but only at much higher doses than reasonable for intake as a sugar substitute.

USES
Stevia enjoys wide use as a noncaloric sweetening agent in Japan and several other countries. However, stevia has not received approval for use under this designation in the United States; nonetheless, it is used widely as a sweetener without claiming it as such. Concentrated steviosides at far higher doses are beginning to be used by people with hypertension; such use may be expected to increase in the future.

ADMINISTRATION
Approximately one-sixth teaspoon of ground stevia (or two to four drops of stevia liquid extract) equals the sweetness of 1 teaspoon of ordinary sugar. This supplies approximately 30 mg steviosides. For hypertension, the dose used in clinical trials was 250 to 500 mg concentrated steviosides three times daily. Maximum safe doses in pregnant or nursing women, young children, and individuals with severe hepatic or renal disease are not established.

SIDE EFFECTS
Stevia is generally regarded as a safe herb, but animal studies suggest that high doses may have antifertility actions in both males and females. The widespread use of stevia in Japan suggests reasonable safety in children and pregnant women.

DENTAL CONSIDERATIONS
Patients may be using stevioside-sweetened products to avoid caries, a use that may be reasonable.

DRUG INTERACTIONS
If a person is accustomed to consuming 25 teaspoons of sugar per day, the equivalent in stevia might produce an antihypertensive effect. Certain more susceptible people might respond at a lower dose. This suggests the possibility of potentiation interactions with antihypertensives, but no such interactions have yet been reported.

valerian
(Valeriana officinalis, Valerianae radix)

OTHER NAMES:
Valerian root, Indian valerian

CLASS:
Herbal remedy

MAJOR INGREDIENTS
Valepotriates (isovaltrate and others), a volatile oil (bornyl isovalerenate and isovalerenic acid), sesquiterpenes, and multiple other substances. Pharmacologically active components are not identified with any certainty but may be isovaleric acid and related derivatives. The fresh underground parts and roots are used medicinally.

CLAIMED ACTIONS
Sedation, reduction in nervousness, sleep promoting, and antispasmodic. Laboratory data suggest valerian

may increase GABA levels at synapses.

USES

Evidence from several RCTs suggests that valerian can improve sleep, especially with continued use. Other proposed uses of valerian lacking meaningful supporting evidence include treatment of restlessness, reduction in nervousness (anxiolytic), agitation associated with menstruation, colic, stomach cramps, and uterine spasticity. Antispasmodic properties are not well defined. It has been used externally by adding to bath water.

ADMINISTRATION

Available for oral use as a variety of products, including tinctures, infusions, and extracts.

SIDE EFFECTS

Generally not observed in usual doses. GI complaints, headache, sleeplessness, mydriasis, excitability, and cardiac disturbances may occur with long-term use.

DENTAL CONSIDERATIONS

Ask why the product is being used.

DRUG INTERACTIONS

Although no interactions are reported, monitor patients for increased sedation when using other CNS depressants. May potentiate CNS depressants.

xylitol

CLASS:
Nonherbal remedy

MAJOR INGREDIENTS

Xylitol is a polyol with the same intensity of sweetness as sucrose, but it cannot serve as a metabolic base for oral microbes.

CLAIMED ACTIONS

Xylitol inhibits the growth of *Streptococcus mutans* and on this basis has been proposed as a prophylactic agent against dental caries. Xylitol may also inhibit growth of *Streptococcus pneumoniae* and thereby reduce the risk of respiratory infections caused by this organism.

USES

In several large RCTs, children who used gums, lozenges, syrups, toothpastes, or candies containing xylitol experienced a reduced incidence of caries compared with control groups. Use of xylitol by nursing mothers may confer some protection to the child, presumably because infants receive their initial *S. mutans* colonization from their mothers. Other RCTs suggest that xylitol use by children may reduce the incidence of otitis media. Xylitol has been suggested as a prophylactic for periodontal disease, but this use has not yet undergone significant study.

ADMINISTRATION

Typical dose of xylitol used in clinical trials for caries prevention was 4.3 to 10 g daily. Higher doses appear to be more effective than lower doses.

SIDE EFFECTS

High consumption of xylitol can cause mild GI distress and possibly diarrhea, especially in children.

DENTAL CONSIDERATIONS

Patients should be reminded that xylitol gum and related products should be used in addition to standard dental hygiene recommendations, not as a substitute for them.

DRUG INTERACTIONS

No dental drug interactions are reported.

yohimbe bark

(Pausinystalia yohimbe)

OTHER NAMES:

Yohimbe cortex

CLASS:

Herbal remedy

MAJOR INGREDIENTS

The principal alkaloid is yohimbine (quebrachine), with lesser amounts of stereoisomers of yohimbine along with other indole alkaloids including corynantheidine and allo-yohimbine. It also contains a variety of plant tannins. The dried bark of the trunk and branches of the tree are the parts used medicinally.

CLAIMED ACTIONS

The major effects of this drug are due to yohimbine. Do not confuse the prescription drug yohimbine with yohimbe. Yohimbine has α_2-adrenergic antagonist activity. Presynaptic α_2-adrenergic receptors regulate norepinephrine release. In a feedback-type action, antagonism of these receptors is associated with greater norepinephrine release. It may also dilate blood vessels; claims are made for a calcium channel blocking action and inhibition of MAO enzymes.

USES

Has been used to treat erectile dysfunction, as an aphrodisiac, for exhaustion, and even for orthostatic hypotension. Limited data concern yohimbine and not yohimbe. Yohimbine has not been approved for this application. According to the German Commission E monographs, yohimbe's effectiveness is not documented, and it is not recommended.

ADMINISTRATION

Limited products are available and usually in combination with other ingredients.

CONTRAINDICATIONS

Not recommended for use by patients with hepatic or renal impairment or with psychiatric disorders.

SIDE EFFECTS

Usual doses produce few side effects. However, significant adverse effects are reported with large doses and include increased salivation, anxiety, hallucinations, exanthema, nervousness, irritability, tachycardia, and sweating. Other effects also are possible. Cardiac failure, possibly fatal, is reported.

DENTAL CONSIDERATIONS

Ask why the product is being used.

DRUG INTERACTIONS

No specific dental drug interactions are reported, but it may have MAO inhibitory action. Avoid use of indirect-acting sympathomimetics and tricyclic antidepressants.

BIBLIOGRAPHY

Blake S: *Alternative remedies CD-ROM,* St Louis, 2001, Mosby.

Blumenthal M et al: *The complete German Commission E monographs,* Austin, 1998, American Botanical Council.

Miller LG: Herbal medicinals: selected clinical considerations focusing on known or potential drug-herb interactions, *Arch Intern Med* 158:2200–2211, 1998.

Mosby's drug consult 2004: the comprehensive reference for generic and brand name drugs, ed 14, St Louis, 2004, Mosby.

Mosby's handbook of herbs and supplements and their therapeutic uses, St Louis, 2003, Mosby.

Natural medicines comprehensive database, Stockton, CA, 2004, Pharmacist's Letter/Prescriber's Letter, Therapeutic Research Faculty.

Nonherbal dietary supplements, *Pharmacist's Letter* 98(4), 1998.

O'Hara MA et al: A review of 12 commonly used medicinal herbs, *Arch Fam Med* 7:523–536, 1998.

PDR for herbal remedies, Montvale, NJ, 1998, Medical Economics.

Therapeutic use of herbs, continuing education booklets part 1 and part 2, Stockton, CA, 1998, Pharmacist's Letter.

Appendix A Abbreviations

ā before

aa of each

ab antibody

abd abdomen

ABGs arterial blood gases

ac before meals *(ante cibum)*

ACE angiotensin-converting enzyme

ACEI angiotensin converting enzyme inhibitor

Ach acetylcholine

ACT activated clotting time

ACTH adrenocorticotropic hormone

ad lib as desired

ADH antidiuretic hormone

ADP adenosine diphosphate

ADR adverse drug reaction

AIDS acquired immunodeficiency syndrome

aka also known as

ALT alanine aminotransferase, serum

ama against medical advice

amb ambulation

amp ampule

ANA antinuclear antibody

ant anterior

ANUG acute necrotizing ulcerative gingivitis

AP anteroposterior

APAP *N*-acetyl-para-aminophenol (acetaminophen)

APB atrial premature beat

aPTT activated partial thromboplastin time

ARC AIDS-related complex

AROM active range of motion

ASA acetylsalicylic acid (aspirin)

asap as soon as possible

ASHD arteriosclerotic heart disease

AST aspartate aminotransferase, serum

AV atrioventricular

BAC blood alcohol concentration

bid twice per day *(bis in die)*

BM bowel movement

BMR basal metabolic rate

bol bolus

BP blood pressure

BPH benign prostatic hypertrophy

bpm beats per minute

BS blood sugar

BUN blood urea nitrogen

Bx biopsy

c̄ with

C Celsius (centigrade)

C section cesarean section

CA cancer

Ca calcium

CAD coronary artery disease

cAMP cyclic adenosine monophosphate

cap capsule

cath catheterization or catheterize

CBC complete blood count

CCB calcium channel blocker

CC chief complaint

cc cubic centimeter

cGMP cyclic guanosine monophosphate

CHD coronary heart disease

CHF congestive heart failure

cm centimeter

CML chronic myeloid leukemia

CMV cytomegalovirus I

CNS central nervous system

CO_2 carbon dioxide

CoA coenzyme A

c/o complains of

CO cardiac output

COMT catechol-*O*-methyltransferase

con rel controlled release

conc concentration

COPD chronic obstructive pulmonary disease

COX2 cyclooxygenase-2

CPAP continuous positive airway pressure

CPK creatinine phosphokinase

CPR cardiopulmonary resuscitation

CrCl creatinine clearance

CRD chronic respiratory disease

CRF chronic renal failure

C&S culture and sensitivity

CSF cerebrospinal fluid

CTZ chemoreceptor trigger zone

CV cardiovascular

CVA cerebrovascular accident

CVP central venous pressure

$CysLT_1$ cysteinyl leukotriene receptor

D&C dilation and curettage

del rel delayed release

DIC disseminated intravascular coagulation

DM diabetes mellitus

DMARD disease-modifying antirheumatic drug

DNA deoxyribonucleic acid

DOB date of birth

dr dram

dsg dressing

DVT deep vein thrombosis

D_5W 5% glucose in distilled water

dx diagnosis

EBV Epstein-Barr virus

ECG electrocardiogram (EKG)

EEG electroencephalogram

EENT ear, eye, nose, and throat

elix elixir, hydroalcoholic solution containing an active drug(s)

ENDO endocrine systems

EPO erythropoietin

EPS extrapyramidal symptoms

ESR erythrocyte sedimentation rate

ext rel extended release

F Fahrenheit

FBS fasting blood sugar

FHT fetal heart tones

FIO_2 inspired oxygen concentration

FSH follicle-stimulating hormone

fx fracture

g gram

GABA γ-aminobutyric acid

gal gallon

GERD gastroesophageal reflux disease

GGTP γ-glutamyl transpeptidase

GHb glycosylated hemoglobin

GI gastrointestinal

G6PD glucose-6-phosphate dehydrogenase

gr grain

GR glucocorticoid receptor

gtt drop

GTT glucose tolerance test

GU genitourinary

Gyn gynecology

HbA_{1c} laboratory test for glycosylated hemoglobin

Hct hematocrit

HCG human chorionic gonadotropin

HDL high-density lipoprotein

HEMA hematologic system

Hgb hemoglobin

HIV human immunodeficiency virus

H&H hematocrit and hemoglobin

H&P history and physical examination

5-HIAA 5-hydroxyindole-acetic acid

HMG-CoA 3-hydroxy-3-methyl-glutaryl–coenzyme A reductase

5-HT 5-hydroxytryptamine (serotonin)

H_2O water

HPA hypothalamic-pituitary-adrenocortical axis

HR heart rate

HRT hormone replacement therapy

hr hour

hs at bedtime *(hora somni)*

HSV herpes simplex virus

HSV-2 herpes genitalis

hypo hypodermically

Hx history

IBS irritable bowel syndrome

ICP intracranial pressure

ICU intensive care unit

IDDM insulin-dependent diabetes mellitus

I&D incision and drainage

IgG immunoglobulin G

IL-2 interleukin-2

IM intramuscular

immed rel immediate release

inf infusion

inh inhalation

inj injection

INR international normalized ratio

INTEG relating to integumentary structures

IOP intraocular pressure

IPPB intermittent positive-pressure breathing

ITP idiopathic thrombocytopenic purpura

IU international unit

IUD intrauterine contraceptive device

IV intravenous

IVP intravenous piggyback

K potassium

kg kilogram

L or l left; liter

lat lateral

lb pound

LDH lactic dehydrogenase

LDL low-density lipoprotein

LDL-C low-density lipoprotein–cholesterol

LE lupus erythematosus

LFT liver function test

LH luteinizing hormone

LHRH luteinizing hormone-releasing hormone

liq liquid

LLQ left lower quadrant

LMP last menstrual period

LOC loss of consciousness

lot lotion

loz lozenge

LR lactated Ringer's solution

LRI lower respiratory infection

LVD left ventricular dysfunction

m meter

m^2 square meter

MAC *Mycobacterium avium* complex

MAO monoamine oxidase

MAOI monoamine oxidase inhibitor

max maximum

META metabolic

mEq milliequivalent

mg milligram

µg microgram

MI myocardial infarction

min minute

mixt mixture

ml milliliter

mm millimeter

mo month

MPA mycophenolic acid

MS musculoskeletal

MVA motor vehicle accident

Na sodium

NC nasal cannula

neg negative

ng nanogram

NIDDM non–insulin-dependent diabetes mellitus

NKA no known allergies

NMDA *N*-methyl-*D*-aspartate

NMI no middle initial

noc nocturnal (night)

NPH neutral protamine Hagedorn

NPO nothing by mouth *(nil per os)*

NS normal saline

NSAID nonsteroidal antiinflammatory drug

NV neurovascular

O_2 oxygen

OBS organic brain syndrome

OC oral contraceptive

OD right eye *(oculus dexter)*

oint ointment

OOB out of bed

ophth ophthalmic

OR operating room

ORIF open reduction, internal fixation

os left eye *(ocular sinister)*

OTC over the counter

ou each eye *(oculus uterque)*

oz ounce

p̄ after (post)

p pulse

PABA para-aminobenzoic acid

PAC premature atrial contraction

pCO_2 arterial carbon dioxide tension (pressure tore)

pO_2 arterial oxygen tension (pressure tore)

PAT paroxysmal atrial tachycardia

PBI protein-bound iodine

PBP penicillin binding protein

pc after meals *(post cibum)*

PCA patient-controlled analgesia

PCN penicillin

PE physical examination

PG prostaglandin

pH hydrogen ion concentration

PMDD premenstrual dysphoric disorder

PMS premenstrual syndrome

PNS peripheral nervous system

PO by mouth *(per os)*

postop postoperatively

PP postprandial

ppm parts per million

preop preoperatively

prep preparation

prn as needed *(pro re nata)*

PSA prostate-specific antigen

PT prothrombin time

PTSD posttraumatic stress disorder

PTT partial thromboplastin time

PVC premature ventricular contraction

PVD peripheral vascular disease

q every

qAM every morning

qd every day

qh every hour

qid four times per day

qod every other day

qPM every night

qt quart

q2h every 2 hours

q3h every 3 hours

q4h every 4 hours

q6h every 6 hours

q12h every 12 hours

qwk every week

r right

rap disintegr rapidly disintegrating

RAR retinoic acid receptor

RBC red blood count or cell

RDA recommended dietary allowance

rec rectal

REM rapid eye movement

RESP respiratory system

rhPDGF-BB recombinant human platelet–derived growth factor

RNA ribonucleic acid

R/O rule out

ROAD reversible obstructive airway disease

ROM range of motion

RTI respiratory tract infection

Rx therapy, treatment, or prescription

s̄ without

SA sinoatrial

SAN sinoatrial node

SC subcutaneous

sec second

SERM selective estrogen receptor modulator

SGOT serum glutamic-oxaloacetic transaminase (now AST)

SGPT serum glutamic pyruvate transaminase (now ALT)

SIADH syndrome of inappropriate antidiuretic hormone

sig patient dosing instructions on prescription label

SL sublingual

SLE systemic lupus erythematosus

slow rel slow release

SMBG self-monitored blood glucose

SMZ sulfamethoxazole

SOB short of breath

sol solution

ss semis (one half)

SSRI selective serotonin reuptake inhibitor

stat at once

STD sexually transmitted disease

surg surgical

sus rel sustained-release dose form

supp suppository

Sx symptoms

syr syrup, a highly concentrated sucrose solution containing a drug(s)

T temperature

$T_{1/2}$ drug half-life

T_3 triiodothyronine

T_4 thyroxine

tab tablet

TB tuberculosis

TBG thyroxine-binding globulin

tbsp tablespoon

TCA tricyclic antidepressant

TD transdermal

temp temperature

TG total triglycerides

TIA transient ischemic attack

tid three times per day *(ter in die)*

time rel time-release dose form

tinc tincture, alcoholic solution of a drug

TMD temporomandibular dysfunction

TMJ temporomandibular joint

TMP trimethoprim

TNF tumor necrosis factor

top topical

tPA tissue plasminogen activator

APPENDIX A

TPN total parenteral nutrition

TPR temperature, pulse, respirations

TSH thyroid-stimulating hormone

tsp teaspoon

TT thrombin time

Tx treatment

U unit

UA urinalysis

ULDL ultra-low-density lipoprotein

URI upper respiratory infection

USP United States Pharmacopeia

UTI urinary tract infection

UV ultraviolet

vag vaginal

visc viscous

VD venereal disease

VHDL very-high-density lipoprotein

VLDL very-low-density lipoprotein

VO verbal order

vol volume

VPB ventricular premature beat

VS vital signs

WBC white blood cell, white blood cell count

WHO World Health Organization

wk week

WNL within normal limits

wt weight

yr year

> greater than

< less than

≠ not equal

↑ increase

↓ decrease

2° secondary

From Gage TW, Pickett FA: *Mosby's dental drug reference 2005,* ed 7, St. Louis, 2005, Mosby.

Appendix B Anesthetics

Anesthetics: general

Uses	Action
IV anesthetic agents are used to induce general anesthesia. The general anesthetic state consists of unconsciousness, amnesia, analgesia, immobility, and attenuation of autonomic responses to noxious stimuli. *Volatile inhalation agents* produce all the components of the anesthetic state but are administered through the lungs via an anesthesia machine. Agents for use include desflurane, enflurane, halothane, isoflurane, and sevoflurane. They're used in practice to maintain general anesthesia.	*IV anesthetic agents* act on the γ–aminobutyric acid (GABA) receptor complex to produce central nervous system (CNS) depression. GABA is the primary inhibitory neurotransmitter in the CNS. Ketamine produces dissociation between the thalamus and the limbic system. *Volatile inhalation agents* are not fully understood but may disrupt neuronal transmission throughout the CNS. These agents may either block excitatory or enhance inhibitory transmission through axons or synapses.

TABLE B–1
Anesthetics: general

Name	Availability	Uses	Dosage range	Side effects
Etomidate (Amidate)	I: 2 mg/ml	IV induction	0.2–0.6 mg/kg	Myoclonus, pain on injection, nausea, vomiting, respiratory depression
Ketamine (Ketalar)	I: 10 mg/ml, 50 mg/ml, 100 mg/ml	Analgesia, sedation, IV induction	1–4.5 mg/kg	Delirium, euphoria, nausea, vomiting
Methohexital (Brevital)	Powder for injection: 500 mg	IV induction, sedation	50–120 mg	Cardiovascular depression, myoclonus, nausea, vomiting, respiratory depression
Midazolam (Versed)	I: 1 mg/ml, 5 mg/ml	Anxiolytic, amnesic, sedation	1–5 mg titrated slowly	Respiratory depression
Propofol (Diprivan)	I: 10 mg/ml	Sedation IV induction maintenance	0.5 mg/kg 2–2.5 mg/kg 100–200 mcg/kg/min	Cardiovascular depression, delirium, euphoria, pain on injection, respiratory depression
Thiopental (Pentothal)	Powder for injection: 2.5% (25 mg/ml)	IV induction	Titrate vs. pt response. Average: 50–75 mg	Cardiovascular depression, nausea, vomiting, respiratory depression

I, Injection.

TABLE B–2
Anesthetics: local

Uses	Action
Local anesthetics suppress pain by blocking impulses along axons. Suppression of pain does not cause generalized depression of the entire nervous system. Local anesthetics may be given topically and by injection (local infiltration, peripheral nerve block [axillary], IV regional [Bier block], epidural, and spinal).	Most local anesthetics fall into one of two groups: esters or amides. Both provide anesthesia and analgesia by reversibly binding to and blocking sodium (Na) channels. This slows the rate of depolarization of the nerve action potential; thus, propagation of the electrical impulses needed for nerve conduction is prevented.

Name	Uses	Onset (min)	Duration (hr)	Side effects
Esters				
Chloroprocaine (Nesacaine)	Local infiltrate Nerve block Spinal	6–12	0.25–0.5	Excitation (e.g., seizures) followed by decreased level of consciousness (drowsiness to unconsciousness), bradycardia, heart block, decreased myocardial contractile force, hypotension, hypersensitivity reaction
Procaine (Novocaine)	Local infiltrate Nerve block Spinal	2–5	0.25–1	Same as above
Tetracaine	Topical spinal	15	2–3	Same as above
Amides				
Bupivacaine (Marcaine, Sensorcaine)	Local infiltrate Nerve block Epidural Spinal	5	2–4	Same as above
Etidocaine (Duranest)	Local infiltrate Nerve block Epidural	3–5	5–10	Same as above
Levobupivacaine (Chirocaine)	Nerve block Epidural	–	–	Same as above
Lidocaine	Local infiltrate Nerve block Spinal Epidural Topical IV regional	<2	0.5–1	Same as above
Mepivacaine (Carbocaine, Polocaine)	Local infiltrate Nerve block Epidural	3–5	0.75–1.5	Same as above
Ropivacaine (Naropin)	Local infiltrate Nerve block Epidural Spinal	1–15	2–6	Same as above

Note: Most side effects are manifestations of excessive plasma concentrations.
From *Mosby's 2006 drug consult for nurses*, St Louis, 2006, Mosby.

TABLE B–3
Contraindications for local anesthetics

Medical problem	Drugs to avoid	Type of contraindication	Alternative drug
Local anesthetic allergy, documented	All local anesthetics in same chemical class (e.g., esters)	Absolute	Local anesthetics in a different chemical class (e.g., amides)
Bisulfate allergy	Vasoconstrictor–containing local anesthetics	Absolute	Any local anesthetic without vasoconstrictor
Atypical plasma cholinesterase	Esters	Relative	Amides
Methemoglobinemia, idiopathic or congenital	Prilocaine	Relative	Other amides or esters
Significant liver dysfunction (ASA III–IV)	Amides	Relative	Amides or esters, but judiciously
Significant renal dysfunction (ASA III–IV)	Amides or esters	Relative	Amides or esters, but judiciously
Significant cardiovascular disease (ASA III–IV)	High concentrations of vasoconstrictors (as in racemic epinephrine gingival retraction cords)	Relative	Local anesthetics with epinephrine concentrations of 1:200,000 or 1:100,000 or mepivacaine 3% or prilocaine 4% (nerve blocks)
Clinical hyperthyroidism (ASA III–IV)	High concentrations of vasoconstrictors (as in racemic epinephrine gingival retraction cords)	Relative	Local anesthetics with epinephrine concentrations of 1:200,000 or 1:100,000 or mepivacaine 3% or prilocaine 4% (nerve blocks)

ASA, American Society of Anesthesiologists' classification.
From Malamed SF: *Handbook of local anesthesia,* ed 5, St Louis, 2004, Mosby.

TABLE B–4
Hydrochloride

Proprietary name	Manufacturer	Percent local anesthetic	Vasoconstrictor	Duration of analgesia (min)		MRD–m and MRD–a
				Pulpal	Soft tissue	
Articaine Hydrochloride (United States) Septocaine	Septodont	4	Epinephrine 1:100,00	60–75	180–360	7 mg/kg
(Canada) Septanest SP Astracaine Ultracaine D-S forte	Septodont Dentsply Hoechst					3.2 mg/lb 500 mg absolute maximum
(Canada)Septanest N Astracaine Ultracaine D-S	Septodont Dentsply Hoechst	4	Epinephrine 1:200,000	45–60	120–300	7 mg/kg 3.2 mg/lb 500 mg absolute maximum
Bupivacaine Hydrochloride Marcaine	Kodak	0.5	Epinephrine 1:200,00	90–180	240–540 (reports up to 720)	1.3 mg/kg 0.6 mg/lb 90 mg absolute maximum
Lidocaine Hydrochloride Lidocaine HCl Alphacaine Xylocaine	Many generics Carlisle Labs Dentsply	2	–	5–10	60–120	4.4 mg/kg 2.0 mg/lb 300 mg absolute maximum

Lidocaine HCl Alphacaine Lignospan Octocaine Xylocaine	Many generics Carlisle Labs Septodont Novocol Chemical Dentsply	2	Epinephrine 1:50,000	60	180–300	6.6 mg/kg 3.0 mg/lb 500 mg absolute maximum	4.4 mg/kg 2.0 mg/lb 300 mg absolute maximum
Lidocaine HCl Alphacaine Lignospan Octocaine Xylocaine	Many generics Carlisle Labs Septodont Novocol Chemical Dentsply	2	Epinephrine 1:50,000	60	180–300	6.6 mg/kg 3.0 mg/lb 500 mg absolute maximum	4.4 mg/kg 2.0 mg/lb 300 mg absolute maximum
Mepivacaine Hydrochloride							
Mepivacaine HCl Arestocaine Carbocaine Isocaine Polocaine Scandonest	Many generics Carlisle Labs Kodak Novocol Dentsply Septodont	3	–	20–40 (20 for infiltration; 40 for nerve block)	120–180	6.6 mg/kg 3.0 mg/lb 400 absolute maximum	4.4 mg/kg 2.0 mg/lb 300 absolute maximum
Mepivacaine HCl Arestocaine Isocaine Polocaine Scandonest Carbocaine	Many generics Carlisle Labs Dentsply Kodak Septodent Novocol	2	Levonordefrin 1:20,000 Neo–Cobefrin 1:20,000	60	180–300	6.6 mg/kg 3.0 mg/lb 400 absolute maximum	4.4 mg/kg 2.0 mg/lb 300 absolute maximum
Carbocaine	Kodak	2	Epinephrine 1:200,000	45–60	120–240	6.6 mg/kg 3.0 mg/lb 400 absolute maximum	4.4 mg/kg 2.0 mg/lb 300 absolute maximum

Continued

TABLE B-4—CONT'D
Hydrochloride

Proprietary name	Manufacturer	Percent local anesthetic	Vasoconstrictor	Duration of analgesia (min)		MRD–m and MRD–a	
				Pulpal	Soft tissue		
Scandonest 2% Special	Septodont	2	Epinephrine 1:200,000	60	120–300	6.6 mg/kg 3.0 mg/lb 400 absolute maximum	4.4 mg/kg 2.0 mg/lb 300 absolute maximum
Prilocaine Hydrochloride							
Prilocaine HCl Citanest Plain	Generic Dentsply	4		10–15 (infiltration) 40–60 (nerve block)	90–120 (inf) 120–240 (nb)	6 mg/kg 2.7 mg/lb 400 mg absolute maximum	
Prilocaine HCl + epinephrine 1:20,000 Citanest Forte	Generic Dentsply	4	Epinephrine 1:200,000	60–90	180–480	6 mg/kg 2.7 mg/lb 400 mg absolute maximum	

*In mid–2003, local anesthetics containing levonordefrin (Neo–Cobefrin) were removed from the market in North America because of difficulties in obtaining the product. It is believed that levonordefrin will become available again in 2004–2005.

MRD, Maximum recommended dose.

From Malamed SF: *Handbook of local anesthesia,* ed 5, St Louis, 2004, Mosby.

TABLE B–5
Mandibular teeth and available local anesthetic techniques

Teeth	Pulpal anesthesia	Soft tissue: Buccal	Soft tissue: Palatal
Incisors	Incisive (Inc) Inferior alveolar (IANB) Gow–Gates (GG) Vazirani–Akinosi (VA) Periodontal ligament (PDL) injection Intraseptal (IS) Intraosseous (IO) Infiltration (lateral incisor only)	IANB GG VA Inc IS Mental PDL Inf IO	IANB GG VA PDL IS Inf IO
Canines	Inferior alveolar Gow–Gates Vazirani–Akinosi Incisive Periodontal ligament injection Intraseptal Intraosseous	IANB GG VA Inc PDL IS IO Inf Mental	IANB GG VA PDL IS Inf IO
Premolars	Inferior alveolar Gow–Gates Vazirani–Akinosi Incisive Periodontal ligament injection Intraseptal Intraosseous	IANB GG VA Inc PDL IS IO Mental Inf	IANB GG VA PDL IS IO Inf
Molars	Inferior alveolar Gow–Gates Vazirani–Akinosi Periodontal ligament injection Intraseptal Intraosseous	IANB GG VA PDL IS IO Inf	IANB GG VA PDL IS IO Inf

From Malamed SF: *Handbook of local anesthesia,* ed 5, St Louis, 2004, Mosby.

TABLE B-6
Maxillary teeth and available local anesthetic

Teeth	Pulpal anesthesia	Soft tissue: Buccal	Soft tissue: Palatal
Incisors	Infraorbital (IO) Infiltration AMSA P–ASA V_2	Infraorbital (IO) Infiltration AMSA P–ASA V_2	Nasopalatine Infiltration AMSA P–ASA V_2
Canines	Infraorbital Infiltration AMSA P–ASA V_2	Infraorbital Infiltration AMSA P–ASA V_2	Nasopalatine Infiltration AMSA P–ASA V_2
Premolars	Infraorbital Infiltration MSA ASA V_2	Infraorbital Infiltration MSA ASA V_2	Greater palatine Infiltration AMSA V_2
Molars	PSA Infiltration V_2	PSA Infiltration V_2	Greater palatine Infiltration V_2

From Malamed SF: *Handbook of local anesthesia,* ed 5, St Louis, 2004, Mosby.

Appendix C Controlled Substances

Controlled substances chart

Drugs	United States	Canada
Heroin, LSD, peyote, marijuana, mescaline, phencyclidine	Schedule I (CI)	Schedule H
Opium, fentanyl, morphine, meperidine, methadone, oxycodone (and its combinations), hydromorphone, codeine (single-drug entity), and cocaine	Schedule II (CII)	Schedule N
Short-acting barbiturates	Schedule II	Schedule C
Amphetamine and methylphenidate	Schedule II	Schedule G
Codeine combinations, hydrocodone combinations, glutethimide, paregoric, phendimetrazine, thiopental, testosterone, and other androgens	Schedule III (CIII)	Schedule F
Benzodiazepines (diazepam, midazolam, etc.), chloral hydrate, meprobamate, phenobarbital, propoxyphene (and combinations), pentazocine (and combinations), and methohexital	Schedule IV (CIV)	Schedule F
Antidiarrheals and antitussives with opioid derivatives	Schedule V (CV)	

LSD, Lysergic acid diethylamide.

Appendix D Disorders and Conditions

TABLE D-1
Asthma medications

Agent	Indication	Mechanism of action	Example
Inhaled β_2-agonist (short-acting)	Acute exacerbation, used in all categories.	Bronchodilator: Smooth muscle relaxation following adenylate cyclase activation, resulting in an increase in cyclic AMP activating protein kinase A, which lowers the needed intracellular calcium for smooth muscle contraction	Albuterol Metaproterenol
Inhaled β_2-agonist (long-lasting)	Longer-term prevention usually added to antiinflammatory therapy.	Bronchodilator (see above)	Salmeterol
Oral β_2-agonist (long-lasting)	Longer term prevention usually added to antiinflammatory therapy.	Bronchodilator (see above)	Albuterol (sustained-release)
Inhaled corticosteroids	Longer-term prevention. Daily medication in all persistent forms. Low-, medium-, high-dose formulations depending on asthma severity/control.	Antiinflammatory: Inhibits cytokine production and adhesion protein activation Reverses β_2 down-regulation Suppresses recruitment of airway eosinophils	Beclomethasone Flunisolide Fluticasone Budesonide Triamcinolone

Systemic corticosteroids	Acute exacerbation, used in all categories. Long-term prevention in severe persistent asthma.	Antiinflammatory (see above)	Methylprednisolone Prednisolone Prednisone
Anticholinergics	Acute exacerbation, used in patients intolerant to short-acting β_2-agonists.	Bronchodilator: Competitive inhibition of muscarinic cholinergic receptors	Ipratropium bromide Cromolyn Nedocromil Theophylline (sustained-release)
Leukotriene modifiers	Long-term control and prevention in Step 2 mild persistent.	Antiinflammatory: Leukotriene receptor antagonist (competitive inhibition) = Zafirlukast/Montelukast 5-Lipooxygenase inhibitor interfering with leukotriene synthesis = Zileuton	Zafirlukast Montelukast Zileuton

* All medications have side effects with which the dentist should be familiar.
* Medication usage/discontinuance based on step-up, step-down fashion relating to symptoms.
* Specific dosage/delivery of medication tailored to patient/severity.
* Children <5 years old have different regimens.

From Sollecito TP, Tino G: *Oral Surg Oral Med Oral Pathol Oral Radiol Endod* 92:486–487, 2001.

TABLE D-2
Drugs used for treatment of seizure disorders

Drug	Pharmacologic category	Adverse effects
Carbamazepine (Epitol, Tegretol)	Tricyclic	Sedation, dizziness, fatigue, confusion, ataxia, nausea, blood dyscrasias, hepatotoxicity
Clonazepam (Klonopin)	Benzodiazepine	Tachycardia, drowsiness, fatigue, anxiety, ataxia, headache, dizziness, blurred vision, xerostomia
Ethosuximide (Zarontin)	Succinimide	Ataxia, sedation, dizziness, hallucinations, behavioral changes, headache, Stevens-Johnson syndrome, systemic lupus erythematosus, nausea, anorexia
Gabapentin (Neurontin)	Neurotransmitter	Somnolence, dizziness, ataxia, fatigue, nystagmus
Phenobarbital (Barbita, Luminal, Solfoton)	Barbiturate	Dizziness, light-headedness, sedation, ataxia, impaired judgement, skin rashes
Phenytoin (Dilantin)	Hydantoin	Dizziness, drowsiness, confusion, ataxia, nausea, gingival hyperplasia, megaloblastic anemia, leukopenia
Primidone (Mysoline)	Barbiturate derivative	Drowsiness, vertigo, ataxia, behavioral changes, headache, nausea
Topiramate (Topamax)	Sulfamate-substituted monosaccharide	Acidosis (may decrease serum bicarbonate concentrations), increased risk of kidney stones, hyperthermia, paresthesias, sedation, confusion, psychomotor slowing, mood disturbances
Valproic acid, sodium valproate (Depakene, Depakote)	Carboxylic acid	Anorexia, diarrhea, nausea, drowsiness, ataxia, irritability, confusion, headache, hepatotoxicity leukopenia, thrombocytopenia resulting in prolonged bleeding time

From Hupp: *Dental clinical advisor,* ed 1, St Louis, 2006, Elsevier.

TABLE D-3

Drugs used for management of oral candidosis

Medication	Dosage and directions[a]
Chlorhexidine 0.12% oral rinse (Peridex, PerioGard)[b] or 0.2% alcohol-free aqueous[c]	15 ml mouthrinse and expectorate tid. NPO 1/2 hr after use.
Nystatin oral suspension 100,000 units/ml[d]	5 ml mouthrinse 1 min and expectorate[e] qid (pc and hs). NPO 1/2 hr after use.
Clotrimazole 10 mg/ml suspension[f]	Swab 1-2 ml on affected area qid (pc and hs). NPO 1/2 hr after use.
Ketoconazole 2% cream (Nizoral) or clotrimazole 1% cream (Lotrimin)	Apply thin film to inner surface of denture(s) and/or corners of mouth qid (pc and hs). NPO 1/2 hr after use.
Clotrimazole 200-mg vaginal tablets (Gyne-Lotrimin)	Dissolve 1/2 tablet slowly in mouth bid. NPO 1/2 hr after use.
Clotrimazole 10-mg oral troches (Mycelex)	Dissolve one troche slowly in mouth 5 × daily. NPO 1/2 hr after use.
Ketoconazole 200-mg tablets (Nizoral)	One tablet PO qd for 7–10 days. Do not take antacids within 2 hr of this medication.[g]
Fluconazole 100-mg tablets (Diflucan)	One tablet PO bid for first day, then one tablet PO qd for 10–14 days.

[a]In most patients, decreased frequency and dosages can be used if maintenance therapy is required.
[b]High alcohol content (11.6%) will irritate mucosa and enhance xerostomia. Should not be prescribed for recovering alcoholics.
[c]Must be prepared by experienced compounding pharmacist. Many formulas include flavorings that decrease efficacy.
[d]High sucrose content. Not first-line choice.
[e]May be swallowed for pharyngeal involvement.
[f]Compounded in confectioners glycerin.
[g]Acidic environment is required for absorption.
From Kleinegger CL: Diseases of the mouth. In Rakel RE, Bope ET, editors: *Conn's current therapy 2002.* Philadelphia, 2002, WB Saunders.

Appendix E Pregnancy and Pediatrics

TABLE E-1
FDA drug pregnancy risk category descriptions

Pregnancy risk category	Description	Application in dentistry
A	Drug has been studied in humans. Evidence supports its safe use. Remote possibility of fetal harm.	Can be appropriately administered during pregnancy
B	Animal studies demonstrate no fetal risk. Inadequate studies in pregnant women. Slightly increased fetal risk.	
C	Teratogenic risk cannot be ruled out. Animal studies show potential adverse fetal effects. Potential benefits may outweigh risks.	Can be used with caution
D	Drug demonstrates risk in humans. Potential benefits may outweigh risks.	Should be avoided
X	Drug demonstrates harm in mother or fetus. Risk clearly outweighs benefit.	

From Hupp: *Dental clinical advisor*, ed 1, St Louis, 2006, Elsevier.

TABLE E-2
FDA drug pregnancy risk category and use during breast-feeding

Generic name	Brand name	FDA pregnancy risk category	Use during breast-feeding
Antimicrobials			
Amoxicillin	Amoxil; Polymox	B	Yes
Cephalexin	Keflex	B	Yes
Clindamycin	Cleocin	B	Yes
Doxycycline	Doryx; Vibramycin; Atridox; Periostat	D	No
Tetracycline	Actisite; Achromycin	D	No
Erythromycin†	Ery-Tab; E-Mycin; E.E.S.; PCE	B	Yes
Metronidazole	Flagyl	B	Caution
Penicillin V Potassium	V-Cillin K; V-Pen	B	Yes
Amoxicillin + clavulanic acid	Augmentin	B	Yes
Azithromycin	Zithromax	B	Yes
Nystatin	Mycostatin	B	Yes
Ketoconazole	Nizoral	C	No
Fluconazole	Diflucan	C	No
Chlorhexidine	Peridex	B	Yes
Analgesics			
Acetaminophen	Tylenol	B	Yes
Aspirin	Bayer	C/D3	No
Ibuprofen	Advil; Motrin	B/D3	Yes
Celecoxib/valdecoxib	Celebrex / Bextra	C/D3	Unknown
Naproxen	Aleve; Anaprox	B/D3	Unknown
Codeine	*Various combinations*	C/D*	Yes
Hydrocodone	*Various combinations*	C/D*	Caution
Oxycodone	*Various combinations*	C/D*	Caution
Sedatives			
Hydroxyzine	Atarax/Vistaril	C	Unknown
Midazolam	Versed	D	No
Diazepam	Valium	D	No
Lorazepam	Ativan	D	No
Triazolam	Halcion	X	No
Chloral hydrate	Somnote	C	Yes
Nitrous oxide	N/A	None‡	Controversial

Continued

TABLE E-2
FDA drug pregnancy risk category and use during breast-feeding—Cont'd

Generic name	Brand name	FDA pregnancy risk category	Use during breast-feeding
Local Anesthetics			
Lidocaine	Xylocaine	B	Yes
Etidocaine	Duranest	B	Yes
Prilocaine	Citanest	B	Yes
Mepivacaine	Carbocaine	C	Yes
Bupivacaine	Marcaine	C	Yes
Articaine	Septocaine	C	Unknown
Vasoconstrictors			
Epinephrine 1:100,000;	N/A	C*	Yes
1:200,000	Neo-Cobefrin	None	Yes
Levonordefrin 1:20,000			
Topical Anesthetics			
Benzocaine	Anbesol; Hurricaine	C	Yes
Lidocaine	Xylocaine; DentiPatch	B	Yes
Tetracaine	Pontocaine	C	Yes

C/D3, Pregnancy risk category D during the third trimester.
C/D*, Pregnancy risk category D in high doses at term or with prolonged use.
C*, Pregnancy risk category C in high doses.
†Avoid estolate form.
‡Best used in the second and third trimesters and for <30 min with at least 50% O2; consult physician.
Modified from Hilgers K, Douglass J, Mathieu G: *Pediatr Dent* 25:459–467, 2003.

TABLE E-3
Drug usage in pediatric dentistry

Drug	Route	Dose	Frequency	Notes
Antibiotics				
Amoxycillin	PO	25–50 mg/kg/day	tds	Syrup or chewable tablets for young children
	IV	100–400 mg/kg/day	tds	
	PO, IV	50 mg/kg up to adult dose 3 g	1 hour before	Endocarditis prophylaxis. For highly susceptible patients, half dose 6 hours later
Amoxycillin plus clavulanic acid	PO	20–40 mg/kg/day	tds	For beta-lactam resistant organisms only
Ampicillin	IV	50–100 mg/kg/day	qid	
	IV	50 mg/kg	stat	Endocarditis prophylaxis
Benzylpenicillin	IV	15–350 mg/kg/day 20,000–500,000 U/kg/day	qid	First IV drug of choice for odontogenic infections
Penicillin VK	PO	<5 years 500 mg/day >5 years 1–2 g/day	qid	Give 1 hour before meals
Cephalexin	PO	25–50 mg/kg/day	qid	
Cephalothin IV	IV	40–80 mg/kg/day	qid	Not in pregnancy
Cephalozin	IV	25–50 mg/kg/day		
Erythromycin	PO	25–40 mg/kg/day	qid	Ethylsuccinate is readily absorbed
Metronidazole	IV	22.5 mg/kg/day	tds	Not in pregnancy
	PO	10–15 mg/kg/day	tds	
Gentamicin	IV	2.5 mg/kg (children) up to 80 mg maximum	stat	Endocarditis prophylaxis, highly susceptible patients. In conjunction with ampicillin. Follow-up dose of ampicillin or amoxycillin required 6 hours later.

Continued

TABLE E-3
Drug usage in pediatric dentistry—Cont'd

Drug	Route	Dose	Frequency	Notes
Antibiotics				
Clindamycin	PO, IV	15–40 mg/kg/day	qid	Risk of pseudomembranous colitis
	PO, IV	10 mg/kg up to adult dose 600 mg	oral 1 hour before, IV stat	Endocarditis prophylaxis, susceptible patients Follow-up dose half initial dose, 6 hours later (5 mg/kg up to 300 mg)
Vancomycin	IV	20 mg/kg up to adult dose 1 g	infused over 1 hour	Endocarditis prophylaxis, susceptible patients allergic to penicillin
Antifungals				
Nystatin	Tablets	500,000 U	tds	
	Mixture	100,000 U/mL	6-hrly	Apply to affected area
Amphotericin B	Lozenges	10 mg	6-hrly	Apply to affected area
	Suspension	100 mg/mL	6-hrly	Apply to affected area
	Ointment	3%	6-hrly	Apply to affected area
Analgesics and sedatives				
Aspirin				Should not be used in children younger than 12 years of age because of the risk of Reye's syndrome
Paracetamol	PO, PR	15 mg/kg	4-hrly	Hepatotoxic if overdose
Codeine phosphate	PO	1–1.5 mg/kg single dose 1–3 mg/kg/day	4–6 divided doses	Similar side effects to narcotics, including nausea and constipation
Pethidine	IV, IM	1 mg/kg	3–4 hrly	Maximum 100 mg
Morphine	IV, IM	0.1–0.2 mg/kg	6-hrly	Should only be used in admitted patients
Naloxone	IM, IV	1–10 μg/kg	stat	May be repeated at 2–3 minute intervals if necessary

Midazolam	IV, IM	0.1–0.2 mg/kg	single dose	Sedation, may be given intranasally
Chloral hydrate	PO	30–50 mg/kg/day, 15–20 mg/kg single dose	4–6 hrly	Sedation
Trimeprazine	PO	3–4 mg/kg	single dose	Vallergan, sedation
Metoclopramide	PO, IM	3–5 years 2 mg 5–9 years 2.5 mg 9–14 years 5 mg 15–19 years 10 mg	single dose	Single dose after narcotic if vomiting or nausea. Maxolon. Dystonic reactions may occur
Other medications				
Kenalog in Orabase	Ointment	Triamcinolone 0.1%	4–6 hrly	Recurrent severe oral ulceration in children, apply to ulcer but do not rub ointment in
Ipecac syrup	PO	0–1 years 5–10 mL 1–12 years 15 mL	>12 years or adult 30 mL	Give copious water. Used for ingestion of noncorrosive poisons. For information contact Poisons Information Service
ε aminocaproic acid	IV	30 mg/kg		Antifibrinolytic, loading dose of 100 mg/kg
Tranexamic acid	PO	15–20 mg/kg	qid	Antifibrinolytic
DDAVP	IV	0.3 μg/kg		Infused over 1 hour before surgery
Heparin	IV	50–100 U/kg	4–6 hrly	Anticoagulant
Tetanus toxoid	IM	0.5 mL	single dose	If immunization protocol not complete, course should be given. Otherwise, a booster may be required for tetanus-prone wounds if >2 years since last booster

From Cameron AC, Widmer RP: *Handbook of pediatric dentistry*, ed 2, London, 2003, Mosby.
The table which forms Table K–2 is a guide to the administration of commonly used drugs in pediatric dentistry. Medications for children should always be prescribed in relation to weight. It is of utmost importance that clinicians understand the contraindications and precautions relevant to the drugs they are prescribing and should consult prescribing information supplied by the pharmaceutical manufacturers and relevant pharmacopeia. In the table PO = oral, IV = intravenous, IM = intramuscular, tds = x3 daily, quid = x4 daily and stat = immediately.

Appendix F Prescription Examples

This appendix illustrates a number of prescriptions that can be used as a guide to help you write prescriptions for dental patients. They can be used as written or modified to address each patient's specific needs and your personal preferences. They are not a substitute for your clinical judgment. The process of selecting and prescribing a medication for a patient usually is straightforward, but it can be challenging in some cases. It is important for the prescribing dentist to be completely knowledgeable about any drug prescribed. Complete prescribing information should be consulted before selecting a drug. This means knowing how the drug acts, its intended use, the dose and dose forms, how frequently the drug should be taken, and adverse effects and drug interactions. These essential drug facts are tools for the profession. In the following examples, prescriptions for brand name drugs are for illustrative purposes only and do not constitute a recommendation for that particular product. In an era of expensive brand name products, generics are generally the less expensive way to prescribe medications, but in some cases (especially for new drugs or specialty products) only brand name products are available.

Before prescribing or recommending (in the case of OTC products) a medication for a patient, it is strongly suggested that the dentist adhere to the following protocol:

A. Examine and evaluate the patient, leading to a diagnosis.
B. Obtain the patient's medical and drug histories (including use of OTC drugs, illegal drugs, and herbal or nonherbal remedies).
C. Determine the duration of drug therapy and the required number of doses.
D. Assess the patient's prior experience with drugs, including drug allergy.
E. Research the potential side effects and drug interactions.
F. Adhere to all federal and state laws regulating drug use in practice.
G. Consider the cost to the patient if less expensive alternatives are available.
H. Consider the patient's ability to use more complex dose forms or to follow complex instructions for use.
I. Have an alternative selection in mind in the event a patient cannot tolerate the prescribed drug.

I. ANALGESICS

Controlled Substances (Requires State and Drug Enforcement Administration [DEA] Registration to Prescribe, with DEA Number Included on the Prescription)

Prescription examples are for acute pain without regard to pain intensity. Because acute pain is generally managed within 3 to 4 days, prescriptions should limit the number of doses to be dispensed. In given situations, more than 10 or 12 doses may be required. *If the analgesic product you are using is not illustrated, don't worry. These are merely examples provided for guidance in prescription writing and are not inclusive of all analgesic products, which number into the hundreds.* For illustrative purposes, both brand and generic names are used. Note that the directions for use indicate a specific time interval for optimum response; prn use is avoided to ensure more appropriate dosing intervals for the analgesic. By-the-clock dosing is much more effective than as-needed doses. The cautions of sedation, hazard of operating an automobile, and avoidance of alcohol are appropriate for each product.

Rx

darvocet-N 100*

Disp: 12 (twelve) tabs

Sig: Take 1 (one) tab PO q4h for pain relief.

*The maximum recommended dose for propoxyphene napsylate is 600 mg/day. Do not take with alcohol, and reduce the dose or select another drug if significant liver or renal failure is present.

Rx

empirin with Codeine No. 4*

Disp: 12 (twelve) tabs

Sig: Take 1 (one) tab PO q4h for pain relief.

*This product contains 60 mg codeine phosphate, a preferable oral adult dose; the No. 3 product contains 30 mg codeine phosphate.

Rx

fiorinal with Codeine 30 mg*

Disp: 12 (twelve) caps

Sig: Take 1 (one) cap PO q4–6h for pain relief.

*This product contains a short-acting barbiturate. Fioricet with Codeine 30 mg contains acetaminophen instead of aspirin.

Rx

lortab 5/500

Disp: 12 (twelve) tabs

Sig: Take 1 (one) tab PO q6h for pain relief.

Rx

percodan

Disp: 10 (ten) tabs

Sig: Take 1 (one) tab PO q6h for pain relief.

Rx

tylenol with Codeine Elixir*

Disp: 90 ml (volume may vary with duration and patient's age)

Sig: Take 5 ml (one teaspoonful) q6–8h for pain relief.

*This is an example for a child age 3–6 yr. For a child age 7–12 yr, the dose is 10 ml, and for adults the dose is 15 ml. Be sure you know the quantities of acetaminophen and codeine phosphate contained in each 5-ml dose. This product also contains alcohol. Your pharmacist can increase the amount of codeine in each 5-ml dose unit; consult your pharmacist for instructions.

Rx

tylenol with Codeine No. 4*

Disp: 12 (twelve) tabs

Sig: Take 1 (one) tab PO q4h for pain relief.

*This product contains 60 mg codeine phosphate, a preferable oral adult dose; the No. 3 product contains 30 mg codeine phosphate.

Rx

vicodin

Disp: 10 (ten) tabs

Sig: Take 1 (one) tab PO q6h for pain relief.

Rx

zydone 5/400*

Disp: 10 (ten) tabs

Sig: Take 1 (one) or 2 (two) tabs PO q4–6h for pain relief.

*Because Zydone is available in several strengths, the prescription must be specific as shown in the example.

nonnarcotics or analgesics not classified as controlled substances

Doses for aspirin and acetaminophen for both adults and children are given in the respective monographs. For consistent dose levels and effects, it is important to prescribe NSAIDs by the clock rather than prn.

Rx

diclofenac sodium 50-mg tabs (immediate-release type)

Disp: 9 (nine) tabs

Sig: Take 1 (one) tab PO q8h for pain relief.

Rx
diflunisal 500-mg tabs*
Disp: 7 (seven) tabs
Sig: Take 2 (two) tabs PO the first dose; then 1 (one) tab PO q12h for pain relief.
*The 250-mg tabs may be sufficient for some patients. The initial dose is 500 mg; do not exceed doses of 1.5 g/day.

Rx
etodolac 400-mg tabs*
Disp: 16 (sixteen) tabs
Sig: Take 1 (one) tab PO q6–8h for pain relief.
*The 200-mg tabs may be sufficient for some patients. Dose limit is 1200 mg/day.

Rx
ibuprofen* 400-mg tabs†
Disp: 24 (twenty-four) tabs
Sig: Take 1 tab PO q4h for pain relief.
*Special preparations for children, such as Children's Motrin with specified doses, are available for toothaches; doses are printed on the package.
†If larger doses are preferred, the time interval between doses must be adjusted to reflect the larger dose; for example, 600 mg every 6 hours. Another option is to recommend OTC ibuprofen in 200-mg tablets and tell the patient to take 2 tabs every 4 hours. For some patients, a prescription may be required to ensure a desirable patient benefit. Ibuprofen also can be used for chronic pain.

Rx
ketoprofen 25-mg caps (or 50-mg caps)*
Disp: 12 (twelve) caps
Sig: Take 1 (one) cap PO q6–8h for pain relief.
*The larger dose may be required for some patients. Select the smaller dose for the elderly and patients with severe renal or hepatic disease; also available OTC in 12.5-mg tabs.

Rx
meclofenamate sodium* 50-mg caps
Disp: 18 (eighteen) caps
Sig: Take 1 (one) cap PO q4–6h for pain relief.
*Total daily dose is limited to 400 mg.

Rx
naproxen sodium 550-mg tabs
Disp: 10 (ten) tabs
Sig: Take 1 (one) tab PO q12h for pain relief.
Naproxen sodium also can be used for chronic pain.

Rx
ultram 50-mg tabs*
Disp: 12 (twelve) tabs
Sig: Take 1 (one) tab PO q4–6h for pain relief.
*For more severe pain, the 100-mg tabs can be prescribed. Do not exceed the daily dose limit of 400 mg.

Rx
vioxx 50-mg tabs
Disp: 5 (five) tabs
Sig: Take 1 (one) tab PO daily for pain relief.

II. ANTIINFECTIVES

The primary considerations when selecting an antiinfective drug include potential causative organisms, severity of infection, age of infection (cellulitis vs. pus formation), patient's prior history of antiinfective drug use, and immunologic status of the patient. The duration of antiinfective drug therapy differs among clinicians, ranging from 5 to 10 days. Certainly surgical intervention or removal of a necrotic pulp makes a significant difference not only in resolution but also in the duration of infection. The examples are provided for illustration purposes and show doses calculated to cover the patient for 7 to 10 days. Examples include both generic and brand name products.

One or two examples of prescriptions for children are shown; doses were calculated using milligram per kilogram of body weight and reflect manufacturers' or USP recommended doses. Antiinfectives should be prescribed to be taken at specific intervals, such as every 6 hours. Using symbols, such as qid for four times per day, may not allow for proper intervals between doses. However, for some drugs, such as rinses or lozenges, abbreviations such as qid or tid are satisfactory. *Note that these prescriptions are intended to help you develop your own prescription as dictated by the patient's need and circumstance.*

Rx

amoxicillin trihydrate 500-mg caps*

Disp: 21 (twenty-one) caps

Sig: Take 1 (one) cap PO q8h for infection until all are taken.

*Some may prefer to give an initial loading dose of 1000 mg followed by the 500-mg doses.

Rx

penicillin V potassium 500-mg tabs*

Disp: 28 (twenty-eight) tabs

Sig: Take 1 (one) tab PO q6h for infection until all are taken.

*Some may prefer to give an initial loading dose of 1000 mg followed by the 500-mg doses.

Rx for Prophylaxis Against Bacterial Endocarditis for Three Different Appointments

Rx

amoxicillin trihydrate 500-mg caps

Disp: 12 (twelve) caps

Sig: Take 4 (four) caps PO 1 hour before each dental appointment.

Rx for a Child Weighing 30 kg (66 lb)

The package insert dose for children is 20 mg/kg/day (in equal doses given every 8 hours) for mild/moderate infections and 40 mg/kg/day (in equal doses given every 12 hours) for severe infections. The example chosen is 20 mg/kg/day; this means the total daily dose will be 600 mg, or 200 mg every 8 hours in individual doses.

Rx

amoxicillin for oral suspension 200 mg/5 ml

Disp: 150 ml*

Sig: Take 5 ml PO q8h for infection until all is taken.

*This is sufficient volume to provide doses for 10 days.

Rx

cefadroxil 500-mg caps

Disp: 14 (fourteen) caps

Sig: Take 1 (one) cap PO q12h for infection until all are taken.

Rx for Prophylaxis Against Bacterial Endocarditis for a Single Appointment

Rx

cefadroxil 1-g tabs*

Disp: 2 (two) tabs

Sig: Take 2 (two) tabs PO 1 hour before appointment.

*Alternatively, 500-mg caps can be used, noting that 4 caps are required for a single use.

Rx

clindamycin hydrochloride 300-mg caps*

Disp: 28 (twenty-eight) caps

Sig: Take 1 (one) cap PO q6h for infection until all are taken.

*Doses of 150 mg also are used, depending on severity of the infection.

Rx

azithromycin 250-mg caps

Disp: 6 (six) caps

Sig: Take 2 (two) caps PO the first day, then 1 (one) cap daily for infection until all are taken.

Take 1 hour ac or 2 hours pc.

Rx

biaxin 250-mg tabs*

Disp: 20 (twenty) tabs

Sig: Take 1 (one) tab PO q12h for infection until all are taken.

*The 500-mg dose may be required for some infections, such as maxillary sinusitis subsequent to loss of root tip in the sinus cavity.

Rx for Prophylaxis Against Bacterial Endocarditis for Six Appointments

Rx

clindamycin hydrochloride 300-mg caps

Disp: 12 (twelve) caps

Sig: Take 2 (two) caps PO 1 hour before each appointment.

Rx

doxycycline 100-mg caps

Disp: 11 (eleven) caps

Sig: Take 1 (one) cap PO q12h the first day, then take 1 (one) cap PO daily for infection until all are taken.

Rx

ery-tab 250-mg tabs*

Disp: 40 (forty) tabs

Sig: Take 1 (one) tab PO q6h for infection until all are taken.

*This is an erythromycin base; other dose options depending on the dose form selected include 333 mg q8h or 500 mg q12h.

Rx

erythromycin ethyl succinate 400-mg tabs

Disp: 40 (forty) tabs

Sig: Take 1 (one) tab PO q6h for infection until all are taken.

Rx

metronidazole 250-mg tabs

Disp: 21 (twenty-one) tabs

Sig: Take 1 (one) tab PO q8h for infection until all are taken; avoid use of alcohol products.

III. ANTIFUNGAL ANTIINFECTIVES

These are examples (not all products are illustrated) of prescriptions for drugs for *Candida* infections of the oral cavity; the drugs usually are prescribed for use over 14 days. Remember that patient evaluation, history, and diagnosis always precede drug selection.

Rx

clotrimazole 10-mg troches

Disp: 70 troches

Sig: Slowly dissolve 1 (one) troche in your mouth five times per day while awake until all are used.

Rx

fluconazole 50-mg tabs*

Disp: 15 (fifteen) tabs

Sig: Take 2 (two) tabs PO the first day, then take 1 (one) tab PO daily for infection until all are taken.

*The 100-mg dose may be required for more severe infections or for immunocompromised patients.

Rx

nystatin ointment*

Disp: 15 (fifteen) g

Sig: Apply a small amount to affected areas after each meal and at bedtime.

*Possible use in angular cheilitis associated with candidiasis.

Rx

nystatin oral suspension (100,000 units/ml)

Disp: 320 ml

Sig: Rinse for 1 min with 5 ml of solution q6h while awake and then expectorate. One rinse should be used just before bedtime.*

*Dentures also should be carefully cleaned and then soaked in the oral solution for approximately 15 min each day during treatment. Although some sugar is contained in the commercial preparation of nystatin oral suspension, it still is effective against candidiasis. An alternative choice for oral nystatin rinse when sugar is not desirable for the patient is shown in the following example. Be sure to check labels for sugar content in all locally acting oral products.

Rx

nystatin extemporaneous powder

Disp: 50 million units*

Sig: Add $^1/_8$ tsp (500,000 units) to 1 cup water (8 oz) and rinse qid for 2 weeks.
*This is the smallest container of powder available; it supplies enough powder for 25 days of use.

IV. OTHER DENTAL PRESCRIPTIONS

The following prescriptions are examples for a variety of dental diseases. They are grouped according to their usual applications. *Again, there may be many choices for treatment that are not shown; these are examples for assistance in prescription writing.*

Recurrent Aphthous Stomatitis

Rx
aphthasol oral paste 5%
Disp: 5 (five) g
Sig: Dab a small amount of paste on ulcer qid, pc, and hs.

Rx
benadryl elixir 40 ml*
Kaopectate 80 ml
Water qs ad 240 ml
Sig: Rinse with 5 ml for 1 to 2 min prn for comfort and then expectorate.
*A 50/50 mixture of Benadryl/Kaopectate also can be used. Benadryl Elixir alone also serves as a palliative rinse, but it contains alcohol; when alcohol is to be avoided use Children's Benadryl, which is alcohol-free.

Rx
chlorhexidine rinse 0.12% or write peridex
Disp: 16 (sixteen) oz
Sig: Rinse with 15 ml twice daily after brushing.*
*Optional application route: moisten a cotton-tipped applicator and dab on aphthous ulcer bid.

Rx
fluocinonide gel 0.05% or write lidex gel
Disp: 15 (fifteen) g
Sig: Apply small amount (dab on or use cotton-tipped applicator) to ulcers bid.

Rx
xylocaine viscous 2%
Disp: 100 ml
Sig: Rinse with 5 ml for 1 to 2 min q4h.
Optional choice: rinse before meals and at bedtime.

Desquamative Lesions (Lichen Planus, Pemphigoid)

Rx
diprolene gel 0.05%*
Disp: 15 (fifteen) g
Sig: Apply a small amount to lesions tid. Apply the last dose at bedtime.
*This is a very-high-potency glucocorticoid; consider switching to a high-potency gel once severe lesions are under control.

Rx
lidex gel 0.05%*
Disp: 30 (thirty) g
Sig: Apply a small amount to lesions tid. Apply the last dose at bedtime.
*This is a high-potency topical glucocorticoid. Alternatively, if the lesions are small, dab a small amount directly on the lesions.

Rx
prednisone 5-mg tabs
Disp: 44 (forty-four) tabs
Sig: Take 2 (two) tabs PO AM and PM for 2 days, then reduce by 1 (one) tab each day until all are taken.

Drugs Affecting Salivary Flow

Prescriptions to reduce salivary flow (using four appointments as an example, because the number of tablets to dispense depends on the number of appointments)

Rx
atropine sulfate 0.40mg tabs
Disp: 4 (four) tabs
Sig: Take 1 tab PO 30 to 60 min before appointment.

Rx
pro-banthine 15-mg tabs
Disp: 4 (four) tabs
Sig: Take 1 (one) tab PO 45–60 min before appointment.
*Many pharmacies may no longer stock this particular drug.

Prescription to stimulate salivary flow in selected patients

Rx
evoxac 30-mg caps
Disp: 42 (forty-two) caps*
Sig: Take 1 (one) cap PO three times per day.
*Larger doses increase risk of side effects; enough doses are ordered for a 2-week period to evaluate patient response.

drugs for herpes labialis

Rx
acyclovir 200-mg caps
Disp: 35 (thirty-five) caps
Sig: Take 1 (one) cap PO five times per day.

Rx
acyclovir cream 5%
Disp: 3 (three) g
Sig: At the first sign of lesion, apply a small amount to affected areas six times per day for 1 week.

Rx
denavir cream 1%
Disp: 2 (two) g
Sig: At first sign of lesion, apply a small amount to affected area q2h (while awake) for 4 days.

Mild Allergic Reactions

Rx
benadryl 25-mg caps*
Disp: 15 (fifteen) caps
Sig: Take 1 (one) cap q4–8h for symptom relief.
Caution: Sedation.
*Adults can take up to 50 mg per dose. Alternative long-acting, nonsedating antihistamines are available, as well as other rapid-onset, short-acting, sedating antihistamines. However, for immediate hypersensitive reactions, rapid-acting drugs are preferred.

Rx
medrol dosepak 4-mg tabs
Disp: 1 (one) unit
Sig: Follow labeled directions on package for use.
Note: One pack contains 21 tabs.

Other Dental Prescriptions

Fluoride toothpaste

Rx
1.1% neutral sodium fluoride toothpaste*
Disp: 2 (two) tubes
Sig: Apply thin ribbon to dry toothbrush and brush for 2 min. Spit out excess; do not eat, drink, or rinse for 30 min after use.
*You may prefer to write Previ-Dent 5000 Plus.

From Gage TW, Pickett FA: *Mosby's dental drug reference 2005*, ed 7, St Louis, 2005, Mosby.

Appendix G Preventing Medication Errors and Improving Medication Safety

Medication safety is a high priority for the health care professional. Prevention of medication errors and improved safety for the patient are important, especially in today's health care environment when today's patient is older and sometimes sicker and the drug therapy regimen can be more sophisticated and complex.

A medication error is defined by the National Coordinating Council for Medication Error Reporting and Prevention (NCC MERP) as "any preventable event that may cause or lead to inappropriate medication use or patient harm while the medication is in the control of the health care professional, patient, or consumer."

Most medication errors occur as a result of multiple, compounding events as opposed to a single act by a single individual.

Use of the wrong medication, strength, or dose; confusion over sound-alike or look-alike drugs; administration of medications by the wrong route; miscalculations (especially when used in pediatric patients or when administering medications intravenously); errors in prescribing and transcription all can contribute to compromising the safety of the patient. The potential for adverse events and medication errors is definitely a reality and is potentially tragic and costly in both human and economic terms.

Health care professionals must take the initiative to create and implement procedures to prevent medication errors and implement methods to reduce medication errors. The first priority in preventing medication errors is to establish a multidisciplinary team to improve medication use. The goal for this team would be to assess medication safety and implement changes that would make it difficult or impossible for mistakes to reach the patient. Some important criteria in making improved medication safety successful include the following:

- Promote a nonpunitive approach to reducing medication errors
- Increase the detection and the reporting of medication errors, near misses, and potentially hazardous situations that may result in medication errors
- Determine root causes of medication errors
- Educate about the causes of medication errors and ways to prevent these errors
- Make recommendations to allow organization-wide, system-based changes to prevent medication errors
- Learn from errors that occur in other organizations and take measures to prevent similar errors

Some common causes and ways to prevent medication errors and improve safety include the following:

Handwriting: Poor handwriting can make it difficult to distinguish between two medications with similar names. Also, many drug names sound similar, especially when the names are spoken over the telephone, poorly enunciated, or mispronounced.

- Take time to write legibly.
- Keep phone or verbal orders to a minimum to prevent misinterpretation.
- Repeat back orders taken over the telephone.
- When ordering a new or rarely used medication, print the name.
- Always specify the drug strength, even if only one strength exists.

- Print generic and brand names of look-alike or sound-alike medications.

Zeros and decimal points: Hastily written orders can present problems even if the name of the medication is clear.

- Never leave a decimal point "naked." Place a zero before a decimal point when the number is less than a whole unit (e.g., use 0.25 mg or 250 mcg, **not**.25 mg).
- Never have a trailing zero following a decimal point (e.g., use 2 mg, **not** 2.0 mg).

Abbreviations: Errors can occur because of a failure to standardize abbreviations. Establishing a list of abbreviations that should never be used is recommended.

- Never abbreviate unit as "U," spell out "unit."
- Do not abbreviate "once daily" as od or qd, or "every other day" as qod; spell it out.
- Do not use D/C, as this may be misinterpreted as either discharge or discontinue.
- Do not abbreviate drug names; spell out the generic and/or brand names.

Ambiguous or incomplete orders: These types of orders can cause confusion or misinterpretation of the writer's intention. Examples include situations where the route of administration, dose, or dosage form has not been specified.

- Do not use slash marks—they are read as the number one (1).
- When reviewing an unusual order, verify the order with the person writing the order to prevent any misunderstanding.
- Read over orders after writing.
- Encourage that the drug's indication for use be provided on medication orders.
- Provide complete medication orders—do not use "resume preop" or "continue previous meds."

High-alert medications: Medications in this category have an increased risk of causing significant patient harm when used in error. Mistakes with these medications may or may not be more common but may be more devastating to the patient if an error occurs. A list of high-alert medications can be obtained from the Institute for Safe Medication Practices (ISMP) at *www.ismp.org*.

Technology available today that can be used to address and help to solve potential medication problems or errors include the following:

- *Electronic prescribing systems*—This refers to computerized prescriber order entry systems. Within these systems is the capability to incorporate medication safety alerts (e.g., maximum dose alerts, allergy screening). Additionally, these systems should be integrated or interfaced with pharmacy and laboratory systems to provide drug–drug and drug–disease interactions alerts and include clinical order screening capability.
- *Bar codes*—These systems are designed to use bar-code scanning devices to validate identity of patients, verify medications administered, document administration, and provide safety alerts.
- *"Smart" infusion pumps*—These pumps allow users to enter drug infusion protocols into a drug library along with predefined dosage limits. If a dosage is outside the limits established, an alarm is sounded and drug delivery is halted, informing the clinician that the dose is outside the recommended range.

- *Automated dispensing systems/point-of-use dispensing system*—These systems should be integrated with information systems, especially pharmacy systems.
- *Pharmacy order entry system*—This should be fully integrated with an electronic prescribing system with the capability of producing medication safety alerts. Additionally, the system should generate a computerized medication administration record (MAR), which would be used by a nursing staff while administering medications.

From *Mosby's 2006 Drug Consult for Nurses,* St Louis, 2006, Mosby.

Appendix H English-Spanish Drug Phrase Translator

TAKING THE MEDICATION HISTORY

- Are you allergic to any medications? (If yes:)
  ¿Es alérgico a algún medicamento? (sí:)
  (Ehs ah-lehr-hee-koh ah ahl-goon meh-dee-kah-mehn-toh) (see:)
  —Which medications are you allergic to?
  ¿A cuál medicamento es alérgico?
  (ah koo-ahl meh-dee-kah-mehn-toh ehs ah-lehr-hee-koh)
  —What happens when you develop an allergic reaction?
  ¿Qué le pasa cuando desarrolla una reacción alérgica?
  (Keh leh pah-sah koo-ahn-doh deh-sah-roh-yah oo-nah reh-ahk-see-ohn ah-lehr-hee-kah)
  —What did you do to relieve or stop the allergic reaction?
  ¿Qué hizo para aliviar o detener la reacción alérgica?
  (Keh ee-soh pah-rah ah-lee-bee-ahr oh deh-teh-nehr lah reh-ahk-see-ohn ah-lehr-hee-kah)
- Do you take any over-the-counter, prescription, or herbal medications? (If yes:)
  ¿Toma medicamentos sin receta, con receta, o naturistas (hierbas medicina-les)? (sí:)
  (Toh-mah meh-dee-kah-mehn-tohs seen reh-seh-tah, kohn reh-seh-tah, oh nah-too-rees-tahs [ee-ehr-bahs meh-dee-see-nah-lehs]) (see:)
  —Why do you take each medication?
  ¿Porqué toma cada medicamento?
  (Pohr-keh toh-mah kah-dah meh-dee-kah-mehn-toh)
  —What is the dosage for each medication?
  ¿Cuál es la dosis de cada medicamento?
  (Koo-ahl ehs lah doh-sees deh kah-dah meh-dee-kah-mehn-toh)
  —How often do you take each medication?
  ¿Con qué frequencia toma cada medicamento?
  (Kohn keh freh-koo-ehn-see-ah toh-mah kah-dah meh-dee-kah-mehn-toh)

Once per day?	¿Una vez por día; diariamente? (Oo-nah behs pohr dee-ah; dee-ah-ree-ah-mehn-teh)
Twice per day?	¿Dos veces por día? (dohs beh-sehs pohr dee-ah)
Three times per day?	¿Tres veces por día? (Trehs beh-sehs pohr dee-ah)
Four times per day?	¿Cuatro veces por día? (Koo-ah-troh beh-sehs pohr-dee-ah)
Every other day?	¿Cada tercer día? (Kah-dah tehr-sehr dee-ah)
Once per week?	¿Una vez por semana? (Oo-nah behs pohr seh-mah-nah)

- How does each medication make you feel?
  ¿Como le hace sentir cada medicamento?
  (Koh-moh leh ah-seh sehn-teer kah-dah meh-dee-kah-mehn-toh)
  —Does the medication make you feel better?

¿Le hace sentir mejor el medicamento?
(Heh ah-seh sehn-teer meh-hohr ehl meh-dee-kah-mehn-toh)
—Does the medication make you feel the same or unchanged?
¿Le hace sentir igual o sin cambio el medicamento?
(Leh ah-seh sehn-teer ee-goo-ahl oh seen kam-bee-oh ehl meh-dee-kah-mehn-toh)
—Does the medication make you feel worse? (If yes:)
¿Se siente peor con el medicamento? (si:)
(Seh see-ehn teh peh-ohr kohn ehl meh-dee-kah-mehn-toh) (see:)
What do you do to make yourself feel better?
¿Qué hace para sentirse mejor?
(Keh ah-seh pah-rah sehn-teer-seh meh-hohr)

PREPARING FOR TREATMENT TO MEDICATION THERAPY

Medication Purpose

This medication will help relieve:
Este medicamento le ayudaráaaliviar:
(Ehs-teh meh-dee-kah-mehn-toh leh ah-yoo-dah-rah ah ah-lee-bee-ahr)

English	Spanish	Pronunciation
abdominal gas	gases intestinales	(gah-sehs een-tehs-tee-nah-lehs)
abdominal pain	dolor intestinal; dolor en el abdomen	(doh-lohr een-tehs-tee-nahl; doh-lohr ehn ehl ahb-doh-mehn)
chest congestion	congestión del pecho	(kohn-hehs-tee-ohn dehl peh-choh)
chest pain	dolor del pecho	(doh-lohr dehl peh-choh)
constipation	constipación; estrñeimiento	(kohns-tee-pah-see-ohn; Ehs-treh nyee-mee-ehn-toh)
cough	tos	(tohs)
headache	dolor de cabeza	(doh-lohr-deh kah-beh-sah)
muscle aches and pains	achaques musculares y dolores	(ah-chah-kehs moos-koo-lah-rehs ee doh-loh-rehs)
pain	dolor	(doh-lohr)

This medication will prevent:
Este medicamento prevendrá:
(Ehs-teh meh-dee-kah-mehn-toh preh-behn-drah)

English	Spanish	Pronunciation
blood clots	coágulos de sangre	(koh-ah-goo-lohs deh sahn-greh)
constipation	constipación; estreñimiento	(kohns-tee-pah-see-ohn; ehs-treh-nyee-mee-ehn-toh)
contraception	contracepción; embarazo	(kohn-trah-sehp-see-ohn; ehm-bah-rah-soh)
diarrhea	diarrea	(dee-ah-reh-ah)
infection	infección	(een-fehk-see-ohn)
seizures	convulciónes; ataque epilé ptico	(kohn-bool-see-ohn-ehs; ah-tah-keh eh-pee-lehp-tee-koh)

Continued

English	Spanish	Pronunciation
shortness of breath	respiración corta; falta de aliento	(rehs-pee-rah-see-ohn kohr-tah; fahl-tah deh ah-lee-ehn-toh)
wheezing	el resollar; la respiración ruidosa, sibilante	(ehl reh-soh-yahr; lah rehs-pee-rah-see-ohn roo-ee-doh-sah, see-bee-lahn-teh)

This medication will increase your:
Este medicamento aumentarásu:
(Ehs-teh meh-dee-kah-mehn-toh ah-oo-mehn-tah-rah soo:)

English	Spanish	Pronunciation
ability to fight infections	habilidad a combatir infecciones	(ah-bee-lee-dahd ah kohm-bah-teer een-fehk-see-oh-nehs)
appetite	apetito	(ah-peh-tee-toh)
blood iron levels	nivel de hierro en la sargre	(nee-behl deh ee-eh-roh ehn lah sahn-greh)
blood sugar	azúcar en la sangre	(ah-soo-kahr ehn lah sahn-greh)
heart rate	pulso; latido	(pool-soh; lah-tee-doh)
red blood cell count	cuenta de cé lulas rojas	(koo-ehn-tah deh seh-loo-lahs roh-hahs)
thyroid hormone levels	niveles de hormona tiroide	(nee-beh-lehs deh ohr-moh-nah tee-roh-ee-deh)
urine volume	volumen de orina	(boh-loo-mehn deh oh-ree-nah)

This medication will decrease your:
Este medicamento reducirásu:
(Ehs-teh meh-dee-kah-mehn-toh reh-doo-see-rah soo:)

English	Spanish	Pronunciation
anxiety	Ansiedad	(ahn-see-eh-dahd)
blood cholesterol level	nivel de colesterol en la sangre	(nee-behl deh koh-lehs-teh-rohl ehn lah sahn-greh)
blood lipid level	nivel de lípido en la sangre	(nee-behl deh lee-pee-doh ehn lah sahn-greh)
blood pressure	presión arterial; de sangre	(preh-see-ohn ahr teh-ree-ahl; deh sahn-greh)
blood sugar level	nivel de azúcar en la sangre	(nee-behl deh ah-soo-kahr ehn lah sahn-greh)
heart rate	pulso; latido	(pool-soh; lah-tee-doh)
stomach acid	ácido en el estó mago	(ah-see-doh ehn ehl ehs-toh-mah-goh)
thyroid hormone levels	niveles de hormona tiroide	(nee-beh-lehs deh ohr-moh-nah tee-roh-ee-deh)
weight	peso	(peh-soh)

This medication will treat:
Este medicamento sirve para:
(Ehs-teh meh-dee-kah-mehn-toh seer-beh pah-rah)

English	Spanish	Pronunciation
cancer of your _____	cancer de su _____	(kahn-sehr deh soo)
depression	depresión	(deh-preh-see-ohn)
HIV infection	infección de VIH	(een-fehk-see-ohn deh beh ee ah-cheh)
inflammation	infamación	(een-flah-mah-see-ohn)
swelling	hinchazón	(een-chah-sohn)
the infection in your _____	la infección en su _____	(lah een-fehk-see-ohn ehn soo)
your abnormal heart rhythm	su ritmo anormal de corazón	(soo reet-moh ah-nohr-mahl deh koh-rah-sohn)
your allergy to _____	su alergia a _____	(soo eh-lehr-hee-ah ah)
your rash	su erupción; sarpullido	(soo eh-roop-see-ohn; sahr-poo-yee-doh)

ADMINISTERING MEDICATION

- Swallow this medication with water or juice.
  Tragüe este medicamento con agua o jugo.
  (Trah-geh ehs-teh meh dee-kah-mehn-toh kohn ah-goo-ah oh hoo-goh)
- If you cannot swallow the medication whole, I can crush it and put it in food.
  Si no puede tragar el medicamento entero puedo aplastarlo (triturarlo) y ponerlo en el alimento.
  (See noh poo-eh-deh trah-gahr ehl meh-dee-kah-mehn-toh ehn-teh-roh poo-eh-doh ah-plahs-tahr-loh [tree-too-rahr-loh] ee poh-nehr-loh ehn ehl ah lee-mehn-toh)
- I need to mix this medication with water or juice before you drink it.
  Necesito mezclar este medicamento en agua o jugo antes de que lo tome.
  (Neh-seh-see-toh mehs-klahr ehs-teh meh-dee-kah-mehn-toh ehn ah-goo-ah oh hoo-goh ahn-tehs deh keh loh toh-meh)
- Do not chew this medication. Swallow it whole.
  No mastique este medicamento. Tragüelo entero.
  (Noh mahs-tee-keh ehs-teh meh-dee-kah-mehn-toh. Trah-geh-loh ehn-teh-roh)
- Gargle with this medication and then swallow it.
  Haga gargaras con este medicamento y luego tragüelo.
  (Ah-gah gahr-gah-rahs koh ehs-teh meh-dee-kah-mehn-toh ee loo-eh-goh trah-geh-loh)
- Place this medication under your tongue and let it dissolve.
  Ponga este medicamento bajo la lengua y deje que se disuelva.
  (Pohn-gah ehs-teh meh-dee-kah-mehn-toh bah-hoh lah lehn-goo-ah ee deh-heh keh seh dee-soo-ehl-bah)
- I would like to give this injection in your:
  Quiero aplicar esta injección en su:
  (Kee-eh-roh ah-plee-kahr ehs-tah een-yehk-see-ohn ehn soo:)

—abdomen	abdomen (ahb-doh-mehn)
—arm	brazo (brah-soh)
—buttocks	nalga (nahl-gah)
—hip	cadera (kah-deh-rah)
—thigh	muslo (moos-loh)

- I will give you this medication through your intravenous line.
  Le daré este medicamento por el tubo de suero intravenoso.
  (Leh dah-reh ehs-teh meh-dee-kah-mehn-toh pohr ehl too-boh deh soo-eh-roh een-trah-beh-noh-soh)
- Let me know if you feel burning or pain at the intravenous site.
  Digame si siente ardor o dolor en el sitio del suero intravenoso.
  (Dee-gah-meh see see-ehn-teh ahr-dohr oh doh-lohr ehn ehl see-tee-oh dehl soo-eh-roh een-trah-beh-noh-soh)
- I need to insert this suppository into your rectum (or vagina).
  Necesito meter este supositorio en el recto (o vagina).
  (Neh-seh-see-toh meh-tehr ehs-teh soo-poh-see-toh-ree-oh ehn ehl rehk-toh [oh bah-hee-nah])
- I need to put this medication into each ear; left ear; right ear.
  Necesito poner este medicamento en cada oreja; oreja izquierda; oreja derecha.
  (Neh-seh-see-toh poh-nehr ehs-teh meh-dee-kah-mehn-toh ehn kah-dah oh-reh-hah; oh-reh-hah ees-kee-ehr-dah; -oh-reh-hah deh-reh-chah)
- I need to put this medication into each eye; left eye; right eye.
  Necesito poner este medicamento en cada ojo; ojo izquierdo; ojo derecho.
  (Neh-seh-see-toh poh-nehr ehs-teh meh-dee-kah-mehn-toh ehn kah-dah oh-hoh; oh-hoh ees-kee-ehr-doh; oh-hoh deh-reh-choh)

PREPARING FOR DISCHARGE

- The generic name for this medication is _____.
  El nombre genérico (sin marca) de este medicamento es _____.
  (Ehl nohn-breh heh-neh-ree-koh [seen mahr-kah] deh ehs-teh meh-dee-kah-mehn-toh ehs _____)
- The trade name for this medication is _____.
  El nombre comercial de este medicamento es _____.
  (Ehs nohm-breh koh-mehr-see-ahl deh ehs-teh meh-dee-kah-mehn-toh ehs _____)
- Take the medication exactly as prescribed.
  Tome el medicamento exactamente como se receta.
  (Toh-meh ehl meh-dee-kah-mehn-toh ehx-ahk-tah-mehn-teh koh-moh seh reh-seh-tah)
- You can safely break a scored tablet in half.
  Puede partir por la mitad la tableta que tiene una muesca (marca).
  (Poo-eh-deh pahr-teer pohr lah mee-tahd lah tah-bleh-tah keh tee-eh-neh oo-nah moo-ehs-kah [mahr-kah])
- Do not crush or chew enteric-coated, extended-release, or sustained-release tablets or capsules.
  No aplaste (triture) o mastique una tableta con capa entérica, de acción prolongada o de mantenimiento.

(Noh ah-plahs-teh [tree-too-reh] oh mahs-tee-keh oo-nah tah-bleh-tah kohn-kah-pah ehn-teh-ree-kah, deh ahk-see-ohn proh-lohn-gah-dah oh deh mahn-teh-nee-mee-ehn-toh)

- If you miss a dose:
  Si pierde una dosis:
  (See pee-ehr-deh oo-nah doh-sees:)
  - —take it as soon as you remember it.
    tómela tan pronto se acuerde.
    (toh-meh-lah tahn prohn-toh seh ah-koo-ehr-deh)
  - —wait until the next dose.
    espere hasta la siguiente dosis.
    (ehs-peh-reh ahs-tah lah see-ghee-ehn-teh doh-sees)
  - —do not double the next dose.
    No doble la siguiente dosis.
    (noh doh-bleh lah see-ghee-ehn-teh doh-sees)
  - —contact your physician.
    llame a su médico.
    (yah-meh ah soo meh-dee-koh)
- Do not stop taking your medication without first speaking with your physician.
  No deje de tomar su medicamento sin hablar primero con su médico.
  (Noh deh-heh deh toh-mahr soo meh-dee-kah-ehn-toh seen ah-blahr pree-meh-roh kohn soo meh-dee-koh)
- Do not drink alcohol while taking this medication.
  No tome alcohol cuando tome este medicamento.
  (Noh toh-meh ahl-kohl koo-ahn-doh toh-meh ehs-teh meh-dee-kah-mehn-toh)
- Do not drive or operate machinery while taking this medication.
  No maneje o use maquinaria cuando toma este medicamento.
  (Noh mah-neh-heh oh oo-seh mah-kee-nah-ree-ah koo-ahn-doh toh-mah ehs-teh meh-dee-kah-mehn-toh)
- Notify your physician right away if you experience a dangerous side effect.
  Llame a su médico inmediatamente si tiene efectos secundarios peligrosos.
  (Llah-meh ah soo meh-dee-koh een-meh-dee-ah-tah-mehn-teh see tee-eh-neh eh-fehk-tohs seh-koon-dah-ree-ohs peh-lee-groh-sohs)
- Check with your physician before taking any over-the-counter medications.
  Cheque con su médico antes de tomar medicamentos sin receta.
  (Cheh-keh kohn soo meh-dee-koh ahn-tehs deh toh-mahr meh-dee-kah-mehn-tohs seen reh-seh-tah)
- Notify your physician if you are pregnant or are planning to become pregnant while taking this medication.
  Dígale a su médico si estáembarazada o planea el embarazo cuando toma este medicamento.
  (Dee-gah-leh ah soo meh-dee-koh see ehs-tah ehm-bah-rah-sah-dah oh plah-neh-ah ehl ehm-bah-rah-soh koo-ahn-doh toh-mah ehs-teh meh-dee-kah-mehn-toh)
- Notify your physician if you are breast-feeding while taking this medication.
  Dígale a su médico si está amamantando (dando de pecho) cuando toma este medicamento.

(Dee-gah-leh ah soo meh-dee-koh see ehs-tah ah-mah-mahn-tahn-doh [dahn-doh deh peh-choh] koo-ahn-doh toh-mah ehs-teh meh-dee-kah-mehn-toh)

- Refill your prescription right away unless you no longer need it.
  Rellene su receta inmediatamente, a menos que no la necesite.
  (Reh-yeh-neh soo reh-seh-tah een-meh-dee-ah-tah-mehn-teh, ah meh-nohs keh noh lah neh-seh-see-teh)

PROPER MEDICATION STORAGE

- Discard expired medications because they may become dangerous or ineffective.
  Tire los medicamentos con fecha vencida (caducados) porque pueden ser peligrosos o inefectivos.
  (Tee-reh lohs meh-dee-kah-mehn-tohs kohn feh-chah behn-see-dah [kah-doo-kah-dohs] pohr-keh poo-eh-dehn sehr peh-lee-groh-sohs oh een-eh-fehk-tee-bohs)
- Keep all medications out of the reach of children at all times.
  Guarde todos los medicamentos fuera del alcance de los niños todo el tiempo.
  (Goo-ahr-deh toh-dohs lohs meh-dee-kah-mehn-tohs foo-eh-rah dehl ahl-kahn-seh deh lohs nee-nyohs toh-doh ehl tee-ehm-poh)
- Store the medication:
  Almacene (guarde) el medicamento:
  (Ahl-mah-seh-neh [goo-ahr-deh] ehl meh-dee-kah-mehn-toh:)
  —in its original container.
  en su empaque original.
  (ehn-soo ehm-pah-keh oh-ree-hee-nahl)
  —in a cool, dry place.
  en un lugar fresco y seco.
  (ehn oon loo-gahr frehs-koh ee seh-koh)
  —away from heat.
  lejos del calor.
  (leh-hohs dehl kah-lohr)
  —at room temperature.
  a temperatura ambiente.
  (ah tehm-peh-rah-too-rah ahm-bee-ehn-teh)
  —out of direct sunlight.
  fuera de la luz directa del sol.
  (foo-eh-rah deh lah loos dee-rehk-tah dehl sohl)
  —in the refrigerator.
  en el refrigerador.
  (ehn ehl reh-free-heh-rah-dohr)

SELECTED DRUG CLASSES

Clasificación de Drogas Selectas (Medicamentos Selectos)

(Klah see-fee-kah-see-ohn deh droh-gahs seh-lehk-tahs [Meh-dee-kah-mehn-tohs Seh-lehk-tohs])

English	Spanish	Pronunciation
Analgesic (narcotic, nonnarcotic)	Analgésico (narcótico, no narcótico)	(Ah-nahl-heh-see-koh [nahr-koh-tee-koh, noh nahr-koh-tee-koh])
Antacid	Antiácido	(Ahn-tee-ah-see-doh)
Antianginal	Antianginoso	(Ahn-tee-ahn-hee-noh-soh)
Antianxiety	Ansiolítico	(Ahn-see-oh-lee-tee-koh)
Antiarrhythmic	Antiarritmico	(Ahn-tee-ah-reet-mee-koh)
Antibiotic	Antibiótico	(Ahn-tee-bee-oh-tee-koh)
Anticoagulant	Anticoagulante	(Ahn-tee-koh-ah-goo-lahn-teh)
Anticonvulsant	Anticonvulsivo	(Ahn-tee-kohn-bool-see-boh)
Antidepressant	Antidepresivo	(Ahn-tee-deh-preh-see-boh)
Antidiarrheal	Antidiarréicos	(Ahn-tee-dee-ah-reh-ee-kohs)
Antifungal	Antimicótico	(Ahn-tee-mee-koh-tee-koh)
Antihistamine	Antihistamínico	(Ahn-tee-ees-tah-mee-nee-koh)
Antihyperlipemic	Antihiperlipémico	(Ahn-tee-ee-pehr-lee-peh-mee-koh)
Antihypertensive	Antihipertensivo	(Ahn-tee-ee-pehr-tehn-see-boh)
Antiinflammatory	Antiinflamatorio; Contra la inflamación	(Ahn-tee-een-flah-mah-toh-ree-oh; kohn-trah lah een-flah-mah-see-ohn)
Antimigraine	Antimigrañoso	(Ahn-tee-mee-grah-nyoh-soh)
Antiparkinsonian	Contra el Parkinson	(Kohn-trah ehl Pahr-keen-sohn)
Antipsychotic	Medicamentos sicóticos	(Meh-dee-kah-mehn-tohs see-koh-tee-kohs)
Antipyretic	Antitérmicos	(Ahn-tee-tehr-mee-kohs)
Antiseptic	Antiséptico	(Ahn-tee-sehp-tee-koh)
Antispasmodic	Antiespasmódico	(Ahn-tee-ehs-pahs-moh-dee-koh)
Antithyroid	Antitiroideos	(Ahn-tee-tee-roh-ee-deh-ohs)
Antituberculosis	Antifímicos	(Ahn-tee-fee-mee-kohs)
Antitussive	Antitusígenos	(Ahn-tee-too-see-heh-nohs)
Antiviral	Antivirales	(Ahn-tee-bee-rah-lehs)
Appetite suppressant	Antisupresivos del apetito	(Ahn-tee-soo-preh-see-bohs dehl ah-peh-tee-toh)
Appetite stimulant	Estimulantes del apetito	(Ehs-tee-moo-lahn-tehs dehl ah-peh-tee-toh)
Bronchodilator	Bronquiolíticos	(Brohn-kee-oh-lee-tee-kohs)
Cancer chemotherapy	Quimioterapia de cancer	(Kee-mee-oh teh-rah-pee-ah deh kahn-sehr)

English	Spanish	Pronunciation
Decongestant	Anticongestivo	(Ahn-tee-kohn-hehs-tee-boh)
Digestant	Digestible	(Dee-hehs-tee-bleh)
Diuretic	Diurético	(Dee-oo-reh-tee-koh)
Emetic	Emético	(Eh-meh-tee-koh)
Fertility	Inductor de la Ovulación	(Een-doohk-tohr deh lah Oh-boo-lah-see-ohn)
Herbal	Medicamentos Naturales; Hierbas Medicinales	(Meh-dee-kah-mehn-tohs Nah-too-rah-lehs, Ee-ehr-bhas Meh-dee-see-nah-lehs)
Hypnotic	Hipnótico	(Eep-noh-tee-koh)
Insulin	Insulina	(Een-soo-lee-nah)
Laxative	Laxante	(Lahx-ahn-teh)
Mineral	Mineral	(Mee-neh-rahl)
Muscle relaxant	Relajante muscular	(Reh-lah-hahn-teh moos-koo-lahr)
Oral contraceptive	Anticonceptivos orales	(Ahn-tee-kohn-sehp-tee-bohs oh-rah-lehs)
Oral hypoglycemic	Hipoglicémico oral	(Ee-poh-glee-seh-mee-koh oh-rahl)
Sedative	Sedantes	(Seh-dahn-tehs)
Steroid	Esteroide	(Ehs-teh-roh-ee-deh)
Thyroid hormone	Tiroideos, hormona tiroide	(Tee-roh-ee-deh-ohs, ohr-moh-nah tee-roh-ee-deh)
Vaccine	Vacuna	(Bah-koo-nah)

ADMINISTRATION ROUTES

Modo de Uso

(Moh-doh deh Oo-soh)

English	Spanish	Pronunciation
By mouth	Oral	(Oh-rahl)
Intradermal	Intradermica	(Een-trah-dehr-mee-kah)
Intramuscular	Intramuscular	(Een-trah-moos-koo-lahr)
Intravenous	Intravenosa	(Een-trah-beh-noh-sah)
Nasal	Nasal	(Nah-sahl)
Oral	Oral	(Oh-rahl)
Otic	Ótica	(Oh-tee-kah)
Patch	Parche	(Pahr-cheh)
Rectal	Rectal	(Rehk-tahl)
Subcutaneous	Subcutanea	(Soob-koo-tah-neh-ah)
Sublingual	Sublingual	(Soob-leen-goo-ahl)
Topical	Topical, Local	(Toh-pee-kahl, Loh-kahl)
Vaginal	Vaginal	(Bah-hee-nahl)

DRUG PREPARATIONS

Presentación del Medicamento

(Preh-sehn-tah-see-ohn dehl Meh-dee-kah-mehn-toh)

English	Spanish	Pronunciation
Capsule	Cápsula	(Kahp-soo-lah)
Cream	Crema	(Kreh-mah)
Drops	Gotas	(Goh-tahs)
Elixir	Elixir, Jarabe	(Eh-leex-eer, Hah-rah-beh)
Fluid	Líquido	(Lee-kee-doh)
Gel	Gel, Jalea	(Hehl, Hah-leh-ah)
Inhaler	Inhalador*	(Een-ah-lah-dohr)
Injection	Inyección	(Een-yehk-see-ohn)
Liquid	Líquido	(Lee-kee-doh)
Lotion	Loción	(Loh-see-ohn)
Lozenge	Trocisco, pastilla	(Troh-sees-koh, Pahs-tee-yah)
Ointment	Ungüento	(Oon-goo-ehn-toh)
Pill	Píldora, Pastilla	(Peel-doh-rah, Pahs-tee-yah)
Powder	Polvo	(Pohl-boh)
Spray	Spray	(Sp-rah-ee)
Suppository	Supositorio	(Soo-poh-see-toh-ree-oh)
Syrup	Jarabe	(Hah-rah-beh)
Tablet	Tableta	(Tah-bleh-tah)

*The h is silent.

ADMINISTRATION FREQUENCY

Frecuencia de la Administración

(Freh-koo-ehn-see-ah deh lah Ahd-mee-nees-trah-see-ohn)

English	Spanish	Pronunciation
Once per day	Una vez por día; diariamente	(Oo-nah behs pohr dee-ah; dee-ah-ree-ah-mehn-teh)
Twice per day	Dos veces por día	(Dohs beh-sehs pohr dee-ah)
Three times per day	Tres veces por día	(Trehs beh-sehs pohr dee-ah)
Four times per day	Cuatro veces por día	(Koo-ah-troh beh-sehs pohr dee-ah)
Every other day	Cada tercer día	(Kah-dah tehr-sehr dee-ah)
Once per week	Una vez por semana	(Oo-nah behs pohr seh-mah-nah)
Every 4 hours	Cada cuatro horas	(Kah-dah koo-ah-troh oh-rahs)
Every 6 hours	Cada seis horas	(Kah-dah seh-ees oh-rahs)
Every 8 hours	Cada ocho horas	(Kah-dah oh-choh oh-rahs)
Every 12 hours	Cada doce horas	(Kah-dah doh-seh oh-rahs)
In the morning	En la mañana	(Ehn lah mah-nyah-nah)

Continued

English	Spanish	Pronunciation
In the afternoon	En la tarde	(Ehn lah tahr-deh)
In the evening	En la noche	(Ehn lah noh-cheh)
Before bedtime	Antes de acostarse	(Ahn-tehs deh ah-kohs-tahr-seh)
Before meals	Antes de la comida; Antes del alimento	(Ahn-tehs deh lah koh-mee-dah; Ahn-tehs dehl ah-lee-mehn-toh)
With meals	Con los alimentos; Con la comida	(Kohn lohs ah-lee-mehn-tohs; Kohn lah koh-mee-dah)
After meals	Después de los alimentos; Despusé de la comida	(Dehs-poo-ehs deh lohs ah-lee-mehn-tohs; Dehs-poo-ehs deh lah koh-mee-dah)
Only when you need it	Solo cuando la necesite	(Soh-loh koo-ahn-doh lah neh-seh-see-teh)
When you have _____ (pain)	Cuando tiene _____ (dolor)	(Koo-ahn-doh tee-eh-neh _____) (doh-lohr)

50 COMMON SIDE EFFECTS

Cincuenta Efectos Secundarios Com˙nes

(Seen-koo-ehn-tah Eh-fehk-tohs Seh-koon-dah-ree-ohs Koh-moo-nehs)

English	Spanish	Pronunciation
Abdominal cramps	Retorcijón abdominal	(Reh-tohr-see-hohn ahb-doh-mee-nahl)
Abdominal pain	Dolor abdominal	(Doh-lohr ahb-doh-mee-nahl)
Abdominal swelling	Inflamación abdominal	(Een-flah-mah-see-ohn ahb-doh-mee-nahl)
Anxiety	Ansiedad	(Ahn-see-eh-dahd)
Blood in the stool	Sangre en el excremento	(Sahn-greh ehn ehl ehx-kreh-mehn-toh)
Blood in the urine	Sangre en la orina	(Sahn-greh ehn la oh-ree-nah)
Bone pain	Dolor de hueso*	(Doh-lohr deh oo-eh-soh)
Chest pain	Dolor de pecho	(Doh-lohr deh peh-choh)
Chest pounding	Palpitación; latidos fuertes en el pecho	(Pahl-pee-tah-see-ohn; lah-tee-dohs foo-ehr-tehs ehn ehl peh-choh)
Chills	Escalofrío	(Ehs-kah-loh-free-oh)
Confusion	Confusión	(Kohn-foo-see-ohn)
Constipation	Constipación, estreñimiento	(Kohns-tee-pah-see-ohn, ehs-treh-nyee-mee-ehn-toh)
Cough	Tos	(Tohs)
Mental depression	Depresión mental	(Deh-preh-see-ohn mehn-tahl)
Diarrhea	Diarrea	(Dee-ah-reh-ah)
Difficult urination	Dificultad al orinar	(Dee-fee-kool-tahd ahl oh-ree-nahr)
Difficulty breathing	Dificultad al respirar	(Dee-fee-kool-tahd ahl rehs-pee-rahr)
Difficulty sleeping	Dificultad al dormir	(Dee-fee-kool-tahd ahl dohr-meer)

English	Spanish	Pronunciation
Dizziness	Mareos; vahídos	(Mah-reh-ohs; bah-ee-dohs)
Dry mouth	Boca seca	(Boh-kah seh-kah)
Easy bruising	Fragilidad capilar; le salen moretones confacilidad	(Frah-hee-lee-dahd kah-pee-lahr; leh sah-lehn moh-reh-toh-nehs kohn fah-see-lee-dahd)
Faintness	Desvanecimiento; sintióun vahído	(Dehs-bah-neh-see-mee-ehn-toh; seen-tee-oh oon bah-ee-doh)
Fatigue	Fatiga, cansancio	(Fah-tee-gah, kahn-sahn-see-oh)
Fever	Fiebre	(Fee-eh-breh)
Frequent urination	Orina frecuente	(Oh-ree-nah freh-koo-ehn-teh)
Headache	Dolor de cabeza	(Doh-lohr deh kah-beh-sah)
Impotence	Impotencia	(Eem-poh-tehn-see-ah)
Increased appetite	Aumento en el apetito	(Ah-oo-mehn-toh ehn ehl ah-peh-tee-toh)
Increased gas	Flatulencia	(Flah-too-lehn-see-ah)
Increased perspiration	Aumento en el sudor	(Ah-oo-mehn-toh ehn ehl soo-dohr)
Indigestion	Indigestión	(Een-dee-hehs-tee-ohn)
Itching	Comezón	(Koh-meh-sohn)
Loss of appetite	Pérdida en el apetito	(Pehr-dee-dah ehn ehl ah-peh-tee-toh)
Menstrual changes	Cambios en la menstruación; Cambio en el ciclo menstrual	(Kahm-bee-ohs ehn la mehns-truh-ah-see-ohn; Kahm-bee-oh ehn ehl see-kloh mehns-truh-ahl)
Mood changes	Cambio en el humor; Cambio en la disposición	(Kahm-bee-oh ehn ehl oo-mohr, Kahm-bee-oh ehn lah dees-poh-see-see-ohn)
Muscle aches	Achaques musculares	(Ah-chah-kehs moos-koo-lah-rehs)
Muscle cramps	Calambre muscular	(Kah-lahm-breh moos-koo-lahr)
Muscle pain	Dolores musculares	(Doh-loh-rehs moos-koo-lah-rehs)
Nasal congestion	Congestión nasal	(Kohn-hehs-tee-ohn nah-sahl)
Nausea	Nausea	(Nah-oo-seh-ah)
Ringing in the ears	Zumbido en los oidos	(Soom-bee-doh ehn lohs oh-ee-dohs)
Skin rash	Erupción en la piel	(Eh-roop-see-ohn ehn lah pee-ehl)
Swelling on the hands, legs or feet	Hinchazón en las manos, piernas, o pies	(Een-chah-sohn ehn lahs mah-nohs, pee-ehr-nahs, oh pee-ehs)
Vaginal bleeding	Sangrado vaginal	(Sahn-grah-doh bah-hee-nahl)
Vision changes	Cambios en la visión; cambios en la vista	(Kahm-bee-ohs ehn lah bee-see-ohn; cahm-bee-ohs ehn lah bees-tah)
Vomiting	Vomitando	(Boh-mee-tahn-doh)
Weakness	Debilidad	(Deh-bee-lee-dahd)

Continued

English	Spanish	Pronunciation
Weight gain	Aumento de peso	(Ah-oo-mehn-toh deh peh-soh)
Weight loss	Pérdida de peso	(Pehr-dee-day deh peh-soh)
Wheezing	Resollar; respiración sibilante	(Reh-soh-yahr; rehs-pee-rah-see-ohn see-bee-lahn-teh)

*The h is silent.
From *Mosby's 2006 Drug Consult for Nurses,* St Louis, 2006, Mosby.

Appendix I Top 200 Drugs

The following list is a compilation of the top 200 drugs for 2005 ranked by number of prescriptions.

Rank (Rx volume)	Generic drug name	Brand name
200	Phenazopyridine HCl	Generic
199	Oxybutynin Chloride Extended-Release	Ditropan XL
198	Desogestrel; Ethinyl Estradiol	Apri
197	Chlorpheniramine Maleate; Hydrocodone	Tussionex
196	Donepezil	Aricept
195	Propranolol Long-Acting	Inderal LA
194	Diclofenac Sodium	Generic
193	Human Insulin Regular/Isophane (Recombinant)	Humulin 70/30
192	Pimecrolimus	Elidel
191	Ferrous Sulfate	Generic
190	Tizanidine HCl	Generic
189	Nortriptyline	Generic
188	Phenytoin Sodium Extended	Dilantin Kapseals
187	Ethinyl Estradiol; Levonorgestrel	Trivora-28
186	Aspirin; Enteric-Coated	Generic
185	Benzonatate	Generic
184	Atomoxetine	Strattera
183	Cetirizine; Pseudoephedrine	Zyrtec-D
182	Polyethylene Glycol 3350	MiraLax
181	Captopril	Generic
180	Clotrimazole; Betamethasone	Generic
179	Paroxetine	Generic
178	Olopatadine	Patanol
177	Fentanyl Transdermal	Duragesic
176	Ciprofloxacin HCl	Generic
175	Insulin Lispro	Humalog
174	Nifedipine Extended-Release	Generic
173	Mupirocin	Bactroban
172	Lovastatin	Generic
171	Clarithromycin Extended-Release	Biaxin XL
170	Acyclovir	Generic
169	Cefprozil	Cefzil
168	Ethinyl Estradiol; Levonorgestrel	Aviane
167	Medroxyprogesterone Tablets	Generic

Continued

Rank (Rx volume)	Generic drug name	Brand name
166	Fosinopril	Monopril
165	Diltiazem Extended-Release	Cartia XT
164	Triamcinolone Acetonide Nasal	Nasacort AQ
163	Ezetimibe	Zetia
162	Diltiazem CD	Generic
161	Propranolol HCl	Generic
160	Buspirone HCl	Generic
159	Terazosin	Generic
158	Budesonide Nasal	Rhinocort Aqua
157	Tolterodine long-acting	Detrol LA
156	Human Insulin Isophane (Recombinant)	Humulin N
155	Carvedilol	Coreg
154	Glipizide	Generic
153	Sumatriptan Oral	Imitrex Oral
152	Omeprazole	Prilosec
151	Famotidine	Generic
150	Acetaminophen; Butalbital; Caffeine	Generic
149	Nitrofurantoin	Macrobid
148	Irbesartan	Avapro
147	Topiramate	Topamax
146	Amoxicillin; Potassium Clavulanate	Augmentin ES-600
145	Cefdinir	Omnicef
144	Insulin Glargine	Lantus
143	Acetaminophen; Oxycodone	Endocet
142	Estrogens; conjugated; Medroxyprogesterone	Prempro
141	Bisoprolol; Hydrochlorothiazide	Generic
140	Acetaminophen; Tramadol	Ultracet
139	Metaxalone	Skelaxin
138	Azithromycin	Zithromax
137	Clindamycin Systemic	Generic
136	Minocycline	Generic
135	Levothyroxine	Levothroid
134	Codeine; Promethazine	Generic
133	Divalproex Sodium	Depakote
132	Meclizine HCl	Generic
131	Metoclopramide	Generic
130	Triamcinolone Acetonide Topical	Generic

Continued

Rank (Rx volume)	Generic drug name	Brand name
129	Gemfibrozil	Generic
128	Cetirizine Syrup	Zyrtec Syrup
128	Quetiapine	Seroquel
127	Hydroxyzine	Generic
126	Valacyclovir	Valtrex
125	Metronidazole Tablets	Generic
124	Doxazosin	Generic
123	Digoxin	Lanoxin
122	Latanoprost	Xalatan
121	Risedronate	Actonel
120	Drospirenone; Ethinyl Estradiol	Yasmin 28
119	Spironolactone	Generic
118	Albuterol; Ipratropium	Combivent
117	Glyburide; Metformin	Glucovance
116	Glimepiride	Amaryl
115	Fenofibrate	TriCor
114	Losartan; Hydrochlorothiazide	Hyzaar
113	Temazepam	Generic
112	Fluticasone Inhalation	Flovent
111	Raloxifene	Evista
110	Estradiol Oral	Generic
109	Amphetamine; Dextroamphetamine Extended-Release	Adderall XR
108	Oxycodone	OxyContin
107	Promethazine Tablets	Generic
106	Amoxicillin	Amoxil
105	Tamsulosin	Flomax
104	Olanzapine	Zyprexa
103	Methylphenidate	Concerta
102	Fexofenadine; Pseudoephedrine	Allegra-D
101	Metformin Extended-Release	Glucophage XR
100	Benazepril	Lotensin
99	Warfarin	Coumadin
98	Rabeprazole	AcipHex
97	Digoxin	Digitek
96	Mometasone Nasal	Nasonex
95	Risperidone	Risperdal
94	Folic Acid	Generic

Continued

Rank (Rx volume)	Generic drug name	Brand name
93	Lisinopril; Hydrochlorothiazide	Generic
92	Rosiglitazone	Avandia
91	Ciprofloxacin	Cipro
90	Valsartan; Hydrochlorothiazide	Diovan HCT
89	Albuterol Nebulizer Solution	Generic
88	Losartan	Cozaar
87	Pioglitazone	Actos
86	Allopurinol	Generic
85	Clonidine	Generic
84	Paroxetine HCl Controlled-Release	Paxil CR
83	Methylprednisolone Tablets	Generic
82	Glyburide	Generic
81	Isosorbide Mononitrate	Generic
80	Valdecoxib	Bextra
79	Ethinyl Estradiol; Norelgestromin	Ortho Evra
78	Doxycycline	Generic
77	Verapamil Sustained-Release	Generic
76	Desloratadine	Clarinex
75	Carisoprodol	Generic
74	Azithromycin	Zithromax Suspension
73	Tramadol	Generic
72	Potassium Chloride	Klor-Con
71	Glipizide Extended-Release	Glucotrol XL
70	Acetaminophen; Oxycodone	Generic
69	Penicillin VK	Generic
68	Amlodipine; Benazepril	Lotrel
67	Valsartan	Diovan
66	Ramipril	Altace
65	Fluconazole	Diflucan
64	Diazepam	Generic
63	Quinapril	Accupril
62	Omeprazole	Generic
61	Enalapril	Generic
60	Naproxen	Generic
59	Cyclobenzaprine	Generic
58	Levofloxacin	Levaquin
57	Trazodone HCl	Generic

Continued

Rank (Rx volume)	Generic drug name	Brand name
56	Trimethoprim/Sulfa	Generic
55	Pravastatin	Pravachol
54	Clopidogrel	Plavix
53	Escitalopram	Lexapro
52	Fluticasone	Flonase
51	Fluticasone; Salmeterol	Advair Diskus
50	Warfarin	Generic
49	Pantoprazole	Protonix
48	Clonazepam	Generic
47	Amitriptyline	Generic
46	Paroxetine HCl	Paxil
45	Ranitidine HCl	Generic
44	Amoxicillin; Potassium Clavulanate	Generic
43	Bupropion Sustained-Release	Wellbutrin SR
43	Amoxicillin	Trimox
42	Citalopram	Celexa
41	Potassium Chloride	Generic
40	Gabapentin	Neurontin
39	Sildenafil	Viagra
38	Venlafaxine Extended-Release	Effexor XR
37	Alendronate	Fosamax
36	Rofecoxib	Vioxx
35	Montelukast	Singulair
34	Cetirizine	Zyrtec
33	Lorazepam	Generic
32	Metoprolol Tartrate	Generic
31	Acetaminophen; Codeine	Generic
30	Esomeprazole	Nexium
29	Ethinyl Estradiol; Norgestimate	Ortho Tri-Cyclen
28	Celecoxib	Celebrex
27	Fexofenadine	Allegra
26	Fluoxetine	Generic
25	Levothyroxine	Levoxyl
24	Zolpidem	Ambien
23	Metformin	Generic
22	Prednisone Oral	Generic
21	Estrogens; Conjugated	Premarin Tabs

Continued

Rank (Rx volume)	Generic drug name	Brand name
20	Triamterene; Hydrochlorothiazide	Generic
19	Ibuprofen	Generic
18	Lansoprazole	Prevacid
17	Simvastatin	Zocor
16	Acetaminophen; Propoxyphene-N	Generic
15	Cephalexin	Generic
14	Metoprolol Succinate	Toprol XL
13	Azithromycin	Zithromax Z-Pak
12	Sertraline	Zoloft
11	Amlodipine	Norvasc
10	Alprazolam	Generic
9	Albuterol Aerosol	Generic
8	Furosemide Oral	Generic
7	Hydrochlorothiazide	Generic
6	Lisinopril	Generic
5	Amoxicillin	Generic
4	Atenolol	Generic
3	Levothyroxine	Synthroid
2	Atorvastatin	Lipitor
1	Acetaminophen; Hydrocodone	Generic

From *Mosby's 2006 Drug Consult for Nurses*, St Louis, 2006, Mosby.

Appendix J Selected References

American Dental Association: Anesthesia color code revision, *ADA News* 24:12, 2003.

American Dental Association, American Academy of Orthopedic Surgeons: Advisory statement on antibiotic prophylaxis for dental patients with total joint replacements, *J Am Dent Assoc* 134:895–899, 2003.

Borea G et al: Tranexamic acid as a mouthwash in anticoagulant-treated patients undergoing oral surgery, *Oral Surg Oral Med Oral Pathol* 75:29–31, 1993.

Cohen DM, Bhattacharyya I, Lydiatt WM: Recalcitrant oral ulcers caused by calcium channel blockers: diagnosis and treatment considerations, *J Am Dent Assoc* 130:1611–1618, Nov 1999.

Cupp MJ, Tracy TS: Role of the cytochrome P450 3A subfamily, *US Pharmacists* 22:HS9–HS21, 1997.

Dajani AS et al: Prevention of bacterial endocarditis: recommendations by the American Heart Association, *JAMA* 277:1794–1801, 1997.

DePaola LG: Managing the care of patients infected with blood borne diseases, *J Am Dent Assoc* 134:350–358, 2003.

Drug interaction facts, updated quarterly, St Louis, Facts and Comparisons.

Facts and comparisons, updated monthly, St Louis, Facts and Comparisons.

Fye KH et al: Celecoxib-induced Sweet's syndrome, *J Am Acad Dermatol* 45:300–302, 2001.

Gahart BL: *2000 intravenous medications*, ed 16, St Louis, 1999, Mosby.

Halevy S, Shai A: Lichenoid drug eruptions, *J Am Acad Dermatol* 29:249–255, 1993.

Hardman JG et al: *Goodman and Gilman's the pharmacological basis of therapeutics*, ed 10, New York, 2002, Mosby.

Little JW, Falace DA: *Dental management of the medically compromised patient*, ed 6, St Louis, 2002, Mosby.

Mancano MA: Drug interactions with protease inhibitors: part I, *Pharmacy Times*, 67:14–17, 2001.

Marx RE, Sawatari Y, Fortin M, Broumand V. Bisphosphonate-induced exposed bone (osteonecrosis/osteopetrosis) of the jaws: Risk factors, recognition, prevetion and treatment, *J Oral Maxillofac, Surg* 63:1581, 2005.

The Medical Letter handbook of adverse drug interactions, New Rochelle, NY, 1999, The Medical Letter.

Melo MD, Obeid G. Osteonecrosis of the Jaws in patients with a history of receiving bisphosphonate therapy, *J Amer Dent Assoc* 136:1675–1681, 2005.

Mosby's drug consult 2004: the comprehensive reference for generic and brand name drugs, ed 14, St Louis, 2004, Mosby.

Pharmacist's Letter 18, 2002.

Pharmacist's Letter 19, 2003.

Physician's desk reference, ed 58, Montvale, NJ, 2004, Medical Economics.

Rees TD: Oral effects of drug abuse, *Crit Rev Oral Biol Med* 3:163–184, 1992.

Rees TD: Systemic drugs as a risk factor for periodontal disease initiation and progression, *Compendium* 16:20–42, 1995.

Shulman JD, Wells LM: Acute fluoride toxicity from ingesting home-use dental products in children birth to 6 years of age, *J Public Health Dent* 57:150–158, 1997.

Skidmore-Roth L: *Mosby's 2002 nursing drug reference*, St Louis, 1999, Mosby.

Taylor SE: New drugs and product approval from 2002, *Tex Dent J* 120:1160–1169, 2003.

Taylor SE, Gage TW: New drugs and products approved from 2000, *Tex Dent J* 118:1070–1081, 2001.

United States Pharmacopeial Convention: *Drug information for the health care professionals USPDI*, ed 24, Englewood, CO, 2004, Micromedex.

United States Pharmacopeial Convention: *USP dictionary of USAN and international drug names 2001*, Rockville, MD, 2001, United States Pharmacopeial Convention.

Valsecchi R, Cainelli T: Gingival hyperplasia induced by erythromycin, *Acta Derm Venereol* 72:157, 1992.

Westbrook P et al: Reversal of nifedipine-induced gingival hyperplasia by the calcium channel blocker, isradipine, *J Dent Res* 74(S1):208, 1995.

Westbrook SD, Paunovich ED, Freytes CO: Adult hemopoietic stem cell transplantation, *J Am Dent Assoc* 127:625–638, 1996.

Whal MJ: Altering anti-coagulant therapy: a survey of physicians, *J Am Dent Assoc* 127:625–638, 1996.

Whal MJ: Myths of dental surgery in patients receiving anticoagulant therapy, *J Am Dent Assoc* 131:77–81, 2000.

Wright JM: Oral manifestations of drug reactions, *Dent Clin North Am* 28:529–543, 1984.

Zelickson BD, Rogers RS: Oral reactions, *Dermatol Clin* 5:695–708, 1987.

From Gage TW, Pickett FA: *Mosby's dental drug reference 2005*, ed 7, St Louis, 2005, Mosby.

Therapeutic/Pharmacologic Index

DRUGS CLASSIFIED BY USUAL THERAPEUTIC/ PHARMACOLOGIC CATEGORY

This section of the book features drugs classified by primary therapeutic or pharmacologic group, or both. Thus you can locate drugs by knowing their primary therapeutic use or general pharmacologic class. This arrangement makes it easy to find the matching drug monograph by using the generic name. The individual drug monographs are arranged by generic name in alphabetical order and can simply be found in the appropriate alphabet section. Colored tabs on the side of the book mark the alphabetical sections. This arrangement allows the book user to see other drugs in the same classification that are included in this volume.

For example, take the case of a patient using a drug for depression and having difficulty recalling the drug name. Find the *Antidepressants* section. All of the antidepressants listed in this volume can be seen and may help stimulate the patient to recall the drug currently used. Or if you want to know which drugs are calcium channel antagonists, go to the *Antihypertensives* section and find the subtopic of calcium channel antagonists. The calcium channel antagonists included in this volume are listed. As you identify the drug, use the generic name to quickly tab to the appropriate alphabet section.

ADRENERGIC AGONISTS
- apraclonidine HCl (Iopidine)
- bitolterol (Tormalate)
- brimonidine tartrate (Alphagan)
- dipivefrin HCl (Propine C)
- dobutamine hydrochloride
- dopamine hydrochloride (Dobutrex)
- ephedrine (Pretz-D)
- epinephrine HCl (Adrenalin)
- epinephryl borate (Epifrin)
- isoetharine HCl (Isoethaine)
- isoproterenol HCl (Isuprel)
- levalbuterol HCl (Xopenex)
- mephentermine sulfate (Wyamine Sulfate)
- metaproterenol sulfate (Alupent)
- metaraminol (Aramine)
- midodrine (Amatine)
- norepinephrine bitartrate (Levophed)
- salmeterol (Serevent Diskus)
- terbutaline sulfate (Brethine)

ALZHEIMER'S
- donepezil HCl (Aricept)
- memantine HCl (Namenda)
- tacrine HCl (Cognex)

AMINOGLYCOSIDES
- gentamicin sulfate (Alcomicin)
- kanamycin sulfate (Kantrex)
- tobramycin sulfate (Tobrex)

AMYOTROPHIC LATERAL SCLEROSIS
- riluzole (Rilutek)

ANALGESICS (NONOPIOID)
- acetaminophen (Tylenol)
- aspirin (Bayer)
- pentosan polysulfate
- salsalate (Anaflex)
- ziconotide (Prialt)

ANALGESICS (NSAIDS)
- (see nonsteroidal antiinflammatory drugs)

ANALGESICS (OPIOIDS)
- buprenorphine HCl (Buprenex)
- butorphanol tartrate (Stadol)
- codeine phosphate/codeine sulfate (Actacode)
- hydrocodone (Anexia)
- hydromorphone HCl (Dilaudid)
- meperidine HCl (Demerol)
- methadone HCl (Dolophine)
- morphine sulfate (MS Contin)
- nalbuphine hydrochloride
- oxycodone HCl (Roxicodone)
- pentazocine HCl (Talwin Nx)
- pentazocine hydrochloride; naloxone hydrochloride (Talwin Nx)

propoxyphene hydrochloride/
propo-xyphene napsylate (Darvon)
propoxyphene napsylate
(Darvon-N)
tramadol HCl (Ultram)

ANESTHETICS (GENERAL)
ketamine (Ketalar)
midazolam HCl (Versed)
propofol (Diprivan)

ANESTHETICS (LOCAL)
articaine HCl (Septocaine)
bupivacaine HCl (Marcaine)
cocaine hydrochloride (Cocaine)
levobupivacaine (Chirocaine)
lidocaine HCl (Xylocaine)
lidocaine hydrocloride (Liboderm)
mepivacaine HCl (local)
mepivacaine HCl (Carbocaine)
procaine (Novocaine)

ANESTHETICS (TOPICAL)
benzocaine (Hurricaine)
lidocaine HCl (Xylocaine)
tetracaine HCl (Pontocaine)

ANTACIDS
magaldrate (Riopan)

ANTAGONISTS
disulfiram (Antabuse)
flumazenil (Romazicon)
naloxone HCl (Narcan)
naltrexone HCl (ReVia, Trexan)

ANTIANGINALS
Nitrates
isosorbide (Isordil)
isosorbide dinitrate/isosorbide
mononitrate (Isordil)
nitroglycerin (Transderm-Nitro)
Beta-adrenergic antagonists
atenolol (Tenormin)
metoprolol tartrate (Lopressor)
nadolol (Corgard)
propranolol HCl (Inderal)
Calcium channel antagonists
bepridil (Vascor)
diltiazem HCl (Cardizem)
felodipine (Plendil)
nicardipine HCl (Cardene)
nifedipine (Procardia)
nimodipine (Nimotop)
verapamil (Calan)
Others
amyl nitrite (Amyl Nitrite)
papaverine (Papacon)

ANTIANEMIC
darbepoetin alfa (Aranesp)
epoetin alfa (Procrit)

ANTIANXIETY/SEDATIVE-HYPNOTICS
Barbiturates
pentobarbital (Nembutal)
phenobarbital (Luminal)
secobarbital (Seconal)
Benzodiazepines
alprazolam (Xanax)
chlordiazepoxide HCl (Librium)
clorazepate dipotassium (Tranxene)
diazepam (Valium)
estazolam (ProSom)
flurazepam HCl (Dalmane)
lorazepam (Ativan)
midazolam (Versed)
oxazepam (Serax)
quazepam (Doral)
temazepam (Restoril)
triazolam (Halcion)
Antihistamines
brompheniramine (Brovex)
carbinoxamine maleate (Carboxine)
chlorpheniramine (Aller-Chlor)
dexchlorpheniramine (Polaramine)
diphenhydramine HCl (Benadryl)
hydroxyzine HCl (Atarax, Vistaril)
promethazine HCl (Phenergan)
Others
buspirone HCl (BuSpar)
butabarbital sodium (Butisol)
chloral hydrate (Aquachloral)
doxepin HCl (Sinaquan)
meprobamate (Equanil, Miltown)
zaleplon (Sonata)
zolpidem tartrate (Ambien)

ANTIASTHMATICS
(see bronchodilators)

ANTICHOLELITHICS
ursodiol (Actigall)

ANTICHOLINERGICS
atropine sulfate (Sal-Tropine)
biperidin (Akineton)
cyclopentolate hydrochloride
(AK-Pentolate)

dicyclomine HCl (Bentyl)
glycopyrrolate (Robinul)
hyoscyamine (Anaspaz)
ipratropium bromide (Atrovent)
methscopolamine (Carbacot)
orphenadrine (Norflex)
oxybutynin (Ditropan)
propantheline (Pro-Banthine)
propantheline bromide (Pro-Banthine)
scopolamine (Trans-Dam Scop)
tiotropium bromide (Spiriva)
tolterodine tartrate (Detrol)

ANTICOAGULANTS
argatroban (Acova)
bivalirudin (Angiomax)
dalteparin sodium (Fragmin)
danaparoid (Orgaran)
enoxaparin sodium (Lovenox)
fondaparinux sodium (Arixtra)
heparin sodium (Heparin)
lepirudin (Refludon)
tinzaparin sodium (Innohep)
tirofiban (Aggrastat)
warfarin sodium (Coumadin)

ANTICONVULSANTS
acetazolamide (Diamox)
carbamazepine (Tegretol)
clonazepam (Klonopin)
diazepam (Valium)
divalproex (Depakote)
ethosuximide (Zarontin)
felbamate (Felbatol)
fosphenytoin (Cerebyx)
gabapentin (Neurontin)
lamotrigine (Lamictal)
levetiracetam (Keppra)
mephobarbital (Mebaral)
methsuximide (Celontin)
oxcarbazepine (Trileptal)
phenobarbital (Luminal)
primidone (Mysoline)
tiagabine HCl (Gabitril)
topiramate (Topamax)
valproic acid/valproate sodium/ divalproex sodium (Depakene)
zonisamide (Zonegran)

ANTIDEPRESSANTS
Atypical
bupropion HCl (Wellbutrin)
nefazodone HCl (Serzone)
trazodone HCl (Desyrel)
venlafaxine HCl (Effexor)
Monoamine oxidase inhibitors
isocarboxazid (Marplan)
phenelzine sulfate (Nardil)
tranylcypromine sulfate (Parnate)
Serotonin-specific reuptake inhibitors
escitalopram (Lexapro)
fluoxetine (Prozac)
fluvoxamine maleate (Luvox)
paroxetine (Paxil)
sertraline (Zoloft)
Tetracyclics
maprotiline HCl (Ludiomil)
mirtazapine (Remeron)
Tricyclics
amitriptyline HCl(Elavil)
amoxapine (Asendin)
clomipramine (Anafranil)
desipramine HCl (Norpramin)
doxepin (Sinequan)
imipramine HCl (Tofranil)
nortriptyline HCl (Pamelor)
protriptyline HCl (Vivactil)
trimipramine (Surmontil)

ANTIDIABETICS
acarbose (Precose)
acetohexamide (Dymelor)
chlorpropamide (Diabinese)
glimepiride (Amaryl)
glipizide (Glucotrol)
glyburide (DiaBeta)
insulin glargine (Lantus)
insulin glulisine (Apidra)
metformin HCl (Glucophage)
miglitol (Glyset)
nateglinide (Starlix)
pioglitazone (Actos)
repaglinide (Prandin)
rosiglitazone maleate (Avandia)
tolazamide (Tolinase)
tolbutamide (Orinase)

ANTIDIARRHEALS
bismuth subsalicylate (Pepto-Bismol)
loperamide HCl (Imodium-AD)
octreotide acetate (Sandostatin)
paregoric

ANTIDIURETIC HORMONE
ANTIDOTES
protamine sulfate (Protamine)

ANTIDYSRHYTHMICS (ANTIARRHYTHMICS)
adenosine (Adenocard)
amiodarone HCl (Cordarone)
digoxin (Lanoxin)
diltiazem (Cardizem)
disopyramide phosphate
dofetilide (Tikosyn)
flecainide (Tambocor)
ibutilide fumarate (Corvert)
lidocaine (Xylocaine Cardiac)
lidocaine hydrocloride
mexiletine HCl (Mexitil)
moricizine (Ethmozine)
propafenone (Rythmol)
propranolol HCl (Inderal)
quinidine (Quinaglute)
sotalol (Betapace)
tocainide HCl (Tonocard)

ANTIEMETICS
aprepitant (Emend)
chlorpromazine (Thorazine)
dimenhydrinate (Dramamine)
dolasetron (Anzemet)
dronabinol (Marinol)
droperidol (Inapsine)
granisetron (Kytril)
meclizine HCl (Bonine)
metoclopramide (Reglan)
palonosetron hydrochloride
prochlorperazine (Compazine)
promethazine (Phenergan)
scopolamine (Transderm-Scop)
thiethylperazine (Torecan)
trimethobenzamide (Tigan)

ANTIFUNGALS (TOPICAL)
amphotericin B (Fungizone)
butoconazole (Gynazole-1)
butenafine (Mentax)
ciclopirox (Loprox)
clotrimazole (Mycelex)
itraconazole (Sporanox)
miconazole (Femizol-m)
naftifine HCl (Naftin)
nystatin (Mycostatin)
oxiconazole (Oxistat)
sertaconazole (Ertacco)
sulconazole nitrate (Exelderm)
terbinafine HCl (Lamisil)
terconazole (Terazol)
tioconazole (Vagistat)

ANTIFUNGALS (SYSTEMIC)
amphotericin B, lipid-based (Abelect)
caspofungin acetate (Cancidas)
fluconazole (Diflucan)
flucytosine (Ancobon)
griseofulvin (Fulvicin)
itraconazole (Sporanox)
ketoconazole (Nizoral)
terbinafine HCl (Lamisil)

ANTIGOUTS
allopurinol (Zyloprim)
colchicine (Colchicine)

ANTIHISTAMINES (H_2) ANTAGONISTS
cimetidine (Tagamet)
famotidine (Pepcid)
nizatidine (Axid)
ranitidine hydrochloride/ranitidine bismuth citrate (Zantac)

ANTIHISTAMINES (H_1) ANTAGONISTS
azatadine maleate (Optimine)
azelastine HCl (Astelin, Optivar)
buclizine (Bucladin-S)
cetirizine HCl (Zyrtec)
clemastine fumarate (Tavist Allergy)
cyclizine (Marezine)
cyproheptadine HCl (Periactin)
desloratadine (Clarinex)
dimenhydrinate (Dramamine)
diphenhydramine (Benadryl)
fexofenadine HCl (Allegra)
hydroxyzine (Atarax, Vistaril)
ketotifen fumarate (Zaditor)
levocabastine (Livostin)
loratadine (Claritin)
meclizine (Bonine)
olopatadine HCl (Patanol)
promethazine (Phenergan)

ANTIHYPERCALCEMICS (OSTEOPOROSIS)
alendronate sodium (Fosamax)
etidronate disodium (Didronel)
calcitonin (Calcimar)
ibandronate sodium (Boniva)
pamidronate disodium (Aredia)
raloxifene (Evista)
risedronate sodium (Actonel)
teriparatide (Forteo)
tiludronate (Skelid)
zoledronic acid (Zometa)

ANTIHYPERLIPIDEMICS
atorvastatin calcium (Lipitor)
cholestyramine resin (Nova-Cholamine)
clofibrate (Atromid-S)
colesevelam HCl (Welchol)
colestipol HCl (Colestid)
ezetimibe; simvastatin
fenofibrate (Tricor)
fluvastatin (Lescol)
fluvastatin sodium (Lescol)
gemfibrozil (Lopid)
lovastatin (Mevacor)
niacin, nicotinic acid
pravastatin (Pravachol)
rosuvastatin calcium (Crestor)
simvastatin (Zocor)

ANTIHYPERTENSIVES
(also see diuretics)
Aldosterone antagonists
eplerenone (Inspra)
spironolactone (Aldactone)
Alpha-adrenergic antagonists
doxazosin mesylate (Cardura)
phenoxybenzamine (Dibenzylre)
phentolamine (Regitine)
prazosin HCl (Minipress)
terazosin (Hytrin)
Alpha/beta-adrenergic antagonists
labetalol (Normodyne)
Angiotensin-converting enzyme inhibitors
benazepril (Lotensin)
captopril (Capoten)
enalapril maleate (Vasotec)
fosinopril (Monopril)
lisinopril (Prinivil, Zestril)
moexipril HCl (Univasc)
perindopril erbumine (Aceon)
quinapril (Accupril)
ramipril (Altace)
trandolapril (Mavik)
Angiotensin II receptor antagonists
candesartan cilexetil (Atacand)
eprosartan (Teveten)
irbesartan (Avapro)
losartan (Cozaar)
olmesartan medoxomil (Benicar)
telmisartan (Micardis)
valsartan (Diovan)
Beta-adrenergic antagonists
Selective
atenolol (Tenormin)
betaxolol (Kerlone)
bisoprolol fumarate (Zebeta)
metoprolol tartrate (Lopressor)
nadolol (Corgard)
Nonselective
carteolol HCl (Cartrol)
carvedilol (Coreg)
penbutolol (Levatol)
pindolol (Visken)
propranolol HCl (Inderal)
timolol maleate (Blocadren)
Calcium channel antagonists
bepridil HCl (Vascor)
diltiazem (Cardizem)
felodipine (Plendil)
isradipine (DynaCirc)
nicardipine HCl (Cardene)
nifedipine (Procardia XL)
nislodipine (Sular)
verapamil (Calan)
Centrally acting
clonidine (Catapres)
guanabenz (Wytensine)
guanfacine (Tenex)
methyldopa (Aldomet)
Other
bosentan (Tracleer)
guanadrel sulfate (Hylorel)
hydralazine HCl (Apresoline)
minoxidil (Loniten)
reserpine (Serpasil)
Other
guanethidine monosulfate (Ismelin)
metyrosine (Demser)

ANTIHYPOGLYCEMIC
glucagon (Glucagon Emergency Kit)

ANTIINFECTIVES (MISCELLANEOUS)
adefovir (Hepsera)
albendazole (Albenza)
aztreonam (Azactam)
clofazimine (Lamprene)
dapsone (Dapsone)
daptomycin (Cubicin)
linezolid (Zyvox)
mebendazole (Vermox)
metronidazole (Flagyl)
nitazoxanide (Alinia)
paromomycin (Humatin)

pentamidine (Nebupent)
pentamidine isethionate (Nebupent)
polymyxin B (Aerosporin)
thiabendazole (Mintezol)

ANTIINFECTIVES (SYSTEMIC)
(see specific class: penicillins, cephalosporins, etc.)

ANTIINFECTIVES (TOPICAL)
bacitracin (Baciguent)
chlorhexidine gluconate (Peridex, PerioGard)
chlorhexidine gluconate (PerioChip)
erythromycin (Erytroderm)
mafenide (Sulfamylon)
mupirocin (Bactroban)
nitrofurazone (Furacin)
silver sulfadiazine (Silvadene)
sulfacetamide (Isopto)

ANTIINFLAMMATORY ANTIARTHRITICS
allopurinol (Zyloprim)
anakinra (Kinera)
aspirin (Bayer)
aurothioglucose/gold sodium thiomalate (Gold-50)
celecoxib (Celebrex)
colchicine (Colchicine)
diflunisal (Dolobid)
etanercept (Enbrel)
etodolac (Lodine)
fenoprofen calcium (Nalfon)
flavocoxid (Limbrel)
ibuprofen (Motrin)
indomethacin (Indocin)
infliximab (Remicade)
ketoprofen (Orudis)
leflunomide (Arava)
methotrexate (Rheumatrex)
methotrexate sodium
nabumetone (Relafen)
naproxen sodium (Anaprox)
oxaprozin (Daypro)
probenecid (Benemid)
rofecoxib (Vioxx)
salsalate (Anaflex)
sulindac (Clinoril)
valdecoxib (Bextra)

ANTIMALARIALS
chloroquine/chloroquine phosphate (Aralen Hydrochloride)
hydroxychloroquine sulfate (Plaquenil)
mefloquine (Lariam)
primaquine (Primacin)
pyrimethamine (Daraprim)
quinine

ANTIPARKINSONIANS
amantadine HCl (Symmetrel)
cabergoline (Dostinex)
benztropine (Cogentin)
biperiden HCl (Akineton)
bromocriptine mesylate (Parlodel)
diphenhydramine (Benadryl)
entacapone (Comtan)
levodopa (Larodopa)
pergolide mesylate (Permax)
pramipexole (Mirapex)
procyclidine HCl (Kemadrin)
ropinirole HCl (ReQuip)
selegiline HCl (Eldepryl)
tolcapone (Tasmar)
trihexyphenidyl HCl (Artane)

ANTIPLATELETS
abciximab (c7E3 Fab, ReoPro)
clopidogrel (Iscover)
eptifibatide (Integrilin)
tirofiban (Aggrastat)

ANTIPSYCHOTICS
Phenothiazines
chlorpromazine HCl (Thorazine)
fluphenazine decanoate (Prolixin)
mesoridazine besylate (Serentil)
perphenazine (Trilafon)
prochlorperazine (Compazine)
thioridazine HCl (Mellaril)
trifluoperazine HCl (Stelazine)
Butyrophenone
haloperidol (Haldol)
Thioxanthene
thiothixene (Navane)
Others
aripiprazole (Abilify)
clozapine (Clozaril)
loxapine HCl (Loxitane)
molindone HCl (Moban)
olanzapine (Zyprexa)
pimozide (Orap)
quetiapine (Seroquel)
risperidone (Risperdal)
ziprasidone HCl (Geodon)
Bipolar disease
lithium carbonate/lithium citrate (Lithobid)
valproic acid (Depakene)

INDEX

dexmethylphenidate HCl (Focalin)
methylphenidate (Ritalin)

BARBITURATES
pentobarbital (Nembutal)
phenobarbital (Luminal)
secobarbital (Seconal)

BRONCHODILATORS
albuterol (Proventil, Ventolin)
aminophylline (Truphylline)
bitolterol (Tormalate)
dyphylline (Dilor)
ephedrine (Pretz-D)
epinephrine HCl (Adrenalin)
formoterol fumarate (Foradil)
ipratropium bromide (Atrovent)
isoproterenol HCl (Isuprel)
levalbuterol (Xopenex)
metaproterenol sulfate (Alupent)
pirbuterol (Maxair)
salmeterol (Serevent Diskus)
theophylline (Theo-Dur)
tiotropium bromide (Spiriva)

CANCER CHEMOTHERAPY
alemtuzumab (Campath)
aminoglutethimide (Cytadren)
anastrozole (Arimadex)
bevacizumab (Avastin)
bexarotene (Targretin)
bicalutamide (Casodex)
bleomycin sulfate (Blenamax)
busulfan (Myleran)
capecitabine (Xeloda)
carboplatin (Paraplatin)
carmustine (BiCNU)
cetuximab (Erbitux)
cisplatin (Platinol-AQ)
cyclophosphamide (Cytoxan)
cytarabine (Ara-C)
daunorubicin citrate liposome (DaunoXome)
docetaxel (Taxotere)
doxorubicin (Doxil)
epirubicin (Ellecin)
erlotinib (Tarreva)
estramustine phosphate sodium (Emeyt)
etoposide, VP-16 (Etopophos)
exemestane (Aromasin)
fludarabine phosphate (Fludara)
fluorouracil, 5FU (Adrucil)
flutamide (Eulexin)
gefitinib (Iressa)
gemcitabine hydrochloride (Gemzar)
hydroxyurea (Hydrea)
idarubicin hydrochloride (Idamycin PFS)
ifosfamide (Ifex)
interferon alfa-2a (Roferon-A)
interferon alfa-2a/2b (Roferon-A)
interferon alfa-2b (Intron-A)
imatinib mesylate (Gleevec)
Interleukin-2 (aldesleukin)
letrozole (Femara)
leucovorin calcium (Wellcovorin)
lomustine (CeeNU)
megestrol acetate (Megace)
melphalan (Alkeran)
mercaptopurine (Purinethol)
mesna (Mesnex)
methotrexate (Rheumatrex)
methotrexate sodium
mitotane (Lysodren)
mitoxantrone (Novantrone)
nilutamide (Nilandron)
oprelvekin (interleukin-2, IL-2)
oxaliplatin (Eloxatin)
paclitaxel (Taxol)
peginterferon alfa-2a (Pegasys)
pentostatin (Nipent)
procarbazine HCl (Matulane)
rituximab (Rituxan)
tamoxifen citrate (Nolvadex)
temozolomide (Temodar)
teniposide (Vumon)
thiotepa (Thioplex)
topotecan (Hycamtin)
toremifene citrate (Fareston)
trastuzumab (Herceptin)
triptorelin pamoate (Trelstar Depot)
valrubicin (Valstar)
vinblastine sulfate (Velban)
vincristine sulfate (Oncovin)
vinorelbine (Navelbine)

CARBAPENEMS
ertapenem (Ivanz)
meropenem (Merrem IV)

CARDIAC GLYCOSIDES
digoxin (Lanoxin)

CENTRAL NERVOUS SYSTEM STIMULANTS
dextroamphetamine sulfate (Dexedrine)
methylphenidate (Ritalin)
methamphetamine (Desoxyn)
modafinil (Provigil)
pemoline (Cylert)

CEPHALOSPORINS
cefaclor (Ceclor)
cefadroxil (Duricef)
cefaditoren pivoxil (Spectracef)
cefazolin sodium (Ancef)
cefdinir (Omnicef)
cefepime (Maxipime)
cefixime (Suprax)
cefonicid sodium (Monocid)
cefoperazone (Cefobid)
cefotaxime sodium (Claforan)
cefotetan disodium (Apatef)
cefoxitin sodium (Mefoxin)
cefpodoxime proxetil (Vantin)
cefprozil (Cefzil)
ceftazidime (Ceptaz)
ceftibuten (Cedax)
ceftizoxime sodium (Cefizox)
ceftriaxone sodium (Rocephin)
cephalexin (Keflex)
cephradine (Velosef)
loracarbef (Lorabid)

CHOLESTEROL LOWERING AGENTS
atorvastatin calcium (Lipitor)
cholestyramine resin (Nova-Cholamine)
ezetimibe; simvastatin (Vytorin)
fluvastatin (Lescol)
fluvastatin sodium (Lescol)
lovastatin (Mevacor)
niacin, nicotinic acid (Niacon)
rosuvastatin calcium (Crestor)

CHOLINERGIC AGONISTS
acetylcholine chloride (Michol-E)
bethanechol chloride (Urecholine)
cabergoline (Dostinex)

CHOLINESTRASE INHIBITORS
ambenonium (Mytelase)
physostigmine (Anti lirium)
pyridostigmine (Mestinon)

COLONY STIMULATING FACTORS
filgrastim (Neupogen)
pegfilgrastim (Neulastin)
sargramostim (granulocyte macrophage colony-stimulating factor, GM-CSF)

DECONGESTANTS
oxymetazoline HCl (Afrin)
phenylephrine HCl (Neo-Synephrine)
pseudoephedrine (Sudafed)

DEMENTIA/ALZHEIMER'S
donepezil (Aricept)
ergoloid mesylate (Hydergine)
galantamine (Reminyl)
rivastigmine tartrate (Exelon)
tacrine (Cognex)

DERMATOLOGICS
acitretin (Soriatane)
adapalene (Differin)
alefacept (Amevive)
alitretinoin (Panretin)
azelaic acid (Azelex)
benzoyl peroxide (Acetoxy)
capsaicin (Zostrix)
doxepin HCl (Zonalon)
isotretinoin (Accutane)
minoxidil (Rogaine)
pimecrolimus (Elidel)
podofilox (Condyline)
podophyllum (Podocon-25)
sulfacetamide (Isopto Cetamide)
tacrolimus (Protopic)
tazarotene (Tazorac)
tretinoin (Retin-A)
zinc oxide/zinc sulfate (Balmax)

DIURETICS
Loop diuretics
bumetanide (Bumex)
furosemide (Lasix)
torsemide (Demadex)
Potassium sparing
amiloride HCl (Midamor)
spironolactone (Aldactone)
triamterene (Dyrenium)
Thiazides
bendroflumethiazide (Naturetin-5)
benzthiazide (Exna)
chlorothiazide (Diuril)
hydrochlorothiazide (HydroDIURIL)
hydroflumethiazide (Diucardin)
Thiazide-like
chlorthalidone (Hygroton)
indapamide (Lozol)
metolazone (Zaroxolyn)
Others
acetazolamide (Diamox)
dorzolamide HCl (Trusopt)
methazolamide (Neptazane)

ENDOCRINE
danazol (Danocrine)
desmopressin (DDAVP)
dutasteride (Avodart)

estradiol (Estradot)
estrogens, conjugated;
medroxyprogesterone acetate (Premphase)
estropipate (Ogen)
finasteride (Proscar)
fluoxymesterone (Halotestin)
glucagon (Glucagon Emergency Kit)
levothyroxine (Synthroid)
liothyronine (T3)
liotrix (Euthroid)
medroxyprogesterone acetate (Provera)
methyltestosterone (Android)
norethindrone (Aygestin)
norgestrel (Ovrette)
oxandrolone (Oxandrin)
oxymetholone (Anadrol)
progesterone (Crinone)
propylthiouracil (Propylthiouracil)
raloxifene HCl (Evista)
teriparatide (Forteo)
testosterone (Depo-Testosterone)
thyroid (Armour Thyroid)
vasopressin (Pitressin)

ERECTILE DYSFUNCTION
alprostadil (Caverject)
sildenafil citrate (Viagra)
tadalafil (Cialis)
vardenafil HCl (Levitra)

ERGOT ALKALOIDS
(see migraine)

ERGOT ALKALOIDS AND DERIVATIVES
methylergonovine (Methergine)

ERGOTAMINE TARTRATE/ DIHYDROERGOTAMINE

EXPECTORANT
guaifenesin (Humibid)

FLUOROQUINOLONES
ciprofloxacin HCl (Cipro)
gatifloxacin (Tequin)
gemifloxacin mesylate (Factive)
levofloxacin HCl (Levaquin)
lomefloxacin (Maxaquin)
moxifloxacin HCl (Avelox)
norfloxacin (Noroxin)
ofloxacin (Floxin)
sparfloxacin (Zagam)

FREE RADICAL SCAVENGER
amifostine (Ethyol)

GASTROESOPHAGEAL REFLUX DISEASE
esomeprazole (Nexium)
lansoprazole (Prevacid)
omeprazole (Prilosec)
rabeprazole sodium (Aciphex)
ranitidine hydrochloride/
ranitidine bismuth citrate (Zantac)

GASTROINTESTINAL DRUGS
balsalazide (Colazol)
bisacodyl (Alophen)
docusate (Docusate)
infliximab (Remicade)
lansoprazole (Prevacid)
mesalamine/5 aminosalicylic acid(5-ASA)
metoclopramide HCl (Reglan)
misoprostol (Cytotec)
octreotide acetate (Sandostatin)
olsalazine sodium (Dipentum)
pancreatin/pancrelipase
rabeprazole (Aciphex)
rabeprazole sodium (Aciphex)
ranitidine hydrochloride/ranitidine bismuth citrate (Zantac)
simethicone (Mylanta)
sucralfate (Carafate)
sulfasalazine (Azulfidine)
tegaserod (Zelnorm)

GLAUCOMA TREATMENT
acetazolamide (Diamox)
apraclonidine (Iopidine)
betaxolol HCl (Betoptic)
bimatoprost (Lumigan)
brinzolamide (Azopt)
cabergoline (Dostinex)
carteolol (Ocupress)
demecarium bromide (Humorsol)
dipivefrin HCl (Propine)
dorzolamide (Trusopt)
ectothiophate iodide (Phospohline Iodide)
emedastine (Emadine)
epinephryl borate (Betaxon)
latanoprost (Xalatan)
levobetaxolol hydrochloride
levobunolol HCl (Betagan)
methazolamide (Neptazane)
metipranolol hydrochloride
pilocarpine (Isopto-Carpine)
timolol maleate (Timoptic)

travoprost (Travatan)
unoprostone isopropyl (Rescula)

GLUCOCORTICOIDS

Inhalant sprays

budesonide (Rhinocort Inh)
flunisolide (Aerobid Inh)
fluticasone propionate (Flonase)
mometasone furoate monohydrate (Novasone)
triamcinolone acetonide (Azmacort)

Systemic

betamethasone (Celestone)
cortisone acetate (Cortone)
dexamethasone (Dexadron)
dexamethasone sodium phosphate
fludrocortisone (Florinef)
hydrocortisone (Cortef)
methylprednisolone (Medrol)
methylprednisolone acetate (Medrol)
methylprednisolone sodium succinate (Depo-Medrol)
prednisolone (Delta-Cortef)
prednisolone sodium phosphate (Pediapred)
prednisone (Meticorten)
triamcinolone acetonide (Aristocort)
triamcinolone/triamcinolone acetonide/ triamcinolone diacetate/ triamcinolone hexacetonide (Aristocort)

Topical

alclometasone (Aclovate)
amcinonide (Cylocort)
betamethasone (Diprolene)
clobetasol (Alti-Clobetasol)
clobetasol propionate (Olux)
clocortolone (Alti-Clobetasol)
desonide (DesOwen)
desoximetasone (Topicort)
dexamethasone (Decaderm)
diflorasone (Florone)
fluocinolone acetonide (Capex)
fluocinonide (Lidex)
flurandrenolide (Cordran)
fluticasone propionate (Cutivate)
halcinonide (Halog)
halobetasol (Ultravate)
hydrocortisone (Allercort)
mometasone furoate monohydrate
rimexolone (Vexol)
triamcinolone/triamcinolone acetonide/triamcinolone diacetate/triamcinolone hexacetonide (Aristocort)

HEMOSTATICS

aminocaproic acid (Amicar)
oxidized cellulose (Surgicel)
thrombin, topical (thrombinar, thrombin-JMI, thrombostat, etc.)
tranexamic acid (Cyklokapron)

HORMONAL AGENTS

abarelix (Plenaxis)
estradiol (Estradot)
estrogens, conjugated; medroxyprogesterone acetate (Premphase)
goserelin acetate (Zoladex)
leuprolide acetate (Lupron)
methyltestosterone (Android)
nafarelin (Synarel)
pegvisomant (Somavert)
progesterone (Crinone)
teriparatide (Forteo)
triptorelin pamoate (Trelstar)
vasopressin (Pitressin)

IMMUNOMODULATORS

imiquimod (Aldara)
interferon alfa-2a (Roferon-A, Pegasys)
interferon alfa-2a/2b
interferon alfa-2b (Intron-A)
interferon beta-1A (Avonex)
interferon gamma-1B (Actimmune)
peginterferon alfa-2a (Pegasys)
peginterferon alfa-2B (PEG-Intron)
thalidomide (Thalomide)

IMMUNOSUPPRESSANTS

azathioprine (Imuran)
cyclosporine (Sandimmune, Neoral)
daclizumab (Zenapax)
mycophenolate mofetil (CellCept)
prednisone (Meticorten)
sirolimus (Rapamune)
tacrolimus (Prograf)
tacrolimus (Protopic)

IRRITABLE BOWEL SYNDROME

alosetron (Lotronex)
tegaserod (Zelnorm)

LEUKOTRIENE PATHWAY INHIBITOR

zileuton (Zyflo)

LEUKOTRIENE RECEPTOR ANTAGONIST

zafirlukast (Accolate)

LINCOSAMIDES
clindamycin HCl (Cleocin)
lincomycin (Lincocin)
lincomycin HCl (Bactramycin)

MACROLIDES
azithromycin (Zithromax)
clarithromycin (Biaxin)
dirithromycin (DynaBac)
erythromycin (Erythrocin)

MALE PATTERN BALDNESS
finasteride (Propecia)
minoxidil (Rogaine)

MAST CELL STABILIZERS
cromolyn sodium (Intal)
lodoxamide (Alomide)
nedocromil sodium (Tilade)
pemirolast potassium (Alamast)

MIGRAINE
(see ergot alkaloids)
almotriptan malate (Axert)
eletriptan (Relpax)
ergotamine tartrate/
dihydroergotamine (Ergostat)
frovatriptan (Frovan)
naratriptan HCl (Amerge)
propranolol HCl (Inderal)
rizatriptan benzoate (Maxalt)
sumatriptan (Imitrax)
timolol (Blocadren)
valproic acid/valproate
sodium/divalproex sodium
zolmitriptan (Zomig)

MINERALS
ferrous fumarate/ferrous
gluconate/ferrous sulfate (Feostat)
potassium acetate/potassium
bicarbonate-citrate/
potassium chloride/
potassium gluconate (Kaon)
potassium chloride (Micro-K)
zinc oxide/zinc sulfate

MONOCLONAL ANTIBODIES
adalimumab (Humira)
alemtuzumab (Campath)
bevacizumab (Avastin)
efalizumab (Raptiva)
omalizumab (Xolair)
rituximab (Rituxan)
trastuzumab (Herceptin)

MUCOLYTIC
acetylcysteine (Acetadote, Mucomyst)
dornase alfa (Pulmozyme)

MULTIPLE SCLEROSIS
glatiramer (Copaxone)

MYASTHENIA GRAVIS
ambenonium (Mytelase)
neostigmine (Prostigmin)
pyridostigmine bromide (Mestinon)

MYDRIATIC
atropine sulfate (optic) (Isopto Atropine)
cyclopentolate hydrochloride
(AK-Pentolate)
tropicamide (Opticyl)

NARCOTICS
(see analgesics [opioid])

NATRIURETIC PEPTIDE
nesiritide (Natrecor)

NITROIMIDAZOLE
metronidazole (Flagyl)

NONSTEROIDAL ANTIINFLAMMATORY DRUGS
celecoxib (Celebrex)
diclofenac (Voltaren)
diflunisal (Dolobid)
etodolac (Lodine)
flurbiprofen (Ansaid)
ibuprofen (Motrin)
indomethacin (Indocin)
ketoprofen (Orudis)
ketorolac tromethamine
meclofenamate (Mecclomen)
mefenamic acid (Ponstel)
meloxicam (Mobic)
nabumetone (Relafen)
naproxen (Naprosyn)
naproxen/naproxen sodium
naproxen sodium (Anaprox)
oxaprozin (Daypro)
piroxicam (Feldene)
rofecoxib (Vioxx)
sulindac (Clinoril)
suprofen (Profenal)
tolmetin (Tolectin)
valdecoxib (Bextra)

OBESITY MANAGEMENT
diethylpropion (Tenuate)

methamphetamine (Desoxyn)
orlistat (Xenical)
phendimetrazine (Prelu-2)
phentermine (Ionamin)
sibutramine (Merida)

OPHTHALMICS

acetylcholine chloride (Michol-E)
atropine sulfate (optic) (Isopto Atropine)
azelastine HCl (Optivar)
betaxolol HCl (Betoptic)
bimatoprost (Lumigan)
cabergoline (Dostinex)
carteolol (Occupres)
ciprofloxacin (Ciloxan)
cyclopentolate hydrochloride (AK-Pentolate)
cyclosporine (Restasis)
dapiprazole hydrochloride (Rev-Eyes)
dexamethasone sodium phosphate; neomycin sulfate (Ocu-dex)
dipivefrin (Propine)
ectothiophate iodide (Phospohline Iodide)
epinastine HCl (Elestat)
epinephryl borate (Epifrin)
erythromycin (Ilotycin)
fluorometholone
gentamicin sulfate; prednisolone acetate (Gentak)
homatropine hydrobromide (optic) (Isopto Homatropine)
hydrocortisone acetate; oxytetracycline hydrochloride (Terra-Cortril)
hydrocortisone; neomycin sulfate; polymyxin B sulfate (Cortisporin)
levobetaxolol hydrochloride (Betaxon)
levocabastine HCl (Livostin)
levofloxacin HCl (Quixin)
lodoxamide (Alomide)
loteprednol (Lotemax, Alrex)
loteprednol etabonate; tobramycin (Zylin)
medrysone (HMS Liquifilm)
metipranolol hydrochloride (OptiPranolol)
moxifloxacin HCl (Vigamox)
naphazoline HCl (Naphcon)
ofloxacin (Ocuflox)
olopatadine (Patanol)
pemirolast potassium
permirolast (Alamast)
phenylephrine hydrochloride; sulfacetamide sodium (Mydfrin)
polymyxin B sulfate; trimethoprim sulfate (Polytrim)
prednisolone acetate (Prednisol)
prednisolone acetate; sulfacetamide sodium (Vasocidin)
prednisolone sodium phosphate (Pediapred)
prednisolone sodium phosphate; sulfacetamide sodium
sulfacetamide (Sulfair)
suprofen (Profenal)
tobramycin (Tobrex)
travoprost (Travatan)
trifluridine (Viroptic)
tropicamide (Opticyl)
unoprostone isopropyl (Rescula)
vidarabine (Vira-A)

ORPHAN DRUGS

miglustat (Zavesca)

OTIC DRUGS

carbamide peroxide (Auro Ear Drops)
gatifloxacin (Zymar)
hydrocortisone; neomycin sulfate; polymyxin B sulfate (Cortisporin)
ofloxacin (Floxin Otic)

OVARIAN STUMULANTS

clomiphene (Clomhexal)

PENICILLINS

amoxicillin/clavulanate potassium (Augmentin)
ampicillin (Alpovex)
ampicillin sodium (Omnipen)
ampicillin/sulbactem sodium (Alphacin)
dicloxacillin (Polaramine)
oxacillin (Prostaphlin)
penicillin G benzathine (Bicillin)
penicillin G potassium (Pfizerpen)
penicillin V potassium (V-Cillin K)
ticarcillin (Ticar)
ticarcillin disodium/clavulanate potassium (Timentin)

PEPTIDE ANTIINFECTIVE

vancomycin HCl (Vancocin)

PERIODONTAL SPECIALTY PRODUCTS

doxycycline hyclate (Atridox)
minocycline HCl (Arestin)

PERIPHERAL VASCULAR DISEASE

isoxsuprine HCl (Vasodilan)

papaverine HCl (Pavabid)
pentoxifylline (Trental)

PHOSPHATE BINDERS
lanthanum carbonate (Fosrenol)
sevelamer hydrochloride (Renagel)

PLATELET AGGREGATION INHIBITORS
aspirin (Bayer)
dipyridamole (Persantine)
eptifibatide (Integrilin)
ticlopidine (Ticlid)
tirofiban (Aggrastat)
treprostinil sodium (Remodulin)

PLATELET REDUCING AGENT
anagrelide HCl (Agrylin)

PNEUMOCYSTIC PNEUMONITIS
atovaquone (Mepron)
pentamidine (Pentam 300)
trimetrexate (Neutrexin)

PROSTAGLANDIN
alprostadil (Caverject)
bimatoprost (Lumigan)
epoprostenol sodium, prostacyclin (Flolan)
latanoprost (Xalatan)
misoprostol (Cytotec)
travoprost (Travatan)
treprostinil sodium (Remodulin)

PROSTATE HYPERPLASIA
alfuzosin HCl (Uroxatral)
dutasteride (Avodart)
finasteride (Proscar)
tamsulosin HCl (Flomax)
terazosin HCl (Hytrin)

RESPIRATORY INHALANTS AND INTANASAL STEROIDS
acetylcysteine (Acetadote, Mucomyst)

SALIVARY STIMULANTS (SIALOGOGUES)
amifostine (Ethyol)
cevimeline (Evoxac)
pilocarpine HCl (Salagen)

SELECTIVE SEROTONIN ANTAGONIST
alosetron HCl (Lotronex)

SKELETAL MUSCLE RELAXANTS
baclofen (Lioresal)
carisoprodol (Soma)
chlorzoxazone (Paraflex)
cyclobenzaprine HCl (Flexeril)
dantrolene sodium (Dantrium)
metaxalone (Skelexan)
methocarbamol (Robaxin)
orphenadrine (Norflex)

SMOKING CESSATION
bupropion HCl (Zyban)
nicotine (Lescol)

STATINS- CHOLESTEROL-LOWERING
ezetimibe; simvastatin (Vytorin)
fluvastatin (Lescol)
lovastatin (Mevacor)
pravastatin sodium (Pravachol)
simvastatin (Zocor)

SULFONAMIDES
sulfacetamide (Sulfair)
sulfacetamide sodium (Sulamyd Sodium)
sulfamethoxazole/trimethoprim (Septra, Bactrim)
sulfisoxazole (Gantrisin)

TETRACYCLINES
demeclocycline HCl (Declomycin)
doxycycline (Periostat)
doxycycline hyclate (Atridox)
doxycycline hyclate (Periostat)
minocycline HCl (Minocin, Arestin)
tetracycline (Achromycin)

THROMBOLYTICS
alteplase, recombinant (Activase, Actilyse)
reteplase, recombinant (Retavase)
tenecteplase (TNKase)

URICOSURIC
probenecid (Benemid)
sulfinpyrazone (Anturane)

URINARY TRACT AGENTS
cysteamine bitatrate (Cystagon)

URINARY TRACT INFECTIONS
flavoxate HCl (Urispas)
fosfomycin tromethamine (Monurol)

Generic and Trade Name Index

Entries can be identified as follows: generic name, Trade Name/Trade Name[Region], DRUG CATEGORY, *Combination Product*

INDEX

G

M

O

P

INDEX

Q

INDEX

T

U

MINIMUM SYSTEM REQUIREMENTS

This CD will run on both PC and Mac.

Microsoft Windows Users

To function properly, your computer should support at least an 800 × 600 pixels screen resolution, 256 colors, and 128 MB RAM, and it should operate on the Windows 98 SE, 2000, or XP operating system. Additionally, be sure your browser has "Show pictures" enabled. For Internet Explorer users, you will find the "Show pictures" option by selecting the following from your menu: Tools > Internet Options > Advanced > Multimedia. If the "Show pictures" box is not checked, do so.

This software is designed to run with Internet Explorer 6.0, Netscape 7 or later, and Firefox 1.x.

Use MS PowerPoint to view the ".ppt" files. These files can also be viewed using MS PowerPoint file viewer.

Macintosh Users

Your computer should meet the following minimum requirements: 800 × 600 pixels screen resolution, 256 colors, 128 MB RAM, and MAC OS 10.2 or later operating system.

This software is designed to run with Safari 1.3 or later and Firefox 1.x. Refer to the help files for problems specific to the browser.

INSTALLATION INSTRUCTIONS

Windows

1. If your system does not support Autorun, click on MDCDP.exe to begin.
2. To use the Search feature, install the Java Runtime Environment, version 1.4.1 (available in the software folder). You should have administrator privileges for this installation. After installation, start the application by clicking MDCDP.exe.
3. For Windows 98 users, the Visual Basic 6.0 Service Pack 5 Run-Time Redistribution Pack (VBRun60sp5.exe) is provided on the CD. Install it from the software folder.
4. PowerPoint viewer (ppviewer2003.exe) can be installed from the software folder of the CD.

Macintosh

1. Click on the CD icon that appears on your desktop; then select MDCDP to open the application.
2. The CD requires the installation of MRJ 2.2.5 in order to use the Search feature (available in the software folder). If manually installed, start the application by clicking on MDCDP.
3. If the browser does not launch after clicking on the "I Agree" button from the MDCDP application or by clicking on the "Start" button on the MServerX applet, open Index.htm to launch the Home page.

4. PowerPoint viewer (PPT98VW.hqx) can be installed from the software folder of the CD.

MINIMUM SOFTWARE REQUIREMENTS

MS PowerPoint/MS Office

Some of the content in this product is available in PPT format. To view this content you will need a copy of MS PowerPoint/MS Office or any other product that can read the PPT file format.

(NOTE: You can also use other File Viewer applications to view PPT files.)

KNOWN ISSUES

1. To get the program to launch in your default browser:

Macintosh Users

Control-click the Home.htm file, select "Get Info," and then select the default browser from the "Opens With" drop-down menu.

Windows Users

Shift-Right-click the Home.htm file, select "Open With," and then select the default browser from the "Choose Program..." menu.

2. If Active Content warning is displayed while running the product, please do the following:
   On Tools > Internet Options > Advanced tab > in Security > Select "Allow active content from CDs to run on my Computer."
3. While using Netscape 8, ensure that "Open requested Pop-ups in New Tab" option is deselected. If not, select the Site Controls icon on the tab and deselect this option.

TECHNICAL SUPPORT

Technical support for this product is available between 7:30 a.m. and 7 p.m. CST, Monday through Friday. Before calling, be sure that your computer meets the minimum system requirements to run this software. Inside the United States and Canada, call 1-800-692-9010. Outside North America, call 314-872-8370. You may also fax your questions to 314-523-4932.

You may also contact Technical Support via e-mail at: technical.support@elsevier.com.

For access to a list of Frequently Asked Questions (FAQ), as well as troubleshooting tips, please visit our website at http://www.us.elsevierhealth.com/TechSupport

Part Number: 9996025888

Pentium, Windows, Adobe, and Macintosh are registered trademarks.

American Dental Association Advisory Statement for Patients with Total Joint Replacement

PATIENTS AT POTENTIAL INCREASED RISK OF EXPERIENCING HEMATOGENOUS TOTAL JOINT INFECTION

- All patients during the first 2 years following joint replacement

IMMUNOCOMPROMISED/IMMUNOSUPPRESSED PATIENTS

- Inflammatory arthropathies such as rheumatoid arthritis, systemic lupus erythematosus
- Drug- or radiation-induced immunosuppression

PATIENTS WITH COMORBIDITIES

- Previous prosthetic joint infections
- Malnourishment
- Hemophilia
- HIV infection
- Insulin-dependent (type 1) diabetes
- Malignancy
- Conditions shown for patients in this category are examples only; there may be additional conditions that place such patients at risk of experiencing hematogenous total joint infections.

Advisory Statements from ADA and AAOS: Antibiotic Prophylaxis for Dental Patients with Total Joint Replacements, *JADA* 134(7):895–899, July 2003. Adapted 2006 with permission of the American Dental Association. Based on Ching and colleagues,[1] Brause,[2] Murray and colleagues,[3] Poss and colleagues,[4] Jacobson and colleagues,[5] Johnson and Bannister,[6] Jacobson and colleagues[7] and Berbari and colleagues.[8]

1. Ching DW, Gould IM, Rennie JA, Gibson PI. Prevention of late haematogenous infection in major prosthetic joints. J Antimicrob Chemother 1989;23:676–80.
2. Brause BD. Infections associated with prosthetic joints. Clin Rheum Dis 1986;12:523–35.
3. Murray RP, Bourne MH, Fitzgerald RH Jr. Metachronous infection in patients who have had more than one total joint arthroplasty. J Bone Joint Surg Am 1991;73(10):1469–74.
4. Poss R, Thornhill TS, Ewald FC, Thomas WH, Batte NJ, Sledge CB. Factors influencing the incidence and outcome of infection following total joint arthroplasty. Clin Orthop 1984;182:117–26.